PHYSICIANS' GUIDE TO RARE DISEASES

PHYSICIANS' GUIDE TO RARE DISEASES

Jess G. Thoene, M.D., Editor

Doris C. Smith, Managing Editor

DOWDEN PUBLISHING COMPANY INC.
MONTVALE, N.J.

Prepared in association with
the National Organization for Rare Disorders

Dowden Publishing Company
110 Summit Avenue
Montvale, NJ 07645
Telephone (201) 391-9100   Fax (201) 391-2778

Library of Congress Catalog Card Number 92-71122
ISBN 0-9628716-0-5
ISSN 1053-9727

First Edition

Design by Philip Denlinger

CONTENTS

EDITOR

JESS G. THOENE, M.D.

Professor of Pediatrics
Associate Professor of Biological Chemistry
Chief, Pediatric Biochemical Genetics and Metabolism
The University of Michigan Medical Center
Ann Arbor, Michigan

President
National Organization for Rare Disorders

Chair
National Commission on Orphan Diseases

MANAGING EDITOR

DORIS C. SMITH

EDITORIAL DIRECTOR

LEWIS A. MILLER

ACKNOWLEDGMENTS

The National Organization for Rare Disorders (NORD) is grateful to the corporations, trade groups, foundations and other philanthropic benefactors without whom NORD's Rare Disease Database and this book would not have been possible:

- Catt Family Foundation
- Generic Pharmaceutical Industry Association (GPIA)
- Hugh J. Andersen Foundation
- March of Dimes
- Pharmaceutical Manufacturers Association (PMA)
- Revco Drug Stores Foundation
- Robert Leet & Clara Guthrie Patterson Trust

The editors express their gratitude to Waldo Bibb for his consummate knowledge of computers and his support during emergencies; to Patrice McSherry, Karen McWilliams, and Kay Genus for their indispensable editorial help; and to the following professional editors and writers: Lynn Alperin, Jean Arbeiter, Peggy Ann Collins, Dennis Connaughton, Elisabeth Cotton, M.D., Nancy D'Epiro, Buffy Gilfoil, Elaine Gomez, Carol Hoidra, Carolyn Lamb, Janice L. Lowry, William Marden, Karen A. Moline, Brita M. O'Carroll, Marjorie Pannell, David Petechuk, Nance A. Seiple, and Esther T. Silverman.

—*Doris C. Smith*

EDITOR'S PREFACE

The physician caring for a person with a rare disease (one affecting fewer than 200,000 Americans) often is hard pressed to find accurate and timely information about the condition. In a busy practice, an encounter with such a patient can be burdensome. Not in the common stream of daily events, the person's symptoms may be perplexing and the diagnostic tests required may not be readily available. A survey by the National Commission on Orphan Diseases of the rare disease experiences of 247 physicians demonstrated that between 20 percent and 40 percent of physicians could neither find information on the availability or location of appropriate treatment or on the existence of support groups, nor access printed information for patients regarding rare diseases.

The National Commission on Orphan Diseases studied the problems of persons with these rare conditions for two years. Their findings demonstrated that about one-third of these patients do not receive correct diagnoses for over five years. Fifteen percent of these persons went without a diagnosis for over six years. Furthermore, persons with rare diseases desperately want and need information on research projects for patient participation, knowledge of new treatments and research advances, easy-to-understand written information about their rare conditions, and details of the location of treatment centers. None of these is readily available, although the National Organization for Rare Disorders has attempted to meet this need with the introduction of the Rare Disease Database on CompuServe, providing comprehensible information in lay terms on over 800 rare diseases. Additionally, through its networking function, NORD assists patients with rare diseases in finding other persons with the same conditions, and maintains a registry of treatment centers.

To address the problem of providing more and better information to physicians, NORD and Dowden Publishing Company have collaborated to produce this first edition of Physicians' Guide to Rare Diseases. This work is an adaptation of the rare disease database entries for close to 700 rare diseases, and has been revised to address the concerns of physicians in primary care specialties. The intent of the volume is not to provide specialists in rare diseases with comprehensive data about these conditions, but rather to assist someone who encounters rare diseases infrequently by providing ready access to signs and symptoms for help in differential diagnosis, to availability of therapy, and to the location of support groups for these patients.

Each major section of the Guide opens with an overview article by a specialist on the Editorial Board. This introduction is intended as a helpful guide to the diseases covered in that section. Because of its synoptic nature, this book is necessarily inadequate with regard to the details of pathophysiology, diagnosis, and treatment. However, by identifying the rare condition and its major presenting symptomatology, it should shorten the time needed to achieve a correct diagnosis, as well as provide ready access for further information and the location of support groups. This last feature is unique to this book, and we hope it will be most helpful to the practicing physician.

Also featured in this first edition of the Guide is a full-color atlas of visual diagnostic signs; a directory of "orphan" drugs organized by use and providing the name of a key contact person at each research center; and a detailed index of symptoms and key words.

The reader's comments will be most welcome, so that we can make the next edition of The Physicians' Guide to Rare Diseases even more valuable. Please address these to me care of the publisher, Dowden Publishing Company, 110 Summit Avenue, Montvale, New Jersey 07645.

I am grateful to the Editorial Board, who undertook to review each article for medical accuracy, and for the outstanding support of Doris

Smith, managing editor, and Carroll Dowden, president of Dowden Publishing Company, who pushed the project along most rapidly. Finally, Abbey Meyers, executive director of NORD, has been the driving force on behalf of rare disease patients in this country for many years, and without her none of this project would have been realized.

—*Jess G. Thoene, M.D.*
Editor
President, National Organization for Rare Disorders
Chair, National Commission on Orphan Diseases

RARE DISEASES:
WHAT PATIENTS NEED

Isolation. Hopelessness. Despair. These are the emotions that permeate the lives of rare disease patients in the United States. An estimated 20 million Americans affected by more than 5,000 rare "orphan" diseases find themselves medically disenfranchised, and falling through the cracks of the health care system because their afflictions are not identified as major public health threats warranting targeted research efforts.

How could these problems be documented so that the magnitude of this human tragedy would raise the profile of research on new treatments for rare conditions? As one patient put it, "Orphan diseases are not important, unless you happen to have one yourself."

In the 1985 amendments to the Orphan Drug Act, Congress mandated the National Commission on Orphan Diseases to study all problems related to rare diseases and make recommendations as to how they may be solved. After several years of intensive study, including surveys of the patient and medical communities, the Commission submitted its report to Congress in February, 1989. Following are some of its findings.

Patients and Families

- 31 percent of patients took between 1 and 5 years to receive a proper diagnosis, and 15 percent went undiagnosed 6 or more years.

• 45 percent of patients said their individual illnesses caused extreme financial hardship on themselves and their families; and 42 percent reported that their diseases prevent them from working or attending school.

Research Findings

• During 1987 the United States government spent $1.3 billion on rare disease research; the pharmaceutical industry spent $51.6 million; and foundations spent $41.6 million. Of the $1.3 billion spent by the federal government on rare disease research, over half was spent on approximately 200 rare forms of cancer. This left only $640 million for the remaining 4,800 orphan diseases.

• Biomedical researchers working on both rare and common diseases feel that it is harder to get funding for rare disease research than for research on a prevalent disease, and that the lack of funds is the single greatest barrier to discovery of treatments for rare illnesses. The Commission found that many of the barriers to progress on research and treatments for rare diseases are caused by both lack of funding and a lack of coordination of existing resources.

• 47 percent of researchers reported that it is difficult to find a sufficient number of patients to participate in a research project on a rare disease. In contrast, 76 percent of rare disease patients reported that it is difficult to obtain information about research projects in which they might want to participate.

In a survey of practicing physicians conducted by the Commission in conjunction with the American Medical Association, the Commission found the following:

• 42 percent of doctors say they need, but are unable to find, printed information to give to their rare disease patients concerning their illnesses.

• 39 percent of these physicians had used an investigational drug or device for at least one of their patients; of these, 92 percent said they would do so again. Of those physicians who had never used an experimental treatment, 72 percent said they would not consider using them.

• The sources of information most frequently used by physicians for diagnosing and treating rare disease patients are pharmaceutical companies (46 percent), the Centers for Disease Control (41 percent), and the National Institutes of Health (39 percent).

• A survey of 106 foundations that fund biomedical research indicated that only 12 foundations funded rare disease research grants, representing only 1.3 percent of their medical research budget.

• A survey of rare disease voluntary health agencies indicated that 48 percent of such agencies fund biomedical research grants on orphan diseases. Half of the agencies estimated that the cost of medical care for patients with the disease they represent ranges from $9,500 to $115,000 per year (1988 figures).

Obviously, the Commission's report defined many problems, aside from orphan drug development, that affect patients, families, biomedical researchers, and practicing physicians. The tools that clinicians have to identify and treat orphan diseases are few, and the frustrations of patients are many. Today, many issues remain unresolved.

A most important issue is the increasingly acute problem of inadequate health insurance coverage. When a child is diagnosed with a hereditary disease, his siblings (and the affected child) are at risk of losing their health insurance. Expensive treatments can consume a family's health insurance and reach a lifetime ceiling, leaving the patient uninsurable for the rest of his life. When a breadwinner changes jobs, the new employer's health insurance may not cover the preexisting health condition of a spouse or child. If it does cover it, the premiums may be greater than the employee's wages!

Even federal health care programs such as Medicare and Medicaid can present obstacles to appropriate patient care. Hospitals are now reimbursed according to DRGs (Diagnosis Related Groups); but there are no DRGs for the vast majority of orphan diseases. And Social Security Disability or SSI benefits can be denied if a patient's disease is not included in the Social Security Administration's Listing of Impairments. Few rare diseases are listed.

The National Organization for Rare Disorders (NORD) evolved out of a coalition of national voluntary health agencies and support groups who worked together for passage of the Orphan Drug Act of 1983. In the battle to pass the legislation during the late 1970s and early 1980s, publicity about the orphan drug dilemma resulted in significant influxes of mail from patients and families, asking for information about their disorders and referrals to agencies and clinics where they could be treated.

Their letters and phone calls had common threads which persist today: years of misdiagnosis; absent or ineffective treatment; isolation due to the uniqueness of their symptoms; despair because little or no research was being pursued. Researchers were hesitant to investigate these rare ailments because they felt it would be too difficult to win a grant from the National Institutes of Health (NIH) for an unknown disease. Moreover, they didn't know whether and where they could find sufficient numbers of patients to conduct a clinical trial, and if they were lucky enough to discover a treatment for one of these diseases, they could not find a pharmaceutical company willing to commercialize it. Indeed, in several cases, academic investigators had to manufacture their drugs by hand in their university laboratories for many years, wondering what would happen to their patients if anything were to happen to them.

Today the picture is not so bleak. By the end of 1990, the FDA had designated over 400 orphan drugs and approved 49 orphan products for treatment of 58 orphan diseases, representing significant advancement in the amelioration of many painful and tragic conditions. The Orphan Drug Act has effectively encouraged development of new treatments for rare diseases. Scientists are encouraged by the FDA's orphan drug grant program. Practicing physicians have a larger armamentarium to assist in the diagnosis and treatment of orphan diseases, as well as easier access to crucial intervention.

The future holds the promise of astonishing breakthroughs that will benefit both rare and prevalent disease patients because of America's efforts to develop orphan drugs. Enzyme replacement therapies, drugs to treat AIDS, and human gene therapy are realities today because the government, industry, academia, and patient groups worked together to insure the success of the Orphan Drug Act. But diagnosis still remains a primary problem, and it can only be solved by clinicians who recognize symptoms early and know where resources are available to affect the course of the disease. To orphan disease patients, however, the major difference between this decade and the past can be summed up in one word: hope.

—*Abbey S. Meyers*
Executive Director
National Organization for Rare Disorders

PHYSICIANS' GUIDE TO RARE DISEASES

1 | GENETIC DISEASES AND DYSMORPHIC SYNDROMES
By Angelo M. DiGeorge, M.D.

In this section are included a few disorders readily recognizable by physicians and lay persons alike, such as Down syndrome; and others so recondite that thus far only a few affected patients have been described. Even physicians with a special interest in rare disorders cannot be expected to instantly recognize or be knowledgeable about every one of them. After 40 years of clinical practice in a busy children's hospital, I have personally seen only 78 percent of the disorders in this chapter. Since about half of these have been described just in the past three decades, I have missed my share of diagnoses. Gorlin's encyclopedic monograph describes about 700 syndromes which involve the head and neck[1], and new entities are being reported in the medical journals every year.

How can the practicing pediatrician or family physician be expected to diagnose such a growing hodgepodge of esoteric conditions? For the serious student of dysmorphology, I recommend Dr. Jon M. Aase's recent book on the systematic approach to the diagnosis of the dysmorphology syndromes[2].

The most important requirement of physicians who seek to enhance their diagnostic acumen is an abiding curiosity about unusual clinical findings. One cannot repeat too often the importance of a detailed history and complete physical examination. Dr. John A. Kolmer, one of my professors in medical school, was fond of admonishing us over and over again, "More mistakes are made in medicine by not looking than by not knowing." Even after assembling the abnormal historical and physical findings, the physician should not be surprised that in many instances these do not immediately conjure up a diagnosis. The next step, as I tell my students, is to "look it up."

Where does one start? Begin with the symptoms index in this compendium. But do not begin by looking up minor or prevalent abnormalities such as micrognathia, low-set ears, cleft lip, scoliosis, or clinodactyly. These manifestations are common to many disorders and are likely to lead you to a jumble of a differential diagnosis. Always begin by looking up the most uncommon, odd, strange, or unfamiliar finding. For example, a low-pitched growling cry will lead you to Cornelia de Lange syndrome; a kitten-like mewing cry leads to cri du chat syndrome, deletion of the short arm of chromosome 5. Likewise, freckles on the lips leads to Peutz-Jeghers syndrome, and freckling of the axilla to type I neurofibromatosis. Unusual abnormalities of the eyes are particularly helpful in zeroing in on a diagnosis. Aniridia (Wilms tumor association), heterochromia of the irides (Waardenburg syndrome), dislocated lens (Marfan syndrome and homocystinuria), and optic nerve hypoplasia (septo-optic dysplasia) are examples of this bull's-eye approach to diagnosis. Similarly, clear to yellow or brown nodules on the surface of the iris (Lisch nodules) are diagnostic of type I neurofibromatosis; and retinal angiomatosis is often the only manifestation in children with von Hippel-Lindau disease. This is, of course, an oversimplified approach which only works for about 25 percent of these disorders, but I have seen children whose diagnoses were unduly delayed for lack of physician curiosity, and failure of even the most cursory inquiry.

Only about a dozen of the more common chromosomal disorders are included here. The phenotypes of Down, trisomy 13, trisomy 18, or cri du chat syndromes can be recognized in the neonatal period and diagnosis readily confirmed cytogenetically. Many girls with Turner syndrome can also be detected in the newborn period if lymphedema is present; and if not, short stature with or without other associated abnormalities should suggest the diagnosis in childhood. On the other hand, males with Klinefelter syndrome are often not recognized until they present as adults with small testes, gynecomastia, and/or infertility.

The physician who uses this compendium should be aware that

another 80 or more chromosomal syndromes have been delineated which are not included here; although each is very rare, their large number obliges chromosomal analysis in all patients with an undiagnosed constellation of congenital anomalies, dysmorphism, and/or mental retardation. Moreover, small chromosomal deletions or duplications are cytogenetically recognizable in only a proportion of patients with certain syndromes described in this section; examples include the Prader-Willi (del 15q11q13), Angelman (del 15q11q13), DiGeorge (del 22q11), trichorhinophalangeal type I (del 8q24.12) and type II (del 8q24.11-24.13), and Beckwith (dup 11p15.5) syndromes.

Imaging is another important diagnostic tool for this group of patients. Radiographs are required for patients with disproportionate short stature and skeletal anomalies and for assessment of osseous maturation. Computerized tomography and magnetic resonance are essential for imaging of the central nervous system and other organs. These technologies are particularly important for the detection of tumors in patients having syndromes with a known predisposition to malignancy such as neurofibromatosis types I and II, and von Hippel-Lindau, Peutz-Jeghers, Beckwith, and Sotos syndromes.

Genetic counseling is obligatory for most of these conditions. The most comprehensive single source of information for the physician is McKusick's catalogue[3]. However, unraveling some of these arcane entities presents a challenge even for the expert geneticist because of the heterogeneity of many similar-appearing syndromes. Two examples of heterogeneity are chondrodysplasia punctata, which occurs in X-linked dominant, X-linked recessive, and autosomal recessive forms with each having markedly different prognoses; and the oral-facial-digital syndrome, which has been subdivided into seven different phenotypes.

Other persuasive reasons to seek expert genetic counseling are the quickening rate at which it is becoming possible to establish diagnoses at the DNA level for some of these conditions and, more importantly, the revision of cherished genetic dogma, emanating from meticulous study of certain selected syndromes.

The recent discovery that an identical gene may behave quite differently depending on whether it was inherited from the mother or the father, has shaken the long-held precept that there is no difference whether a given gene comes from mother or father. The clearest evidence of this is provided by the Prader-Willi and Angelman syndromes; about 60 and 40 percent of each, respectively, have an identical cytogenetic deletion of chromosome 15 but surprisingly have markedly different phenotypes. It has been established that in Prader-Willi syndrome the deletion occurs on the paternally derived chromosome 15; whereas in Angelman syndrome the deletion occurs on the maternally derived chromosome 15. These findings implicate genetic imprinting, a phenomenon in which the expression of genes is influenced by their parental origin.

Genetic imprinting has also been invoked to explain the bizarre genetics of fragile X syndrome, the most common cause of familial mental retardation. Initially, the disorder was thought to be inherited in the classical X-linked recessive fashion; males with the abnormal X are retarded and females heterozygous for the abnormal X chromosome are normal. However, it was subsequently learned that 20 percent of males having the fragile X mutation are asymptomatic and that 30 percent of carrier females show some mental retardation. Most recently, it has become clear that although the daughters of asymptomatic males are themselves normal, in the next generation the children of these daughters, both male and female, may have the syndrome. To explain this enigma, some investigators have invoked the phenomenon of genomic imprinting, wherein genes inherited from the mother behave differently from those inherited from the father as a result of different modification in the two parents[4,5].

Treatment is the short suit of dysmorhology. For most of these conditions there are as yet no known specific treatment modalities. However, by the application of corrective surgical procedures and supportive, medical, and paramedical technology, a large proportion of affected patients can lead normal and productive lives. Another important way the physician can help these individuals and their families is by remembering to make them aware of the many voluntary organizations dedicated to specific diseases; this manual is one of the most complete sources of such information. These groups consist of caring, compassionate individuals skilled in teaching patients about their conditions and with firsthand knowledge of coping mechanisms and available resources. In addition, they promote physicians' and public education programs; they raise funds for research; and they lobby government agencies for increased research funding, and pharmaceutical companies for development of orphan drugs.

Finally, a word of caution to the young physician. In your lifetime the number of rare diseases will almost surely double. The function of only a small percentage of all the genes is known. Every patient with a rare disease cannot be pigeonholed into one of the known entities. Always be alert to the possibility of a "new" rare disease.

References

1. Syndromes of the Head and Neck, 3rd ed.: R.J. Gorlin, M.M. Cohen, Jr., L.S. Levin; Oxford University Press, 1990.
2. Diagnostic Dysmorphology: J.M. Aase; Plenum Publishing Corporation, 1990.
3. Mendelian Inheritance in Man, 9th ed.: V.A. McKusick; The Johns Hopkins University Press, 1990.
4. Instability of a 550-based pair DNA segment and abnormal methylation in fragile X syndrome: I. Oberle, F. Rousseau, D. Heitz, et al.; Science, 252:1097, 1991.
5. Fragile X genotype characterized by an unstable region of DNA: S. Yu, M. Pritchard, E. Kremer, et al.; Science, 252:119, 1991.

GENETIC DISEASES AND DYSMORPHIC SYNDROMES
Listings in This Section

11Q- SYNDROME

Description 11q- syndrome is a rare genetic disorder affecting the long arm of chromosome 11. Characteristics include a narrow prominent forehead, abnormally shaped nose and mouth, ocular disorders, and mental retardation. Related chromosome 11 disorders are deletion on the short arm of chromosome 11 and partial trisomy of 11q.

Synonyms
Deletion on Long Arm of Chromosome 11

Signs and Symptoms Hypertelorism, strabismus, and ptosis are the ocular manifestations of 11q- syndrome. Other facial abnormalities include a narrow protruding forehead, broad nasal root, short upturned tip of the nose, fish-like mouth, and receding chin. The ears may be misshapen and there may be simian creases in the hands. Mental retardation is also present. Various congenital heart defects are common.

Etiology 11q- syndrome results from a deletion on the long arm (q) of chromosome 11. The cause of the chromosome break is unknown; its size and location determine the disorder's severity and forms of abnormality.

Epidemiology A rare disorder, 11q- syndrome is present at birth, and over 80 percent are female. About 25 percent die under the age of 2 years.

Related Disorders See *Trisomy 13 Syndrome; Trisomy 18 Syndrome; Down Syndrome.*

Deletion on the short arm of 11p13 is associated with aniridia and, in 50 percent of patients, with Wilms tumor, the most common form of renal cancer in children. (See *Aniridia; Wilms Tumor.*)

Partial trisomy 11q characteristics may include severe psychomotor retardation, microcephaly, cleft palate, large beaked nose, micrognathia, short hands, and displaced thumbs.

Treatment—Standard Symptomatic treatment with special education, physical therapy, and vocational services is appropriate. Genetic counseling is advised.

Treatment—Investigational Please contact the agencies listed under Resources, below, for the most current information.

Resources
For more information on 11q- syndrome: National Organization for Rare Disorders (NORD); Support Organization for Trisomy (S.O.F.T) and Other Related Disorders; Association for Retarded Citizens; National Institute of Child Health and Human Development (NICHHD).

For genetic information and genetic counseling referrals: March of Dimes Birth Defects Foundation; NIH/National Center for Education in Maternal and Child Health (NCEMCH).

References
Syndromes of the Head and Neck, 3rd ed.: R.J. Gorlin, et al.; Oxford University Press, 1990, p. 85.

13Q- SYNDROME

Description 13q- syndrome, a chromosomal disorder caused by a partial deletion of the long arm of chromosome 13, is characterized primarily by mental and growth deficiencies; other abnormalities include microcephaly and retinoblastoma. Syndromes that involve other deviations of chromosome 13 are 13q-mosaicism; monosomy 13; inversion (insertion) 13; ring 13; translocation 13; trisomy 13.

Synonyms
13q- Chromosomal Syndrome

Signs and Symptoms Abnormalities of infants born with 13q- syndrome include microcephaly, trigonocephaly, holoprosencephaly, large low-set ears, a prominent nasal bridge, hypertelorism, ptosis, coloboma, retinoblastoma, microphthalmia, a prominent maxilla, micrognathia, and a short webbed neck. Digital abnormalities, including small or absent thumbs, clinodactyly, and short big toes may occur. The soles of the feet may be permanently flexed, so that walking is done on the toes. Genitourinary anomalies in males include cryptorchidism and hypospadias. In females, the urethra may open into the vagina. There may be cardiac, pelvic, and renal defects.

Etiology Partial deletion of the long arm (q) of chromosome 13 is the cause of 13q- syndrome. The severity and type of abnormalities depend on the size and location of the missing genetic information.

Epidemiology This rare congenital disorder affects males and females in equal numbers.

Related Disorders See *Trisomy 13 Syndrome (Patau); Wolf-Hirschhorn Syndrome; Cri du Chat Syndrome; 18p- Syndrome.*

13q- mosaicism is a disorder in which some cells of the body have a partial deletion in the long arm of chromosome 13 while other cells are normal. 13q-mosaicism has features similar to those of 13q- syndrome but with a greater variability in type and severity because of the presence of normal cells.

Monosomy 13 may refer to any deletion of chromosome 13, or to the absence of one of the pair of chromosomes. Features may be similar to those of 13q- syndrome.

Intrachromosomal insertion of chromosome 13 involves the breaking off of a section of chromosome 13 and its subsequent reattachment in a different way, e.g., inversion. Mental deficiency, personality defects, psychosis, and other symptoms and signs may occur.

In 13 ring chromosome, chromosome 13 has a ringlike shape. When parts of the chromosome are missing, abnormalities can be similar to those of 13q- syndrome.

Translocation 13 is identified by the exchange of parts between chromosome 13 and another chromosome. Some characteristics are similar to those of 13q- syndrome, including retinoblastoma and developmental delay.

18q- syndrome characteristics include microcephaly, midfacial hypoplasia, mental deficiency, hypotonia and impaired coordination, and short stature. There may be hypertelorism, epicanthic folds, and nystagmus; low-set ears; deafness; cleft palate; and simian creases on the palms. The soles of the feet may be permanently flexed so that walking is done on the toes. Cryptorchidism in males and underdeveloped labia minora in females may be present.

Treatment—Standard Special education classes and physical therapy may benefit these patients. Genetic counseling is advised.

Treatment—Investigational Please contact the agencies listed under Resources, below, for the most current information.

Resources

For more information on 13q- syndrome: National Organization for Rare Disorders (NORD); Support Group for Trisomy 18/13 (S.O.F.T.) and Other Related Disorders; NIH/National Institute for Child Health & Human Development (NICHHD).

For genetic information and genetic counseling referrals: March of Dimes Birth Defects Foundation; NIH/National Center for Education in Maternal and Child Health (NCEMCH).

References

Smith's Recognizable Patterns of Human Malformation, 4th ed.: K.L. Jones; W.B. Saunders Company, 1988, pp. 54–55, 38–41, 56–59.

Interstitial Del (13)(q21.3q31) Associated with Psychomotor Retardation, Eczema, and Absent Suck and Swallowing Reflex: P.J. Peet et al.; J. Med. Genet., December 1987, issue 24(12), pp. 786–788.

Intrachromosomal Insertion of Chromosome 13 in a Family with Psychosis and Mental Subnormality: S.H. Roberts, et al.; J. Ment. Defic. Res., September 1986, issue 30(part 3), pp. 227–232.

18p- Syndrome

Description Among the primary features of 18p- syndrome (deletion of the short arm of chromosome 18) are unusual facial characteristics and mild-to-severe mental retardation.

Synonyms

Short Arm 18 Deletion Syndrome

Signs and Symptoms Physical characteristics include hypertelorism, ptosis, epicanthal folds, low nasal bridge, downturned mouth, a rounded face, micrognathia, and large protruding ears. Microcephaly and mental retardation, a tendency towards hypotonia, and mild-to-moderate growth deficiency are also usually present. The patient often has an IQ averaging between 45 to 50, although some patients have no mental deficiency at all. The ability to speak simple sentences may be delayed until 7 years of age, or older. Poor concentration, emotional lability, and restlessness may be characteristic. Other features that may be present include relatively small hands and feet, depression of the breastbone, and a high occurrence of dental caries.

Etiology 18p- syndrome is caused by the deletion of the short arm (p) of chromosome 18.

Epidemiology Symptoms are apparent at birth. Females are affected at least twice as often as males. Older parental age may be related to the occurrence of 18p- syndrome in offspring.

Related Disorders See *Down Syndrome; Trisomy 13 Syndrome; Trisomy 18 Syndrome.*

Partial trisomy 14 results in mental, motor, and growth retardation. Ptosis, malformed ears, and cardiac and genital anomalies may also be present. Seizures may occur.

Treatment—Standard Affected children may benefit from early intervention programs in special education and language development, along with physical therapy. Genetic counseling is recommended.

Treatment—Investigational Please contact the agencies listed under Resources, below, for the most current information.

Resources

For more information on 18p- syndrome: National Organization for Rare Disorders (NORD); The Chromosome 18 Registry and Research Society; S.O.F.T. and Other Related Disorders (Support Organization for Trisomy); National Institute of Child Health and Human Development (NICHHD); Association for Retarded Citizens (ARC).

For genetic information and genetic counseling referrals: March of Dimes Birth Defects Foundation; NIH/National Center for Education in Maternal and Child Health (NCEMCH).

References
Smith's Recognizable Patterns of Human Malformation, 4th ed.: K.L. Jones; W.B. Saunders Company, 1988, pp. 56–57.
Duplication 18p- With Mild Influence on the Phenotype: B. Johansson, et al.; Am. J. Med. Genet., April 29, 1988, vol. 4, pp. 871–874.

AARSKOG SYNDROME

Description The characteristic features of the rare Aarskog syndrome include stunted growth and abnormalities of the face, hands, and genitals, often accompanied by mild mental retardation.

Synonyms

Faciodigitogenital Syndrome
Faciogenital Dysplasia

Signs and Symptoms Facial abnormalities include ocular hypertelorism, ptosis, a short, broad nose, broad philtrum, and low-set, floppy ears. Dental deformities may be present. The chest may be depressed. Hands are short and broad, joints are highly extendible, and feet are short, broad, and flat. Characteristic genital abnormalities include cryptorchidism and a shawl scrotum, and there may be an inguinal hernia.

Growth deficiency may or may not be apparent at birth, but is usually evident by ages 1 to 3 years. A mild mental deficiency may be present.

Etiology Inheritance is thought to be sex-linked dominant, but father-to-son transmission has also been reported. The genetic defect is located on the Xq13 chromosome.

Epidemiology Males are affected more often and more severely than females.

Related Disorders See *Oral-Facial-Digital Syndrome.*

Juberg-Hayward syndrome (orocraniodigital syndrome) is characterized by short stature resulting from growth hormone deficiency. Affected individuals have microcephaly, cleft lip and palate, and deformities of the thumbs and toes.

Nager acrofacial dysostosis (mandibulofacial dysostosis) consists of cleft lip and palate, and defective development of the maxilla, the mandible, and the bones of the upper extremities. Thumbs are abnormally small.

Treatment—Standard Surgical correction of some abnormalities may be required, as may orthodontic treatment. Genetic counseling is advised.

Treatment—Investigational Research is in progress to locate the causative gene. Families with this disorder having 2 generations of affected individuals should contact Richard A. Lewis, M.D., Departments of Ophthalmology, Medicine, Pediatrics, and the Institute for Molecular Genetics, Baylor College of Medicine, One Baylor Plaza, NC-206, Houston, Texas 77030; (713) 798-3030.

Please contact the agencies listed under Resources, below, for the most current information.

Resources

For more information on Aarskog syndrome: National Organization for Rare Disorders (NORD); NIH/National Institute of Child Health & Human Development (NICHHD).

For genetic information and genetic counseling referrals: March of Dimes Birth Defects Foundation; NIH/National Center for Education in Maternal and Child Health (NCEMCH).

References

Mendelian Inheritance in Man, 9th ed.: V.A. McKusick; The Johns Hopkins University Press, 1990, pp. 3, 1171, 1591–1592.

Smith's Recognizable Patterns of Human Malformation, 4th ed.: K.L. Jones; W.B. Saunders Company, 1988, pp. 110–111.

Autosomal Dominant Inheritance of the Aarskog Syndrome: R.E. Grier, et al.; Am. J. Med. Genet., May 1983, issue 15(1), pp. 39–46.

The Aarskog (Facio-Digital-Genital) Syndrome in South Africa. A Report of Three Families: M. de Saxe, et al.; S. Afr. Med. J., February 1984, issue 65(8), pp. 299–303.

AASE-SMITH SYNDROME

Description Aase-Smith syndrome is characterized by congenital hypoplastic anemia accompanied by triphalangeal thumb and other abnormalities.

Synonyms
> Anemia-Congenital Triphalangeal Thumb Syndrome
> Triphalangeal Thumb Syndrome

Signs and Symptoms Features of the syndrome are present at birth. Skin pallor is accompanied by anemia and variable leukocytopenia. There is a mild growth deficiency. Associated abnormalities include triphalangeal thumbs, hypoplastic radii, narrow shoulders, and late closure of fontanelles. Possible cardiac anomalies include ventricular septal defect. Hepato- and splenomegaly may be present. The anemia often diminishes as the child grows.

Etiology The cause is unknown. An autosomal recessive inheritance has been suggested.

Epidemiology Both males and females appear to be affected.

Treatment—Standard Hypoplastic anemia is treated by bone marrow transplantation from HLA-compatible siblings. Blood transfusions and, in some cases, corticosteroid therapy may also be appropriate.

Treatment—Investigational Please contact the agencies listed under Resources, below, for the most current information.

Resources
   For more information on Aase-Smith syndrome: National Organization for Rare Disorders (NORD); NIH/National Heart, Lung and Blood Institute (NHLBI); Human Growth Foundation (HGF); NIH/National Institute of Child Health and Human Development.
   For genetic information and genetic counseling referrals: March of Dimes Birth Defects Foundation; National Center for Education in Maternal and Child Health (NCEMCH).

References
   Smith's Recognizable Patterns of Human Malformation, 4th ed.: K.L. Jones; W.B. Saunders Company, 1988, p. 277.

Mendelian Inheritance in Man, 9th ed.: V.A. McKusick; The Johns Hopkins University Press, 1990, pp. 1031–1032.

ACHONDROPLASIA

Description Achondroplasia is a hereditary, congenital disorder that results in short stature because of an impairment of endochondral bone formation. Craniofacial abnormalities are among the associated conditions.

Signs and Symptoms The vault of the skull is usually large in order to accommodate the enlarged brain, making the forehead broad. Hydrocephalus may be present. Brain-stem compression may occur and result in death in young children.

A low nasal bridge is characteristic. The limbs are short; the trunk appears longer than the extremities. The hands are short and broad, with a trident appearance. A dorsal kyphosis is usually present, and the legs may be bowed. Most adult males are under 4½ feet tall, and females are about 3 inches shorter.

Achondroplasia does not cause any mental deficiencies, and life expectancy in infants who survive their first year is normal.

Etiology Achondroplasia is inherited as an autosomal dominant trait, but 90 percent of cases are caused by fresh mutations. Children of fathers of advanced age are more likely to be born with a fresh achondroplasia mutation.

Epidemiology Onset occurs during gestation. Achondroplasia is one of the most common forms of congenital bone disturbances present from birth, but may not be evident until deficiency of normal growth is apparent.

Related Disorders Achondroplasia is one of the chondrodystrophies.

Treatment—Standard Ultrasonography of the brain in infancy is done to determine the presence of hydrocephalus. Orthopedic surgery may be beneficial. Genetic counseling is useful. Little People of America is an organization providing social contact for persons with achondroplasia. The organization also acts as an advocate on their behalf.

Treatment—Investigational Please contact the agencies listed under Resources, below, for the most current information.

Resources

For more information on achondroplasia: National Organization for Rare Disorders (NORD); The National Arthritis and Musculoskeletal and Skin Diseases Information Clearinghouse; Little People of America; Human Growth Foundation; Short Stature Foundation.

For genetic information and genetic counseling referrals: March of Dimes Birth Defects Foundation; National Center for Education in Maternal and Child Health (NCEMCH).

References

Smith's Recognizable Patterns of Human Malformation, 4th ed.: K.L. Jones; W.B. Saunders Company, 1988, pp. 298–303.

Mendelian Inheritance in Man, 9th ed.: V.A. McKusick; The Johns Hopkins University Press, 1990, pp. 9–11.

ACRODYSOSTOSIS

Description Acrodysostosis is a very rare genetic disorder primarily characterized by short stature, mental retardation, and bony deformities of the face and extremities.

Synonyms
Peripheral Dysostosis

Signs and Symptoms Short stature is apparent at birth, and growth retardation continues over the years. The head is brachycephalic, and facial characteristics include hypertelorism, a short and flattened nose, underdeveloped maxilla, prognathism, and malaligned teeth. The hands and feet are short and stubby, with broad, short nails. Bones in the arms, legs, and elbows are deformed, and early fusion of these bones occurs. Mental deficiency is present in most cases.

Etiology The cause is not known; an autosomal dominant inheritance is suggested. It has been found that the parents of these patients are usually older than normal.

Epidemiology Acrodysostosis is a very rare disorder that affects females twice as often as males.

Related Disorders Reported cases of acrodysostosis may represent other disorders such as pseudohypoparathyroidism.

Treatment—Standard Plastic surgery may be required in severe cases of acrodysostosis. Genetic counseling may be beneficial.

Treatment—Investigational Please contact the agencies listed under Resources, below, for the most current information.

Resources

For more information on acrodysostosis: National Organization for Rare Disorders (NORD); International Center for Skeletal Dysplasia; NIH/National Institute of Child Health and Human Development (NICHHD); Human Growth Foundation (HGF); Parents of Dwarfed Children.

For genetic information and genetic counseling referrals: March of Dimes Birth Defects Foundation; NIH/National Center for Education in Maternal and Child Health (NCEMCH).

References

Mendelian Inheritance in Man, 9th ed.: V.A. McKusick; The Johns Hopkins University Press, 1990, p. 15.

Smith's Recognizable Patterns of Human Malformation, 4th ed.: K.L. Jones; W.B. Saunders Company, 1988, pp. 392–393.

ADAMS-OLIVER SYNDROME

Description Adams-Oliver syndrome is a very rare genetic disorder in which congenital scalp and skull defects occur, along with peripheral skeletal abnormalities.

Synonyms
> Absence Defect of Limbs, Scalp, and Skull
> Hemimelia and Scalp-Skull Defects
> Scalp-Skull and Limbs, Absence Defect of

Signs and Symptoms Bald, ulcerated areas on the vertex of the scalp, usually with underlying bony defects of the skull, are present at birth. These skull and scalp abnormalities usually heal spontaneously during the first few months of life, but in a few cases plastic surgery may be necessary.

Severity of the limb abnormalities varies. Digits may be short or absent, and metacarpals may be missing. In the most severe cases, lower extremities below mid-calf may also be absent.

Etiology Adams-Oliver syndrome is transmitted through autosomal dominant inheritance.

Epidemiology The syndrome is present at birth and is extremely rare. Males and females are affected equally.

Related Disorders See *Holt-Oram Syndrome; Split-Hand Deformity.*

Aplasia cutis congenita is localized failure of development of the skin, most commonly at the vertex of the scalp but also rarely of the trunk and limbs, particularly the lower part of the legs. The affected skin may be covered by a membrane and may ulcerate, leaving in a few weeks a hairless scar.

Treatment—Standard Healing of skin defects generally occurs spontaneously; surgical repair of ulcerated areas may, however, be necessary. Other treatment is symptomatic and supportive. Genetic counseling is advised.

Treatment—Investigational Please contact the agencies listed under Resources, below, for the most current information.

Resources

For more information on Adams-Oliver syndrome: National Organization for Rare Disorders (NORD); The National Arthritis and Musculoskeletal and Skin Diseases Information Clearinghouse.

For genetic information and genetic counseling referrals: March of Dimes Birth Defects Foundation; NIH/National Center for Education in Maternal and Child Health (NCEMCH).

References

Congenital Scalp Defects with Distal Limb Reduction Anomalies: J.P. Fryns; J. Med. Genet., August 1987, issue 24(8), pp. 493–496.

Mendelian Inheritance in Man, 9th ed: V.A. McKusick; The Johns Hopkins University Press, 1990, pp. 4–5.

AMELOGENESIS IMPERFECTA

Description Amelogenesis imperfecta is a rare genetic disorder in which formation of dental enamel is defective. Several distinct forms of the condition have been identified: hypocalcified (hypomineralized), hypomaturation (snow-capped teeth), and hypoplastic (hypoplastic-explastic).

Synonyms

  Brown Enamel, Hereditary

Signs and Symptoms The disorder is characterized by defective or missing tooth enamel. Secondary effects include early tooth loss, heightened susceptibility to periodontal and alveolar disease, and increased sensitivity to hot and cold. The dental pulp (pulpa) in the root canal is exposed in some cases, and an open bite may occur because the upper and lower jaws do not align properly. Psychological problems can arise because of the unsightly teeth.

  Hypocalcified type: Suspected autosomal recessive cases of this form of amelogenesis imperfecta are more severe than those resulting from autosomal dominant inheritance. Unerupted and newly erupted teeth are covered by a light yellow-brown enamel. After eruption, the enamel turns brown or black from food stains. The enamel crumbles easily and wears off rapidly, so that by the ages of 10 to 12 years only the cores of the teeth, consisting of dentin, remain. Enamel of the cervical portion of the teeth may be better calcified. Incomplete closing of the upper and lower jaws produces an anterior open bite. The teeth are overly sensitive to temperature changes. On x-ray the enamel appears less dense than the dentin of the core. The crown of the affected tooth appears to have small irregular holes, with a dense line of calcified enamel at the neck of the tooth. The hypocalcified type of amelogenesis imperfecta is the most frequently occurring variant of the disorder.

  Hypomaturation type (snow-capped teeth): In this sex-linked recessive form of amelogenesis imperfecta, the enamel of the primary teeth in males looks white and has the appearance of ground glass. The enamel of the permanent teeth is mottled and yellow. The soft enamel can be penetrated by a sharp dental instrument under pressure. In females, the enamel of the primary teeth shows vertical bands of abnormal white enamel that looks like ground glass randomly alternating with bands of translucent normal enamel. The enamel of the permanent teeth shows vertical bands of either opaque white or opaque yellow enamel randomly alternating with bands of translucent normal enamel.

  Pigmented autosomal recessive hypomaturation type: Both primary and secondary teeth are involved. The enamel is clear-to-cloudy light brown and of normal thickness. It is, however, softer than normal, can be penetrated by a sharp dental instrument, and tends to break off from the dentin core. X-rays show a lack of contrast between enamel and dentin.

  Hypoplastic types: In the **pitted autosomal dominant hypoplastic type,** the enamel is thin with random pits from pinpoint to pinhead size primarily on the surfaces of permanent teeth facing the lips or cheeks (labial or buccal). In both primary and permanent dentition, some teeth may be normal. X-rays show a normal contrast between the enamel and the dentin core of the teeth. In the **rough autosomal dominant hypoplastic type,** the enamel is thin, brown, and very hard, with a granular vitreous surface. There is lack of contact between adjacent teeth. On x-ray the teeth appear outlined by a thin layer of enamel. A high contrast between enamel and dentin is seen. In the **rough autosomal recessive hypoplastic type,** the tooth surface is rough, grainy, and light yellow-brown in color. Lack of contact between adjacent teeth occurs. X-rays show the lack of enamel. Many teeth are unerupted and partially resorbed into the jaws. Microscopically, the only evidence of enamel is the laminated agatelike glassy calcification on the surface of the tooth core.

In the **smooth autosomal dominant hypoplastic type** of amelogenesis imperfecta, the enamel is thin, brown, smooth, and glossy, except where it is hypocalcified at contact points. Lack of contact occurs between adjacent teeth. X-rays show many unerupted teeth with resorption of the crowns in the jaw bones. Small calcified spots may be seen adjacent to unerupted teeth. In the **smooth sex-linked dominant hypoplastic form,** both males and females are affected. In males, the enamel is thin, brown or yellow-brown, smooth, and shiny. In females, alternating vertical bands of normal and abnormal enamel (Lyon effect) occur. These bands are visible on x-ray. In the **local autosomal dominant hypoplastic** variant, only the baby teeth are affected. Pits and grooves of hypoplastic enamel occur horizontally across the middle third of a tooth. Defective enamel may be present in all or only some of the teeth. The most frequently affected teeth are the incisors, or the baby molars.

Diagnosis of amelogenesis imperfecta is usually made by x-ray examination at the time the teeth erupt. By 1 to 2 years of age, the diagnosis can be made by visual examination.

Etiology As noted above, amelogenesis imperfecta is inherited through various modes of transmission. The structural defect in enamel formation during development of the embryo is thought to be the result of the inhibition of crystallization in the interrod region related to the craniofacial development. Poor oral hygiene can aggravate symptoms.

Epidemiology Amelogenesis imperfecta affects between 1:14,000 to 1:16,000 children in the United States. Some 40 percent of them have the hypocalcified dominant type. The autosomal dominant and recessive forms of the disorder affect males and females in equal numbers. The sex-linked dominant type of the disorder affects twice as many males as females. The sex-linked recessive type affects only males.

Related Disorders See *Trichodentoosseous Syndrome.*

The genetic disorder **taurodontism,** which may be a form of trichodentoosseous syndrome, is characterized by large cavities in the jaw bones in which the tooth pulp rests. Molars are usually the most severely affected. The disorder is most often found in Eskimos who use their teeth for cutting hides.

Treatment—Standard The condition may be corrected with orthodontics and restorative procedures. Desensitizing toothpaste can prevent painful sensitivity to heat and cold. Good oral hygiene is important. Genetic counseling is recommended for families of affected children.

Treatment—Investigational Please contact the agencies listed under Resources, below, for the most current information.

Resources
For more information on amelogenesis imperfecta: National Organization for Rare Disorders (NORD); National Foundation for Ectodermal Dysplasias; NIH/National Institute of Dental Research.

For genetic information and genetic counseling referrals: March of Dimes Birth Defects Foundation; National Center for Education in Maternal and Child Health (NCEMCH).

References
Mendelian Inheritance in Man, 9th ed.: V.A. McKusick; The Johns Hopkins University Press, 1990, pp. 54, 1028, 1562–1563.
A New Classification of Heritable Human Enamel Defects and a Discussion of Dentin Defects: E.D. Shields; Birth Defects, 1983, issue 19(1), pp. 107–127.
A Clinical, Genetic, and Ultrastructural Study of Snow-Capped Teeth: Amelogenesis Imperfecta, Hypomaturation Type: V.H. Escobar, et al.; Oral Surgery, December 1981, issue 52(6), pp. 607–614.

AMNIOTIC BANDS

Description When the fetus is constrained in its fetal habitat, a variety of extrinsic deformations may be produced in an otherwise normal fetus. Important causes of fetal constraint are serious deficiency of amniotic fluid and pregnancy in a bicornuate uterus. When constrictive amniotic bands occur late in pregnancy, they may result in defective development of limbs or parts of limbs, whereas when they occur early in pregnancy, they often cause deformities of the spine, chest, and face, and even may result in fetal death.

Synonyms
Early Constraint Defects
Oligohydramnios Sequence

Signs and Symptoms Compression of the chest in utero can result in underdevelopment of the lungs, making the infant incapable of independent breathing. Vascular constriction may cause reduction in the size of limbs. Compression of legs or arms may result in joint stiffness and dislocations. Scoliosis and clubfeet are common deformations. Craniofacial deformities include flattening of the nose and ears.

Premature rupture of the amniotic sac may cause problems during delivery, since the neonate cannot maneuver properly.

Decreased amniotic fluid may be detected early in the 2nd trimester by alpha-fetoprotein screening.

Etiology Early rupture of the amniotic sac can occur idiopathically; rarely, it is the result of amniocentesis. Oligohydramnios can also result from a fetal kidney disorder, since in the later stages of pregnancy fetal urine comprises a large portion of the amniotic fluid. Bilateral renal agenesis is the most common cause of oligohydramnios. When oligohydramnios is the result of insufficient fetal urine output, first-degree family members should be checked for hereditary kidney disease.

Epidemiology Both males and females are affected. Infants with amniotic bands are more commonly born to young women with preeclampsia.

Related Disorders See *Pierre Robin Syndrome; Clubfoot; Renal Agenesis, Bilateral.*

Potter syndrome (oligohydramnios tetrad) is characterized by facial anomalies, pulmonary hypoplasia, limb deformities, and hypoplastic or absent kidneys. The disorder results from inadequate urinary output from the fetus, or from chronic leakage of amniotic fluid.

Treatment—Standard Treatment is symptomatic and supportive. Genetic counseling may benefit families of infants with certain forms of inherited kidney disease that can cause amniotic bands.

Treatment—Investigational Artificial instillation of amniotic fluid is being investigated for treatment of women with severe oligohydramnios, when conservative measures have proved ineffective.

Please contact the agencies listed under Resources, below, for the most current information.

Resources

For more information on amniotic bands: National Organization for Rare Disorders (NORD); NIH/National Institute of Child Health and Human Development.

For genetic information and genetic counseling referrals: March of Dimes Birth Defects Foundation; NIH/National Center for Education in Maternal and Child Health (NCEMCH).

References

Smith's Recognizable Patterns of Human Malformation, 4th ed.: K.L. Jones; W.B. Saunders Company, 1988, pp. 572–573.

Artificial Instillation of Amniotic Fluid as a New Technique for the Diagnostic Evaluation of Cases of Oligohydramnios; U. Gembruch, et al.; Prenat. Diagn., January 1988, issue 8(1), pp. 33–45.

Acute Development of Oligohydramnios in a Pregnancy Complicated by Chronic Hypertension and Superimposed Pre-Eclampsia: P.J. Weinbaum, et al.; Am. J. Perinatol., January 1986, issue 3(1), pp. 47–49.

Oligohydramnios; Clinical Associations and Predictive Value for Intrauterine Growth Retardation: E.H. Philipson, et al.; Am. J. Obstet. Gynecol., June 1, 1983, issue 146(3), pp. 271–278.

Elevated Maternal Serum Alpha-Fetoprotein, Second-Trimester Oligohydramnios, and Pregnancy Outcome: W.L. Koontz, et al.; Obstet. Gynecol., September 1983, issue 62(3), pp. 301–304.

ANENCEPHALY

Description Anencephaly is a developmental brain disorder characterized by the absence of the cranial vault. The cerebral hemispheres are missing or grossly defective.

Signs and Symptoms Because of the absence of brain tissue, infants cannot perform basic functions, such as movement, and do not survive more than a few days or weeks. Amniocentesis and ultrasound examination can detect anencephaly.

Etiology Anencephaly is the result of defective closure of the anterior portion of the neural tube. Both autosomal and X-linked recessive inheritances have been reported.

Epidemiology Both males and females are affected.

Related Disorders See *Spina Bifida.*

Treatment—Standard Counseling concerning medical intervention is beneficial.

Treatment—Investigational Please contact the agencies listed under Resources, below, for the most current information.

Resources
  For more information on anencephaly: National Organization for Rare Disorders (NORD); Fighters for Encephaly Support; NIH/National Institute of Neurological Disorders and Stroke (NINDS).
  For genetic information and genetic counseling referrals: March of Dimes Birth Defects Foundation; National Center for Education in Maternal and Child Health (NCEMCH).

References
  Mendelian Inheritance in Man, 9th ed.: V.A. McKusick; The Johns Hopkins University Press, 1990, pp. 1034, 871–872, 1564.
  Smith's Recognizable Patterns of Human Malformation, 4th ed.: K.L. Jones; W.B. Saunders Company, 1988, pp. 548–549, 659–660.
  When Is Termination of Pregnancy during the Third Trimester Morally Justifiable?: F.A. Chervenak, et al.; New Eng. J. Med., February 1984, 310(8), pp. 501–504.
  Diagnostic Effectiveness of Ultrasound in Detection of Neural Tube Defect. The South Wales Experience of 2509 Scans (1977-1982) in High-Risk Mothers: C.J. Roberts, et al.; Lancet, November 1983, pp. 1068–1069.
  Neural Tube Defect-Specific Acetylcholinesterase: Its Properties and Quantitation in the Detection of Anencephaly and Spina Bifida: J.R. Bonham, et al.; Clin. Chim. Acta, November 1987, 170(1), pp. 69–77.

ANGELMAN SYNDROME

Description Angelman syndrome is characterized by severe congenital mental retardation, and unusual facies and muscular abnormalities that were first unfortunately described as the happy puppet syndrome.

Signs and Symptoms Characteristic features are microcephaly with an occipital groove, a protruding mandible, and an open mouth with a visible tongue. Patients seem to smile continually and they laugh excessively, features which do not seem to occur because of happiness but may be a result of a brain stem defect. Mental retardation is severe, and speech is absent. Motor development is slowed and muscle tone decreased, and jerky limb movements and hand flapping are characteristic. Patients also have poor balance. Epilepsy develops in the early years of life; it may decrease with age.

Etiology About 40 percent of patients with Angelman syndrome have a cytogenetic deletion of chromosome 15q11q13. The deletion occurs on the maternally derived chromosome 15. In these patients the risk of recurrence is very low.

In the nondeletion cases the risk of recurrence is unknown. All familial cases have had cytogenetically normal chromosomes.

In a few patients with normal chromosomes both chromosomes 15 have been paternal in origin (paternal unipaternal disomy).

The identical cytogenetic deletion occurs in Prader-Willi syndrome. Chromosomal imprinting appears to be critical in the expression of these 2 syndromes.

Epidemiology Males and females are affected equally.

Treatment—Standard Multidisciplinary evaluations should include neurologists, orthopedists, physical therapists, nutritionists, social workers, educators, ophthalmologists, psychologists or psychiatrists, and dentists. Family and individual psychiatric counseling, as well as genetic counseling, may be beneficial. Other treatment is symptomatic and supportive.

Treatment—Investigational Please contact the agencies listed under Resources, below, for the most current information.

Resources

For more information on Angelman syndrome: National Organization for Rare Disorders (NORD); Angelman Research Group; Angelman Syndrome Support Group; NIH/National Institute of Child Health and Human Development (NICHHD).

For genetic information and genetic counseling referrals: March of Dimes Birth Defects Foundation; National Center for Education in Maternal and Child Health (NCEMCH).

References

Mendelian Inheritance in Man, 9th ed.: V.A. McKusick; The Johns Hopkins University Press, 1990, pp. 1231–1232.

Smith's Recognizable Patterns of Human Malformation, 4th ed.: K.L. Jones; W.B. Saunders Company, 1988, pp. 168–169.

Syndromes of the Head and Neck, 3rd ed.: R.J. Gorlin, et al.; Oxford University Press, 1990, pp. 616–617.

The Angelman or "Happy Puppet" Syndrome. Clinical and Electroencephalographic Features and Cerebral Blood Flow: I. Bjerre, et al.; Acta Paediatr. Scand., May 1984, 73(3), pp. 398–402.

Happy-Puppet Syndrome: S. Pelc, et al.; Helv. Paediatr. Acta, August 1976, 319(2), pp. 183–188.
The Angelman ("Happy Puppet") Syndrome: C.A. Williams, et al.; Am. J. Genet., April 1982, 11(4), pp. 453–460.

ANODONTIA

Description Anodontia is a genetic condition in which all or most of the primary and secondary teeth are missing. It is usually associated with a group of nonprogressive syndromes called ectodermal dysplasias, in which the skin, skin appendages, and mucous membranes are affected.

Synonyms
> Anodontia Vera
> Complete Anodontia
> Partial Anodontia (Hypodontia)

Signs and Symptoms Anodontia may be either complete or partial. Children who have complete anodontia do not develop either primary or secondary teeth. This form of the disease is usually accompanied by abnormal development of sweat glands, hair, and nails. In partial anodontia, only some teeth are missing.

Etiology When the disorder is associated with ectodermal dysplasia, it is inherited either as an X-linked recessive or autosomal recessive trait.

Epidemiology Anodontia is congenital. In the X-linked disorder, about 60 to 75 percent of female carriers are minimally affected and can be ascertained by careful clinical evaluation.

Related Disorders Ectodermal dysplasia syndromes are hereditary and nonprogressive. They affect the skin and other organs that develop from the ectodermal germ layer during gestation. Respiratory infection is a common serious complication that develops because those affected tend to exhibit a weakened immune system and impaired respiratory mucus glands.

Treatment—Standard Complete anodontia is treated by fitting the patient with dentures. Partial anodontia that results in missing front teeth can be treated with a bridge that consists of an acrylic tooth that is attached to 3 orthodontic wires, which form a support for the device.

Treatment—Investigational Please contact the agencies listed under Resources, below, for the most current information.

Resources
> **For more information on anodontia:** National Organization for Rare Disorders (NORD); National Foundation for Ectodermal Dysplasias; NIH/National Institute of Dental Research.
>
> **For genetic information and genetic counseling referrals:** March of Dimes Birth Defects Foundation; National Center for Education in Maternal and Child Health (NCEMCH).

References
Prevalence of Tooth Agenesis Correlated with Jaw Relationship and Dental Crowding: L.R. Dermaut, et al.; Am. J. Orthod. Dentofacial Orthop., September 1986, issue 90(3), pp. 204–210.

A Review of Tooth Formation in Children with Cleft Lip/Palate: R. Ranta; Am. J. Orthod. Dentofacial Orthop., July 1986, issue 90(1), pp. 11–18.

New Technique for Semipermanent Replacement of Missing Incisors: J. Artun, et al.; Am. J. Orthod. Dentofacial Orthop., May 1984, issue 85(5), pp. 367–375.

ANTLEY-BIXLER SYNDROME

Description The very rare Antley-Bixler syndrome is characterized by multiple skeletal fusions, especially of the skull, the hip bones, and part of the arm bones.

Synonyms
Multisynostotic Osteodysgenesis
Craniosynostosis, Choanal Atresia, Radiohumeral Synostosis
Trapezoidocephaly-Multiple Synostosis Syndrome

Signs and Symptoms Craniofacial abnormalities include craniosynostosis, frontal bossing, and midface hypoplasia, with a depressed nasal bridge, proptosis, and choanal atresia. Ear development is abnormal. Other characteristics include radiohumeral synostosis and femoral bowing and fractures.

Prenatal diagnosis can be made with ultrasound.

Etiology The cause is not known; an autosomal recessive inheritance is suspected.

Epidemiology Males and females are both affected.

Related Disorders The **camptomelic syndrome** is characterized by osteochondrodysplasia, and is associated with a flat face, bowed tibia with skin dimpling, hypoplastic scapulae, and short vertebrae.

Features of **acrocephalosyndactyly syndromes** include abnormalities related to craniosynostosis, and syndactyly.

Treatment—Standard Treatment for Antley-Bixler syndrome is symptomatic and supportive.

Treatment—Investigational Please contact the agencies listed under Resources, below, for the most current information.

Resources
For more information on **Antley-Bixler syndrome:** National Organization for Rare Disorders (NORD); National Association for the Craniofacially Handicapped; Society for the Rehabilitation of the Facially Disfigured, Inc.; National Craniofacial Foundation; About Face; NIH/National Institute of Dental Research.

For genetic information and genetic counseling referrals: March of Dimes Birth Defects Foundation; National Center for Education in Maternal and

Child Health (NCEMCH).

References
Smith's Recognizable Patterns of Human Malformation, 4th ed.: K.L. Jones; W.B. Saunders Company, 1988, pp. 378–379.
Mendelian Inheritance in Man, 9th ed.: V.A. McKusick; The Johns Hopkins University Press, 1990, pp. 1036–1037.

APERT SYNDROME

Description Apert syndrome is an inherited disorder in which characteristic malformations of the head, fingers, and toes occur, along with mental deficiency.

Synonyms
> Acrocephalosyndactyly, Type I
> Syndactylic Oxycephaly
> Vogt Cephalodactyly

Signs and Symptoms Acrocephaly (resulting from craniostenosis) and syndactyly are the key identifying features of the syndrome. Other symptoms may include hypertelorism, exophthalmos, cataracts, and a high, pointed palate. Vertebral deformities and radioulnar synostosis may occur. In about 50 percent of mentally retarded patients with Apert syndrome, the IQ is above 70.

Etiology The disorder is autosomal dominant; however, a large number of cases are considered to be fresh mutations. Above-average parental age has been associated with sporadic cases.

Epidemiology Both males and females may be affected by Apert syndrome.

Related Disorders See *Carpenter Syndrome; Crouzon Disease; Pfeiffer Syndrome; Saethre-Chotzen Syndrome.*

Treatment—Standard Syndactyly and vertebral deformities may be corrected surgically. Reconstructive surgery is performed for facial and cranial deformities. Special education classes are necessary.

Treatment—Investigational Please contact the agencies listed under Resources, below, for the most current information.

Resources
For more information on Apert syndrome: National Organization for Rare Disorders (NORD); NIH/National Institute of Child Health and Human Development (NICHHD).

For genetic information and genetic counseling referrals: March of Dimes Birth Defects Foundation; National Center for Education in Maternal and Child Health (NCEMCH).

References

Smith's Recognizable Patterns of Human Malformation, 4th ed.: K.L. Jones; W.B. Saunders Company, 1988, pp. 372–373.

Mendelian Inheritance in Man, 9th ed.: V.A. McKusick; The Johns Hopkins University Press, 1990, pp. 13–14.

ARTHROGRYPOSIS MULTIPLEX CONGENITA (AMC)

Description AMC is characterized by hypomobility of multiple joints due to fibrous ankylosis. This is a heterogeneous group of disorders which includes neurogenic AMC, myopathic AMC, Guerin-Stern syndrome, and amyoplasia congenita.

Synonym
> Congenital Multiple Arthrogryposis
> Fibrous Ankylosis of Multiple Joints

Signs and Symptoms The deformities are present at birth. The primary feature of typical AMC is limited or fixed flexion contracture of joints. Soft tissue webbing may have developed over the flexed joints, and the muscles may be hypoplastic. The long bones of the skeleton are exceptionally slender, but skeletal x-rays are otherwise normal. Cleft palate and cryptorchidism may be present. Intelligence usually is normal.

Etiology The cause is unknown. Most types of AMC are not hereditary, but autosomal recessive inheritance has been reported in one large inbred Arabic kindred in Israel.

There is evidence of nervous system involvement, and electromyographic studies show muscle fiber changes, suggesting a myopathic origin.

Epidemiology Males and females are affected equally.

Related Disorders **Pterygium syndrome** is an autosomal recessive disorder in which winglike webbing may occur around multiple joints.

Popliteal pterygium syndrome is an autosomal dominant disorder characterized by popliteal webbing, pits in the lower lip, cleft lip and palate, and genital and digital anomalies.

In **amyoplasia congenita,** a generalized lack of muscular development is accompanied by multiple joint contractures.

Treatment—Standard Physiotherapy in the newborn period and early infancy is beneficial. Splints can be made to augment the stretching exercises to increase range of motion. Removable splints for the knees and feet that permit regular muscle exercise are recommended. Surgery may be required on ankles, knees, hips, elbows, or wrists to achieve better position or greater range of motion. In some cases, tendon transfers have been performed.

Treatment—Investigational Please contact the agencies listed under Resources,

below, for the most current information.

Resources
For more information on AMC: National Organization for Rare Disorders (NORD); Support Group for Arthrogryposis Multiplex Congenita; Arthrogryposis Support Group; The National Arthritis and Musculoskeletal and Skin Diseases Information; Human Growth Foundation; Short Stature Foundation.

For genetic information and genetic counseling referrals: March of Dimes Birth Defects Foundation; National Center for Education in Maternal and Child Health (NCEMCH).

References
Mendelian Inheritance in Man, 9th ed.: V.A. McKusick; The Johns Hopkins University Press, 1990, pp. 107–108, 155–156, 1044–1046, 1567.

Smith's Recognizable Patterns of Human Malformation, 4th ed.: K.L. Jones; W.B. Saunders Company, 1988, pp. 140–141.

ASPHYXIATING THORACIC DYSTROPHY (ATD)

Description ATD is a very rare genetic disorder affecting development of the thoracic bone structure. Major features include a small thoracic cage, shortened bones of the arms and legs, and renal dysfunction.

Synonyms
Asphyxiating Thoracic Dysplasia
Jeune Syndrome
Thoracic-Pelvic-Phalangeal Dystrophy

Signs and Symptoms The characteristic bell-shaped chest cavity in the newborn leaves the infant unable to breathe properly and susceptible to pulmonary infections. Other findings include hypertension, pancreatic cysts, and polydactyly. These patients have insufficient growth of the pelvic bones, and shortened long bones of the arms and legs. Problems in respiration, and chronic nephritis leading to renal failure are the most serious complications.

Prenatal diagnosis of ATD can be made using ultrasound imaging.

Etiology ATD is caused by hardening of the endochondral bone in the fetal thorax. It is inherited as an autosomal recessive trait.

Epidemiology About 1:120,000 live births are affected. Males and females are affected in equal numbers.

Related Disorders Chondroectodermal dysplasia is characterized by shortened extremities and short stature. Polydactyly, fused wrists, and dystrophy of the fingernails are seen, along with lip abnormalities and heart defects.

Metatrophic short stature, noticed in infancy, is characterized by a long narrow thorax, flattening of the vertebral bones, and relatively short limbs. Progressive deformity of the bones of the thorax and spine causes kyphoscoliosis and a marked shortening of the trunk, resulting in short-spine short stature and severe skeletal dysplasia.

Treatment—Standard To facilitate breathing, the chest may be surgically expanded by removal of cartilage in the sternum or by implantation of an acrylic device to expand the rib cage. Renal dysfunction is managed with dialysis or transplantation. Genetic counseling may benefit families affected by this disorder. Other treatment is symptomatic and supportive.

Treatment—Investigational Please contact the agencies listed under Resources, below, for the most current information.

Resources

For more information on ATD: National Organization for Rare Disorders (NORD); The National Arthritis and Musculoskeletal and Skin Diseases Information Clearinghouse; International Center for Skeletal Dysplasia; Human Growth Foundation (HGF).

For genetic information and genetic counseling referrals: March of Dimes Birth Defects Foundation; NIH/National Center for Education in Maternal and Child Health (NCEMCH).

References

Smith's Recognizable Patterns of Human Malformation, 4th ed.: K.L. Jones; W.B. Saunders Company, 1988, pp. 292–295.

A Thoracic Expansion Technique for Jeune's Asphyxiating Thoracic Dystrophy: D.W. Todd, et al.; J. Pediatr. Surg., February 1986, issue 21(2), pp. 161–163.

Asphyxiating Thoracic Dysplasia. Clinical, Radiological, and Pathological Information on Ten Patients: R. Oberklaid, et al.; Arch. Dis. Child, October 1977, issue 52(10), pp. 758–765.

The Jeune Syndrome (Asphyxiating Thoracic Dystrophy) in an Adult: J.M. Friedman, et al.; Am. J. Med., December 1975, issue 59(6), pp. 857–862.

BECKWITH-WIEDEMANN SYNDROME

Description Beckwith-Wiedemann syndrome is a rare congenital disorder characterized by macroglossia, omphalocele, macrosomia, and ear creases.

Synonyms

Exomphalos-Macroglossia-Gigantism Syndrome.

Signs and Symptoms Although some patients with Beckwith-Wiedemann syndrome have few or no symptoms, a variety of signs and symptoms are possible. Among the more severe expressions are omphalocele; macroglossia, which may cause feeding and breathing difficulties; and hypoglycemia, which is present in about one-third of cases and requires immediate treatment to prevent neurologic complications. Mild-to-moderate mental retardation, polycythemia, and microcephaly may also occur.

Other characteristics include hemihypertrophy and unusual facial features such as ear deformities, hypoplasia of the midface, frontal bossing, and moles. Cardiovascular defects include cardiomegaly.

Male children may have cryptorchidism; females, enlarged clitoris, uterus, or bladder.

Both malignant and benign tumors may develop. Malignant tumors occur in 5 to 10 percent of patients. The most common types are Wilms tumor, adrenocortical carcinoma, hepatoblastoma, rhabdomyosarcoma, gonadoblastoma, and neuroblastoma. Benign tumors include adenoma of the adrenal cortex, cardiac hamartoma, umbilical myxoma, and ganglioneuroma.

As children with Beckwith-Wiedemann syndrome grow older, the characteristics of the disorder are less noticeable. Excess growth rate often slows after the first few years of life.

Etiology An autosomal dominant inheritance has been suggested. The locus of the mutations is at 11p15.5.

Epidemiology Males and females are affected equally. Over 200 cases of the disorder have been reported in the medical literature since 1963.

Treatment—Standard Treatment may include surgery to repair omphalocele and hypospadias. If malignant or benign tumors develop, they must be treated and/or removed through surgery. Neonatal hypoglycemia, if present, is usually transient and is treated by intravenous glucose. If left untreated, hypoglycemia can be life-threatening and can cause mental retardation.

Beckwith-Wiedemann patients should be screened at 3-month intervals by abdominal ultrasound examination to monitor the growth of internal organs and tumors; and alpha-fetoprotein measurements should be monitored until patients are 7 years old.

Genetic counseling may benefit patients and their families. Other treatment is symptomatic and supportive.

Treatment—Investigational Please contact the agencies listed under Resources, below, for the most current information.

Resources

For more information on Beckwith-Wiedemann syndrome: National Organization for Rare Disorders (NORD); Beckwith-Wiedemann Support Group; NIH/National Institute of Child Health and Human Development (NICHHD).

For genetic information and genetic counseling referrals: March of Dimes Birth Defects Foundation; NIH/National Center for Education in Maternal and Child Health (NCEMCH); Barbara Biesecker, Genetic Counselor, University of Michigan Medical School.

References

Mendelian Inheritance in Man, 9th ed.: V.A. McKusick; The Johns Hopkins University Press, 1990, pp. 292–294.

Smith's Recognizable Patterns of Human Malformation, 4th ed.: K.L. Jones; W.B. Saunders Company, 1988, pp. 136–139.

Genetic Linkage of Beckwith-Wiedemann Syndrome to 11p15: A.J. Ping, et al.; Am. J. Hum. Genet., issue 44, 1989, pp. 720–723.

BLOOM SYNDROME

Description Bloom syndrome is an inherited disorder characterized by short stature, facial telangiectasia, photosensitivity, and susceptibility to infections and, later in life, to malignancies. Except for the susceptibility to infections and cancer, affected persons generally have good health, particularly in infancy and childhood.

Synonyms

Short Stature, Telangiectatic Erythema of the Face

Signs and Symptoms Affected infants are small at birth. Normal size is not achieved, but body proportions are normal. The face is often small and narrow, and is characteristically covered with telangiectasia during the first year. Areas of abnormal pigmentation may occur on the rest of the body. The skin is highly photosensitive, especially on the affected areas on the face. Typically there are immunologic abnormalities that lead to vulnerability to infection. In addition, almost 50 percent of patients eventually develop a wide variety of malignancies, especially leukemia and squamous cell carcinoma. Occasionally, abnormalities of the eyes, ears, hands, and feet may be present.

Etiology Bloom syndrome is inherited as an autosomal recessive trait. Cytogenetic characteristics include chromosomal breakage and sister chromatid exchanges.

Epidemiology The syndrome most often affects persons of Ashkenazic Jewish ancestry. A slight male predominance is unexplained.

Treatment—Standard Sunscreen should be used. Treatment is symptomatic, with antibiotics and cancer therapy as necessary.

Treatment—Investigational Please contact the agencies listed under Resources, below, for the most current information.

Resources

For more information on Bloom syndrome: National Organization for Rare Disorders (NORD); NIH/National Institute of Child Health and Human Development; Bloom Syndrome Registry; Human Growth Foundation (HGF); National Foundation for Jewish Genetic Diseases.

For genetic information and genetic counseling referrals: March of Dimes Birth Defects Foundation; National Center for Education in Maternal and Child Health (NCEMCH).

References

Mendelian Inheritance in Man, 9th ed.: V.A. McKusick; The Johns Hopkins University Press, 1990, pp. 1066–1068.

Cecil Textbook of Medicine, 18th ed.: J.B. Wyngaarden and L.H. Smith, Jr., eds.; W.B. Saunders Company, 1988, pp. 168, 1113, 1001, 1096.

Smith's Recognizable Patterns of Human Malformation, 4th ed.: K.L. Jones; W.B. Saunders Company, 1988, pp. 94–95.

BLUE RUBBER BLEB NEVUS

Description Blue rubber bleb nevus is a very rare congenital vascular disorder that affects the skin and internal organs. The primary feature is multiple distinctive hemangiomas, which are rubbery and blisterlike. The tumors vary in color, size, shape, number, and site. They may be tender and are usually benign.

Synonyms

Bean Syndrome

Signs and Symptoms Blue rubber bleb nevus is characterized by soft, tender, elevated blue, blue-black, or purplish-red hemangiomas, some of which are present at birth. They are blood-filled and compressible, refilling immediately after compression. Hyperhidrosis may occur in the surrounding areas, and nocturnal pain is common. External hemangiomas are usually located on the upper arms or trunk. Internal hemangiomas may be found in the liver, lungs, spleen, gallbladder, kidney, and skeletal muscles. Nevi in the gastrointestinal tract may produce bleeding and chronic anemia; in the brain, they may result in hemorrhage and increased cranial pressure.

Etiology Blue rubber bleb nevus is inherited as an autosomal dominant trait.

Epidemiology Males and females are affected in equal numbers.

Related Disorders See *Maffucci Syndrome; von Hippel-Lindau Syndrome.*

Treatment—Standard Carbon dioxide laser surgery is recommended for removal of external hemangiomas. For internal hemangiomas, conventional surgery usually is necessary. Surgical resection may be required to treat growths in the gastrointestinal tract. Genetic counseling may benefit patients and their families. Other treatment is symptomatic and supportive.

Treatment—Investigational Please contact the agencies listed under Resources, below, for the most current information.

Resources

For more information on blue rubber bleb nevus: National Organization for Rare Disorders (NORD); NIH/National Institute of Arthritis, Musculoskeletal and Skin Diseases (NIAMS) Clearinghouse.

For genetic information and genetic counseling referrals: March of Dimes Birth Defects Foundation; NIH/National Center for Education in Maternal and Child Health (NCEMCH).

References

Mendelian Inheritance in Man, 9th ed.: V.A. McKusick; The Johns Hopkins University Press, 1990, p. 141.

Blue Rubber Bleb Nevus Syndrome Presenting with Recurrence: K.S. Sandhu, et al.; Dig. Dis. Sci., February 1987, issue 32(2), pp. 214–219.

Central Nervous System Involvement in Blue Rubber Bleb Nevus Syndrome: S. Satya-Murti, et al.; Arch. Neurol., November 1986, issue 43(11), pp. 1184–1186.

CARPENTER SYNDROME

Description Carpenter syndrome is a rare genetic disorder in which characteristic anomalies of the head, hands, and genitalia occur. Mental retardation is also present in affected individuals.

Synonyms

Acrocephalopolysyndactyly II

Signs and Symptoms Carpenter syndrome is a form of craniosynostosis. In addition to skull deformities, brachydactyly with webbing, duplication of the big toe, and cryptorchidism are present. Down-slanting eyes, a flattened nose, low-set ears, and mandibular hypoplasia are characteristic features, along with obesity and cardiac anomalies. Mental retardation is common, but intelligence is normal in some patients.

Etiology Carpenter syndrome is inherited as an autosomal recessive trait.

Epidemiology Males and females are affected in equal numbers.

Related Disorders See *Oral-Facial-Digital Syndrome; Apert Syndrome.*

Goodman syndrome (acrocephalopolysyndactyly type IV) is a mild form of Carpenter syndrome in which mental retardation does not occur and hand deformities are less pronounced than in Carpenter syndrome.

Nager acrofacial dysostosis (mandibulofacial dysostosis) is a rare hereditary disorder in which cleft lip and palate and mandibular hypoplasia occur. Smaller-than-normal thumbs are also observed in affected individuals.

In **Sakati syndrome (acrocephalopolysyndactyly type III)**, characteristic head and digital anomalies are accompanied by short legs with bowed femurs, hypoplastic ears, alopecia, dry skin, cryptorchidism, microphallus, inguinal hernias, and congenital heart disease.

Treatment—Standard Early craniofacial surgery may relieve intracranial pressure and limit the severity of mental retardation, as well as correct the characteristic facial anomalies. Additional surgical intervention is indicated for the correction of cardiac and digital abnormalities. Genetic counseling is advised.

Treatment—Investigational Please contact the agencies listed under Resources, below, for the most current information.

Resources

For more information on Carpenter syndrome: National Organization for Rare Disorders (NORD); NIH/National Institute of Child Health and Human Development (NICHHD); FACES—National Association for the Craniofacially Handicapped; National Craniofacial Foundation; Institute of Reconstructive Plastic Surgery.

For genetic information and genetic counseling referrals: March of Dimes Birth Defects Foundation; NIH/National Center for Education in Maternal and Child Health (NCEMCH).

References
Mendelian Inheritance in Man, 9th ed.: V.A. McKusick; The Johns Hopkins University Press, 1990, pp. 998–999.
Acrocephalopolysyndactyly Type II Carpenter Syndrome; Clinical Spectrum and Attempt at Unification with Goodman and Summit Syndromes: D.M. Cohen; Am. J. Med. Genet., October 1987, issue 28(2), pp. 311–324.
Carpenter Syndrome; Natural History and Clinical Spectrum: L.K. Robinson; Am. J. Med. Genet., March 1985, issue 20(3), pp. 461–469.

CEREBRO-COSTO-MANDIBULAR SYNDROME

Description Cerebro-costo-mandibular syndrome is a rare genetic disorder in which severe micrognathia and palatal defects are present, along with multiple rib abnormalities. Mental retardation may also occur.

Synonyms
> Cerebrocostomandibular Syndrome
> Rib Gap Defects with Micrognathia

Signs and Symptoms The syndrome is characterized by severe micrognathia, glossoptosis, abnormalities of the palate, and multiple rib defects, particularly between the 3rd and 7th pairs. The thorax is small and bell-shaped with gaps between the posterior ossified and anterior cartilaginous ribs. Rarely, hearing loss may result from a defect of the middle ear, and speech development may be delayed. Moderate-to-severe mental retardation occurs in about one-third of patients. Rib fractures and pseudarthrosis of the ribs usually improve with age.

The infant's difficulty with nipple feeding may lead to failure to thrive. Respiratory distress may be a significant problem, and increased susceptibility to respiratory infections may be life-threatening. Pneumonia and otitis media often recur. Almost half of the children die in the first year.

Etiology The inheritance pattern is not established. The syndrome appears to have been transmitted through autosomal recessive inheritance in one family, and as an autosomal dominant trait in others.

Epidemiology Males and females tend to be affected in equal numbers.

Related Disorders See *Pierre Robin Syndrome.*

Treatment—Standard Intensive medical intervention may be necessary for respiratory distress, feeding difficulty, and respiratory infections. Surgical correction of the palate may be required. Genetic counseling is advisable.

Treatment—Investigational Please contact the agencies listed under Resources, below, for the most current information.

Resources
> **For more information on cerebro-costo-mandibular syndrome:** National Organization for Rare Disorders (NORD); National Craniofacial Foundation;

FACES—National Association for the Craniofacially Handicapped; Craniofacial Family Association; NIH/National Institute of Child Health and Human Development (NICHHD).

For genetic information and genetic counseling referrals: March of Dimes Birth Defects Foundation; National Center for Education in Maternal and Child Health (NCEMCH).

References

Mendelian Inheritance in Man, 9th ed.: V.A. McKusick; The Johns Hopkins University Press, 1990, p. 180.

Smith's Recognizable Patterns of Human Malformation, 4th ed.: K.L. Jones; W.B. Saunders Company, 1988, pp. 534–535.

Cerebrocostomandibular Syndrome. Case Report and Literature Review: K.G. Smith, et al.; Clin. Pediatr. (Phila.), April 1985, issue 24(4), pp. 223–225.

The Course of the Cerebrocostomandibular Syndrome: D.J. Harris, et al.; Birth Defects, 1977, issue 13(3C), pp. 117–130.

CHARGE ASSOCIATION

Description CHARGE is the acronym for a very rare disorder that results from several defects in early fetal development. A minimum of 4 of the following characteristics are necessary for the diagnosis: **C**oloboma of the eye; **H**eart defects; **A**tresia of the choanae; **R**etardation of growth and development, and central nervous system abnormalities; **G**enital hypoplasia in males; and **E**ar abnormalities and loss of hearing.

Signs and Symptoms Coloboma is present in over three-fourths of CHARGE patients. About 80 percent of affected individuals have cardiac abnormalities. These include ventricular and atrial septal defects, patent ductus arteriosus, and tetralogy of Fallot. Choanal atresia occurs in over half of patients, and retarded growth and development as well as mental deficiency and/or central nervous system abnormalities are present in about 90 percent. Approximately three-fourths of males with CHARGE association have microphallus and testicular hypoplasia. Close to 90 percent of patients have ear abnormalities: the ears may be short, wide, and cup-shaped, and may differ in shape. There may be mild to severe hearing loss.

In addition to those anomalies included in the CHARGE acronym, affected infants may also have feeding difficulties, microcephaly, micrognathia, cleft lip and palate, and tracheoesophageal fistulas. There may also be rib and renal anomalies. Some patients have features of the DiGeorge syndrome (see *DiGeorge Syndrome*).

Etiology Most instances are sporadic. The etiology is heterogeneous. In some cases the disorder is transmitted as an autosomal recessive trait. Recurrences of certain abnormalities have been observed within families.

Epidemiology CHARGE association is very rare, affecting only approximately 200 persons in the United States. Females are affected twice as often as males.

Treatment—Standard A full heart evaluation is recommended for all children with coloboma or choanal atresia in whom CHARGE association is a possible diagnosis. All patients with conotruncal or aortic arch defects and abnormalities in other parts of the body should be evaluated for CHARGE association and DiGeorge syndrome.

Surgery to correct cardiac and other anomalies may be appropriate.

Treatment—Investigational Please contact the agencies listed under Resources, below, for the most current information.

Resources

For more information on CHARGE association: National Organization for Rare Disorders (NORD); NIH/National Institute of Child Health and Human Development (NICHHD).

For genetic information and genetic counseling referrals: March of Dimes Birth Defects Foundation; National Center for Education in Maternal and Child Health (NCEMCH).

References

Mendelian Inheritance in Man, 9th ed.: V.A. McKusick; The Johns Hopkins University Press, 1990, pp. 1093–1094.

Smith's Recognizable Patterns of Human Malformation, 4th ed.: K.L. Jones; W.B. Saunders Company, 1988, pp. 606–608.

The Pattern of Cardiovascular Malformation in Charge Association: A.E. Lin, et al.; Am. J. Dis. Child, September 1987, issue 141(9), pp. 1010–1013.

The CHARGE Association. How Well Can They Do?: E. Goldson, et al.; Am. J. Dis. Child, September 1986, issue 140(9), pp. 918–921.

Familial Charge Syndrome: Clinical Report with Autopsy Findings: L.A. Metlay, et al.; Am. J. Med. Genet., March 1987, issue 26(3), pp. 577–581.

CLEFT LIP AND CLEFT PALATE

Description Cleft lip and cleft palate are common congenital malformations. A cleft is defined as an incomplete closure of palate or lip, or both. The defect is caused when the maxillae do not fuse properly during embryonic development. The cleft may be barely noticeable or result in severe deformity requiring surgery.

Synonyms

Cheiloschisis

Hare lip

Signs and Symptoms There are several varieties of cleft malformations, and over 200 syndromes have cleft lip and/or palate as a feature. The most severe types involve the lip, gum, bone, and soft and hard palates. Less inclusive clefts may involve only one of these structures. Clefts may occur uni- or bilaterally.

Affected individuals usually have a flat nose and splayed lips, abnormalities of tooth development (absent, supernumerary, or deformed teeth), abnormal growth of the ipsilateral alar nasal cartilage, and mild ocular hypertelorism, and are at increased risk for otitis media and hearing loss. Speech may be impaired.

Etiology When cleft lip and cleft palate occur as part of a syndrome, the etiology is that of the syndrome. When they occur in isolation, the etiology is less clear. Both a genetic mutation and environmental factors may be involved.

Epidemiology Cleft lip and palate affect more than 5500 newborns each year in the United States. The frequency in neonates is 1:700, but this ratio varies according to race. Orientals are most likely to be affected; blacks, least likely. Males are at least twice as likely as females to be affected by cleft lip, but females are more prone to cleft palate.

Treatment—Standard Initial treatment must ensure that the newborn can feed. Obturators used for this purpose must be replaced as the dental arches grow. Therapy requires the coordinated efforts of a team of specialists, including pediatricians, dental specialists, surgeons, speech pathologists, and psychologists.

Cleft lip can be corrected by surgery, usually when the child is still an infant. Later a second cosmetic procedure may be indicated. Cleft palate may also be treated surgically or by a prosthesis. More than one surgical procedure may be required, the first usually being performed during the toddler years. Speech and hearing should also be assessed by a speech pathologist during this time. Both may improve from therapy and surgery. Braces usually are effective to treat dental complications; sometimes dental prosthetics are needed to replace missing teeth.

Treatment—Investigational New surgical and dental corrective procedures are being researched and developed. Other studies concentrate on facial and psychological development.

Although a cleft palate is closed during early childhood, difficulties may persist if the palate is excessively short in relation to the pharynx. For information on the use, in children 8 years and older, of a material applied to the rear of the pharynx that brings the pharynx and palate into the proper relationship, please contact William N. Williams, D.D.S., University of Florida, College of Dentistry, Box J-424, Gainesville, Florida 32610; (904) 392-4370.

Please contact the agencies listed under Resources, below, for the most current information.

Resources

For more information on cleft lip and cleft palate: National Organization for Rare Disorders (NORD); FACES—National Association for the Craniofacially Handicapped; National Craniofacial Foundation; Craniofacial Family Association; The Cleft Palate Foundation, Inc.; Society for the Rehabilitation of the Facially Disfigured, Inc.; About Face; NIH/National Institute of Dental Research.

For genetic information and genetic counseling referrals: March of Dimes Birth Defects Foundation; NIH/National Center for Education in Maternal and Child Health (NCEMCH).

References

Syndromes of the Head and Neck, 3rd ed.: R.J. Gorlin, et al.; Oxford University Press, 1990, pp. 693–784.

Mendelian Inheritance in Man, 9th ed.: V.A. McKusick; The Johns Hopkins University Press, 1990, pp. 196–198, 1000, 1100–1101, 1392, 1576.

Smith's Recognizable Patterns of Human Malformation, 4th ed.: K.L. Jones; W.B. Saunders Company, 1988, pp. 196–199.

Nelson Textbook of Pediatrics, 13th ed.: R.E. Behrman and V.C. Vaughan, III, eds.; W.B. Saunders Company, 1987, pp. 804–805.

CLUBFOOT

Description The term "clubfoot" is a word used to describe several kinds of congenital ankle and foot deformities. The defect can be mild or severe, unilateral or bilateral.

Synonyms

Calcaneal Valgus
Calcaneovalgus
Metatarsus Varus
Talipes Calcaneus
Talipes Equinovarus
Talipes Equinus
Talipes Valgus
Talipes Varus
Valgus Calcaneus

Signs and Symptoms The several types of clubfoot are shown in the synonyms, above. In the most common form, **calcaneal valgus,** the heel turns outward from the midline and the anterior part of the foot is elevated. In **equinovarus,** the heel turns inward from the midline of the leg; the foot is plantar flexed, and the Achilles tendon is very tight. In **metatarsus adductus,** the forefoot deviates toward the midline. In **metatarsus varus,** the inner border of the foot does not reach the ground, so that the patient must walk on the outer border of the foot. Clubfoot is not painful and causes no difficulties until the infant begins to stand and walk. At that point, the defect forces the child to walk as if on a peg leg. If both feet are affected, the child usually walks on the balls of the feet. In severe cases, the child may walk on the sides or even the dorsum of the feet. Without the protection of the thick skin of the sole of the foot, the sides and dorsum may become ulcerated. Growth of the entire extremity may be affected.

Etiology The cause is unclear. The most likely explanation is a combination of hereditary factors and environmental influences such as infection, drugs, and disease, which may affect prenatal growth.

It has been suggested that 2 etiologic types of clubfoot may occur. One is characterized by an even sex ratio, normal maternal age curve, recurrence risk of about 10 percent, and probable dominant inheritance with about 40 percent penetrance. The other group is described as born to younger mothers; affected persons are predominantly male and show no clear pattern of inheritance.

Uterine constraint may be associated with clubfoot (see **Amniotic Bands**). Children with spina bifida (see **Spina Bifida)** sometimes develop a form of clubfoot. In such cases, muscle imbalance or spasticity may cause twisting of a normal foot.

Epidemiology Clubfoot is usually present at birth. In the United States, it affects approximately 9,000 infants (about 1:400 live births). Boys are affected twice as often as girls.

Treatment—Standard Treatment of clubfoot is begun soon after birth. Serial casting for 3 to 6 months is usually required, with frequent follow-up by an orthopedist. In milder cases, splinting and night bracing may be sufficient. Surgical correction is required in more severe cases, especially when heel cord lengthening is needed.

When initiated early, conservative treatment is successful in more than half of cases. With expert early treatment, most patients are able to wear regular shoes, participate in sports, and lead active lives. Left untreated, however, the deformity becomes fixed, and growth of the entire extremity may be affected. Surgery after infancy may successfully treat the foot, but the rest of the leg may be permanently deformed.

Treatment—Investigational Please contact the agencies listed under Resources, below, for the most current information.

Resources

For more information on clubfoot: National Organization for Rare Disorders (NORD); NIH/National Institute of Child Health & Human Development (NICHHD).

For genetic information and genetic counseling referrals: March of Dimes Birth Defects Foundation; National Center for Education in Maternal and Child Health (NCEMCH).

References

Mendelian Inheritance in Man, 9th ed.: V.A. McKusick; The Johns Hopkins University Press, 1990, p. 198.

Clubfoot: Public Health Education Information Sheet, Health Education Information Sheet, March of Dimes (1983).

COCKAYNE SYNDROME

Description Cockayne syndrome is a progressive disorder with characteristics that include growth retardation, photosensitivity, and a prematurely aged appearance.

Synonyms

Progeroid Nanism

Signs and Symptoms Infants affected by Cockayne syndrome generally appear normal at birth, with features of the disorder manifesting during the 2nd year of life. A few cases of prenatal onset have been reported.

Craniofacial abnormalities include microcephaly, a thin nose, sunken eyes, lack of subcutaneous facial fat, and prognathism. Dental caries may occur. The individual will be short of stature but have disproportionately long arms and legs, and large hands and feet. Joints may be large and habitually flexed, and there may be kyphosis. The extremities may feel cold and have a bluish color, and the patient may experience tremor and unsteady gait. Affected individuals are highly photosensitive and may be mentally deficient and partially deaf. Ocular involvement includes optic atrophy with retinal pigmentation, and cataracts. Hepatomegaly may occur. Older patients may be sexually underdeveloped.

Etiology Cockayne syndrome has autosomal recessive inheritance. Cells from these patients show defective repair of damage due to ultraviolet radiation.

Epidemiology Over 70 cases of the syndrome have been reported.

Related Disorders See *Hutchinson-Gilford Syndrome,* some aspects of which are similar to Cockayne syndrome.

Treatment—Standard Treatment is symptomatic and supportive.

Treatment—Investigational Please contact the agencies listed under Resources, below, for the most current information.

Resources

For more information on Cockayne syndrome: National Organization for Rare Disorders (NORD); NIH/National Institute of Child Health and Human Development; Human Growth Foundation (HGF); Research Trust for Metabolic Diseases in Children.

For genetic information and genetic counseling referrals: March of Dimes Birth Defects Foundation; National Center for Education in Maternal and Child Health (NCEMCH).

References

Syndromes of the Head and Neck, 3rd ed.: R.J. Gorlin, et al.; Oxford University Press, 1990, pp. 492–494.

Smith's Recognizable Patterns of Human Malformation, 4th ed.: K.L. Jones; W.B. Saunders Company, 1988, pp. 122–123.

Mendelian Inheritance in Man, 9th ed.: V.A. McKusick; The Johns Hopkins University Press, 1990, pp. 1101–1103.

COFFIN-LOWRY SYNDROME

Description Coffin-Lowry syndrome is characterized by short stature, mental retardation, hypotonia, and various facial and skeletal abnormalities.

Synonyms

Coffin Syndrome

Mental Retardation with Osteocartilaginous Anomalies

Signs and Symptoms Affected individuals have a prominent square forehead and narrow temples, and prominent chin and ears; hypertelorism and downslanting palpebral fissures; a broad nose with thick alar cartilage; thick lips; and an open mouth. There may be feeding and respiratory problems.

Patients are short in stature. Hands are large and soft, with thick, tapering fingers and prominent hypothenar. Pectus carinatum or pectus excavatum may be present. An awkward gait is characteristic in both males and females. In males, the skin is loose and easily stretched. Affected males are severely mentally retarded. Only 20 percent of females are severely mentally deficient, and 20 percent are normal.

Etiology Coffin-Lowry syndrome has X-linked inheritance; the gene is on the short arm of the X chromosome (Xp22.2). Female heterozygotes are usually less severely affected.

Epidemiology Males and females seem to be affected in equal numbers, but symptoms may be more severe in males and usually progress with age.

Treatment—Standard Treatment for Coffin-Lowry disease is symptomatic and supportive. Genetic counseling will be helpful for patients and their families.

Treatment—Investigational Please contact the agencies listed under Resources, below, for the most current information.

Resources

For more information on **Coffin-Lowry syndrome:** National Organization for Rare Disorders (NORD); NIH/National Institute of Neurological Disorders & Stroke (NINDS); The National Arthritis and Musculoskeletal and Skin Diseases Information Clearinghouse.

For **genetic information and genetic counseling referrals:** March of Dimes Birth Defects Foundation; National Center for Education in Maternal and Child Health (NCEMCH).

References
Smith's Recognizable Patterns of Human Malformation, 4th ed.: K.L. Jones; W.B. Saunders Company, 1988, pp. 236–237.

Syndromes of the Head and Neck, 3rd ed.: R.J. Gorlin, et al.; Oxford University Press, 1990, pp. 827–829.

Brief Clinical Report: Early Recognition of the Coffin-Lowry Syndrome: W.G. Wilson, et al.; Am. J. Med. Genet., 1981, issue 8(2), pp. 215–220.

Early Clinical Signs in Coffin-Lowry Syndrome: J.S. Vles, et al.; Clin. Genet., November 1984, issue 26(5), pp. 448–452.

Forearm Fullness in Coffin-Lowry Syndrome: A Misleading Yet Possible Early Diagnostic Clue: J.H. Hersh, et al.; Am. J. Med. Genet., June 1984, issue 18(2), pp. 195–199.

COFFIN-SIRIS SYNDROME

Description Coffin-Siris syndrome is a congenital disorder in which mental retardation, short stature, and malformations of the 5th digit are present from birth in affected individuals. Feeding problems and frequent respiratory infections are typical.

Synonyms
> Fifth Digit Syndrome
> Mental Retardation with Hypoplastic 5th Fingernails and Toenails
> Short Stature—Onychodysplasia

Signs and Symptoms Characteristic facies includes a wide nose and/or mouth, low nasal bridge, and thick lips. Scalp hair may be sparse or excessive. Nails on the 5th finger and toe may be hypoplastic or absent. Short stature and mental deficiency are typical, and there may be joint laxity (dislocated elbows are common) and mild-to-severe hypotonia. Dental and motor development may be retarded. Feeding problems, vomiting, and recurrent respiratory infections are early manifestations. Occasionally, patients have variable skin, skeletal, genital, and cardiac defects, as well as Dandy-Walker syndrome.

Etiology The cause is unknown; an autosomal recessive inheritance may be involved.

Epidemiology Females are affected 4 times as frequently as males; lethality in males is suspected.

Related Disorders See *Dandy-Walker Syndrome.*

Treatment—Standard Treatment is symptomatic and supportive.

Treatment—Investigational Please contact the agencies listed under Resources, below, for the most current information.

Resources
> **For more information on Coffin-Siris syndrome:** National Organization for Rare Disorders (NORD); NIH/National Institute of Child Health and Human Development (NICHHD); Short Stature Foundation; Human Growth Foundation (HGF).

References
> Smith's Recognizable Patterns of Human Malformation, 4th ed., K.L. Jones; W.B. Saunders Company, 1988, pp. 522–523.
> Mendelian Inheritance in Man, 9th ed.: V.A. McKusick; The Johns Hopkins University Press, 1990, pp. 336–337.

CONRADI-HÜNERMANN SYNDROME

Description Conradi-Hünermann syndrome, a form of chondrodysplasia punctata, affects infants and young children and is characterized by facial abnormalities, mild-to-moderate growth deficiencies, large skin pores, and sparse but coarse hair.

Synonyms
Chondrodysplasia Punctata
Chondrodystrophia Calcificans Congenita
Conradi Disease
Dysplasia Epiphysialis Punctata

Signs and Symptoms Affected children have a short neck and a broad, flat nose. Large pores in the skin, resembling orange peel, may occur on the body, and scalp hair tends to be coarse and sparse. Ichthyotic skin lesions may be present (see *Ichthyosis*). Epiphyseal calcification slows growth in the extremities, and scoliosis may occur even in infancy. Buildup of fibrous tissue around joints may limit mobility. Cataracts may develop, and a small percentage of patients may be mentally retarded.

Etiology Conradi-Hünermann syndrome is the X-linked dominant form of chondrodysplasia punctata.

Epidemiology This extremely rare syndrome is present at birth and seems to affect only females, since the gene defect is lethal for hemizygous males.

Related Disorders Chondrodysplasia (rhizomelic type) is a form of chondrodysplasia punctata inherited as an autosomal recessive trait. Affected individuals may have facial anomalies, cardiac and vision disorders, and a predisposition to recurrent infections. Spasticity and mental retardation are also present. Calcifications of hip and shoulder joints inhibit growth in the extremities. The condition is usually lethal in the first year of life.

Fetal warfarin syndrome has features similar to those of Conradi-Hünermann syndrome, including growth deficiency, unusual facies, and recurrent infection, along with mental retardation. The condition results from maternal use of warfarin during pregnancy.

Treatment—Standard Orthopedic surgery may be useful in the correction of problems associated with bone growth abnormalities, and problems with vision may be treated surgically or with corrective lenses. Dermatologic conditions should be treated symptomatically. Genetic counseling is advised.

Treatment—Investigational Please contact the agencies listed under Resources, below, for the most current information.

Resources
For more information on Conradi-Hünermann syndrome: National Organization for Rare Disorders (NORD); The National Arthritis and Musculoskeletal and Skin Diseases Information Clearinghouse; NIH/National Eye Institute; International Center for Skeletal Dysplasias; Human Growth Foundation (HGF); Parents of Dwarfed Children; Little People of America; Short Stature Foundation.
For more information on scoliosis: National Scoliosis Foundation, Inc.
For more information on ichthyosis: National Ichthyosis Foundation.

For genetic information and genetic counseling referrals: March of Dimes Birth Defects Foundation; National Center for Education in Maternal and Child Health (NCEMCH).

References
Syndromes of the Head and Neck, 3rd ed.: R.J. Gorlin, et al.; Oxford University Press, 1990, pp. 188–190.

Mendelian Inheritance in Man, 9th ed.: V.A. McKusick; The Johns Hopkins University Press, 1990, p. 190.

Smith's Recognizable Patterns of Human Malformation, 4th ed.: K.L. Jones; W.B. Saunders Company, 1988, pp. 338–339.

CORNELIA DE LANGE SYNDROME

Description Individuals with Cornelia de Lange syndrome greatly resemble each other. Major characteristics include skeletal and facial anomalies, excessive hairiness, and severe mental retardation.

Synonyms
> Amsterdam Dwarf Syndrome of de Lange
> Brachmann-de Lange Syndrome

Signs and Symptoms Neonates have low birth weight (under 5 pounds) and feeding difficulties. Typical craniofacial features include microcephaly; a small, broad nose; thin, downturned lips; thick, bushy eyebrows; and long eyelashes. Cleft palate may occur. Hands and feet are small, and limb abnormalities include phocomelia and oligodactyly. Other characteristics include hirsutism, hearing loss, seizures, and cardiac and gastrointestinal abnormalities. Stature is small. Mental retardation is severe and speech may be impaired.

Etiology The syndrome is suspected to be genetic in origin, but the mode of transmission is unknown. Most cases are sporadic.

Epidemiology Males and females appear to be affected in equal numbers. There is a 2 to 4 percent recurrence rate within families. The syndrome is estimated to occur in between 1:10,000 and 1:30,000 births.

Treatment—Standard Physical and occupational therapy, special education, hearing aids, and prosthetic limbs may all be beneficial. Genetic counseling is recommended.

Treatment—Investigational Please contact the agencies listed under Resources, below, for the most current information.

Resources
For more information on Cornelia de Lange syndrome: National Organization for Rare Disorders (NORD); Cornelia de Lange Syndrome Foundation; NIH/National Institute of Child Health and Human Development (NICHHD).

For genetic information and genetic counseling referrals: March of Dimes Birth Defects Foundation; NIH/National Center for Education in Maternal and Child Health (NCEMCH).

References

Mendelian Inheritance in Man, 9th ed.: V.A. McKusick; The Johns Hopkins University Press, 1990, pp. 230–232.

Smith's Recognizable Patterns of Human Malformation, 4th ed.: K.L. Jones; W.B. Saunders Company, 1988, pp. 80–83.

Normal Language Skills and Normal Intelligence in a Child with De Lange Syndrome: T.H. Cameron, et al.; J. Speech Hear. Discord., May 1988, 53(2), pp. 219–222.

Mild Brachmann-de Lange Syndrome: Changes of Phenotype with Age: F. Greenberg, et al.; Am. J. Med. Genet., January 1989, issue 32(1), pp. 90–92.

CRANIOMETAPHYSEAL DYSPLASIA

Description Craniometaphyseal dysplasia is a rare genetic disorder in which characteristic craniofacial and skeletal anomalies occur, accompanied by hearing loss.

Synonyms
Osteochondroplasia

Signs and Symptoms The disorder is usually evident at birth, and is characterized by hyperostosis of the bones of the cranial vault, face, and mandible. The thickening is especially evident at the nasal bridge, and the nasal passages are abnormally small as a result of bony encroachment. Hypertelorism and proptosis occur, and there may be mandibular malocclusion. If cranial pressure is not relieved, facial paralysis, deafness, and loss of vision may occur. The limbs may be affected by sclerosis or metaphyseal splaying. Intelligence is usually normal.

Etiology The cause is not known. Both autosomal dominant and recessive forms have been described, but they cannot be distinguished on clinical grounds alone.

Epidemiology Males and females are equally affected.

Related Disorders See *Osteopetrosis.*

Pyle disease (metaphyseal dysplasia), often confused with craniometaphyseal dysplasia, is a rare genetic disorder with few clinical findings, and the skull is only mildly affected. It is characterized by marked splaying of the long bones, which is more severe than that seen in craniometaphyseal dysplasia.

Frontometaphyseal dysplasia is a rare genetic disorder characterized by a wide nasal bridge, incomplete development of the sinuses, hypertelorism, supraorbital bossing, micromandible, and multiple deformities of the teeth and bones. Mental retardation may also occur.

Treatment—Standard Early surgical treatment to relieve cranial pressure and correct the facial deformities may also help eliminate vision and hearing complications. Genetic counseling may be beneficial.

Treatment—Investigational Please contact the agencies listed under Resources, below, for the most current information.

Resources

For more information on craniometaphyseal dysplasia: National Organization for Rare Disorders (NORD); NIH/National Institute of Child Health and Human Development (NICHHD); National Craniofacial Foundation; National Foundation for Facial Reconstruction; National Association for the Craniofacially Handicapped.

For genetic information and genetic counseling referrals: March of Dimes Birth Defects Foundation; NIH/National Center for Education in Maternal and Child Health (NCEMCH).

References

Mendelian Inheritance in Man, 9th ed.: V.A. McKusick; The Johns Hopkins University Press, 1990, pp. 235, 1113.

Smith's Recognizable Patterns of Human Malformation, 4th ed.: K.L. Jones; W.B. Saunders Company, 1988, p. 349.

Optic Atrophy and Visual Loss in Craniometaphyseal Dysplasia: C. Puliafito, et al.; Am. J. Ophthalmol., November 1981, issue 92(5), pp. 696–701.

Autosomal Dominant Craniometaphyseal Dysplasia. Clinical Variability: A. Carnevale, et al.; Clin. Genet., January 1983, issue 23(1), pp. 17–22.

CRI DU CHAT SYNDROME

Description Cri du chat syndrome is characterized in infants by a high, shrill, mewing, kitten-like cry that fades in later infancy. Other abnormalities are present.

Synonyms

5p- Syndrome
Cat's Cry Syndrome
Chromosome 5p- Syndrome
Le Jeune Syndrome

Signs and Symptoms The characteristic cry is present during the first weeks of life. Birth weight usually is low, and growth is slow. Almost all patients are microcephalic and mentally deficient. The typical infant has a round face with hypertelorism, epicanthal folds, strabismus, low-set and/or malformed ears, a small chin, prominent nose, and facial asymmetry. Simian creases are common. Over three-quarters of infants are hypotonic; as infants grow older this is replaced with hyperreflexia.

Abnormalities that occur less frequently include myopia, cleft lip and cleft palate, bifid uvula, clinodactyly, hemivertebra, inguinal hernia, cryptorchidism, absent kidney and spleen, clubfoot, and flat feet. Seven of 13 adults in one study had scoliosis and 11 patients had short metacarpals and metatarsals.

Etiology A partial deletion of the short arm of chromosome 5 causes cri du chat syndrome. The more severe the deletion, the more severe the effect on intelligence, height, and weight.

Epidemiology Cri du chat syndrome was first described in 1963; since then over 100 cases have been reported. It has been estimated that the syndrome occurs in about 1:50,000 births and accounts for approximately 1 percent of institutionalized mentally retarded patients.

Treatment—Standard Treatment for cri du chat syndrome is symptomatic and supportive.

Treatment—Investigational Please contact the agencies listed under Resources, below, for the most current information.

Resources

For more information on cri du chat syndrome: National Organization for Rare Disorders (NORD); Cri-du-Chat Society; 5p- Society; NIH/National Institute of Child Health and Human Development.

For genetic information and genetic counseling referrals: March of Dimes Birth Defects Foundation; National Center for Education in Maternal and Child Health (NCEMCH).

References

Syndromes of the Head and Neck, 3rd ed.: R.J. Gorlin, et al.; Oxford University Press, 1990, pp. 48–49.

Smith's Recognizable Patterns of Human Malformation, 4th ed.: K.L. Jones; W.B. Saunders Company, 1988, pp. 40–41.

Psychomotor Development in 65 Home-reared Children with Cri-du-chat Syndrome: L.E. Wilkins, et al.; J. Pediatr., 1980, issue 97, p. 401.

CROUZON DISEASE

Description Crouzon disease is a form of craniosynostosis in which characteristic facial anomalies occur, accompanied by mental retardation and disturbances in vision and hearing.

Synonyms
  Acrocephalosyndactyly II
  Craniofacial Dysostosis
  Crouzon Craniofacial Dysostosis

Signs and Symptoms Acrocephaly, hypertelorism, exophthalmos, strabismus, a parrot-beaked nose with deviated septum, hypoplastic maxilla, and mandibular prognathism are present in affected individuals. In more than 50 percent of cases, progressive vision loss and conductive hearing loss occur. Mental retardation is evident, and spinal anomalies are present in about one-third of patients. Abnormal cranial growth begins in the first year of life and is completed by age 3 years. Life expectancy is normal.

Etiology The disease is inherited as an autosomal dominant trait.

Epidemiology Males and females are affected in equal numbers.

Related Disorders See *Apert Syndrome (Acrocephalosyndactyly Type I); Carpenter Syndrome (Acrocephalosyndactyly Type II); Saethre-Chotzen Syndrome.*

Treatment—Standard Surgery is indicated to relieve intracranial pressure and to correct craniofacial anomalies. Vision loss may be treated with corrective lenses or with ophthalmic surgical procedures. Genetic counseling is recommended.

Treatment—Investigational Please contact the agencies listed under Resources, below, for the most current information.

Resources

For more information on Crouzon disease: National Organization for Rare Disorders (NORD); National Craniofacial Foundation; FACES—National Association for the Craniofacially Handicapped; Society For the Rehabilitation of the Facially Disfigured, Inc.; About Face.

For genetic information and genetic counseling referrals: March of Dimes Birth Defects Foundation; National Center for Education in Maternal and Child Health (NCEMCH).

References

Developmental Abnormalities: A.B. Baker and R.J. Joynt; *in* Clinical Neurology, revised edition, Harper & Row, 1986, pp. 71–74.

Premature Closure of the Cranial Sutures: L.P. Roland and C. Kennedy; *in* Merritt's Textbook of Neurology, 7th ed., Lea & Febiger, 1984, pp. 376–379.

Three-Dimensional Cat Scan Reconstruction—Pediatric Patients: K.E. Salyer, et al.; Clin. Plast. Surg., July 1986, issue 13(3), pp. 463–474.

The Encyclopedia of Genetic Disorders and Birth Defects, J. Wynbrandt and M.D. Ludman, eds.; Facts on File, 1991, pp. 88–89.

CYSTIC HYGROMA

Description Cystic hygroma, a cystic lymphangioma, usually occurs at the nape of the neck.

Synonyms

Cystic Lymphangioma
Fetal Cystic Hygroma
Hygroma Colli

Signs and Symptoms Cystic hygroma may be present at birth or can begin during early childhood. The sac, filled with lymphatic fluid and cells, is thin-walled and compressible, and it grows rapidly upward toward the ear, or down toward the axilla. Rarely it may originate in the axilla, groin, retroperitoneal cavity, chest wall, hip, or the coccygeal region. Surgical or drug treatment usually prevents the cyst from greatly enlarging; however, it may become progressive, causing hydrops.

Cystic hygroma can be detected during pregnancy through ultrasonography and testing for a greatly elevated level of alpha-1-fetoprotein in the amniotic fluid.

Etiology Cystic hygroma is probably inherited through autosomal recessive genes. The hygroma is thought to be caused by a failure of the lymph system to properly connect with the cervical blood vessels.

Epidemiology Males and females are affected in equal numbers.

Related Disorders Cystic hygroma may be seen in persons with *Turner Syndrome*. See also *Cavernous Lymphangioma*.

Treatment—Standard Treatment may include surgery as well as use of bleomycin in a microsphere-in-oil emulsion. Recurrence of the hygroma is possible after treatment. Genetic counseling may be helpful.

Treatment—Investigational Please contact the agencies listed under Resources, below, for the most current information.

Resources

For more information on cystic hygroma: National Organization for Rare Disorders (NORD); National Lymphatic & Venous Diseases Foundation, Inc.; American Cancer Society; NIH/National Cancer Institute PDQ (Physician Data Query) phoneline.

For genetic information and genetic counseling referrals: March of Dimes Birth Defects Foundation; National Center for Education in Maternal and Child Health (NCEMCH).

References
Mendelian Inheritance in Man, 9th ed.: V.A. McKusick; The Johns Hopkins University Press, 1990, pp. 1388–1389.
Fetal Cystic Hygroma Colli: Antenatal Diagnosis, Significance, and Management: A.S. Garden, et al.; Am. J. Obstet. Gynecol., February 1986, issue 154(2), pp. 221–225.
Treatment of Cystic Hygroma and Lymphangioma with the use of Bleomycin Fat Emulsion: N. Tanigawa, et al.; Cancer, August 15, 1987, issue 60(4), pp. 741–749.
Fetal Cystic Hygroma and Turner's Syndrome: R.F. Carr, et al.; Am. J. Dis. Child., June 1986, issue 140(6), pp. 580–583.

DENTIN DYSPLASIA, CORONAL

Description Coronal dentin dysplasia is a genetic disorder characterized by opalescent deciduous teeth and normal-appearing, but abnormal, secondary dentition.

Synonyms
Anomalous Dysplasia of Dentin
Dentin Dysplasia, Type II
Pulp Stones
Pulpal Dysplasia

Signs and Symptoms The deciduous teeth have a brownish-blue opalescent look. On x-ray, they show obliterated pulp chambers and reduced root canals. The permanent teeth are normal in color but contain flame-shaped pulp chambers, often with an extension reaching into the root, and numerous pulp stones. Root formation in the permanent teeth is usually normal.

Etiology Coronal dentin dysplasia is inherited as an autosomal dominant trait.

Epidemiology Males and females are affected in equal numbers.

Related Disorders See *Dentin Dysplasia, Radicular; Dentinogenesis Imperfecta, Type III.*

Treatment—Standard Coronal dentin dysplasia may be treated by curettage around the tips of the roots and retrograde amalgam seal, or by more conventional root canal therapy. However, preventive dental care provides the best available means of maintaining the teeth.

Genetic counseling is recommended for families of children with coronal dentin dysplasia.

Treatment—Investigational Please contact the agencies listed under Resources, below, for the most current information.

Resources

For more information on coronal dentin dysplasia: National Organization for Rare Disorders (NORD); National Foundation for Ectodermal Dysplasias; NIH/National Institute of Dental Research.

For genetic information and genetic counseling referrals: March of Dimes Birth Defects Foundation; National Center for Education in Maternal and Child Health (NCEMCH).

References
Mendelian Inheritance in Man, 9th ed.: V.A. McKusick; The Johns Hopkins University Press, 1990, p. 257.

A Scanning Electron Microscopic Study of Dentin Dysplasia Type II in Primary Dentition: J.R. Jasmin, et al.; Oral Surg., July 1984, issue 58(1), pp. 57–63.

Dentinal Dysplasia: A Clinicopathological Study of Eight Cases and Review of the Literature: N.E. Steidler, et al.; Br. J. Maxillofac. Surg., August 1984, issue 22(4), pp. 274–286.

DENTIN DYSPLASIA, RADICULAR

Description Radicular dentin dysplasia is a genetic disorder characterized by atypical formation of the dentin, resulting in abnormal roots and pulp chambers.

Synonyms
Dentin Dysplasia, Type I
Radicular Dentin Dysplasia
Rootless Teeth

Signs and Symptoms The teeth generally are of normal shape and color, although in some cases there is an opalescent shine. X-rays reveal half-moon–shaped or obliterated pulp chambers in the roots. Areas around the abnormally short roots may appear radiolucent.

Both the deciduous and permanent teeth are affected. The teeth are often poorly aligned and can be chipped easily. Without treatment, persons with radicular dentin dysplasia may lose their teeth by age 30 to 40 years.

Etiology Radicular dentin dysplasia is inherited as an autosomal dominant disorder.

Epidemiology Radicular dentin dysplasia affects about 1:100,000 persons. Males and females are affected in equal numbers.

Related Disorders See *Dentin Dysplasia, Coronal; Dentinogenesis Imperfecta, Type III.*

Treatment—Standard Filling the tips of the root canals permits the teeth to remain in their natural positions. Sometimes the affected teeth must be extracted and replaced with dentures.

Genetic counseling is recommended for families of children with radicular dentin dysplasia.

Treatment—Investigational Please contact the agencies listed under Resources, below, for the most current information.

Resources

For more information on radicular dentin dysplasia: National Organization for Rare Disorders (NORD); National Foundation for Ectodermal Dysplasias; NIH/National Institute of Dental Research.

For genetic information and genetic counseling referrals: March of Dimes Birth Defects Foundation; National Center for Education in Maternal and Child Health (NCEMCH).

References
Mendelian Inheritance in Man, 9th ed.: V.A. McKusick; The Johns Hopkins University Press, 1990, p. 257.

Dentin Dysplasia Type I: A Clinical Report: J.A. Petrone, et al.; J. Am. Dent. Assoc., December 1981, issue 103(6), pp. 891–893.

Dentin Dysplasia Type I: A Scanning Electron Microscopic Analysis of the Primary Dentition: M. Melnick, et al.; Oral Surg., October 1980, issue 50(4), pp. 335–340.

DENTINOGENESIS IMPERFECTA, TYPE III

Description Dentinogenesis imperfecta, type III, is an inherited dental disorder in which the primary and secondary teeth erode early and the pulp is revealed. Other genetic anomalies often occur concomitantly with this dental disorder.

Synonyms

Brandywine Type Dentinogenesis Imperfecta
Dentinogenesis Imperfecta, Shields Type III

Signs and Symptoms The crowns of both primary and secondary teeth decay, sometimes exposing the pulp. The pulp is smooth and amber-colored and reflects an iridescent light. Secondary teeth may be characterized by absent or partially absent pulp chambers and root canals, whereas those of the primary teeth may be larger than normal. Secondary teeth may also be pitted.

The teeth of carriers may appear normal, but the pulp chamber may be larger than normal, and the enamel may be quite thin. This condition is referred to as shell teeth.

Etiology Dentinogenesis imperfecta is inherited through an autosomal dominant gene, which is thought to be on chromosome 4q13—q21.

Epidemiology First diagnosed in the Brandywine, Maryland community, dentino-genesis imperfecta, type III, is also found in the Ashkenazi Jewish population.

Related Disorders See *Dentin Dysplasia, Radicular; Dentin Dysplasia, Coronal.*

Dentinogenesis imperfecta, type I (DGI 1; opalescent dentin; opalescent teeth without osteogenesis imperfecta; dentinogenesis imperfecta, Shields type II; capdepont teeth; hereditary brown teeth) is a genetic condition in which the teeth are bluish-gray or amber-colored and reflect an iridescent light, without concomitant brittle bones. The teeth have bulbous crowns. Roots, root canals, and pulp chambers are absent or too small. Bringing the teeth together, as occurs when chewing, causes the enamel to separate from the ivory.

Treatment—Standard Children are fitted with dental crowns as early as possible for cosmetic benefit; adults may undergo tooth extraction and replacement with dentures.

Families of affected children may benefit from genetic counseling.

Treatment—Investigational Please contact the agencies listed under Resources, below, for the most current information.

Resources

For more information on dentinogenesis imperfecta, type III: National Organization for Rare Disorders (NORD); National Foundation for Ectodermal Dysplasias; NIH/National Institute of Dental Research.

For genetic information and genetic counseling referrals: March of Dimes Birth Defects Foundation; National Center for Education in Maternal and Child Health (NCEMCH).

References

Dentinogenesis Imperfecta in the Brandywine Isolate (DI Type III): Clinical, Radiologic, and Scanning Electron Microscopic Studies of the Dentition: L.S. Levin, et al.; Oral Surg., September 1983, issue 56(3), pp. 267–274.

An Autosomal-Dominant Form of Juvenile Periodontitis: Its Localization to Chromosome 4 and Linkage to Dentinogenesis Imperfecta and Gc; J. Craniofac. Genet. Dev. Biol., 1986, issue 6(4), pp. 341–350.

An Unusual Presentation of Opalescent Dentin and Brandywine Isolate Hereditary Opalescent Dentin in an Ashkenazic Jewish Family: A. Heimler, et al.; Oral Surg. Oral Med. Oral Pathol., June 1985, issue 59(6), pp. 608–615.

DIASTROPHIC DYSPLASIA

Description Diastrophic dysplasia is a hereditary growth disorder characterized by short limbs, abnormally curved bones, joint and hand deformities, and clubfeet. Intelligence is usually normal.

Synonyms
Chondrodystrophy with Clubfeet

Signs and Symptoms Onset is prenatal. Infants are short in stature. Abnormalities of the spine generally include scoliosis, kyphosis, and cervical spina bifida. Pelvic bones, the femoral head, and the coccyx may be malformed. On weight-bearing, the hip and knee joints tend to dislocate. The thumb is extended in a characteristic hitchhiker position, and synostosis of proximal interphalangeal joints is present. Severe bilateral clubfeet may occur.

Craniofacial abnormalities include cleft palate (about 25 percent of patients) and occasionally a beak-shaped nose and facial hemangioma. In early infancy the pinna of the ear may have cystlike swellings; later these may develop into cauliflowerlike shapes with or without ossification.

Etiology The genetic defect, transmitted by autosomal recessive genes, affects the manner in which cartilage is converted to bone.

Epidemiology Males and females are affected in equal numbers.

Related Disorders See *Achondroplasia; Arthrogryposis Multiplex Congenita.*

Treatment—Standard Treatment consists of orthopedic management, including surgery, braces, casts, and manipulations. Dental treatment and surgical closure of the cleft palate are used when necessary. Corticosteroids are injected into the ear to treat the cartilage deformity. Genetic counseling is recommended.

Treatment—Investigational Please contact the agencies listed under Resources, below, for the most current information.

Resources
For more information on diastrophic dysplasia: National Organization for Rare Disorders (NORD); The National Arthritis and Musculoskeletal and Skin Diseases Information Clearinghouse; Little People of America; Human Growth Foundation (HGF); Short Stature Foundation; International Center for Skeletal Dysplasia.

For genetic information and genetic counseling referrals: March of Dimes Birth Defects Foundation; National Center for Education in Maternal and Child Health (NCEMCH).

References
Mendelian Inheritance in Man, 9th ed.: V.A. McKusick; The Johns Hopkins University Press, 1990, p. 1142.
Smith's Recognizable Patterns of Human Malformation, 4th ed.: K.L. Jones; W.B. Saunders Company, 1988, pp. 326–327.

Disorders of the Spine in Diastrophic Dwarfism: D. Bethem, et al.; J. Bone Joint Surg. (Am.), 1980, issue 62(4), pp. 529–536.

DiGeorge Syndrome

Description DiGeorge syndrome results from developmental defects of the 3rd and 4th pharyngeal pouches (fetal thymus and parathyroids) and, often, the 4th branchial arch. The thymus and parathyroids may be hypoplastic or absent. Expression of the defects is highly variable.

Synonyms
> Third and Fourth Pharyngeal Pouch Syndrome
> Thymic Aplasia
> Thymic Hypoplasia

Signs and Symptoms Hypoparathyroidism is often the initial sign, and may result in seizures during the first few days of life.

Patients with a severely underdeveloped thymus will develop frequent infections from viruses, fungi, *Pneumocystis carinii,* and certain bacteria. Chronic nasal infections, diarrhea, oral candidiasis, and *Pneumocystis* pneumonia are very common. In the majority of patients some thymic tissue is present and immunodeficiency is minimal or absent.

Facial characteristics associated with DiGeorge syndrome include hypertelorism, antimongoloid eye slant, notched and low-set ears, and micrognathia. The most common associated cardiovascular anomalies include truncus arteriosus, interrupted aortic arch, and tetralogy of Fallot.

Gastrointestinal tract anomalies and a variable but generally moderate mental deficiency are sometimes seen.

Etiology Most often the condition occurs sporadically, but a few instances of autosomal dominant inheritance have been reported. In 5 to 10 percent of cases, deletion of the long arm of chromosome 22 is found. The syndrome occurs in some infants of diabetic mothers and occasionally in infants with the fetal alcohol syndrome. It occurs concurrently with a variety of other syndromes, such as the CHARGE association. DiGeorge syndrome also occurs in infants with retinoic acid embryopathy. Faulty development of the cephalic neural crest is believed to be the common pathogenetic mechanism involved in all of these conditions.

Epidemiology Males and females seem to be affected in equal numbers.

Related Disorders See *Nezelof Syndrome; Severe Combined Immunodeficiency; Wiskott-Aldrich Syndrome.*

Treatment To control infantile seizures, blood calcium levels must be increased. Orally administered calcium and vitamin D are indicated. Immunodeficiency usually improves spontaneously after the first few years of life unless the thymus is completely absent. Transplantation of fetal thymus tissue, bone marrow transplantation, and administration of various thymic hormones have been used to treat severe cases. Optimal treatment is still evolving.

When infections occur, they must be treated vigorously with antifungal, antibiotic, and supportive measures. Trimethoprim-sulfamethoxazole and the orphan drug, pentamidine isethionate, are used to treat *P. carinii.* Cytomegalovirus and generalized herpes simplex infections are treated with antiviral agents.

Patients with severe immunodeficiency must be protected as much as possible from infectious agents. They should not be immunized with live viral vaccines. Corticosteroids and immunosuppressant drugs must be avoided. Should blood transfusions be necessary, the blood must be irradiated or "washed" to remove all viable lymphocytes that might cause graft-versus-host disease (GVHD).

Cardiac surgery is often necessary for life-threatening heart defects.

Please contact the agencies and persons listed under Resources, below, for the most current information.

Resources

For more information on DiGeorge syndrome: National Organization for Rare Disorders (NORD); NIH/National Institute of Child Health and Human Development; Immune Deficiency Foundation; Angelo M. DiGeorge, M.D., St. Christopher's Hospital for Children, Philadelphia, Pennsylvania; Frank Greenberg, M.D., Baylor College of Medicine; Craig B. Langman, M.D. and Samuel S. Gidding, M.D., Children's Memorial Hospital, Chicago, Illinois.

For genetic information and genetic counseling referrals: March of Dimes Birth Defects Foundation; National Center for Education in Maternal and Child Health (NCEMCH).

References

Mendelian Inheritance in Man, 9th ed.: V.A. McKusick; The Johns Hopkins University Press, 1990, pp. 916–917.

Smith's Recognizable Patterns of Human Malformation, 4th ed.: K.L. Jones; W.B. Saunders Company, 1988, pp. 556–557.

Immunodeficiency: R.H. Buckley; J. Allergy. Clin. Immunol., December 1983, issue 6(72), pp. 627–641.

DOWN SYNDROME

Description Down syndrome is the most common and readily identifiable genetic condition associated with mental retardation. Facial, skeletal, and frequently cardiac anomalies are among the more than 50 clinical signs seen in the syndrome, although it is rare to find all or even most of them in one person.

Synonyms
Mongolism
Trisomy 21 Syndrome

Signs and Symptoms Some common characteristics include microcephaly; small mouth; flat nasal bridge; Brushfield spots in the iris; epicanthal folds; small ears sometimes folded over at the tops; short neck; a simian crease on the palm; and poor muscle tone.

All children with Down syndrome have some degree of mental retardation, usually in the mild-to-moderate range, but sometimes profound.

Approximately 50 percent of affected children have congenital heart disease. They are prone to respiratory, eye, and ear problems. They are 20 times more likely to develop leukemia than the general population, but it is believed that leukemia itself is not inherited but results from an increased genetic susceptibility to leukemia-causing environmental factors. Life expectancy is close to normal.

Etiology In Down syndrome, the mental and physical abnormalities are caused by the presence of an extra chromosome contributed by either the egg or sperm cell; i.e., a total of 47 chromosomes instead of the normal 46. Trisomy 21, with 3 chromosomes 21, is the most common form of Down syndrome.

Epidemiology Approximately 1:800 live births, or 7000 children with Down syndrome are born in the United States each year. The incidence is higher for children born to women and men over 35. The most common forms of the syndrome do not usually occur more than once in a family. All races and societal economic levels are affected equally.

Treatment—Standard The basic neurologic disorder cannot be altered, but early intervention can benefit affected children (see Resources, below, for organizations such as the Association for Children with Down Syndrome, which can recommend helpful programs). Education of both parent and child can begin in the postnatal period. Learning, language, mobility, self care, and socialization skills can be developed early, followed up by toddler and preschool programs. Many of the children can be educated in the public schools, learn basic academic and prevocational skills with special training, and perform many daily living activities independently.

Treatment—Investigational Please contact the agencies listed under Resources, below, for the most current information.

Resources

For more information on Down syndrome: National Organization for Rare Disorders (NORD); Association for Children with Down Syndrome; National Down Syndrome Congress; National Association for Down Syndrome; National Down Syndrome Society; National Center for Down Syndrome; NIH/National Institute of Child Health and Human Development; Children's Brain Diseases Foundation; National Association for Retarded Citizens.

For genetic information and genetic counseling referrals: March of Dimes Birth Defects Foundation; National Center for Education in Maternal and Child Health (NCEMCH); National Institute of Mental Retardation (Canadian Association for the Mentally Retarded).

References

Smith's Recognizable Patterns of Human Malformation, 4th ed.: K.L. Jones; W.B. Saunders Company, 1988, pp. 10–15, 659–661.

DUBOWITZ SYNDROME

Description Dubowitz syndrome, a very rare developmental disorder, is characterized by short stature and an unusual facies.

Synonyms
Intrauterine Short Stature

Signs and Symptoms Onset is intrauterine or immediately postnatal. Affected children have low birth weight, usually about 5 lbs at full term. Short stature is a prominent feature. Facial abnormalities include a relatively high nasal bridge, hypoplasia of supraorbital ridges, ocular hypertelorism, ptosis, blepharophimosis, prominent ears, delayed eruption of teeth as well as dental decay, abnormalities of the jaw area (zygoma, malar eminence, mandible), and, occasionally, cleft palate. The voice is often high-pitched, the hair is sparse, and eczema may be present on the face, knees, and elbows. Intelligence is usually normal, with some memory deficits or learning disabilities, although some patients are mildly retarded and speech usually is impaired. These children may be hyperactive.

Etiology The condition is considered to be autosomal recessive. The genetic defect causes intrauterine or postnatal growth retardation.

Epidemiology Males and females are equally affected.

Related Disorders See *Bloom Syndrome.*

Treatment—Standard Treatment is symptomatic and supportive.

Treatment—Investigational Please contact the agencies listed under Resources, below, for the most current information.

Resources
For more information on Dubowitz syndrome: National Organization for Rare Disorders (NORD); NIH/National Institute of Child Health and Human Development; Human Growth Foundation (HGF); Short Stature Foundation.

For genetic information and genetic counseling referrals: March of Dimes Birth Defects Foundation; National Center for Education in Maternal and Child Health (NCEMCH).

References
Smith's Recognizable Patterns of Human Malformation, 4th ed.: K.L. Jones; W.B. Saunders Company, 1988, pp. 92–93.
Mendelian Inheritance in Man, 9th ed.: V.A. McKusick; The Johns Hopkins University Press, 1990, p. 1150.

DYSPLASIA EPIPHYSEALIS HEMIMELICA

Description Dysplasia epiphysealis hemimelica is characterized by overgrowth of the epiphyseal cartilage of one or more of the carpal or tarsal bones. Less often, the cartilage on other bones, e.g., the ankle, knee, or hip joint, can be affected.

Synonyms
> Chondrodystrophy, Epiphyseal
> Epiphyseal Osteochondroma, Benign
> Tarsoepiphyseal Aclasis
> Tarsomegaly
> Trevor Disease

Signs and Symptoms Onset of symptoms usually is between 2 and 4 years of age. Pain and discomfort occur because of the excessive cartilage growth. Usually only one limb is involved, and the limbs may be unequal in length.

Etiology The cause is unknown. No familial cases have been reported.

Epidemiology The disorder primarily affects males.

Related Disorders Chondrodysplasia punctata consists of a group of disorders characterized by a pug nose, scaly skin lesions, and abnormalities in epiphyseal cartilage. See **Conradi-Hünermann Syndrome,** an X-linked dominant form of chondrodysplasia punctata that affects infants and young children.

Treatment—Standard Treatment consists of surgical removal of cartilage overgrowth in joints where it causes pain and discomfort. Other treatment is symptomatic and supportive.

Treatment—Investigational Please contact the agencies listed under Resources, below, for the most current information.

Resources
> For more information on dysplasia epiphysealis hemimelica: National Organization for Rare Disorders (NORD); National Arthritis, Musculoskeletal & Skin Disease (NIAMS) Information Clearinghouse.

References
> Mendelian Inheritance in Man, 9th ed.: V.A. McKusick; The Johns Hopkins University Press, 1990, p. 276.
> The Variable Manifestations of Dysplasia Epiphysealis Hemimelica: E.M. Azouz, et al.; Pediatr. Radiol., 1985, issue 15(1), pp. 44–49.
> Dysplasia Epiphysealis Hemimelica: R. Cruz-Conde, et al.; J. Pediatr. Orthop., September 1984, issue 4(5), pp. 625–629.
> Dysplasia Epiphysealis Hemimelica. A Clinical and Genetic Study: J.M. Horan, et al.; J. Bone Joint Surg. (Br.), May 1983, issue 65(3), pp. 350–354.

ENGELMANN DISEASE

Description The major features of Engelmann disease, a rare genetic bone disorder, include diaphyseal dysplasia, muscle weakness, bone pain, an unusual gait, extreme fatigue, and anorexia, leading to a malnourished appearance.

Synonyms

Camurati-Engelmann Disease
Osteopathia Hyperostotica Multiplex Infantilis
Progressive Diaphyseal Dysplasia

Signs and Symptoms Onset is usually in childhood. Normal muscle development is lacking, and weakness in the leg muscles results in an unusual waddling walk. Bone pain is severe, especially in the femur. The bones at the base of the skull, the bones of the hands and feet, and rarely the jaw bone may be affected. Overgrowth of the bones near the eye sockets may occur, and can result in loss of vision. Fatigue, headache, and poor appetite may be present.

Etiology Engelmann disease is inherited as an autosomal dominant trait.

Epidemiology Males and females are affected in equal numbers.

Related Disorders See *Paget's Disease of Bone; Myotonic Dystrophy; Muscular Dystrophy, Becker; Muscular Dystrophy, Duchenne; Muscular Dystrophy, Emery-Dreifuss.*

Treatment—Standard Treatment usually involves corticosteroids such as cortisone or prednisone for relief of symptoms. Eye surgery to decompress the optic nerves is most often ineffective and usually not recommended. Genetic counseling may benefit patients and their families. Other treatment is symptomatic and supportive.

Treatment—Investigational Please contact the agencies listed under Resources, below, for the most current information.

Resources

For more information on Engelmann disease: National Organization for Rare Disorders (NORD); NIH/National Arthritis and Musculoskeletal and Skin Diseases Information Clearinghouse.

For genetic information and genetic counseling referrals: March of Dimes Birth Defects Foundation; NIH/National Center for Education in Maternal and Child Health (NCEMCH).

References

Mendelian Inheritance in Man, 9th ed.: V.A. McKusick; The Johns Hopkins University Press, 1990, pp. 299–300.

Smith's Recognizable Patterns of Human Malformation, 4th ed.: K.L. Jones; W.B. Saunders Company, 1988, pp. 428–429.

Progressive Diaphyseal Dysplasia: Evaluation of Corticosteroid Therapy: Y. Naveh, et al.; Pediatrics, February 1985, issue 75(2), pp. 321–323.

Clinical and Scintigraphic Evaluation of Corticosteroid Treatment in a Case of Progressive Diaphyseal Dysplasia: L.A. Verbruggen, et al.; J. Rheumatol., August 1985, issue 12(4), pp. 809–813.

Progressive Diaphyseal Dysplasia (Camurati-Engelmann): Radiographic Follow-up and CT Findings: J.K. Kaftori, et al.; Radiology, September 1987, issue 164(3), pp. 777–782.

FAIRBANK DISEASE

Description Fairbank disease is sometimes characterized by small, irregular, mottled epiphyses. Although the patient may not experience symptoms during early childhood, subsequent developmental hip abnormalities may cause pain in the hips, knees, or ankles, and restrict movement.

Synonyms
Multiple Epiphyseal Dysplasia

Signs and Symptoms The disease manifests between 2 and 5 years of age when patients begin to waddle or walk awkwardly. Patients 5 to 14 years of age may experience pain in hips, knees, or ankles because of continuing alterations in bone structure.

The most prominent symptom involves the hips and may be confused with bilateral Legg-Perthe disease. Less commonly involved are the bones of the shoulders, feet, or hands. Vertebrae are usually normal but may be affected slightly. The femur, including the cartilage, can change shape and density and then recover. Although bone tissue reforms, the bones may be slightly shorter and mild short stature results.

Etiology Fairbank disease is an inherited dominant trait.

Epidemiology Males and females are affected in equal numbers.

Related Disorders See *Conradi-Hünermann Syndrome.*

Treatment—Standard Hip surgery may alleviate restricted movement, and physical therapy and genetic counseling may be beneficial. Other treatment is symptomatic and supportive.

Treatment—Investigational Please contact the agencies listed under Resources, below, for the most current information.

Resources
For more information on Fairbank disease: National Organization for Rare Disorders (NORD); International Center for Skeletal Dysplasia; Human Growth Foundation (HGF); Little People of America; Parents of Dwarfed Children; Short Stature Foundation; NIH/National Institute of Child Health and Human Development.

For genetic information and genetic counseling referrals: March of Dimes Birth Defects Foundation; National Center for Education in Maternal and Child Health.

References
Multiple Epiphyseal Dysplasia: A Family Study: T. Gibson, et al.; Rheumatol. Rehabil., November 1979, 18(4), pp. 239–242.
The Epiphyseal Dysplasias: J. Spranger; Clin. Orthop., January–February 1976, 114, pp. 46–59.

FETAL ALCOHOL SYNDROME (FAS)

Description Fetal alcohol syndrome refers to a wide range of mental and physical birth defects that affect the offspring of mothers who consume alcohol while pregnant.

Synonyms
> Alcoholic Embryopathy
> Alcohol-Related Birth Defects

Signs and Symptoms Characteristics of FAS infants include smaller-than-normal length, low birth weight, and microcephaly. Failure to thrive and physical and mental retardation are common.

The infants have a characteristic facies, including protruding forehead, short palpebral fissures, epicanthal folds, short upturned nose with a flattened bridge, retracted upper lip, micrognathia, cleft palate, and abnormally shaped ears. Some minor joint and limb abnormalities may occur, including a palmar simian crease. Cardiac complications consist mainly of septal defects.

Alcohol withdrawal occurs within the first 24 hours of life. Symptoms associated with withdrawal include irritability, tremors and convulsions, increased muscle tone, opisthotonos, rapid breathing, abdominal distention, and vomiting.

Infants may exhibit all or only some of these symptoms. There is a direct relationship between the severity of symptoms and the level of alcohol consumption.

Etiology It is not certain whether alcohol itself or a breakdown product causes the syndrome.

Epidemiology The incidence of FAS in the United States is 1 or 2:1,000 live births. Although the majority of Americans know about the risk of consuming alcohol during pregnancy, the incidence of FAS is not declining significantly.

Related Disorders FAS may be associated with upper respiratory abnormalities that contribute to the development of apnea, lung hypertension, and sudden infant death syndrome.

Treatment—Standard The syndrome can be prevented by total abstinence from alcohol by the pregnant woman during her pregnancy.

Treatment is generally symptomatic and supportive. Agencies that treat alcohol addiction, special education services, and agencies that provide services to mentally retarded individuals and their families may be beneficial.

Treatment—Investigational Research is under way to study the effects of alcohol on fetuses, to find a treatment and prevention for alcoholism, and to determine the stages of pregnancy during which alcohol-related birth defects are most likely to occur. Other studies are seeking ways to prevent FAS and other alcohol-related birth defects.

Please contact the agencies listed under Resources, below, for the most current information.

Resources
   For more information on fetal alcohol syndrome: National Organization for Rare Disorders (NORD); Fetal Alcohol Education Program; U.S. Dept. of Health and Human Services Public Health Service; National Clearinghouse for Alcohol Information; Alcoholics Anonymous; NIH/National Institute of Mental Health.

References
   Alcohol Research: Meeting the Challenge: NIAAA, National Clearinghouse for Alcohol Information (NCALI). For sale by the Superintendent of Documents, U.S. Government Printing Office, Washington, D.C., p. 11.
   Upper Airway Obstruction in Infants with Fetal Alcohol Syndrome: A.G. Usowicz, et al.; Am. J. Dis. Child, October 1986, issue 140(10), pp. 1039–1041.

FRAGILE X SYNDROME

Description Fragile X syndrome is an X chromosome defect that causes mental retardation and a wide range of associated signs and symptoms.

Synonyms
   FRAXA
   Marker X Syndrome
   Martin-Bell Syndrome
   X-Linked Mental Retardation and Macroorchidism

Signs and Symptoms The face is typically long and narrow, and a high arched palate, large ears, otitis media, strabismus, and dental problems are present. Other common characteristics include hyperextensible joints, hypotonia, and heart problems including mitral valve prolapse. In males abnormally large testes are a distinctive feature.
   In young children, delayed motor development, hyperactivity, behavioral problems, toe walking, and occasional seizures can occur. Autism is suggested by poor eye contact, hand flapping, hand biting, and self-stimulating behaviors. (See *Autism.*)
   Poor sensory skills and mathematical ability are sometimes found in conjunction with good reading skills. Speech and language problems can include echolalia, perseveration, poor language content, and cluttering (dropping of letters or syllables when speaking). Affected girls tend to be shy and socially withdrawn, and to have particular difficulty with mathematics.

Etiology The condition results from a defect on the X chromosome near the end of the long arm (Xq27.3). In karyotyping, the tip of the X chromosome is susceptible to breakage under certain conditions (fragile site). A special cell culture must be used when searching for this defect in cytogenetic studies.

Epidemiology Fragile X syndrome occurs with more frequency and severity among males than females (4 to 1). It is estimated that 1:1000 males and 1:700 females have the fragile X chromosome. About 20 percent of males who inherit the mutation have no clinical manifestations of the disorder. About one-third of carrier females have some evidence of mental retardation. About 1:350 persons carries the fra(X) mutation. Affected individuals do not reproduce. The explanation for these puzzling findings is not clear, but this is a very active subject of research.

Related Disorders **Renpenning syndrome** is a form of inherited X-linked mental retardation caused by the presence of the genetic defect at a different site than that of fragile X (marXq28). This disorder occurs more frequently in males, although some females may also be affected.

Treatment—Standard Treatment includes special education; speech, occupational, and sensory integration training; and behavior modification programs. Surgical correction of heart defects is sometimes necessary. Genetic counseling will benefit families of affected persons. Other treatment is symptomatic and supportive.

Treatment—Investigational Folic acid has been found to improve hyperactivity and attention deficits in some preadolescent males with fragile X syndrome. However, further study of this treatment is warranted to determine longterm benefits and possible side effects.

Families with children who have the fragile X chromosome and who wish to participate in clinical research may contact Valerie Simon, Michael Reiss, M.D., and Lisa Freund, Ph.D., The Kennedy Institute, Behavioral Genetics Unit, Room 103, 707 North Broadway Avenue, Baltimore, Maryland 21205; (301) 550-9321 or (301) 550-9313 (collect).

Please contact the agencies listed under Resources, below, for the most current information.

Resources

For more information on fragile X syndrome: National Organization for Rare Disorders (NORD); Fragile X Foundation; Fragile X Association of Michigan; Fragile X Syndrome Support Group; Institute for Basic Research in Developmental Disabilities; NIH/National Institute of Child Health & Human Development (NICHHD).

For genetic information and genetic counseling referrals: March of Dimes Birth Defects Foundation; NIH/National Center for Education in Maternal and Child Health (NCEMCH).

References

Mendelian Inheritance in Man, 9th ed.: V.A. McKusick; The Johns Hopkins University Press, 1990, pp. 1670–1673.

Genetics and Expression of the Fragile X Syndrome: W.T. Brown, et al.; Ups. J. Med. Sci. (Supp.), 1986, issue 44, pp. 137–154.

Folic Acid as an Adjunct in the Treatment of Children with the Autism Fragile-X Syndrome (AFRAX): C. Gillberg, et al.; Dev. Med. Child. Neurol., October 1986, issue 28(5), pp. 624–627.

FRASER SYNDROME

Description Fraser syndrome is a rare genetic disorder characterized by multiple physical abnormalities that include craniofacial anomalies, renal malformation or agenesis, and incomplete development of the sexual organs.

Synonyms
Cryptophthalmos-Syndactyly Syndrome

Signs and Symptoms Craniofacial abnormalities include cryptophthalmos, malformation of the lacrimal ducts, a broad nose with a flattened bridge, high or cleft palate, a malformed or absent larynx, and deformities of the middle and outer ear. Hair growth may extend from the forehead to the eyebrows. Other characteristics may include syndactyly, malformed or absent kidneys, a displaced navel, widely spaced nipples, and malformation of the pubic bones. In males, there may be hypospadias or cryptorchidism; in females, clitorimegaly, fused labia, bicornuate uterus, or malformed fallopian tubes.

Mental deficiency may be present.

Etiology Fraser syndrome is an autosomal recessive genetic disorder.

Epidemiology Males and females are affected in equal numbers.

Related Disorders See *Renal Agenesis, Bilateral.*

Cat-eye syndrome is characterized by coloboma of the iris and anal atresia. Other abnormalities may include renal agenesis, severe psychomotor retardation, and congenital heart disease.

Melnick-Fraser syndrome (branchio-oto-renal syndrome) is a genetic disorder characterized by hearing loss and kidney malformations, including renal agenesis.

Treatment—Standard Treatment may include surgical correction of some malformations. Other treatment is symptomatic and supportive. Genetic counseling may benefit families of affected children.

Treatment—Investigational Please contact the agencies listed under Resources, below, for the most current information.

Resources

For more information on Fraser syndrome: National Organization for Rare Disorders (NORD); NIH/National Institute of Child Health & Human Development; National Kidney Foundation; American Kidney Fund; National Craniofacial Foundation; National Association for the Craniofacially Handicapped; National Foundation for Facial Reconstruction.

For genetic information and genetic counseling referrals: March of Dimes Birth Defects Foundation; NIH/National Center for Education in Maternal and Child Health (NCEMCH).

References

Mendelian Inheritance in Man, 9th ed.: V.A. McKusick; The Johns Hopkins University Press, 1990, pp. 1115–1116.

Smith's Recognizable Patterns of Human Malformation, 4th ed.: K.L. Jones; W.B. Saunders Company, 1988, pp. 204–205.

The Clinical Spectrum of the Fraser Syndrome: Report of Three New Cases and Review: J. Gattuso, et al.; J. Med. Genet., September 1987, issue 24(9), pp. 549–555.

Fraser Syndrome (Cryptophthalmos-Syndactyly Syndrome). A Review of Eleven Cases with Postmortem Findings: P. Boyd, et al.; Am. J. Med. Genet., September 1988, issue 31(1), pp. 159–168.

ENT Abnormalities Associated with Fraser Syndrome: Case Report and Literature Review: M. Mina, et al.; J. Otolaryngol., August 1988, issue 17(5), pp. 233–236.

FREEMAN-SHELDON SYNDROME

Description Freeman-Sheldon syndrome, a very rare genetic disorder that is present at birth, is characterized by abnormal muscle and skeletal development. The face, eyes, hands, and feet are most often affected. Patients usually have normal intelligence, although mental deficiency can occur.

Synonyms

Craniocarpotarsal Dystrophy
Whistling Face Syndrome
Whistling Face-Windmill Vane Hand Syndrome

Signs and Symptoms Patients have stiffened muscles. Abnormalities in the interior bone structure of the skull are often present. Other characteristics include a round forehead (sometimes with ridges across the lower portion); a flat, expressionless face with full cheeks and a small mouth, giving a typical whistling appearance; and a small nose with flared nostrils and a broadened bridge. The tongue is small, the roof of the mouth is high, and speech has a nasal quality. The patient may have deep-set eyes and strabismus, a long philtrum, and an H-shaped dimple on the chin. Infants may fail to thrive because of dysphagia and vomiting.

The 2nd through 5th fingers are permanently flexed toward contracted thumbs, and the skin is thickened over the first finger. Clubfeet with contracted toes may occur, and occasionally spina bifida. (See *Clubfoot; Spina Bifida.*) In males, an inguinal hernia or cryptorchidism may be present. Low birth weight, small stature, scoliosis, or dislocation of the hip may be present in some children.

Etiology Freeman-Sheldon syndrome is usually inherited as an autosomal dominant trait, but autosomal recessive inheritance has been reported in a few families.

Epidemiology Males and females are affected in equal numbers. Over 65 cases of Freeman-Sheldon syndrome have been identified worldwide since the disorder was first recognized in 1938.

Related Disorders See *Arthrogryposis Multiplex Congenita.*

Treatment—Standard Treatment usually involves multiple surgical procedures (which can be difficult because of muscle stiffness and thickened tissues) or the use of splints or casts to improve bent fingers or feet. Correction of the thumb deformity may be the first surgery in the longterm treatment of many cases. Cosmetic facial or hand and foot restructuring surgery can improve appearance. Genetic counseling will benefit patients and their families. Other treatment is symptomatic and supportive.

Treatment—Investigational Please contact the agencies listed under Resources, below, for the most current information.

Resources

For more information on Freeman-Sheldon syndrome: National Organization for Rare Disorders (NORD); Freeman-Sheldon Parent Support Group; The National Arthritis and Musculoskeletal and Skin Diseases Information Clearinghouse.

For genetic information and genetic counseling referrals: March of Dimes Birth Defects Foundation; National Center for Education in Maternal and Child Health (NCEMCH).

References

Mendelian Inheritance in Man, 9th ed.: V.A. McKusick; The Johns Hopkins University Press, 1990, pp. 978–979.

Smith's Recognizable Patterns of Human Malformation, 4th ed.: K.L. Jones; W.B. Saunders Company, 1988, pp. 182–183.

Ocular Abnormalities in the Freeman-Sheldon Syndrome: M. O'Keefe, et al.; Am. J. Ophthalmol., September 1986, issue 102(3), pp. 346–348.

New Evidence for Genetic Heterogeneity of the Freeman-Sheldon (FS) Syndrome: M. Sanchez, et al.; Am. J. Med. Genet., November 1986, issue 25(3), pp. 507–511.

Freeman-Sheldon Syndrome: A Disorder of Congenital Myopathic Origin?: J. Vanek, et al.; J. Med. Genet., June 1986, issue 23(3), pp. 231–236.

GOLDENHAR SYNDROME

Description Goldenhar syndrome encompasses a wide spectrum of ear, eye, facial, vertebral, and other congenital malformations. The disorder is almost always more severe on one side.

Synonyms

Auriculo-Oculo-Vertebral Syndrome
Facio-Auriculo-Vertebral Anomaly
First and Second Branchial Arch Syndrome
Goldenhar-Gorlin Syndrome
Mandibulofacial Dysostosis with Epibulbar Dermoids
Oculo-Auriculo-Vertebral Spectrum

Signs and Symptoms The syndrome is commonly associated with varying combinations of the following abnormalities, many of which are often asymmetric and unilateral: macrostomia; malar, maxillary, and mandibular hypoplasia; absent or closed nares; frontal bossing; microtia; middle ear anomalies; deafness; anomalies of the tongue and soft palate; hemivertebra.

Less common abnormalities associated with Goldenhar syndrome include epibulbar dermoid, strabismus, microphthalmia, inner ear anomalies, cleft lip, and cleft palate. Neurologic, cardiac, pulmonary, renal, and gastrointestinal anomalies occur.

Hemifacial microsomia (HFM), now thought to be part of the spectrum of Goldenhar syndrome, is characterized by facial abnormalities that may be bilateral but are always quite asymmetrical, and by the fairly frequent finding of facial nerve paralysis. The wide variety of features in HFM includes mandibular hypoplasia with tilting of the jaw to one side, macrostomia, unilateral microtia, and variable hypoplasia of the cheek and eye on the affected side.

Etiology The etiology of Goldenhar syndrome is not known. Most cases are sporadic, some familial. Expression within a family may be variable.

Epidemiology Goldenhar syndrome occurs in 1:5000 to 1:25,000 newborn infants. Approximately 70 percent of cases occur in males.

Related Disorders See *Treacher-Collins Syndrome; Spina Bifida.*

Treatment—Standard Spinal and/or facial deformities may be managed surgically. Speech and language therapy and special education may be beneficial. The child may also benefit from supportive counseling.

Treatment—Investigational Advances in tissue and bone grafts currently under investigation may be useful in treating Goldenhar syndrome.

Please contact the agencies listed under Resources, below, for the most current information.

Resources

For more information on Goldenhar syndrome: National Organization for Rare Disorders (NORD); The Hemifacial Microsomia/Goldenhar Syndrome Family Support Network; International Center for Skeletal Dysplasia; Society for the Rehabilitation of the Facially Disfigured, Inc.; FACES—National Association for the Craniofacially Handicapped; National Craniofacial Foundation; Orofacial Guild; About Face; NIH/National Institute of Child Health and Human Development (NICHHD).

For genetic information and genetic counseling referrals: March of Dimes Birth Defects Foundation; National Center for Education in Maternal and Child Health (NCEMCH).

References

Syndromes of the Head and Neck, 3rd ed.: R.J. Gorlin, et al.; Oxford University Press, 1990, pp. 641–649.

Smith's Recognizable Patterns of Human Malformation, 4th ed.: K.L. Jones; W.B. Saunders Company, 1988, pp. 584–587.

Goldenhar's Syndrome: A Case Study: L. Belenchia; J. Commun. Disord., October 1985, issue 18(5), pp. 383–392.

Congenital Absence of the Portal Vein in Oculoauriculovertebral Dysplasia (Goldenhar Syndrome): J.H. Seashore, et al., Pediatr. Radiol., 1986, issue 16(5), pp. 437–439.

The Use of Microvascular Free Flaps for Soft Tissue Augmentation of the Face in Children with Hemifacial Microsomia: La Rossa; Cleft Palate J., April 1980, issue 17(2), pp. 138–143.

GORDON SYNDROME

Description Gordon syndrome, one of a group of genetic musculoskeletal disorders called the distal arthrogryposes, is characterized by camptodactyly, a cleft palate, and clubfoot. Other developmental abnormalities may also occur.

Synonyms
> Arthrogryposis Multiplex Congenita, Distal, Type IIA
> Camptodactyly-Cleft Palate-Clubfoot
> Distal Arthrogryposis, Type IIA

Signs and Symptoms Major features are one or two permanently flexed fingers, a cleft palate, and clubfoot. An affected fetus usually has limited movement in utero. An omphalocele is sometimes present at birth, and there may be cutaneous syndactyly and abnormalities in the fingerprints. Fertility of adults with Gordon syndrome may be lessened or absent.

Etiology The syndrome has autosomal dominant inheritance.

Epidemiology Onset is in utero. Females and males are affected in equal numbers.

Related Disorders See *Arthrogryposis Multiplex Congenita.*

Treatment—Standard Gordon syndrome can be diagnosed in utero. Abnormalities associated with this disorder can often be corrected through surgery and physical therapy.

Treatment—Investigational Please contact the agencies listed under Resources, below, for the most current information.

Resources
  For more information on Gordon syndrome: National Organization for Rare Disorders (NORD); AVENUES, a National Support Group for Arthrogryposis; The National Arthritis and Musculoskeletal and Skin Diseases Information Clearinghouse.

References
Mendelian Inheritance in Man, 9th ed.: V.A. McKusick; The Johns Hopkins University Press, 1990, pp. 155–156.
Three Distinct Types of X-Linked Arthrogryposis Seen in 6 Families: J.G. Hall, et al.; Clin. Genet., February 1982, issue 21(2), pp. 81–97.
The Gordon Syndrome: Autosomal Dominant Cleft Palate, Camptodactyly, and Club Feet: M. Robinow, et al.; Amer. J. Med. Genet., 1981, issue 9(2), pp. 139–146.

GOTTRON SYNDROME

Description Gottron syndrome is a mild form of **progeria** in which the extremities remain unusually small. The prognosis for a normal life is good.

Synonyms
>Acrogeria, Familial

Signs and Symptoms From infancy on, patients seem older than their age as a result of thin, parchment-like skin on their hands and feet, which remain small into adulthood. Veins on the chest are prominent because of the small amount of subcutaneous fat.

Etiology Gottron syndrome appears to be familial, but the inheritance pattern is not understood.

Epidemiology Males and females are affected equally.

Related Disorders See *Hutchinson-Gilford Syndrome,* a more severe form of progeria that affects children; and *Werner Syndrome,* another form of progeria that affects adults.

Treatment—Standard Treatment is symptomatic and supportive.

Treatment—Investigational Please contact the agencies listed under Resources, below, for the most current information.

Resources
>**For more information on Gottron syndrome:** National Organization for Rare Disorders (NORD); The Progeria Foundation; The Progeria International Registry (PIR); NIH/National Institute of Child Health and Human Development; Sunshine Foundation. (The Sunshine Foundation raises funds to bring all children with progeria together each year so that their progress can be studied while the children socialize in a vacation atmosphere.)

>**For genetic information and genetic counseling referrals:** March of Dimes Birth Defects Foundation; National Center for Education in Maternal and Child Health (NCEMCH).

References
>Mendelian Inheritance in Man, 9th ed.: V.A. McKusick; The Johns Hopkins University Press, 1990, p. 1000.
>Cecil Textbook of Medicine, 18th ed.: J.B. Wyngaarden and L.H. Smith, Jr., eds.; W.B. Saunders Company, 1988, p. 2035.

GREIG CEPHALOPOLYSYNDACTYLY SYNDROME (GCPS)

Description Greig cephalopolysyndactyly is a rare genetic disorder characterized by macrocephaly, an unusual facies, and multiple physical deformities of the hands and feet.

Synonyms
> Greig Syndrome
> Greig Polysyndactyly Craniofacial Dysmorphism Syndrome

Signs and Symptoms Craniofacial characteristics include macrocephaly, a high, prominent forehead, broad nose, and ocular hypertelorism. Polysyndactyly, syndactyly, and enlarged thumbs and great toes are usually present. Occasionally there is camptodactyly as well as hydrocephalus and mild mental retardation.

Etiology GCPS is believed to be inherited as an autosomal dominant genetic trait. The location of the defective gene has been established to be on the short arm of chromosome 7.

Epidemiology The syndrome is very rare. Males and females are affected in equal numbers.

Related Disorders See *Apert Syndrome.*

Treatment—Standard Corrective surgery may be performed for the syndactyly. Genetic counseling may benefit patients and their families. Other treatment is symptomatic and supportive.

Treatment—Investigational Please contact the agencies listed under Resources, below, for the most current information.

Resources
> **For more information on Greig cephalopolysyndactyly syndrome:** National Organization for Rare Disorders (NORD); National Craniofacial Foundation; Society for the Rehabilitation of the Facially Disfigured, Inc.; FACES—National Association for the Craniofacially Handicapped; National Institute of Child Health & Human Development (NICHHD).
>
> **For genetic information and genetic counseling referrals:** March of Dimes Birth Defects Foundation; NIH/National Center for Education in Maternal and Child Health (NCEMCH).

References
> Mendelian Inheritance in Man, 9th ed.: V.A. McKusick; The Johns Hopkins University Press, 1990, pp. 775–776.
> Smith's Recognizable Patterns of Human Malformation, 4th ed.: K.L. Jones; W.B. Saunders Company, 1988, pp. 376–377.
> Greig Cephalopolysyndactyly: Report of 13 Affected Individuals in Three Families: M. Baraiter, et al.; Clin. Genet., October 1983, issue 24(4), pp. 257–265.
> Chromosomal Localisation of a Developmental Gene in Man: Direct DNA Analysis Demonstrates that Greig Cephalopolysyndactyly Maps to 7p13 L: Brueton, et al.; Am. J. Med. Genet., December 1988, issue 31(4), pp. 799–804.
> The Greig Cephalopolysyndactyly Syndrome: Report of a Family and Review of the Literature: T. Gallop, et al.; Am. J. Med. Genet., September 1985, issue 22(1), pp. 59–68.
> Evaluation of a Uniform Operative Technique to Treat Syndactyly: D. Keret, et al.; J. Hand Surg., September 1987, issue 12(5 pt. 1), pp. 727–729.

HALLERMANN-STREIFF SYNDROME

Description The syndrome is characterized by proportionate short stature and bony abnormalities of the calvaria, face, and jaw.

Synonyms

> François Dyscephalic Syndrome
> Hallermann-Streiff-François Syndrome
> Mandibulo-Oculo-Facial Dyscephaly
> Oculomandibulodyscephaly
> Oculomandibulofacial Syndrome

Signs and Symptoms Children are born with a birdlike face: a receding jaw, narrow, beaked nose, and thinned or absent hair overlying the skull sutures. Eyebrows may be absent or underdeveloped. The eyeballs and corneas are abnormally small, and cataract or glaucoma, or both, may be present. Dental abnormalities include the presence of teeth at birth, or, at a few weeks of age, the eruption of teeth that are not well anchored in the jaw and often fall out. Permanent teeth, which normally erupt during childhood, are usually absent except for the first permanent molars. Abnormalities of the skull and face may predispose some patients to respiratory disorders. Additionally, motor and mental retardation (15 percent), progeroid appearance, and atrophy of the elastic tissue of the skin may occur. There is proportionate short stature.

Etiology The cause is uncertain. In practically all instances chromosomal studies have been normal. Almost all cases have been sporadic. A few familial cases suggest autosomal recessive inheritance, but these are not accepted by all dysmorphologists.

Epidemiology Males and females are affected in equal numbers. Since the disorder was first identified in 1948, about 150 cases have been reported.

Related Disorders See *Treacher Collins Syndrome; Seckel Syndrome.*

Treatment—Standard Treatment is symptomatic and supportive. Vision problems can be successfully treated. Infections should be guarded against. A tracheostomy may be necessary for severe respiratory distress. Services that assist physically and mentally retarded individuals are helpful. Genetic counseling will benefit patients and their families.

Treatment—Investigational Please contact the agencies listed under Resources, below, for the most current information.

Resources

   For more information on Hallermann-Streiff syndrome: National Organization for Rare Disorders (NORD); Hallermann-Streiff Parent Association; International Center for Skeletal Dysplasia; FACES—National Association for the Craniofacially Handicapped; Society for the Rehabilitation of the Facially Disfigured; National Craniofacial Foundation; About Face; NIH/National Child Health

& Human Development (NICHHD).

For genetic information and genetic counseling referrals: March of Dimes Birth Defects Foundation; National Center for Education in Maternal and Child Health (NCEMCH).

References

Mendelian Inheritance in Man, 9th ed.: V.A. McKusick; The Johns Hopkins University Press, 1990, pp. 1229–1230.

Smith's Recognizable Patterns of Human Malformation, 4th ed.: K.L. Jones; W.B. Saunders Company, 1988, pp. 102–103.

Airway Management in Hallermann-Streiff Syndrome: R.T. Sataloff, et al.; Am. J. Otolaryngol., January–February 1984, issue 5(1), pp. 64–67.

Hallermann-Streiff Syndrome: Report of a Case: A.J. Malerman, et al.; ASDC J. Dent. Child., July–August 1986, issue 53(4), pp. 287–292.

Dento-Alveolar Abnormalities in Oculomandibulodyscephaly (Hallermann-Streiff Syndrome): P.J. Slootweg, et al.; J. Oral. Pathol., April 1984, issue 13(2), pp. 147–154.

HOLT-ORAM SYNDROME (HOS)

Description Holt-Oram syndrome is a genetic disorder consisting primarily of congenital heart disease and upper limb abnormalities, typically of the forearm, fingers, and wrist.

Synonyms

Atriodigital Dysplasia

Heart-Hand Syndrome

Upper Limb-Cardiovascular Syndrome

Signs and Symptoms The most common congenital cardiac findings are atrial and ventricular septal defects, although other anomalies may be present.

The shoulders are narrow and not proportioned, and there may be forearm hypoplasia. The thumbs may be hypoplastic or absent, and there may be finger syndactyly and camptodactyly. The thenar eminence on the palm of the hand may be abnormally flat. The skeletal defects often occur bilaterally, but may be somewhat more severe on the left side. Abnormalities of the carpal bones appear to occur more often than those of the thumb.

There is a range of severity in Holt-Oram syndrome, and bony abnormalities may also be quite mild.

Pregnant women at risk of having an affected child may undergo ultrasound imaging procedures prenatally to evaluate fetal development as early as 14 weeks into pregnancy.

Etiology The syndrome is inherited as an autosomal dominant trait. There is not a clear correlation in the severity of features between parents and children; parents with only mild skeletal defects may pass a severe form to their offspring. HOS has been observed to occur in more than one person in a family.

Epidemiology Approximately 200 hundred cases have been identified worldwide since the disorder was first described in 1960. All ethnic groups and races can be affected. Males and females are affected in equal numbers.

Related Disorders See *Thrombocytopenia-Absent Radius Syndrome.*

Treatment—Standard Treatment is by surgical correction where necessary, both of the heart and skeletal problems. Services that benefit the physically handicapped may be helpful in some cases. Other treatment is symptomatic and supportive. Genetic counseling is recommended for patients and their families.

Treatment—Investigational Please contact the agencies listed under Resources, below, for the most current information.

Resources

For more information on Holt-Oram syndrome: National Organization for Rare Disorders (NORD); American Heart Association.

For cardiac symptoms information: NIH/National Heart, Lung and Blood Institute (NHLBI).

For bone symptoms information: The National Arthritis and Musculoskeletal and Skin Diseases Information Clearinghouse; International Center for Skeletal Dysplasia.

For genetic information and genetic counseling referrals: March of Dimes Birth Defects Foundation; National Center for Education in Maternal and Child Health (NCEMCH).

References

Mendelian Inheritance in Man, 9th ed.: V.A. McKusick; The Johns Hopkins University Press, 1990, pp. 468–469.

Smith's Recognizable Patterns of Human Malformation, 4th ed.: K.L. Jones; W.B. Saunders Company, 1988, p. 272.

Cross-Sectional Echocardiographic Imaging of Supracardiac Total Anomalous Pulmonary Venous Drainage to a Vertical Vein in a Patient with Holt-Oram Syndrome: K.Z. Zhang, et al.; Chest, January 1981, issue 79(1), pp. 113–115.

HUTCHINSON-GILFORD SYNDROME

Description In this progeria syndrome, children age rapidly, are very short of stature, and have characteristic facies. Intelligence is normal.

Synonyms

> Gilford Syndrome
> Premature Senility Syndrome
> Progeria (Childhood)
> Souques-Charcot Syndrome

Signs and Symptoms Birthweight is normal, and the growth rate does not plateau until about 1 year of age. At 10 years, most affected children have the height of the average 3-year-old. Lifetime height rarely exceeds that of a normal 5-year-old.

Craniofacial characteristics include a relatively large head but a small face, with a sharp, beaklike nose and receding chin. Because of the small size of the jaw, the teeth are often crowded and irregular. The eyes protrude and may have bluish sclerae and cloudy corneas. Patients may have no eyebrows and eyelashes and no hair on the scalp, revealing prominent veins; alternatively, the hair may turn gray.

The skin is dry, thin, and wrinkled, and often is a brownish color. Scarcity of subcutaneous fat leads to the wrinkling and appearance of age. The long bones are decalcified and thin, and the chest is narrow. The abdomen protrudes. There may be splenomegaly and umbilical or inguinal hernias. The sex organs remain undeveloped.

In adolescence, the patient becomes susceptible to strokes, atherosclerosis, occlusion of the coronary artery, and angina. These and assorted other complications are associated with high levels of blood lipoprotein. Very rarely, amino acids are lost in the urine. Life-threatening heart disease or stroke may occur.

Etiology The cause is unclear. There seems to be no familial pattern. High paternal age has been implicated in some studies but this finding has not been conclusive.

Epidemiology The syndrome is very rare. Boys and girls are affected equally, and usually survive into their teens.

Related Disorders See **Werner Syndrome,** an adult form of progeria.

In **Gottron Syndrome** (acrogeria), only the hands and feet are involved; these remain unusually small and age much more rapidly than the rest of the body.

Treatment—Standard Treatment is supportive. Symptomatic therapy of heart conditions, stroke, etc., may be necessary.

Treatment—Investigational Please contact the agencies listed under Resources, below, for the most current information.

Resources

For more information on Hutchinson-Gilford syndrome: National Organization for Rare Disorders (NORD); Progeria Foundation; The Progeria International Registry (PIR); NIH/National Institute of Child Health and Human Development (NICHHD); Sunshine Foundation. (The Sunshine Foundation raises funds to bring all children with progeria together once each year so that their medical progress can be studied while the children socialize in a vacation atmosphere.)

References
Mendelian Inheritance in Man, 9th ed.: V.A. McKusick; The Johns Hopkins University Press, 1990, pp. 797–798.
Smith's Recognizable Patterns of Human Malformation, 4th ed.: K.L. Jones; W.B. Saunders Company, 1988, pp. 118–119.
Syndromes of the Head and Neck, 3rd ed.: R.J. Gorlin, et al.; Oxford University Press, 1990, pp. 482–485.

HYPOCHONDROPLASIA

Description Hypochondroplasia is a type of chondrodystrophy characterized by short stature. It becomes evident during mid childhood.

Synonyms
> Achondroplasia Tarda
> Atypical Achondroplasia

Signs and Symptoms At birth, those affected appear normal. Arms and legs do not develop properly, however, and the body becomes thick and shorter than normal. The patient has a normal-sized head; but arms, legs, hands, and feet, although shaped normally, are disproportionately small. Elbow flexibility is limited. Arms and legs are not usually bowed. Motor abilities may develop slowly, but intelligence is usually normal.

Hypochondroplasia can be distinguished from other forms of short-limbed short stature by clinical and radiological examination of the skull and long bones of the arms and legs.

Etiology The disorder is inherited as an autosomal dominant trait.

Epidemiology Females appear to be affected more often than males.

Related Disorders See *Achondroplasia.*

Kozlowski spondylometaphyseal dysplasia is usually diagnosed by the time the patient is 2 years old, although onset generally occurs during the first year. The bones are affected, especially the spine and pelvis, by a reduction of calcification. The neck and trunk are short, the legs are bowed, and there is a waddling gait. Patients experience pain and a limited range of motion. Males and females are affected equally.

Treatment—Standard Treatment of hypochondroplasia may consist of orthopedic corrections and physical therapy. Pregnant patients may require caesarean section. Genetic counseling may benefit patients and their families. Other treatment is symptomatic and supportive.

Treatment—Investigational Please contact the agencies listed under Resources, below, for the most current information.

Resources

For more information on hypochondroplasia: National Organization for Rare Disorders (NORD); International Center for Skeletal Dysplasia; NIH/National Arthritis, Musculoskeletal and Skin (NIAMS) Information Clearinghouse; Human Growth Foundation (HGF); Parents of Dwarfed Children.

For genetic information and genetic counseling referrals: March of Dimes Birth Defects Foundation; NIH/National Center for Education in Maternal and Child Health (NCEMCH).

References
Mendelian Inheritance in Man, 9th ed.: V.A. McKusick; The Johns Hopkins University Press, 1990, p. 502.
Achondroplasia and Hypochondroplasia. Clinical Variation and Spinal Stenosis: R. Wynne-Davies, et al., J. Bone Joint Surg. (Br.), 1981, issue 63B(4), pp. 508–515.

IMPERFORATE ANUS

Description Imperforate anus is a congenital disorder in which the anus is missing or abnormally located. An associated anomaly is the presence of a fistula that connects the vagina or bladder to the rectum or colon.

Synonyms
Anal Atresia
Anal Stenosis
Anorectal Malformations

Signs and Symptoms Imperforate anus is congenital and is identified by an abnormal or absent anus. The rectum may open into the vagina in females or near the scrotum in males.

Etiology The disorder may be inherited either through autosomal recessive or through X-linked genes.

Epidemiology The incidence of imperforate anus in the United States is approximately 1:5,000 births. Six males are affected for every 4 females.

Related Disorders Since imperforate anus occurs as one manifestation in a number of multiple malformation syndromes, affected neonates must be carefully examined for other abnormalities.

Treatment—Standard Imperforate anus is surgically corrected by dilating, enlarging, or repositioning the external opening to allow for elimination of feces. Genetic counseling may benefit patients and their families.

Treatment—Investigational Please contact the agencies listed under Resources, below, for the most current information.

Resources
  For more information on imperforate anus: National Organization for Rare Disorders (NORD); National Digestive Diseases Information Clearinghouse; United Ostomy Association, Inc.
  For genetic information and genetic counseling referrals: March of Dimes Birth Defects Foundation; National Center for Education in Maternal and Child Health (NCEMCH).

References
The Genital Tract in Female Children with Imperforate Anus: R. Hall, et al.; Am. J. Obstet. Gynecol., January 15, 1985, issue 151 (2), pp. 169–171.
Imperforate Anus with Long but Apparent Low Fistula in Females: F.G. Cigerroa, et al.; J. Pediatr. Surg., January 1988, issue 23 (1 pt. 2), pp. 42–44.

The Genitourinary System in Patients with Imperforate Anus: G.A. McLorie, et al.; J. Pediatr. Surg., December 1987, issue 22(12), pp. 1100–1104.

IVEMARK SYNDROME

Description Ivemark syndrome is a rare progressive disorder characterized primarily by congenital asplenia or, sometimes, splenic hypoplasia or polysplenia, as well as malformations of the cardiovascular system and situs inversus.

Synonyms
Asplenia with Cardiovascular Anomalies
Bilateral Rightsidedness Sequence

Signs and Symptoms Cardiovascular abnormalities may result in cyanosis and heart failure. Pulmonary involvement is characterized by isomerism, with both lungs resembling a normal right lung in asplenia; in polysplenia, leftsidedness predominates. The stomach may be displaced to the right or left side of the body, and the bowel may be rotated improperly and may have a volvulus. Renal anomalies may be present, and physical and mental development may be retarded. The patient is vulnerable to increased infection, especially of the skin and respiratory system.

Diagnosis of asplenia is confirmed by the presence of Heinz or Howell-Jolly bodies in erythrocytes. Prenatal diagnosis can be made by ultrasound examination.

Etiology Autosomal recessive inheritance is suggested.

Epidemiology Ivemark syndrome is a rare disorder that affects males 3 times more often than females.

Treatment—Standard Infections are treated with antibiotics. Surgery may be indicated to relieve some of the associated signs or abnormalities.

Genetic counseling may benefit patients and their families. Other treatment is symptomatic and supportive.

Treatment—Investigational Please contact the agencies listed under Resources, below, for the most current information.

Resources
For more information on Ivemark syndrome: National Organization for Rare Disorders (NORD); NIH/National Institute of Child Health and Human Development (NICHHD).

For genetic information and genetic counseling referrals: March of Dimes Birth Defects Foundation; NIH/National Center for Education in Maternal and Child Health (NCEMCH).

References
Mendelian Inheritance in Man, 9th ed.: V.A. McKusick; The Johns Hopkins University Press, 1990, pp. 1049–1050.

Smith's Recognizable Patterns of Human Malformation, 4th ed.: K.L. Jones; W.B. Saunders Company, 1988, p. 543.

Prenatal Diagnosis of Asplenia/Polysplenia Syndrome: D. Chitayat, et al.; Am. J. Obstet. Gynecol., May 1988, issue 158(5), pp. 1085–1087.

Prolonged and Functional Survival with the Asplenia Syndrome: M. Wolfe, et al.; Am. J. Med., December 1986, issue 81(6), pp. 1089–1091.

JARCHO-LEVIN SYNDROME

Description Multiple deformities, including those of the face and head, hands, thorax, and spine, characterize Jarcho-Levin syndrome.

Synonyms
  Spondylocostal Dysplasia—Type I
  Spondylothoracic Dysplasia

Signs and Symptoms Craniofacial anomalies include a large occiput, wide nasal bridge, antiverted nares, and upwardly slanted eyelids. Syndactyly and campodactyly with long digits are also characteristic. The thorax is small, causing respiratory problems that are often fatal. Spinal abnormalities include neural defects and hemivertebrae. The neck and trunk are characteristically short. Genitourinary tract anomalies may be present. Occasionally, distention of the stomach and pelvis may occur as a result of bladder obstruction.

Etiology The inheritance is autosomal recessive. Autosomal dominant inheritance has also been reported.

Epidemiology Jarcho-Levin syndrome affects males and females equally. Most cases have occurred in Puerto Rican children.

Related Disorders Features of **thanatophoric dysplasia** include vertebral abnormalities, a narrow thorax and short pelvis, short limbs with short digits, hypotonia, and a large cranium, low nasal bridge, and small facies.

Treatment—Standard Treatment is symptomatic and supportive. Genetic counseling may be beneficial.

Treatment—Investigational Please contact the agencies listed under Resources, below, for the most current information.

Resources
  For more information on Jarcho-Levin syndrome: National Organization for Rare Disorders (NORD); National Institute of Child Health and Human Development (NICHHD).

  For genetic information and genetic counseling referrals: March of Dimes Birth Defects Foundation; NIH/National Center for Education in Maternal and Child Health (NCEMCH).

References

Mendelian Inheritance in Man, 9th ed.: V.A. McKusick; Johns Hopkins University Press, 1990, pp. 1525–1526.

Smith's Recognizable Patterns of Human Malformation, 4th ed.: K.L. Jones; W.B. Saunders Company, 1988, p. 536.

Prenatal Findings in a Case of Spondylocostal Dysplasia I (Jarcho-Levin) Syndrome; R. Romero, et al.; Obstet. Gynecol., June 1988, 6(2), p. 988.

Neural Defects in Jarcho-Levin Syndrome: M.G. Reyes, et al.; J. Child Neurol., January 1989, 4(1), p. 51.

KARTAGENER SYNDROME

Description Kartagener syndrome is a genetic disorder characterized by sinusitis, bronchiectasis, and situs inversus.

Synonyms

Chronic Sinobronchial Disease and Dextrocardia
Dextrocardia, Bronchiectasis, and Sinusitis
Immotile Cilia Syndrome
Kartagener Triad
Primary Ciliary Dyskinesia
Situs Inversus, Bronchiectasis, and Sinusitis

Signs and Symptoms Kartagener syndrome is a congenital disease that usually manifests during infancy. The major symptoms—sinusitis, bronchiectasis, and situs inversus—persist into adulthood. Mucus accumulation in the sinuses leads to sinusitis; mucus accumulation in the lungs results in coughing, bronchitis, and bronchiectasis. Chronic ear infections and possible abnormalities of the inner ear may lead to hearing loss. Situs inversus is diagnosed by x-ray; if it is complete, cardiac complications may occur.

Reproductive complications can also be associated with Kartagener syndrome. Reduced sperm motility produces sterility in males, and slow movement of the egg through the fallopian tubes may cause infertility in females.

Etiology Kartagener syndrome is inherited as an autosomal recessive trait with incomplete penetrance.

Epidemiology Kartagener syndrome affects approximately 1:30,000 to 1:60,000 individuals.

Related Disorders Bronchiectasis is characterized by enlarged bronchial tubes. Congenital bronchiectasis is the result of abnormal fetal development. Acquired bronchiectasis may be caused by a variety of disorders, such as measles, sinusitis, chronic bronchitis, pneumonia, cystic fibrosis, emphysema, lung abscess, silicosis, lung cancer, or the presence of foreign substances in the lungs.

Patients may exhibit either a dry or mucus-producing cough from the accumulation of mucus in the bronchioles. The sputum is thick and has a foul odor. Infection and inflammation is usually partial; only rarely does it involve an entire lung. Antibiotic drugs are indicated to prevent deterioration of bronchial tubes and spread of infection.

Polynesian bronchiectasis (immotile cilia syndrome) is a type of ciliary dyskinesia that results in bronchial tube complications and reduced motility of cilia. The syndrome is primarily confined to Samoans and the Maoris of New Zealand. It is differentiated from Kartagener syndrome through laboratory evaluation of the cilia.

Fibrosing alveolitis is characterized by abnormalities of fibrous tissue between the alveoli, which results in inflammation. Coughing and rapid breathing develop when the patients exercises moderately. Cyanosis results from lack of circulating oxygen. Infection, emphysema, or cardiac complications may also develop.

Treatment—Standard Patients usually require daily postural drainage. Fever and systemic symptoms are treated with antibiotic therapy. Surgery may be indicated to correct abnormalities in circulation.

Other treatment is symptomatic and supportive. Genetic counseling is recommended for patients and their families.

Treatment—Investigational Please contact the agencies listed under Resources, below, for the most current information.

Resources

For more information on Kartagener syndrome: National Organization for Rare Disorders (NORD); American Lung Association; NIH/National Heart, Lung and Blood Institute (NHLBI).

For genetic information and genetic counseling referrals: March of Dimes Birth Defects Foundation; National Center for Education in Maternal and Child Health (NCEMCH).

References

Mendelian Inheritance in Man, 9th ed.: V.A. McKusick; The Johns Hopkins University Press, 1990, pp. 1283–1284.

Internal Medicine, 2nd ed.: J.H. Stein, ed.; Little, Brown and Company, 1987, p. 691.

Kartagener's Syndrome with Motile Cilia and Immotile Spermatozoa: Axonemal Ultrastructure and Function: L.J. Wilton, et al.; Am. Rev. Respir. Dis., December 1986, issue 40(4), pp. 1233–1236.

KLINEFELTER SYNDROME (47, XXY)

Description The classic form of Klinefelter syndrome is the most common cause of primary hypogonadism in males. It is characterized by the presence of an extra X chromosome. It is usually not diagnosed until after puberty.

Signs and Symptoms Abnormally small testes have sclerosed tubules and are azoospermic. Gynecomastia often occurs. Secondary sexual characteristics may be attenuated, resulting in a high-pitched voice and diminished facial and body hair. Muscles are underdeveloped. Mental retardation generally is not present, although affected persons may not achieve higher education levels. Personality disorder may occur.

Many other variants occur, such as 46,XY/47,XXY (mosaic); 48,XXXY; and 48,XXYY.

Etiology Klinefelter syndrome results from the presence of an extra X chromosome, which is paternal in origin in 33 percent of patients and maternal in origin in 67 percent of patients.

Epidemiology Klinefelter syndrome occurs in 1:1000 newborn males.

Treatment—Standard Androgens, such as testosterone enanthate or cypionate, are given to promote virilization. Affected patients are infertile. Patients may achieve cosmetic benefit from mastectomy.

Treatment—Investigational Please contact the agencies listed under Resources, below, for the most current information.

Resources
For more information on Klinefelter syndrome: National Organization for Rare Disorders (NORD); Klinefelter's Syndrome Association of America; NIH/National Institute of Child Health and Human Development (NICHHD).

For genetic information and genetic counseling referrals: March of Dimes Birth Defects Foundation; National Center for Education in Maternal and Child Health (NCEMCH).

References
Cecil Textbook of Medicine, 18th ed.: J.B. Wyngaarden and L.H. Smith, Jr., eds.: W.B. Saunders Company, 1988, pp. 167–170, 1412–1413.

KLIPPEL-FEIL SYNDROME

Description Klippel-Feil syndrome is a congenital disorder that affects the spine. Associated complications include hearing loss and neurologic, cardiac, renal, and respiratory problems. The syndrome is categorized into types I, II, and III.

Synonyms
Congenital Cervical Synostosis

Signs and Symptoms The 3 types of Klippel-Feil syndrome are all characterized by scoliosis, fusion of neck vertebrae, and low hairline at the nape.

In type I, the neck and upper back vertebrae are fused into bony blocks. In type II, fusion occurs at only one or 2 disks. Patients with type III disease exhibit fusion in the neck and back or lower back. The presence of craniocervical fusion increases the risk for injury to the head and neck. Neurologic, cardiac, and respiratory complications result from compressed vertebrae. In some families, the disorder may be associated with sensorineural hearing loss. In 4 isolated cases, the disorder was associated with absent vagina and conductive deafness.

Etiology The syndrome is inherited as an autosomal dominant trait.

Epidemiology The syndrome is rare. Males and females are affected in equal numbers.

Related Disorders **Wildervanck syndrome** is congenital, and is characterized by fusion of the cervical vertebrae, congenital perceptive deafness, and ocular palsy. The syndrome is almost completely limited to females.

Treatment—Standard Treatment is supportive and symptomatic. Genetic counseling may benefit patients and their families.

Treatment—Investigational Please contact the agencies listed under Resources, below, for the most current information.

Resources
For more information on **Klippel-Feil syndrome:** National Organization for Rare Disorders (NORD); NIH/National Arthritis and Musculoskeletal and Skin Diseases (NIAMS) Information Clearinghouse.

For **genetic information and genetic counseling referrals:** March of Dimes Birth Defects Foundation; NIH/National Center for Education in Maternal and Child Health (NCEMCH).

References
Mendelian Inheritance in Man, 9th ed.: V.A. McKusick; The Johns Hopkins University Press, 1990, p. 552.

Aural Abnormalities in Klippel-Feil Syndrome: I. Ohtani, et al.; Am. J. Otolaryngol., November 1985, issue 6(6), pp. 468–471.

KLIPPEL-TRENAUNAY SYNDROME

Description Klippel-Trenaunay syndrome is a vascular disorder characterized by cutaneous hemangiomata with hypertrophy of the related soft tissues and bone. Severity of disease and associated complications may vary widely in patients.

Synonyms
Angio-Osteohypertrophy Syndrome
Congenital Dysplastic Angiectasia
Elephantiasis Congenita Angiomatosa
Klippel-Trenaunay-Weber Syndrome
Hemangiectatic Hypertrophy
Osteohypertrophic Nevus Flammeus

Signs and Symptoms The most common sign is a congenital nevus flammeus, which is apparent at birth, may extend over a large area, and usually deepens in color over time.

Vascular lesions consisting of masses of veins, lymph vessels, and capillaries can be detected in utero by ultrasonography. These obstructive lesions lead to development of varicose veins during infancy and early childhood. All or part of the limbs and digits may be affected, and enlarged, as may the trunk. Edema may develop rarely in response to compression or malformations of lymph vessels. Atrophy may occur in an affected limb.

Other associated features are adactyly, polydactyly, dilated pulmonary veins, partial overgrowth of the face without nevus flammeus, absence of an ear canal opening, thrombocytopenia, hypofibrinogenemia, spina bifida, congenital dislocation of the hips, larger-than-normal feet, and bilateral cryptorchidism. Skin ulcerations associated with constrictive blood flow can occur, as can eczema, flesh-colored warts, cellulitis, scoliosis, and hyperhidrosis. Thrombophlebitis may be present, but is usually stationary.

Hemorrhage may occur because abnormal blood vessels do not contain sufficient clotting factor. Dilation of abdominal veins may lead to bleeding in the rectum, vagina, or vulva. In some cases, hypertrophy in the bladder or colon may cause bleeding, and compressing growths near the spinal cord may result in partial paralysis.

Parkes-Weber syndrome, a subdivision of Klippel-Trenaunay syndrome, is characterized by arteriovenous shunts.

Etiology The cause is unknown.

Epidemiology Klippel-Trenaunay syndrome is a rare disorder that affects males and females in equal numbers.

Related Disorders See *Sturge-Weber Syndrome.*

Treatment—Standard Treatment is symptomatic. Argon, yellow light, or carbon dioxide laser surgery may lighten or remove the nevus flammeus. Blood vessel abnormalities in the colon may require intestinal resection. Lesions in the bladder may be removed with a high-frequency electrical current, using a cystoscope. Pain from varicose veins may be relieved by wearing elastic support stockings.

Surgery to correct leg length discrepancy is usually not indicated in children if the difference is less than 1 cm. Instead, scoliosis may be prevented with the use of a compensating shoe lift. Leg length discrepancy should be monitored through x-ray every 6 months and surgically corrected if it becomes significant. Surgery is not indicated in children to treat varicose veins because of the risk of complications and recurrence.

Patients with cellulitis, thrombophlebitis, recurrent bleeding, or anemia may be treated with diuretics, antibiotics, or iron supplements. Ulcerations or eczema may require topical medication.

Treatment—Investigational The flashlamp-pulsed tunable dye laser is showing promising results for treating nevus flammeus in children under 18.

Please contact the agencies listed under Resources, below, for the most current information.

Resources

For more information on Klippel-Trenaunay syndrome: National Organization for Rare Disorders (NORD); Klippel-Trenaunay Syndrome Support Group; NIH/National Institute of Neurological Disorders & Stroke (NINDS); The

National Congenital Port Wine Stain Foundation; Sturge-Weber Support Group.

For genetic information and genetic counseling referrals: March of Dimes Birth Defects Foundation; National Center for Education in Maternal and Child Health (NCEMCH).

References

CT Findings in Splenic Hemangiomas in the Klippel-Trenaunay-Weber Syndrome: R.L. Pakter, et al.; J. Comput. Assist. Tomogr., January–February 1987, issue 11(1), pp. 88–91.

A Retromedullary Arteriovenous Fistula Associated with the Klippel Syndrome: A Clinicopathologic Study: N. Benhaiem-Sigaux, et al.; Acta Neuropathol. (Berl.), 1985, issue 66(4), pp. 318–324.

Correction of Leg Inequality in the Klippel-Trenaunay-Weber Syndrome: M. Peixinho, et al.; Int. Orthop., 1982, issue 6(1), pp. 45–47.

Surgical Implications of Klippel-Trenaunay Syndrome: Peter P. Gloriezk, et al.; Ann. Surg., March 1983, issue 197, p. 353.

LARSEN SYNDROME

Description Larsen syndrome is a congenital, genetic disorder that affects many systems of the body. Characteristics include dislocations and abnormalities of the bones, an abnormally high foot arch, unusual facies, and cylindrical fingers.

Synonyms

Sinding-Larsen-Johansson Disease

Signs and Symptoms Features of the syndrome include a prominent forehead, upturned nose with a flattened bridge, hypertelorism, and low-set ears. Dislocations of bones in the knees, hips, and elbow are common. Patients may have mild scoliosis or osteoporosis. The fingers are usually cylindrical in shape and may be syndactylic. Pes cavus and clubbing are common abnormalities of the feet.

Congenital heart or respiratory complications may occur. Some males may have cryptorchidism.

Etiology Larsen syndrome is inherited as an autosomal dominant trait; many sporadic cases are also known. Symptoms are thought to result from a gestational embryonic disorder of the mesenchyma.

Epidemiology Larsen syndrome affects males and females equally. As of 1983, only about 80 cases had been described in the United States.

Related Disorders See *Arthrogryposis Multiplex Congenita* and *Ehlers-Danlos Syndrome.*

Treatment—Standard Infants should be managed by manipulation of joints and casts or traction. Older children may benefit from orthopedic surgery to correct bone deformities or dislocations. Reconstructive surgery may be appropriate to repair heart valve and spinal abnormalities, or cleft palate or cleft lip. Speech therapy and services for physically or mentally impaired patients and their families may be helpful.

Genetic counseling may benefit patients and their families. Other treatment is symptomatic and supportive.

Treatment—Investigational Please contact the agencies listed under Resources, below, for the most current information.

Resources

For more information on Larsen syndrome: National Organization for Rare Disorders (NORD); NIH/National Institute of Child Health and Human Development (NICHHD); The National Arthritis and Musculoskeletal and Skin Diseases Information Clearinghouse.

For genetic information and genetic counseling referrals: March of Dimes Birth Defects Foundation; National Center for Education in Maternal and Child Health (NCEMCH).

References

Mendelian Inheritance in Man, 7th ed.: V.A. McKusick; The Johns Hopkins University Press, 1986, pp. 451, 1079.

Spinal Deformities in Larsen's Syndrome: J.R. Bowen, et al.; Clin Orthop., July–August 1985, issue 197, pp. 159–163.

Severe Cardiac Anomalies in Sibs with Larsen Syndrome: P. Strisciuglio, et al.; J. Med. Genet., December 1983, issue 20(6), pp. 422–424.

Cardiovascular Manifestations in the Larsen Syndrome: E.A. Kiel, et al.; Pediatrics, June 1983, issue 20(6), pp. 422–424.

Sinding-Larsen-Johansson Disease. Its Etiology and Natural History: R.C. Medlar, et al.; J. Bone Joint Surg. [Am.], December 1978, issue 60(8), pp. 1113–1116.

LAURENCE-MOON-BIEDL SYNDROME (LMBS)

Description Laurence-Moon-Biedl syndrome is an inherited disorder characterized by hypogonadism, retinitis pigmentosa, mental retardation, polydactyly, and obesity. Most investigators suggest that this syndrome actually consists of 2 distinct syndromes, Laurence-Moon and Bardet-Biedl.

Synonyms

    Adipogenital-Retinitis Pigmentosa-Polydactyly Syndrome
    Bardet-Biedl Syndrome
    Laurence-Biedl Syndrome
    Laurence-Moon-Bardet-Biedl Syndrome
    Laurence-Moon Syndrome

Signs and Symptoms Obesity is one of the earliest signs, occurring before age 4 years. Onset of retinitis pigmentosa may be soon after, and cataracts, strabismus, and microphthalmos are common. Hypogonadism is accompanied by delayed onset of puberty and development of secondary sex characteristics. Boys may be sterile and develop breastlike tissue; girls may be amenorrheic and fail to develop breasts.

Besides the obesity and the ocular and gonadal manifestations, the other cardinal features are mental retardation and polydactyly. The presence of retinal degeneration and at least 3 of the cardinal features confirms the diagnosis.

Various other abnormalities may also occur. Neuromuscular complications are ataxia, muscle paralysis, and rigidity or spasticity. Kidney disease is common, including structural and functional abnormalities. Diabetes may also occur. Congenital heart defects are rare.

Etiology Laurence-Moon-Biedl syndrome is thought to be transmitted by 2 autosomal recessive genes on the same chromosome.

Epidemiology Almost 600 cases have been reported. Boys are affected twice as often as girls. The incidence is greatest among Kuwaiti Arabs.

Related Disorders See *Prader-Willi Syndrome.*

Alstrom syndrome is similar to LMB, but without mental retardation or polydactyly. Syndrome features are nerve deafness, baldness, and diabetes mellitus.

Weiss syndrome is characterized by deafness, obesity, hypogonadism, and mental retardation.

Biemond II syndrome resembles LMB except that eye abnormalities affect the iris, not the retina.

Treatment—Standard Surgery may be indicated to correct polydactyly. Visual aids may help those who have retained some useful vision. A strictly controlled diet may help manage appetite and control weight. Endocrine therapy may be required in hypogonadal individuals.

Treatment—Investigational Research is being conducted at the Cullen Eye Institute of the Baylor College of Medicine in Houston, Texas, on the subject of inherited retinal diseases including Laurence-Moon-Biedl syndrome. Families with at least 2 affected members and both parents living are needed to participate in the program.

Please contact the agencies listed under Resources, below, for the most current information.

Resources

For more information on Laurence-Moon-Biedl syndrome: National Organization for Rare Disorders (NORD); Laurence-Moon-Biedl Support Network; NIH/National Institute of Child Health and Human Development; NIH/National Institute of Neurological Disorders & Stroke (NINDS).

For services to persons visually impaired: American Council of the Blind, Inc. (ACB); American Foundation for the Blind (AFB); American Printing House for the Blind; National Association for Parents of the Visually Impaired (NAPVI); National Library Service for the Blind and Physically Handicapped; National Society to Prevent Blindness; Vision Foundation, Inc.

References

The Spectrum of Renal Disease in Laurence-Moon-Biedl Syndrome: J.D. Harnett, et al.; N. Engl. J. Med., September 8, 1988, issue 319(10), pp. 615–618.

Bardet-Biedl Syndrome and Related Disorders: A.P. Schachat and I.H. Maumenee; Arch. Ophthalmol., February 1982, issue 100(2), pp. 285–288.

LEPRECHAUNISM

Description Leprechaunism is a progressive hereditary endocrine disorder characterized by pancreatic hyperplasia, insulin resistance, and excessive amounts of estrogens. It may be associated with abnormal carbohydrate metabolism, and hepatic siderosis. Physical and sometimes mental retardation occur, and abnormalities of the face and external genitalia are also seen.

Synonyms
Donohue Syndrome

Signs and Symptoms Growth retardation begins in utero. Arms and legs are short, but hands and feet tend to be large. Subcutaneous fatty tissue usually disappears with advancing age. Affected children have an elfin face, with sunken cheeks, a pointed chin, a flat broad nose, low-set ears, and ocular hypertelorism. Other features include hirsutism and dark pigmentation in skin creases. In girls, the nipples and clitoris may be enlarged, and ovaries may be enlarged and cystic. In boys, the penis may be larger than normal. Mental development is sometimes retarded.

Patients with leprechaunism have hypoglycemia and hyperinsulinemia after fasting. They are also more susceptible to infections.

Etiology It has been established that the disorder is inherited as an autosomal recessive trait, and that parents of affected children are often consanguineous. The disorder has recently been proven to be caused by a defect in the gene coding for the insulin receptor.

Epidemiology Leprechaunism has been reported in about 50 patients, with twice as many females as males.

Related Disorders See *Williams Syndrome.*

The **Patterson-David syndrome** is a very rare disorder that has been confused with leprechaunism. Affected children may have a normal birth weight, hyperpigmentism, loose skin on the hands and feet, unusual facies, severe mental retardation, bony deformities, and skeletal dysplasia.

Treatment—Standard Treatment is symptomatic and supportive. Genetic counseling may benefit families of affected children. Infections should be guarded against and aggressively treated.

Treatment—Investigational Please contact the agencies listed under Resources, below, for the most current information.

Resources
For more information on leprechaunism: National Organization for Rare Disorders (NORD); National Institute of Diabetes, Digestive & Kidney Diseases

Information Clearinghouse; Research Trust for Metabolic Disorders in Children.

For genetic information and genetic counseling referrals: March of Dimes Birth Defects Foundation; National Center for Education in Maternal and Child Health (NCEMCH).

References
Mendelian Inheritance in Man, 9th ed.: V.A. McKusick; The Johns Hopkins University Press, 1990, pp. 1293–1295.

Smith's Recognizable Patterns of Human Malformation, 4th ed.: K.L. Jones; W.B. Saunders Company, 1988, p. 537.

The Patterson Syndrome, Leprechaunism, and Pseudoleprechaunism: T.J. David, et al.; J. of Med. Genetics, August 1981, issue 18(4), pp. 294–298.

Insulin Resistance in an Infant with Leprechaunism: H. Kashiwa, et al.; Acta Paediatrica Scandinavica, September 1984, issue 73(5), pp. 701–704.

MACROGLOSSIA

Description Macroglossia is a disorder in which the tongue is too large for the mouth, sometimes causing it to protrude. Macroglossia may be either congenital or acquired.

Synonyms
> Enlarged Tongue
> Giant Tongue

Signs and Symptoms In infants, macroglossia can complicate feeding. As the child matures, speech may be affected, and the jaw and teeth may not develop properly, resulting in dental abnormalities. The tip of the tongue may become ulcerative or necrotic.

Etiology Macroglossia may be associated with a wide variety of congenital and acquired syndromes and diseases, including the following: mandibulofacial dysostosis, Apert syndrome, cretinism, Greig hypertelorism, amyloidosis, myxedema, type 2 glycogen storage disease, congenital hypothyroidism, Sturge-Weber syndrome, acromegaly, neurofibromatosis, Down syndrome, craniofacial dysostosis, Hurler syndrome, Beckwith-Wiedemann syndrome, and lymphangiomas.

Epidemiology Males and females are affected equally.

Related Disorders The tongue may become enlarged in persons who have lost their teeth and have not replaced them with dentures.

Treatment—Standard Congenital macroglossia may resolve as the child matures so that the tongue is relative in size to other oral structures.

Macroglossia in edentulous persons may resolve if the patient is fitted with dentures.

The tongue may be reduced in size by orthodontic procedures or by surgery with remodeling of the mouth.

Treatment—Investigational Please contact the agencies listed under Resources, below, for the most current information.

Resources

For more information on macroglossia: National Organization for Rare Disorders (NORD); Association for Glycogen Storage Diseases; NIH/National Institute of Dental Research; Clinical Smell and Taste Research Center; Connecticut Chemosensory Clinical Research Center, Department of Oral Biology.

References

Macroglossia: Etiologic Considerations and Management Techniques: F.M. Rizer, et al.; Int. J. Pediatr. Otorhinolaryn., July 1985, issue 9(5), pp. 189–194.

Spontaneous Regression of Anterior Open Bite Following Treatment of Macroglossia: Maisels; Br. J. Plastic Surg., October 1979, issue 32(4), pp. 309–314.

MAFFUCCI SYNDROME

Description Maffucci syndrome is a congenital disorder characterized by hemangioma and enchondromatosis that may be present at birth or appear later in infancy or childhood.

Synonyms

Dyschondrodysplasia with Hemangiomas
Enchondromatosis with Multiple Cavernous Hemangiomas
Hemangiomatosis Chondrodystrophica
Kast Syndrome
Multiple Angiomas and Endochondromas

Signs and Symptoms The skin lesions, cavernous or capillary hemangiomas, are unilateral in almost half of patients, and when bilateral, differ in size. Lesions may occur in some viscera, and in the mucous membranes, commonly the mouth but also the esophagus, ileum, and anus. The skin lesions do not necessarily overlie those of bone.

Endochondral involvement results in dyschondroplasia of the long bones. During early childhood, endochondromas may also develop in the small bones of the hands and feet.

Patients are usually short, and scoliosis may develop where there is severe unilateral enchondromatosis. Bone fractures are common.

At least one-fourth of patients develop malignancies, especially chondrosarcomas. Other connective tissue neoplasms include gliomas, fibrosarcomas, angiosarcomas, lymphangiosarcomas, mesenchymal ovarian tumors, and pancreatic adenocarcinomas.

Etiology The syndrome is inherited as an autosomal dominant trait.

Epidemiology Maffucci syndrome affects males and females in equal numbers. First identified in 1881, the syndrome is very rare. Fewer than 105 cases have been documented in the United States.

Related Disorders See *Ollier Disease; Blue Rubber Bleb Nevus; Klippel-Trenaunay Syndrome.*

Treatment—Standard Because there are so many different symptoms and signs, an individual approach to treatment is necessary. Orthopedic treatment or surgery may be appropriate to correct differences in leg length, scoliosis, and bone deformities. There is some question as to the effectiveness of reconstructive surgery for the hemangiomas and enchondromas. Malignant neoplasms may respond to radiation therapy, chemotherapy, surgery, or a combination of these.

Treatment—Investigational Please contact the agencies listed under Resources, below, for the most current information.

Resources

   For more information on Maffucci syndrome: National Organization for Rare Disorders (NORD); The National Arthritis and Musculoskeletal and Skin Diseases Information Clearinghouse; NIH/National Heart, Lung and Blood Institute (NHLBI); American Cancer Society; NIH/National Cancer Institute PDQ (Physician Data Query) phoneline.

   For genetic information and genetic counseling referrals: March of Dimes Birth Defects Foundation; National Center for Education in Maternal and Child Health (NCEMCH).

References

   Chondrosarcoma in Maffucci's Syndrome: T.C. Sun, et al.; J. Bone Joint Surg. (Am.), October 1985, issue 67(8), pp. 1214–1219.

   Angiosarcoma Arising in a Patient with Maffucci Syndrome: T.I. Davidson, et al.; Eur. J. Surg. Oncol., December 1985, issue 11(4), pp. 381–384.

MALIGNANT HYPERTHERMIA

Description Malignant hyperthermia is a pharmacogenetic disorder in which the patient develops a rapid, high fever after anesthesia administration or some muscle relaxants. Offending drugs include halothane, cyclopropane, or succinylcholine.

Synonyms

   Fulminating Hyperpyrexia
   Hyperthermia of Anesthesia
   Malignant Fever
   Malignant Hyperpyrexia

Signs and Symptoms Patients may have been previously unaffected by anesthesia or injection of muscle relaxants, although a few may have reported previous episodes of muscle cramps or weakness. After anesthetic drugs or muscle relaxants are administered, the patient quickly develops a high fever, sometimes as high as 110 degrees. Muscles are characterized by twitching and rigidity. Headache, nausea, vomiting, hypotension, tachycardia, and cardiac arrhythmias may be present.

Major complications include skeleton muscle degeneration (rhabdomyolysis), renal failure, pulmonary edema, and disruption of blood clotting mechanisms. Levels of creatine phosphokinase are elevated.

Etiology Persons may inherit a predisposition to malignant hyperthermia through an autosomal dominant pattern. It may be related to an increase in the level of sarcoplasmic calcium.

Epidemiology Malignant hyperthermia is extremely rare. Males and females are affected equally.

Related Disorders Boys affected with **King syndrome** (characteristics include slanted eyes, low-set ears, receding chins, webbed necks, cryptorchidism, spinal abnormalities, and short stature), and perhaps *Noonan Syndrome,* may also experience malignant hyperthermia.

Treatment—Standard Immediate rapid treatment is indicated, with cooling of the body, support of respiration, and bicarbonate for metabolic acidosis. The antispasmodic, dantrolene sodium, is effective. Procaine and verapamil may be useful.

Prevention includes elucidation of a history of abnormal response to involved drugs. Biopsy of the thigh muscle can aid diagnosis. Dantrolene sodium given the day before anesthesia has prevented malignant hyperthermia. Regional or local anesthesia may be indicated for at-risk individuals.

Treatment—Investigational Research is ongoing to develop a less invasive diagnostic test and more effective therapies.

The offending gene for malignant hyperthermia has been identified on chromosome 19. When the gene is found, a genetic test will be developed to identify the exact biochemical defect that is triggered by the gene in the hope of developing a cure.

Please contact the agencies listed under Resources, below, for the most current information.

Resources

For more information on malignant hyperthermia: National Organization of Rare Disorders (NORD); Malignant Hyperthermia Association of the United States; The North American MH Registry.

For names of on-call physicians available 24 hours/day to treat MH emergencies: Medic Alert Foundation International.

For genetic information and genetic counseling referrals: March of Dimes Birth Defects Foundation; National Center for Education in Maternal and Child Health (NCEMCH).

For malignant hypothermia clinics: Mayo Clinic, Dept. of Anesthesiology, 200 1st St. SW, Rochester, MN 55905, (507) 285-5601; University of Texas, Medical Branch at Galveston, Dept. of Anesthesiology, Galveston, TX 77550, (409) 761-1906; Hahnemann University Medical School, Dept. of Anesthesiology, Broad and Vine Streets, Philadelphia, PA 19102, (215) 448-7960; Massachusetts General Dept. of Anesthesiology, Room ACC3, Fruit Street, Boston, MA 02114, (617) 726-8800; University of Toronto, MH Investigatory Unit, Room 5268, Medical Sciences Building, Toronto, Ontario M5S-1A, Canada.

References
Mendelian Inheritance in Man, 8th ed.: V.A. McKusick; The Johns Hopkins University Press, 1986, pp. 406–407.
Internal Medicine, 3rd ed.: J.H. Stein, ed.-in-chief; Little, Brown and Company, 1990, p. 2416.

MARFAN SYNDROME

Description Marfan syndrome is an inherited disorder that affects the connective tissues of the cardiovascular and musculoskeletal systems, and the eyes.

Synonyms
Arachnodactyly

Signs and Symptoms Affected persons are tall and thin. Both the face and limbs are abnormally long. Other features include excessive joint mobility, flat feet, hypotonia, a protruding or indented sternum, and scoliosis. Teeth may be crowded because of an abnormally high palate. Striae may appear on the skin.

Significant cardiovascular problems may be present. The most common is mitral valve prolapse, which is often asymptomatic. Enlargement and degeneration of the aorta, aortic aneurysm, and aortic regurgitation are also common, and account for most deaths.

The major ocular findings are severe myopia, ectopia lentis (about 50 percent of patients), increased axial globe length, corneal flatness, and occasionally retinal detachment.

Emphysema develops in almost all patients with Marfan syndrome. Pneumothorax occurs in about 5 percent of patients, either spontaneously or traumatically, and requires prompt treatment.

Etiology Marfan syndrome is transmitted through a single mutant autosomal dominant gene on chromosome 15. Penetrance is complete but expression of clinical manifestations may be variable. The nature of the connective tissue derangement is unknown.

Epidemiology The syndrome affects males and females in equal numbers. In the United States, about 25,000 to 30,000 persons are affected, many of whom have not been diagnosed.

Related Disorders See *Ehlers-Danlos Syndrome; Homocystinuria; Acromegaly.*

Treatment—Standard Treatment is symptomatic. Beta-adrenergic blocking agents (e.g., propranolol and atenolol) are used to treat cardiovascular symptoms. Because early mortality is usually the result of aortic dilation, patients should have annual electrocardiography. Malfunctioning valves may be treated medically, but surgical replacement of the aorta may eventually become necessary. Patients should minimize stress on the aorta by avoiding activities such as heavy lifting and sports.

Scoliosis and chest deformity are the most serious complications of the skeletal system. An orthopedic surgeon should be consulted if curvature of more than 10 degrees develops. Some children, especially girls, have been treated with estrogens in order to reduce the length of time of susceptibility to curvature. This therapy produces minimal physical side effects and may actually reduce final height, but may produce psychological problems as the child copes with early sexual maturation. Deformities of the sternum can be corrected surgically, but should be postponed until mid adolescence if the problem is solely cosmetic.

Failure to detect any of the ocular abnormalities may result in permanent visual disability. Increased risk of retinal detachment warrants special care, and patients should be counseled to avoid activities that may result in a blow to the eye.

Treatment—Investigational Other beta-adrenergic blocking drugs are being investigated as possible therapies to treat cardiovascular symptoms. Basic research continues on the etiology of the syndrome, including studies of the biochemistry of connective tissue and of the location and nature of the genetic defect.

Please contact the agencies listed under Resources, below, for the most current information.

Resources

For more information on Marfan Syndrome: National Organization for Rare Disorders (NORD); National Marfan Foundation; The National Arthritis and Musculoskeletal and Skin Diseases Information Clearinghouse.

For genetic information and genetic counseling referrals: March of Dimes Birth Defects Foundation; NIH/National Center for Education in Maternal and Child Health (NCEMCH).

References

Internal Medicine, 3rd ed.: J.H. Stein, ed.-in-chief; Little, Brown and Company, 1990, pp. 226–227.

Mendelian Inheritance in Man, 9th ed.: V.A. McKusick; The Johns Hopkins University Press, 1990, pp. 599–601, 1309, 206.

MECKEL SYNDROME

Description Meckel syndrome is a rare inherited disorder with a wide variety of manifestations, the most common of which are sloping forehead, posterior encephalocele, polydactyly, and polycystic kidney. Liver abnormalities are also common. Infants rarely live more than a few days or weeks.

Synonyms

Dysencephalia Splanchnocystica
Gruber Syndrome
Meckel-Gruber Syndrome

Signs and Symptoms Characteristic features are posterior encephalocele and other brain abnormalities, renal cysts, and abnormalities of the bile ducts of the liver. Polydactyly and shortening or bowing of the long bones of the arms and legs are common. In males the testicles may contain abnormal cysts and may fail to descend or grow properly.

Etiology Meckel syndrome is inherited as an autosomal recessive trait.

Epidemiology Males and females are affected in equal numbers. Estimates of the incidence of this syndrome vary in different populations from 1:140,000 to 1:9,000 births. The incidence appears to be higher in India, Finland, and among the Tatars in the Soviet Union.

Related Disorders See *Smith-Lemli-Opitz Syndrome.*

Potter syndrome is a rare hereditary disorder marked by congenital cysts of the kidneys and liver. Patients also suffer from cerebral hemorrhage, aortic aneurysm, and hypertension.

Ullrich-Feichtiger syndrome exhibits the same symptoms as Meckel syndrome with the addition of some facial deformities that include small jaws and cleft palate.

Treatment—Standard Meckel syndrome can be identified in pregnant women during the 5th month of pregnancy either through ultrasound testing or amniocentesis. Treatment is symptomatic and supportive. Genetic counseling is recommended for families affected by this disorder.

Treatment—Investigational Please contact the agencies listed under Resources, below, for the most current information.

Resources

For more information on Meckel syndrome: National Organization for Rare Disorders (NORD); NIH/National Institute of Child Health and Human Development.

For genetic information and genetic counseling referrals: March of Dimes Birth Defects Foundation; NIH/National Center for Education in Maternal and Child Health (NCEMCH).

References
Mendelian Inheritance in Man, 9th ed.: V.A. McKusick; The Johns Hopkins University Press, 1990, pp. 1310–1311.

Smith's Recognizable Patterns of Human Malformation, 4th ed.: K.L. Jones; W.B. Saunders Company, 1988, pp. 152–153.

Are Bowing of Long Tubular Bones and Preaxial Polydactyl Signs of the Meckel Syndrome? F. Majewski, et al.; Hum. Genet., 1983, issue 65(2), pp. 125–133.

The Meckel Syndrome: Clinicopathological Findings in 67 Patients; R. Salonen, et al.; Am. J. Med. Genet., August 1984, issue 18(4), pp. 671–689.

A New Syndrome with Features of the Smith-Lemli-Opitz and Meckel-Gruber Syndromes in a Sibship with Cerebellar Defects: A.C. Casamassima, et al.; Am. J. Med. Genet., February 1987, issue 26(2), pp. 321–336.

Studies on the Elevated Amniotic Fluid sp 1 in Meckels' Syndrome; Modified Glycosylation of sp 1; M. Heikinheimo, et al.; Placenta, July–August 1987, issue 8(4), pp. 427–432.

MELNICK-NEEDLES SYNDROME

Description Melnick-Needles syndrome is a disorder in which bones develop abnormally. Patients are characterized by hypertelorism, bowed arm and leg bones, and micrognathia.

Synonyms
> Melnick-Needles Osteodysplasty
> Osteodysplasty of Melnick and Needles

Signs and Symptoms Patients with this syndrome exhibit unique facial characteristics, including hypertelorism, micrognathia, small facial bones, a slow-developing skull, and an abnormal bite. The syndrome also affects the limbs. The humerus, phalanges, radius, fibula, and tibia may be shorter than normal, bowed, and flared.

Although patients usually achieve a normal height, their gait may be unusual, a result of the presence of coxa valga.

The upper trunk may also be affected. The thoracic cage may be smaller than normal, the ribs irregular, and the shoulders narrowed. Other symptoms include pectus excavatum, longer-than-normal vertebrae, and flared ilium. These deformities make the patients more susceptible to respiratory infections.

The pelvis may also be involved, and the hip may become dislocated. Osteoarthritis may affect the hip and spine. Complications relating to childbirth and kidney malfunction may also occur.

Etiology Melnick-Needles syndrome is a genetically transmitted disorder. The exact genetic mechanism is not known, but X-linked dominance with lethality in males appears most likely.

Epidemiology Melnick-Needles syndrome occurs at birth and affects females more often than males.

Related Disorders Multiple epiphyseal dysplasia is an inherited disorder that affects the bones. It is usually diagnosed when the patient is between 2 and 5 years and begins to exhibit an unusual gait. Osteoarthritis may develop in the joints. Patients reach normal height, but exhibit smaller-than-normal hands and feet. Males and females are affected equally.

Treatment—Standard Treatment is symptomatic and supportive. Genetic counseling may benefit patients and their families.

Treatment—Investigational Please contact the agencies listed under Resources, below, for the most current information.

Resources
  For more information on Melnick-Needles syndrome: National Organization for Rare Disorders (NORD); International Center for Skeletal Dysplasia; NIH/National Institute of Child Health and Human Development (NICHHD).
  For genetic information and genetic counseling referrals: March of Dimes Birth Defects Foundation; NIH/National Center for Education in Mater-

nal and Child Health (NCEMCH).

References
Smith's Recognizable Patterns of Human Malformation, 4th ed.: K.L. Jones; W.B. Saunders Company, 1988. pp. 528–529.

Melnick-Needles Syndrome in Males: M. Krajewska-Walasek, et al.; Am. J. Med. Genet., May 1987, issue 27(1), pp. 153–158.

METAPHYSEAL CHONDRODYSPLASIA, MCKUSICK TYPE

Description Metaphyseal chondrodysplasia (McKusick type) is a progressive genetic disorder characterized by short-limbed short stature caused by abnormal development of long-bone cartilage.

Synonyms
Cartilage-Hair Hypoplasia
Cartilage-Hair Hypoplasia with Short-Limbed Dwarfism

Signs and Symptoms Metaphyseal chondrodysplasia (McKusick type) primarily affects the peripheral bones, resulting in short-limbed short stature. Adult height is about 120 cm. The range of symptoms is wide and includes abnormalities of the spine; hypermobile fingers; and fine, thin hair on the head, eyebrows, and eyelashes.

Etiology The disorder is inherited through autosomal recessive genes.

Epidemiology Metaphyseal chondrodysplasia (McKusick type) is rare. It is most often diagnosed in Finland, although it was first described in the Amish communities of the United States. Males and females are affected equally.

Related Disorders See *Hypochondroplasia.*

Metaphyseal chondrodysplasia, Jansen type (chondrodysplasia, Murk-Jansen type) is another type of short-limbed short stature, which is inherited through an autosomal dominant pattern. Distortion of the spine, pelvis, and lower legs is present. The skull bones, including those of the inner ear, are sclerosed, causing deafness. Patients also exhibit a receding chin and abnormally short fingers.

Metaphyseal chondrodysplasia (Schmid type) is a rare progressive disorder characterized by bowed legs, a waddling gait, and moderately short stature. Adult height is about 140 cm.

Treatment—Standard Some patients may benefit from physiotherapy and orthopedic treatment. Genetic counseling may be helpful for patients and their families.

Treatment—Investigational Please contact the agencies listed under Resources, below, for the most current information.

Resources

For more information on metaphyseal chondrodysplasia, McKusick type: National Organization for Rare Disorders (NORD); Human Growth Foundation (HGF); Little People of America; Parents of Dwarfed Children; Short Stature Foundation.

For genetic information and genetic counseling referrals: March of Dimes Birth Defects Foundation; National Center for Education in Maternal and Child Health (NCEMCH).

References

Mendelian Inheritance in Man, 9th ed.: V.A. McKusick; The Johns Hopkins University Press, 1990, pp. 1322–1323.

The Jansen Type of Metaphyseal Chondrodysplasia: Confirmation of Dominant Inheritance and Review of Radiographic Manifestations in the Newborn and Adult: J. Charrow, et al.; Am. J. Med. Genet., June 1984, issue 18(2), pp. 321–327.

Metaphyseal Chondrodysplasia, Schmid Type. Clinical and Radiographic Delineation with a Review of the Literature: R.S. Lachman, et al.; Pediatr. Radiol., 1988, issue 18(2), pp. 93–102.

MOEBIUS SYNDROME

Description Moebius syndrome is an inherited type of facial paralysis caused by absent or decreased 6th and 7th nerve development. Abnormalities of the facial muscles and jaw develop. Central nervous system abnormalities may also occur. Mental retardation is present in about 10 percent of cases.

Synonyms

Congenital Facial Diplegia Syndrome
Congenital Oculofacial Paralysis
Sixth and Seventh Nerve Palsy

Signs and Symptoms From birth, patients exhibit a masklike expression, especially when crying or laughing. Nerve and muscle abnormalities cause the mouth and eyes to remain open during sleep, resulting in ocular ulcerations. Feeding during infancy is difficult. Speech problems may develop. Fluid secretions of the mouth may be breathed into the lungs, resulting in bronchopneumonia. Epicanthal folds, microphthalmos, and malformations of the jaw and tongue may also occur.

Many abnormalities of the hands and feet may be present, including polydactyly, oligodactyly, and clubfeet. Congenital dislocation of the hip may also occur.

Etiology Moebius syndrome is thought to be inherited as an autosomal dominant trait, but most often occurs sporadically.

Epidemiology The syndrome is very rare. Males and females are affected in equal numbers.

Related Disorders Facioscapulohumoral muscular dystrophy (Landouzy-Dejerine muscular dystrophy) is characterized by muscle weakness and atrophy of the face, shoulders, and arms. A genetic disorder, it usually manifests between 9 and 20 years of age, although onset can be much earlier. The face is flat and mask-like. Patients may not be able to raise their arms above the head; later, the pelvis and legs develop weakness.

Treatment—Standard Medical therapy may be indicated for dry or ulcerated eyes. Parenteral tube feeding may be necessary during infancy, and later, patients may require a special diet to avoid aspirating food into the lungs. Speech may improve with therapy and vocal cord surgery. Other surgery involving muscle transfer may be necessary to correct abnormalities of the eye, face, hands, or feet.

Other treatment is symptomatic and supportive. Genetic counseling will benefit patients and their families.

Treatment—Investigational Please contact the agencies listed under Resources, below, for the most current information.

Resources

For more information on Moebius syndrome: National Organization for Rare Disorders (NORD); NIH/National Institute of Neurological Disorders & Stroke (NINDS); FACES—National Association for the Craniofacially Handicapped; Society for the Rehabilitation of the Facially Disfigured, Inc.; About Face.

For genetic information and genetic counseling referrals: March of Dimes Birth Defects Foundation; National Center for Education in Maternal and Child Health (NCEMCH).

References

Extraocular Muscle Aplasia in Moebius Syndrome: E.I. Traboulsi, et al.; J. Pediatr. Ophthalmol. Strabismus, May–June 1986, issue 23(3), pp. 120–122.

Abnormal B.A.E.P. in a Family with Moebius Syndrome: Evidence for Supranuclear Lesion: M. Stabile, et al.; Clin. Genet., May 1984, issue 25(5), pp. 459–463.

Moebius Syndrome. Case Report of a 30-Year Follow-up: D.C. Morello, et al.; Plast. Reconstr. Surg., September 1977, issue 60(3), pp. 451–453.

NAIL-PATELLA SYNDROME

Description Nail-patella syndrome is a rare genetic disorder characterized primarily by nail dysplasia, bone deformities, and, in some cases, renal abnormalities.

Synonyms

Fong Syndrome
Hereditary Onychoosteodysplasia
Turner-Kieser Syndrome

Signs and Symptoms The nails, especially the thumbs, are hypoplastic with splitting, ridges, discoloration, and abnormal moons. The patellae are hypoplastic or absent, and there often are abnormalities of the elbows affecting range of movement, ilia (iliac spurs, seen in almost three-quarters of patients), and scapulae.

About half of patients have a cloverleaf pigmentation of the iris, and one-third of patients have renal signs (proteinuria, abnormal urinary sediment). The renal disease is usually benign, although it occasionally leads to early fatality. Other, less frequent, abnormalities are skeletal, ocular, muscular, and neurologic.

Etiology The syndrome is inherited as an autosomal dominant trait linked to the ABO blood group locus.

Related Disorders See *Alport Syndrome.*

   Nail-patella–like renal disease involves the kidneys without apparent bone and nail abnormalities. However, electron microscopy reveals histopathologic changes similar to nail-patella syndrome.

Treatment—Standard Renal dialysis and possibly kidney transplantation may be indicated in the treatment of kidney complications. Genetic counseling may be of benefit for patients and their families. Other treatment is symptomatic and supportive.

Treatment—Investigational Please contact the agencies listed under Resources, below, for the most current information.

Resources

   For more information on nail-patella syndrome: National Organization for Rare Disorders (NORD); National Kidney Foundation; National Kidney and Urologic Diseases Information Clearinghouse.

   For genetic information and genetic counseling referrals: March of Dimes Birth Defects Foundation; National Center for Education in Maternal and Child Health (NCEMCH).

References
Mendelian Inheritance in Man, 9th ed.: V.A. McKusick; The Johns Hopkins University Press, 1990, pp. 643–644, 1370.

Smith's Recognizable Patterns of Human Malformation, 4th ed.: K.L. Jones; W.B. Saunders Company, 1988, pp. 386–387.

An Autosomal Recessive Disorder, with Glomerular Basement Membrane Abnormalities Similar to Those Seen in the Nail Patella Syndrome; Report of a Kindred: J.R. Salcedo; Am. J. Med. Genet., 1984, issue 19, pp. 579–584.

NEUROFIBROMATOSIS (NF)

Description The term neurofibromatosis is used to describe what are now known to be two distinctly different disorders, the more common type 1 neurofibromatosis (NF 1), and the less common type 2 (NF 2). Both disorders are transmitted in an autosomal dominant fashion, but the genes involved are on separate chromosomes. Both conditions are characterized by the occurrence of multiple neurofibromas. In the recent past, great lay interest in neurofibromatosis has been sparked by the Broadway show and the movie based on the book by Sir Frederick Treves, *The Elephant Man and Other Reminiscences.* Lamentably, this led to the vogue of referring to NF 1 as Elephant Man disease; not only is this odious but it now appears that Treves' patient had Proteus syndrome rather than NF 1. (See **Proteus Syndrome.**)

Synonyms
Bilateral Acoustic Neurofibromatosis (NF 2)
Central Neurofibromatosis (NF 2)
Neurofibroma, Multiple
Recklinghausen Disease (NF 1)

Signs and Symptoms NF 1 usually has its onset during childhood. The disease is progressive and tends to become more active at puberty and during pregnancy. Although the course and symptoms of NF vary and are unpredictable, brown (café-au-lait) spots are usually the first sign. These spots measure approximately 0.5 cm in diameter in children and grow to 1.5 cm in diameter in adults. Six or more 0.5 café-au-lait macules and two or more neurofibromas are diagnostic in a child. Axillary or inguinal freckling or two or more Lisch nodules in the iris are other important diagnostic criteria.

The most common tumors, neurofibromas, occur in NF 1 and can form under the skin or in deeper areas in the body. Pain may or may not occur. Tumors can produce disfigurement and orthopedic problems, including scoliosis and pseudoarthrosis. Sexual development may be delayed or precocious, and learning disabilities may develop. Optic glioma, hamartomas, and other CNS lesions are common.

NF 2 develops later than NF 1, usually in the teens and 20s. Fewer café-au-lait spots and cutaneous neurofibromas develop. It is characterized by bilateral acoustic neuromas and may be associated with brain and spinal cord tumors. Buzzing or ringing in the ears and loss of hearing are the clinical manifestations of these neuromas.

Etiology NF 1 and 2 have autosomal dominant inheritance; however, about half of all cases are due to new mutations. The gene for NF 1 is on chromosome 17 (17q11.2). The gene for NF 2 is on chromosome 22 (22q).

A localized (unilateral and not crossing the midline) form of neurofibromatosis appears to be caused by a somatic mutation, with little risk of recurrence.

Epidemiology NF affects approximately 100,000 Americans, both male and female. NF 1 affects 1:4,000 individuals; NF 2 affects 1:50,000.

Treatment—Standard Once diagnosis is established, a systematic monitoring program of follow-up is indicated. Quantitation of specific signs, such as café-au-lait macules, neurofibromas, and Lisch nodules is indicated. Tests, such as computed tomography, magnetic resonance imaging, and electroencephalography, are dictated by clinical findings. About 50 percent of patients require surgery to remove troublesome neurofibromas. Surgical indications for optic gliomas, acoustic neuromas, and other tumors must be individualized. Since management options are evolving, physicians managing these patients must be aware of current consensus regarding treatment.

Treatment—Investigational Neurofibromatosis research is ongoing and includes recombinant DNA and nerve growth factor. Recent identification of chromosome markers for both types of NF may lead to genetic testing.

Families with one or more members who have central neurofibromatosis (NF 2) with bilateral acoustic neuromas are being sought for a clinical research study at the National Institute of Neurological Disorders and Stroke (NINDS) in Bethesda, MD. The study's goal is to establish methods for early detection and diagnosis. Clinicians who wish to refer potential candidates or obtain additional information should contact Donald Wright, M.D., Surgical Neurology Branch, NINDS, Building 10A, Room 3E68, Bethesda, MD 20892, (301) 496-2921.

Researchers are also investigating learning disabilities and neurologic changes in NF children from birth to 18 years of age. A controlled study is under way of NF children and siblings who do not have the disorder. Testing is being performed in conjunction with Children's Hospital, 111 Michigan Avenue NW, Washington, DC 20010; (202) 745-2187.

Ongoing research is directed toward understanding the genetic changes in tumor formation in neurofibromatosis. Known or suspected malignancy tissue is requested. Samples of neurofibromas from female patients are also requested. Please contact Gary R. Skuse, M.D., or Peter T. Rowley, M.D., University of Rochester Medical Center, Division of Genetics, Box 641, 601 Elmwood Ave., Rochester, NY 14642; (716) 275-3461.

Please also contact the agencies listed under Resources, below, for current information.

Resources

For more information on neurofibromatosis: National Organization for Rare Disorders (NORD); Neurofibromatosis, Inc.; The National Neurofibromatosis Foundation, Inc.; NIH/National Institute of Neurological Disorders & Stroke (NINDS).

For genetic information and genetic counseling referrals: March of Dimes Birth Defects Foundation; National Center for Education in Maternal and Child Health (NCEMCH).

Clinical facilities:

Massachusetts General Hospital Neurofibromatosis Clinic, Department of Neurosurgery, 15 Parkman Street, Room 312, Boston, MA 02114; (617) 726-3776, Attention of Robert Marthuza, M.D.

Children's Hospital Neurofibromatosis Clinic, 111 Michigan Avenue NW, Washington, DC 20010; (202) 745-2187, Attention of Kenneth Rosenbaum, M.D.

Children's Hospital Neurofibromatosis Clinic, 34th and Civic Center Blvd., Room 9028, Phila., PA 19104; (215) 596-9645, Attention of Anna Meadows, M.D.

Baylor College of Medicine Neurofibromatosis Clinic, One Baylor Plaza, Houston, Texas 77030; (713) 799-6103, Attention of Vincent Riccardi, M.D.

Mount Sinai School of Medicine Neurofibromatosis Clinic, 100th Street and Madison Avenue, New York, NY 10029; (212) 650-6500, Attention of Alan Rubinstein, M.D.

References

Mendelian Inheritance in Man, 9th ed.: V.A. McKusick; The Johns Hopkins University Press, 1990, pp. 12–13, 650–656.

Smith's Recognizable Patterns of Human Malformation, 4th ed.: K.L. Jones; W.B. Saunders Company, 1988, pp. 452–453.

Neurofibromatosis 1 (Recklinghouse Disease) and Neurofibromatosis 2 (Bilateral Acoustic Neurofibromatosis). An Update: J.J. Mulvihill, et al.; Ann. Int. Med., 1990, vol. 113(1), pp. 39–52.

NOONAN SYNDROME

Description Noonan syndrome is characterized by congenital heart defects, short stature, broad or webbed neck, and droopy eyelids.

Synonyms
Turner-like Syndrome

Signs and Symptoms The most common cardiac defects are pulmonary valvular stenosis or atrial septal defect, occurring in two-thirds of patients. Average adult height of males is 64 inches, and that of females, 60 inches. A characteristic facies includes hypertelorism, epicanthus, an antimongoloid palpebral slant, ptosis, micrognathia, and ear abnormalities. Other findings include webbing of the neck, pectus carinatum or pectus excavatum, cubitum valgum, and in males, undescended testes. Puberty usually occurs normally, but is delayed 2 years on average.

Etiology Noonan syndrome is inherited primarily through an autosomal dominant pattern, with highly variable expression. Many cases appear to be sporadic.

Epidemiology The syndrome is thought to occur in approximately 1:1,000 to 1:2,500 persons. The wide variety of symptoms may contribute to significant underdiagnosis and misdiagnosis.

Related Disorders See *Turner Syndrome.* See also *Malignant Hyperthermia.*

Treatment—Standard Cryptorchidism should be treated by 2 to 3 years of age. Severe ptosis can be surgically corrected. Severe pulmonary stenosis may require surgery or balloon dilation.

Genetic counseling is useful for families of children with Noonan syndrome.

Treatment—Investigational Human growth hormone treatment for the short stature of Noonan syndrome is at the investigational stage.

Please contact the agencies listed under Resources, below, for the most current information.

Resources

For more information on Noonan syndrome: National Organization for Rare Disorders (NORD); Noonan Syndrome Support Group; NIH/National Institute of Child Health and Human Development (NICHHD); Human Growth Foundation (HGF).

For genetic information and genetic counseling referrals: March of

Dimes Birth Defects Foundation; National Center for Education in Maternal and Child Health (NCEMCH).

References

Percutaneous Balloon Vulvoplasty for Pulmonary Valve Stenosis in Infants and Children: I.D. Sullivan, et al.; Br. Heart J., October 1985, issue 54(4), pp. 435–441.

Noonan Syndrome: The Changing Phenotype: J.E. Allanson, et al.; Am. J. Med. Gen., July 1985, issue 21(3), pp. 507–514.

Mendelian Inheritance in Man, 9th ed.: V.A. McKusick; The Johns Hopkins University Press, 1990, pp. 664–665.

ORAL-FACIAL-DIGITAL SYNDROME (OFD)

Description OFD syndrome is characterized by neuromuscular disturbances, mental disturbances, cleft palate and other facial malformations, shortened limbs, and hands and feet deformities. It is categorized into types I-IV.

Synonyms

Mohr Syndrome (Type II OFD)

Orofaciodigital Syndrome

Signs and Symptoms Symptoms common to all 4 types of the syndrome include neuromuscular disturbances; clefts of the tongue, jaw, and lip; overgrowth of the frenulum of the tongue; epicanthal folds; broad-based nose; syndactyly, brachydactyly, and clinodactyly; and extra divisions between skull sections.

In type I, those affected have coarse, thin hair, skin lesions, and unilateral polysyndactyly.

Type II is similar to type I, but polysyndactyly of the toes is bilateral.

Type III is characterized by the presence of extra teeth and jaw-winking.

Type IV patients have shortened limbs. Also present may be psychomotor retardation, clefts and other abnormalities of the jaw and tongue, and tooth malformations. Ocular manifestations include see-saw winking and exotropia.

Etiology OFD is believed to be inherited in types II, III, and IV as an autosomal recessive trait. Type I is X-linked dominant, and lethal in males.

Epidemiology The syndrome is very rare. Except for Type I, males and females are affected in equal numbers.

Related Disorders See *Joubert Syndrome.*

Juberg-Hayward syndrome (orocraniodigital syndrome) is a rare hereditary disorder characterized by cleft lip and palate, microcephaly, thumb and toe abnormalities, and short stature due to growth hormone deficiency.

Nager acrofacial dysostosis (mandibulofacial dysostosis) is a rare hereditary disorder characterized by cleft lip and palate, abnormalities of jaw and arm bones, and abnormally small thumbs.

Treatment—Standard Reconstructive surgery for facial clefts may be necessary. Other treatment is symptomatic and supportive. Genetic counseling is recommended for patients and their families.

Treatment—Investigational Please contact the agencies listed under Resources, below, for the most current information.

Resources
   For more information on oral-facial-digital syndrome: National Organization for Rare Disorders (NORD); NIH/National Institute of Dental Research; FACES—National Association for the Craniofacially Handicapped; About Face; National Foundation for Facial Reconstruction.
   For information on cleft palate: American Cleft Palate Cranial Facial Association; National Cleft Palate Association; National Foundation of Dentistry for the Handicapped.
   For genetic information and genetic counseling referrals: March of Dimes Birth Defects Foundation; National Center for Education in Maternal and Child Health (NCEMCH).

References
   Mendelian Inheritance in Man, 9th ed.: V.A. McKusick; The Johns Hopkins University Press, 1990, p. 1697.
   The Spectrum of the Oro-Facial-Digital Syndrome: O.M. Fenton, et al.; Br. J. Plast. Surg., October l985, issue 38(4), pp. 532–539.
   Mohr Syndrome in Two Siblings: A. Gencik, et al.; J. Genet. Hum., December l983, issue 31(4), pp. 307–315.
   Prenatal Diagnosis of Mohr Syndrome by Ultrasonography: M. Iaccarino, et al.; Prenat. Diagn., November–December l985, issue 5(6), pp. 415–418.
   Orocraniodigital (Juberg-Hayward) Syndrome with Growth Hormone Deficiency: H.M. Kingston, et al.; Arch. Dis. Child, October 1982, issue 57(10), pp. 790–792.
   A Case of The Orocraniodigital (Juberg-Hayward) Syndrome: N.C. Nevin, et al.; J. Med. Genet., December 1981, issue 18(6), pp. 478–481.
   Syndrome of Acrofacial Dysostosis, Cleft Lip/Palate, and Triphalangeal Thumb in a Brazilian Family: A. Richieri-Costa, et al.; Am. J. Med. Genet., 1983, issue 14, pp. 225–229.

OSTEOGENESIS IMPERFECTA (OI)

Description Osteogenesis imperfecta is characterized by unusually fragile bones that fracture easily. There are generally considered to be 4 types, some with subtypes. The congenital form, type II, is the most severe; affected infants are either stillborn or die soon after birth of respiratory insufficiency.

Synonyms
   Brittle Bone Disease
   Lobstein Disease (Type I)
   Vrolik Disease (Type II)

Signs and Symptoms Fractures, especially of the long bones of the legs, are common even after minimal trauma.
   Type I is characterized by blue sclera, little or no deformity, normal stature, and hearing loss in about 50 percent of patients.

Type II is lethal in the newborn period. Infants are born with multiple fractures, marked long bone deformities, and compressed fractures.

Patients with type III have short stature and only a variable scleral hue. Hearing loss and dentinogenesis are common. Deformation of bones tends to be progressive.

Patients with type IV have normal sclera, mild bone deformity, and variable short stature. Dentinogenesis is common, but hearing loss is rare.

Etiology The most common form of inheritance is autosomal dominant, but a recessive pattern has been identified in a few patients. More than 50 mutations in the genes that encode the chains of type I collagen have been delineated. The nature of the mutation determines the phenotype.

Epidemiology Osteogenesis imperfecta occurs in 1:20,000 to 1:50,000 births in the United States.

Treatment—Standard Treatment is generally symptomatic. Physical therapy and hydrotherapy help strengthen muscles, increase weight-bearing capacity, and reduce the tendency to fracture.

Metal rods surgically placed in the long bones (rodding) can help prevent fracture. Plastic braces are preferable to plaster casts as protective devices because they permit greater mobility and are water-resistant. Inflatable suits can provide protection, especially to young children.

Treatment—Investigational Please contact the agencies listed under Resources, below, for the most current information.

Resources

For more information on osteogenesis imperfecta: National Organization for Rare Disorders (NORD); Osteogenesis Imperfecta Foundation; The National Arthritis and Musculoskeletal and Skin Diseases Information Clearinghouse.

Clinic: Michael P. White, M.D., Medical Director, Metabolic Research Unit, Shriners' Hospital for Crippled Children, 2001 Lindbergh Boulevard, St. Louis, MO 63131.

For genetic information and genetic counseling referrals: March of Dimes Birth Defects Foundation; National Center for Education in Maternal and Child Health (NCEMCH).

References

Mendelian Inheritance in Man, 9th ed.: V.A. McKusick; The Johns Hopkins University Press, 1990, pp. 205–206, 691–696, 1399–1401.

Cecil Textbook of Medicine, 18th ed.: J.B. Wyngaarden and L.H. Smith, Jr., eds.; W.B. Saunders Company, 1988, pp. 1180–1181, 1982.

Smith's Recognizable Patterns of Human Malformation, 4th ed.: K.L. Jones; W.B. Saunders Company, 1988, pp. 432–437.

Brittle Bones–Fragile Molecules: Disorders of Collagen Gene Structure and Expression: P.H. Byers; Trends in Genetics, 1990, vol. 6, pp. 293–300.

OSTEOPETROSIS

Description Osteopetrosis is characterized by increased bone density and brittle bones, resulting in frequent fractures. Skeletal and other abnormalities may also be present. There is a severe, lethal form seen at birth and a milder form (Albers-Schönberg syndrome) with delayed manifestations.

Synonyms
 Albers-Schönberg Syndrome
 Generalized Congenital Osteosclerosis
 Ivory Bones
 Marble Bones

Signs and Symptoms The severe, lethal form of the disease is evident at birth and is diagnosed by skeletal x-rays. There is an increased density in bone and decreased density in marrow. Craniofacial abnormalities include macrocephaly, a deformity of the base of the skull, and delayed fontanelle closure. Dental defects, cataracts, deafness, chest deformity, growth retardation, pancytopenia, and brain damage may occur. Death usually occurs in infancy or childhood. A subtype of this form of osteopetrosis is associated with renal tubular acidosis and carbonic anhydrase II deficiency.

The delayed form **(Albers-Schönberg syndrome)** is milder and may not be diagnosed until adolescence or adulthood when spinal pain or multiple bone fractures arouse suspicion. Vision problems, facial paralysis, and anemia may be present.

Etiology Lethal osteopetrosis is inherited as an autosomal recessive trait. The delayed form is generally considered to be autosomal dominant, but an autosomal recessive form has been described.

Epidemiology Males and females are equally affected in both forms of osteopetrosis.

Related Disorders See *Osteogenesis Imperfecta.*

Melorheostosis is a rare form of osteosclerosis or hyperostosis caused by a lack of calcium density in the bone. A genetic inheritance has not been established. The disorder results in shortening or deformity of at least one limb with accompanying pain and restricted movement. Prognosis is guardedly favorable.

Osteopoikilosis ("spotted bones") is a rare autosomal dominant disorder that may occur concomitantly with melorheostosis, usually between the ages of 15 and 60. Although the disorder is often asymptomatic, joint pain and skin lesions may be present. Osteopoikilosis can be diagnosed by the presence of spotty shadows on x-rays of most bones.

Treatment—Standard For the severe form, bone marrow transplantation is curative for the bone disorder; brain damage secondary to compression persists but is not progressive. For mild forms, treatment is symptomatic and supportive. Physical therapy may be beneficial in some cases. Genetic counseling may be helpful in families of patients.

Treatment—Investigational Please contact the agencies listed under Resources, below, for the most current information.

Resources

For more information on osteopetrosis: National Organization for Rare Disorders (NORD); The National Arthritis and Musculoskeletal and Skin Diseases Information Clearinghouse; Research Trust for Metabolic Diseases in Children.

For genetic information and genetic counseling referrals: March of Dimes Birth Defects Foundation; National Center for Education in Maternal and Child Health (NCEMCH).

References

Mendelian Inheritance in Man, 9th ed.: V.A. McKusick; The Johns Hopkins University Press, 1990, pp. 698, 1402–1404.

Smith's Recognizable Patterns of Human Malformation, 4th ed.: K.L. Jones; W.B. Saunders Company, 1988, pp. 353–355.

Juvenile Osteopetrosis: Effects on Blood and Bone of Prednisone and a Low Calcium, High Phosphate Diet: L.M. Dorantes, et al.; Arch. Dis. Child, July 1986, issue 61(7), pp. 666–670.

Bone Marrow Transplantation: Research Report; U.S. Dept. of Health and Human Services, National Cancer Institute, September 1986, NIH publication No. 86-1178.

PALLISTER-KILLIAN SYNDROME

Description Features of Pallister-Killian syndrome include severe retardation, seizures, hypotonia, and distinctive facies.

Synonyms

Isochromosome 12p Mosaicism
Killian Syndrome
Mosaic Tetrasomy 12p
Pallister Mosaic Aneuploidy
Pallister Mosaic Syndrome
Teschler-Nicola/Killian Syndrome
Teschler-Nicola Syndrome

Signs and Symptoms Congenital manifestations are hypertelorism and distinctive facies. Growth deficiency, balding, and hypotonia develop during infancy and early childhood. Later in childhood, contractures, seizures, and severe delay in psychomotor development occur.

Etiology Karyotype of peripheral lumphocytes is usually normal, but cultured fibroblasts and direct bone marrow analysis will show tetrasomy for 12p.

Epidemiology The syndrome is very rare, and little is known.

Treatment—Standard Treatment of Pallister-Killian syndrome is symptomatic and supportive. Patients can benefit from early intervention programs for the mildly to moderately mentally retarded that emphasize educational, verbal, mobility, self-care, and social skills.

Surgical procedures, including plastic septum correction and functional septorhinoplasty, may be beneficial.

Genetic counseling is recommended for families of children with Pallister-Killian syndrome.

Treatment—Investigational Research is directed toward mosaicism of the short arm of chromosome 12 (isochromosome 12p) with the eventual goal of developing a prenatal test.

Please contact the agencies listed under Resources, below, for the most current information.

Resources

For more information on Pallister-Killian syndrome: National Organization for Rare Disorders (NORD); NIH/National Institute for Child Health & Human Development (NICHHD).

For genetic information and genetic counseling referrals: March of Dimes Birth Defects Foundation; National Center for Education in Maternal and Child Health (NCEMCH).

References

Mosaic Tetrasomy 12p: Four New Cases, and Confirmation of the Chromosomal Origin of the Supernumerary Chromosome in One of the Original Pallister-Mosaic Syndrome Cases: D. Warburton, et al.; Am. J. Med. Genet., June 1987, issue 27(2), pp. 275–283.

Isochromosome 12p Mosaicism (Pallister Mosaic Aneuploidy or Pallister-Killian Syndrome): Report of 11 Cases: J.F. Reynolds, et al.: Am. J. Med. Genet., June 1987, issue 27(2), pp. 257–274.

Chromosomal Mosaicism in the Killian/Teschler-Nicola Syndrome: L.J. Raffel, et al.; Am. J. Med. Genet., August 1986, issue 24(4), pp. 607–611.

PARRY-ROMBERG SYNDROME

Description Parry-Romberg syndrome is characterized by unilateral soft tissue atrophy of the face. The syndrome can resolve spontaneously or worsen slowly and then stabilize.

Synonyms

Facial Hemiatrophy
Progressive Hemifacial Atrophy
Romberg Syndrome
Romberg Hemifacial Atrophy

Signs and Symptoms Parry-Romberg syndrome is characterized by abrupt unilateral atrophy of facial tissue, which can spread to the tongue, soft palate, and mucous membranes of the gums. Muscle and bone are rarely affected. On the affected side there may be sensory impairment, hyperhidrosis, and tear duct dysfunction. Facial features may shift to the affected side, and the eye and cheek may become sunken. Some cases are accompanied by pain, similar to that which occurs with trigeminal neuralgia. Facial hair may turn white and fall out. Contralateral Jacksonian (focal) epilepsy may occur.

Etiology The etiology of Parry-Romberg syndrome is not known. Possible causes include injury, irritation, neuritis in the peripheral sympathetic nervous system, or a trigeminal nerve lesion. Some cases may be a type of scleroderma. Nearly all cases have been sporadic.

Epidemiology Parry-Romberg syndrome is a rare disorder that affects males and females in equal numbers. Onset is usually during the 20s.

Related Disorders See *Scleroderma; Trigeminal Neuralgia.*

Horner syndrome (cervical sympathetic paralysis syndrome) is characterized by ptosis, miosis, exophthalmos, and anhidrosis that involves only the face and neck. The etiology is not known, but hypotheses include inheritance and injury to the cervical sympathetic ganglia.

Treatment—Standard Treatment of Parry-Romberg syndrome is by reconstructive or microvascular surgery. Some cases may respond to fat cell injection or silicone implantation. Muscle or bone grafts may also be helpful. Other treatment is symptomatic and supportive.

Treatment—Investigational Please contact the agencies listed under Resources, below, for the most current information.

Resources

For more information on Parry-Romberg syndrome: National Organization for Rare Disorders (NORD); FACES—National Association for the Craniofacially Handicapped; Society for the Rehabilitation of the Facially Disfigured, Inc.; National Craniofacial Foundation; NIH/National Institute of Neurological Disorders & Stroke (NINDS); NIH/National Institute of Dental Research.

References

Mendelian Inheritance in Man, 9th ed.: V.A. McKusick; The Johns Hopkins University Press, 1990, p. 392.

Progressive Hemifacial Atrophy (Parry-Romberg Disease): M.T. Miller, et al.; J. Pediatr. Ophthalmol. Strabismus, January–February 1987, issue 24(1), pp. 27–36.

Liposuction Fat Grafts in Face Wrinkles and Hemifacial Atrophy: A. Chajchir, et al.; Aesthetic Plast. Surg., 1986, issue 10(2), pp. 115–117.

The Use of Free Revascularized Grafts in the Amelioration of Hemifacial Atrophy: M.J. Jurkiewicz, et al.; Plast. Reconstr. Surg., July 1985, issue 76(1), pp. 44–55.

Hemifacial Atrophy. A Review of an Unusual Craniofacial Deformity with a Report of a Case: D.D. Dedo; Arch. Otolaryngol., September 1978, issue 104(9), pp. 538–541.

PFEIFFER SYNDROME

Description Pfeiffer syndrome is an inherited disorder primarily characterized by coronal craniostenosis and abnormalities of the face as well as of the hands and feet.

Synonyms
Acrocephalosyndactyly V

Signs and Symptoms Craniofacial features include acrobrachycephaly, hypertelorism, and slightly slanted eyelid folds. Elevated intracranial pressure may occur, but intelligence is usually normal. An underdeveloped maxilla, high arched palate, and prominent mandible may be apparent. Maleruption of the teeth may cause malocclusion. The facial appearance usually improves with age.

Partial syndactyly characterizes the toes and fingers, sometimes with broad, short thumbs and big toes. The small phalanges in the thumb may be either triangular or trapezoid in shape and occasionally fused with the distal phalanx so that the thumb points away from the other fingers. A varus deformity may also be present. A mild hearing loss due to a defect in the middle ear may occur.

Etiology Pfeiffer syndrome is inherited as an autosomal dominant trait.

Epidemiology This rare disorder affects males and females equally.

Related Disorders See *Apert Syndrome; Saethre-Chotzen Syndrome; Crouzon Disease.*

Treatment—Standard Treatment is symptomatic and supportive. Early childhood interventions include surgery to relieve intracranial pressure and the "Le Fort III advancement surgery" to prevent progressive malformation of the upper jaw. Genetic counseling may be beneficial.

Treatment—Investigational Please contact the agencies listed under Resources, below, for the most current information.

Resources
For more information on Pfeiffer syndrome: National Organization for Rare Disorders (NORD); NIH/National Institute of Child Health and Human Development (NICHHD); FACES—National Association for the Craniofacially Handicapped; National Craniofacial Foundation; Society for the Rehabilitation of the Facially Disfigured, Inc.; About Face.

For genetic information and genetic counseling referrals: March of Dimes Birth Defects Foundation; National Center for Education in Maternal and Child Health (NCEMCH).

References
Mendelian Inheritance in Man, 9th ed.: V.A. McKusick; The Johns Hopkins University Press, 1990, p. 15.

Smith's Recognizable Patterns of Human Malformation, 4th ed.: K.L. Jones; W.B. Saunders Company, 1988, pp. 368–369.

Variable Expression in Pfeiffer Syndrome: H.M. Sanchez, et al.; J. Med. Genet., February 1981, 18(1), pp. 73–75.

Maxillary Growth Following Le Fort III Advancement Surgery in Crouzon, Apert, and Pfeiffer Syndromes: D.I. Bachmayer, et al.; Am. J. Orthod. Dentofacial Orthop., November 1986, 90(5), pp. 420–430.

Hearing Loss in Pfeiffer's Syndrome: C.W. Cremers; Int. J. Pediatr. Otorhinolaryngol., December 1981, 3(4), pp. 343–353.

PIERRE ROBIN SYNDROME

Description Pierre Robin syndrome is characterized by micrognathia, glossoptosis, and cleft soft palate. The latter 2 signs may be consequences of the underdevelopment of the jaw prior to 9 weeks' gestation.

Synonyms
Pierre Robin Anomalad
Pierre Robin Complex
Pierre Robin Sequence
Robin Anomalad
Robin Sequence
Robin Syndrome

Signs and Symptoms The placement of the tongue may obstruct normal breathing. This in turn can result in failure to thrive, dysphagia, and apneic spells. Cyanosis may be evident. Respiratory disturbances may lead to cor pulmonale, pulmonary hypertension, and possibly congestive heart failure. Infants may vomit and develop sleep disturbances that persist into adulthood.

Etiology The appearance of Pierre Robin syndrome with no underlying disorder may indicate autosomal recessive inheritance. The syndrome may also result from mechanical constraint of the fetus in the womb; e.g., the chin may be compressed in such a way as to limit its normal development. Recent research also suggests that the development of Pierre Robin syndrome may be influenced by drugs taken by a woman during pregnancy.

Epidemiology Pierre Robin syndrome affects males and females equally. In about one-third of cases it occurs as a feature in a multiple defect disorder such as trisomy 18 syndrome, Stickler syndrome, or a number of other syndromes.

Related Disorders See *Stickler Syndrome; Cerebro-Costo-Mandibular Syndrome; Treacher Collins Syndrome.*

Treatment—Standard Pierre Robin syndrome can be detected in utero using ultrasound imaging.

Affected infants should be observed closely for breathing difficulties. Intubation or tracheostomy may be necessary.

Since spontaneous closure of the cleft soft palate may occur, surgical correction may be postponed for a few years. Surgery to improve the appearance of the jaw may be beneficial.

Genetic counseling may be helpful for patients and their families. Other treatment is symptomatic and palliative.

Treatment—Investigational Please contact the agencies listed under Resources,

below, for the most current information.

Resources
For more information on Pierre Robin syndrome: National Organization for Rare Disorders (NORD); FACES–National Association for the Craniofacially Handicapped; National Craniofacial Foundation; Forward Face.

For information about local cleft palate teams: American Cleft Palate Cranial Facial Association; National Cleft Palate Association; NIH/National Institute of Child Health & Human Development (NICHHD).

For genetic information and genetic counseling referrals: March of Dimes Birth Defects Foundation; NIH/National Center for Education in Maternal and Child Health (NCEMCH).

References
Smith's Recognizable Patterns of Human Malformation, 4th ed.: K.L. Jones; W.B. Saunders Company, 1988, pp. 196–199.

Glossoptosis-Apnea Syndrome in Infancy: F. Cozzi and A. Pierro; Pediatrics, May 1985, issue 75(5), pp. 836–843.

The Pierre Robin Syndrome Reassessed in the Light of Recent Research: J.R. Edwards and D.R. Newall; Br. J. Plast. Surg., July 1985, issue 38(3), pp. 339–342.

POLAND SYNDROME

Description Poland syndrome is a congenital developmental disorder with variable unilateral involvement of chest muscles combined with syndactyly and other abnormalities of the hand, arm, and wrist.

Synonyms
Poland Anomaly
Poland Syndactyly

Signs and Symptoms Unilateral hypoplasia or absence of the pectoralis major muscle, along with ipsilateral syndactyly, characterizes the syndrome. In 75 percent of cases, the abnormality affects the right side of the body. Other chest muscles and the cartilage and ribs, and the breast and areola may be absent or abnormally developed on the affected side. Beside the ipsilateral syndactyly, other abnormalities of the hand, arm, forearm, and wrist may be present. Occasionally there are renal anomalies and hemivertebrae.

Etiology The cause of Poland syndrome is not known. Current theories include sporadic mutation or a genetic cause, although the mode of transmission is not understood.

Epidemiology Poland syndrome affects males 3 times as often as females. Incidence is about 1:30,000 births. Approximately 10 percent of patients with hand syndactyly may have Poland syndrome.

Treatment—Standard Reconstructive surgery is performed to replace absent chest muscles, correct hand abnormalities, and graft ribs into place.

Treatment—Investigational Please contact the agencies listed under Resources, below, for the most current information.

Resources

For more information on Poland syndrome: National Organization for Rare Disorders (NORD); The National Arthritis and Musculoskeletal and Skin Diseases Information Clearinghouse.

For genetic information and genetic counseling referrals: March of Dimes Birth Defects Foundation; National Center for Education in Maternal and Child Health (NCEMCH).

References

Mendelian Inheritance in Man, 9th ed.: V.A. McKusick; The Johns Hopkins University Press, 1990, pp. 759–760.

Smith's Recognizable Patterns of Human Malformation, 4th ed.: K.L. Jones; W.B. Saunders Company, 1988, pp. 260–261.

Early Reconstruction of Poland's Syndrome Using Autologous Rib Grafts Combined with a Latissimus Muscle Flap: J.A. Haller, Jr., et al.; J. Pediatr. Surg, August 1984, 19(4), pp. 423–429.

Poland's Syndrome: Correction of Thoracic Anomaly Through Minimal Incisions: P. Santi, et al.; Plast. Reconstr. Surg., October 1985, 76(4), pp. 639–641.

Early Correction of the Thoracic Deformity of Poland's Syndrome in Children with the Latissimus Dorsi Muscle Flap: Long Term Follow-up of Two Cases: H. Anderl, et al.; Br. J. Plast. Surg., April 1986, 39(2), pp. 167–172.

PRADER-WILLI SYNDROME

Description Prader-Willi syndrome is a multisystem disorder diagnosed more often in males born after a prolonged gestation period, often in the breech position. The disease's primary features include infantile hypotonia, failure to thrive, hypogonadism, short stature, and impaired intellectual and behavioral functioning. Hyperphagia leads to obesity in early childhood.

Synonyms

Hypogenital Dystrophy with Diabetic Tendency
Hypotonia-Hypomentia-Hypogonadism-Obesity Syndrome
Labhart-Willi Syndrome
Prader-Labhart-Willi Syndrome
Willi-Prader Syndrome

Signs and Symptoms Early symptoms include decreased fetal movement, low birth weight, hypotonia, sleepiness, weak cry, poor sucking ability, acromicria, narrow bifrontal forehead diameter, strabismus, almond-shaped palpebral fissures, and developmental delays in head control and ability to crawl.

Hyperphagia develops between 1 and 3 years of age. If left uncontrolled, obesity can lead to life-threatening heart and lung complications.

Sexual development may begin early but stops before puberty. Cryptorchidism and micropenis occur frequently in boys, and hypoplastic labia are seen less frequently in girls. Patients are mentally retarded, most with IQs between 40 and 60. Patients tend to be fair and blue-eyed. They are sun-sensitive and frequently scratch or pick at sores and insect bites.

Etiology About 60 percent of persons with Prader-Willi syndrome have a cytogenetic deletion of chromosome 15q11q13. The deletion always occurs on the paternally derived chromosome 15; these are sporadic *de novo* deletions, since the father of affected persons has normal chromosomes. There is less than 1:1000 risk of recurrence when a cytogenetic deletion is found.

An identical cytogenetic deletion is seen in patients with Angelman syndrome, but the involved chromosome is always of maternal origin. These findings suggest that chromosomal imprinting may be critical in the expression of these 2 syndromes.

Some patients with Prader-Willi syndrome who do not have a cytogenetic deletion have been found by DNA markers to have inherited both chromosomes from the mother (maternal uniparental disomy).

Epidemiology The syndrome is more common in males than females.

Treatment—Standard High resolution prometaphase chromosome analysis is recommended. Treatment is symptomatic. Physical therapy may be necessary to develop walking pattern and improve muscle size and tone. Extreme hyperphagia requires strict diet, nutrition, and exercise programs, including a 60 percent caloric intake reduction.

Treatment—Investigational Please contact the agencies listed under Resources, below, for the most current information.

Resources

For more information on Prader-Willi syndrome: National Organization for Rare Disorders (NORD); Prader-Willi Syndrome Association; NIH/National Institute of Child Health and Human Development (NICHHD).

For genetic information and genetic counseling referrals: March of Dimes Birth Defects Foundation; National Center for Education in Maternal and Child Health (NCEMCH).

References

Cecil Textbook of Medicine, 18th ed.: J.B. Wyngaarden and L.H. Smith Jr., eds.; W.B. Saunders Company, 1988, p. 1203.

Smith's Recognizable Patterns of Human Malformation, 4th ed.: K.L. Jones; W.B. Saunders Company, 1988, pp. 170–173.

Mendelian Inheritance in Man, 9th ed.: V.A. McKusick; The Johns Hopkins University Press, 1990, pp. 783–786.

PROTEUS SYNDROME

Description Proteus syndrome is a rare hereditary disorder characterized by abnormal, asymmetric growth in any system, and diverse abnormalities involving the skin, face, eyes, ears, lungs, muscles, and nerves.

Signs and Symptoms Although infants may appear normal at birth, symptoms become apparent during the first year. Hemihypertrophy, macrocephaly, and scoliosis are characteristic. Skin lesions resembling nevi may occur, as well as hemangiomas, lipomas, and lymphangiomas. Morbidity resulting in amputation is common. Areas of the tongue can become enlarged with longer-than-normal papillae. Abnormal growths in the abdominal cavity may occur in some cases. Infrequent abnormalities include mental deficiency, seizures, strabismus, myopia, external auditory canal hyperostosis, pulmonary cystic malformations.

Etiology The cause is unknown; all instances have been sporadic. Joseph Merrick, the famous Elephant Man, is believed to have had this disorder rather than neurofibromatosis.

Epidemiology Proteus syndrome affects males and females in equal numbers.

Related Disorders See *Klippel-Trenaunay Syndrome; Maffucci Syndrome; Neurofibromatosis.*

Bannayan-Zonana syndrome encompasses macrocephaly, multiple lipomas, and hemangiomas. The syndrome is hereditary.

Cowden syndrome is characterized by multiple nodules, often hamartomas. It is hereditary.

Nevus sebaceus of Jadassohn, a port wine lesion on the scalp or face, often enlarges during puberty or early adulthood. Rarely, it may be the precursor of other growths, including basal carcinoma.

Treatment—Standard Some growths and bone malformations can be removed or corrected surgically. Other treatment is symptomatic and supportive.

Treatment—Investigational Please contact the agencies listed under Resources, below, for the most current information.

Resources

For more information on Proteus syndrome: National Organization for Rare Disorders (NORD); International Center for Skeletal Dysplasia; The National Arthritis and Musculoskeletal and Skin Diseases Information Clearinghouse.

For genetic information and genetic counseling referrals: March of Dimes Birth Defects Foundation; National Center for Education in Maternal and Child Health (NCEMCH).

References

Smith's Recognizable Patterns of Human Malformation, 4th ed.: K.L. Jones; W.B. Saunders Company, 1988, pp. 458–459.

Mendelian Inheritance in Man, 9th ed.: V.A. McKusick; The Johns Hopkins University Press, 1990, pp. 808–809.

Proteus Syndrome: The Elephant Man Diagnosed: J.A.R. Tibbles, et al.; Br. Med. J., 1986, issue 293, pp. 683–685.

The Proteus Syndrome: Partial Gigantism of the Hands and/or Feet, Nevi, Hemihypertrophy, Subcutaneous Tumors, Macrocephaly or Other Skull Anomalies and Visceral Afflictions: H.R. Wiedemann, et al.; Eur. J. Pediatr., 1983, issue 140, pp. 5–12.

Proteus Syndrome: Report of Two Cases with Pelvic Lipomatosis: T. Costa, et al.; Pediatrics, 1985, issue 76, pp. 984–989.

Proteus Syndrome or Another Hamartosis?: B.G. Kousseff; J. Clin. Dysmorphol., 1984, 2(3), pp. 23–26.

ROBERTS SYNDROME

Description Roberts syndrome is a very rare genetic disorder characterized by severe defects in facial and limb development, growth deficiency, and mental retardation.

Synonyms
> Hypomelia-Hypotrichosis-Facial Hemangioma Syndrome
> Pseudothalidomide Syndrome

Signs and Symptoms Patients frequently are missing bones in their limbs. The bones that are present are often extremely short, and phocomelic.

A low birth weight, growth deficiency, and mental retardation are common, as are microbrachiocephaly; sparse, silvery hair; cleft lip with or without cleft palate; hypertelorism; malformed ears; micrognathia, and cryptorchidism. Less common signs include brain hernia, hydrocephaly, unusually small eyes, cataracts, clouding of the cornea, cardiac and renal anomalies, and thrombocytopenia.

Etiology Roberts syndrome is inherited as an autosomal recessive trait. Premature centromere separation is a common cytogenetic finding.

Epidemiology Males and females are affected in equal numbers.

Related Disorders See *Thrombocytopenia-Absent Radius Syndrome.*

Treatment—Standard Individuals with Roberts syndrome may benefit from surgery for facial and limb defects. Prosthetic devices can also reduce problems associated with missing limbs. Other treatment is symptomatic and supportive. Genetic counseling may be helpful for patients and their families.

Treatment—Investigational Please contact the agencies listed under Resources, below, for the most current information.

Resources
For more information on Roberts syndrome: National Organization for Rare Disorders (NORD); International Center for Skeletal Dysplasia; Association of Children's Prosthetic and Orthotic Clinics (ACPOC); FACES—National Association for the Craniofacially Handicapped; National Craniofacial Foundation; NIH/National Institute of Child Health and Human Development (NICHHD).

For genetic information and genetic counseling referrals: March of Dimes Birth Defects Foundation; NIH/National Center for Education in Maternal and Child Health (NCEMCH).

References

Mendelian Inheritance in Man, 9th ed.: V.A. McKusick; The Johns Hopkins University Press, 1990, pp. 1464–1465.

Smith's Recognizable Patterns of Human Malformation, 4th ed.: K.L. Jones; W.B. Saunders Company, 1988, pp. 256–257.

ROBINOW SYNDROME

Description The characteristic features of Robinow syndrome include a typical facies, short stature, and hypoplasia of the genitals.

Synonyms

Fetal Face Syndrome

Signs and Symptoms The head is macrocephalic, and the child has a flattened profile. Hypertelorism, a prominent forehead, depressed nasal bridge, triangular mouth, and micrognathia are characteristic. The forearms and fingers are short, hemivertebrae may be present, and there is mild-to-moderate short stature. Males have micropenis and cryptorchidism; females, small clitoris and labia. Occasional symptoms include seizures, navel and inguinal hernias, cleft palate, other digital anomalies, and speech and walking difficulties.

Etiology Both autosomal dominant and autosomal recessive inheritances have been reported. The recessive type is said to be more severe, but the 2 forms usually cannot be separated.

Epidemiology Robinow syndrome affects males and females in equal numbers.

Related Disorders See *Aarskog Syndrome.*

Treatment—Standard Treatment for Robinow syndrome includes surgery to correct physical abnormalities. Genetic counseling may be beneficial. Other treatment is symptomatic and supportive.

Treatment—Investigational Please contact the agencies listed under Resources, below, for the most current information.

Resources

For more information on Robinow syndrome: National Organization for Rare Disorders (NORD); NIH/National Institute of Child Health and Human Development (NICHHD); Human Growth Foundation (HGF).

For genetic information and genetic counseling referrals: March of Dimes Birth Defects Foundation; NIH/National Center for Education in Maternal and Child Health (NCEMCH).

References

Mendelian Inheritance in Man, 9th ed.: V.A. McKusick; The Johns Hopkins University Press, 1990, p. 847.

Smith's Recognizable Patterns of Human Malformation, 4th ed.: K.L. Jones; W.B. Saunders Company, 1988, pp. 112–113.

Robinow Syndrome: Report of Two Patients and Review of Literature: M. Butler, et al.; Clin. Genet., February 1987, 31(2), pp. 77–85.

Craniofacial Pattern Similarities and Additional Orofacial Findings in Siblings with Robinow Syndrome: H. Israel, et al.; J. Craniofac. Genet. Dev. Biol., 1988, 8(1), pp. 63–73.

RUBINSTEIN-TAYBI SYNDROME

Description Rubinstein-Taybi syndrome is a rare genetic disorder associated with multiple abnormalities that include characteristic facial features and abnormally wide fingers and toes.

Synonyms

Rubinstein Syndrome

Broad Thumb-Hallux Syndrome

Signs and Symptoms The syndrome is present at birth. Craniofacial abnormalities include a small skull, narrow and prominent forehead, beaked nose, unusually high and narrow palate, low-set and abnormally shaped ears, and eye defects such as strabismus and blocked or missing tear ducts.

The fingertips and toes are typically broad. Other abnormalities include hirsutism, scoliosis, and congenital heart disease, and cryptorchidism and an angulated penis in males. A small, irregularly shaped pelvis, and kidney and lung defects may occur in some individuals.

Respiratory problems and eye and ear infections are common. Also typical are difficulties with feeding, such as regurgitation, gagging, and choking, as well as diarrhea and chronic constipation. These problems seem to improve for many children as they grow, after about 4 or 5 years of age.

Mental retardation of some degree is present.

Etiology The cause of Rubinstein-Taybi syndrome is not known. Most cases have been sporadic, although in some instances autosomal dominant or autosomal recessive inheritance is suggested. It is possible that some sporadic cases may represent new dominant mutations.

Epidemiology Since the syndrome was first described in 1963, more than 250 cases have been reported in the medical literature in the United States. According to one study, the disorder may affect approximately 1:300 to 1:500 institutionalized persons with mental retardation in the United States. There is no estimate for the prevalence among noninstitutionalized patients. Males and females are affected equally.

Related Disorders See *Hallermann-Streiff Syndrome; Seckel Syndrome; Treacher Collins Syndrome.*

Treatment—Standard Drugs or surgery may improve some associated symptoms, and antibiotics may be needed. Treatment otherwise is symptomatic and supportive. Patients may benefit from services for mentally retarded individuals. Speech therapy, sign language lessons, or an alternative method of communication should be taught as soon as possible. Genetic counseling will be beneficial.

Treatment—Investigational Please contact the agencies listed under Resources, below, for the most current information.

Resources

For more information on Rubinstein-Taybi syndrome: National Organization for Rare Disorders (NORD); Rubinstein-Taybi Parent Support Group; Rubinstein-Taybi Support Group; National Institute of Child Health and Human Development (NICHHD).

For case documentation of Rubinstein-Taybi syndrome patients: Jack H. Rubinstein, Director, Cincinnati Center for Developmental Disorders, Cincinnati, Ohio 45229-2899.

For genetic information and genetic counseling referrals: March of Dimes Birth Defects Foundation; National Center for Education in Maternal and Child Health (NCEMCH).

References

Mendelian Inheritance in Man, 9th ed.: V.A. McKusick; The Johns Hopkins University Press, 1990, pp. 1466–1467.

Smith's Recognizable Patterns of Human Malformation, 4th ed.: K.L. Jones; W.B. Saunders Company, 1988, pp. 84–87.

Rubinstein-Taybi Syndrome: Further Evidence of a Genetic Aetiology: D.R. Gillies, et al.; Dev. Med. Child. Neurol., December 1985, issue 27(6), pp. 751–755.

Dominant Inheritance of a Syndrome Similar to Rubinstein-Taybi: P. Cotsirilos, et al.; Am. J. Med. Genet., January 1987, issue 26(1), pp. 85–93.

Rubinstein-Taybi Syndrome in the Neonate: R. Gambon, et al.; Helv. Paediatr. Acta, August 1984, issue 39(3), pp. 279–283.

RUSSELL-SILVER SYNDROME

Description Russell-Silver syndrome is commonly thought of as a disorder of short stature, although some affected persons attain normal height in adulthood.

Synonyms

Russell Syndrome
Silver-Russell Syndrome
Silver Syndrome

Signs and Symptoms Full-term infants with Russell-Silver syndrome are usually small at birth, and many individuals remain short throughout life. Craniofacial features include a normal-sized head that may appear large in comparison to the rest of the body, a small triangular face with down-turned corners of the mouth, and a prominent forehead. Light-brown spots may occur on the skin. The arms are unusually short, 5th fingers may be short and incurved, and there is syndactyly of the toes. Cryptorchidism as well as precocious puberty may occur. Intelligence is often normal; however, mental retardation is possible. Some developmental abnormalities tend to improve with age.

Lateral organ asymmetry may occur (Silver syndrome). When the organs are of equal size bilaterally, the disorder is sometimes termed Russell syndrome.

The syndrome can be diagnosed in utero.

Etiology The cause is unknown. Inheritance as either an X-linked or dominant trait with incomplete penetrance has been suggested, as has fetal disturbance at 6 to 7 weeks' gestation, or defects in the body's ability to manufacture or use human growth hormone.

Epidemiology Onset is in utero. Males and females are affected in equal numbers; however, males are usually more severely affected than females.

Treatment—Standard Some gains in overall body growth may occur with use of human growth hormone. Other treatment is symptomatic and supportive.

Treatment—Investigational Please contact the agencies listed under Resources, below, for the most current information.

Resources

For more information on Russell-Silver syndrome: National Organization for Rare Disorders (NORD); Association for Children with Russell-Silver Syndrome; The National Arthritis and Musculoskeletal and Skin Diseases Information Clearinghouse; Human Growth Foundation (HGF); Parents of Dwarfed Children; Little People of America; International Center for Skeletal Dysplasia; Short Stature Foundation.

For genetic information and genetic counseling referrals: March of Dimes Birth Defects Foundation; National Center for Education in Maternal and Child Health (NCEMCH).

References

Mendelian Inheritance in Man, 9th ed.: V.A. McKusick; The Johns Hopkins University Press, 1990, pp. 1476–1477, 1716.

Smith's Recognizable Patterns of Human Malformation, 4th ed.: K.L. Jones; W.B. Saunders Company, 1988, pp. 88–89.

Treatment of Silver-Russell Type Dwarfism with Human Growth Hormone: Effects on Serum Somatomedin-C Levels and on Longitudinal Growth Studied by Knemonetry: C.J. Partsch, et al.; Acta Endocrinol. [Suppl.] (Copenh.), 1986, issue 279, pp. 139–146.

Reevaluation of Russell-Silver Syndrome: R.A. Pagon, et al.; J. Pediatr., November 1985, issue 107(5), pp. 733–737.

X-linked Short Stature with Skin Pigmentation: Evidence for Heterogeneity of the Russell-Silver Syndrome: M.W. Partington; Clin. Genet., February 1986, issue 29(2), pp. 151–156.

SAETHRE-CHOTZEN SYNDROME

Description Saethre-Chotzen syndrome is a congenital disorder characterized by various craniofacial and skeletal malformations. Short stature may be present, as well as skin abnormalities of the fingers and toes. Intelligence is usually normal, but mild-to-moderate mental retardation may develop.

Synonyms

Acrocephalosyndactyly Type III
Chotzen Syndrome

Signs and Symptoms The craniofacial abnormalities, some of which are related to the coronal craniostenosis characteristic of this disorder, include brachycephaly, skull asymmetry, hypertelorism, ptosis, and strabismus, as well as an unusually shaped ear with a prominent crus. Syndactyly is often present; brachydactyly and clinodactyly may occur. Some cardiac and renal problems can develop.

Etiology The syndrome is thought to be inherited as an autosomal dominant trait.

Epidemiology Both males and females can be affected.

Related Disorders See *Apert Syndrome; Pfeiffer Syndrome.*

Treatment—Standard Treatment is symptomatic and supportive. Patients should be monitored closely for cardiac or renal problems, and signs of infection. A medical evaluation may be appropriate for family members because of the possibility of developing a milder, less debilitating form of the syndrome. Genetic counseling also may be worthwhile.

Treatment—Investigational Please contact the agencies listed under Resources, below, for the most current information.

Resources

For more information on Saethre-Chotzen Syndrome: National Organization for Rare Disorders (NORD); National Craniofacial Foundation; FACES—National Association for the Craniofacially Handicapped; Society for the Rehabilitation of the Facially Disfigured, Inc.; About Face; NIH/National Institute of Child Health and Human Development.

For genetic information and genetic counseling referrals: March of Dimes Birth Defects Foundation; NIH/National Center for Education in Maternal and Child Health (NCEMCH).

References

Mendelian Inheritance in Man, 9th ed.: V.A. McKusick; The Johns Hopkins University Press, 1990, pp. 14–15.

Smith's Recognizable Patterns of Human Malformation, 4th ed.: K.L. Jones; W.B. Saunders Company, 1988, pp. 364–367.

Dermatoglyphics in Saethre-Chotzen Syndrome: A Family Study: L. Borbolla, et al.; Acta Paediatr. Acad. Sci. Hung., 1983, issue 24(3), pp. 269–279.

The Saethre-Chotzen Syndrome: O.A. Pantke, et al.; Birth Defects, 1975, issue 11(2), pp. 190–225.

SECKEL SYNDROME

Description Seckel syndrome is primarily characterized by marked intrauterine and postnatal growth failure, mental retardation, and a typical facies that gave rise to the adjective *bird-headed*.

Synonyms
Nanocephaly

Signs and Symptoms Craniofacial abnormalities include microcephaly and micrognathia and a resulting prominence of the midface and beaklike nose. The ears are low-set and malformed and the eyes large. Other congenital conditions include hypoplasia of the proximal radius, simian crease, clinodactyly of the 5th finger, hip dislocation, hypoplasia of the proximal fibula, and cryptorchidism in the male. Among the abnormalities that are present in some cases are facial asymmetry, scoliosis, and hypoplastic external genitalia.

The height of affected persons reaches 3 to 3.5 ft. (91 to 106 cm.). Mental deficiency is moderate to severe.

Etiology Seckel syndrome is an inherited autosomal recessive trait.

Epidemiology Incidence is very slightly higher in females, but severity of the syndrome is equal in the sexes.

Related Disorders See *Anemia, Fanconi; Hallermann-Streiff Syndrome.*

Treatment—Standard Treatment of Seckel syndrome is symptomatic and supportive. Genetic counseling may be beneficial.

Treatment—Investigational Please contact the agencies listed under Resources, below, for the most current information.

Resources
   For more information on Seckel syndrome: National Organization for Rare Disorders (NORD); International Center for Skeletal Dysplasia; Human Growth Foundation (HGF); Little People of America; Parents of Dwarfed Children; NIH/National Institute of Child Health and Human Development (NICHHD).
   For genetic information and genetic counseling referrals: March of Dimes Birth Defects Foundation; National Center for Education in Maternal and Child Health (NCEMCH).

References
   Mendelian Inheritance in Man, 9th ed.: V.A. McKusick; The Johns Hopkins University Press, 1990, p. 1065.
   Syndromes of the Head and Neck, 3rd ed.: R.J. Gorlin, et al.; Oxford University Press, 1990, pp. 313–316.
   Smith's Recognizable Patterns of Human Malformation, 4th ed.: K.L. Jones; W.B. Saunders Company, 1988, pp. 100–101.
   Pigmentary Changes in Seckel's Syndrome: A. Fathizadeh, et al.; J. Am. Acad. Dermatol., July 1979, 1(1), pp. 52–54.

Seckel Syndrome: An Overdiagnosed Syndrome: E. Thompson, et al.; J. Med. Genet., June 1985, 22(3), pp. 192–201.

Microcephaly, Micrognathia, and Bird-headed Dwarfism: Prenatal Diagnosis of a Seckel-like Syndrome: D.F. Majoor-Krakauer, et al.; Am. J. Med. Genet., May 1987, 27(1), pp. 183–188.

SEPTO-OPTIC DYSPLASIA

Description Septo-optic dysplasia is a birth defect characterized by hypoplastic optic disks and pituitary deficiencies. Often, the anterior horns of the brain's lateral ventricles are separated because of the absence of the septum pellucidum.

Synonyms
De Morsier Syndrome

Signs and Symptoms Features of septo-optic dysplasia are present at birth. The primary sign is visual impairment, including amblyopia and nystagmus. Pupil response to light may vary. Esotropia and exotropia sometimes occur.

Hypopituitarism of varying degree may be present early or develop later and, if not treated during childhood, will result in stunted growth. Jaundice occasionally occurs at birth. Mental retardation or learning disabilities may also occur.

Etiology The cause is not known.

Epidemiology Septo-optic dysplasia is rare. Affected children are often the first-born of young mothers. Males and females are affected equally.

Related Disorders Absent septum pellucidum with porencephaly is a rare congenital disorder characterized by hemiatrophy, nystagmus, seizures, and short stature.

Treatment—Standard Therapy is symptomatic and supportive. Pituitary hormones deficiencies may be treated by hormone replacement therapy.

Treatment—Investigational Please contact the agencies listed under Resources, below, for the most current information.

Resources
For more information on septo-optic dysplasia: National Organization for Rare Disorders (NORD); NIH/National Institute of Neurological Disorders & Stroke (NINDS).

For genetic information and genetic counseling referrals: March of Dimes Birth Defects Foundation; National Center for Education in Maternal and Child Health (NCEMCH).

References
Hormonal, Metabolic, and Neuroradiologic Abnormalities Associated with Septo-Optic Dysplasia: S.A. Arslanian, et al.; Acta Endocrinol. (Copenh.), October 1984, 107(2), pp. 282–288.

Absence of the Septum Pellucidum. Overlapping Clinical Syndromes: S.A. Morgan, et al.; Arch. Neurol., August 1985, 42(8), pp. 769–770.

SIRENOMELIA SEQUENCE

Description Sirenomelia sequence is a congenital disorder characterized by a single lower extremity.

Synonyms
Mermaid Syndrome

Signs and Symptoms Abnormal development of the lower limbs results in a single lower extremity or 2 legs that are joined together. Accompanying spine and skeletal malformations, with either absent or defective vertebrae, commonly occur. The internal and external sex organs, rectum, kidneys, and bladder may also be missing or underdeveloped. An imperforate anus and other abnormalities of the lower gastrointestinal tract may be present. Ultrasonography can detect sirenomelia sequence during the 2nd trimester of pregnancy.

Etiology The cause of sirenomelia sequence is unknown, but irregularities in early embryonic vascular development produce the defects. Instead of the 2 umbilical arteries that normally branch out of the lower part of the aorta and carry blood to the caudal end of the embryo, a single large artery arises from high in the abdominal cavity. Referred to as a vitelline artery steal, this process diverts blood and nutrients away from the embryo's caudal region to the placenta.

Epidemiology Sirenomelia sequence occurs once in every 60,000 to 100,000 births.

Related Disorders Caudal regression syndrome (caudal dysplasia sequence) is characterized by abnormal development of the embryo's caudal region. Resulting abnormalities include marked growth deficiency in the caudal area, incomplete vertebral development, and incontinence. In some cases microcephaly, cleft lip and palate, renal agenesis, and imperforate anus may occur. Although the etiology has not been determined, it is thought that the cause of caudal regression syndrome is not vascular, as in the case of sirenomelia sequence. About one-fifth of all cases occur in infants of diabetic mothers.

Treatment—Standard Surgical separation of the joined legs has been successful. Prognosis depends on the involvement of the gastrointestinal system, vertebrae, and other structural deformities. Other treatment is symptomatic and supportive.

Treatment—Investigational Please contact the agencies listed under Resources, below, for the most current information.

Resources
For more information on sirenomelia sequence: National Organization for Rare Disorders (NORD); NIH/National Institute of Child Health and Human

Development.

For genetic information and genetic counseling referrals: March of Dimes Birth Defects Foundation; NIH/National Center for Education in Maternal and Child Health (NCEMCH).

References

Smith's Recognizable Patterns of Human Malformation, 4th ed.: K.L. Jones; W.B. Saunders Company, 1988, pp. 574–575.

Prenatal Diagnosis of Sirenomelia: M. Sitori, et al.; J. Ultrasound Med., February 1989, 8(2), pp. 83–88.

Sirenomelia. Angiographic Demonstration of Vascular Anomalies: G. Malinger, et al.; Arch. Pathol. Lab. Med., July 1982, 106(7), pp. 347–348.

Vascular Steal: The Pathogenetic Mechanism Producing Sirenomelia and Associated Defects of the Viscera and Soft Tissues: R.E. Stevenson, et al.; Pediatrics, September 1986, 78(3), pp. 451–457.

SMITH-LEMLI-OPITZ SYNDROME

Description Smith-Lemli-Opitz syndrome is a hereditary developmental disorder characterized by craniofacial, limb, and genital abnormalities as well as failure to thrive and mental retardation. Two forms exist: type II is more severe than type I.

Synonyms

Lowry-Miller-MacLean Syndrome (Type II)

Signs and Symptoms In the severe form of the disorder (type II), stillbirth is common; infants are often born in breech position and may not survive the neonatal period.

Physical characteristics of the less severe form (type I) include a small, abnormally long and narrow head; ptosis, epicanthal folds, and strabismus; a broad nasal tip with anteverted nostrils; and broad lateral ridges in the palate and a moderately small mandible. Palms and soles frequently have a simian crease; webbing often appears between the 2nd and 3rd toes. Fingertips frequently show whorl dermatoglyphic patterns. Cryptorchidism, hypospadias, and hypogonadism may be present; in severe cases, sex-reversal occurs (XY males have female external genitalia).

Other characteristics include low birth weight and subsequent failure to thrive; vomiting in early infancy and tendency toward a shrill cry; moderate-to-severe mental retardation; and early hypotonia that later becomes hypertonic.

Occasional features of Smith-Lemli-Opitz syndrome include a broad nasal bridge, cleft palate, a clenched hand with the index finger overlying the 3rd finger, an asymmetric short thumb, and distal palmar axial triradius. The forefoot may deviate toward the metatarsus adductus, and a hip may be dislocated. The child may also have a deep sacral dimple, a pit anterior to the anus, nipples that are wide apart, inguinal hernia, pyloric stenosis, dilated renal calices, and a cardiac defect.

Etiology Smith-Lemli-Opitz syndrome is an autosomal recessive inherited disorder.

Epidemiology Over 120 type I and 50 type II cases have been recorded. Males are affected more often than females; however, the syndrome may be more easily diagnosed in males because of the apparent genital abnormalities.

Treatment—Standard Twenty percent of those who survive past the early neonatal period die from pneumonia within the first year. This complication is treated with appropriate antibiotics. Other treatment of Smith-Lemli-Opitz syndrome is symptomatic and supportive. Special education services, physical therapy, and genetic counseling are recommended.

Treatment—Investigational Please contact the agencies listed under Resources, below, for the most current information.

Resources

For more information on **Smith-Lemli-Opitz syndrome:** National Organization for Rare Disorders (NORD); NIH/National Institute of Child Health and Human Development (NICHHD); J.M. Opitz, M.D., Shodar Children's Hospital, P.O. Box 5539, Helena, MT 59604.

For **genetic information and genetic counseling referrals:** March of Dimes Birth Defects Foundation; National Center for Education in Maternal and Child Health (NCEMCH).

References

Smith's Recognizable Patterns of Human Malformation, 4th ed.: K.L. Jones; W.B. Saunders Company, 1988, pp. 104–105.

SOTOS SYNDROME

Description Sotos syndrome is a rare hereditary disorder characterized by excessive growth over the 90th percentile during the first 2 to 3 years of life. Mild mental retardation may be present.

Synonyms

Cerebral Gigantism

Signs and Symptoms The primary symptoms of Sotos syndrome are large birth weight and excessive growth during the first 2 to 3 years of life. By 10 years of age, the patient reaches a height age of 14 or 15 years. Physical characteristics include a disproportionately large and long head with a slightly protrusive forehead, large hands and feet, hypertelorism, and downslanting eyes. Not all of these features occur in every patient. Mild developmental retardation is common. Other characteristics include clumsiness and an awkward gait as well as unusual aggressiveness or irritability.

Persons with this disorder have abnormal dermatoglyphics. Bone and dental ages tend to be 2 to 4 and 1 to 2 years advanced, respectively.

Differential diagnosis should include XYY and fragile X syndromes. Endocrine evaluation usually reveals no abnormalities. Children should be tested for elevated growth hormone levels to rule out a growth hormone-secreting pituitary tumor.

Less than 5 percent of patients have developed benign or malignant tumors.

Etiology The great majority of cases are sporadic. A dominant hereditary pattern also has been documented in some cases. The disorder has been ascribed to impaired function of the hypothalamic-pituitary axis, but thus far all functional pituitary tests have been normal.

Epidemiology Sotos syndrome affects males and females equally.

Related Disorders See *Acromegaly.*

Treatment—Standard Initial abnormalities resolve as growth rate becomes normal after the first 2 to 3 years of life. Medical treatment is symptomatic and supportive.

Treatment—Investigational Please contact the agencies listed under Resources, below, for the most current information.

Resources

For more information on Sotos syndrome: National Organization for Rare Disorders (NORD); Sotos Syndrome USA Support Group; Juan Sotos, M.D., Children's Hospital, Columbus, Ohio; Sotos Syndrome Support Group of Great Britain; NIH/National Institute of Child Health and Human Development (NICHHD).

For genetic information and genetic counseling referrals: March of Dimes Birth Defects Foundation; National Center for Education in Maternal and Child Health (NCEMCH).

References

Smith's Recognizable Patterns of Human Malformation, 4th ed.: K.L. Jones; W.B. Saunders Company, 1988, pp. 128–129.

Syndromes of the Head and Neck, 3rd ed.: R.J. Gorlin, et al.; Oxford University Press, 1990, pp. 332–336.

SPLIT-HAND DEFORMITY

Description Split-hand deformity is a genetic disorder characterized by the absence of fingers or parts of fingers, often occurring with a cleft of the hand. When a cleft does occur, both hands and both feet usually are affected. Many types and combinations of deformities occur in this disorder.

Synonyms

    Ectrodactilia
    Ectrodactyly
    Ektrodactylie
    Karsch-Neugebauer Syndrome
    Lobster Claw Deformity

Signs and Symptoms There are 2 typical patterns of characteristics in split-hand deformity. In one type, in which the hand has a lobster-claw appearance, the 3rd digit is absent and replaced with a cone-shaped cleft that tapers toward the wrist, dividing the hand into 2 parts. The remaining fingers or parts of fingers on each side of the cleft are often joined or webbed. If the cleft is present, it generally is found on both hands, and the feet are usually similarly affected.

In the 2nd variety of split-hand deformity, only the 5th digit is present and there is no cleft. Severity varies between these types, and cases of each type occasionally are found in the same family.

Affected individuals usually have normal intelligence and live normal life spans, although with varying degrees of disability related to the severity of the deformity.

Etiology Split-hand deformity is an autosomal dominant inherited trait. Occasionally split-hand deformity will skip a generation.

Epidemiology Males and females are affected equally. Frequency is estimated at 1:90,000 births.

Treatment—Standard Reconstructive surgery when applicable may improve the deformity, and prosthetics are available to help achieve normal functioning. Genetic counseling may benefit patients and their families. Other treatment is symptomatic and supportive.

Treatment—Investigational Please contact the agencies listed under Resources, below, for the most current information.

Resources
For more information on split-hand deformity: National Organization for Rare Disorders (NORD); International Center for Skeletal Dysplasia; NIH/National Institute of Arthritis and Musculoskeletal and Skin Diseases Clearinghouse; Association of Children's Prosthetic and Orthotic Clinics.

For genetic information and genetic counseling referrals: March of Dimes Birth Defects Foundation; NIH/National Center for Education in Maternal and Child Health (NCEMCH).

References
Mendelian Inheritance in Man, 9th ed.: V.A. McKusick; The Johns Hopkins University Press, 1990, pp. 874–875, 998, 1720.
Monodactylous Splithand-Splitfoot: A Malformation Occurring in Three Distinct Genetic Types: G. Bujdoso, et al.; Eur. J. Pediatr., May 1980, issue 133(3), pp. 207–215.

SPONDYLOEPIPHYSEAL DYSPLASIA CONGENITA

Description Congenital spondyloepiphyseal dysplasia is a rare hereditary disorder characterized by short stature, abnormal bone development, and ocular abnormalities.

Signs and Symptoms Symptom manifestations vary greatly. These include flat facial features, myopia or retinal detachment, short-trunk small stature, and barrel-chestedness. Knees tend to be misaligned, pointing either outward or inward, resulting in late onset of walking and a waddling gait. Hands and feet appear normal, and patients usually have normal intelligence. Patients may reach an adult height of 84 cm (33 inches) to 128 cm (50.4 inches).

In some cases complications ensue, e.g., retinal detachment resulting in severe vision impairment or blindness. Stress on the lax ligaments may cause spinal cord compression. Kyphoscoliosis, hyperextensible finger joints, and joint dislocation may also occur.

Etiology The disorder appears to be an autosomal dominant inherited trait.

Epidemiology Incidence is about 1:100,000 live births. Males and females are equally affected.

Related Disorders See *Morquio Syndrome; Mucopolysaccharidosis; Spondyloepiphyseal Dysplasia Tarda.*

Treatment—Standard Treatment includes early symptomatic correction of clubfoot deformity, closure of the cleft palate, and prevention or treatment of retinal detachment. Lifelong orthopedic care is often necessary. Genetic counseling is recommended for further family planning.

Treatment—Investigational Please contact the agencies listed under Resources, below, for the most current information.

Resources

For more information on congenital spondyloepiphyseal dysplasia: National Organization for Rare Disorders (NORD); NIH/National Institute of Child Health and Human Development; Human Growth Foundation (HGF); Little People of America; Short Stature Foundation.

For genetic information and genetic counseling referrals: March of Dimes Birth Defects Foundation; National Center for Education in Maternal and Child Health (NCEMCH).

References

Smith's Recognizable Patterns of Human Malformation, 4th ed.: K.L. Jones; W.B. Saunders Company, 1988, pp. 310–311.

SPONDYLOEPIPHYSEAL DYSPLASIA TARDA

Description Spondyloepiphyseal dysplasia tarda is a hereditary disorder characterized by short stature and skeletal abnormalities.

Synonyms

X-Linked Spondyloepiphyseal Dysplasia

Signs and Symptoms Symptoms occur between 5 and 10 years of age, at which point spinal growth appears to stop. Shoulders become hunched, and kyphosis and scoliosis develop. The neck appears to shorten, and the chest broadens. During adolescence, skeletal abnormalities may cause pain in the back, hips, shoulders, knees, and ankles. Adult patients are short of stature; height usually ranges from 130 cm (51 inches) to 158 cm (62 inches). The trunk is short, the chest cage is large, and the limb length is relatively normal.

Etiology In most cases, the disorder is inherited as an X-linked recessive trait, although autosomal dominant and recessive inheritances have also been demonstrated.

Epidemiology Males are affected more often than females.

Related Disorders See *Morquio Syndrome; Mucopolysaccharidosis; Spondyloepiphyseal Dysplasia Congenita.*

Multiple epiphyseal dysplasia is characterized by development of a waddling gait in affected children between the ages of 2 and 5 years. Osteoarthritic joint changes cause pain. Patients have an almost normal body size, with disproportionately small hands and feet. Males and females are affected equally. The disorder is inherited as an autosomal dominant trait.

Treatment—Standard Treatment of spondyloepiphyseal dysplasia tarda is supportive and symptomatic. Physical therapy is recommended for joint stiffness and pain. Severely debilitating osteoarthritis of the hips may occur by age 60 and require total hip replacement. Genetic counseling is recommended for further family planning.

Treatment—Investigational Please contact the agencies listed under Resources, below, for the most current information.

Resources

For more information on **spondyloepiphyseal dysplasia tarda:** National Organization for Rare Disorders (NORD); NIH/National Institute of Child Health and Human Development; Human Growth Foundation (HGF); Little People of America; Short Stature Foundation; National Cleft Palate Association.

For **genetic information and genetic counseling referrals:** March of Dimes Birth Defects Foundation; National Center for Education in Maternal and Child Health (NCEMCH).

References

Smith's Recognizable Patterns of Human Malformation, 4th ed.: K.L. Jones; W.B. Saunders Company, 1988, pp. 328–329.

STICKLER SYNDROME

Description Stickler syndrome is characterized by micrognathia, cleft palate, and congenital abnormalities of the eye. Bone abnormalities and degenerative changes in some joints may occur early in life. Expressivity of the syndrome may be mild, moderate, or severe. With early treatment the prognosis may be favorable.

Synonyms

Arthro-Ophthalmopathy
Epiphyseal Changes and High Myopia
Ophthalmoarthropathy
Weissenbacher-Zweymuller Syndrome

Signs and Symptoms Craniofacial abnormalities include a broad, flat, sunken bridge of the nose, giving a flattened appearance to the face, and cleft palate and small jaw (the Pierre Robin anomaly). Both sensorineural and conductive deafness may develop. Ocular abnormalities may include severe myopia, astigmatism, and changes of the optic disk. Cataracts, detachment of the retina, and blindness may develop during the first decade of life. Glaucoma simplex may also occur.

Bony abnormalities are usually present in joints such as the ankles, knees, and wrists. Affected children may be stiff and sore after strenuous exercise. Sometimes swelling, redness, and warmth may be present and result in crepitation and temporary locking of joints. X-rays may show irregularities of the joint surfaces, especially in the vertebral column and the knees. Subluxation of the hips is another frequent finding. Abnormalities of the epiphyseal plate may occur, and cartilage fragments may be present within the joint. There may be hyperextensibility of the finger, knee, and elbow joints. Fingers may be tapered.

Etiology Stickler syndrome is inherited as an autosomal dominant trait.

Epidemiology Both males and females are affected.

Related Disorders See *Spondyloepiphyseal Dysplasia Congenita.*

Wagner syndrome is inherited as an autosomal dominant disorder that may be mild, moderate, or severe. It is characterized by facial abnormalities, an underdeveloped jaw, saddle nose, cleft palate, and vision abnormalities. Hip deformities and joint hyperextensibility in the fingers, elbows, and knees may also occur. Differentiation from the Stickler syndrome is difficult, and some experts believe they are the same condition.

Treatment—Standard Avoidance of excessive physical exertion including contact sports may prevent joint stiffness and soreness in the ankles, knees, and wrists. Detached retinas may be surgically corrected. Genetic counseling will be helpful to families of affected children.

Treatment—Investigational Please contact the agencies listed under Resources, below, for the most current information.

Resources

For more information on Stickler syndrome: National Organization for Rare Disorders (NORD); The National Arthritis and Musculoskeletal and Skin Diseases Information Clearinghouse; NIH/National Eye Institute.

References

Mendelian Inheritance in Man, 9th ed.: V.A. McKusick; The Johns Hopkins University Press, 1990, pp. 108–110.

Smith's Recognizable Patterns of Human Malformation, 4th ed.: K.L. Jones; W.B. Saunders Company, 1988, pp. 242–245.

Management of Retinal Detachment in the Wagner-Stickler Syndrome: B.M. Billington, et al.; Transactions Ophthalmol. Soc. U.K., 1985, issue 104(pt. 8), pp. 875–879.

Stickler's Syndrome or Hereditary Progressive Arthro-Ophthalmopathy: M. Vallat, et al.; J. Fr. Ophthalmol., 1985, issue 8(4), pp. 301–307.

The Wagner-Stickler Syndrome–A Study of 22 Families: R.M. Liberfarb, et al.; J. Pediatrics, September 1981, issue 99(3), pp. 394–399.

STURGE-WEBER SYNDROME

Description Sturge-Weber syndrome is characterized by leptomeningeal angiomas, intracranial calcifications, and seizures. A facial nevus flammeus may be present. Intraocular angiomas may result in glaucoma.

Synonyms

Encephalofacial Angiomatosis
Encephalotrigeminal Angiomatosis
Leptomeningeal Angiomatosis
Meningeal Capillary Angiomatosis
Sturge-Kalischer-Weber Syndrome
Sturge-Weber Phakomatosis
Sturge-Weber-Dimitri Syndrome

Signs and Symptoms Usually, but not always, a unilateral nevus flammeus develops along the site of the trigeminal nerve. As the patient ages, the stain deepens and elevations may also develop. On the same side of the face as the nevus are leptomeningeal angiomas and intracranial calcifications.

Nevi are bilateral in about 37 percent of patients and unilateral in 50 percent. They involve the limbs and trunk in about 36 percent of patients, and lips and oral mucosa in about 25 percent.

Seizures, which are common, begin during the first year and worsen with age. Over half of patients experience mental deficiencies; and 30 percent, either hemiparesis or hemiplegia.

Ocular complications occur in about 40 percent of patients; they do not develop in individuals who do not have port wine stains. The affected eye is always on the same side of the head as the nevus. Glaucoma and buphthalmos occur in about 30 percent of patients, often at birth; onset, however, may be anytime during the first 2 years. Other ocular complications include angiomas in the conjunctiva, choroid, and cornea; different-colored eyes; hydrophthalmos; hemianopia; lens opacification or displacement; retinal detachment; angioid streaks; optic atrophy; and cortical blindness.

Other syndromes that may occur in association with Sturge-Weber syndrome include Klippel-Trenaunay syndrome, tuberous sclerosis, neurofibromatosis, and Wyburn-Mason syndrome.

Etiology The etiology is unknown. All cases have been sporadic, so no evidence of heredity has been proven.

Epidemiology Sturge-Weber syndrome is a rare congenital disease. Only a few thousand cases have been reported in the United States. Males and females are equally affected.

Related Disorders See *Neurofibromatosis; Tuberous Sclerosis; von Hippel-Lindau Syndrome.*

Treatment—Standard Treatment is symptomatic and supportive. Until recently, the argon laser was used to try to remove or lighten the port wine stain. This procedure was associated with crusting, scabbing, and scarring, and sufficient pain to require a local anesthetic. The flash pump dye laser has replaced the argon laser as a more effective means of removing or lessening the stain. Children as young as 1 month can be treated with this laser, because pain is minimal and skin is not damaged. The flash pump dye laser is available at NYU Medical Center, Duke University Medical Center, UCLA School of Medicine, Thomas Jefferson University Hospital, Northwestern University Hospital, Boston University Medical Center, Massachusetts General Hospital, and elsewhere.

Anticonvulsant medications may be prescribed to control seizures; phenytoin, however, tends to aggravate oral tissue hypertrophy. Special education services, genetic counseling, and physical therapy may benefit patients and their families.

Treatment—Investigational Children under the age of 1 year with Sturge-Weber syndrome and seizures are being examined with the positron emission tomography (**PET**) scan by Harry T. Chugani, M.D., under a grant from the National Institutes of Health. Dr. Chugani is seeking to identify patients with controlled seizures who might benefit from hemispherectomy. For more information: Dr. Harry T. Chugani, UCLA Medical Center, Department of Pediatric Neurology, 10833 LeConte, Los Angeles, CA 90024-1752; (215) 825-5946.

Research is being conducted to evaluate whether the tunable dye laser is effective in treating the port wine stain. Patients as young as 1 month of age are being accepted for treatment. For more information on this and other types of lasers and treatment, contact the Sturge-Weber Foundation.

Research on port wine stains is also being pursued by Dr. Odile Enjolras, Dept. of Dermatology, Hospital Tarnier, Paris, France.

Please contact the agencies listed under Resources, below, for the most current information.

Resources

For more information on Sturge-Weber syndrome: National Organization for Rare Disorders (NORD); Sturge-Weber Foundation; Sturge-Weber Support Group; National Congenital Port Wine Stain Foundation; NIH/National Institute of Neurological Disorders & Stroke (NINDS).

For genetic information and genetic counseling referrals: March of Dimes Birth Defects Foundation; National Center for Education in Maternal and Child Health (NCEMCH).

References
Mendelian Inheritance in Man, 9th ed.: V.A. McKusick; The Johns Hopkins Press, 1990, p. 883.
Birth Defects Compendium, 2nd ed.: Daniel Bergsma; March of Dimes, 1979, 1987.

THROMBOCYTOPENIA-ABSENT RADIUS (TAR) SYNDROME

Description TAR syndrome is a genetic disorder characterized by thrombocytopenia and the absence or underdevelopment of the radius.

Synonyms
> Radial Aplasia-Amegakaryocytic Thrombocytopenia Syndrome
> Radial Aplasia-Thrombocytopenia Syndrome

Signs and Symptoms The thrombocytopenia is most severe during early infancy, and may cause excessive bleeding from the skin or mucous membranes, or intracranially. Other blood disorders such as absent or underdeveloped megakaryocytes; eosinophilia; granulocytosis; and anemia may occur. TAR infants are said to be more likely to develop an intolerance to cow's milk.

The radius is absent or underdeveloped, usually bilaterally. Also present may be underdevelopment of the ulna and defects of the hands, legs, and feet.

Short stature, bowed legs, shortened humerus, underdeveloped shoulder girdle, and dislocation of the hip may occur, as well as spina bifida and kidney or heart defects. A nevus flammeus may be present on the forehead.

Etiology TAR syndrome is inherited as an autosomal recessive trait.

Epidemiology The disorder occurs at birth. Males and females are affected in equal numbers.

Related Disorders See *Anemia, Fanconi.*

Treatment—Standard Early management is necessary for the various blood conditions of these patients. Braces and/or surgical correction may be required for related bone malformations. Genetic counseling is suggested for patients and their families. Other treatment is symptomatic and supportive.

Treatment—Investigational Please contact the agencies listed under Resources, below, for the most current information.

Resources
For more information on **TAR syndrome:** National Organization for Rare Disorders (NORD); Thrombocytopenia-Absent Radius Syndrome Association (TARSA); NIH/National Institute of Child Health and Human Development.

For **genetic information and genetic counseling referrals:** March of Dimes Birth Defects Foundation; NIH/National Center for Education in Maternal and Child Health (NCEMCH).

References
Mendelian Inheritance in Man, 9th ed.: V.A. McKusick; The Johns Hopkins University Press, 1990, pp. 1504–1505.

Smith's Recognizable Patterns of Human Malformation, 4th ed.: K.L. Jones; W.B. Saunders Company, 1988, pp. 276.

Thrombocytopenia-Absent Radius Syndrome: A.G. Aledo, et al.; An. Esp. Pediatr., January 1982, issue 16(1), pp. 82–87.

TOOTH AND NAIL SYNDROME

Description Tooth and nail syndrome is characterized by absent teeth and poorly formed nails.

Synonyms
Dysplasia of Nails with Hypodontia
Witkop Tooth-Nail Syndrome

Signs and Symptoms Signs of tooth and nail syndrome include lack of mandibular incisors, second molars, maxillary canines, and other permanent teeth. Finger- and toenails are hypoplastic and slow-growing.

Etiology The syndrome appears to be inherited as an autosomal dominant trait in some families.

Epidemiology Males and females are affected equally.

Treatment—Standard Treatment is symptomatic and supportive; dentures may be helpful. Genetic counseling may be beneficial.

Treatment—Investigational Please contact the agencies listed under Resources, below, for the most current information.

Resources
For more information on tooth and nail syndrome: National Organization for Rare Disorders (NORD); National Foundation for Ectodermal Dysplasias; NIH/National Institute of Child Health and Human Development (NICHHD).

For genetic information and genetic counseling referrals: March of Dimes Birth Defects Foundation; National Center for Education in Maternal and Child Health (NCEMCH).

References
Syndromes of the Head and Neck, 3rd ed.: R.J. Gorlin, et al.; Oxford University Press, 1990, pp. 863–864.

TREACHER COLLINS SYNDROME

Description Treacher Collins syndrome is a rare genetic disorder characterized by slanted eyes, dysphagia, deafness, and deformities of the maxilla, mandible, and ears.

Synonyms

Francheschetti-Klein Syndrome

Mandibulofacial Dysostosis

Signs and Symptoms A patient with Treacher Collins syndrome typically has an especially long face, a beaklike nose, and receding chin. Other characteristic features include slanted eyes and notching of the lower eyelids. Malar and maxillary as well as mandibular hypoplasia may cause dysphagia or respiratory problems for the newborn. The pinna and external acoustic meatus may be malformed, and the tympanic membrane may be replaced with a bony plate. Almost 50 percent of patients have conductive deafness.

Etiology The syndrome, whose gene locus may possibly reside on the long arm of chromosome 5, is inherited as an autosomal dominant trait. A positive family history is found in fewer than half of new Treacher Collins patients. Thus, it is suspected that approximately 60 percent of cases represent genetic mutations.

Epidemiology Males and females are affected in equal numbers.

Related Disorders See *Goldenhar Syndrome (oculo-auriculo-vertebral syndrome); Oral-Facial-Digital Syndrome.*

Nager acrofacial dysostosis is marked by defective development of bones of the jaw and arms, cleft lip and palate, ear deformities and hearing loss, and abnormally small thumbs. The disorder is inherited and is rare.

Juberg-Hayward syndrome (oro-cranio-digital syndrome) is a rare hereditary disorder also characterized by cleft lip and palate and by deformities of the thumbs as well as the toes. The head is microcephalic. Growth hormone deficiency resulting in short stature has been reported in one boy.

Treatment—Standard During infancy, insertion of feeding or breathing tubes may be required. Early hearing evaluation is indicated. The need for surgery or hearing aids will depend on the type of deafness present. Speech and language difficulties may require appropriate therapy. Surgery to improve the appearance of the jaw and ears may be appropriate.

The age of the child determines the type of surgical treatment. During infancy, attention is directed toward the upper airway. A tracheostomy may be needed. The notched lower eyelid can be repaired in the infant's first year, and slanting eyelids and flat cheek bones, during the preschool and early school years. Correction of the jaws and malocclusion is usually done in stages, with the final corrections being performed in teenage years, along with orthodontic therapy.

For external ear abnormalities, minor anomalies can be surgically corrected before the child starts school. If the major portion of the ear is missing, it is best to wait until age 6 so that sufficient rib cartilage is available for framework and grafting.

Genetic counseling may benefit patients and their families. Other treatment is symptomatic and supportive.

Treatment—Investigational Various surgical methods to improve the appearance of Treacher Collins patients are being studied.

Please contact the agencies listed under Resources, below, for the most current information.

Resources

For more information on Treacher Collins syndrome: National Organization for Rare Disorders (NORD); Treacher Collins Family Support Network; National Institute of Child Health & Human Development (NICHHD); FACES–National Association for the Craniofacially Handicapped; National Craniofacial Foundation; Forward Face; American Society for Deaf Children; Deafness Research Foundation; Craniofacial Centre Children's Hospital.

For genetic information and genetic counseling referrals: March of Dimes Birth Defects Foundation; NIH/National Center for Education in Maternal and Child Health (NCEMCH).

References

Mendelian Inheritance in Man, 9th ed.: V.A. McKusick; The Johns Hopkins University Press, 1990, p. 598.

Smith's Recognizable Patterns of Human Malformation, 4th ed.: K.L. Jones; W.B. Saunders Company, 1988, pp. 210–211.

Psychosocial Adjustment of 20 Patients with Treacher Collins Syndrome Before and After Reconstructive Surgery: E.M. Arndt, et al.; Br. J. Plast. Surg., November 1987, issue 40(6), pp. 605–609.

Anthropometric Evaluation of Dysmorphology in Craniofacial Anomalies; Treacher Collins Syndrome: J.C. Kolar, et al.; Am. J. Phys. Anthropol., December 1987, issue 74(4), pp. 441–451.

Familial Treacher Collins Syndrome: P.S. Murty, et al.; J. Laryngol. Otol., July 1988, issue 102(7), pp. 620–622.

TRICHODENTOOSSEOUS SYNDROME (TDOS)

Description TDOS is one of the ectodermal dysplasias and primarily affects teeth, hair, and bones. Intelligence and life span are usually unaffected.

Synonyms
Curly Hair Osteosclerosis

Signs and Symptoms Infants are born with kinky hair that may straighten with age, and curly eyelashes. Nails are thin and likely to peel or break.

Dental abnormalities, including abscessed teeth during the first years of life, are a major feature of TDOS. Tooth enamel may become yellow-brown, thin, and pitted. X-rays reveal taurodontia and mild-to-moderate increased bone density. Since teeth may not grow appropriately during infancy, TDOS children may lose teeth and have delayed dentition.

Unlike most other ectodermal dysplasias, TDOS does not affect the respiratory tract.

Etiology TDOS is inherited as an autosomal dominant trait. Symptoms are caused by a defect in ectodermal cells involving the formation and structure of teeth, hair, and nails.

Epidemiology TDOS affects males and females equally and can occur in conjunction with other hereditary disorders.

Treatment—Standard Dental treatment involves early restoration of teeth with jacket crowns and/or prosthetic replacement. Genetic counseling may be beneficial.

Treatment—Investigational Please contact the agencies listed under Resources, below, for the most current information.

Resources

For more information on trichodentoosseous syndrome: National Organization for Rare Disorders (NORD); National Foundation for Ectodermal Dysplasias; NIH/National Institute of Dental Research.

For genetic information and genetic counseling referrals: March of Dimes Birth Defects Foundation; National Center for Education in Maternal and Child Health (NCEMCH).

References

Smith's Recognizable Patterns of Human Malformation, 4th ed.: K.L. Jones; W.B. Saunders Company, 1988, pp. 482–483.

A Tricho-Odonto-Onychial Subtype of Ectodermal Dysplasia: H. Kresbach, et al.; Z. Hautkr., May 1984, 59(9), pp. 601–613.

Tricho-Dento-Osseous Syndrome: Heterogeneity or Clinical Variability: S.D. Shapiro, et al.; Am. J. Med. Genet., October 1983, 16(2), pp. 225–236.

TRICHORHINOPHALANGEAL SYNDROME (TRPS)

Description Trichorhinophalangeal syndrome occurs in 2 forms: types I and II. Type II **(Langer-Giedion syndrome)** is the more severe. Both I and II are forms of ectodermal dysplasia, and are characterized by thin, brittle hair, a bulbous nose, cone-shaped epiphyses, and varying degrees of growth retardation. Fingers are abnormally developed and facial appearance is unusual.

Synonyms

Langer-Giedion Syndrome (Type II)

Signs and Symptoms TRPS type I is characterized primarily by hair and bone abnormalities. Scalp hair is fine, brittle, and sparse. Some individuals may become completely bald. Eyebrows are thick near the nose, but extremely thin nearer the temples. The tip of the nose is bulbous, and the upper lip is thin and the philtrum long. These facial abnormalities often subside at adolescence. Thin nails and extra teeth occur in some cases. Abnormalities of the skeletal system include cone-shaped epiphyses in some fingers and toes, pectus carinatum, and scoliosis. Intelligence is usually normal.

In TRPS type II (Langer-Giedion syndrome), facies and hair and epiphyseal abnormalities are similar to type I. Distinguishing features for Langer-Giedion syndrome are multiple exostoses, mild microcephaly, and mild-to-moderate mental retardation. The exostoses occur primarily near the ends of the tubular arm and leg bones and usually develop by age 3 or 4. Other bones may also be affected. Delayed onset of speech, and, less frequently, hearing loss have occurred. An increased susceptibility to respiratory infections and hip dislocations may be present.

Etiology Both types I and II have been traced to band 8q24. Type II is the result of a larger deletion which includes band q23 or other subbands.

Epidemiology Both forms of trichorhinophalangeal syndrome are very rare.

Treatment—Standard Treatment is symptomatic and supportive. Surgery may correct limb deformities. Genetic counseling may be beneficial.

Treatment—Investigational Please contact the agencies listed under Resources, below, for the most current information.

Resources

For more information on trichorhinophalangeal syndrome: National Organization for Rare Disorders (NORD); National Foundation for Ectodermal Dysplasias; NIH/National Institute of Child Health and Human Development (NICHHD).

For genetic information and genetic counseling referrals: March of Dimes Birth Defects Foundation; National Center for Education in Maternal and Child Health (NCEMCH).

References
Mendelian Inheritance in Man, 9th ed.: V.A. McKusick; The Johns Hopkins University Press, 1990, pp. 942, 558–560.

Syndromes of the Head and Neck, 3rd ed.: R.J. Gorlin, et al.; Oxford University Press, 1990, pp. 806–812.

Trichorhinophalangeal Dysplasia (Gideon Syndrome). A Case Report: G.B. Kuna, et al.; Clin. Pediatr. (Phila.), January 1978, 17(1), pp. 96–98.

New Clinical Observations in the Trichorhinophalangeal Syndrome: R.M. Goodman, et al.; J. Craniofac. Genet. Dev. Biol., 1981, 1(1), pp. 15–29.

Clinical and Scanning Electron Microscopic Findings in a Solitary Case of Trichorhinophalangeal Syndrome Type I: E.P. Prens, et al.; Acta Derm. Venereol. (Stockh.), 1984, 64(3), pp. 2449–2453.

TRIPLOID SYNDROME

Description Triploid syndrome is an extremely rare disorder in which a complete extra set of chromosomes is present. Affected infants usually are lost through early miscarriage. Some are stillborn or live only a few days, and a few infants have survived as long as 5 months. These infants have severely retarded fetal growth and many other prenatal abnormalities.

Synonyms
Chromosome Triploidy Syndrome
Triploidy

Signs and Symptoms Associated abnormalities include an unusually large placenta, lack of prenatal skeletal growth, and craniofacial characteristics such as ocular hypertelorism, low nasal bridge, low-set malformed ears, and micrognathia. There may be syndactyly of the 3rd and 4th fingers, and simian creases of the hands. Congenital defects of the heart and sex organs may be present, as well as abnormal brain development and renal and adrenal hypoplasia. Less often there are an unusually shaped skull, cleft lip or palate, meningomyelocele, and hernias. There may also be liver and gallbladder deformities and twisted colon.

The pregnant mother may experience preeclampsia.

Etiology Triploid syndrome is caused by a complete extra set of chromosomes, i.e., 69 rather than 46. Triplication of the chromosomes is most often the result of double fertilization of an egg. The disorder is not inherited, and there is no evidence of increased risk of recurrence.

Epidemiology Parental age does not seem to be a factor. Males and females are affected in equal numbers.

Related Disorders See *Down Syndrome; 11q- Syndrome; 18p- Syndrome.*

Treatment—Standard Treatment of triploid syndrome is symptomatic and supportive.

Treatment—Investigational Please contact the agencies listed under Resources, below, for the most current information.

Resources
For more information on triploid syndrome: National Organization for Rare Disorders (NORD); NIH/National Institute of Child Health and Human Development (NICHHD).

For genetic information and genetic counseling referrals: March of Dimes Birth Defects Foundation; NIH/National Center for Education in Maternal and Child Health (NCEMCH).

References
Smith's Recognizable Patterns of Human Malformation, 4th ed.: K.L. Jones; W.B. Saunders Company, 1988, pp. 32–35.
Syndromes of the Head and Neck, 3rd ed.: R.J. Gorlin, et al.; Oxford University Press, 1990, pp. 64–65.
Diplospermy II Indicated as the Origin of a Live Born Human Triploid (69, XXX): B.M. Page, et al.; J. Med. Genet., October 1981, issue 18(5), pp. 386–389.
Morphologic Anomalies in Triploid Liveborn Fetuses: N. Doshi, et al.; Hum. Pathol., August 1983, issue 14(4), pp. 716–723.
Midtrimester Preeclamptic Toxemia in Triploid Pregnancies: R. Toaff, et al.; Isr. J. Med. Sci., March 1976, issue 12(3), pp. 234–239.

TRISOMY

Description Trisomies are very rare genetic disorders in which an extra chromosome is added to one of the normal pairs. The triplication of the chromosome may be partial; i.e., either an extra short arm (p) or an extra long arm (q) is present. Defects are classified by the name of the abnormal chromosome pair and the portion of the chromosome affected. In general, the most common symptom of the trisomies is mental retardation. (There are, however, many causes of mental retardation, and most are genetic anomalies that are not trisomies.)

Synonyms
Chromosomal Triplication

Signs and Symptoms Following is a description of a few trisomy disorders not further discussed in the PHYSICIANS' GUIDE TO RARE DISEASES. See also *Trisomy 13 Syndrome; Trisomy 18 Syndrome; Down Syndrome (Trisomy 21)*.

Partial trisomy 6p is characterized by a triplicated section of the short arm of the 6th chromosome. Manifestations include mental retardation, multiple facial abnormalities, and malformations of the lungs and kidney. Two kidneys may be present on one side of the body, with crossed ureters.

Trisomy 8 patients are typically slender and of normal height. The ears are low-set and malformed, and the eyes tend to be down-slanted. Bone and joint abnormalities may involve the ribs, spine, and kneecaps; joint contractures are common. Deep creases are seen in the palms of the hands and soles of the feet. Mental and motor retardation is mild to moderate, often associated with delayed and hard-to-understand speech. Most patients with trisomy 8 are chromosomal mosaics (i.e., they have 2 or more cell types that have different numbers of chromosomes).

Trisomy 9p is identified by an extra short arm of chromosome 9, leading to abnormalities in the hands, feet, and pelvic bones. The pattern of bone structures in x-rays of patients with trisomy 9p appears to be unique among patients with chromosomal abnormalities. Other typical features include down-turned corners of the mouth, a large rounded nose, slightly wide and deep-set slanted eyes, unusual fingerprints, and mental retardation.

Trisomy 10q is characterized by a triplication of part of the long arm of the 10th chromosome. Predominant manifestations include dolichocephaly, prominent forehead, and abnormally open seams and fontanelles on the skull at birth. A broad nose, cleft palate, ptosis, posteriorly rotated ears, congenital heart defects, and severe mental retardation also occur.

Partial trisomy 22 (cat-eye syndrome) is characterized by coloboma of the iris and by anal atresia. Severe mental and physical retardation, wide-set slanted eyes, and tags or fistulas in front of the ears may develop. Congenital heart disease may occur. A few cases with full trisomy have been reported in patients with similar symptoms and signs, but micrognathia and hypotonia distinguish them from the partial trisomy.

Etiology The trisomies are inborn abnormalities of the chromosomes. In some cases the chromosome abnormalities are related to advanced maternal or paternal age.

Epidemiology Some trisomies might affect a few hundred or a few thousand children per year; some only a handful of children in the United States. The most common trisomy is Down syndrome (trisomy 21), affecting approximately 7000 newborn infants each year.

Related Disorders There are many trisomy disorders with a wide range of manifestations.

Treatment—Standard Genetic counseling will be helpful to families of patients with a trisomy disorder. Some genetic counselors suggest that pregnant women over the age of 35 should undergo amniocentesis, since many trisomies can be detected before birth.

Parent and infant education can begin immediately after birth. Children with mental retardation usually benefit from early intervention programs and special education. The individual child should receive direct service programming to develop learning, language, mobility, self-care, and socialization skills. Toddler and preschool programs can further enhance the acquisition of skills to enable persons with mental retardation to reach their maximum potential.

Treatment—Investigational Please contact the agencies listed under Resources, below, for the most current information.

Resources

For more information on trisomy: National Organization for Rare Disorders (NORD); Support Organization for Trisomy 18/13 (SOFT 18/13); Association for Retarded Citizens; National Down Syndrome Congress.

For genetic information and genetic counseling referrals: March of Dimes Birth Defects Foundation; National Center for Education in Maternal and Child Health (NCEMCH).

References
Smith's Recognizable Patterns of Human Malformation, 4th ed.: K.L. Jones; W.B. Saunders Company, 1988, pp. 10–79.

TRISOMY 13 SYNDROME

Description Trisomy 13 syndrome is a genetic disorder with varied characteristics that include gross defects of the brain; midline anomalies; cleft lip or cleft palate, or both; polydactyly; and cardiac defects.

Synonyms
>D Trisomy Syndrome
>Patau Syndrome
>Trisomy 13-15 Syndrome

Signs and Symptoms Newborns are usually small and have severe abnormalities:

microcephaly and a sloping forehead; wide sutures and patent fontanelles; often a myelomeningocele (not quite one-half of cases); holoprosencephaly; and cleft lip and/or cleft palate. Other defects include capillary hemangiomas, especially on the forehead in the midline, dermal sinuses on the scalp, and loose folds of skin over the back of the neck. The ears are low-set and malformed. Infants are often apneic, appear to be deaf, and have severe mental retardation.

Ocular anomalies frequently include microphthalmia, coloboma, and retinal dysplasia. Shallow supraorbital ridges and slanted palpebral fissures are characteristic. The hands are polydactylic, with flexed fingers that may or may not overlap; narrow, spherical fingernails; and a palmar simian crease. There may be polydactyly of the feet, and the heels are prominent.

Other common congenital anomalies include atrial and ventricular septal defects, a patent ductus arteriosus, defects of the pulmonary and aortic valves, and dextrocardia, as well as abnormal genitalia in both sexes, including cryptorchidism and bicornuate uterus.

Etiology An additional chromosome 13 causes the abnormalities.

Epidemiology Trisomy 13 syndrome occurs in 1:12,000 live births. Approximately one percent of all spontaneous abortions have trisomy 13. About half of affected infants die during the first months and about 90 percent during the first year. Males and females of all nationalities and races are affected equally.

Treatment—Standard Treatment is symptomatic and supportive.

Treatment—Investigational Please contact the agencies listed under Resources, below, for the most current information.

Resources

For more information on trisomy 13 syndrome: National Organization for Rare Disorders; Support Organization for Trisomy 18/13 (SOFT 18/13); NIH/National Institute of Child Health and Human Development (NICHHD); Association for Retarded Citizens; National Institute of Mental Retardation (Canada).

For genetic information and genetic counseling referrals: March of Dimes Birth Defects Foundation; National Center for Education in Maternal and Child Health (NCEMCH).

References

Smith's Recognizable Patterns of Human Malformation, 4th ed.: K.L. Jones; W.B. Saunders Company, 1988, pp. 20–25.

Syndromes of the Head and Neck, 3rd ed.: R.J. Gorlin, et al.; Oxford University Press, 1990, pp. 40–43.

Trisomy 18 Syndrome

Description Trisomy 18 syndrome is a genetic disorder with onset in utero. Infants have multiple congenital anomalies, appear thin and frail, have difficulty feeding, fail to thrive, and show generalized hypertonicity with rigidity in flexion of the limbs. Mental retardation also is present.

Synonyms
> Edwards Syndrome

Signs and Symptoms Danger signals may occur in utero, with weak fetal activity and hydramnios. There is often just one umbilical artery and a small placenta, and the infant may be premature or small for gestational age with a feeble cry and a lowered sound response. Skeletal muscle and subcutaneous fat are hypoplastic. The head is microcephalic, with a prominent occiput and small jaw and mouth, creating a pinched look. Epicanthal folds, cleft lip or cleft palate (or both), low-set and malformed ears, and redundant skin folds, especially over the back of the neck, are common. Mental retardation is usually severe.

The hand characteristically makes a clenched fist, the index finger overlapping the 3rd and 4th fingers; the fingernails are hypoplastic; and the thumbs are absent or hypoplastic. The distal crease on the 5th finger is often absent, and a low-arch dermal ridge fingertip pattern is common. Abnormalities of the feet include syndactyly, clubfeet, and a shortened and often dorsiflexed big toe.

Congenital anomalies often occur in the lungs and diaphragm; other frequent abnormalities include a patent ductus arteriosus, ventricular and atrial septal defects, and pulmonary and aortic valve defects. The kidneys and ureters are often affected, and hernias, separation of the rectus muscles of the abdominal wall, and cryptorchidism are also common.

Etiology The syndrome is caused by the presence of a 3rd chromosome 18, which is responsible for the physical and mental abnormalities of this developmental disorder.

Epidemiology Female infants are 4 times more likely than male infants to have trisomy 18 syndrome. It occurs in 1:5000 to 1:7000 newborn infants. Maternal age is usually above average. About half of affected infants die by 2 months and fewer than 10 percent survive one year.

Treatment—Standard Treatment is symptomatic and supportive.

Treatment—Investigational Please contact the agencies listed under Resources, below, for the most current information.

Resources
> **For more information on trisomy 18 syndrome:** National Organization for Rare Disorders; Support Organization for Trisomy 18/13 (SOFT 18/13); NIH/National Institute of Child Health and Human Development (NICHHD); Association for Retarded Citizens; National Institute of Mental Retardation (Canada).

> **For genetic information and genetic counseling referrals:** March of Dimes Birth Defects Foundation; National Center for Education in Maternal and Child Health (NCEMCH).

References

Smith's Recognizable Patterns of Human Malformation, 4th ed.: K.L. Jones; W.B. Saunders Company, 1988, pp. 16–19.
Syndromes of the Head and Neck, 3rd ed.: R.J. Gorlin, et al.; Oxford University Press, 1990, pp. 43–46.

TURNER SYNDROME

Description Turner syndrome is a genetic disorder of females in which there is a lack of sexual development at puberty. Other characteristics include small stature, a webbed neck, heart defects, and various other abnormalities. About half of individuals have a 45,X karyotype; others are 45,X/46,XX mosaics or have other X chromosome defects.

Synonyms

45,X Syndrome
Bonnevie-Ulrich Syndrome
Gonadal Dysgenesis (45,X)
Monosomy X

Signs and Symptoms Affected individuals have female characteristics, but do not undergo puberty or develop secondary sexual characteristics (breasts, and pubic and axillary hair) because they have immature (streak) ovaries and cannot produce estrogen.

Growth is slowed and adults are almost always under 5 feet tall. Intelligence is usually normal. Visual-spatial deficits may be present. Lowered self-esteem may occur during adolescence.

Congenital abnormalities include a narrow, arched palate; small mandible; broad chest; and, at the nape of the neck, loose skin folds, webbing, and low hairline. Typical cardiac defects may include coarctation of the aorta and other left side anomalies. Urinary tract abnormalities include horseshoe kidney and double ureters. Patients with mosaicism (45,X/46,XX) have attenuated clinical manifestations.

Etiology The syndrome is caused by an absence or defect of the X chromosome. The karyotype is 45,X in 50 percent of cases, lacking one of the X chromosomes; in 30 to 40 percent, there is mosaicism (45,X/46,XX). In the remainder of cases, the 2nd X chromosome is present but shows a variety of abnormalities (isochromosomes, deletions, rings, etc.).

Epidemiology The disorder occurs in about 1:3000 live-born females. The 45,X karyotype at conception is about 1.5 percent, but the majority are spontaneously aborted. Cystic hygroma is common in these aborted fetuses.

Related Disorders See *Noonan Syndrome.*

Treatment—Standard There is no cure, but certain measures can provide a more normal life. Genetically engineered growth hormone has proven helpful in many cases. At puberty, replacement therapy with estrogen allows normal development of breasts, labia, vagina, uterus, and fallopian tubes, although patients are infertile. In vitro fertilization with a donor egg, and pregnancy, are possible.

Treatment—Investigational The National Institutes of Health request the cooperation of physicians in referring patients (age 4 to 12 years) with Turner syndrome. Patients will be offered enrollment in a longterm treatment protocol to assess the effect of treatment with low-dose estrogen and growth hormone on adult height. Referring physicians will receive a complete summary of all evaluations, and patients will continue to be followed in conjunction with their referring physicians. For more information, contact Gordon B. Cutler, Jr., M.D., National Institutes of Health, 9000 Rockville Pike, Building 10, Room 10N260, Bethesda, Maryland 20892; or Judith Levine Ross, M.D., Medical College of Pennsylvania, Philadelphia.

Please contact the agencies listed under Resources, below, for the most current information.

Resources

For more information on Turner syndrome: National Organization for Rare Disorders (NORD); Turner Syndrome Support Group of New England; Turner Syndrome Society of the United States; Turner Syndrome Society; NIH/National Institute of Child Health and Human Development (NICHHD).

For genetic information and genetic counseling referrals: March of Dimes Birth Defects Foundation; National Center for Education in Maternal and Child Health (NCEMCH).

References

Turner Syndrome: R.G. Rosenfeld and M.M. Grumbach, eds.; Marcel DeKles, Inc., 1989, pp. 1–552.

Smith's Recognizable Patterns of Human Malformation, 4th ed.: K.L. Jones; W.B. Saunders Company, 1988, pp. 75–79.

VACTERL ASSOCIATION

Description VACTERL association is an acronym for (**V**)ertebral anomalies; (**A**)nal atresia; congenital (**C**)ardiac disease; (**T**)racheo(**E**)sophageal fistula; (**R**)enal anomalies; radial dysplasia and other (**L**)imb defects. These features can be combined in various ways, and can be manifestations of several recognized disorders. Related conditions such as the **REAR** syndrome (see below) and the **VATER** association, which have some of the same characteristics, have been expanded into the VACTERL association.

Signs and Symptoms The abnormalities of VACTERL association are present at birth.

Vertebral anomalies can include divided spinal disks, incomplete or half-developed spinal disks, and developmental abnormalities of the sacrum.

Anal atresia may be present, as may fistulas involving the rectum, urethra, and vagina.

The most common cardiac abnormality is ventricular septal defect (see **Ventricular Septal Defects**).

Tracheoesophageal fistula can be present. Occasionally the esophagus may be absent.

The most common renal abnormality is agenesis; however, the renal tissue can be overdeveloped.

Radial limb dysplasia can include hypoplasia and triphalangism in the thumb, polydactyly, and absence of some of the fingers.

Some persons with VACTERL association may not grow at a normal rate, but mental development is usually normal.

Etiology The abnormalities of VACTERL association are presumed to be defects in the mesodermal layer of the embryo during fetal development. The developmental abnormalities are thought to occur sporadically; however, some scientists believe some cases to be genetic.

Epidemiology VACTERL association is very rare. Males are affected in slightly greater numbers than females.

Related Disorders See *Holt-Oram Syndrome.*

REAR syndrome is an acronym for (**R**)enal anomalies, deformed external (**E**)ars and perceptive deafness, (**A**)nal stenosis, and (**R**)adial dysplasia. Underdeveloped kidneys are the most common renal abnormalities. The external ears are malformed and deafness is present at birth. The anus is constricted or smaller than normal, and other anal abnormalities can occur. Abnormal tissue development is present in the area of the radius or humerus.

Townes-Brocks syndrome is characterized by congenital anal atresia and hand, foot, and ear abnormalities. These include triphalangeal thumb, an extra thumb, fusion of the metatarsals or absence of some bones in the feet, exceptionally large external ears, and mild sensorineural deafness.

Treatment—Standard Treatment of VACTERL association by successive surgical rehabilitation of malformations is often useful. Other treatment is symptomatic and supportive.

Treatment—Investigational Please contact the agencies listed under Resources, below, for the most current information.

Resources

For more information on VACTERL association: National Organization for Rare Disorders (NORD); National Center for Child Health and Human Development.

For genetic information and genetic counseling referrals: March of Dimes Birth Defects Foundation; National Center for Education in Maternal and Child Health (NCEMCH).

References

Mendelian Inheritance in Man, 9th ed.: V.A. McKusick; The Johns Hopkins University Press, 1990, pp. 963, 88.

Smith's Recognizable Patterns of Human Malformation, 4th ed.: K.L. Jones; W.B. Saunders Company, 1988, pp. 602–603.

Tracheal Agenesis and Associated Malformations: A Comparison with Tracheoesophageal Fistula and the VACTERL Association: J.A. Evans, et al.; Am. J. Med. Genet., May 1985, issue 21(1), pp. 21–38.

A Population Study of the VACTERL Association: Evidence for Its Etiologic Heterogeneity: M.J. Khoury, et al.; Pediatrics, May 1983, issue 71(5), pp. 815–820.

Townes Syndrome. A Distinct Multiple Malformation Syndrome Resembling VACTERL Association: J.H. Hersh, et al.; Clin. Pediatr., February 1986, issue 25(2), pp. 100–102.

VON HIPPEL-LINDAU SYNDROME

Description The von Hippel-Lindau syndrome is a hereditary disorder characterized by angiomata of the retina and hemangioblastoma of the cerebellum. Other parts of the brain as well as the spinal cord may be affected.

Synonyms
>
> Angiomatosis Retina
> Cerebelloretinal Hemangioblastomatosis
> Retinocerebral Angiomatosis

Signs and Symptoms Onset usually is during young adulthood, but manifestations may appear as early as the age of 8. These include headaches, dizziness, ataxia, and behavioral abnormalities caused by neurologic disturbances. Retinal angiomas usually appear by the 3rd decade. Later in life, patients may develop angiomatous tumors in the cerebellum, spinal cord, lungs, liver, and elsewhere. Ophthalmoscopic examination reveals subretinal yellow spots and star-shaped material. Tumors of the retina may be associated with benign, slowly growing hemangioblastomas, usually located in the cerebellum. Other areas of the central nervous system are affected rarely.

Benign pheochromocytomas of the adrenal glands in about 15 percent of patients may cause chronic hypertension, headache, cold hands and feet, and excessive sweating. Blood pressure may return to normal as the patient ages. Renal cysts and tumors occur in about one-third of patients and pancreatic cysts and tumors in one-fifth.

Etiology The syndrome is inherited as an autosomal dominant genetic trait; the defective gene has been mapped to chromosome 3p25. Patients may have a mild, moderate, or severe form of the disease because of highly variable expressivity. The syndrome is also characterized by almost complete penetrance; almost all patients who carry the gene will eventually have clinical manifestations of the disorder.

Epidemiology Males and females are affected equally.

Related Disorders See *Neurofibromatosis; Sturge-Weber Syndrome; Tuberous Sclerosis.*

Treatment—Standard Laser and cryotherapy can destroy retinal lesions smaller than 2.5 cm. Larger lesions respond best to cryotherapy.

Genetic counseling may be of benefit; other treatment is symptomatic and supportive.

Treatment—Investigational The role of oncogenes in tumors from persons with von Hippel-Lindau syndrome is being investigated by Gary Skuse, M.D. and Peter Rowley, M.D. of the Division of Genetics, University of Rochester School of Medicine. They request notification of surgery for tumors in this condition so that arrangements can be made to receive tissue samples. Please call Dr. Rowley, Dr. Skuse, or Barbara Kosciolek at (716) 275-3461.

Please contact the agencies listed under Resources, below, for the most current information.

Resources

For more information on von Hippel-Lindau syndrome: National Organization for Rare Disorders (NORD); NIH/National Institute of Neurological Disorders & Stroke; NIH/National Eye Institute; Eye Research Institute of Retina Foundation; National Cancer Institute PDQ (Physician Data Query) phoneline.

For genetic information and genetic counseling referrals: March of Dimes Birth Defects Foundation; National Center for Education in Maternal and Child Health (NCEMCH).

References

Smith's Recognizable Patterns of Human Malformation, 4th ed.: K.L. Jones; W.B. Saunders Company, 1988, p. 455.

WAARDENBURG SYNDROME

Description Waardenburg syndrome is a hereditary disorder with characteristics that include abnormalities of the face and hair as well as deafness. The syndrome occurs in 2 forms: types I and II.

Synonyms

Klein-Waardenburg Syndrome
Van der Hoeve-Halbertsma-Waardenburg-Gualdi Syndrome
Waardenburg-Klein Syndrome

Signs and Symptoms Type I is characterized by lateral displacement of the medial canthi and of the inferior lacrimal puncta. This leads to shortening of the eyelids and reduced visibility of the medial parts of the sclera, giving the impression of strabismus and hypertelorism. Other characteristics include partial or total heterochromia of the irides, a white forelock or premature graying of the hair, congenital sensorineural deafness, prominence of the medial portion of the eyebrows, a thin nose, and full lips.

Type II is characterized by the pigmentary disorder and deafness, but lateral displacement of the medial canthi is absent.

Aganglionic megacolon (Hirschsprung's disease) has been reported in association with Waardenburg syndrome in several dozen patients.

Etiology Waardenburg syndrome is inherited through dominant genes with complete penetrance and variable expressivity. Within a family, all degrees of severity, from mild to severe, may be encountered. All the defects in this disorder are thought to result from a defect of migration of cells of the anterior neural crest.

Epidemiology The syndrome occurs in 1:4000 live births. Males and females are affected equally.

Related Disorders See *Albinism; Vitiligo.*

Vogt-Koyanagi syndrome (uveo-oto-cutaneous syndrome) is characterized by poliosis, premature graying of the hair, baldness, vitiligo of the hands, face, neck, and trunk, hearing impairment and tinnitus, uveitis, and retinitis. The syndrome primarily affects Orientals.

Harada syndrome is similar to the Vogt-Koyanagi syndrome except that in some cases skin and hair symptoms are absent. Any skin and hair lesions that are present may disappear with time, and hearing and vision may partially recover spontaneously. Harada syndrome also mostly affects persons of Oriental heritage.

Treatment—Standard Recognition of the syndrome in infancy can lead to early detection of deafness.

Treatment is symptomatic and supportive. A hearing aid, sign language and lip-reading techniques, and special schooling may be helpful. Genetic counseling may aid families of affected children.

Treatment—Investigational Please contact the agencies listed under Resources, below, for the most current information.

Resources

For more information on Waardenburg syndrome: National Organization for Rare Disorders (NORD); National Craniofacial Foundation; FACES—National Association for the Craniofacially Handicapped; Craniofacial Family Association; NIH/National Institute of Dental Research; NIH/National Eye Institute; Alexander Graham Bell Association for the Deaf; Self-Help for Hard-of-Hearing People, Inc. (SHHH); National Information Center on Deafness; National Association of the Deaf; Eye Research Institute of Retina Foundation; National Federation of the Blind; American Council of the Blind; National Organization for Albinism and Hypopigmentation (NOAH); National Vitiligo Foundation.

For genetic information and genetic counseling referrals: March of Dimes Birth Defects Foundation; National Center for Education in Maternal and Child Health (NCEMCH).

References

Waardenburg's Syndrome: A.M. DiGeorge, et al.; J. Pediatrics, November 1960, vol. 57(5), pp. 649–669.

Smith's Recognizable Patterns of Human Malformation, 4th ed.: K.L. Jones; W.B. Saunders Company, 1988, pp. 208–209.

GENETIC DISEASES AND DYSMORPHIC SYNDROMES | 151

Syndromes of the Head and Neck, 3rd ed.: R.J. Gorlin, et al.; Oxford University Press, 1990, pp. 466–469.

WERNER SYNDROME

Description Werner syndrome is a form of premature aging which begins in adolescence or early adulthood and results in the appearance of old age by 30 to 40 years.

Synonyms
  Progeria of Adulthood

Signs and Symptoms Affected individuals appear normal until adolescence or young adulthood. The syndrome progresses steadily. Stature typically is short. Facial characteristics include a nose that becomes beaked and thin, prominent eyes, and thinned eyebrows and lashes. Cataracts often develop by about age 25 to 30 years. By age 20 the patient may have graying hair, and baldness may ensue. The torso tends to be stocky and the abdomen may protrude. Subcutaneous fat and muscle mass are lost, resulting in extreme thinness of the arms and legs. The hands and feet are small, and the fingers short and deformed.

The skin, especially on the face, legs, and feet, undergoes scleroderma-like changes that leave it taut and shiny. There may be ulcerations on the legs and feet. Hypogonadism may be present, and secondary sex characteristics such as pubic, axillary, and facial hair are absent or regress.

Diabetes mellitus, arteriosclerosis, and osteoporosis may develop. Calcification occurs in the extremities and the heart, particularly the valves and coronary arteries. Other potentially fatal complications include cerebral stroke and cancers.

Werner syndrome can occur in partial forms, exhibiting only a few of the symptoms described, and having a milder, slower course.

Etiology The syndrome appears to be hereditary, with an autosomal recessive mode of transmission. It is also theorized that chromosomal instability is responsible for the premature aging.

The biochemical defect or defects responsible for Werner syndrome are not known. Urinary hyaluronic acid has been found to be elevated.

Epidemiology Incidence in the United States appears to be between 1:one million and 20:one million cases. Males and females over the age of about 14 years are affected.

Related Disorders See *Hutchinson-Gilford Syndrome; Gottron Syndrome (acrogeria).*

Treatment—Standard Available treatments for Werner syndrome are supportive and symptomatic. They include surgery for cataracts and skin grafting for ulcerations.

Treatment—Investigational Please contact the agencies listed under Resources,

below, for the most current information.

Resources
For more information on Werner syndrome: National Organization for Rare Disorders (NORD); Progeria Foundation; The Progeria International Registry (PIR); The National Arthritis and Musculoskeletal and Skin Diseases Information Clearinghouse.

References
Syndromes of the Head and Neck, 3rd ed.: R.J. Gorlin, et al.; Oxford University Press, 1990, pp. 485–487.

Mendelian Inheritance in Man, 9th ed.: V.A. McKusick; The Johns Hopkins University Press, 1990, pp. 1532–1533.

Smith's Recognizable Patterns of Human Malformation, 4th ed.: K.L. Jones; W.B. Saunders Company, 1988, pp. 120–121.

Cecil Textbook of Medicine, 18th ed.: J.B. Wyngaarden and L.H. Smith, Jr., eds.; W.B. Saunders Company, 1988, p. 1202.

WILLIAMS SYNDROME

Description Williams syndrome is a rare congenital disorder characterized by elfin facies, exceptionally sensitive hearing, developmental delays, short stature, and an impulsive, outgoing personality. Cardiovascular anomalies and/or infantile hypercalcemia are often present.

Synonyms
> Beuren Syndrome
> Hypercalcemia-Supravalvar Aortic Stenosis
> Infantile Hypercalcemia Syndrome, Idiopathic
> Williams-Beuren Syndrome

Signs and Symptoms Some children have a low birth weight and fail to thrive. Vomiting, gagging, diarrhea, and constipation are common in infancy. Blood calcium may be elevated; when this sign occurs, it persists only during the first year of life, then disappears.

The face at birth is characteristically elfin-like, with a small head, broad forehead, puffiness around the eyes, depressed nasal bridge, wide mouth, and full lips. Children whose eyes are blue or green (unlike those with brown eyes) may have a star-like pattern in the iris. Highly sensitive hearing often results in patients overreacting to loud and high-pitched sounds. Motor development, e.g., sitting and walking, and language and gross and fine motor skills may be delayed. Puberty may be premature.

Heart disorders occur in 75 percent of cases. Most common findings are supravalvar aortic stenosis and pulmonary artery stenosis. Umbilical or inguinal hernias may occur.

The personality is friendly and talkative. Mild mental retardation may occur, but some children have average intelligence with severe learning disabilities. These children may exhibit attention-deficit behaviors, but generally have good longterm memory.

Etiology The cause is unknown; with the possible exception of very few instances, the condition has been sporadic.

Epidemiology Infants of both sexes and all races are affected. The disorder occurs in about 1:20,000 births.

Related Disorders See *Noonan Syndrome,* known to be an inherited disorder, which is also associated with pulmonary artery stenosis.

An elevated blood calcium in infancy, without a known cause or any other symptoms, may be due to **idiopathic infantile hypercalcemia.**

Supravalvar aortic stenosis (narrowing of the aorta above the aortic valve) may occur alone, or in conjunction with other disorders.

Treatment—Standard To treat elevated blood calcium levels in affected infants, excessive vitamin D in the diet should be avoided and calcium should be restricted to 25 to 100 mg/day. For severe hypercalcemia, hydrocortisone analog therapy may be considered on a temporary basis. An endocrinologist should be consulted. After a child is a few months old, calcium levels will return to normal even in untreated patients.

For the physical and mental developmental deficiencies, centers for developmentally disabled children and special education services in schools may be needed. Medical help from specialists, speech and language therapy, occupational and physical therapy, and vocational training can all be beneficial.

Treatment—Investigational Please contact the agencies listed under Resources, below, for the most current information.

Resources

For more information on Williams syndrome: National Organization for Rare Disorders (NORD); Williams Syndrome Association; Infantile Hypercalcaemia Foundation Ltd.; NIH/National Institute of Child Health and Human Development.

For genetic information and genetic counseling referrals: March of Dimes Birth Defects Foundation; National Center for Education in Maternal and Child Health (NCEMCH).

References

Smith's Recognizable Patterns of Human Malformation, 4th ed.: K.L. Jones; W.B. Saunders Company, 1988, pp. 106–107.

Mendelian Inheritance in Man, 9th ed.: V.A. McKusick; The Johns Hopkins University Press, 1990, pp. 979–961.

Facts About Williams Syndrome: Williams Syndrome Association.

WOLF-HIRSCHHORN SYNDROME (WHS)

Description Wolf-Hirschhorn syndrome is a chromosomal defect disorder with the manifestations discussed below.

Synonyms
> 4p- Syndrome
> Chromosome Number 4 Short Arm Deletion Syndrome
> Wolf Syndrome

Signs and Symptoms The most frequently occurring features of the syndrome are low birth weight, hypotonia, physical and mental retardation, microcephaly, high forehead, wide nasal bridge with a broad or beaked nose, epicanthal folds, and hypertelorism. Cardiac and renal defects and seizures occur in about one-half of patients. Hypospadias and cryptorchidism are common in males; in females, the urethra may open into the vagina.

Other facial involvement includes strabismus, ptosis, coloboma of the eye, arched eyebrows, cleft lip, cleft palate, short philtrum, downturned mouth, micrognathia, and low-set ears.

Etiology Wolf-Hirschhorn syndrome is a genetic disorder caused by a deletion of the 4p16 band of chromosome 4. Most instances are *de novo* defects, but in 10 to 15 percent the condition is inherited as a translocation defect.

Epidemiology Incidence has been reported to be 1:50,000. Twice as many females as males are affected. About one-third of patients die in the first 2 years of life.

Related Disorders See *Cri du Chat Syndrome; Down Syndrome; Trisomy; Trisomy 13 Syndrome; Trisomy 18 Syndrome.*

Treatment—Standard Reconstructive surgery is indicated in some cases. Special education, physical therapy, vocational services, and genetic counseling may be beneficial. Other treatment is symptomatic and supportive.

Treatment—Investigational Please contact the agencies listed under Resources, below, for the most current information.

Resources

For more information on Wolf-Hirschhorn syndrome: National Organization for Rare Disorders (NORD); National Institute of Child Health and Human Development (NICHHD).

For genetic information and genetic counseling referrals: March of Dimes Birth Defects Foundation; NIH/National Center for Education in Maternal and Child Health (NCEMCH).

References
Mendelian Inheritance in Man, 9th ed.: V.A. McKusick; The Johns Hopkins University Press, 1990, p. 985.

Syndromes of the Head and Neck, 3rd ed.: R.J. Gorlin, et al.; Oxford University Press, 1990, pp. 46–48.

WYBURN-MASON SYNDROME

Description Wyburn-Mason syndrome is a rare genetic disorder that usually affects the brain, eyes, and skin. Major symptoms may include nevi and brain and eye aneurysms.

Synonyms
>   Cerebroretinal Arteriovenous Aneurysm
>   Bonnet-Dechaume-Blanc Syndrome

Signs and Symptoms Wyburn-Mason syndrome is usually present at birth but is not evident until the 4th decade. Onset of symptoms can be either sudden or gradual. Vision is usually lost in one eye, accompanied by severe headache, vomiting, and sudden bulging of the affected eye. Nevi also usually occur around the affected eye. A midbrain aneurysm may produce signs of neurologic deterioration, including a stiff neck, loss of consciousness, tinnitus, deafness, and aphasia.

Etiology The cause is not known; the syndrome may be inherited as an autosomal dominant trait.

Epidemiology Wyburn-Mason syndrome affects males more often than females.

Related Disorders See *Sturge-Weber Syndrome; von Hippel-Lindau Syndrome.*

Treatment—Standard Treatment is symptomatic and supportive. Surgery may be recommended to repair brain or eye aneurysms. Genetic counseling may be beneficial.

Treatment—Investigational Please contact the agencies listed under Resources, below, for the most current information.

Resources

   For more information on Wyburn-Mason syndrome: National Organization for Rare Disorders (NORD); NIH/National Institute of Neurological & Communicative Disorders and Stroke (NINCDS).

   For genetic information and genetic counseling referrals: March of Dimes Birth Defects Foundation; NIH/National Center for Education in Maternal and Child Health (NCEMCH).

References
Wyburn-Mason Syndrome Subcutaneous Angioma Extirpation After Preliminary Embolisation: R.J. de Keizer, et al.; Doc. Ophthalmol., March 1981, 50(2), pp. 263–273.
Combined Phakomatoses; A Case Report of Sturge-Weber and Wyburn-Mason Syndrome Occurring in the Same Individual: J.B. Ward, et al.; Ann. Ophthalmol., December 1983, 15(12), pp. 1112–1116.

2 | INBORN ERRORS OF METABOLISM
By Jess G. Thoene, M.D.

The term "inborn errors of metabolism" was introduced by Dr. A.E. Garrod in the early part of this century. His exciting discoveries regarding the nature of inheritance of alcaptonuria led to a proliferation of knowledge over the ensuing eight decades such that now the standard reference textbook, *The Metabolic Basis of Inherited Disease*, lists over 100 separate chapter headings in two volumes devoted to the description of known inborn errors of metabolism. These errors of metabolism cover a wide range of metabolic pathways resulting in a diversity of conditions that extend from phenylketonuria to diseases not normally thought of in this sense, such as diabetes mellitus.

The human genome is comprised of more than 100,000 genes, and is susceptible to mutation at each locus. Interruption in the DNA sequence coding for an enzyme leads to failure for the chemical reaction mediated by that enzyme to proceed at the proper rate. This produces adverse consequences resulting from underproduction of an essential metabolite, accumulation of unmetabolized precursors, or overproduction of compounds which normally exist in minute amounts. Symptoms range from catastrophic overwhelming disease in infancy (disorders of the urea cycle) to kidney stones (cystinuria) or osteoarthritis and pigmented cartilage in old age (alcaptonuria).

Most inborn errors of metabolism are rare, with an incidence of 1:10,000 to 1:100,000 in the general population. Most are inherited via an autosomal recessive pattern. This means that both parents of the affected individual are carriers (obligate heterozygotes) but usually are clinically unaffected. The risk of two carriers having another such affected (homozygous) individual is 1:4 for each pregnancy. A few inborn errors are inherited as X-linked traits. In X-linked conditions, half of a carrier female's daughters will also be carriers, half of her sons will be affected (hemizygotes), and half of her sons and daughters will be unaffected. Typical X-linked traits include Lesch-Nyhan syndrome, ornithine transcarbamylase deficiency, and Hunter syndrome.

The diagnosis of inborn errors of metabolism requires access to a laboratory skilled in the performance of analysis of body fluids for the metabolites of interest, such as assays for amino acids and organic acids in plasma and urine. The diagnosis of storage disorders usually requires direct tissue assay of the suspected defective enzyme, e.g., lysosomal enzymes. Disorders of carbohydrate metabolism, heavy metals, steroid metabolism, and other disorders may require shipping samples to specific reference laboratories as well. The physician can determine a center able to provide the required analysis by querying the resource agencies listed at the end of each rare disease discussion in this chapter.

The infant with catastrophic overwhelming illness is a frequent dilemma in neonatal intensive care units. Although a majority of the time these infants' illnesses derive from sepsis, or disorders of the respiratory or cardiovascular system, a proportion are due to an inborn error of metabolism. The diagram accompanying this chapter shows an approach to sorting out the various diagnostic possibilities. It is essential to remember to measure the infant's electrolytes and bicarbonate initially. Demonstration of an increased anion gap (the sum of the sodium and potassium minus the sum of the chloride and bicarbonate >18 mEq/L) is a strong indication of the presence of an organic acidemia. In this case, analysis of urine for organic acids is essential.

Finding abnormalities in urinary organic acids should lead directly to a diagnosis. Some of these are listed in the figure. Among them are maple syrup urine disease **(MSUD),** beta-ketothiolase deficiency, propionic and methylmalonic aciduria, isovaleric acidemia **(IVA),** medium-chain acyl-CoA dehydrogenase deficiency (MCAD), glutaricacidurias types I and II, oxoprolinuria, and a number of other rare disorders. Other clinical signs suggesting an organic acidemia in the newborn peri-

Figure 2.1. An approach to diagnosis of infants with inborn errors of metabolism.

(Expanded from Urea Cycle Enzymes, Figure 20-4, p. 640, by S.W. Brusilow and A.L. Horwich; *in* The Metabolic Basis of Inherited Disease, 6th ed.: C.R. Scriver, et al., eds. Copyright McGraw-Hill, 1989. Used with permission.)

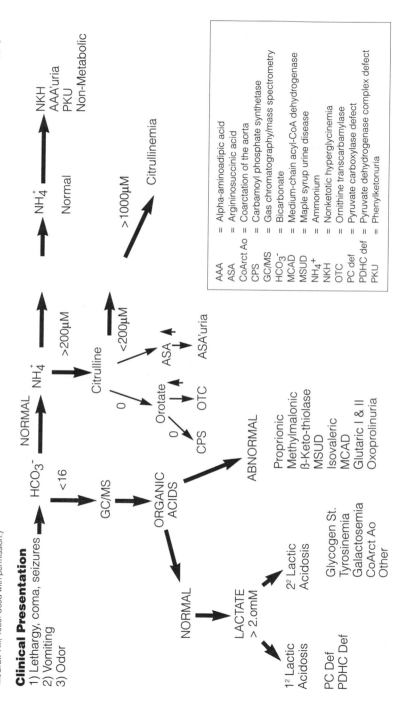

od include thrombocytopenia and/or neutropenia, elevations of plasma lactate, or a peculiar odor. Several organic acidemias such as MSUD and IVA result in an excretion of compounds that are very pungent.

If the organic acids are normal and an increased anion gap is present, then plasma lactate should be measured. Urinary lactate is unstable and may not show up on a urinary organic acid determination. Elevation in plasma lactate above 2 mM suggests either primary or secondary lactate acidosis. Secondary lactic acidosis may be the result of shock or a number of inborn errors of metabolism, including the glycogen storage diseases, tyrosinemia, galactosemia, and non-metabolic diseases such as coarctation of the aorta. Primary lactic acidoses include defects in the enzymes pyruvate carboxylase and pyruvate dehydrogenase complex.

If the acid-base balance is normal and the ammonia is elevated, then plasma citrulline should be determined. This distinguishes the various disorders in the urea cycle including carbamoyl phosphate synthetase (CPS) deficiency, ornithine transcarbamylase (OTC) deficiency, argininosuccinic aciduria (ASA), or citrullinemia. If both the organic acids and ammonia are normal, then only a few inborn errors of metabolism are likely to produce this clinical picture, including nonketotic hyperglycinemia (NKH) and alpha-aminoadipic aciduria.

Mucopolysaccharidoses may be detected by finding an increase in the urinary excretion of mucopolysaccharides. Other storage disorders do not produce excretion of characteristic metabolites in the urine. These patients require either skin biopsy or other measurement of tissue enzyme deficiency for diagnosis.

The physical examination is usually normal in patients with disorders of amino acid metabolism and urea cycle defects, except for neurologic symptoms. Findings suggestive of a storage disorder include ocular changes with either retinal pigmentation, cherry red spots, or cataracts. Coarse facies, enlargement of liver and spleen, abnormal thickening of the skin, joint limitation, and bony abnormalities also are hallmarks of a number of storage disorders.

Inborn errors have been diagnosable but not treatable until very recently. Effective therapy for many disorders of amino acid metabolism and of carbohydrate metabolism as well as some other inborn errors is becoming available. Most disorders of amino acid metabolism can be partially treated by limiting intake of the offending metabolite. These children may not be able to tolerate more than 1 gm/kg/day of dietary protein, which may still permit adequate growth and development. Although most infants in America are fed a diet containing between 2 and 3 grams/kg/day of protein, many infants of the Third World thrive on much less than that. This dietary limitation can be ameliorated to some extent by increasing the amount of dietary amino acids which are not metabolized via the defective metabolic pathway. Many special infant formulas with specific amino acids deleted are available.

Specific therapy for inborn errors of metabolism also involves alternative means for metabolizing toxic compounds. For example, the treatment of hyperammonemia in urea cycle disorders includes the administration of sodium benzoate and phenylacetate. These agents react with nitrogen-containing compounds to produce alternative means of waste nitrogen (ammonia) excretion. In cystinosis, treatment with cysteamine produces depletion of the accumulation of cystine within lysosomes by altering the cystine to a substance the patient with cystinosis is able to metabolize.

Disorders of organic acid metabolism may respond to vitamin therapy. Many enzymes require cofactors (vitamins) for catalytic activity. In rare instances, the genetic defect involves the region of the enzyme which binds the cofactor. In these cases it is sometimes possible to achieve some improvement in enzyme function by treating the patient with pharmacologic doses of the specific vitamin cofactor needed by that enzyme. An example is B12 therapy in vitamin B12-responsive methylmalonic aciduria.

Plasma carnitine should be measured in patients with metabolic acidosis, particularly if organic acids are abnormal. If the carnitine is low, therapy with carnitine can be instituted with good effect in many instances. Carnitine is required for the oxidation of fatty acids within mitochondria, since fatty acids are conjugated to carnitine prior to their transport into mitochondria. Many organic acidemias result in secondary carnitine deficiency because of the urinary excretion of acylcarnitines, which are the conjugation product between the organic acids that accumulate in the disorder and the body's endogenous carnitine stores. Secondary carnitine deficiency then augments the debility caused by the organic acidemia, since failure to oxidize fatty acids completely in the mitochondria leads to accumulation of ketone bodies and hypoglycemia as well as metabolic acidosis and enhanced lactate production.

A high index of suspicion coupled with rapid referral to an appropriate diagnostic laboratory or tertiary care center will result in ameliorating illness and saving lives for patients with these diseases.

References

The Metabolic Basis of Inherited Disease, 6th ed: C. Scriver, A. Beaudet, W. Sly, D. Valle; McGraw-Hill, 1989.

Disorders of Amino Acid Metabolism: J.G. Thoene; *in* Internal Medicine, 3rd ed.: J.H. Stein, ed.-in-chief; Little, Brown and Company, 1990, pp. 2301–2320.

INBORN ERRORS OF METABOLISM
Listings in This Section

5-OXOPROLINURIA

Description 5-Oxoprolinuria is caused by an inborn error of glutathione metabolism, which may result in central nervous system impairment.

Synonyms
Pyroglutamicaciduria

Signs and Symptoms Massive amounts of 5-oxoproline (pyroglutamic acid) are excreted in the urine, and abnormally high levels of this acid and lactic acid are found in the blood and cerebrospinal fluid. Metabolic acidosis usually is present. Without treatment, mental retardation, impaired muscle coordination (cerebellar ataxia), and seizures may occur.

Etiology 5-Oxoprolinuria, inherited as an autosomal recessive trait, is the result of a deficiency of the enzyme glutathione synthetase.

Epidemiology The disorder is very rare. It can be present at birth, and affects males and females equally.

Related Disorders The inborn **5-oxoprolinase deficiency** is characterized by excretion of a moderate amount of 5-oxoproline in the urine, and by higher than normal blood levels of this substance. There usually are no other symptoms related to the enzyme deficiency.

Glutathionuria (gamma-glutamyl transpeptidase deficiency) is a very rare, possibly hereditary metabolic disorder. Concentrations of glutathione in blood and urine are excessive. Mild mental retardation and behavioral problems may be present.

Treatment—Standard Bicarbonate therapy is used to compensate for metabolic acidosis. Genetic counseling is recommended for families of affected children.

Treatment—Investigational Please contact the agencies listed under Resources, below, for the most current information.

Resources
    For more information on 5-oxoprolinuria: National Organization for Rare Disorders (NORD); NIH/National Institute of Neurological Disorders & Stroke (NINDS); Research Trust for Metabolic Diseases in Children.
    For genetic information and genetic counseling referrals: March of Dimes Birth Defects Foundation; National Center for Education in Maternal and Child Health (NCEMCH).

References
The Metabolic Basis of Inherited Disease, 6th ed.: C.R. Scriver, et al., eds.; McGraw-Hill, 1989, p. 2353.
Ophthalmological, Psychometric and Therapeutic Investigation in Two Sisters with Hereditary Glutathione Synthetase Deficiency (5-Oxoprolinuria): A. Larsson, et al.; Neuropediatrics, August 1985, issue 16(3), pp. 131–136.
Neonatal 5-Oxoprolinuria: Difficult-to-Diagnose?: I.S. Mendelson, et al.; J. Inherited Metab. Dis., 1983, issue 6(1), pp. 44–48.

The Cerebral Lesions in a Patient with Generalized Glutathione Deficiency and Pyroglutamic Aciduria (5-Oxoprolinuria): K. Skullerud, et al.; Acta Neuropathol. (Berlin), 1980, issue 52(3), pp. 235–238.

ACIDEMIA, ISOVALERIC (IVA)

Description IVA is a hereditary metabolic disorder that usually begins in infancy and occurs in both an acute and a chronic intermittent form.

Synonyms
> Isovaleric Acid-CoA Dehydrogenase Deficiency
> Isovalericacidemia
> Isovaleryl-CoA Carboxylase Deficiency

Signs and Symptoms Onset may be as early as a few days of age or as late as 1 year. The acute form of IVA is characterized by attacks of vomiting, lack of appetite, and listlessness. Infants become increasingly lethargic, have increased neuromuscular irritability, and are often hypothermic. Usually there is a strong odor like that of sweaty feet.

Intermittent episodes are most often triggered by upper respiratory infections or excessive consumption of high-protein foods. Severe acidity and ketoacidosis follow, and coma may ensue. Ketoacidotic episodes tend to occur often in early infancy and young childhood, but their frequency usually diminishes as the patient grows older. Children with IVA often have a natural aversion to protein foods, even at a young age.

IVA can be diagnosed prenatally by measuring the amounts of isovalerylglycine in amniotic fluid.

Etiology IVA is inherited through autosomal recessive genes, as are all known organic acidemias. IVA symptoms are the result of a deficiency of the enzyme isovaleryl co-enzyme A (CoA) dehydrogenase, which is needed for the oxidation of the amino acid leucine.

Many of the effects of the organic acidemias are due to secondary carnitine depletion.

Epidemiology Males and females are affected equally.

Related Disorders See *Acidemia, Methylmalonic; Acidemia, Propionic; Glutaricaciduria II; Maple Syrup Urine Disease; Nonketotic Hyperglycinemia.*

Treatment—Standard IVA is treated with moderate dietary restriction of the amino acid leucine and supplementation of L-carnitine. Oral administration of glycine at 150 to 300 mg/kg/day is lifesaving and may permit normal growth and development. Other treatment is symptomatic and supportive. Genetic counseling is recommended for families of affected children.

With treatment and a low-protein diet the disorder becomes chronically intermittent, and a nearly normal life is possible.

Treatment—Investigational

Please contact the agencies listed under Resources, below, for the most current information.

Resources

For more information on IVA: National Organization for Rare Disorders (NORD); British Organic Acidemia Association; National Institute of Diabetes, Digestive & Kidney Diseases Information Clearinghouse; Research Trust for Metabolic Diseases in Children.

For genetic information and genetic counseling referrals: March of Dimes Birth Defects Foundation; National Center for Education in Maternal and Child Health (NCEMCH).

References

The Metabolic Basis of Inherited Disease, 6th ed.: C.R. Scriver, et al., eds.; McGraw-Hill, 1989, pp. 795–798.

The Response to L-Carnitine and Glycine Therapy in Isovaleric Acidaemia: C. de Sousa, et al.; European J. Pediatr., February 1986, issue 144(5), pp. 451–456.

Stable Isotope Dilution Analysis of Isovalerylglycine in Amniotic Fluid and Urine and its Application for the Prenatal Diagnosis of Isovaleric Acidemia: D.G. Hine, et al.; Pediatr. Res., March 1986, issue 20(3), pp. 222–226.

ACIDEMIA, METHYLMALONIC

Description The methylmalonic acidemias are caused by an enzymatic defect in the oxidation of amino acids. The resultant abnormally high levels of acid in the blood and body tissues and concomitant metabolic acidosis cause the symptoms described below.

Synonyms

Methylmalonic Aciduria

Signs and Symptoms Onset usually is during the first few months of life. Acutely, drowsiness, coma, and seizures may occur, with mental retardation a longterm consequence. Symptoms may also include lethargy, failure to thrive, recurrent vomiting, dehydration, respiratory distress, diminished muscle tone, and an enlarged liver.

Laboratory findings include an abnormally high amount of methylmalonic acid in the blood and urine. Metabolic acidosis is present. The blood or urine may show elevated levels of ketone bodies such as acetone, as well as excessive levels of the amino acid glycine. Hyperammonemia may also be present. The concentration of white blood cells, blood platelets, and red blood cells may be lower than normal. Hypoglycemia may occur.

Etiology The methylmalonic acidemias, which segregate into 4 complementation groups, all inherited as autosomal recessive traits, may be caused by a defect in the enzyme methylmalonyl-CoA mutase, or in adenosylcobalamin synthetic enzymes.

Many of the effects of the organic acidemias are worsened because of secondary carnitine depletion.

Related Disorders See *Acidemia, Propionic.*

Epidemiology Each of the methylmalonic acidemias occurs at a rate of about 1:50,000 to 1:100,000 live births.

Treatment—Standard The diet must be carefully controlled. Treatment includes a low-protein regimen and restriction of the amino acids isoleucine, valine, and threonine. To assure a balanced diet, certain medical foods must be fed to affected children. Pharmacologic doses of vitamin B12 are indicated in the B12-responsive variants.

Carnitine supplementation at 100 to 300 mg/kg/day is recommended for associated carnitine deficiency.

Genetic counseling is recommended for the families of affected children.

Treatment—Investigational Please contact the agencies listed under Resources, below, for the most current information.

Resources

For more information on the methylmalonic acidemias: National Organization for Rare Disorders (NORD); British Organic Acidemia Association; Research Trust for Metabolic Diseases in Children.

For genetic information and genetic counseling referrals: March of Dimes Birth Defects Foundation; National Center for Education in Maternal and Child Health (NCEMCH).

References

Clinical Heterogeneity in Cobalamin C Variant of Combined Homocystinuria and Methylmalonic Aciduria: G.A. Mitchell, et al.; J. Pediatr., March 1986, issue 108(3), pp. 410–415.

The Metabolic Basis of Inherited Disease, 6th ed.: C.R. Scriver, et al., eds.; McGraw-Hill, 1989, pp. 832–840.

ACIDEMIA, PROPIONIC

Description Propionic acidemia, an inherited disorder that is caused by a deficiency of the biotin-requiring enzyme propionyl-CoA carboxylase **(PCC),** usually results in catastrophic illness beginning in the newborn period.

Synonyms

Hyperglycinemia with Ketoacidosis and Leukopenia
Ketotic Glycinemia
Propionyl-CoA Carboxylase (PCC) Deficiency

Signs and Symptoms Initial signs in affected infants are protein intolerance, vomiting, failure to thrive, lethargy, and profound metabolic acidosis. Intercurrent infections may prove fatal.

Other characteristics may include diminished muscle tone, thrombocytopenia, and liver abnormalities such as fatty infiltration. The blood exhibits an elevated concentration of glycine and a massive amount of propionate. EEG abnormalities are possible, and affected patients may experience slowed development and mental retardation.

Amniocentesis to test for PCC activity in amniocytes is possible. An alternative is to measure the concentration of methylcitrate in the amniotic fluid.

When the disorder is suspected in patients and relatives of patients who may be carriers, definitive diagnosis requires measurement of PCC activity in leukocytes or fibroblasts.

Without treatment, the acidosis and ketosis can cause dehydration, lethargy, and vomiting. Brain damage, including coma, generalized seizures, and death result if the disorder is left untreated.

Etiology Propionic acidemia is an autosomal recessive disorder, one of the organic acidemias. The parents of affected patients may show consanguinity.

Symptoms and signs are due to metabolic acidosis caused by a deficiency of PCC, which is needed for metabolism of the amino acids isoleucine, valine, threonine, and methionine.

Many of the adverse effects of organic acidemia are due to secondary carnitine depletion.

Epidemiology Males and females are affected equally.

Related Disorders See *Acidemia, Methylmalonic.*

Treatment—Standard Treatment requires fluid and electrolyte therapy. Sodium bicarbonate is used to resolve the acidosis. This also can be accomplished either by peritoneal dialysis or exchange transfusions. Treatment must begin as soon as acidosis is recognized.

Longterm treatment involves maintenance of a diet low in protein through use of special formulas low in the amino acids isoleucine, valine, threonine, and methionine. On these restricted diets patients can experience good metabolic control with acceptable growth and development if adequate general nutrition is maintained through use of medical foods.

Patients with propionic acidemia develop secondary carnitine deficiency because of loss of propionyl-carnitine and other acyl-carnitines in the urine. In **carnitine deficiency syndromes,** the transport of fatty acids into mitochondria for oxidation and energy production is impaired. Because large amounts of glucose must be used to meet the patient's metabolic requirements, hypoglycemia often results.

Treatment—Investigational It is possible that patients with propionic acidemia could respond to biotin treatment. A therapeutic trial of this coenzyme of PCC can be performed.

Please contact the agencies listed under Resources, below, for the most current information.

Resources

For more information on propionic acidemia: National Organization for

Rare Disorders (NORD); British Organic Acidemia Association; Research Trust for Metabolic Diseases in Children; National Institute of Diabetes, Digestive & Kidney Diseases Information Clearinghouse.

For genetic information and genetic counseling referrals: March of Dimes Birth Defects Foundation; National Center for Education in Maternal and Child Health (NCEMCH).

References
The Metabolic Basis of Inherited Disease, 6th ed.: C.R. Scriver, et al., eds.; McGraw-Hill, 1989, pp. 821–845.

Mendelian Inheritance in Man, 9th ed.: V.A. McKusick; The Johns Hopkins University Press, 1990, pp. 1211–1213.

ADRENOLEUKODYSTROPHY (ALD)

Description ALD is characterized by cerebral demyelination and adrenal atrophy. The disease has 2 inheritance patterns and appears in 3 different forms categorized by age of onset (X-linked, occurring as adult-onset and childhood-onset; and autosomal recessive, with neonatal onset).

Synonyms
Addison Disease with Cerebral Sclerosis
Addison-Schilder Disease
Adrenomyeloneuropathy
Encephalitis Periaxialis Diffusa
Flatau-Schilder Disease
Myelinoclastic Diffuse Sclerosis
Schilder Disease
Schilder Encephalitis
Siewerling-Creutzfeldt Disease
Sudanophilic Leukodystrophy

Signs and Symptoms All forms of ALD, including 85 percent of heterozygotes, are characterized by greatly increased blood plasma and tissue levels of very long chain fatty acids **(VLCFAs)**, which accumulate in the cerebral white matter and the adrenal glands. A few persons with elevated VLCFA levels may have mild symptoms or none at all. In others, the disease may progress very slowly.

Women who are heterozygotic for childhood or adult-onset ALD but are not symptomatic during childhood may have elevated levels of VLCFAs. At age 30 years, symptoms and signs may begin; these may include progressive spastic paraparesis, ataxia, hypertonia, mild peripheral neuropathy, abnormal reflexes of the plantar extensors, and urinary problems. There are no adrenal symptoms, however, and mental and sensory functions are unimpaired.

Childhood ALD, the most common form of the disorder, affects only males. The first symptoms appear between the ages of 4 and 8 years. Females may be carriers of childhood ALD but are asymptomatic. Behavioral changes such as poor memory, deteriorating school work, increasing loss of emotional control, and dementia may be the first signs. A spastic gait, hyperreflexia, hemiparesis, speech disorders, hearing loss, and vision problems including visual agnosia are also seen in children with this disorder.

Manifestations of decreased adrenal gland function usually appear later than the neurologic features. These adrenocortical symptoms and signs can include hypotension, weakness, fatigue, dehydration, weight loss, microcardia, increased skin pigmentation, and decreased secretion of adrenal hormones in response to adrenocorticotropic hormone (ACTH). More advanced neurologic signs can include a progressive optic atrophy and brain demyelination. MRI examination shows lesions in the posterior occipital and parietal lobe white matter. In the adrenal cortex, distended cells can be found in the inner and the thick middle layers.

Adolescent or adult-onset ALD (adrenomyeloneuropathy) may affect the spinal cord. It too affects only males, although females can be carriers. Symptoms and signs, which usually first appear between the ages of 21 and 35, may include progressive leg stiffness, spastic paraparesis of the lower extremities, and ataxia. Sensory changes indicate that involvement of the spinal tracts and peripheral nerves has occurred. Decreased function of the adrenal cortex and testes may be present. ALD should be suspected, even in the absence of neurologic manifestations, in males who have decreased adrenal function with a family history of Addison disease (see also *Addison Disease*). Although adult-onset ALD progresses more slowly than the childhood form, it too can ultimately result in deterioration of brain function.

Neonatal ALD is inherited as an autosomal recessive disorder, and therefore both males and females are affected. It has different pathologic findings. Symptoms and signs appear in the newborn period and include mental retardation, facial abnormalities, seizures, polymicrogyria, retinal degeneration, hypotonia, hepatomegaly, and adrenal insufficiency. In addition to demyelination of the brain's white matter, there may also be gray matter involvement. Hepatic peroxisomes are decreased or absent, and plasma pipecolic acid may be increased. This form of ALD tends to be quickly progressive. Persons who are heterozygotic for neonatal ALD exhibit no neurologic or adrenal symptoms.

CT scan or magnetic resonance imaging (MRI) will show changes in the brain. Laboratory tests for VLCFAs are the most definitive diagnostic procedures. Female carriers and newborn infants at high risk for ALD are detected by measuring the level of long chain fatty acids in plasma or fibroblast cultures. Prenatal diagnosis can be made through amniocentesis and culture of amniotic cells or by study of cultured chorion villus biopsy.

Etiology Abnormal or absent peroxisomes lead to the accumulation of VLCFAs in these conditions, but the precise enzyme deficiency preventing breakdown of VLCFAs is not known. The excess of saturated and unsaturated fatty acid chains is distributed throughout the tissues of the entire body, but tends to accumulate more in the brain's white matter and the adrenal cortex.

Epidemiology Childhood ALD usually begins before age 10 (most often around 7 years). Onset of adult ALD is usually between ages 21 and 35. Female heterozygotes for ALD rarely have manifestations of the disorder, but if these do occur they commonly appear after the age of 30 years.

Related Disorders See *Addison Disease; Leukodystrophy, Canavan; Leukodystrophy, Metachromatic; Refsum Syndrome; Zellweger Syndrome.*

Treatment—Standard Adrenal steroids are given for the adrenocortical deficiency symptoms of ALD, which are the same as in Addison disease. Treatment for neurologic symptoms associated with ALD is symptomatic and supportive. Seizures usually respond well to anticonvulsants. The severe discomfort of spasticity has been managed with some success with baclofen.

Physical therapy, psychological support, special education, and visiting nurse services are often required to help the patient and family cope with the effects of childhood ALD. Genetic counseling for families affected by the disorder is suggested.

Treatment—Investigational Current research is directed toward the identification of the gene that causes ALD.

Hugo W. Moser, M.D., at the Kennedy Institute in Baltimore, Maryland, has been awarded a grant from the Office of Orphan Products Development, Food and Drug Administration, for research in treating ALD with glycerol trioleate. A recent modification in which dietary VLCFA restriction is combined with oral glycerol trioleate does lower VLCFA levels. Its clinical efficacy is being tested.

Lorenzo's oil (erucic acid) is being tested in conjunction with triolein oil as a possible treatment for patients with rapidly progressive childhood ALD. Because of the possible toxicity of this agent, careful monitoring is required.

Bone-marrow transplantation also is being tested as a treatment for childhood ALD; this procedure, however, is not recommended for patients with relatively advanced neurologic symptoms.

Please contact the agencies listed under Resources, below, for the most current information.

Resources

For more information on ALD: National Organization for Rare Disorders (NORD); United Leukodystrophy Foundation; ALD Project, Hugo W. Moser, M.D.; NIH/National Institute of Neurological Disorders & Stroke (NINDS); Children's Brain Diseases Foundation for Research; Research Trust for Metabolic Diseases in Children.

For genetic information and genetic counseling referrals: March of Dimes Birth Defects Foundation; National Center for Education in Maternal and Child Health (NCEMCH).

References
Disorders of Peroxisome Biogenesis: P.B. Lazarow and H.W. Moser; *in* Metabolic Basis of Inherited Disease, 6th ed.: C.R. Scriver, et al., eds.; McGraw-Hill, 1989, pp. 1479–1509.

Adrenoleukodystrophy (X-Linked): H.W. Moser and A.B. Moser; *in* Metabolic Basis of Inherited Disease, 6th ed.: C.R. Scriver, et al., eds.; McGraw-Hill, 1989, pp. 1511–1532.

Adrenoleukodystrophy: Extracts from "Adrenoleukodystrophy in Children and Adults–Diagnosis and Genetic Counseling": H.W. Moser; Newsletter of Research Trust for Metabolic Diseases in Children (1986), pp. 5–7.

Adrenoleukodystrophy: Survey of 303 Cases: Biochemistry, Diagnosis, and Therapy: H.W. Moser, et al.; Annals of Neurology, December 1984, issue 16(6), pp. 628–641.

ALCAPTONURIA

Description Patients with alcaptonuria excrete large amounts of dark-colored urine, the result of spontaneous oxidation of homogentisic acid, which also accumulates in the tissues. In normal functioning, the amino acid tyrosine is metabolized into homogentisic acid, and further into maleylacetoacetic acid. In alcaptonuria, the pathway is not completed because of a deficiency of the enzyme homogentisic acid oxidase, and further metabolism of homogentisic acid is prevented. Accumulation of the acid leads to severe degeneration of the cartilage of the spine and other major joints, and osteoarthritis.

Synonyms
Alcaptonuric Ochronosis
Hereditary Alcaptonuria
Homogentisicacidura

Signs and Symptoms In their late 20s or 30s, patients develop discoloration of the nose, outer ears, and sclera of the eye. The urine may be dark, or may darken upon standing. Somewhat later, patients develop stiffness, pain, and restricted motion in the hips, knees, and shoulders. Still later, symptoms include more severely restricted motion of the spine; thickened ear cartilages; and darkened middle and inner ear structures.

Patients with alcaptonuria who also have kidney disease, and thus an impaired excretion of homogentisic acid, become symptomatic earlier and symptoms tend to be more severe.

Etiology Deficiency of the enzyme homogentisic acid oxidase is inherited as an autosomal recessive trait.

Epidemiology Males and females are affected in equal numbers, although symptoms tend to be more severe in males. Alcaptonuria is unusually prevalent in Czechoslovakia and the Dominican Republic.

Treatment—Standard Occupations that place stress on the large joints should be avoided. Attempts to prevent symptoms through diets low in tyrosine or high in ascorbic acid have had no effect. Other treatment is symptomatic and supportive.

Treatment—Investigational Please contact the agencies listed under Resources, below, for the most current information.

Resources
For more information on alcaptonuria: National Organization for Rare Dis-

orders (NORD); The National Arthritis and Musculoskeletal and Skin Diseases Information Clearinghouse; Bert N. La Du, M.D., Department of Pharmacology, University of Michigan School of Medicine; Research Trust for Metabolic Diseases in Children.

For genetic information and genetic counseling referrals: March of Dimes Birth Defects Foundation; National Center for Education in Maternal and Child Health (NCEMCH).

References

The Metabolic Basis of Inherited Disease, 6th ed.: C.R. Scriver, et al., eds.; McGraw-Hill, 1989, pp. 775–790.

Internal Medicine, 3rd ed.: J.H. Stein, ed.-in-chief; Little, Brown and Company, 1990, pp. 2301–2310.

ALPHA-1-ANTITRYPSIN (AAT) DEFICIENCY

Description A deficiency of AAT allows proteolytic enzymes to attack various tissues of the body, causing emphysema and also affecting the liver, joints, and blood.

Alpha-1-antitrypsin is a nonspecific serum protease inhibitor (antiprotease) of proteolytic enzymes released by neutrophils in response to infection, or in the inflammatory process. A relative deficiency of AAT results in uncontrolled protease activity, especially in the basilar regions of the lung.

Synonyms

Homozygous Alpha-1-Antitrypsin Deficiency
Serum Protease Inhibitor Deficiency

Signs and Symptoms The most common manifestation of AAT deficiency is progressive panacinar emphysema. In persons who are homozygous for the condition the initial symptoms may be seen as early as the 2nd decade, with clinical disease developing by the time the individual reaches the 30s or early 40s. In patients with intermediate levels of antitrypsin, symptoms onset occurs during the 40s. The earliest symptom is most often progressive shortness of breath, but chronic cough or frequent respiratory infections may also be present. Full clinical disease develops by the mid to late 50s.

Other early signs, also frequently seen in asymptomatic AAT-deficient persons, suggest hyperinflation and loss of elastic recoil in the lungs: low forced expiratory volume, low diffusing capacity, and abnormalities seen on lung scan. Arterial hypoxemia without carbon dioxide retention is also present. The perfusion defects are most often seen in the basilar areas of the lung, particularly early in the disease course. Also helpful for diagnosis are a missing or greatly reduced alpha-1-globulin peak, and low serum AAT levels.

Hepatic symptoms of AAT deficiency may appear during the neonatal period, childhood, or adolescence. Infants may have jaundice and ascites and feed poorly. Affected children and adolescents experience fatigue, decreased appetite, swelling of the legs or abdomen, and hepatomegaly. About 25 percent of infants with hepatic symptoms experience no further complications, and liver involvement seems to end after infancy. In the rest (estimated at a small percentage of all cases) cirrhosis eventually develops. The resulting increased intrahepatic venous pressure is associated with nosebleeds, bruising, ascites, gastric and esophageal varices, and occasional internal bleeding. All tests of hepatic function will probably have abnormal results. Later in the course of the cirrhosis, drowsiness may occur after protein-rich meals, as the liver is unable to synthesize urea. Susceptibility to infection may also complicate later stages of the disease.

Hepatic cellular pathology findings in adults with AAT deficiency emphysema are similar to those of infants with symptomatic hepatic involvement, but no hepatic symptoms seem to result in these cases.

Other less common manifestations of AAT deficiency include erosive joint destruction and hematologic abnormalities involving clotting mechanisms.

Etiology Alpha-1-antitrypsin phenotypes result from a number of different alleles at the alpha-1-antitrypsin locus on chromosome 14. For this reason there is great variability of the enzyme, with about 60 different genetic variants recorded so far. Serum deficiencies result from impaired release of AAT from the liver cells after synthesis. Normally levels of AAT are low, rising quickly in response to physiologic stress. AAT-deficient patients appear to have close to normal antiprotease levels until infection, surgery, pregnancy, or other stressful conditions occur; then they are unable to release enough of the protein to meet their needs. Liver involvement seems to result from impairment in storage or release of antiprotease in the hepatocyte. It is not known why only some persons with AAT deficiency have liver involvement.

Epidemiology Deficiencies of AAT are most common in persons of North and Central European descent. The condition may be suspected when emphysema occurs in a woman, a relatively young man, a nonsmoker, or someone with a family history of emphysema.

Related Disorders Other disorders of protease-antiprotease imbalance include adult respiratory distress syndrome, chronic bronchitis, certain pneumonias, and pancreatitis.

Treatment—Standard Symptomatic treatment for AAT-associated emphysema includes oxygen therapy and antibiotics for the frequent respiratory infections. Exercise programs help increase the person's overall functioning.

Treatment of hepatic disease is also symptomatic. Phenobarbital or cholestyramine are directed against jaundice and itching, and diuretics and potassium are used to maintain electrolyte balance. Proper nutrition is essential. Surgically created shunts to lower intrahepatic venous pressure may become necessary. Liver transplantations have been attempted, but with limited success.

The orphan biological product, alpha-1-proteinase inhibitor (Prolastin—Cutter Biological, Miles, Inc.), inhibits the action of alpha-1-proteinase and thus replaces the deficient alpha-1-antitrypsin.

Treatment—Investigational Research is under way to determine if hepatic release of AAT can be induced with danazol, a modified synthetic testosterone. This approach has increased serum levels to 50 percent of normal, which is low but may be sufficient to prevent tissue damage in otherwise healthy nonsmoking individuals.

Other agents being investigated include synthetic neutrophil elastase inhibitors, certain acylating agents, sulfonyl fluorides, short chain fatty acids, and chloromethyl ketone peptides.

An AAT deficiency registry has been established by the National Heart, Lung and Blood Institute at 22 clinical centers throughout the country. Patients who participate in the registry are seen every 6 months during a 5-year period.

Please contact the agencies listed under Resources, below, for the most current information.

Resources

For more information on AAT deficiency: National Organization for Rare Disorders (NORD); Alpha-1 Support Group Newsletter; American Lung Association; American Liver Foundation; NIH/National Heart, Lung and Blood Institute (NHLBI); Children's Liver Foundation.

To locate AAT registry clinics: Alpha-1-Antitrypsin Deficiency Registry.

For genetic information and genetic counseling referrals: March of Dimes Birth Defects Foundation; National Center for Education in Maternal and Child Health (NCEMCH).

References

The Metabolic Basis of Inherited Disease, 6th ed.: C.R. Scriver, et al., eds.; McGraw-Hill, 1989, pp. 2417–2420.

Alpha-1-Antitrypsin Deficiency: J. Lieberman; Med. Clin. of N. Amer., 1973, vol. 57(3), pp. 691–706.

ANDERSEN DISEASE

Description Andersen disease, one of the glycogen storage diseases, is characterized by cirrhosis and possible liver failure.

Synonyms

> Amylopectinosis
> Andersen Glycogenosis
> Brancher Deficiency
> Glycogen Storage Disease IV
> Glycogenosis Type IV

Signs and Symptoms A newborn with Andersen disease appears to be normal. In a few months the infant seems not to be thriving, with little weight gain, a lack of muscle tone, and nonspecific gastrointestinal problems. The liver and spleen progressively enlarge. The course of Andersen disease is marked by progressive cirrhosis of the liver, edema, and sometimes ascites. Besides the hypotonia, neurologic abnormalities include muscular atrophy and decreased tendon reflexes. Diagnosis can be made prenatally.

Etiology The disease is inherited as an autosomal recessive trait. Symptoms are caused by lack of the brancher enzyme amyl-transglucosidase, and by abnormal glycogen.

Epidemiology Andersen disease is one of the rarest of the glycogen storage diseases, comprising less than 5 percent of all patients with these conditions. It usually begins during infancy, and affects males and females in equal numbers. All glycogen storage diseases together affect fewer than 1:40,000 persons in the United States.

Related Disorders See *von Gierke Disease; Forbes Disease; Hers Disease.*

Treatment—Standard Treatment primarily focuses at managing the cirrhosis and associated problems. A low-protein diet and salt restriction can be helpful for edema or ascites. Further treatment is symptomatic and supportive. Genetic counseling for families of affected children is essential.

Treatment—Investigational Liver transplantation has been used experimentally as an intervention for Andersen disease. More research is needed before this procedure can be recommended as a useful therapy, since other tissues are involved.

Please contact the agencies listed under Resources, below, for the most current information.

Resources

For more information on Andersen disease: National Organization for Rare Disorders (NORD); NIH/National Institute of Diabetes, Digestive & Kidney Diseases Information Clearinghouse; Association for Glycogen Storage Diseases; Research Trust for Metabolic Diseases in Children.

For genetic information and genetic counseling referrals: March of Dimes Birth Defects Foundation; National Center for Education in Maternal and Child Health (NCEMCH).

References
The Metabolic Basis of Inherited Disease, 6th ed.: C.R. Scriver, et al., eds.; McGraw-Hill, 1989, pp. 441–443.

Liver-Spleen Scintigraphy in Glycogen Storage Disease (Glycogenoses): S. Heyman; Clin. Nucl. Med., December 1985, issue 10(12), pp. 839–843.

A Juvenile Variant of Glycogenosis IV (Andersen Disease): A.S. Guerra, et al.; Eur. J. Pediatr., August 1986, issue 145(3), pp. 179–181.

Nervous System Involvement in Type IV Glycogenosis: K.R. McMaster, et al.; Arch. Pathol. Lab. Med., March 1979, issue 103(3), pp. 105–111.

ARGINASE DEFICIENCY

Description Arginase deficiency is 1 of the 6 urea cycle disorders, caused by a deficiency of one of the biosynthetic enzymes needed for the conversion of ammonia to urea, which is then normally excreted in the urine. These enzymatic deficiencies cause an excess of ammonia in the blood and body tissues.

Synonyms
> Argininemia
> Inborn Errors of Urea Synthesis
> Urea Cycle Disorder

Signs and Symptoms Onset of symptoms may occur at birth, but also may not be noticeable until some weeks or months of age. The disorder is characterized in infants by progressive mental retardation, seizures, and spasticity. Symptoms also include lack of appetite, vomiting, and hepatomegaly. If left untreated, the disorder may progress to serious and permanent central nervous system dysfunction. A life-threatening elevation of ammonia in the blood is rare, however.

The diagnosis is suspected in the presence of an elevated level of arginine in the blood with concomitant hyperammonuria, and normal plasma concentrations of other amino acids.

Etiology Arginase deficiency has an autosomal recessive inheritance, and results from deficiency of the enzyme arginase.

Epidemiology The deficiency is very rare, with fewer than 1000 known cases in the United States. Males and females are affected equally.

Related Disorders See *Reye Syndrome.*

The following urea cycle disorders are all characterized by deficiencies of enzymes that are needed for different steps in the synthesis of urea from ammonia. See *N-Acetyl Glutamate Synthetase (NAGS) Deficiency; Ornithine Transcarbamylase (OTC) Deficiency; Carbamyl Phosphate Synthetase (CPS) Deficiency; Citrullinemia; Argininosuccinic Aciduria.* The symptoms of all urea cycle disorders include hyperammonemia, in different degrees of severity.

Treatment—Standard Diagnostic testing should be done immediately when a urea cycle disorder is suspected. Tests should include measurement of plasma levels of ammonia, amino acids, and bicarbonate.

Treatment should be started when hyperammonemia is noted, to prevent coma and brain damage. The orphan drug benzoate/phenylacetate (Ucephan—McGaw Laboratories, Inc.) was approved in 1988 for use in the prevention and treatment of hyperammonemia in patients with urea cycle enzymopathy due to enzyme deficiencies.

Arginase deficiency may respond to restriction of dietary protein, and Ucephan therapy.

Genetic counseling is vital for families of children with urea cycle disorders.

Treatment—Investigational A new investigational drug, sodium (or calcium) phenylbutyrate, which does not have an offensive smell, is being developed by Saul Brusilow, M.D. at The Johns Hopkins Hospital. This drug is intended to enhance waste nitrogen excretion and prevent ammonia buildup in the blood.

Enzyme replacement therapy shows potential promise for treatment of urea cycle disorders. A preliminary regimen consisting of acute hemodialysis followed by a restricted intake of protein, plus sodium benzoate, sodium phenylacetate, and arginine or citrulline is being used on an experimental basis for other causes of hyperammonemia.

Please contact the agencies listed under Resources, below, for the most current information.

Resources

For more information on arginase deficiency: National Organization for Rare Disorders (NORD); National Urea Cycle Disorders Foundation; National Institute of Diabetes, Digestive & Kidney Diseases Information Clearinghouse; Research Trust for Metabolic Diseases in Children; Saul Brusilow, M.D., Professor of Pediatrics, Johns Hopkins Hospital; Steve Cederbaum, M.D., Professor of Pediatrics, UCLA Medical School.

For genetic information and genetic counseling referrals: March of Dimes Birth Defects Foundation; National Center for Education in Maternal and Child Health (NCEMCH).

References

Urea Cycle Enzymes: S.W. Brusilow and A.L. Horwich; *in* The Metabolic Basis of Inherited Disease, 6th ed.: C.R. Scriver, et al., eds.; McGraw-Hill, 1989, pp. 629–665.

Symptomatic Inborn Errors of Metabolism in the Neonate: S.W. Brusilow and D.L. Vallee; Current Therapy in Neonatal-Perinatal Medicine, Marcel Decker, 1985, pp. 207–212.

ARGININOSUCCINIC ACIDURIA

Description Argininosuccinic aciduria is 1 of 6 hereditary urea cycle disorders, which are caused by deficiency of the enzymes required for the synthesis of urea from ammonia. The deficiencies result in an excess of ammonia in the blood and body tissues.

Synonyms
Argininosuccinase Deficiency
Inborn Errors of Urea Synthesis
Urea Cycle Disorder

Signs and Symptoms Argininosuccinic aciduria is characterized by hyperammonemia in early infancy. The onset usually is at birth, but symptoms and signs may not be noticeable for days or weeks. Manifestations include lethargy, lack of appetite, vomiting, seizures, and coma. Hepatomegaly may be present. The plasma level of citrulline is moderately elevated (about 100 micromolar). The markedly increased plasma level of argininosuccinic acid is the basis for the diagnosis (see the illustration in the Introduction to Inborn Errors of Metabolism). Immediate treatment after diagnosis in newborns is imperative. If left untreated, brain damage, coma, and death will occur.

Etiology The disorder has an autosomal recessive inheritance. Deficiency of the enzyme argininosuccinase causes the accumulation of excess ammonia.

Epidemiology Argininosuccinic aciduria is very rare, affecting fewer than 1000 persons in the United States. Males and females are affected equally.

Related Disorders The symptoms of all urea cycle disorders result from hyperammonemia, in different degrees of severity. See *N-Acetyl Glutamate Synthetase Deficiency; Ornithine Transcarbamylase Deficiency; Carbamyl Phosphate Synthetase Deficiency; Citrullinemia; and Arginase Deficiency.*

Organic acidemias are characterized by hyperammonemia associated with metabolic acidosis, with an anion gap, and sometimes ketonuria. These disorders are also of genetic origin and affect the urea cycle as a secondary phenomenon.

See also *Reye Syndrome.*

Treatment—Standard Diagnostic testing should be done immediately when a urea cycle disorder is suspected. Tests should include measurement of plasma levels of ammonia, amino acids, and bicarbonate. Before the results of these tests are available, however, treatment of hyperammonemia should begin, to prevent coma or brain damage.

The drug benzoate/phenylacetate (Ucephan—McGaw Laboratories, Inc.) has been approved for use in the prevention and treatment of hyperammonemia in patients with urea cycle enzymopathy due to enzyme deficiencies.

Genetic counseling is imperative for the family of children with argininosuccinase deficiency.

Treatment—Investigational A regimen being used on an experimental basis consists of acute hemodialysis followed by a restricted intake of protein and administration of sodium benzoate, sodium phenylacetate, and arginine or citrulline.

Enzyme replacement therapy shows potential promise for treatment of urea cycle disorders, including argininosuccinase deficiency. Research on this type of therapy is in a preliminary stage.

Two new investigational drugs, sodium (or calcium) benzoate and sodium (or calcium) phenylacetate, are used to enhance waste nitrogen excretion and thus prevent toxic ammonia buildup in the blood. These orphan drugs have been developed by Saul Brusilow, M.D., of Johns Hopkins Hospital. Dr. Brusilow is also developing sodium (or calcium) phenylbutyrate, which does not have an offensive smell.

Please contact the agencies listed under Resources, below, for the most current information.

Resources

For more information on argininosuccinic aciduria: National Organization for Rare Disorders (NORD); National Urea Cycle Disorders Foundation; National Institute of Diabetes, Digestive & Kidney Diseases Information Clearinghouse; The National Kidney Foundation; Research Trust for Metabolic Diseases in Children; Saul Brusilow, M.D., Johns Hopkins Hospital.

For genetic information and genetic counseling referrals: March of

Dimes Birth Defects Foundation; National Center for Education in Maternal and Child Health (NCEMCH).

References

Urea Cycle Enzymes, S.W. Brusilow and A.L. Horwich *in* The Metabolic Basis of Inherited Disease, 6th ed.: C. Scriver, et al., eds.; McGraw-Hill, 1989, pp. 629–665.

Symptomatic Inborn Errors of Metabolism in the Neonate: S.W. Brusilow and D.L. Vallee; Current Therapy in Neonatal-Perinatal Medicine, Marcel Decker, 1985, pp. 207–212.

BLUE DIAPER SYNDROME

Description Blue diaper syndrome is a metabolic disorder characterized by digestive disturbances, fever, bluish urine, and visual difficulties. Kidney disease may eventually develop in some cases.

Synonyms

> Drummond Syndrome
> Hypercalcemia
> Indicanuria Syndrome

Signs and Symptoms The syndrome is generally detected in infants only when the urine stains their diapers blue. Other general findings include irritability, failure to thrive, constipation, poor appetite, and vomiting. Infections and fevers are frequent. The child typically has poor vision resulting from ocular abnormalities.

Because blood levels of calcium are elevated, nephrocalcinosis develops, which may lead to eventual kidney failure.

Etiology Blue diaper syndrome has an autosomal recessive mode of inheritance. The biochemical nature of the defect remains uncertain, although it is thought to relate to a defect in the intestinal absorption of tryptophan. Intestinal bacteria convert the excessive tryptophan into indican and related derivatives; it is these substances that color the urine blue.

Treatment—Standard Ingestion of calcium should be kept to a relatively low level to prevent kidney damage. The use of antibiotics for intestinal bacteria, and administration of nicotinic acid may be beneficial.

Treatment—Investigational Please contact the agencies listed under Resources, below, for the most current information.

Resources

For more information on blue diaper syndrome: National Organization for Rare Disorders (NORD); The National Kidney Foundation; National Institute of Diabetes, Digestive & Kidney Diseases Information Clearinghouse; Research Trust for Metabolic Diseases in Children.

For genetic information and genetic counseling referrals: March of Dimes Birth Defects Foundation; National Center for Education in Maternal and Child Health (NCEMCH).

References
Mendelian Inheritance in Man, 8th ed.: V.A. McKusick; Johns Hopkins University Press, 1986, p. 841.

CARBAMYL PHOSPHATE SYNTHETASE (CPS) DEFICIENCY

Description In CPS deficiency, 1 of 6 hereditary urea cycle disorders, the enzyme lacking is carbamyl phosphate synthetase, needed for the synthesis of urea from ammonia. The result is an excess of ammonia in the blood and body tissues. If untreated, brain damage, coma, and death may ensue.

Synonyms
Hyperammonemia
Inborn Errors of Urea Synthesis
Urea Cycle Disorder

Signs and Symptoms Onset of the symptoms occurs at birth. Manifestations in infants are hyperammonemia, lethargy, coma, and seizures. Other symptoms and signs include disinterest in eating, vomiting, and hepatomegaly. The diagnosis is based on severe hyperammonemia with normal citrulline in plasma, and absent orotate in the urine. (See the illustration in the Introduction to Inborn Errors of Metabolism.) For these infants, immediate treatment after diagnosis is imperative.

Etiology This condition is inherited as an autosomal recessive trait.

Epidemiology The disorder is very rare; fewer than 1000 persons in the United States are affected, males and females equally.

Related Disorders See *Reye Syndrome.*
The symptoms of all urea cycle disorders result from hyperammonemia, in varying degrees of severity. See *N-Acetyl Glutamate Synthetase Deficiency; Ornithine Transcarbamylase Deficiency; Citrullinemia; Argininosuccinic Aciduria; Arginase Deficiency.*
Organic acidemias are characterized by hyperammonemia associated with metabolic acidosis, with an anion gap, and, sometimes, ketonuria. These disorders are also of genetic origin and affect the urea cycle as a secondary phenomenon.

Treatment—Standard Diagnostic testing should be done as soon as a urea cycle disorder is suspected. Tests should include measurement of plasma levels of ammonia, amino acids, and bicarbonate.
Treatment should be started before test results are known, to prevent coma or brain damage. As soon as hyperammonemia due to CPS deficiency is diagnosed in a newborn, dialysis or exchange transfusion should be started. If hyperammonic coma is present shortly after birth, a combined treatment, which may include hemodialysis, must be started as soon as possible.
The drug benzoate/phenylacetate (Ucephan—McGaw Laboratories, Inc.) has

been approved for use in the prevention and treatment of hyperammonemia in patients with urea cycle enzymopathy due to enzyme deficiencies.

Genetic counseling is imperative for the family of children with CPS deficiency.

Treatment—Investigational Preliminary research on enzyme replacement therapy seems promising for treatment of urea cycle disorders, including CPS deficiency. A regimen being used on an experimental basis consists of acute hemodialysis followed by a restricted intake of protein, plus sodium benzoate, sodium phenylacetate, and arginine or citrulline.

Two new investigational drugs, sodium (or calcium) benzoate, and sodium (or calcium) phenylacetate, are used to enhance waste nitrogen excretion. These orphan drugs have been developed by Saul Brusilow, M.D., Johns Hopkins Hospital, who is also developing sodium (or calcium) phenylbutyrate, which does not have an offensive smell.

Please contact the agencies listed under Resources, below, for the most current information.

Resources

   For more information on carbamyl phosphate synthetase deficiency: National Organization for Rare Disorders (NORD); National Urea Cycle Disorders Foundation; National Institute of Diabetes, Digestive & Kidney Diseases Information Clearinghouse; The National Kidney Foundation; Research Trust for Metabolic Diseases in Children; Saul Brusilow, M.D., Johns Hopkins Hospital.

   For genetic information and genetic counseling referrals: March of Dimes Birth Defects Foundation; National Center for Education in Maternal and Child Health (NCEMCH).

References

Urea Cycle Enzymes: S.W. Brusilow and A.L. Horwich; *in* The Metabolic Basis of Inherited Disease, 6th ed.: C.R. Scriver, et al., eds.; McGraw-Hill, 1989, pp. 629–663.

Symptomatic Inborn Errors of Metabolism in the Neonate: S.W. Brusilow and D.L. Vallee; *in* Current Therapy in Neonatal-Perinatal Medicine, Marcel Decker, 1985, pp. 207–212.

CARNITINE DEFICIENCY SYNDROMES, HEREDITARY

Description A deficiency in carnitine, which is normally synthesized in the liver and kidneys, results in muscle weakness and other manifestations described below.

Signs and Symptoms Muscle weakness is the primary symptom. Intermittent shortages of energy supply in muscle tissue may result in rhabdomyolyis. Urinary myoglobin loss may also be associated.

Systemic carnitine deficiency differs from myopathic carnitine deficiency by the presence of low carnitine concentrations in tissues other than muscle, as well as in blood and urine. Central nervous system, hepatic, and myocardial involvement may be present. Degenerative encephalopathy may lead to episodes of vomiting, confusion, and stupor, progressing to coma.

Carnitine deficiency may also be associated with hypoglycemia, and damage to the heart muscle may result in chronic cardiomyopathy.

Etiology Excessive urinary loss is believed to be the cause of carnitine deficiency in most individuals. In some instances total carnitine levels may be normal but are nonetheless insufficient to meet metabolic needs because of the presence of another associated disorder.

Carnitine deficiency usually occurs in conjunction with organic acidemias such as isovaleric, methylmalonic, and propionic acidemias. It may also rarely be present where there is severe liver disease or renal tubular dysfunction.

Epidemiology Males and females are equally affected. Individuals with any of the organic acidemias, severe liver disease, or renal tubular dysfunction are at risk of developing the deficiency.

Related Disorders See *Acidemia, Isovaleric; Acidemia, Propionic; Acidemia, Methylmalonic.*

Treatment—Standard Carnitine deficiency may be corrected by oral L-carnitine and, to some degree, by certain changes in diet. Consumption of foods high in carnitine content, such as red meat and dairy products, should be encouraged. High oral doses of L-carnitine may cause an extremely unpleasant fishlike body odor; this disappears with dosage reduction. Diarrhea may occasionally occur in some patients.

Synthetic L-carnitine is available in tablet and liquid form.

Treatment—Investigational Please contact the agencies listed under Resources, below, for the most current information.

Resources

For more information on carnitine deficiency: National Organization for Rare Disorders (NORD); National Institute of Diabetes, Digestive & Kidney Diseases Information Clearinghouse; Research Trust for Metabolic Diseases in Children; British Organic Acidemia Association.

For genetic information and genetic counseling referrals: March of Dimes Birth Defects Foundation; NIH/National Center for Education in Maternal and Child Health (NCEMCH).

References

Cecil Textbook of Medicine, 18th ed.: J.B. Wyngaarden and L.H. Smith, Jr., eds.; W.B. Saunders Company, 1988, pp. 2278–2279.

Mendelian Inheritance in Man, 8th ed.: V.A. McKusick; The Johns Hopkins University Press, 1986, p. 849.

The Metabolic Basis of Inherited Disease, 6th ed.: C.R. Scriver, et al., eds.; McGraw-Hill, 1989, pp. 894–898.

Carnitine: Metabolism And Clinical Chemistry: N. Siliprandi, et al.; Clin. Chim. Acta, July 31, 1989, issue 183(1), pp. 3–11.

Decreased Fasting Free Fatty Acids with L-Carnitine in Children with Carnitine Deficiency: W.F. Schwenk, et al.; Pediatr. Res., May 1988, issue 23(5), pp. 491–494.

Transport of Carnitine into Cells in Hereditary Carnitine Deficiency: B.O. Eriksson, et al.; J. of Inherited Metab. Disease, 1989, issue 12(2), pp. 108–111.

CARNOSINEMIA

Description Carnosinemia is a hereditary metabolic disorder typically characterized by neurologic abnormalities that include severe mental retardation and myoclonic seizures.

Synonyms
Carnosinase Deficiency
Hyper-Beta Carnosinemia

Signs and Symptoms In some patients with carnosinemia, seizures occur at less than one year of age. Growth and motor and mental development are slow. As neurologic damage progresses, myoclonic jerks involving the head and limbs occur. By the age of 2 years, signs of mental retardation may be apparent. Other patients with low serum carnosinase are normal.

Etiology Carnosinemia is an autosomal recessive hereditary metabolic disorder. The biochemical mechanisms are not clear. There is defective metabolism of carnosine (beta-alanyl-L-histidine), a dipeptide usually found in muscle tissue, by the enzyme carnosinase. Patients usually have carnosinuria and deficient serum carnosinase.

Epidemiology Carnosinemia is a very rare disorder that affects males and females equally.

Related Disorders See *Phenylketonuria.*

Treatment—Standard Treatment is symptomatic and supportive. Intravenous replacement of carnosinase and low carnosine diets are being evaluated. More research is necessary to determine if these treatments will be safe and effective, or necessary in all instances.

Treatment—Investigational Please contact the agencies listed under Resources, below, for the most current information.

Resources
For more information on carnosinemia: National Organization for Rare Disorders (NORD); National Institute of Diabetes, Digestive and Kidney Diseases Information Clearinghouse; Research Trust for Metabolic Diseases in Children.

For genetic information and genetic counseling referrals: March of Dimes Birth Defects Foundation; National Center for Education in Maternal and Child Health (NCEMCH).

References
The Metabolic Basis of Inherited Disease, 6th ed.: C.R. Scriver, et al., eds.; McGraw-Hill, 1989, pp. 755–771.

CITRULLINEMIA

Description Citrullinemia is 1 of 6 hereditary urea cycle disorders that are caused by a deficiency of one of the enzymes needed for the synthesis of urea from ammonia. In citrullinemia, the deficient enzyme is argininosuccinic acid synthetase. Untreated citrullinemia is characterized by hyperammonemia, which may lead to brain damage, coma, and death.

Synonyms
Argininosuccinic Acid Synthetase Deficiency
Urea Cycle Disorder
Inborn Errors of Urea Synthesis

Signs and Symptoms The onset of symptoms usually is at birth. The hyperammonemia is accompanied by lack of appetite, vomiting, listlessness, seizures, and coma. Diagnosis is based on hyperammonemia plus the absence of argininosuccinate and its anhydrides in plasma, and a plasma concentration of citrulline greater than 1000 micromolar (markedly elevated). The disorder must be treated immediately upon diagnosis. If left untreated, brain damage, coma, and death occur in the first weeks of life.

Etiology Citrullinemia is an autosomal recessive hereditary disorder. Deficient activity of argininosuccinic acid synthetase causes an accumulation of excess ammonia in blood and body tissues.

Epidemiology The disorder is very rare, affecting fewer than 1000 persons in the United States. Males and females are affected equally.

Related Disorders See *Reye Syndrome.*
The urea cycle disorders are all characterized by deficiencies of enzymes needed for varying steps in the synthesis of urea from ammonia. See *N-Acetyl Glutamate Synthetase Deficiency; Ornithine Transcarbamylase Deficiency; Carbamyl Phosphate Synthetase Deficiency; Argininosuccinic Aciduria; Arginase Deficiency.*

Organic acidemias are characterized by hyperammonemia associated with metabolic acidosis, with an anion gap, and sometimes with ketonuria. These disorders are also of genetic origin and affect the urea cycle as a secondary phenomenon.

Treatment—Standard Diagnostic testing should be done as soon as a urea cycle disorder is suspected. Tests should include measurement of plasma levels of ammonia, amino acids, and bicarbonate.
Treatment of hyperammonemia should be started before test results are available, to prevent coma or brain damage. The drug benzoate/phenylacetate

(Ucephan—McGaw Laboratories, Inc.) has been approved for use in preventing and treating hyperammonemia in patients with urea cycle enzymopathy due to enzyme deficiencies.

Genetic counseling is imperative for the family of children with citrullinemia.

Treatment—Investigational Two new investigational drugs, sodium (or calcium) benzoate, and sodium (or calcium) phenylacetate, are being used to enhance waste nitrogen excretion, and prevent toxic ammonia buildup in the blood. These orphan drugs have been developed by Saul Brusilow, M.D., Johns Hopkins Hospital, who is also developing sodium (or calcium) phenylbutyrate, which does not have an offensive smell.

Preliminary results with enzyme replacement therapy show promise for treatment of urea cycle disorders, including citrullinemia. One experimental regimen consists of acute hemodialysis followed by a restricted intake of protein, plus administration of sodium benzoate, sodium phenylacetate, and arginine or citrulline.

Please contact the agencies listed under Resources, below, for the most current information.

Resources

For more information on citrullinemia: National Organization for Rare Disorders (NORD); National Urea Cycle Disorders Foundation; National Institute of Diabetes, Digestive & Kidney Diseases Information Clearinghouse; The National Kidney Foundation; Research Trust for Metabolic Diseases in Children; Saul Brusilow, M.D., Johns Hopkins Hospital.

For genetic information and genetic counseling referrals: March of Dimes Birth Defects Foundation; National Center for Education in Maternal and Child Health (NCEMCH).

References

Urea Cycle Enzymes: S.W. Brusilow and A.L. Horwich; in The Metabolic Basis of Inherited Disease, 6th ed.: C.R. Scriver, et al., eds.; McGraw-Hill, 1989, pp. 629–663.
Symptomatic Inborn Errors of Metabolism in the Neonate: S.W. Brusilow and D.L. Vallee; in Current Therapy in Neonatal-Perinatal Medicine, Marcel Decker, 1985, pp. 207–212.

CYSTINOSIS

Description Cystinosis, a hereditary disorder of lysosomal cystine transport, is characterized by the intralysosomal accumulation of cystine. Clinically, 3 forms of the disease are recognized. **Infantile nephropathic cystinosis,** in which symptoms and signs can appear as early as 6 to 12 months of life, is the most severe form of the disease, leading to renal failure by 10 years of age if untreated. In **benign** (or **adult) cystinosis,** crystalline cystine accumulates primarily in the cornea. In the **intermediate** form (also termed **juvenile** or **adolescent cystinosis),** ocular and renal manifestations become significant in the patients' teens or twenties.

One of the major manifestations of cystinosis is the renal **Fanconi syndrome** (see Related Disorders, below).

Synonyms
>   Cystine Storage Disease
>   Fanconi II
>   Lignac-Fanconi Syndrome

Signs and Symptoms Cystine accumulates in the lysosomes of all tissues. Early clinical manifestations involve the kidneys and eyes. Hexagonal or rectangular crystals are present in marrow aspirates, leukocytes, and rectal mucosa, as well as in the cornea and conjunctiva. In heterozygotes for this disorder, there are elevated levels of intracellular cystine, but no clinical manifestations. Cystine accumulation in the kidney results in renal tubular acidosis, hypokalemia, polyuria, polydipsia, hypophosphatemia. The accumulation of cystine crystals in the cornea and conjunctiva causes photophobia, headache, and itching and burning of the eyes. The crystals are visible by slit-lamp examination of the cornea.

Infantile nephropathic cystinosis becomes apparent before the age of 1 year. Ocular findings include patchy depigmentation of the retina and photophobia. Hypophosphatemic (vitamin D-resistant) rickets occurs, as well as poor linear growth, and the child is pale and thin and fails to thrive. Rickets appears as the child grows older. Untreated cystinosis leads to glomerular failure by 10 years of age.

Renal manifestations of intermediate, or juvenile, cystinosis resemble those of the infantile form, although the course is milder. Rickets sometimes occurs.

The adult form of cystinosis is typically benign. This form is primarily characterized by corneal crystals. Renal function remains intact.

Etiology The mode of inheritance for all forms of cystinosis is autosomal recessive.

Related Disorders Fanconi syndrome is characterized by abnormal renal proximal tubular function, particularly involving excessive excretion of glucose, phosphates, amino acids, bicarbonate, water, potassium, calcium, sodium, and carnitine. The syndrome may be associated with other hereditary metabolic conditions including tyrosinemia, galactosemia, fructose intolerance, glycogen storage disease—type I, Wilson·disease, familial nephrosis, and Lowe syndrome. Fanconi syndrome also is associated with iatrogenic and environmental causes, including the use of certain aminoglycosides or outdated tetracycline; and poisoning by heavy metals or other chemicals.

See *Wilson Disease; Lowe Syndrome.*

Treatment—Standard Benign forms of cystinosis require no treatment.

Nephropathic cystinosis is treated symptomatically with fluids and electrolytes to prevent dehydration. Sodium bicarbonate or sodium citrate is administered to maintain normal electrolyte balance. Phosphate and vitamin D are required to correct hypophosphatemia and prevent rickets.

Hemodialysis or renal transplantation is required in endstage renal disease. Renal transplantation is successful in this condition, although little improvement in growth accompanies renal transplantation. Corneal transplantation has been successfully performed using living related donors.

Cystinosis can be detected prenatally by amniocentesis, or via chorionic villus sampling.

Treatment—Investigational The cystine-depleting agents cysteamine and phosphocysteamine are being investigated. Cysteamine has a strong, unpleasant odor, a disadvantage that phosphocysteamine lacks. For more information, contact Jess Thoene, M.D., at the University of Michigan School of Medicine.

Please contact the agencies listed under Resources, below, for the most current information.

Resources

For more information on cystinosis: National Organization for Rare Disorders (NORD); Cystinosis Foundation; National Kidney and Urologic Diseases Information Clearinghouse; Research Trust for Metabolic Diseases in Children.

For genetic information and genetic counseling referrals: March of Dimes Birth Defects Foundation; National Center for Education in Maternal and Child Health; Jess Thoene, M.D., University of Michigan School of Medicine.

References

The Metabolic Basis of Inherited Disease, 6th ed.: C.R. Scriver, et al., eds.; New York, McGraw-Hill, 1989, pp. 2619–2635.

Abnormalities in Amino Acid Metabolism in Clinical Medicine: W.L. Nyhan; Appleton-Century-Crofts, 1984.

CYSTINURIA

Description Cystinuria is marked by inherited abnormal intestinal and kidney transport of the amino acids cystine, lysine, arginine, and ornithine. Excessive cystinuria causes formation of calculi in the kidney, bladder, and ureter. Four subtypes are recognized. In **type I** cystinuria, there is a defect in the active transport of cystine and the dibasic amino acids lysine, arginine, and ornithine in the kidneys and small intestine. Carriers of the defective gene are generally asymptomatic. In **type II** cystinuria, cystine and lysine transport is severely impaired in the kidney and only moderately in the intestines. In **type III** cystinuria, renal transport of cystine and lysine is defective; intestinal transport is normal. Carriers of the defective gene for this variant of the disease typically have slightly elevated levels of cystine and lysine in the urine. In **hypercystinuria,** there is moderate elevation of urinary cystine excretion but normal intestinal absorption of cystine and the dibasic amino acids.

Signs and Symptoms Urinary excretion of cystine is excessively high, exceeding the solubility limit of cystine. Also excreted in massive amounts in the urine are the amino acids lysine, arginine, and ornithine; these, however, are much more soluble in urine than cystine, and produce no associated symptoms.

The initial symptom of cystinuria is usually acute renal colic. Other findings include hematuria, obstruction, and infections of the urinary tract. Frequent recurrences ultimately may lead to kidney damage.

The calculi are usually small, with a jagged crystalline surface. These may be accompanied by urinary "gravel," which consists of yellowish-brown hexagonal crystals.

All patients with urinary calculi should be screened for cystinuria.

Etiology Cystinuria is an autosomal recessive hereditary disorder caused by abnormal transport of cystine and the dibasic amino acids.

Epidemiology Onset of cystinuria symptoms generally occurs between ages 10 and 30 years, although elevated cystine excretion is found from infancy. The disorder occurs in approximately 1:7,000 to 1:10,000 persons; the prevalence varies in different countries. The disease occurs in both sexes.

Related Disorders In **dibasic aminoaciduria,** transport of lysine, arginine, and ornithine is impaired, resulting in increased urinary levels of these amino acids. In **lysinuria,** lysine transport alone is defective, with ensuing large amounts of urinary lysine. Disease carriers tend to have increased levels of the relevant amino acids.

Treatment—Standard The primary objective is reduction of cystine concentration in the urine. Consumption of large amounts of fluid both day and night maintains a high volume of urine and reduces cystine concentration. Alkalinization of the urine increases the solubility of cystine and therefore helps prevent stone formation. Agents used include sodium bicarbonate, citrate, and acetazolamide.

Another approach is administration of D-penicillamine, although there is some risk of side effects with this drug. D-penicillamine promotes mixed-disulfide formation, which is more soluble in the urine and is excreted. Side effects may include fever and rash, and other allergic reactions.

The orphan drug alpha-mercaptopropionylglycine (Thiola—manufactured by Mission Pharmacal of San Antonio, Texas) has been approved by the FDA as a treatment for cystinuria. This agent lowers the level of urinary cystine.

Kidney and bladder surgery sometimes becomes necessary, but calculi commonly recur. Small stones may be removed by endoscopic basket extraction, and laser techniques and ultrasound have been used to dissolve stones.

Treatment—Investigational Please contact the agencies listed under Resources, below, for the most current information.

Resources

For more information on cystinuria: National Organization for Rare Disorders (NORD); The National Kidney Foundation; Charles Y.C. Pak, M.D., University of Texas Health Science Center at Dallas.

For genetic information and genetic counseling referrals: March of Dimes Birth Defects Foundation; National Center for Education in Maternal and Child Health (NCEMCH).

References

The Metabolic Basis of Inherited Disease, 6th ed.: C. Scriver, et al., eds.; McGraw-Hill, 1989, pp. 2479–2496.

Mendelian Inheritance in Man., 8th ed., V.A. McKusick; The Johns Hopkins University Press, 1988, p. 891.

Percutaneous Catheter Dissolution of Cystine Calculi: S.P. Dretler, et al.; J. of Urology, February 1984, issue 131(2), pp. 216–219.

FABRY DISEASE

Description Fabry disease is a disorder of lipid metabolism in which products of glycolipids accumulate in various tissues.

Synonyms
Alpha-Galactosidase Deficiency
Angiokeratoma Corporis Diffusum
Glycolipid Lipidosis
Hemorrhagic Nodular Purpura
Hereditary Dystopic Lipidosis

Sign and Symptoms
Wart-like angiokeratomas typically appear over the lower trunk. Abdominal pain may develop, similar to that seen in appendicitis. There may be pain in the extremities (acroparesthesia) that lasts minutes to days, and episodic fever. Manifestations in the eyes include glycolipid deposits and contortion and dilation of the blood vessels. Symptomatic episodes increase with age, and kidney failure and cardiac or cerebral complications may develop as the patient ages.

The milder form of Fabry disease that develops in women is characterized by corneal opacities.

Etiology Fabry disease is X-linked, inherited as a recessive trait with variable penetrance. The condition is caused by alpha-galactosidase-A enzyme deficiency, which produces an accumulation of glycolipid products, particularly glycosphingolipid, in various tissues of the body.

Epidemiology Fabry disease primarily affects males, but also may affect heterozygous females in a milder form. Prevalence in the United States is estimated at 2500 persons.

Treatment—Standard Replacement of the deficient enzyme by transfusion has been tried but is not generally practical on a longterm basis. Treatment is otherwise symptomatic and supportive.

Treatment—Investigational A biotechnology process is being developed to manufacture the orphan drug ceramide trihexosidase/alpha-galactosidase-A as a treatment for Fabry disease. For more information: Dr. D. Calhoune, Department of Chemistry, City College of New York, Convent Ave. at 138th St., New York, NY 10031.

Please contact the agencies listed under Resources, below, for the most current

information.

Resources
For more information on Fabry disease: National Organization for Rare Disorders (NORD); National Lipid Diseases Foundation; National Tay-Sachs and Allied Diseases Association; NIH/National Institute of Neurological Disorders & Stroke (NINDS); Research Trust for Metabolic Diseases in Children.

For genetic information and genetic counseling referrals: March of Dimes Birth Defects Foundation; National Center for Education in Maternal and Child Health (NCEMCH).

References
Cecil Textbook Of Medicine, 18th ed.: J.B. Wyngaarden and L.H. Smith, Jr., eds.; W.B. Saunders Company, 1988, pp. 1144–1145.

FARBER DISEASE

Description Farber disease is characterized by the inability to produce lysosomal acid ceramidase, causing painful and progressive articular deformities.

Synonyms
Acid Ceramidase Deficiency
Farber Lipogranulomatosis

Signs and Symptoms Symptoms typically appear before 4 months of age. The first signs are swollen joints and a hoarse cry, skin that is sensitive to the touch, and finger flexion. Difficulty in breathing and swallowing, vomiting, and fever may also develop. Cardiac involvement occurs because of nodular growth around the valves. Nodules also are often found in the spleen, intestines, lymph nodes, kidney, tongue, thymus, gallbladder, and liver. The central nervous system is usually involved, and intelligence may or may not be normal.

Etiology The disease is due to deficiency of lysosomal acid ceramidase, and is inherited as an autosomal recessive trait.

Epidemiology Farber disease affects males and females equally.

Related Disorders Symptoms of juvenile rheumatoid arthritis may be similar to those of Farber disease and should be considered in the differential diagnosis.

Treatment—Standard Treatment is symptomatic and supportive. Corticosteroids may provide some relief for joint pain. Tracheostomy may be necessary if breathing passages become blocked by nodular growths. Cosmetic surgery may be desirable for growths in the facial area.

Genetic counseling is appropriate for patients and their families. Prenatal diagnosis by amniocentesis is possible during the 15th to 16th weeks of pregnancy.

Treatment—Investigational Please contact the agencies listed under Resources, below, for the most current information.

Resources

For more information on Farber disease: National Organization for Rare Disorders (NORD); Arthritis Foundation; The National Arthritis and Musculoskeletal and Skin Diseases Information Clearinghouse; Research Trust For Metabolic Diseases in Children.

For genetic information and genetic counseling referrals: March of Dimes Birth Defects Foundation; National Center for Education in Maternal and Child Health (NCEMCH).

References

The Metabolic Basis Of Inherited Disease, 5th ed.: J.B. Stanbury, et al., eds.; McGraw-Hill, 1983, pp. 820–829.

Internal Medicine, 2nd ed.: J.H. Stein, ed.; Little, Brown and Company, 1987, pp. 2073.

Annals of Rheumatic Disease: July 1987, issue 46(7), pp. 559–561.

Diagnosis of Lipogranulomatosis (Farber's Disease) by Use Of Cultured Fibroblasts: J.T.Dulaney, et al.; J. of Pediatr., July 1976, issue 89(1), pp. 59–61.

FORBES DISEASE

Description Forbes disease, a glycogen storage disease, is caused by a lack of the enzyme amylo-1,6-glucosidase. Excessive amounts of glycogen are accumulated in the liver and muscles, and cardiac involvement is seen in some cases.

Synonyms

Amylo-1,6-Glucosidase Deficiency
Cori Disease
Glycogen Storage Disease III
Glycogenosis Type III
Limit Dextrinosis

Signs and Symptoms During the first 4 to 6 years of life, manifestations of Forbes disease may be indistinguishable from those of von Gierke disease, although the latter tends to be more severe. The amount of glycogen in the liver and muscles is abnormally high. The liver is enlarged and the abdomen protrudes. The muscles are often flaccid.

Other findings include hypoglycemia that does not respond to glucagon administration, and hyperlipemia.

Some patients show only the protruding abdomen and enlarged liver. In these patients, the liver decreases in size progressively through adolescence and the symptoms disappear. Growth is slow during childhood and puberty may be delayed, but adult height is usually normal.

Diagnosis is made by detection of elevated glycogen on liver biopsy. White blood cells or fibroblasts can be used to assay for amylo-1,6-glucosidase deficiency.

Etiology Forbes disease is inherited as an autosomal recessive trait. Without activity of amylo-1,6-glucosidase, stored glycogen is only partially metabolized, and the resulting limit dextrin accumulates in liver and muscle tissues, producing the impaired glycemic response.

Epidemiology All glycogen storage diseases together affect fewer than 1:40,000 persons in the United States. Forbes disease usually begins during childhood, and males are found to be affected more often than females.

Related Disorders See *von Gierke Disease; Andersen Disease; Hers Disease.*

Treatment—Standard Treatment is aimed at prevention of hypoglycemia, with frequent small servings of carbohydrates and a high protein diet advised during the day. Nighttime continuous tube feeding of hydrolyzed protein, amino acid, or carbohydrate solutions may be needed to promote normal childhood growth.

Genetic counseling is required for families of children with Forbes disease and other glycogen storage diseases. Affected individuals can expect to live a normal life span, but muscle disorders may develop with age.

Treatment—Investigational Please contact the agencies listed under Resources, below, for the most current information.

Resources

For more information on Forbes disease: National Organization for Rare Disorders (NORD); National Institute of Diabetes, Digestive & Kidney Diseases Information Clearinghouse; Association for Glycogen Storage Diseases; Research Trust for Metabolic Diseases in Children.

For genetic information and genetic counseling referrals: March of Dimes Birth Defects Foundation; National Center for Education in Maternal and Child Health (NCEMCH).

References

Myopathy And Growth Failure In Debrancher Enzyme Deficiency: Improvement With High-Protein Nocturnal Enteral Therapy: A.E. Slonim, et al.; J. of Pediatr., December 1984, issue 105(6), pp. 906–911.

Neuromuscular Involvement In Glycogen Storage Disease Type III: S.W. Moses, et al.; Acta Paediatr. Scand., March 1986, issue 75(2), pp. 289–296.

FRUCTOSE INTOLERANCE, HEREDITARY

Description Hereditary fructose intolerance is an inherited disorder characterized by an inability to metabolize fructose or its precursors. The metabolic error results from a deficiency of the enzyme fructose-1-phosphate aldolase.

Synonyms

Fructose-1-Phosphate Aldolase Deficiency

Fructosemia

Fructosuria

Signs and Symptoms Manifestations of the disease begin shortly after birth. Addition of fructose to the diet of an affected infant will produce prolonged vomiting, failure to thrive, coma, jaundice, and hepatomegaly. A bleeding tendency occurs because of a deficiency in clotting factors. Blood levels of glucose and phosphate are lowered, and levels of fructose in the blood and urine are increased. Patients with hereditary fructose intolerance usually develop an aversion for fruit and sweets.

Early recognition is important to avoid damage to the liver, kidney, and small intestine. There may be intellectual impairment.

Etiology Hereditary fructose intolerance is caused by a deficiency of the enzyme fructose-1-phosphate aldolase. It is inherited as an autosomal recessive trait.

Epidemiology Hereditary fructose intolerance occurs equally in males and females.

Related Disorders See *Fructosuria*.

Treatment—Standard As long as patients with hereditary fructose intolerance do not ingest fructose or fructose-containing sugars, such as sucrose, they can remain asymptomatic.

Treatment—Investigational Please contact the agencies listed under Resources, below, for the most current information.

Resources

For more information on hereditary fructose intolerance: National Organization for Rare Disorders (NORD); National Institute of Diabetes, Digestive & Kidney Diseases Information Clearinghouse.

For genetic information and genetic counseling referrals: March of Dimes Birth Defects Foundation; National Center for Education in Maternal and Child Health (NCEMCH).

References

The Metabolic Basis of Inherited Disease, 6th ed.: C.R. Scriver, et al., eds.; McGraw-Hill, 1989, pp. 399, 407–413.

FRUCTOSURIA

Description Fructosuria, characterized by urinary excretion of fructose, is caused by a deficiency of hepatic fructokinase, which is needed for the synthesis of glycogen from fructose.

Synonyms

Essential Fructosuria
Hepatic Fructokinase Deficiency
Levulosuria

Signs and Symptoms Fructosuria is marked only by the presence of fructose in the urine, which is the basis for the diagnosis. It is a benign heritable trait that causes no symptoms.

Etiology The disorder is rare. It is inherited as an autosomal recessive trait.

Epidemiology Fructosuria affects approximately 1:130,000 persons in the United States, and occurs equally in males and females.

Related Disorders Because fructose in the urine may be mistaken for glucose, fructosuria should be differentiated from diabetes mellitus.

Treatment—Standard Treatment is not required.

Treatment—Investigational Please contact the agencies listed under Resources, below, for the most current information.

Resources

For more information on fructosuria: National Organization for Rare Disorders (NORD); National Institute of Diabetes, Digestive & Kidney Diseases Information Clearinghouse; Research Trust for Metabolic Diseases in Children.

For genetic information and genetic counseling referrals: March of Dimes Birth Defects Foundation; National Center for Education in Maternal and Child Health (NCEMCH).

References

Mendelian Inheritance in Man, 7th ed.: V.A. McKusick; The Johns Hopkins University Press, 1986, p. 978.

Essential Fructosuria, Hereditary Fructose Intolerance, and Fructose-1,6-Diphosphatase Deficiency: R. Gitzelmann, et al.; *in* The Metabolic Basis of Inherited Disease, 5th ed.: J.B. Stanbury, et al.; McGraw-Hill, 1983, pp. 118–140.

GALACTOSEMIA, CLASSIC

Description Classic galactosemia is a disorder in newborns of galactose metabolism. If untreated, the prognosis is poor.

Synonyms

Galactose-1-Phosphate Uridyl Transferase Deficiency

Signs and Symptoms Clinical manifestations appear early in the newborn period and include vomiting, jaundice, hepatomegaly, hypoglycemia, irritability, listlessness, aminoaciduria, ascites, mental retardation, and cataracts. If treatment is not begun when the symptoms first appear, hepatic cirrhosis, severe mental retardation, growth deficiency, and overwhelming infection can ensue.

Girls with galactosemia may develop impaired ovarian function.

Some cases of classic galactosemia are mild, with few symptoms and without severe impairment.

Pregnant women who are asymptomatic carriers can be detected by testing the activity of galactose-1-phosphate uridyl transferase in their red blood cells. Galactosemia can be diagnosed in infants at birth by determining the enzyme activity level in red blood cells.

Etiology Classic galactosemia is inherited as an autosomal recessive trait. Deficiency of the enzyme galactose-1-phosphate uridyl transferase results in the infant's inability to metabolize galactose, and leads to accumulation of galactose-1-phosphate.

Epidemiology The incidence is about 1:50,000. Males and females are affected in equal numbers.

Treatment—Standard After birth, an affected infant's diet should contain galactose and lactose-free milk substitutes and foods such as casein hydrolysates and soy bean products. Strict dietary restriction should be maintained until the child is at least 2 years old, and preferably 6 years of age. Appropriate treatment may be necessary to control intercurrent infections. Emotional effects of the strict diet may require attention throughout childhood. Genetic counseling is recommended for families of galactosemia patients.

Liver and kidney failure, brain damage, and cataracts can be prevented through avoidance of galactose. Children treated with this special diet usually show satisfactory general health and growth, and can make reasonable though often not optimal intellectual progress.

Treatment—Investigational Please contact the agencies listed under Resources, below, for the most current information.

Resources
For more information on galactosemia: National Organization for Rare Disorders (NORD); Parents of Galactosemic Children, Inc.; National Institute of Diabetes, Digestive & Kidney Diseases Information Clearinghouse; Research Trust for Metabolic Diseases in Children.

For genetic information and genetic counseling referrals: March of Dimes Birth Defects Foundation; National Center for Education in Maternal and Child Health (NCEMCH).

References
Nelson Textbook of Pediatrics, 13th ed.: R.E. Behrman and V.C. Vaughan, III, eds.; W.B. Saunders Company, 1987, pp. 308–309.
Galactosemia: How Does Long-Term Treatment Change the Outcome?: R. Gitzelmann, et al.; Enzyme, 1984, issue 32(1), pp. 37–46.

GAUCHER DISEASE

Description Gaucher disease is the most common of the lipid storage diseases, which include Tay-Sachs, Fabry, and Niemann-Pick diseases. There are 3 forms of Gaucher disease: Type I (nonneuronopathic); Type II (acute neuronopathic, or infantile cerebral); Type III (subacute neuronopathic).

Synonyms
Cerebroside Lipidosis
Familial Splenic Anemia

Gaucher-Schlagenhaufer
Glucosyl Ceramide Lipidosis

Signs and Symptoms In **Type I** Gaucher disease, bone deterioration is a prominent finding. Other symptoms and signs include hepatomegaly, splenomegaly, and anemia. Rare manifestations may include renal and pulmonary involvement.

In **Type II,** symptoms and signs include hepatomegaly or splenomegaly and neurologic manifestations such as hyperextension of the head, neck rigidity, apathy, catatonia, strabismus, increased deep reflexes, laryngeal spasm, and mental retardation.

In **Type III,** symptoms and signs are similar to those of Type I but also include central nervous system findings such as seizures, mental retardation, and abnormal movements of the eyes, limbs, and head.

A diagnostic assay is available to detect affected persons and carriers, and the condition can also be diagnosed with amniocentesis.

Etiology All types of Gaucher disease are inherited as autosomal recessive traits and are caused by failure to produce the enzyme glucocerebrosidase. All are characterized by the presence of Gaucher (lipid-laden) cells in the bone marrow and other organs, e.g., the spleen and liver.

Epidemiology Type I affects both men and women, with onset at any age, although most patients are in their late teens. A high proportion of Ashkenazi Jews are affected.

Type II is a rare form of the disease with onset usually in the first few months of life. Both sexes are affected, with a slight prevalence in males. There is no racial prevalence.

Type III, the rarest form of Gaucher disease, may be variable in its age of onset but usually begins during childhood and adolescence. Both sexes are affected.

All types of Gaucher disease together affect between 20,000 and 40,000 people worldwide.

Treatment—Standard Treatment is symptomatic and supportive. When circumstances warrant, total or partial splenectomy and joint replacement may be considered.

The orphan drug Ceredase (glucocerebrosidase/beta-glucosidase) was approved by the FDA in April 1991 for use in Type I Gaucher disease. For further information Genzyme Corporation may be contacted at (800) 332-1042.

Treatment—Investigational The National Institutes of Health **(NIH)** have established a program to study neurogenetic and lysosomal storage disorders. Patients included in these studies may be evaluated at the NIH through the Interinstitute Medical Genetics Clinic as well as the Molecular Neurogenetics Unit, Clinical Neuroscience Branch, National Institute of Mental Health (NIMH); and the Human Genetics Branch, National Institute of Child Health and Human Development (NICHHD). For further information, please contact Patient Care Coordinator, Human Genetics Branch, NIH/National Institute of Child Health and Human Development, Bethesda, Maryland 20892; (301) 496-7661.

For research on replacement enzymes in bone marrow transplantations, contact Robert Desnick, M.D., Division of Medical Genetics, Mount Sinai Hospital, Annenberg Building, Room 17-76, 100th Street and 5th Avenue, New York, NY 10029.

Robert E. Lee, M.D. is compiling a database dealing with the disease. He can be contacted at the University of Pittsburgh Medical School, Department of Pathology, Pittsburgh, Pennsylvania 15261.

Please contact the agencies listed under Resources, below, for the most current information.

Resources

For more information on Gaucher disease: National Organization for Rare Disorders (NORD); National Gaucher Foundation; NIH/National Institute of Neurological Disorders and Stroke; National Lipid Diseases Foundation.

For genetic information and genetic counseling referrals: March of Dimes Birth Defects Foundation; National Center for Education in Maternal and Child Health (NCEMCH).

References

The Metabolic Basis of Inherited Diseases, 6th ed.: C.R. Scriver, et al., eds.; McGraw-Hill, 1989, pp. 1677–1698.

Mendelian Inheritance in Man, 9th ed.: V.A. McKusick; The John Hopkins University Press, 1990, pp. 1200–1204.

GLUTARICACIDURIA I (GA I)

Description GA I is an enzyme deficiency disorder characterized by dystonia and dyskinesia. Mental retardation also may occur.

Synonyms

Glutaricacidemia I
Glutaryl-CoA Dehydrogenase Deficiency

Signs and Symptoms Affected individuals usually appear normal at birth. During the first year of life, disease manifestations may begin to be seen, including vomiting, metabolic acidosis, and hypotonia. Opisthotonus, dystonia, and chronic athetotic and choreic movements are observed in some patients. Mental retardation may be present, and some patients have unusual facies.

Elevated concentrations of glutaric acid, beta-hydroxyglutaric acid, and occasionally glutaconic acid may be found in the urine. Excretion of glutaric acid may exceed 1 gram per day. Glutaric acid concentrations are also elevated in blood serum, cerebrospinal fluid, and body tissues.

Glutaricaciduria can be diagnosed by the finding of excessive glutaric acid in the urine, or by analysis of the deficient enzyme in leukocytes. Fetal detection is possible by testing amniocytes for the enzyme glutaryl-CoA dehydrogenase.

Etiology Glutaricaciduria, one of the organic acidemias, is inherited as an autosomal recessive trait. The condition is caused by a deficiency of the enzyme glutaryl-CoA dehydrogenase. Accumulation of 5-carbon dicarboxylic acids may secondarily impair synthesis of gamma-aminobutyric acid (GABA), which functions as a neurotransmitter in the brain, inhibiting nerve excitation.

Many of the adverse effects of the organic acidemias are due to carnitine depletion.

Epidemiology Males and females are affected equally. There are fewer than 100 cases of this type of organic aciduria known in the United States.

Related Disorders See *Glutaricaciduria II.*

Treatment—Standard See as in *Glutaricaciduria II.*

Peritoneal dialysis or hemodialysis may be necessary. The usefulness of dietary restriction of lysine (which is oxidized via glutaric acid) has not been established. Acute episodes of metabolic acidosis and dehydration are treated with intravenous fluids and bicarbonate.

Patients with suspected secondary carnitine deficiency should have plasma carnitine measured. If a deficiency is present, supplementation with 100-300 mg/kg/day of oral L-carnitine is recommended.

Genetic counseling is mandatory for families of children with glutaricaciduria.

Treatment—Investigational An experimental regimen for the treatment of glutaricaciduria involves a low protein or low lysine diet, and the administration of riboflavin and baclofen, a gamma-aminobutyric acid (GABA) analyst. Diet and riboflavin have had inconsistent effects on the clinical symptoms. Urinary excretion of glutaric acid markedly decreased with this treatment. Some neurologic symptoms improved during treatment with baclofen. Longterm effects of this therapy are unknown.

Please contact the agencies listed under Resources, below, for the most current information.

Resources

For more information on glutaricaciduria I: National Organization for Rare Disorders (NORD); National Urea Cycle Disorders Foundation; Saul Brusilow, M.D., Johns Hopkins Hospital; British Organic Acidemia Association; Research Trust for Metabolic Disorders in Children.

For genetic information and genetic counseling referrals: March of Dimes Birth Defects Foundation; National Center for Education in Maternal and Child Health (NCEMCH).

References

The Metabolic Basis of Inherited Disease: C.R. Scriver, et al., eds.; McGraw-Hill, 1989, pp. 845–853.

Symptomatic Inborn Errors of Metabolism in the Neonate: S.W. Brusilow and D.L. Vallee; *in* Current Therapy in Neonatal-Perinatal Medicine, Marcel Decker, 1985, pp. 24–27.

Treatment of Glutaryl-CoA Dehydrogenase Deficiency (Glutaric Aciduria). Experience with Diet, Riboflavin, and Gaba Analog: N.J. Brandt, et al.; J. of Pediatr., April 1979, issue 94(4), pp. 669–673.

GLUTARICACIDURIA II (GA II)

Description GA II, one of the organic acidemias, manifests in 2 forms. The more serious neonatal form (IIA), with or without congenital anomalies, is characterized by large amounts of glutaric and other acids in blood and urine. Severe disease may cause newborn death within a few weeks. The milder later-onset form (IIB) is associated with metabolic acidosis, and hypoglycemia without ketosis.

Synonyms
Electron Transfer Flavoprotein (ETF) Deficiency
Multiple Acyl-CoA Dehydrogenation Deficiency

Signs and Symptoms The neonatal form, GA IIA, the more severe condition, may or may not be associated with congenital anomalies.

In newborns with congenital anomalies, onset of severe hypoglycemia, metabolic acidosis, hypotonia, hepatomegaly, and, often, the odor of sweaty feet occurs within the first 2 days of life. Congenital anomalies include hypoplastic midface, hypertelorism, low-set ears, abdominal wall defects, and hypospadias. The organic acids glutaric, lactic, butyric, isobutyric, 2-methylbutyric, ethylmalonic, adipic, and isovaleric, are produced during oxidation of amino acids and accumulate in the plasma in very high amounts. These infants may not survive their first week.

Initial symptoms and signs and disease course seen in newborns without congenital anomalies are similar to the above. In some instances manifestations are milder and infants survive for a longer period.

In the later-onset form, GA IIB, initial manifestations may first occur anywhere between a few weeks or years of life to adulthood. A patient with this form presented with vomiting, hypoglycemia, and acidosis at 7 weeks of age. Others have been symptom-free until adulthood, when vomiting, severe hypoglycemia, and fatty infiltration of the liver were seen. One sibling of a woman with GA IIB had only nausea, and a stale odor to her breath, but then developed hypoglycemic coma. Another sibling of this patient had jaundice, hepatomegaly, and hypoglycemia. Excessive amounts of glutaric and ethylmalonic acids were excreted in the urine of the latter 3 related patients.

Glutaricaciduria can be diagnosed by the findings of excessive glutaric acid in the urine, or by analysis of the deficient enzyme in leukocytes. Fetal detection is possible by testing for acyl-CoA dehydrogenase; otherwise, it is imperative that testing be done as soon after birth as possible.

Etiology Each form of GA II is inherited as an autosomal recessive trait, and each is caused by deficiency of an element (electron transfer flavoprotein—**ETF;** or electron transfer flavoprotein ubiquinone oxidoreductase—**ETF-QO**) common to all 3 acyl-CoA dehydrogenase enzymes.

Many of the adverse effects of organic acidemias are due to secondary carnitine depletion.

Epidemiology Males and females are affected equally.

Related Disorders See *Glutaricaciduria I; Medium-Chain Acyl-CoA Dehy-*

drogenase Deficiency.

Treatment—Standard GA IIA is usually fatal for newborns with immediate signs of severe disease, even when there are no congenital anomalies. The usefulness of restricting the amino acids lysine, hydroxylysine, and tryptophan (which generate glutaric acid) has not been established. Acute metabolic acidosis and dehydration are treated with fluids and bicarbonate.

For patients with milder disease, dietary restriction of protein and fat together with administration of riboflavin and carnitine has had some success.

Patients with secondary carnitine depletion should have plasma carnitine measured. If it is deficient, a supplement of 100-300 mg/kg/day of oral L-carnitine should be started.

Genetic counseling is recommended for families of patients with glutaricaciduria II.

Treatment—Investigational Please contact the agencies listed under Resources, below, for the most current information.

Resources
For more information on glutaricaciduria: National Organization for Rare Disorders (NORD); Lactic Acidosis Support Group; National Urea Cycle Disorders Foundation; Saul Brusilow, M.D., Johns Hopkins Hospital; British Organic Acidemia Association; Research Trust for Metabolic Disorders in Children.

For genetic information and genetic counseling referrals: March of Dimes Birth Defects Foundation; National Center for Education in Maternal and Child Health (NCEMCH).

References
The Metabolic Basis of Inherited Disease, 6th ed.: C.R. Scriver, et al., eds.; McGraw-Hill, 1989, pp. 923–931.
Symptomatic Inborn Errors of Metabolism in the Neonate: S.W. Brusilow and D.L. Vallee; *in* Current Therapy in Neonatal-Perinatal Medicine: Marcel Decker, 1985, pp. 24–27.

GLYCOGEN STORAGE DISEASE VII (GSD VII)

Description GSD VII is characterized by a deficiency of the enzyme phosphofructokinase-I in muscle and a partial deficiency of the enzyme in red blood cells. This deficiency prevents the metabolism of glucose into available energy during exercise.

Synonyms
> Glycogen Disease of Muscle
> Glycogenosis Type VII
> Muscle Phosphofructokinase Deficiency
> Phosphofructokinase Deficiency
> Tarui Disease

Signs and Symptoms Patients experience easy fatigability, and on strenuous exercise, muscular pain and cramps and myoglobinuria, which is usually not severe. Hyperuricemia accompanies exercise, and other manifestations include gout and recurrent jaundice. Like McArdle disease, there is no hyperglycemia.

Etiology GSD VII is inherited as an autosomal recessive trait.

Epidemiology Onset is in childhood, and males and females are affected in equal numbers.

Related Disorders See *McArdle Disease; Pompe Disease; Forbes Disease.*

Treatment—Standard Treatment of GSD VII is symptomatic and supportive. Avoidance of strenuous exercise will prevent muscle pain and cramps.

Treatment—Investigational Please contact the agencies listed under Resources, below, for the most current information.

Resources

For more information on GSD VII: National Organization for Rare Disorders (NORD); Association for Glycogen Storage Disease; National Institute of Diabetes, Digestive & Kidney Diseases Information Clearinghouse; Research Trust for Metabolic Diseases in Children.

For genetic information and genetic counseling referrals: March of Dimes Birth Defects Foundation; National Center for Education in Maternal and Child Health (NCEMCH).

References

The Metabolic Basis of Inherited Disease, 6th ed.: C.R. Scriver, et al., eds.; McGraw-Hill, 1989, pp. 445–446.

Excess Purine Degradation in Exercising Muscles of Patients with Muscle Glycogen Storage Disease Types V and VII: I. Mineo, et al.; J. Clin. Invest., August 1985, issue 76(2), pp. 556–560.

Hartnup Disease

Description Hartnup disease is a rare metabolic disorder that involves an error of neutral amino acid transport. Intermittent episodes of skin rash and ataxia are the primary clinical features.

Synonyms

Pellagra-Cerebellar Ataxia-Renal Aminoaciduria Syndrome

Signs and Symptoms The disease is characterized by a red, scaly rash that typically occurs after exposure to sunlight. Sudden attacks of ataxia, double vision, and fainting may occur. If left untreated, retarded mental development, short stature, emotional instability, and dementia may develop. Mild arrhythmias may also occur in untreated cases, but are extremely rare.

Etiology Hartnup disease is an inborn error of renal and intestinal amino acid transport involving tryptophan and the other neutral amino acids. The condition is inherited as an autosomal recessive trait. Genetic evaluation of children born to mothers affected by Hartnup disease suggests that the abnormal metabolism of amino acids in this disorder does not have an adverse effect on the fetus.

Epidemiology Hartnup disease usually begins in childhood and continues into adulthood; males and females seem to be affected equally. The condition occurs in approximately 1:24,000 newborns.

Related Disorders See *Acidemia, Methylmalonic.*

Pellagra results from a deficiency of nicotinic acid. Generalized manifestations of pellagra include anorexia, diarrhea, constipation, weakness, and emotional instability. Cutaneous manifestations of the disorder include burning or stinging after exposure to the sun, scaliness or roughness, and reddish-brown coloration. There also may be soreness of the oral cavity. Pellagra tends to occur in countries where corn is the staple food, and is very rare in the United States.

Treatment—Standard Symptomatic episodes of Hartnup disease can be minimized with good nutrition and 50 to 300 mg/day of nicotinamide. Avoidance of the sun and sulfonamide drugs is also indicated. Treatment of episodes is symptomatic and supportive. Genetic counseling may be appropriate for affected families.

Treatment—Investigational Please contact the agencies listed under Resources, below, for the most current information.

Resources

For more information on Hartnup disease: National Organization for Rare Disorders (NORD); National Institute of Diabetes, Digestive & Kidney Diseases Information Clearinghouse; Research Trust for Metabolic Diseases in Children.

For genetic information and genetic counseling referrals: March of Dimes Birth Defects Foundation; National Center for Education in Maternal and Child Health (NCEMCH).

References
The Metabolic Basis of Inherited Disease, 6th ed.: C.R. Scriver, et al., eds.; 1989, pp. 2516–2527.
Maternal Hartnup Disorder: B.E. Mahon, et al.; Am. J. Med. Genet., July 1986, issue 24(3), pp. 513–518.
Occurrences of Methylmalonic Aciduria and Hartnup Disorder in the Same Family: V.E. Shih, et al.; Clin. Genet., September 1984, issue 26(3), pp. 216–220.

HERS DISEASE

Description Hers disease is a hereditary glycogen storage disease manifested by milder symptoms than most other glycogen storage diseases. Characteristics include hepatomegaly and ketosis, and moderate hypoglycemia and growth retardation. Symptoms and signs may not be apparent during childhood, and affected individuals can often lead normal lives. In some cases, however, symptoms are more severe.

Synonyms

Glycogen Storage Disease VI
Glycogenosis Type VI
Hepatophosphorylase Deficiency Glycogenosis
Liver Phosphorylase Deficiency
Phosphorylase *b* Kinase Deficiency

Signs and Symptoms The mild-to-moderate hypoglycemia of Hers disease can cause faintness, weakness, hunger, and nervousness. Other findings may include hepatomegaly caused by accumulation of glycogen in the liver, and slowing of the growth rate. In many instances, the person can adapt to hypoglycemia and will remain asymptomatic for long periods.

The specific diagnosis can be established by liver biopsy and assay for phosphorylase activity.

Etiology Hers disease is heterogeneous, and is inherited as either an autosomal recessive or X-linked trait. Symptoms result from deficiency of phosphorylase *b* kinase, which leads to hepatic accumulation of glycogen, and hypoglycemia.

Epidemiology All glycogen storage diseases together affect fewer than 1:40,000 persons in the United States. Manifestations of Hers disease may not be noticed until adulthood.

Related Disorders See *von Gierke Disease; Forbes Disease; Andersen Disease.*

Treatment—Standard Symptoms of Hers disease are generally mild, and the patient usually requires no specific treatment. Avoidance of prolonged fasting, and regular monitoring by a physician are recommended. Genetic counseling is mandatory.

Treatment—Investigational Please contact the agencies listed under Resources, below, for the most current information.

Resources

For more information on Hers disease: National Organization for Rare Disorders (NORD); Association for Glycogen Storage Diseases; Research Trust for Metabolic Diseases in Children; National Institute of Diabetes, Digestive & Kidney Diseases Information Clearinghouse.

For genetic information and genetic counseling referrals: March of Dimes Birth Defects Foundation; National Center for Education in Maternal and Child Health (NCEMCH).

References

The Metabolic Basis of Inherited Disease, 6th ed.: C.R. Scriver, et al., eds.; McGraw-Hill, 1989, pp. 444–445.

Cecil Textbook of Medicine, 18th ed.: J.B. Wyngaarden and L.H. Smith, Jr., eds.: W.B. Saunders Company, 1988, p. 425.

HISTIDINEMIA

Description Deficiency of the enzyme histidase, required for oxidation of the amino acid histidine, results in elevated concentrations of histidine in the blood, and excessive amounts of histidine, imidazole pyruvic acid, and other imidazole metabolism products excreted in the urine. Mental retardation and a speech defect have been thought to be associated with some cases of histidinemia, although this is now believed to be an artifact of ascertainment.

Synonyms
Histidase Deficiency

Signs and Symptoms Early cases of histidinemia were identified by such features as mental retardation, speech defects, seizures, unusual behavior, and learning disabilities. It is now known, however, that histidinemia occurs in clinically normal persons.

Etiology The disorder is inherited as an autosomal recessive trait.

Epidemiology Histidinemia occurs in about 1:20,000 births, with males and females affected equally.

Related Disorders Histidinuria, characterized by abnormally high amounts of histidine in the urine, is due to a defect of histidine reabsorption in the renal distal tubules. The disorder is inherited as an autosomal recessive trait, and is very rare.

Treatment—Standard Benign cases of histidinemia require no treatment. Speech therapy can be helpful, if appropriate, and genetic counseling is beneficial.

Treatment—Investigational Please contact the agencies listed under Resources, below, for the most current information.

Resources
   For more information on histidinemia: National Organization for Rare Disorders (NORD); National Institute of Diabetes, Digestive & Kidney Diseases Information Clearinghouse; Research Trust for Metabolic Diseases in Children.
   For genetic information and genetic counseling referrals: March of Dimes Birth Defects Foundation; National Center for Education in Maternal and Child Health (NCEMCH).

References
   The Metabolic Basis of Inherited Disease, 6th ed.; C.R. Scriver, et al., eds.; McGraw-Hill, 1989, pp. 566–572.

HOMOCYSTINURIA

Description Homocystinuria is a metabolic disorder characterized by abnormal amounts of homocystine and methionine in blood, cerebrospinal fluid, and urine.

Synonyms
Homocystinemia
Cystathionine Beta-Synthase Deficiency

Signs and Symptoms Manifestations of homocystinuria include ectopia lentis, zonal cataracts, osteoporosis, seizures, mental retardation, pulmonary embolism, and coronary occlusion. Patients may have the signs and symptoms of Marfan syndrome (e.g., elongated body and extremities, pectus excavatum, and cardiovascular defects—see *Marfan Syndrome).*

Etiology Homocystinuria is inherited as an autosomal recessive trait. Symptoms are caused by an inborn error of amino acid metabolism resulting from deficiency of the enzyme cystathionine beta-synthase.

Epidemiology Onset is at birth. Males and females are affected in equal numbers. Like other inborn errors of metabolism, homocystinuria is a very rare disorder.

Related Disorders Cystathioninuria is a genetic disorder transmitted through autosomal recessive genes. It is characterized by a deficiency of gamma-cystathionase leading to increased amounts of cystathionine in the urine. Mental retardation may occur.

Treatment—Standard Treatment for homocystinuria consists of a methionine-restricted diet supplemented with cystine. Pharmacologic doses of pyridoxine may also be beneficial. Genetic counseling will be helpful for families of affected children.

Treatment—Investigational Betaine treatment for homocystinuria is being investigated.

Please contact the agencies listed under Resources, below, for the most current information.

Resources
For more information on homocystinuria: National Organization for Rare Disorders (NORD); National Institute of Diabetes, Digestive & Kidney Diseases Information Clearinghouse.

For genetic information and genetic counseling referrals: March of Dimes Birth Defects Foundation; National Center for Education in Maternal and Child Health (NCEMCH).

References
The Metabolic Basis of Inherited Disease, 6th ed.: C.R. Scriver, et al., eds.; McGraw-Hill, 1989, pp. 693–699, 715–717.

HUNTER SYNDROME

Description Hunter syndrome (mucopolysaccharidosis type II—**MPS II**) occurs in 2 forms, mild and severe, both with the same enzymatic deficiency of iduronate sulfatase.

Synonyms
Mucopolysaccharidosis Type II

Signs and Symptoms Onset of symptoms in patients with the severe form usually occurs from ages 2 to 4 years, with mental and physical progressive deterioration thereafter. Facial features become coarsened, and a short neck, widely spaced teeth, and hearing loss are also often present. Whitish nodular skin lesions may occur on the arm or back. Hydrocephalus is commonly seen after 4 years of age. Recurrent upper respiratory infections, diarrhea, hepatomegaly, joint stiffness, growth failure, and mental retardation are typical features of the severe form of Hunter syndrome. The syndrome is often fatal between 7 and 10 years of age, usually from neurologic and cardiopulmonary disease.

In the mild form of Hunter syndrome, mental function is usually normal and physical deterioration is greatly reduced. Complications include coronary and valvular disease and hearing impairment. Carpal tunnel syndrome and joint stiffness can result in loss of hand function. Some patients succumb to cardiopulmonary disease as young adults, while others survive into their 70s.

Hunter syndrome can be diagnosed prenatally.

Etiology The syndrome is inherited as an X-linked recessive trait. Deficiency of the enzyme iduronate sulfatase results in an inability to metabolize mucopolysaccharides. The accumulation of large, undegraded mucopolysaccharides in the cells of the body causes the physical and mental deterioration.

Epidemiology Only males are affected. The disorder occurs in 1:100,000 live births.

Related Disorders See *Hydrocephalus.*

The severe form of Hunter syndrome has features similar to those of Hurler syndrome except for the lack of corneal clouding and slower progression of physical involvement and mental retardation. See *Hurler Syndrome.*

The mucolipidoses are a family of similar disorders, producing symptoms very much like those of the mucopolysaccharidoses. See *Mucopolysaccharidosis; Mucolipidosis II; Mucolipidosis III; Mucolipidosis IV.*

Treatment—Standard Treatment of Hunter syndrome is symptomatic and supportive. Hernias may require surgical intervention. Implantation of a ventricular shunt may be needed for hydrocephalus. Hearing devices, physical therapy, and genetic counseling services may be helpful for patients and their families.

Treatment—Investigational Treatments aimed at checking early development of Hunter syndrome are now being studied. Approaches include enzyme replacement therapy and bone marrow transplantation.

Please contact the agencies listed under Resources, below, for the most current information.

Resources
For more information on Hunter syndrome: Joseph Muenzer, M.D., University of Michigan; National Organization for Rare Disorders (NORD); National

MPS Society; MPS (Mucopolysaccharidoses) Research Funding Center, Inc.; Society of Mucopolysaccharide Diseases, Inc.; Society of MPS Diseases; National Institute of Diabetes, Digestive and Kidney Diseases Information Clearinghouse.

For genetic information and genetic counseling referrals: March of Dimes Birth Defects Foundation; National Center for Education in Maternal and Child Health (NCEMCH).

References
The Metabolic Basis of Inherited Disease, 6th ed.: C.R. Scriver, et al., eds.; McGraw-Hill, 1989, pp. 1573–1574.

MPS Society brochure.

MPS Research Funding Center Bulletin.

HURLER SYNDROME

Description Hurler syndrome (mucopolysaccharidosis type I—**MPS I**) appears in 3 forms of varying severity. Hurler syndrome (MPS I-H) is the most severe; Scheie syndrome (MPS I-S) is milder; and Hurler/Scheie syndrome (MPS I-H/S) is considered to be the intermediate form.

Synonyms
Mucopolysaccharidosis Type I

Signs and Symptoms Newborns with Hurler syndrome (MPS I-H) usually appear normal, although inguinal and umbilical hernias may be present. Onset of symptoms occurs from 6 months to 2 years of age. Craniofacial abnormalities occurring at this time include coarse facial features, a prominent forehead, macroglossia, misaligned teeth, and clouding of the cornea. Also evident are recurrent upper respiratory infections, noisy breathing, and a persistent nasal discharge. Hydrocephalus appears after 2 to 3 years of age. Developmental delay becomes apparent from 1 to 2 years of age. The child is short of stature, and mental retardation is progressive thereafter. Joint stiffness is severe, resulting in claw hand, and kyphoscoliosis and hepatomegaly may develop.

Hurler/Scheie syndrome (MPS I-H/S), the intermediate form, is characterized by normal intelligence but progressive physical involvement that is milder than in Hurler syndrome. Corneal clouding, joint stiffness, deafness, and valvular heart disease can develop by the early to mid teens.

In Scheie syndrome (MPS I-S), the mild form, stature, intelligence, and life expectancy are normal. Onset of symptoms such as stiff joints, clouding of the cornea, and aortic valvular disease and/or stenosis usually occurs after 5 years of age, but diagnosis often is not made until the patient is 10 to 20 years.

Diagnosis can be made prenatally.

Etiology The 3 forms of Hurler syndrome described above are autosomal recessive, and all are due to alpha-L-iduronidase deficiency.

Epidemiology Males and females tend to be affected equally. Incidence is approximately 1:100,000 live births.

Related Disorders See *Hydrocephalus; Mucopolysaccharidosis.*

The mucolipidoses are a family of similar disorders, producing symptoms very much like those of MPS. Mucolipidosis II resembles Hurler syndrome; the 2 disorders are very difficult to distinguish. (See *Mucolipidosis II.)*

Treatment—Standard Treatment is symptomatic and supportive. Physical therapy and medical and genetic counseling services may be useful to patient and family.

Treatment—Investigational Treatment approaches for checking early development of MPS are under study. These include enzyme replacement therapy and bone marrow transplantation.

Please contact the agencies listed under Resources, below, for the most current information.

Resources

For more information on Hurler syndrome: National Organization for Rare Disorders (NORD); MPS (Mucopolysaccharidoses) Research Funding Center, Inc.; National MPS Society; National Institute of Diabetes, Digestive & Kidney Diseases Information Clearinghouse; Society of Mucopolysaccharide Diseases, Inc.; Society of MPS Diseases.

For genetic information and genetic counseling referrals: March of Dimes Birth Defects Foundation; National Center for Education in Maternal and Child Health (NCEMCH).

References

The Metabolic Basis of Inherited Disease, 6th ed.: C.R. Scriver, et al., eds.; McGraw-Hill, 1989, pp. 1573–1574.

HYPERCHYLOMICRONEMIA

Description Hyperchylomicronemia is a rare hereditary inborn error of metabolism caused by the absence of the enzyme lipoprotein lipase. The disorder is characterized by a massive accumulation of chylomicrons in blood plasma following consumption of dietary fats, and a corresponding increase of the blood plasma concentration of triglycerides (greater than 2000 mg/dl). The concentration of very low density lipoprotein **(VLDL)** is normal, distinguishing type I from type V chylomicronemia.

Synonyms

Buerger-Gruetz Syndrome
Essential Familial Hyperlipemia
Exogenous Hypertriglyceridemia
Fat-Induced Hyperlipemia
Fredrickson Type I Hyperlipoproteinemia
Hyperlipidemia I
Hyperlipoproteinemia Type I

Retention Hyperlipemia

Signs and Symptoms The disorder initially is characterized by eruptive xanthomas, which are raised, whitish-yellow nodules containing a milky fluid, on a red base. These lesions may vary from 0.1 to 0.3 inches in diameter, but may cluster and form large plaques. The number of nodules can range from few to hundreds. They are generally located on the buttocks, shoulders, and extremities, although sometimes they are also found on the face and mucous membranes. These eruptive xanthomas are neither painful nor itchy, and the patient may mistake them for acne. The nodules typically appear with an increased level of triglycerides in the blood, and disappear when the triglyceride level decreases.

Some patients also experience gastrointestinal symptoms, including anorexia, nausea, abdominal distension, diarrhea, and abdominal pain. Pancreatitis, sometimes with bleeding, often occurs when triglyceride levels are excessively high. Hepatomegaly and splenomegaly may occur, particularly in infants and children. Macrophages that have incorporated chylomicrons are sometimes seen in the spleen and bone marrow of these patients.

Ocular findings include a milky or "tomato juice" appearance in the retinal blood vessels; and the fundus may appear pale pink upon ophthalmologic examination. The retina may contain white fatty deposits, and circulation may be disturbed, with narrowing of the blood vessels and bleeding. Vision can be adversely affected.

Etiology The disorder is transmitted as an autosomal recessive trait. The specific metabolic error is a deficiency of the enzyme lipoprotein lipase.

Epidemiology Hyperchylomicronemia is a very rare disorder, present at birth, which affects males and females in equal numbers. It is estimated to affect 20,000 adults in the United States.

Related Disorders Hyperlipoproteinemia type V (mixed hyperlipemia) is characterized by an excessive amount of chylomicrons in the blood. High levels of prebetalipoproteins are also present. The blood plasma has a milky white appearance, and VLDL is also elevated. The disorder is thought to be inherited as a recessive trait.

Familial apolipoprotein C-II deficiency is a rare autosomal recessive hereditary disorder characterized by a deficiency of apolipoprotein C-II, needed for functioning of the enzyme lipoprotein lipase. An accumulation of chylomicrons and elevated VLDL occurs in blood plasma. Attacks of pancreatitis may recur.

Treatment—Standard Restriction of dietary fat is the most effective management approach. However, adequate intake of essential fatty acids must be maintained, and an increase in carbohydrates will be required. If the patient can tolerate medium-chain-triglyceride supplements, dietary management may be simplified.

Use of alcohol should be discouraged, and drugs such as estrogens that affect triglyceride synthesis should be avoided. During pregnancy, strict dietary control and monitoring will be required, and genetic counseling is recommended for afflicted families.

Treatment—Investigational Please contact the agencies listed under Resources, below, for the most current information.

Resources

    For more information on hyperchylomicronemia: National Organization for Rare Disorders (NORD); National Institute of Diabetes, Digestive & Kidney Diseases Information Clearinghouse; National Lipid Storage Diseases Foundation; Research Trust for Metabolic Diseases in Children.

    For genetic information and genetic counseling referrals: March of Dimes Birth Defects Foundation; National Center for Education in Maternal and Child Health (NCEMCH).

References

The Metabolic Basis of Inherited Disease, 6th ed.: C.R. Scriver, et al., eds.; McGraw-Hill, 1989, pp. 1175–1180.

Mendelian Inheritance in Man, 9th ed.: V.A. McKusick; The Johns Hopkins University Press, 1990, pp. 1256–1257.

HYPEROXALURIA, PRIMARY (PH)

Description PH is an inherited disorder characterized by an excess of oxalic acid, which forms oxalate crystals and urine stones. Two forms are presently recognized, types I and II.

Synonyms

    Lepoutre's Syndrome

    Oxalosis

    Oxaluria

Signs and Symptoms Manifestations usually first appear in childhood, but the onset of symptoms can occur during infancy or occasionally in adulthood. Calcium oxalate crystals and stones can cause renal colic, urinary tract obstruction, and hematuria. The small crystals collect in the kidneys, causing progressive kidney damage and eventual renal failure. Some patients present in endstage renal disease with oliguria or anuria. Calcium oxalate deposition (oxalosis) can occur in the eyes, bones, joints, heart, and other organs.

    Prenatal diagnosis has been obtained by fetal liver biopsy at the 17th week of pregnancy.

Etiology Type I PH, the most common form of the disorder, is inherited as an autosomal recessive trait. Type I is due to a deficiency of peroxisomal alanine: glyoxalate aminotransferase.

    Type II PH, also autosomal recessive, is due to a deficiency of D-glycerate dehydrogenase.

Epidemiology Males and females are affected in equal numbers.

Treatment—Standard The principal treatment for types I and II consists of high fluid intake, large daily doses of pyridoxine (vitamin B6), and supplements of phosphate and magnesium. A low oxalate diet is helpful, one that omits foods high in oxalic acid such as spinach, rhubarb, soybeans, tofu, beets, greens, plantain, Swiss chard, collards, gooseberries, leeks, okra, wheat germ, raspberries, sweet potatoes, peanut butter, and tea.

In patients who still have kidney function, a greatly increased fluid intake helps keep the kidneys flushed out and limits crystal formation. In patients who have lost kidney function, aggressive dialysis is an appropriate treatment until kidney transplantation can be performed. This should be done as soon as possible, since dialysis does not adequately remove oxalate. Previously, kidney transplants were considered inappropriate for patients with PH, but transplantation with therapy to help prevent recurrence is now a successful method of treatment.

Genetic counseling is helpful to families. However, the severity of the disease may be impossible to predict because it varies widely even in the same family.

Treatment—Investigational For type I PH, liver transplantation provides the normal enzyme and corrects the metabolic defect. Combined liver and kidney transplantation has been performed on more than 25 patients with type I PH. Liver transplantation alone has been performed on one patient with adequate residual kidney function.

Please contact the agencies listed under Resources, below, for the most current information.

Resources

For more information on primary hyperoxaluria: National Organization for Rare Disorders (NORD); The Oxalosis and Hyperoxaluria Foundation; National Institute of Diabetes, Digestive & Kidney Diseases Information Clearinghouse; Research Trust for Metabolic Diseases in Children.

For genetic information and genetic counseling referrals: March of Dimes Birth Defects Foundation; National Center for Education in Maternal and Child Health (NCEMCH).

References

Understanding Oxalosis and Hyperoxaluria: Treatment of Renal Failure in the Primary Hyperoxalurias: R.W.E. Watts; Nephron, 1990, vol. 56, pp. 1–5.

Oxalate Metabolism in Relation to Urinary Stone: G.A. Rose, ed.; Springer-Verlag, 1988.

HYPERPROLINEMIA TYPE I

Description Hyperprolinemia type I is a very rare hereditary disorder characterized by an excessive elevation of proline in the blood and urine. The high level of this amino acid is caused by a deficiency in the metabolic activity of the enzyme proline oxidase.

Synonyms

Proline Oxidase Deficiency
Proline Dehydrogenase Deficiency

Signs and Symptoms Diagnosis is established by measurement of plasma proline. The proline concentration in the plasma is between 500 and 2000 micromolar. Other findings associated with hyperprolinemia type I include abnormally high urinary levels of hydroxyproline and glycine. Renal disturbances have also been reported in association with this condition, but are not thought to be causally related.

Etiology Hyperprolinemia type I is transmitted as an autosomal recessive trait.

Epidemiology The disorder is present at birth. Males and females are affected in equal numbers.

Related Disorders See *Hyperprolinemia Type II.*

Treatment—Standard No therapy is indicated.

Resources

For more information on hyperprolinemia type I: National Organization for Rare Disorders (NORD); National Institute of Diabetes, Digestive & Kidney Diseases Information Clearinghouse; Research Trust for Metabolic Diseases in Children.

For genetic information and genetic counseling referrals: March of Dimes Birth Defects Foundation; National Center for Education in Maternal and Child Health (NCEMCH).

References

Mendelian Inheritance in Man, 9th ed.: V.A. McKusick; The Johns Hopkins University Press, 1990, pp. 1261–1262.

The Metabolic Basis of Inherited Disease, 6th ed.: C.R. Scriver, et al., eds.; McGraw-Hill, 1989, pp. 587–588.

HYPERPROLINEMIA TYPE II

Description Hyperprolinemia type II is a very rare hereditary disorder characterized by excessive urinary proline excretion. The high level of this amino acid results from a deficiency of the enzyme delta-1-pyrroline-5-carboxylic acid dehydrogenase.

Synonyms

Pyrroline Carboxylate Dehydrogenase Deficiency

Signs and Symptoms The abnormally high plasma level of proline (greater than 2000 micromolar) is the primary feature of the disorder. In some cases, mild mental retardation and seizures have been reported, but are not thought to be causally related.

Etiology Hyperprolinemia type II is transmitted as an autosomal recessive trait.

Epidemiology The disorder, very rare, is present at birth. Males and females are affected in equal numbers.

Related Disorders See *Hyperprolinemia Type I.*

Treatment—Standard No therapy is indicated.

Resources

For more information on hyperprolinemia type II: National Organization for Rare Disorders (NORD); National Institute of Diabetes, Digestive & Kidney Diseases Information Clearinghouse; Research Trust for Metabolic Diseases in Children.

For genetic information and genetic counseling referrals: March of Dimes Birth Defects Foundation; National Center for Education in Maternal and Child Health (NCEMCH).

References

Mendelian Inheritance in Man, 9th ed.: V.A. McKusick; The Johns Hopkins University Press, 1990, p. 1262.

The Metabolic Basis of Inherited Disease, 6th ed.: C.R. Scriver, et al., eds.; McGraw-Hill, 1989, pp. 577–587.

LACTOSE INTOLERANCE

Description Lactose intolerance is a malabsorption syndrome in which deficiency of the intestinal enzyme lactase causes impaired absorption of nutrients from the small bowel.

Synonyms

Alactasia
Hypolactasia
Lactase Deficiency
Disaccharidase Deficiency
Glucose-Galactose Malabsorption

Signs and Symptoms Children have diarrhea and fail to thrive. Adult symptoms include rumbling noises in the intestines (borborygmi), bloating, and flatus. Abdominal cramps may be present, as well as diarrhea severe enough to interfere with the absorption of other nutrients.

Etiology The enzymatic defect is inherited.

Epidemiology Lactase deficiency is fairly common among all ethnic groups, although Asians, blacks, and individuals of Jewish descent appear to have a somewhat higher incidence of the disorder.

Related Disorders Other rare malabsorption syndromes include **glucose-galactose intolerance,** and **sucrase** and **isomaltase deficiencies.**

Treatment—Standard Lactose intolerance is easily controlled by adherence to a lactose-free diet. This can be accomplished by avoidance of dairy products or by using special reduced-lactose products. Alternatively, enzyme replacement products can be added to dairy products, making them more digestible. For information, please contact Lactaid, Inc., P.O. Box 111, Pleasantville, NJ 08232.

Treatment—Investigational Please contact the agencies listed under Resources, below, for the most current information.

Resources

For more information on lactose intolerance: National Organization for Rare Disorders (NORD); National Institute of Diabetes, Digestive & Kidney Diseases Information Clearinghouse.

References
> The Metabolic Basis of Inherited Disease, 6th ed.: C.R. Scriver, et al., eds.; McGraw-Hill, 1989, pp. 2987–2997.
> Cecil Textbook of Medicine, 18th ed.: J.B. Wyngaarden and L.H. Smith, Jr., eds.; W.B. Saunders Company, 1988, p. 751.

LEIGH DISEASE

Description Leigh disease is a genetic metabolic disorder characterized by lesions of the brain, spinal cord, and optic nerve. Serum levels of lactic acid, pyruvate, and alanine are elevated. Some cases have been associated with a defect in the enzyme pyruvate dehydrogenase phosphatase.

Synonyms
> Ataxia with Lactic Acidosis II
> Encephalomyelopathy
> Leigh Necrotizing Encephalopathy
> Pyruvate Dehydrogenase Phosphatase
> Subacute Necrotizing Encephalopathy

Signs and Symptoms Diagnosis is generally made in infancy, with low body weight, growth retardation, and seizures. Progressive neurologic deterioration follows, with mental retardation and death.

Symptoms of some forms of Leigh disease resemble those of Wernicke encephalopathy, a thiamine deficiency disorder. Cardiomegaly and optic atrophy develop in some cases.

Etiology Leigh disease is thought to be inherited as an autosomal recessive trait.

Epidemiology In 80 percent of known cases, the disease developed in infants. Both sexes are affected.

Related Disorders Wernicke encephalopathy, a degenerative brain disorder associated with a deficiency of thiamine, is marked by ataxia and apathy, confusion, disorientation, or delirium. Various vision dysfunctions may also develop. This disorder often occurs in conjunction with **Korsakoff syndrome,** which involves a thiamine deficiency that is usually caused by alcoholism. Wernicke encephalopathy can be severely disabling and life-threatening if it is not recog-

nized and treated early.
See *Tay-Sachs Disease; Sandhoff Disease.*

Treatment—Standard Genetic counseling is recommended for families, and services which benefit vision-impaired people may be helpful if needed.

Treatment—Investigational Please contact the agencies listed under Resources, below, for the most current information.

Resources
For more information on Leigh disease: National Organization for Rare Disorders (NORD); National Leigh Disease Foundation, Inc.; Lactic Acidosis Support Group; NIH/National Institute of Neurological Disorders & Stroke (NINDS); National Tay-Sachs/Allied Diseases Association; Children's Brain Diseases Foundation for Research.

For genetic information and genetic counseling referrals: March of Dimes Birth Defects Foundation; National Center for Education in Maternal and Child Health (NCEMCH).

For information relating to vision problems: NIH/National Eye Institute; American Council for the Blind, Inc. (ACB); American Foundation for the Blind (AFB); American Printing House for the Blind; National Association for Parents of the Visually Impaired (NAPVI); Research Trust for Metabolic Diseases in Children.

References
Mendelian Inheritance in Man, 9th ed.: V.A. McKusick; Johns Hopkins University Press, 1990, p. 1451.

LESCH-NYHAN SYNDROME

Description Lesch-Nyhan syndrome, a metabolic disorder caused by deficiency of hypoxanthine-guanine phosphoribosyltransferese **(HPRT),** is characterized by hyperuricemia and severe neurologic disturbances.

Synonyms
> Hereditary Hyperuricemia
> Hyperuricemia, Choreoathetosis, Self-Mutilation Syndrome
> Hyperuricemia-Oligophrenia
> Juvenile Gout, Choreoathetosis, Mental Retardation Syndrome
> Nyhan syndrome

Signs and Symptoms Clinical manifestations are first seen at 3 to 6 months of age. Hyperuricemia is usually present, and orange crystals may occasionally be seen in the diapers. Neurologic signs and symptoms begin within the first year with athetosis, or with hypotonia leading to difficulty in holding the head. Mental retardation is usually present and moderate, although evaluation may be difficult because of dysarthria. Nephrolithiasis may develop.

The striking feature of Lesch-Nyhan syndrome, seen in 85 percent of cases, is self-mutilation. The characteristic is quite variable: it can first appear at one year of age or in the mid-teens; can involve biting of lips, fingers, and hands, and beating of the head against hard objects; and can occur for short periods (a day) or long ones (months).

The syndrome can be detected prenatally by amniocentesis or chorionic villus biopsy.

Etiology Lesch-Nyhan syndrome is an X-linked hereditary disorder that results from partial or complete deficiency of HPRT.

Epidemiology Only males are known to be affected, although females are carriers.

Treatment—Standard Allopurinol is used to treat the symptoms related to hyperuricemia. There is no present effective, sustained treatment for the neurologic sequelae, although success has been reported with carbidopa/levodopa as well as behavior modification techniques for the self-mutilating behavior; and diazepam, phenobarbital, and haloperidol for chorea.

Treatment—Investigational Applications of gene replacement therapy are being investigated.

Please contact the agencies listed under Resources, below, for the most current information.

Resources

For more information on Lesch-Nyhan syndrome: National Organization for Rare Disorders (NORD); NIH/National Institute of Neurological Disorders and Stroke (NINDS); William L. Lyhan, M.D., U.C. School of Medicine, San Diego; Research Trust for Metabolic Diseases in Children.

For genetic information and genetic counseling referrals: March of Dimes Birth Defects Foundation; National Center for Education in Maternal and Child Health (NCEMCH).

References

The Metabolic Basis of Inherited Disease, 6th ed.: C.R. Scriver, et al., eds.; McGraw-Hill, 1989, pp. 1007–1028, 1038.

LOWE SYNDROME

Description Lowe syndrome is a rare, inherited metabolic disorder characterized by ocular and bone abnormalities, mental retardation, and renal dysfunction.

Synonyms

        Cerebrooculorenal Dystrophy
        Lowe-Bickel Syndrome
        Lowe-Terry-Machlachlan Syndrome
        Oculocerebrorenal Dystrophy

Signs and Symptoms Manifestations usually are first seen in early infancy, in males. These signs and symptoms include hydrophthalmos, cataracts and glaucoma, epicanthal folds, flabby, areflexic muscles, joint hypermobility, rickets, under-developed testes, excess fatty tissue, and wide-ranging weight and temperature fluctuations. Hyperactivity and mental retardation are commonly found. Female carriers sometimes have opacities in the lens of the eye.

Aminoaciduria and phosphaturia may be present, and renal tubular acidosis may develop. Microscopic studies may show abnormalities in the kidneys, testes, eyes, and brain.

DNA probes are available for carrier and prenatal detection.

Etiology Lowe syndrome is transmitted through an X-linked recessive gene, which has been localized to the Xq25 region.

Epidemiology The syndrome is very rare, and affects only males.

Related Disorders See *Cystinosis; Cystinuria.*

Vitamin D-resistant rickets, caused by abnormal vitamin D metabolism and lower-than-normal blood calcium, occurs most often in infancy and early child-hood. It is characterized by a bending and distortion of the bones, a delayed clos-ing of the fontanelles, and muscular pain.

Treatment—Standard Treatment consists of appropriate medications to reduce or alleviate symptoms and to correct behavioral and renal problems. The low blood level of phosphorus is treated with oral replacement of phosphorus alone, or phos-phorus in combination with vitamin D to prevent rickets. Sodium bicarbonate is often required to correct acidosis. Surgery or drugs may be used to treat eye prob-lems such as cataracts and glaucoma; the cataractous lens can be removed in infancy. Eyeglasses or contact lenses may be necessary. Genetic counseling may be beneficial.

Treatment—Investigational Carnitine is under investigation as a possible treatment. Inherited retinal disease is being studied at Cullen Eye Institute of the Baylor College of Medicine in Houston, Texas. Another investigation is under way at the National Institutes of Child Health and Human Development (NICHHD) under the direction of Lawrence Charnas, M.D., NIH/National Institute of Child Health and Human Development, Building 10, Room 8C-429, Bethesda, Mary-land 20892; (301) 496-6683.

Please contact the agencies listed under Resources, below, for the most current information.

Resources

For more information on Lowe syndrome: National Organization for Rare Disorders (NORD); Lowe Syndrome Association; NIH/National Institute of Child Health and Human Development (NICHHD).

For genetic information and genetic counseling referrals: March of Dimes Birth Defects Foundation; NIH/National Center for Education in Mater-nal and Child Health (NCEMCH).

References

Mendelian Inheritance in Man, 9th ed.: V.A. McKusick; The Johns Hopkins University Press, 1990, 1662–1663.

220 | INBORN ERRORS OF METABOLISM

Smith's Recognizable Patterns of Human Malformation, 4th ed.: K.L. Jones; W.B. Saunders Company, 1988, pp. 180–181.
Oral Carnitine Therapy in Children with Cystinosis and Renal Fanconi Syndrome: W. Gahl, et al.; J. Clin. Invest., February 1988, issue 81(2), pp. 549–560.

MANNOSIDOSIS

Description Mannosidosis is a genetic disorder characterized by a defect in the degradation of glycoproteins, the end result of which is a lysosomal accumulation of oligosaccharides, and a progressive mental and physical deterioration. Two forms occur, primarily differentiated by degree of severity.

Synonyms
Lysosomal Alpha-D-Mannosidase Deficiency

Signs and Symptoms Symptoms of Type I mannosidosis, the more severe form, begin within the first year of life. Findings include rapidly progressive mental retardation, hepatosplenomegaly, and skeletal abnormalities. This form of mannosidosis may be fatal before the child reaches 10 years of age.

The milder form of the disorder, Type II, develops between age 1 year and age 4 years. Mild-to-moderate mental retardation usually is noticed in childhood or adolescence.

Other findings in Types I and II may vary in degree, and include a prominent forehead and jaw, flattening of the nose, widely spaced teeth, and thick tongue and lips. Corneal opacities, cataracts, and hearing loss may develop. Abdominal distention results from the hepatosplenomegaly. Articular and spinal abnormalities may develop, and growth is impaired. Immune system compromise may lead to susceptibility to infection, particularly bacterial infection of the respiratory tract.

Etiology Mannosidosis is inherited as an autosomal recessive trait. The affected individual has an error of enzyme metabolism which leads to accumulation of mannose-rich oligosaccharides.

Epidemiology Mannosidosis probably affects only a few hundred persons, both males and females, in the United States.

Related Disorders See *Mucopolysaccharidosis; Mucolipidosis II (I-cell disease); Mucolipidosis III (pseudo-Hurler polydystrophy).*

Treatment—Standard Treatment of mannosidosis is symptomatic and supportive. Genetic counseling may be beneficial.

Treatment—Investigational Enzyme replacement by means of bone marrow transplantation is under investigation for treatment of the lysosomal storage disorders, including mannosidosis.

Please contact the agencies listed under Resources, below, for the most current information.

Resources

For more information on mannosidosis: National Organization for Rare Disorders (NORD); National Institute of Diabetes, Digestive & Kidney Diseases Information Clearinghouse; Research Trust for Metabolic Diseases in Children.

For genetic information and genetic counseling referrals: March of Dimes Birth Defects Foundation; National Center for Education in Maternal and Child Health (NCEMCH).

References

The Metabolic Basis of Inherited Disease, 6th ed.: C.R. Scriver, et al., eds.; McGraw-Hill, 1989, pp. 1605–1609.

MAPLE SYRUP URINE DISEASE

Description Maple syrup urine disease, a hereditary condition that derives its name from the odor of the patient's urine and sweat, is caused by abnormal metabolism of the branched chain amino acids, leucine, isoleucine, and valine. Catastrophic illness in the newborn period with metabolic acidosis, seizures, coma, and death occur in the untreated patient.

Synonyms

Branched Chain Ketonuria
Ketoaciduria

Signs and Symptoms Newborns begin to develop symptoms and signs several days after birth. Findings include the characteristic sweet odor of the sweat and urine, along with poor feeding, lethargy, and coma. Seizures also may occur. If the infant survives longer than a few months, mental retardation becomes apparent.

Blood tests reveal high levels of leucine, isoleucine, and valine.

Etiology The disease is transmitted as an autosomal recessive trait. A defective enzyme fails to perform decarboxylation of the branched chain keto-acids, derived by transamination of the amino acids leucine, isoleucine, and valine. Their excessive accumulation causes severe metabolic acidosis and neurologic damage.

Epidemiology The disease is extremely rare. Incidence in the United States Caucasian population is estimated at 1:200,000. Males and females are equally affected.

Treatment—Standard Treatment should begin as soon as possible after birth. Acidosis is treated by intravenous bicarbonate, peritoneal dialysis, or exchange transfusions. Children with this disorder must stay on a strict diet established by a physician, limiting the dietary intake of the branched chain amino acids.

Treatment—Investigational Please contact the agencies listed under Resources, below, for the most current information.

Resources

For more information on maple syrup urine disease: National Organization for Rare Disorders (NORD); Families with Maple Syrup Urine Disease; Research Trust for Metabolic Diseases in Children; National Institute of Diabetes, Digestive & Kidney Diseases Information Clearinghouse.

For genetic information and genetic counseling referrals: March of Dimes Birth Defects Foundation; National Center for Education in Maternal and Child Health (NCEMCH).

References

The Metabolic Basis of Inherited Disease, 6th ed.: C.R. Scriver, et al., eds.; McGraw-Hill, 1989, pp. 678–687.

Cecil Textbook of Medicine, 18th ed.: J.B. Wyngaarden and L.H. Smith, Jr., eds.; W.B. Saunders Company, 1988, pp. 1150, 1159.

MAROTEAUX-LAMY SYNDROME

Description There are 3 clinical variants of Maroteaux-Lamy syndrome (mucopolysaccharidosis type VI—**MPS VI**): severe, intermediate, and mild. The severe form of this condition is similar to the severe form of Hurler syndrome, except for the preservation of intelligence in Marotaux-Lamy.

Synonyms

Arylsulfatase-B Deficiency
Mucopolysaccharidosis Type VI
Polydystrophic Dwarfism

Signs and Symptoms Macrocephaly and a prominent chestbone may be present at birth. Other manifestations of Maroteaux-Lamy syndrome usually appear between the 2nd and 3rd year. The most prominent findings are coarse facial features and short stature. Corneal opacities may be present. Bone abnormalities including stubby fingers, joint restrictions and claw hand, lumbar lordosis, and pain in the hip generally occur after ages 3 to 4 years. Carpal tunnel syndrome may develop, as well as a wobbly gait that is the result of inwardly pointed knees and toes. Other typical findings include noisy and strained breathing, deafness, hepatosplenomegaly, and aortic valvular dysfunction. Blindness and hydrocephalus may be complications. The intellect is usually normal.

Etiology The syndrome has an autosomal recessive inheritance. A deficiency of the enzyme arylsulfatase B (N-acetylgalactosamine-4-sulfatase) causes an excess of dermatan sulfate in the urine. The enzyme deficiency results in an inability to metabolize mucopolysaccharides. Accumulation of these large undegraded mucopolysaccharides in body cells causes the physical symptoms and abnormalities.

Epidemiology The incidence is unknown. Maroteaux-Lamy syndrome affects males and females equally.

Related Disorders See *Mucopolysaccharidosis.*

The mucolipidoses are a family of disorders that produce symptoms very much like those of the mucopolysaccharidoses. See *Mucolipidosis II; Mucolipidosis III; Mucolipidosis IV.*

Treatment—Standard Treatment is symptomatic and supportive. Hernias may require surgery. Physical therapy and hearing aids may benefit the patient. Genetic counseling may be helpful to patient and family. Prenatal diagnosis is now possible.

Treatment—Investigational Treatment approaches aimed at checking early development of Maroteaux-Lamy syndrome include enzyme replacement therapy and bone marrow transplantation. The latter procedure was used to treat a young girl with the syndrome, and greatly decreased the size of her enlarged liver and spleen and improved her cardiopulmonary function, joint mobility, and visual acuity. The successful outcome of bone marrow transplantation in this case demonstrates that toxic compounds which accumulate in the tissues can be removed and metabolized by transplanted cells. However, more research is needed before this treatment will be available for general use.

Please contact the agencies listed under Resources, below, for the most current information.

Resources

For more information on Maroteaux-Lamy syndrome: National Organization for Rare Disorders (NORD); MPS (Mucopolysaccharidoses) Research Funding Center, Inc.; National MPS Society; Society of Mucopolysaccharide Diseases, Inc.; Society of MPS Diseases; National Institute of Diabetes, Digestive & Kidney Diseases Information Clearinghouse.

For genetic information and genetic counseling referrals: March of Dimes Birth Defects Foundation; National Center for Education in Maternal and Child Health (NCEMCH).

References

The Metabolic Basis of Inherited Disease, 6th ed.: C.R. Scriver, et al., eds.; McGraw-Hill, 1989, pp. 1576–1577.

MPS Society brochure.

MPS Research Funding Center Bulletin.

MCARDLE DISEASE

Description McArdle disease is a rare glycogen storage disease associated with a deficiency of muscle phosphorylase, normally utilized in the degradation of glycogen to glucose in muscle tissue. Painful cramps occur after strenuous exercise, and kidney failure can rarely develop.

Synonyms

    Glycogenosis Type V
    Glycogen Storage Disease Type V
    Muscle Phosphorylase Deficiency

Myophosphorylase Deficiency

Signs and Symptoms Symptoms of the disease usually do not appear before age 10 years, and development is normal. Muscle function is normal while at rest or during moderate exercise. Painful muscle cramps occur after vigorous exercise, at which time myoglobin can often be detected in the urine. Diagnosis is confirmed by failure to see a rise in blood lactate after exercise. The diagnosis can also be confirmed by muscle biopsy; phosphorylase activity will be reduced or absent in affected patients.

Etiology McArdle disease, inherited as an autosomal recessive trait, is caused by deficiency of the enzyme myophosphorylase.

Epidemiology All glycogen storage diseases together affect fewer than 1:40,000 persons in the United States, with males and females being affected in equal numbers.

Related Disorders See *Pompe Disease; Forbes Disease; Glycogen Storage Disease VII.*

Treatment—Standard Treatment usually consists of the avoidance of strenuous exercise. Oral glucose and fructose supplements have been used but with varied results.

Treatment—Investigational Please contact the agencies listed under Resources, below, for the most current information.

Resources
   For more information on McArdle disease: National Organization for Rare Disorders (NORD); Association for Glycogen Storage Diseases; National Institute of Diabetes, Digestive & Kidney Diseases Information Clearinghouse; Research Trust for Metabolic Diseases in Children.
   For genetic information and genetic counseling referrals: March of Dimes Birth Defects Foundation; National Center for Education in Maternal and Child Health (NCEMCH).

References
   Cecil Textbook of Medicine, 18th ed.: J.B. Wyngaarden and L.H. Smith, Jr., eds.; W.B. Saunders Company, 1988, p. 1135.

MEDIUM-CHAIN ACYL-COA DEHYDROGENASE (MCAD) DEFICIENCY

Description This metabolic disorder, caused by an inherited enzyme deficiency, is characterized by recurrent episodes of metabolic acidosis, hypoglycemia, lethargy, and coma.

Synonyms
   Acyl-CoA Dehydrogenase Deficiency, Medium-Chain

Carnitine Deficiency
Dicarboxylicaciduria
Nonketotic Carnitine Deficiency

Signs and Symptoms Onset of symptoms occurs during infancy or early child-hood. Intermittent hypoglycemia and metabolic acidosis are characteristic after fasting. Coma sometimes ensues. During episodes of hypoglycemia, tests usually show excessive amounts of dicarboxylic acids in the urine (6 to 8 carbon atoms in length). Fatty changes in the liver may also occur. Detection of the compound suberylglycine in the urine appears to be diagnostic for this condition.

Etiology MCAD deficiency is one of the organic acidemias and has an autosomal recessive inheritance. It is caused by a deficiency of the enzyme medium-chain acyl-CoA dehydrogenase, which is needed for the oxidation of medium-chain fatty acids. This enzyme plays a central role in the metabolism of fats.

Many of the effects of organic acidemias are attributed to secondary carnitine depletion.

Epidemiology Incidence is about 1:50,000 live births. Males and females are affected in equal numbers.

Related Disorders See *Glutaricaciduria II.*

Treatment—Standard Prevention of fasting for prolonged periods will help pre-vent symptoms. This may require awakening the child at night for feeding, or nighttime intravenous or enteral feeding. Acute episodes of acidosis and dehydra-tion are treated with fluids and bicarbonate.

Patients with proven carnitine deficiency should be given a supplement of 100 to 300 mg/kg/day of oral L-carnitine. Other treatment is symptomatic and support-ive.

Treatment—Investigational Please contact the agencies listed under Resources, below, for the most current information.

Resources

For more information on **MCAD deficiency:** National Organization for Rare Disorders (NORD); British Organic Acidemia Association; National Institute of Diabetes, Digestive & Kidney Diseases Information Clearinghouse; Research Trust for Metabolic Diseases in Children.

For genetic information and genetic counseling referrals: March of Dimes Birth Defects Foundation; National Center for Education in Maternal and Child Health (NCEMCH).

References

The Metabolic Basis of Inherited Disease, 6th ed.: C.R. Scriver, et al., eds.; McGraw-Hill, 1989, pp. 898–907.
Catalytic Defect of Medium-Chain Acyl-Coenzyme A Dehydrogenase Deficiency: Lack of Both Cofactor Responsiveness and Biochemical Heterogeneity in Eight Patients: B.A. Amendt, et al.; J. Clin. Investi., 1985, issue 76, pp. 963–969.
Dicarboxylic Aciduria: Deficient 1-(14)C-Octanoate Oxidation and Medium-Chain Acyl-CoA Dehydrogenase in Fibroblasts: W.J. Rhead, et al.; Science, 1983, issue 221, pp. 73–75.

MENKES DISEASE

Description Menkes disease is a genetic disturbance of copper metabolism beginning before birth and resulting in deficient copper levels in many body tissues. Structural changes occur in the hair, brain, bones, liver, and arteries. The disease is most often fatal within 3 years.

Synonyms
> Kinky Hair Disease
> Steely Hair Disease
> Trichopoliodystrophy
> X-Linked Copper Deficiency
> X-Linked Copper Malabsorption

Signs and Symptoms Affected individuals are often born prematurely, and hypothermia and hyperbilirubinemia may be present. Neonates appear normal, some with the characteristic pudgy cheeks. At about 6 weeks, the fine neonatal hair loses pigment and eventually becomes kinky, tangled, and sparse. Neurologic deficit is evident by 1 to 3 months of age, with hypertonia, irritability, feeding difficulties, convulsions, and subdural hematoma or cranial thrombosis, with eventual spastic dementia and seizures. At this time developmental delay is apparent. On x-ray, osteoporosis and wormian bones may be seen. Fractures occur often, and the combination of these seen with subdural hematoma have led to the incorrect diagnosis of child abuse.

Other findings in Menkes disease include emphysema, bladder abnormalities, and ocular irregularities.

Etiology Menkes disease is inherited as an X-linked recessive trait.

Epidemiology An Australian study of Menkes disease from 1966 to 1971 suggested an incidence of 1:35,500 live births. A 1980 study modified this figure to 1:90,000 live births. Other estimates place the number of cases at 1:50,000 and 1:100,000.

Related Disorders See *Wilson Disease.*

Indian childhood cirrhosis is a familial and probably genetically determined disease. In this condition, an extremely large amount of copper accumulates in the liver, and the clinical picture is similar to that of Menkes disease.

Treatment—Standard Although copper supplementation has corrected the hepatic and blood serum copper levels, cerebral deterioration continued. The only form of copper absorbed from the intestine is copper nitriloacetate.

Other treatment is symptomatic and supportive.

Treatment—Investigational Attempts are being made to identify a form of copper supplementation that can meet enzymatic requirements, especially in restoring normal copper levels in the brain. The effects of vitamin C on copper metabolism are also being investigated, as well as the use of monoamine oxidase inhibitors in regard to defective catecholamine synthesis, which, it is theorized, may play a role in Menkes disease.

Please contact the agencies listed under Resources, below, for the most current information.

Resources

For more information on Menkes disease: National Organization for Rare Disorders (NORD); Corporation for Menkes Disease; NIH/National Institute of Neurological Disorders & Stroke (NINDS).

For genetic information and genetic counseling referrals: March of Dimes Birth Defects Foundation; NIH/National Center for Education in Maternal and Child Health (NCEMCH).

References

Mendelian Inheritance in Man, 9th ed.: V.A. McKusick; The Johns Hopkins University Press, 1990, pp. 1665–1668.

The Metabolic Basis of Inherited Disease, 6th ed.: C.R. Scriver, et al., eds.; McGraw-Hill, 1989, pp. 1422–1428.

Metallothionein Gene Regulation in Menkes Syndrome: D.H. Hamer; Arch. Dermatol., October 1987, vol. 123(10), pp. 1384a–1385a.

Life-Span and Menkes Kinky Hair Syndrome: Report of a 13-Year Course of this Disease: C. Sander, et al.; Clin. Genet., March 1988, vol. 33(3), pp. 228–233.

Menkes Syndrome in a Girl with X-Autosome Translocation: S. Kapur, et al.; Am. J. Med. Genet., February 1987, vol. 26(2), pp. 503–510.

Genetic Diseases of Copper Metabolism: J.R. Prohaska; Clin. Physiol. Biochem., 1986, vol. 4(1), pp. 87–93.

MORQUIO SYNDROME

Description Morquio syndrome (mucopolysaccharidosis type IV—**MPS IV**) manifests in 2 forms, A and B. Both forms are due to enzyme deficiency, which leads to an accumulation of keratan sulfate. Bony abnormalities of the head, chest, hands, knees, and spine may result. Intellect is preserved. Each form has mild and severe phenotypes.

Synonyms

Morquio Disease

Mucopolysaccharidosis Type IV

Signs and Symptoms Both forms are characterized by short stature with a short trunk and a unique spondyloepiphyseal dysplasia.

The first signs may be detected from 12 months of age to 3.5 years. These include macrocephaly, a broad mouth, small nose, short neck, corneal clouding, and widely spaced and thinly enameled teeth. Other early features are retarded growth, genu valgum, kyphosis, and a short trunk. The child may have a tendency to fall. As development continues, a short barrel chest and disproportionately long arms are evident, along with enlarged and possibly hyperextensible wrists and stubby hands. The misaligned knees and knobby joints may cause a wobbly gait. Joint laxity and bony abnormalities of the spine can result in spinal cord compression. Further findings include hepatomegaly, thoracic kyphoscoliosis, aortic regurgitation, and hearing loss.

Etiology The syndrome is autosomal recessive. Type A results from a deficiency of N-acetyl-galactosamine-6-sulfatase; type B, from deficient beta-galactosidase. Both deficiencies lead to an inability to metabolize mucopolysaccharides. The accumulation of these large undegraded mucopolysaccharides in body cells, and the resultant accumulation of keratan sulfate in the urine, cause the physical symptoms and abnormalities.

Epidemiology Males and females are affected in equal numbers. In the general population, prevalence is fewer than 1:100,000 live births. In the French-Canadian population, Morquio syndrome is the most common type of mucopolysaccharidosis.

Related Disorders See *Mucopolysaccharidosis.*

The mucolipidoses are a family of similar disorders that produce symptoms very much like those of the mucopolysaccharidoses. See *Mucolipidosis II; Mucolipidosis III; Mucolipidosis IV.*

Treatment—Standard When spinal cord compression is present, surgery to stabilize the upper cervical spine, usually by spinal fusion, can be lifesaving. Treatment is otherwise symptomatic and supportive. Physical therapy and special educational services may be useful, and genetic counseling may be helpful to the parents of patients.

Treatment—Investigational Treatments aimed at checking early development of Morquio syndrome are under study. These include enzyme replacement therapy and bone marrow transplantation.

Please contact the agencies listed under Resources, below, for the most current information.

Resources

For more information on Morquio syndrome: National Organization for Rare Disorders (NORD); MPS (Mucopolysaccharidoses) Research Funding Center, Inc.; National MPS Society; National Institute of Diabetes, Digestive & Kidney Diseases Information Clearinghouse; Society of Mucopolysaccharide Diseases, Inc.; Society of MPS Diseases.

For genetic information and genetic counseling referrals: March of Dimes Birth Defects Foundation; National Center for Education in Maternal and Child Health (NCEMCH).

References
The Metabolic Basis of Inherited Disease, 6th ed.: C.R. Scriver, et al., eds.; McGraw-Hill, 1989, pp. 1575–1576.

MUCOLIPIDOSIS II (ML II)

Description ML II is a hereditary metabolic disorder caused by enzyme deficiency. Mucolipids and mucopolysaccharides accumulate in body tissues, resulting in facial and skeletal abnormalities and physical and mental retardation. The disorder is similar to Hurler syndrome, but usually occurs earlier and is more severe.

Synonyms

I-Cell Disease

Inclusion Cell Disease

Leroy Disease

Signs and Symptoms Many features of ML II may be apparent at birth, but onset of manifestations often occurs from 6 to 10 months of age. Craniofacial abnormalities include depression of the nasal bridge, a long and narrow head, and a high forehead. Skeletal features include kyphoscoliosis, gibbus, anterior beaking and wedging of vertebrae, widening of the ribs, and proximal pointing of the metacarpals. Physical and mental retardation may be severe. Inguinal and umbilical hernias, and hepatomegaly accompanied by a protruding abdomen are often seen. Other clinical problems include frequent respiratory infections, gingival hyperplasia, corneal opacities, and severe joint contractures.

Increased urinary excretion of glycosaminoglycans has not been observed with this condition.

Prenatal detection is possible.

Etiology ML II is autosomal recessive. A variety of lysosomal enzymes are deficient in body cells but are strikingly elevated in the blood.

Epidemiology Males and females are affected equally, and siblings have a 1 in 4 chance of being affected.

Related Disorders See *Hurler Syndrome; Mucolipidosis III; Mucopolysaccharidosis.*

Treatment—Standard Treatment is symptomatic and supportive. Antibiotics are often prescribed for respiratory infections, and orthopedic complications are managed as they arise. Genetic counseling is advised for families with this disorder.

Treatment—Investigational Treatments under study for checking early development of ML II include enzyme replacement therapy and bone marrow transplantation.

Please contact the agencies listed under Resources, below, for the most current information.

Resources

For more information on ML II: National Organization for Rare Disorders (NORD); MPS (Mucopolysaccharidoses) Research Funding Center, Inc.; National Lipid Diseases Foundation; The MPS Society, Inc.; Society of Mucopolysaccharide Diseases, Inc.; Society of MPS Diseases; National Institute of Diabetes, Digestive & Kidney Diseases Information Clearinghouse.

For genetic information and genetic counseling referrals: March of Dimes Birth Defects Foundation; National Center for Education in Maternal and Child Health (NCEMCH).

References
The Metabolic Basis of Inherited Disease, 6th ed.: C.R. Scriver, et al., eds.; McGraw-Hill, 1989,
pp. 1590–1591.

MUCOLIPIDOSIS III (ML III)

Description The enzyme deficiencies in ML III result in the accumulation of
mucopolysaccharides and mucolipids in body tissues without excess of
mucopolysaccharides in the urine. Although this form of mucolipidosis is less
severe than that seen in ML II (I-cell disease), most individuals do not survive
past age 30 years.

Synonyms
> Gangliosidosis GM1 Type 1
> Pseudo-Hurler Polydystrophy
> Pseudopolydystrophy

Signs and Symptoms Clinical manifestations appear from age 2 years to 4 years.
Joint stiffness is one of the first symptoms and is progressive, with the child developing scoliosis and claw-hand deformity by age 6. Short stature is also evident by
then. Hip joint deterioration and carpal tunnel syndrome develop. Other characteristics include corneal opacities and minimal-to-moderate coarseness of facial
features. Aortic valve disease is common, and aortic regurgitation may be present.
Mild mental retardation, easy fatigability, congestive heart failure, and dysostosis
multiplex may occur.

Etiology ML III is inherited as an autosomal recessive trait. The disorder is due to
defective mannose-6-phosphate lysosomal recognition markers, resulting in excess
accumulations of ganglioside; these affect the central nervous system, liver, spleen,
renal glomerular epithelium, and bone tissue.

Epidemiology Males and females are affected equally. Siblings of patients have a 1
in 4 chance of developing the disease.

Related Disorders See *Mucolipidosis II (I-cell disease); Marotaux-Lamy Syndrome.*

Treatment—Standard Treatment is symptomatic and supportive. Physical therapy
may be beneficial. It is suggested that hip replacement be performed after puberty. Genetic counseling is recommended for further family planning.

Treatment—Investigational Please contact the agencies listed under Resources,
below, for the most current information.

Resources
For more information on ML III: National Organization for Rare Disorders
(NORD); MPS (Mucopolysaccharidoses) Research Funding Center, Inc.; The
MPS Society, Inc.; Society of Mucopolysaccharide Diseases, Inc.; Society of MPS
Diseases; National Institute of Diabetes, Digestive, & Kidney Diseases Informa-

tion Clearinghouse.

For genetic information and genetic counseling referrals: March of Dimes Birth Defects Foundation; National Center for Education in Maternal and Child Health (NCEMCH).

References

The Metabolic Basis of Inherited Disease, 6th ed.: C.R. Scriver, et al., eds.: McGraw-Hill, 1989, pp. 1591–1598.

MUCOLIPIDOSIS IV (ML IV)

Description ML IV is a metabolic disorder of enzyme deficiency. It is associated with psychomotor deterioration and abnormalities of the eye.

Synonyms

Sialolipidosis

Signs and Symptoms Manifestations generally are seen at birth or during early infancy. The initial finding usually is clouding of the cornea. Retinal degeneration is sometimes seen in the first year. Retardation of physical and mental development usually is not evident until the end of the first year, and progresses gradually. Although a few patients may slowly improve their psychomotor skills, most affected children are severely retarded, physically and mentally. Patients with this condition do not develop hepatomegaly, splenomegaly, or mucopolysacchariduria, and have no skeletal involvement. Cultured fibroblasts show abnormal lysosomal inclusions.

The condition can be detected prenatally through amniocentesis.

Etiology ML IV is transmitted as an autosomal recessive trait. The deficient enzyme is unknown, but is presumed to be a lysosomal enzyme yet to be described.

Epidemiology Children of both sexes are affected. Approximately 50 percent of reported patients are of Ashkenazi Jewish extraction, with ancestors from eastern Europe, especially southern Poland. Fewer than 20 patients have been reported in the medical literature, but the exact incidence is unknown.

Treatment—Standard Treatment is symptomatic and supportive. Genetic counseling is advised for families affected by the disorder.

Treatment—Investigational Treatments involving enzyme replacement therapy and bone marrow transplantation may be beneficial but have not been attempted for ML IV.

Please contact the agencies listed under Resources, below, for the most current information.

Resources

For more information on ML IV: National Organization for Rare Disorders (NORD); Children's Association for Research on Mucolipidosis IV; National Lipid

Diseases Foundation; National Institute of Diabetes, Digestive & Kidney Diseases Information Clearinghouse.

For genetic information and genetic counseling referrals: March of Dimes Birth Defects Foundation; National Center for Education in Maternal and Child Health (NCEMCH).

References

The Metabolic Basis of Inherited Disease, 6th ed.: C.R. Scriver, et al., eds.; McGraw-Hill, 1989, pp. 1803–1805.

MUCOPOLYSACCHARIDOSIS (MPS)

Description The mucopolysaccharidoses are a group of hereditary disorders of lysosomal storage in which enzyme deficiencies result in deposition of undegraded mucopolysaccharides in body tissues and organs. Each deficient enzyme will produce fairly specific clinical manifestations, so that diagnosis rests both on clinical and enzymatic assessment.

Signs and Symptoms The clinical manifestations and degree of severity of the various MPS disorders are varied, but some characteristics are shared by all: unusual facies; a progressive, chronic, and disabling course; multisystem involvement with organ enlargement; and dysostosis multiplex.

When involvement is severe, although newborns may appear normal, at about 12 months signs of growth and mental retardation are evident. Growth may appear to stop after the age of 3 or 4 years. In mild forms of MPS, patients have normal stature.

In many patients vision and hearing are impaired, as are joint mobility and cardiovascular and respiratory function. Hepatosplenomegaly occurs in most patients, and the central nervous system and brain may be affected.

For individual discussions of the following mucopolysaccharidosis disease subdivisions, see **Hurler Syndrome; Hunter Syndrome; Sanfilippo Syndrome; Morquio Syndrome; Marotaux-Lamy Syndrome; Sly Syndrome.**

MPS I-H	Hurler Syndrome—severe form of MPS I
MPS I-S	Scheie Syndrome—mild form of MPS I
MPS I-H/S	Hurler/Scheie Syndrome
MPS II	Hunter Syndrome—severe form of MPS II
(severe)	
MPS II	Hunter Syndrome—mild form of MPS II
(mild)	
MPS III-A	Sanfilippo Syndrome
III-B	
III-C	
III-D	
MPS IV-A	Morquio Syndrome
IV-B	
MPS V	No longer used—formerly, Scheie Syndrome

MPS VI   Maroteaux-Lamy—severe, intermediate, mild
MPS VII   Sly Syndrome

Etiology All the mucopolysaccharidoses have autosomal recessive inheritance except for Hunter syndrome, which is X-linked recessive. Each MPS disorder is caused by deficiency of a specific lysosomal enzyme necessary for the metabolism of dermatan sulfate, heparan sulfate, and/or keratan sulfate. These undegraded mucopolysaccharides accumulate in tissues and organs and are also excreted in the urine.

Epidemiology Males and females are affected equally in the mucopolysaccharidoses except for the X-linked Hunter syndrome, which only affects males.

Related Disorders The mucolipidoses are a family of disorders that produce symptoms and signs very much like those of MPS. See *Mucolipidosis II; Mucolipidosis III; Mucolipidosis IV.*

Treatment—Standard Treatment of all the mucopolysaccharidoses is symptomatic and supportive. If hernias, hydrocephalus, and vision problems occur, corrective surgery may be indicated. Physical therapy may be helpful for joint contractures. Genetic counseling will benefit families of affected patients.

Treatment—Investigational Treatments that are being investigated are enzyme replacement therapy and bone marrow transplantation. Please contact the agencies listed under Resources, below, for the most current information.

Resources

For more information on mucopolysaccharidosis: National Organization for Rare Disorders (NORD); MPS (Mucopolysaccharidoses) Research Funding Center, Inc.; National MPS Society; Society of MPS Diseases; Society of Mucopolysaccharide Diseases, Inc.; National Institute of Diabetes, Digestive & Kidney Diseases Information Clearinghouse.

For genetic information and genetic counseling referrals: March of Dimes Birth Defects Foundation; NIH/National Center for Education in Maternal and Child Health (NCEMCH).

References

The Metabolic Basis of Inherited Disease, 6th ed.: C.R. Scriver, et al., eds.; McGraw-Hill, 1989, pp. 1565–1588.

The Mucopolysaccharidoses and Anaesthesia: A Report of Clinical Experience: I.A. Herrick, et al.; Can. J. Anaesth., January 1988, issue 35(1), pp. 67–73.

Mucopolysaccharidoses and Anaesthetic Risks: P. Sjogren, et al.; Acta Anaesthesiol. Scand., April 1987, issue 31(3), pp. 214–218.

Electroretinographic Findings in the Mucopolysaccharidoses: R.C. Caruso, et al.; Ophthalmology, December 1986, issue 93(12), pp. 1612–1616.

MULTIPLE CARBOXYLASE DEFICIENCY

Description Multiple carboxylase deficiency results from impaired activity of 3 enzymes that are dependent on the vitamin biotin: propionyl CoA carboxylase, beta-methylcrotonyl CoA carboxylase, and pyruvate carboxylase. This impairment causes defective organic acid metabolism. The disorder is treatable.

Synonyms
Biotinidase Deficiency
Carboxylase Deficiency, Multiple (MCD)

Signs and Symptoms Multiple carboxylase deficiency is characterized by the development of an erythematous rash, ataxia, seizures, neuroirritability, and lactic acidosis. Other symptoms and signs that may occur are hypotonia and immune system impairment. Additionally, poor muscle coordination associated with ataxia and impaired physical development are seen. Hearing loss also may develop.

Multiple carboxylase deficiency is diagnosed by testing the urine for metabolites that indicate deficiency in the carboxylase enzymes.

Etiology Multiple carboxylase deficiency is an autosomal recessive hereditary disorder, caused by a defect in the enzyme biotinidase.

Epidemiology The onset of multiple carboxylase deficiency usually occurs at about 3 months of age. Males and females are affected in equal numbers.

Treatment—Standard Treatment is with oral biotin (vitamin H; coenzyme R; part of vitamin B complex) supplements. *It is imperative that treatment be started as soon as the diagnosis is made.* With biotin treatment, symptoms of the disorder disappear.

Genetic counseling is recommended for families of affected children.

Treatment—Investigational Please contact the agencies listed under Resources, below, for the most current information.

Resources
For more information on multiple carboxylase deficiency: National Organization for Rare Disorders (NORD); National Institute of Diabetes, Digestive & Kidney Diseases Information Clearinghouse; Research Trust for Metabolic Diseases in Children.

References
Biotin and Multiple Carboxylase Deficiency: J. Thoene and D. Buchanan; *in* Clinical Studies in Medical Biochemistry: R. Glew and S. Peters, eds.; Oxford University Press, 1987, pp. 89–95.
Ocular Aspects in Biotinidase Deficiency: Clinical and Genetic Original Studies: G. Campana, et al.; Ophthalmic Paediatr. Genetica, June 1987, issue 8(2), pp. 125–129.
Multiple Carboxylase Deficiency due to Deficiency of Biotinidase: L.P. Thuy, et al.; J. of Neurogenet., November 1986, issue 3(6), pp. 357–63.

MULTIPLE SULFATASE DEFICIENCY

Description Multiple sulfatase deficiency is a very rare hereditary metabolic disorder characterized by impairment of several sulfatase enzymes, leading to ichthyosis and corneal opacities, with severe neurologic and skeletal abnormalities also occurring.

Synonyms
Mucosulfatidosis
Sulfatidosis, Juvenile, Austin Type

Signs and Symptoms Manifestations of multiple sulfatase deficiency usually become apparent during the 1st or 2nd year of life. Development of walking and speech are abnormal. Other characteristics include a depressed bridge of the nose, large head circumference, deafness, pectus excavatum, and spinal abnormalities. The sella turcica may be J-shaped, and the phalanges broader than normal. Hepatomegaly and splenomegaly are often seen, and ichthyosis is a common finding.

Laboratory tests show abnormal bone marrow cells and white blood cells. The levels of urinary dermatan sulfate and heparan sulfate are elevated, and deficiencies of various other sulfatase enzymes are observed.

Etiology The disorder is transmitted as an autosomal recessive trait. The metabolic error is deficiency of arylsulfatases A, B, and C, 2 steroid sulfatases, and 4 other sulfatases required for the metabolism of mucopolysaccharides. Possibly the disease results from a mutual post-translational modification of all the affected enzymes.

Epidemiology Multiple sulfatase deficiency is present at birth, although symptoms typically only become noticeable during the first 2 years of life. The rare disorder affects males and females in equal numbers.

Related Disorders See *Maroteaux-Lamy Syndrome; Leukodystrophy, Metachromatic; Ichthyosis.*

Treatment—Standard Orthopedic management is recommended for spinal abnormalities. Dermatologic symptoms can be alleviated by the application of emollients such as petroleum jelly after bathing. Twelve percent ammonium lactate lotion has also been used effectively to treat the skin lesions.

Treatment—Investigational Please contact the agencies listed under Resources, below, for the most current information.

Resources
For more information on multiple sulfatase deficiency: National Organization for Rare Disorders (NORD); NIH/National Institute of Neurological Disorders and Stroke; National Lipid Diseases Foundation; National Tay Sachs/Allied Diseases Association; Research Trust for Metabolic Diseases in Children.

For genetic information and genetic counseling referrals: March of Dimes Birth Defects Foundation; National Center for Education in Maternal and Child Health (NCEMCH); Foundation for Ichthyosis and Related Skin Types, Inc.

References
The Metabolic Basis of Inherited Disease, 6th ed.: C.R. Scriver, et al., eds.; McGraw-Hill, 1989, pp. 1726, 1729, 1736–1737, 1945, 1956, 1959.
Therapeutic Activity of Lactate 12% Lotion in the Treatment of Ichthyosis. Active Versus Vehicle and Active Versus a Petroleum Cream: M. Buxman, et al.; J. Am. Acad. Dermatol., December 1986, vol. 15(6), pp. 1253–1258.

N-ACETYL GLUTAMATE SYNTHETASE (NAGS) DEFICIENCY

Description NAGS deficiency is the most recently described and rarest of the hereditary urea cycle disorders. These disorders are caused by a deficiency of one of the enzymes needed for the synthesis of urea from ammonia. The deficiencies result in hyperammonemia. Untreated, this disorder leads to brain damage, coma, and eventually death.

Synonyms
Inborn Errors of Urea Synthesis
Urea Cycle Disorder

Signs and Symptoms NAGS deficiency is characterized in infants by hyperammonemia. Manifestations include lack of interest in eating; vomiting; and hepatomegaly. The diagnosis is suspected if hyperammonemia is present, citrulline is absent in plasma, and there is a low level of orotic acid in the urine. Confirmation requires measurement of the enzyme in the liver. Immediate treatment after diagnosis in newborns is imperative.

Etiology This condition is inherited as an autosomal recessive hereditary disorder in which the activity of N-acetyl glutamate synthetase is deficient. Its product, N-acetyl-L-glutamate, is required for activation of the enzyme carbamyl phosphate synthetase. This secondary deficiency causes an accumulation of excess ammonia in blood and body tissues.

Epidemiology Only a few instances of this disorder are known.

Related Disorders The symptoms of all urea cycle disorders result from hyperammonemia, in varying degrees of severity. See *Carbamyl Phosphate Synthetase Deficiency; Ornithine Transcarbamylase Deficiency; Citrullinemia; Argininosuccinic Aciduria; Arginase Deficiency.*
See also *Reye Syndrome.*
Organic acidemias are characterized by hyperammonemia associated with metabolic acidosis, with an anion gap, and sometimes ketonuria. These disorders are also of genetic origin and affect the urea cycle as a secondary phenomenon.

Treatment—Standard Diagnostic testing should be done as soon as a urea cycle disorder is suspected. These tests should include measurement of pH and determination of plasma levels of ammonia, amino acids, and bicarbonate.
Treatment of hyperammonemia should be started before test results are known, to prevent coma and brain damage. The drug benzoate/phenylacetate

(Ucephan—McGaw Laboratories, Inc.) has been approved for use in preventing and treating hyperammonemia in patients with urea cycle enzymopathy due to enzyme deficiencies.

Treatment—Investigational Dr. Saul Brusilow of Johns Hopkins Medical School is developing sodium (or calcium) phenylbutyrate, which does not have the offensive smell of phenylacetate.

Please contact the agencies listed under Resources, below, for the most current information.

Resources

For more information on N-acetyl glutamate synthetase deficiency: National Organization for Rare Disorders (NORD); National Urea Cycle Disorders Foundation; National Institute of Diabetes, Digestive & Kidney Diseases Information Clearinghouse; Saul Brusilow, M.D., Johns Hopkins Hospital; The National Kidney Foundation; Research Trust for Metabolic Diseases in Children.

For genetic information and genetic counseling referrals: March of Dimes Birth Defects Foundation; National Center for Education in Maternal and Child Health (NCEMCH).

References

Disorders of the Urea Cycle: S.W. Brusilow; Hospital Practice, October 15, 1985, issue 305, pp. 65–72.

Symptomatic Inborn Errors of Metabolism in the Neonate: S.W. Brusilow and D.L. Vallee; *in* Current Therapy in Neonatal-Perinatal Medicine, Marcel Decker, 1985, pp. 207–212.

NIEMANN-PICK DISEASE

Description Niemann-Pick disease, comprising several disorders of lipid metabolism, is characterized by the accumulation of sphingomyelin and cholesterol in many organs. A recent classification divides the group into 2 major categories based on etiology: Type I, the disorders in which sphingomyelinase is deficient and sphingomyelin and cholesterol are major storage components; and Type II, with a more varied and less certain etiology. Types I and II are further divided into acute, subacute, and chronic forms.

Synonyms

Lipid Histiocytosis

Sphingomyelin Lipidosis

Signs and Symptoms Certain characteristics are shared by both Types I and II: different degrees of hepatosplenomegaly and formation of foam cells in bone marrow, and disparate increased amounts of sphingomyelin, cholesterol, glycosphingolipids, and bis(monoacylglycero)-phosphate in the large thoracic and abdominal organs.

The acute form of Type I, **Type IA,** is the most common. Prenatal lipid storage has occurred. Sphingomyelinase activity is deficient, and hepatosplenomegaly and nervous system abnormalities are evident respectively within 6 months of age to 1 year. Other characteristics include vomiting, diarrhea, failure to thrive, pyrexia, bright red spots in the macula, and skin discoloration. Progression is rapid in Type IA, with death usually occurring by age 5 years.

The subacute form of Type I, **Type IS,** begins in infancy or early childhood with hepatosplenomegaly and sphingomyelinase deficiency. This form is more slowly progressive, and there is in general less nervous system involvement.

The chronic form of Type I, **Type IC,** begins in adulthood with hepato- and/or splenomegaly and the discovery of foam cells. The nervous system may be involved.

The acute form of Type II, **Type IIA,** begins in infancy with hepatosplenomegaly and, sometimes, jaundice. Psychomotor difficulties also begin at this time, from a few days of life to 2 years; these symptoms include hypertonicity of the arms and legs, and ataxia. Respiratory infection is common and is often the cause of death. Type IIA is usually fatal by 8 years of age.

The subacute form of Type II, **Type IIS,** has varied manifestations. Age of onset ranges from infancy to 18 years, and death may occur in infancy up to the mid 30s. Characteristics include hepatosplenomegaly, presence of foam cells, jaundice in infancy, progressive psychomotor retardation, a form of opththalmo-plegia, and seizures.

The chronic form of Type II, **Type IIC,** begins in adulthood. Characteristics include foam cell storage and, possibly, hepatosplenomegaly. There may or may not be cerebral damage; when present, it may include ataxia, progressive dementia, and a form of ophthalmoplegia.

Etiology The inheritance of all forms of Niemann-Pick disease appears to be autosomal recessive.

Epidemiology This group of diseases is rare. It has been identified in persons of all races, but the incidence of Types IA and IS appears to be greater in families of Jewish ancestry.

Treatment—Standard Treatment is supportive and symptomatic.

Treatment—Investigational Bone marrow transplantation is being investigated for some forms of Niemann-Pick disease.

Please contact the agencies listed under Resources, below, for the most current information.

Resources

For more information on Niemann-Pick disease: National Organization for Rare Disorders (NORD); National Tay-Sachs/Allied Diseases Association, Inc.; NIH/National Institute of Neurological Disorders & Stroke (NINDS); National Lipid Diseases Foundation; Research Trust for Metabolic Diseases in Children.

For genetic information and genetic counseling referrals: March of Dimes Birth Defects Foundation; National Center for Education in Maternal and Child Health (NCEMCH).

References
  The Metabolic Basis of Inherited Disease, 6th ed.: C.R. Scriver, et al., eds.; McGraw-Hill, 1989,
    pp. 1655–1671.
  Cecil Textbook of Medicine, 18th ed.: J.B. Wyngaarden and L.H. Smith, Jr., eds.; W.B. Saunders
    Company, 1988, pp. 1147–1149.

NONKETOTIC HYPERGLYCINEMIA

Description Nonketotic hyperglycinemia is a genetic disorder characterized by a defect in glycine metabolism. Severe illness usually occurs soon after birth, and may be fatal. Surviving patients become mentally retarded and may develop seizures.

Synonyms
  Nonketotic Glycinemia

Signs and Symptoms Affected newborns may appear normal for the first day or two, after which they become listless and may have convulsions. Progression is rapid. The neonate feeds poorly, in some cases vomiting occurs, and the patient fails to thrive. Apnea that may develop is fatal without support, and most infants die in these early days. Patients who survive this early period usually develop seizures (generally myoclonic, sometimes grand mal) and are severely mentally retarded, although some patients have a milder course. Other manifestations include opisthotonos and hiccuping.

  The amount of glycine in plasma, urine, and cerebrospinal fluid is extremely high.

Etiology Nonketotic hyperglycinemia is an autosomal recessive disorder caused by impaired catabolism of the amino acid glycine.

Epidemiology Males and females are affected in equal numbers.

Related Disorders See *Acidemia, Isovaleric; Acidemia, Methylmalonic; Acidemia, Propionic; Glutaricaciduria II; Maple Syrup Urine Disease.*

Treatment—Standard Only supportive care including intravenous feeding, assisted ventilation, and anticonvulsant therapy is available. Genetic counseling is recommended for families of affected children.

Treatment—Investigational Strychnine treatment has been of limited success in a few cases of nonketotic hyperglycinemia. Diazepam and sodium benzoate, in combination with choline and folic acid (vitamins of the B complex) can sometimes be beneficial to treat the seizures.

  Please contact the agencies listed under Resources, below, for the most current information.

Resources
  For more information on nonketotic hyperglycinemia: National Organization for Rare Disorders (NORD); National Institute of Diabetes, Digestive & Kid-

ney Diseases Information Clearinghouse; Research Trust for Metabolic Diseases in Children.

For genetic information and genetic counseling referrals: March of Dimes Birth Defects Foundation; National Center for Education in Maternal and Child Health (NCEMCH).

References

The Metabolic Basis of Inherited Disease, 6th ed.: C.R. Scriver, et al., eds.; McGraw-Hill, 1989, pp. 743–753.

The Effectiveness of Benzoate in the Management of Seizures in Nonketotic Hyperglicinemia: J.A. Wolff, et al.; Amer. J. Dis. Child, June 1986, issue 140(6), pp. 596–602.

Nonketotic Hyperglycinemia: Treatment with Diazepam–A Competitor for Glycine Receptors: R. Matalon, et al.; Pediatrics, April 1983, issue 71(4), pp. 581–584.

ORNITHINE TRANSCARBAMYLASE (OTC) DEFICIENCY

Description OTC deficiency is 1 of 6 hereditary urea cycle disorders, which are caused by a deficiency of one of the enzymes needed for the synthesis of urea from ammonia. The deficiencies cause an excess of ammonia in the blood and body tissues.

Synonyms

Hyperammonemia Type II
Inborn Errors of Urea Synthesis
Ornithine Carbamoyl Transferase Deficiency
Ornithine Carbamyl Transferase Deficiency
Urea Cycle Disorder

Signs and Symptoms The disorder is characterized by hyperammonemia, lack of appetite, vomiting, drowsiness, seizures, and coma. Hepatomegaly may be present. Diagnosis is based on finding a high level of orotate in the urine, which distinguishes OTC deficiency from carbamyl phosphate synthetase deficiency. Citrulline is absent in the plasma.

Immediate treatment after diagnosis is imperative. If left untreated, brain damage and coma usually occur, and death may ensue.

Etiology OTC deficiency is an X-linked hereditary disorder. Affected males (hemizygotes) have catastrophic symptoms, whereas heterozygotic females have a much milder course. Approximately one-third of cases may be due to a new mutation in the gene responsible for the deficiency. Deficiency of ornithine transcarbamylase results in an accumulation of excess ammonia in blood and body tissues.

Epidemiology Fewer than 1000 persons in the United States have the disorder. Onset of symptoms in males occurs during the first few days of life. Females who carry the mutant are usually asymptomatic. Some women who are OTC carriers may not experience hyperammonemia until during pregnancy or delivery.

Related Disorders The symptoms of all urea cycle disorders result from hyperammonemia, in varying degrees of severity. See *N-Acetyl Glutamate Synthetase Deficiency; Carbamyl Phosphate Synthetase Deficiency; Citrullinemia; Argininosuccinic Aciduria; Arginase Deficiency.*

See also *Reye Syndrome.*

Organic acidemias are characterized by hyperammonemia associated with metabolic acidosis, with an anion gap, and sometimes ketonuria. These disorders are genetic in origin and affect the urea cycle as a secondary phenomenon.

Treatment—Standard Diagnostic testing should begin as soon as a urea cycle disorder is suspected. These tests should include measurement of pH and determination of plasma levels of ammonia, amino acids, and bicarbonate. Treatment of hyperammonemia should be started before test results are available, to prevent coma or brain damage.

Immediate dialysis or exchange transfusion after diagnosis of OTC deficiency in male newborns is imperative.

The orphan drug benzoate/phenylacetate (Ucephan—McGaw Laboratories, Inc.) has been approved for use in the prevention and treatment of hyperammonemia in patients with urea cycle enzymopathy due to enzyme deficiencies.

Genetic counseling is imperative for the family of children with OTC Deficiency.

Treatment—Investigational Saul Brusilow, M.D., Johns Hopkins Hospital, is developing sodium (or calcium) phenylbutyrate, which does not have the offensive smell of the other drugs used.

Please contact the agencies listed under Resources, below, for the most current information.

Resources

For more information on ornithine transcarbamylase deficiency: National Organization for Rare Disorders (NORD); National Urea Cycle Disorders Foundation; National Institute of Diabetes, Digestive & Kidney Diseases Information Clearinghouse; Saul Brusilow, M.D., Johns Hopkins Hospital; The National Kidney Foundation; British Organic Acidemia Association; Research Trust for Metabolic Diseases in Children.

For genetic information and genetic counseling referrals: March of Dimes Birth Defects Foundation; National Center for Education in Maternal and Child Health (NCEMCH).

References

The Metabolic Basis of Inherited Disease, 6th ed.: C.R. Scriver, et al., eds.; McGraw-Hill, 1989, pp. 629–663.

Disorders of the Urea Cycle: S.W. Brusilow; Hosp. Prac., October 15, 1985, issue 305, pp. 65–72.

Symptomatic Inborn Errors of Metabolism in the Neonate: S.W. Brusilow and D.L. Vallee; *in* Curr. Ther. in Neonatal-Perinatal Med., Marcel Decker, 1985, pp. 207–212.

PHENYLKETONURIA (PKU)

Description PKU is a metabolic disorder caused by a deficiency of the enzyme phenylalanine hydroxylase. The interrupted metabolism of dietary phenylalanine results in accumulation of the amino acid in body fluids with resultant progressive, severe, irreversible mental retardation.

Synonyms

Foelling Disease
Phenylalaninemia
Phenylpyruvic Oligophrenia

Signs and Symptoms Infants are normal at birth, and phenylpyruvic acid, a phenylalanine metabolite, may not be found in the urine during the first days of life. Some neonates may be lethargic and feed poorly. Other manifestations in infants include vomiting, irritability, an eczematoid skin rash, and a musty or mousey body odor that is caused by phenylacetic acid in the urine and perspiration.

In untreated children, retarded development may be evident at several months of age, and patients are often short for their age. Because high concentrations of phenylalanine interfere with melanin production, affected individuals are almost always light-haired with a fair complexion. Craniofacial abnormalities in untreated children include microcephaly, prominent maxilla, widely spaced teeth, and impaired development of dental enamel. Skin coarsening may occur. Occasionally bone decalcification, syndactyly, and flat feet are present.

It is not understood why high levels of phenylalanine cause severe mental retardation in children. The average IQ of untreated children is less than 50, and these patients have to be institutionalized as adults. Heterozygotic children of women with PKU often have severe mental retardation.

Neurologic findings are present only in some patients, and vary. Seizures occur in about 25 percent of older children, and EEG abnormalities in 80 percent. Spasticity, hypertonicity, and increased deep tendon reflexes are among the most frequent neurologic manifestations; about 5 percent of children thus affected become physically disabled. Athetosis and tremors have been seen. Nervous system myelinization seems to be delayed but not absent.

In adulthood, the sperm count of affected males may be low. Females often have spontaneous abortions and intrauterine growth retardation. Children of women with PKU may have microcephaly and congenital heart disease, as well as the mental retardation mentioned above. There appears to be some correlation between the severity of these manifestations and the mother's plasma level of phenylalanine.

Laboratory findings: Plasma levels of phenylalanine are 10 to 60 times normal; plasma tyrosine is low; and levels of phenylalanine metabolites such as phenylpyruvic acid and other phenolic acids excreted in the urine are high. Substances such as dopamine, serotonin, and melanin are reduced.

Many studies demonstrate that PKU patients who are treated with a low phenylalanine diet before 3 months of age do well, with mean IQs of 100 (see Treatment—Standard, below).

There are several variants of PKU (**hyperphenylalaninemias**) which are characterized by elevated plasma phenylalanine levels that are not so high as those in classical PKU. For example, in tetrahydrobiopterin deficiency, neurologic deterioration occurs even when phenylalanine levels are controlled (see Etiology, below).

Prenatal diagnosis is available, and routine neonatal screening is required by law in all 50 states and in virtually all hospitals in developed countries.

Etiology PKU has an autosomal recessive inheritance. The condition is caused by a defect of phenylalanine hydroxylase, a liver enzyme that catalyses the hydroxylation of phenylalanine to tyrosine. The other forms of hyperphenylalaninemia, which are clinically and biochemically distinct from PKU, result from an enzyme complex, of which varying members may be deficient.

The mechanism of mental retardation in PKU is not known. Normal brain development may be disturbed by a high phenylalanine concentration. Impairment of brain myelinization has been suggested, as well as disturbed neuronal migration in the first 6 months of life.

High plasma phenylalanine levels may also be caused by tetrahydrobiopterin deficiency, possibly resulting from insufficient amounts of either biopterin or dihydropterin reductase. Since tetrahydrobiopterin is involved in the production of serotonin, dopamine, and norephrine, for example, a deficiency of these neurotransmitters may be the reason for the continued neurologic deterioration in spite of controlled plasma phenylalanine. (See also ***Tetrahydrobiopterin Deficiencies.***)

Epidemiology Phenylketonuria occurs in 1:11,600 live births in the United States. Males and females are affected equally. The disorder is found in most racial groups, although it is rarer in blacks and Ashkenazi Jews.

Related Disorders Phenylketonuria belongs to the group of disorders caused by defective amino acid metabolism.

Treatment—Standard The goal of treatment, to keep plasma phenylalanine levels within the normal range, can be achieved through diet. Limiting the child's intake of phenylalanine, however, must be done cautiously, because it is an essential amino acid. A carefully maintained dietary regimen can prevent mental retardation and neurologic, behavioral, dermatologic, and EEG abnormalities. Treatment must be started at a very young age (under 3 months), however, or some degree of mental retardation may be expected. If it is begun after the age of 2 or 3 years, only hyperactivity and seizures may be controlled. If patients are subsequently allowed to stop controlling their phenylalanine intake, neurologic changes occur in adolescence and adulthood. Their IQs may decline after a peak at the end of the controlled diet periods. Other problems that may appear and become severe once the patient is off the diet include academic and behavioral problems, poor visual-motor coordination, poor problem-solving skills, low developmental age, and the onset of EEG abnormalities.

There is some controversy over the age at which dietary treatment can be discontinued, but it begins to be clear that high phenylalanine levels continue to harm even after brain myelinization is complete. Phenylalanine intake should therefore probably be limited indefinitely, with possibly some relaxation of dietary control.

Since phenylalanine occurs in almost all natural proteins, maintaining proper nutrition is impossible on a phenylalanine-low diet. Dietary use of special phenylalanine-free preparations is therefore essential. These include Lofenalac (for a low phenylalanine diet) and Phenyl-Free, both from Mead Johnson. Low-protein foods such as fruits, vegetables, and some cereals are allowed.

As mentioned above, phenylalanine intake must not be too severely limited or phenylalanine deficiency may develop, resulting in anorexia, fatigue, aggressive behavior, and sometimes anemia. Both the child's behavior and plasma levels of phenylalanine and its metabolites must be monitored regularly.

Mild forms of PKU appear to require no treatment. See also *Tetrahydrobiopterin Deficiencies.*

Treatment—Investigational See also *Tetrahydrobiopterin Deficiencies.*

Attempts are being made to develop improved medical foods for affected adults.

Trials were begun in 1985 on the use of enzyme reactors for management of PKU. In this procedure, which resembles dialysis, a phenylalanine hydroxylase derived from plant or microbial cells is attached to a fixed matrix and placed in indirect contact with the patient's blood. The enzyme is capable of rapidly metabolizing plasma phenylalanine. This treatment is expected to be useful primarily for pregnant women with PKU and for the treatment of sudden peaks of phenylalanine levels that may occur with infections or other physiologically stressful conditions. For further information concerning this procedure, contact Clara Ambrus, M.D., Ph.D., Children's Hospital, 140 Hodge Avenue, Buffalo, New York 14222; (716) 878-7704.

Please contact the agencies listed under Resources, below, for the most current information.

Resources

For more information on phenylketonuria: National Organization for Rare Disorders (NORD); PKU Parents Group; National PKU Foundation; PKU Collaborative Study; NIH/National Institute of Child Health and Human Development; National Association for Retarded Citizens; National Institute of Mental Retardation.

For genetic information and genetic counseling referrals: March of Dimes Birth Defects Foundation; National Center for Education in Maternal and Child Health (NCEMCH).

References

Biochemical and Neuropsychological Effects of Elevated Plasma Phenylalanine in Patients with Treated PKU: W. Krause, et al.; J. Clin. Inv., January 1985, vol. 75(1), pp. 40–48.

Preliminary Support for the Oral Administration of Valine, Isoleucine and Leucine for Phenylketonuria: M.K. Jordan, et al.; Devel. Med. Child Neurology, 1985, vol. 27, pp. 33–39.

Loss of Intellectual Function in Children with Phenylketonuria after Relaxation of Dietary Phenylalanine Restriction: M. Seashore, et al.; Pediatrics, February 1985, vol. 75(2), pp. 226–232.

Abnormalities in Amino Acid Metabolism in Clinical Medicine: W.L. Nyhan; Appleton-Century-Crofts, 1984.

Tetrahydrobiopterin Deficiencies: Preliminary Analysis from an International Survey: J.L. Dhondt; J. Pediatr., April 1984, vol. 104(4), pp. 501–508.

Phenylketonuria and its Variants: S. Kaufman; Adv. Hum. Genet., 1983, vol. 13, pp. 217–297.

Diet Termination in Children with Phenylketonuria. A Review of Psychological Assessments used to Determine Outcome: S.E. Waisbren, et al.; J. Inherited Metab. Dis., 1980, vol. 3(4), pp. 149–153.

POMPE DISEASE

Description Pompe disease is a glycogen storage disease in which excessive glycogen accumulates in tissue lysosomes, particularly in the muscles. In the infantile form, the clinical result is hypotonia with death due to respiratory and cardiac failure in the first year of life. Other, less severe, variants are known.

Synonyms
Acid Maltase Deficiency
Alpha-1,4-Glucosidase Deficiency
Cardiomegalia Glycogenica Diffusa
Generalized Glycogenosis
Glycogenosis Type II
Lysosomal Alpha-Glucosidase Deficiency

Signs and Symptoms Pompe disease occurs in different degrees of severity, depending on the age at onset.

In the infantile form, symptoms onset usually is at 2 to 5 months of age, but can occur at birth. There are problems with respiration, and severe muscle weakness without muscle wasting is noted. Cardiomegaly, hepatomegaly, and macroglossia also occur. Progressive cardiac deterioration follows, and the condition is usually fatal by 12 to 18 months of age.

In the childhood form, symptoms begin in late infancy or early childhood, and progression is slower than in the early infantile form. The extent of organ involvement varies. Skeletal muscle weakness is usually present, while cardiac involvement is minimal. Children usually survive into their teens.

The adult form usually begins in the 2nd to 4th decade, with muscle weakness typical of other chronic muscle disorders. This form of the disorder is slowly progressive and without cardiac involvement, and life expectancy is usually normal.

Prenatal diagnosis of Pompe disease is possible with amniocentesis. Diagnosis after birth can be made by measuring the level of enzyme activity in white blood cells, and by determining the glycogen content of muscle cells.

Etiology Pompe disease is inherited as an autosomal recessive trait. The metabolic error is an inborn lack of the enzyme acid alpha-1,4-glucosidase.

Epidemiology Pompe disease and all other glycogen storage disorders together affect fewer than 1:40,000 persons in the United States. Males and females are affected in equal numbers, and the infantile and childhood forms are more common than the adult form.

Related Disorders See *McArdle Disease; Glycogen Storage Disease VII; Forbes Disease; Andersen Disease; Werdnig-Hoffman Disease.*

Treatment—Standard Treatment of Pompe disease is symptomatic and supportive. Attempts at enzyme replacement have thus far not been successful. Genetic counseling may be helpful for the families of children with the disease.

Treatment—Investigational Please contact the agencies listed under Resources, below, for the most current information.

Resources

For more information on **Pompe disease:** National Organization for Rare Disorders (NORD); Association for Glycogen Storage Diseases; Research Trust for Metabolic Diseases in Children; National Institute of Diabetes, Digestive & Kidney Diseases Information Clearinghouse; Alfred Slonim, M.D., Center for Inborn Errors of Metabolism.

For **genetic information and genetic counseling referrals:** March of Dimes Birth Defects Foundation; National Center for Education in Maternal and Child Health (NCEMCH).

References

The Metabolic Basis of Inherited Disease, 6th ed.: C.R. Scriver, et al., eds.; McGraw-Hill, 1989, pp. 437–440.

Cecil Textbook of Medicine, 18th ed.: J.B. Wyngaarden and L.H. Smith, Jr., eds.; W.B. Saunders Company, 1988, pp. 361, 1134.

PORPHYRIA

Description The porphyrias are a group of disorders characterized by an overproduction of porphyrin or its precursors. The porphyrias are generally characterized as hepatic or erythropoietic according to the site of porphyrinogenesis. The main clinical manifestations of these disorders are cutaneous and neurologic.

Etiology Four of the major porphyrias are inherited as autosomal dominant traits; one (porphyria cutanea tarda) can be both inherited (autosomal dominant) and acquired; and 3 are autosomal recessive. Various environmental factors, such as drugs, chemicals, food, and exposure to the sun can precipitate acute attacks.

Epidemiology It is unlikely that more than one form of porphyria will occur in the same family, or that someone with one type of porphyria will develop another.

Related Disorders See the separate discussions of the following porphyrias: *Porphyria, Acute Intermittent; Porphyria, ALA-D; Porphyria, Congenital Erythropoietic; Porphyria Cutanea Tarda; Porphyria, Erythropoietic Proto-*

porphyria; Porphyria, Hereditary Coproporphyria; Porphyria, Variegate.

Treatment—Standard Acute attacks are treated by intravenous fluids and the administration of hematin.

In general, drugs which trigger acute attacks in persons with acute intermittent porphyria, variegate porphyria, and hereditary coproporphyria include the barbiturates, some tranquilizers and sedatives, sulfonamides, griseofulvin, anti-epileptic agents, and contraceptive pills.

Treatment—Investigational Please contact the agencies listed under Resources, below, for the most current information.

Resources

For more information on porphyria: National Organization for Rare Disorders (NORD); American Porphyria Foundation; National Institute of Diabetes, Digestive & Kidney Diseases Information Clearinghouse.

For genetic information and genetic counseling referrals: March of Dimes Birth Defects Foundation; National Center for Education in Maternal and Child Health (NCEMCH).

References

The Metabolic Basis of Inherited Disease, 6th ed.: C.R. Scriver, et al., eds.; McGraw-Hill, 1989, pp. 1305–1365.

PORPHYRIA, ACUTE INTERMITTENT (AIP)

Description AIP is one of the hereditary hepatic porphyrias. The enzymatic defect is a lack of porphobilinogen deaminase (PBG-D; uroporphyrinogen I-synthase), but other factors, such as drugs, hormones, and dietary changes contribute to acute attacks.

Synonyms

Pyrroloporphyria
Swedish Porphyria

Signs and Symptoms The manifestations of AIP are varied and can mimic those of numerous other conditions. The finding of an increased level of urinary delta-aminolevulinic acid indicates that an acute porphyria is present; a deficiency of PBG-deaminase in red blood cells usually establishes the diagnosis of AIP (although false positive results can occur).

Severe abdominal pain is a common symptom of the acute attack, with nausea, vomiting, and constipation. There may be pain in the back, arms, and legs, and muscle weakness. Urinary retention may occur, but urinary symptoms may also include frequency, incontinence, dysuria, and urine the color of port wine. Both hypertension and hyponatremia (from the vomiting) may occur during an acute attack. Central nervous system involvement may include confusion, hallucinations, and seizures. Neuropathy is a common symptom, and motor neuropathy may result in respiratory deficiency. The patient may feel depressed, anxious, and paranoid; porphyria has been misdiagnosed as psychosis.

The course of AIP varies; it may be chronic with few acute attacks, or there may be periods of remission alternating with acute attacks. Not all individuals who inherit this condition become symptomatic. The prognosis greatly depends on early detection and careful preventive measures.

Etiology Environmental factors that contribute to precipitation of the acute attack include certain drugs, chemicals, and diet. These factors can greatly influence the severity of symptoms.

Epidemiology Symptomatic AIP is estimated to affect fewer than 1:100,000 persons, most frequently those of Scandinavian, Anglo-Saxon, or German ancestry. Women are affected more often than men; in both, the disorder generally occurs after puberty.

Treatment—Standard The orphan drug hematin (Panhematin) is effective in suppressing acute attacks of AIP. Newer agents such as haem-arginate and Sn-proto-porphyrin appear promising.

Diagnosis is essential before medications are given, since the effects of many commonly used drugs are unknown or unclear in some types of porphyria. Advice from a center specializing in porphyria is recommended regarding drug administration to these patients. A list of these institutions may be obtained from the American Porphyria Foundation. If a person is diagnosed as having acute intermittent porphyria while taking longterm medications such as tranquilizers, antiseizure drugs, or birth control pills, specialist monitoring or withdrawal of the drug may be needed.

Because acute attacks can occur with carbohydrate restriction, patients should be advised not to restrict carbohydrate and calorie intake. If weight loss is desired, consultation with a nutritionist is recommended.

Some women report premenstrual attacks of AIP that resolve with the onset of menstruation. Exogenous steroids have been used in some such cases.

Genetic counseling is recommended for individuals with AIP. Only 50 percent of an affected person's offspring will carry the gene, and most of those with the disease will remain latent for most of their lives. If the condition is identified early, preventive measures can be taken and treatment can be successful in symptom control in most cases.

Patients with symptomatic AIP should wear a Medic Alert bracelet.

Treatment—Investigational Please contact the agencies listed under Resources, below, for the most current information.

Resources

For more information on acute intermittent porphyria: National Organization for Rare Disorders (NORD); American Porphyria Foundation; Porphyria Support Group; National Institute of Diabetes, Digestive & Kidney Diseases Information Clearinghouse.

For genetic information and genetic counseling referrals: March of Dimes Birth Defects Foundation; National Center for Education in Maternal and

Child Health (NCEMCH).

References
The Metabolic Basis of Inherited Disease, 6th ed.: C.R. Scriver, et al., eds.; McGraw-Hill, 1989, pp. 1320–1329.

PORPHYRIA, ALA-D

Description ALA-D porphyria is a recently described acute hepatic porphyria. The enzymatic defect is a lack of delta-aminolevulinic acid dehydratase.

When a patient is diagnosed as having ALA-D, relatives should be examined as well, so that individuals with latent disease can avoid precipitating agents.

Signs and Symptoms Severe abdominal pain is a common symptom of the acute attack, with nausea, vomiting, and constipation. Pain may also affect the extremities, and generalized muscle weakness may be present. There may be paralysis of the extremities and the muscles of the respiratory system.

Determination of elevated urinary ALA indicates that an acute porphyria is present; if the level of ALA-D is deficient (1/2 normal) in red blood cells, the diagnosis of ALA-D porphyria is usually established (although false positive and equivocal results do occur).

Environmental factors that contribute to precipitation of acute attacks may include reduced carbohydrate intake, ingestion of alcohol, and stress.

Etiology The disorder is inherited as an autosomal recessive trait.

Epidemiology ALA-D porphyria is extremely rare. There are only a few known cases.

Related Disorders See *Porphyria, Acute Intermittent.*

Treatment—Standard Because the disorder is so rare, therapeutic experience is not extensive. ALA-D porphyria is similar to acute intermittent porphyria, and treatment should cautiously be the same: elimination of precipitating factors, routine carbohydrate intake, administration of glucose, and use of hematin.

Treatment—Investigational Please contact the agencies listed under Resources, below, for the most current information.

Resources
For more information on ALA-D porphyria: National Organization for Rare Disorders (NORD); American Porphyria Foundation; Porphyria Support Group; National Institute of Diabetes, Digestive & Kidney Diseases Information Clearinghouse.

For genetic information and genetic counseling referrals: March of Dimes Birth Defects Foundation; National Center for Education in Maternal and Child Health (NCEMCH).

References

The Metabolic Basis of Inherited Disease, 6th ed.: C.R. Scriver, et al., eds.; McGraw-Hill, 1989, pp. 1317–1320.

PORPHYRIA, CONGENITAL ERYTHROPOIETIC (CEP)

Description CEP is one of the hereditary erythropoietic porphyrias; the deficient enzyme is uroporphyrinogen III cosynthase. Levels of porphyrins are markedly increased in bone marrow, red blood cells, plasma, urine, and feces, and may also be deposited in the teeth and bones.

Synonyms
> Congenital Porphyria
> Günther Porphyria

Signs and Symptoms As is characteristic of the erythropoietic porphyrias, symptoms usually begin during early infancy, although cases of adult onset have been reported. The initial sign in infancy may be pink to brown diaper staining. Skin photosensitivity may also be an early characteristic; bullae may result in bacterial infection and scarring of the damaged skin. Facial features and fingers may be lost over time. Erythrodontia, hypertrichosis, and alopecia are common. Red blood cells have a shortened life span, and anemia often results. Splenomegaly may be present.

Etiology Congenital erythropoietic porphyria is inherited as an autosomal recessive trait. The metabolic error is a faulty conversion of porphobilinogen (PBG) to uroporphyrinogen in the erythroid cells of the bone marrow. Environmental factors that may aggravate the symptoms or provoke an acute attack include drugs, chemicals, diet, and sun exposure. These factors can greatly influence the severity of symptoms.

Epidemiology CEP is extremely rare. No gender or racial predilections have been established.

Treatment—Standard Sunlight, and trauma to the skin from infection and injury should be avoided. Transfusions with packed erythrocytes and splenectomy have been performed. These procedures have short-term effects on the hemolysis and porphyrin excretion but must be used with caution. Intravenous hematin and oral charcoal have also been used.

Consultation with a medical center specializing in porphyria is advisable concerning the use of drugs by these patients. Genetic counseling may be useful when appropriate.

Treatment—Investigational Please contact the agencies listed under Resources, below, for the most current information.

Resources
For more information on congenital erythropoietic porphyria: National

Organization for Rare Disorders (NORD); American Porphyria Foundation; Porphyria Support Group; National Institute of Diabetes, Digestive & Kidney Diseases Information Clearinghouse.

For genetic information and genetic counseling referrals: March of Dimes Birth Defects Foundation; National Center for Education in Maternal and Child Health (NCEMCH).

References
The Metabolic Basis of Inherited Disease, 6th ed.: C.R. Scriver, et al., eds.; McGraw-Hill, 1989, pp. 1329–1332.

PORPHYRIA CUTANEA TARDA (PCT)

Description PCT results from an inherited or acquired deficiency of the enzyme uroporphyrinogen decarboxylase. The disorder occurs in both children and adults.

Synonyms
    Idiosyncratic Porphyria
    Porphyria Cutanea Symptomatica

Signs and Symptoms Initial symptoms of both inherited and acquired PCT are cutaneous, with blistering on the hands, face, and arms after exposure to sunlight or minor trauma. Hyper- and hypopigmentation, and hirsutism as well as alopecia may develop. Neurologic and abdominal symptoms are not characteristic of PCT. Liver function abnormalities are common but are generally mild.

Etiology PCT may be inherited as an autosomal dominant trait, or it may be acquired. The metabolic error in either case is a deficiency of the enzyme uroporphyrinogen decarboxylase (URO-D). In the inherited form, the enzyme is lacking in all body tissues; when acquired, the deficiency is present only in the liver. Environmental factors may include estrogens, chlorinated hydrocarbons, iron, alcohol, and of course, exposure to the sun.

Epidemiology PCT is the most common of the porphyrias. The inherited form generally is first seen in childhood. Acquired PCT most often occurs in adults and is more prevalent in males, although the number of affected females is increasing.

Treatment—Standard Precipitating factors (see Etiology, above) must be avoided. Phlebotomy or alternatively the use of chloroquine has been used to treat PCT.

Treatment—Investigational Please contact the agencies listed under Resources, below, for the most current information.

Resources
    For more information on porphyria cutanea tarda: National Organization for Rare Disorders (NORD); American Porphyria Foundation; Porphyria Support Group; National Institute of Diabetes, Digestive & Kidney Diseases Information Clearinghouse.

    For genetic information and genetic counseling referrals: March of

Dimes Birth Defects Foundation; National Center for Education in Maternal and Child Health (NCEMCH).

References
The Metabolic Basis of Inherited Disease, 6th ed.: C.R. Scriver, et al., eds.; McGraw-Hill, 1989, pp. 1332–1337.

PORPHYRIA, ERYTHROPOIETIC PROTOPORPHYRIA (EPP)

Description EPP is characterized by a deficiency of ferrochelatase, which leads to an accumulation of protoporphyrin in the bone marrow, red blood cells, and sometimes in the liver. Excess protoporphyrin is excreted by the liver into the bile, which in turn enters the intestine and is excreted in the feces. There are no urinary abnormalities associated with EPP.

Synonyms
Erythrohepatic Protoporphyria
Protoporphyria

Signs and Symptoms Symptoms begin in childhood and are mostly related to photosensitivity. After exposure to artificial light as well as sunlight, patients may experience burning, itching, edema, and erythema. Occasionally, the skin problems occur only after extended sunlight exposure. In some cases lesions occur that persist for days or weeks and leave a scar. Severe sequelae such as bullae, hyperpigmentation, and mutilation are not common. The cutaneous manifestations of EPP tend to be more severe in the summer and can recur throughout life.

Other manifestations of this type of porphyria include gallstones containing protoporphyrin, and occasionally, the development of severe hepatic complications. Some carriers of the genetic abnormality remain asymptomatic and have normal porphyrin levels.

The diagnosis is established by identification of increased protoporphyrin in the red blood cells, plasma, and feces.

Etiology EPP is inherited as an autosomal dominant trait. Protoporphyrin accumulates in erythrocytes, plasma, and feces.

Epidemiology Erythropoietic protoporphyria usually begins in childhood, and males and females are affected equally.

Treatment—Standard Exposure to the sun and some artificial light, especially theater lighting, should be avoided. Beta-carotene may improve sunlight tolerance. Cholestyramine may be photoprotective to some extent and reduces hepatic protoporphyrin.

Hepatic deposits of protoporphyrin may lead to liver abnormalities in patients with EPP. Although hepatic involvement is not common, when it occurs it is severe, and avoidance of hepatotoxic agents is recommended.

It is advisable to consult with a center specializing in the treatment of porphyria before administering any drug to a patient with EPP. Genetic counseling may be useful, since pregnancy is tolerated much better than was formerly believed.

Treatment—Investigational Please contact the agencies listed under Resources, below, for the most current information.

Resources

For more information on erythropoietic protoporphyria: National Organization for Rare Disorders (NORD); American Porphyria Foundation; Porphyria Support Group; National Institute of Diabetes, Digestive & Kidney Diseases Information Clearinghouse.

For genetic information and genetic counseling referrals: March of Dimes Birth Defects Foundation; National Center for Education in Maternal and Child Health (NCEMCH).

PORPHYRIA, HEREDITARY COPROPORPHYRIA (HCP)

Description HCP, an inherited hepatic porphyria, is due to deficiency of coproporphyrinogen oxidase, and is similar to acute intermittent porphyria (AIP), but with milder symptoms and with the additional characteristic in some patients of photosensitivity.

Signs and Symptoms Although the patient is sensitive to sunlight, skin disease is rarely severe in HCP. The characteristic features of AIP are present here in milder form, and include pain in the abdomen and arms and legs; generalized weakness that may result in respiratory paralysis; urinary retention; vomiting; constipation; increased heart rate; confusion; hallucinations; psychosis; and seizures.

The diagnosis is established by identification of excess coproporphyrin in urine and stool.

Etiology HCP is inherited as an autosomal dominant trait. Symptoms are the result of a deficiency of coproporphyrinogen oxidase. Drugs such as barbiturates, tranquilizers, anticonvulsants, and estrogens may precipitate an attack, as may diet and sun exposure.

Epidemiology HCP is the least common of the hepatic porphyrias. Onset may be at any age.

Related Disorders See *Porphyria, Acute Intermittent.*

Treatment—Standard Precipitating factors must be avoided. For treatment information, see *Porphyria, Acute Intermittent.*

Treatment—Investigational Please contact the agencies listed under Resources, below, for the most current information.

Resources

For more information on hereditary coproporphyria: National Organization for Rare Disorders (NORD); American Porphyria Foundation; Porphyria Support Group; National Institute of Diabetes, Digestive & Kidney Diseases Information Clearinghouse.

For genetic information and genetic counseling referrals: March of Dimes Birth Defects Foundation; National Center for Education in Maternal and Child Health (NCEMCH).

References

The Metabolic Basis of Inherited Disease, 6th ed.: C.R. Scriver, et al., eds.; McGraw-Hill, 1989, pp. 1338–1341.

PORPHYRIA, VARIEGATE (VP)

Description VP, a hepatic porphyria produced by a deficiency in protoporphyrinogen oxidase, is characterized by neurologic abnormalities or photosensitivity, or both.

Synonyms

Protocoproporphyria
Royal Malady
South African Genetic Porphyria

Signs and Symptoms The neurologic and visceral features of VP are similar to those seen in acute intermittent porphyria and hereditary coproporphyria. The cutaneous features are identical to those seen in porphyria cutanea tarda **(PCT)**. Differential diagnosis must be made, because the treatment used for PCT is not successful in variegate porphyria. Plasma porphyrin fluorescence is generally seen in VP. When only cutaneous symptoms are present, the urinary 8- and 7-carboxylic porphyrins and isocoproporphyrin seen in porphyria cutanea tarda will differentiate that disorder from variegate porphyria.

Cutaneous symptoms and signs include burning, blistering, and scarring of sun-exposed areas; hyperpigmentation; hypertrichosis; and skin fragility (see *Porphyria Cutanea Tarda)*.

The neurovisceral symptoms and signs include severe abdominal pain, vomiting, and neuropathy (see *Porphyria, Acute Intermittent)*.

Etiology VP is inherited as an autosomal dominant trait. Symptoms are due to an inborn deficiency of protoporphyrinogen oxidase. Factors that may trigger acute neurovisceral attacks are the same as for acute intermittent porphyria and hereditary coproporphyria, and include barbiturates, estrogens, and reduced carbohydrate ingestion. Precipitating factors for the cutaneous symptoms and signs are the same as for porphyria cutanea tarda.

Epidemiology VP may begin between the ages of 10 to 30 years. It is more common in the white population of South Africa than elsewhere in the world. The disorder may affect males and females in equal numbers.

Related Disorders See *Porphyria, Acute Intermittent; Porphyria, Hereditary Coproporphyria; Porphyria Cutanea Tarda.*

Treatment—Standard Precipitating factors must be eliminated. For treatment of acute attacks, see *Porphyria, Acute Intermittent.*

Treatment—Investigational Please contact the agencies listed under Resources, below, for the most current information.

Resources

For more information on variegate porphyria: National Organization for Rare Disorders (NORD); American Porphyria Foundation; Porphyria Support Group; National Institute of Diabetes, Digestive & Kidney Diseases Information Clearinghouse.

For genetic information and genetic counseling referrals: March of Dimes Birth Defects Foundation; National Center for Education in Maternal and Child Health (NCEMCH).

References

The Metabolic Basis of Inherited Disease, 6th ed.: C.R. Scriver, et al., eds.; McGraw-Hill, 1989, pp. 1341–1342.

PSEUDOGOUT

Description Pseudogout is characterized by deposits of calcium pyrophosphate dihydrate (**CPPD**) crystals in one or more joints, causing symptoms and signs that mimic gout and other arthritides.

Synonyms

Articular Chondrocalcinosis
Calcium Pyrophosphate Dihydrate Crystal Deposition Disease

Signs and Symptoms Acute attacks of pseudogout involve swelling, stiffness, warmth, and pain, usually in one joint, most often the knee. Episodes last from 1 day to several weeks and can subside without treatment. They can be severe, but are usually not as disabling or painful as gout itself.

A milder, chronic form of pseudogout produces symptoms similar to the acute episode but less painful.

Etiology The cause of the crystal deposition is unknown. There is evidence that some cases of pseudogout are familial. Associations seem to exist with certain metabolic conditions such as hyperparathyroidism, familial hypocalciuric hypercalcemia, and hemochromatosis, and with surgery or other trauma as well as aging.

Epidemiology Pseudogout appears in mature adults. Some studies indicate a greater prevalence in women; other studies, in men. Asymptomatic articular calcinosis is common in persons over age 50. A familial pattern of incidence has been observed in several countries.

Related Disorders Gout is a recurrent acute arthritis that results from deposition of monosodium urate crystals in a person with hyperuricemia. In most cases gout is responsive to drugs and diet therapy.

Treatment—Standard There is at present no known way to prevent the formation of CPPD crystals, or to satisfactorily remove existing ones.

Acute attacks of pseudogout are treated in several ways. The excess fluid and CPPD crystals are drained from the affected joint. If only one joint is involved, a corticosteroid may be injected locally. Colchicine is effective for treating pseudogout as well as true gout. Aspirin and other nonsteroidal antiinflammatory drugs may be used.

During an attack the affected joint may need rest and protection with splints or canes. Once the episode subsides, or in the milder chronic form, rest should be balanced with carefully monitored appropriate exercise.

Surgical intervention and repair may be needed in rare cases of severe joint damage, pain, instability, or immobility.

Treatment—Investigational Please contact the agencies listed under Resources, below, for the most current information.

Resources

For more information on pseudogout: National Organization for Rare Disorders (NORD); Arthritis Foundation; The National Arthritis and Musculoskeletal and Skin Diseases Information Clearinghouse.

References

Arthritis and Allied Conditions, 11th ed.: D.J. McCarty; Lea & Febiger, 1989, pp. 1711–1731.

Cecil Textbook of Medicine, 18th ed.: J.B. Wyngaarden and L.H. Smith, Jr., eds.; W.B. Saunders Company, 1988, p. 2037.

PYRUVATE DEHYDROGENASE (PDH) DEFICIENCY

Description Pyruvate dehydrogenase deficiency is a disorder of carbohydrate metabolism that results in persistent or recurrent metabolic acidosis, and mental retardation and other neurologic symptoms and signs.

Synonyms

> Alaninuria
> Intermittent Ataxia with Pyruvate Dehydrogenase Deficiency
> Lactic and Pyruvate Acidemia with Carbohydrate Sensitivity
> Lactic and Pyruvate Acidemia with Episodic Ataxia and Weakness

Signs and Symptoms Biochemical abnormalities of PDH deficiency may vary from severe acidosis (due to abnormally high levels of lactic acid) appearing shortly after birth, to mildly elevated levels following a meal high in carbohydrates. Elevation of blood lactate levels and alaninuria may occur only during acute episodes. Diagnosis can be made postnatally by biochemical assay in fibroblast cells.

Recurrent episodes of muscle incoordination are seen, often with upper respiratory infection or other minor stress. The growth rate may be slowed in affected children, and varying degrees of neurologic deficits and mental retardation may occur.

Etiology The disorder is inherited as an autosomal recessive trait. A deficiency of the enzyme pyruvate dehydrogenase causes defective oxidation of pyruvate, and in severe cases, lactic acidosis may be triggered by consumption of a meal high in carbohydrates.

Epidemiology Males appear to be affected in slightly higher numbers than females.

Related Disorders See *Leigh Disease.*

Treatment—Standard Symptoms of this disorder can be controlled to some extent by avoiding carbohydrates and increasing fat in the diet. Avoidance of infection and undue stress is also recommended. Some cases may respond to treatment with thiamine (vitamin B1) or lipoic acid.

Genetic counseling is appropriate for families of affected children.

Treatment—Investigational Please contact the agencies listed under Resources, below, for the most current information.

Resources

For more information on PDH deficiency: National Organization for Rare Disorders (NORD); Lactic Acidosis Support Group; British Organic Acidemia Association; Research Trust for Metabolic Diseases in Children; NIH/National Institute of Neurological Disorders & Stroke (NINDS).

For genetic information and genetic counseling referrals: March of Dimes Birth Defects Foundation; National Center for Education in Maternal and Child Health (NCEMCH).

References

The Metabolic Basis of Inherited Disease, 6th ed.: C.R. Scriver, et al., eds.; McGraw-Hill, 1989, pp. 873–874.

PYRUVATE KINASE DEFICIENCY

Description Pyruvate kinase deficiency, a hereditary blood disorder, is characterized by a deficiency of the enzyme pyruvate kinase and is associated with hemolytic anemia.

Signs and Symptoms The chronic hemolytic anemia that occurs varies from mild to severe. Jaundice, splenomegaly, and gallstones or leg ulcers may develop. The anemia tends to worsen after infections. Onset of anemia and jaundice is usually in infancy or early childhood. If symptoms are first seen in adulthood, the disorder is generally less severe.

Etiology Pyruvate kinase deficiency is inherited as an autosomal recessive trait.

Epidemiology The disorder is rare, with a distribution that appears to be worldwide. Males and females are affected in equal numbers.

Related Disorders See the discussion of **Glucose-6-phosphatase dehydrogenase (G6PD) deficiency** in *Anemia, Hemolytic, Hereditary Nonspherocytic.*

Treatment—Standard The anemia of pyruvate kinase deficiency is usually treated with blood transfusions. In severe cases among infants and young children, splenectomy may be needed. Other treatment is symptomatic and supportive.

Treatment—Investigational Please contact the agencies listed under Resources, below, for the most current information.

Resources

For more information on pyruvate kinase deficiency: National Organization for Rare Disorders (NORD); NIH/National Heart, Lung and Blood Institute (NHLBI).

For genetic information and genetic counseling referrals: March of Dimes Birth Defects Foundation; National Center for Education in Maternal and Child Health (NCEMCH).

References

The Metabolic Basis of Inherited Disease, 6th ed.: C.R. Scriver, et al., eds.; McGraw-Hill, 1989, pp. 2342–2348.

REFSUM SYNDROME

Description Refsum syndrome is a slowly progressive disorder of lipid metabolism characterized by the accumulation of phytanic acid in blood and tissues and associated with neurologic disorders.

Synonyms

Heredopathia Atactica Polyneuritiformis
Hypertrophic Neuropathy of Refsum
Phytanic Acid Storage Disease

Signs and Symptoms The 4 major features of the syndrome are retinitis pigmentosa, peripheral neuropathy, ataxia, and elevated protein in cerebrospinal fluid without pleocytosis. Other characteristics include nystagmus, anosmia, ichthyosis, and epiphyseal dysplasia.

Etiology The syndrome is inherited as an autosomal recessive trait. Deficiency of phytanic acid alpha-hydroxylase leads to an accumulation of phytanic acid in the blood plasma and tissues of the body.

Epidemiology Onset has occurred from early childhood to age 50 years, but symptoms and signs are most often first seen by age 20 years. Males and females are affected in equal numbers.

Related Disorders See *Acanthocytosis; Gaucher Disease.*

Treatment—Standard Dietary restriction of foods containing phytanic acid lowers its plasma concentration. This reduction, however, may not be seen for months, leading to the conclusion that phytanate body stores are being used. With adherence to the diet, peripheral neuropathy is eventually arrested and ichthyosis disappears. It appears that while eye and ear symptoms do not regress, progression is arrested. Foods containing phytanic acid include dairy products; tunafish, cod, and haddock; lamb and stewed beef; white bread, white rice, and boiled potatoes; and egg yolk.

Plasmapheresis as a supplement to a dietary regimen has been effective in providing a positive initial response.

Treatment—Investigational Please contact the agencies listed under Resources, below, for the most current information.

Resources

For more information on Refsum syndrome: National Organization for Rare Disorders (NORD); National Lipid Diseases Foundation; United Leukodystrophy Foundation; RP Foundation Fighting Blindness; NIH/National Institute of Neurological Disorders & Stroke (NINDS); Research Trust for Metabolic Diseases in Children.

For genetic information and genetic counseling referrals: March of Dimes Birth Defects Foundation; National Center for Education in Maternal and Child Health (NCEMCH).

References
The Metabolic Basis of Inherited Disease, 6th ed.: C.R. Scriver, et al., eds.; McGraw-Hill, 1989, pp. 1533–1547.
Heredopathia Atactica Polyneuritiformis (Refsum's Disease) Treated by Diet and Plasma-exchange: F.B. Gibberd, et al.; Lancet, 1986, issue 1(8116), pp. 575–578.

SANDHOFF DISEASE

Description Sandhoff disease is a progressive, inherited, lipid storage disorder that leads to the eventual destruction of the central nervous system as well as involvement of the larger viscera. It is a severe form of Tay-Sachs disease and is not restricted to any particular ethnic group.

Synonyms
Gangliosidosis GM2 Type 2

Signs and Symptoms Initial manifestations usually are seen in the 3rd to the 6th month of life, and include feeding problems, lethargy, and a marked startle response to sound. Cherry red macular spots are usually seen. Motor and mental deterioration may be progressive, and symptoms and signs include motor weakness, spasticity, heart murmurs, myoclonic and generalized seizures, blindness, and splenomegaly. A positive Babinski sign is typical, and the outer toes spread after the side of the sole of the foot has been stroked.

Etiology Sandhoff disease is transmitted as an autosomal recessive condition. It is caused by hexosaminidase beta-subunit deficiency. GM2 ganglioside accumulates in the brain and large viscera.

Epidemiology The disorder is very rare, and is found in persons of all ethnic backgrounds. Males and females are affected equally.

Related Disorders See *Tay-Sachs Disease; Gaucher Disease; Niemann-Pick Disease; Batten Disease; Epilepsy.*

Treatment—Standard Treatment is symptomatic and supportive. Genetic counseling will benefit families of affected persons.

Treatment—Investigational Enzyme replacement therapy is being tested as a possible treatment for Sandhoff disease, but more research is needed to determine the safety and effectiveness of this procedure.

Please contact the agencies listed under Resources, below, for the most current information.

Resources

For more information on Sandhoff disease: National Organization for Rare Disorders (NORD); National Tay-Sachs/Allied Diseases Association; National Lipid Diseases Foundation; NIH/National Institute of Neurological Disorders & Stroke (NINDS).

For genetic information and genetic counseling referrals: March of Dines Birth Defects Foundation; NIH/National Center for Education in Maternal and Child Health (NCEMCH).

References

The Metabolic Basis of Inherited Disease, 6th ed.: C.R. Scriver, et al., eds.; McGraw-Hill, 1989, pp. 331–332.

Internal Medicine, 3rd ed.: J.H. Stein, ed.-in-chief; Little, Brown and Company, 1990, p. 2320.

SANFILIPPO SYNDROME

Description Sanfilippo syndrome (mucopolysaccharidosis type III—**MPS III**) is characterized by severe mental deterioration but only mild physical disease, and urinary excretion of heparan sulfate. The 4 forms of the syndrome are classified according to the specific enzyme lack in the process of eliminating heparan sulfate. Types A and B are the most common.

MPS III-A lacks heparan N-sulfatase.

MPS III-B lacks alpha-N-acetylglucosaminidase.

MPS III-C lacks acetyl-CoA: alpha-glucosaminide acetyltransferase.

MPS III-D lacks N-acetylglucosamine 6-sulfatase.

Synonyms

Mucopolysaccharidosis Type III

Signs and Symptoms Children appear normal at birth; onset of symptoms and signs occurs between 2 and 6 years of age. Initial manifestations include hyperactivity, hirsutism, developmental delay (generally evident by 2 to 3 years of age), and mild hepatosplenomegaly. An unexplained diarrhea may occur but usually disappears in later childhood. There may be mild dysostosis multiplex and mild joint stiffness.

Signs of mental retardation are usually first seen at ages 3 to 5 years, and neurologic deterioration is evident from 6 to 10 years. Between the ages of 3 to 6 years, behavioral disturbances and intellectual decline usually are first seen. Sleep disturbance may be present, and seizures may occur. Speech is often delayed, and some children never acquire the ability to speak. Deafness may be profound in even the moderately affected patient. The child may be able to start school but will often become a behavior problem, with temper tantrums and aggressiveness increasing as dementia progresses.

Etiology All types of Sanfilippo syndrome are autosomal recessive. Deficiency of the enzymes specific to the syndrome results in an inability to metabolize mucopolysaccharides. The accumulation of these large, undegraded mucopolysaccharides in the cells of the body causes the physical symptoms and abnormalities.

Epidemiology The syndrome occurs in about 1:50,000 live births. Males and females are affected equally.

Related Disorders Patients with MPS Type III are more similar to those with MPS Type II (see *Hunter Syndrome*) than to those with other forms.

Treatment—Standard Treatment is symptomatic and supportive. Genetic counseling may be helpful to the parents of affected patients. Prenatal diagnosis is now possible for this disorder.

Treatment—Investigational Treatments aimed at checking early development of Sanfilippo syndrome are now under study. These include enzyme replacement therapy and bone marrow transplantation.

Please contact the agencies listed under Resources, below, for the most current information.

Resources

For more information on Sanfilippo syndrome: National Organization for Rare Disorders (NORD); MPS (Mucopolysaccharidoses) Research Funding Center, Inc.; National MPS Society; Society of Mucopolysaccharide Diseases, Inc.; Society of MPS Diseases; National Institute of Diabetes, Digestive & Kidney Diseases Information Clearinghouse.

For genetic information and genetic counseling referrals: March of Dimes Birth Defects Foundation; National Center for Education in Maternal and Child Health (NCEMCH).

References
The Metabolic Basis of Inherited Disease, 6th ed.: C.R. Scriver, et al., eds.; McGraw-Hill, 1989, pp. 1574–1575.
MPS Society brochure.

SIALADENITIS

Description Sialadenitis, inflammation of a salivary gland, results from obstruction of a salivary gland or duct, and is usually accompanied by painful swelling of the gland and possible bacterial infection.

Signs and Symptoms The affected gland becomes enlarged, tender, and red. Calculi may block secretions from the gland, leading to infection and other complications such as the formation of a salivary fistula or development of an abscess.

Etiology In most cases the cause is unknown. Ingestion of potassium iodide or mercury can lead to sialadenitis because of salivary hypersecretion.

Epidemiology The condition is rare.

Related Disorders See *Sjögren's Syndrome.*

Mixed tumor of the salivary gland (pleomorphic adenoma of the salivary gland) is a slowly growing, benign tumor of unknown origin, usually located in the parotid salivary glands. Onset is slow, but later growth may be rapid. Pain and paralysis of the facial muscles may occur. This disorder tends to be familial.

Periodic sialadenosis (periodic sialorrhea, or recurring salivary adenitis) is a disorder of unknown cause, possibly of autosomal dominant inheritance, characterized by sudden discomfort in the parotid region, and excessive saliva. The outer ear sometimes appears distorted.

Treatment—Standard Initial treatment involves hydration and massage to move the stone out of the gland. Antibiotics and corticosteroids have been used to treat secondary symptoms.

For recurrent infectious sialadenitis, surgical removal of the salivary gland may be necessary. Alternative treatment methods have been used to induce shrinkage of the gland, such as radiation, tying of the salivary duct, or cutting the tympanic nerve.

Treatment—Investigational For treatment of the chronic, recurrent form of sialadenitis a new method is being investigated. The procedure, which has had some success thus far, consists of instilling an amino acid or protein solution into the salivary duct. The solution hardens and causes a reduction or elimination of salivary gland tissue. The hardened protein is later reabsorbed.

Please contact the agencies listed under Resources, below, for the most current information.

Resources

For more information on sialadenitis: National Organization for Rare Disorders (NORD); NIH/National Institute of Dental Research.

References

Salivary Glands: J.R. Saunders, Jr., et al.; Surg. Clin. N. Amer., February 1986, issue 66(1), pp. 59–81.

Parotid Gland Atrophy Induced by Occlusion of the Ductal System with a Protein Solution: G. Rettinger, et al.; Am. J. Otolaryngology, May–June 1984, issue 5(3), pp. 183–190.

SIALIDOSIS

Description Sialidosis, previously called **mucolipidosis I,** is caused by a deficiency in the degradation of glycoproteins due to an inherited defect in the enzyme alpha-neuraminidase. Findings include normal urinary mucopolysaccharides and elevated urinary oligosaccharides containing salic acid.

Two forms of sialidosis are known: type I, characterized by myoclonus and neuropathy; and type II, typified by myoclonus plus mild coarsening of the facial features, skeletal changes, and mild mental retardation.

Synonyms

Mucolipidosis I

Signs and Symptoms Type I symptoms and signs, usually first seen in the teens, include an ocular cherry-red spot, impaired vision, night blindness, myoclonus, and, possibly, ataxia, tremor, nystagmus, and seizures.

Type II is characterized by the visual abnormalities of type I plus manifestations such as a coarse facies, hepatosplenomegaly, dysostosis multiplex, and mental retardation. Time of onset is variable, but affected infants who appear normal at birth will progress to the full type II syndrome.

Carriers of sialidosis can be detected by an enzyme assay in cultured fibroblasts, making prenatal diagnosis possible.

Etiology Sialidosis is an autosomal recessive inherited disorder in which the activity of the enzyme alpha-neuraminidase is deficient.

Epidemiology The disorder is very rare. Males and females are affected equally.

Treatment—Standard Treatment is symptomatic and supportive. Genetic counseling is advised for families affected by this disorder.

Treatment—Investigational Please contact the agencies listed under Resources, below, for the most current information.

Resources

For more information on sialidosis: National Organization for Rare Disorders (NORD); National Lipid Diseases Foundation; MPS (Mucopolysaccharidoses) Research Funding Center, Inc.; The MPS Society, Inc.; Society of Mucopolysaccharide Diseases, Inc.; Society of MPS Diseases; National Institute of

Diabetes, Digestive & Kidney Diseases Information Clearinghouse.

For genetic information and genetic counseling referrals: March of Dimes Birth Defects Foundation; National Center for Education in Maternal and Child Health (NCEMCH).

References

The Metabolic Basis of Inherited Disease, 6th ed.: C.R. Scriver, et al., eds.; McGraw-Hill, 1989, pp. 1611–1614.

SLY SYNDROME

Description Sly syndrome (mucopolysaccharidosis type VII—**MPS VII**) is a metabolic disorder in which there is an excess of urinary dermatan sulfate. Symptomatology is similar to that seen in Hurler syndrome (MPS I). Mental retardation, short stature, and skeletal, intestinal, and corneal abnormalities are characteristic.

Synonyms

Beta-Glucuronidase Deficiency
Mucopolysaccharidosis Type VII

Signs and Symptoms Moderate and nonprogressive mental retardation initially appearing at about 3 years of age seems to be a common feature of Sly syndrome. Patients have unusual facies. Corneal opacities develop at about 8 years of age. Short stature is a common characteristic, and the dysostosis multiplex seen in the mucopolysaccharidoses may be severe, and include joint contractures, dislocated hips, and spinal malformations. Other findings include hepatosplenomegaly, inguinal and umbilical hernias, and aortic regurgitation.

A severe neonatal form exists, the newborns presenting with hydrops fetalis and dysostosis multiplex.

Prenatal diagnosis is now possible for Sly syndrome from the 4th month of pregnancy on.

Etiology The syndrome is inherited as an autosomal recessive trait. The enzyme beta-glucuronidase is deficient.

Epidemiology Fewer than 20 cases have been identified throughout the world. Males and females are affected equally.

Related Disorders See *Mucopolysaccharidosis.*

The mucolipidoses are a family of disorders that produce symptoms very similar to those of the mucopolysaccharidoses. See *Mucolipidosis II; Mucolipidosis III; Mucolipidosis IV.*

Treatment—Standard Treatment of Sly syndrome is symptomatic and supportive. Surgical intervention may be required to correct orthopedic problems, hernias, and ocular and cardiovascular abnormalities. Genetic counseling may be helpful to both patient and family.

Treatment—Investigational Treatments aimed at checking early development of Sly syndrome include enzyme replacement therapy and bone marrow transplantation.

Please contact the agencies listed under Resources, below, for the most current information.

Resources

For more information on Sly syndrome: National Organization for Rare Disorders (NORD); MPS (Mucopolysaccharidoses) Research Funding Center, Inc.; National MPS Society; Society of Mucopolysaccharide Diseases, Inc.; Society of MPS Diseases; National Institute of Diabetes, Digestive & Kidney Diseases Information Clearinghouse.

For genetic information and genetic counseling referrals: March of Dimes Birth Defects Foundation; National Center for Education in Maternal and Child Health (NCEMCH).

References

The Metabolic Basis of Inherited Disease, 6th ed.: C.R. Scriver, et al., eds.; McGraw-Hill, 1989, p. 1577.

TANGIER DISEASE

Description Tangier disease is a slowly progressive inherited metabolic disease marked by decreased or absent plasma concentrations of high density lipoproteins, low plasma cholesterol levels, and accumulation of cholesterol esters in certain body tissues.

Synonyms

> Alpha High-Density Lipoprotein Deficiency
> Familial Alpha-Lipoprotein Deficiency
> Alphalipoproteinemia
> Analphalipoproteinemia
> Familial High-Density Lipoprotein Deficiency

Signs and Symptoms Initial characteristics are severely decreased plasma high density lipoproteins, low plasma cholesterol levels, normal or elevated triglycerides, and large, yellow-orange tonsils and adenoids. The rectum may also have the same color. As the disease progresses, neuropathy, hepatomegaly, splenomegaly, corneal deposits, and coronary artery disease may develop.

Etiology The cause seems to be autosomal inheritance of a defective gene controlling HDL production. The absence of normal amounts of high density lipoproteins in the blood causes the symptoms.

Epidemiology Tangier disease is thought to be present at birth, but symptoms only become apparent during later childhood or adulthood. The disease is very rare; probably fewer than 50 persons are affected worldwide.

Treatment—Standard Treatment of Tangier disease is symptomatic and supportive.

Treatment—Investigational Please contact the agencies listed under Resources, below, for the most current information.

Resources
   For more information on Tangier disease: National Organization for Rare Disorders (NORD); National Lipid Diseases Foundation; NIH/National Institute of Neurological Disorders & Stroke (NINDS); National Tay-Sachs/Allied Diseases Association.
   For genetic information and genetic counseling referrals: March of Dimes Birth Defects Foundation; National Center for Education in Maternal and Child Health (NCEMCH).

References
   The Metabolic Basis of Inherited Disease, 6th ed.: C.R. Scriver, et al., eds.; McGraw-Hill, 1989, pp. 1267–1279.
   Tangier Disease. A Histological and Ultrastructural Study: P. Dechelotte, et al.; Pathol. Res. Pract., October 1985, issue 180(4), pp. 424–430.

TAY-SACHS DISEASE

Description Tay-Sachs disease, a GM2 gangliosidosis, results in progressive destruction of the central nervous system. The disease is generally found among children of Jewish heritage.

Synonyms
      GM2 Gangliosidosis, Type I
      Hexosaminidase Alpha-Subunit Deficiency (Variant B)

Signs and Symptoms Mild motor weakness is usually the initial manifestation, with onset around 3 to 5 months of age. An abnormal startle response and myoclonic jerk may also be seen at this time. Between 6 and 10 months further signs appear, i.e., feeding difficulties, hypotonia, weakness, restlessness, and vision abnormalities such as staring episodes, unusual eye movements, and cherry red macular spots. By the end of the first year there is increasing loss of vision.
   After 12 months the child begins to regress, losing learned skills and coordination. Seizures begin, and deterioration continues, ending with the child flaccid, unresponsive, and paralyzed.
   Tay-Sachs disease can be detected prenatally through amniocentesis, and prospective parents can be tested to determine their carrier status.

Etiology Tay-Sachs is inherited as an autosomal recessive trait, and results in deficient hexosaminidase activity. One of the hexosaminidase subunits (B subunit) has been located on chromosome 5. This deficiency leads to storage of GM2 gangliosides in the central nervous system.

Epidemiology The disease primarily affects persons of Jewish ancestry, especially those of Eastern European Ashkenazi descent. It also is often found in some communities of Italian descent, in Irish Catholics, and in non-Jewish Canadians.

Related Disorders See *Sandhoff Disease,* which is clinically indistinguishable from Tay-Sachs but is found in the general population.

Treatment—Standard Treatment is symptomatic.

Treatment—Investigational Please contact the agencies listed under Resources, below, for the most current information.

Resources

For more information on Tay-Sachs disease: National Organization for Rare Disorders (NORD); National Tay-Sachs/Allied Diseases Association, Inc.; NIH/National Institute of Child Health and Human Development; National Foundation for Jewish Genetic Diseases; National Lipid Diseases Foundation; Research Trust for Metabolic Diseases in Children.

For genetic information and genetic counseling referrals: March of Dimes Birth Defects Foundation; National Center for Education in Maternal and Child Health (NCEMCH).

References
The Metabolic Basis of Inherited Disease, 6th ed.: C.R. Scriver, et al., eds.; McGraw-Hill, 1989, pp. 1807–1839.

Cecil Textbook of Medicine, 18th ed.: J.B. Wyngaarden and L.H. Smith, Jr., eds.; W.B. Saunders Company, 1988, pp. 149, 157, 174.

Mendelian Inheritance in Man, 9th ed.: V.A. McKusick; The Johns Hopkins University Press, 1990, pp. 1492–1497.

TETRAHYDROBIOPTERIN DEFICIENCIES

Description Tetrahydrobiopterin deficiency is a rare genetic, neurologic disorder present at birth. When the coenzyme tetrahydrobiopterin is deficient, an abnormally high blood level of the amino acid phenylalanine occurs and low levels of neurotransmitters result. To avoid irreversible neurologic damage, diagnosis and treatment of this progressive disorder are essential early in life.

Synonyms
Atypical Hyperphenylalaninemia
BH4 Deficiency
Malignant Hyperphenylalaninemia

Signs and Symptoms In general, symptoms of tetrahydrobiopterin deficiencies usually include neurologic disturbances, muscle tone and coordination abnormalities, seizures, and delayed motor development.

Etiology Tetrahydrobiopterin deficiencies are inherited as autosomal recessive traits.

Epidemiology Tetrahydrobiopterin deficiency occurs worldwide and is estimated to affect 1 to 3 percent of infants diagnosed with phenylketonuria (**PKU**) at birth. PKU occurs at a rate of 1:10,000 to 1:20,000 live births in the United States.

Related Disorders See *Phenylketonuria.*

Hyperphenylalaninemia is identified by the presence of abnormally high blood levels of the amino acid phenylalanine in newborns, which may or may not be associated with elevated levels of tyrosine. This disorder may be a type of PKU or it may be associated with short-term deficiencies of phenylalanine hydroxylase or *p*-hydroxyphenylpyruvic acid oxidase.

Treatment—Standard Treatment should be started as early as possible because of the potentially severe neurologic development. A low phenylalanine diet does not control the metabolic imbalance, but may be necessary to keep phenylalanine levels within normal range. Treatment with tetrahydrobiopterin (BH4) is mandatory to normalize blood phenylalanine levels by restoring liver phenylalanine hydroxylase activity.

Genetic counseling is essential for patients and their families.

Treatment—Investigational Treatments being tested for tetrahydrobiopterin deficiencies include administration of l-dopa and 5-hydroxytryptophan. High-dosage tetrahydrobiopterin administration is used with dynamic improvement in some patients. Synthetic forms of tetrahydrobiopterin are also under study.

The Food and Drug Administration has awarded a research grant to Joseph Muenzer, M.D., University of Michigan, Ann Arbor, Michigan, for studies on tetrahydrobiopterin as a treatment for this disorder.

Please contact the agencies listed under Resources, below, for the most current information.

Resources

For more information on tetrahydrobiopterin deficiencies: National Organization for Rare Disorders (NORD); NIH/National Institute of Neurological Disorders & Stroke (NINDS); National Association for Retarded Citizens; National Institute of Mental Retardation; Children's Brain Diseases Foundation for Research; Research Trust for Metabolic Diseases in Children.

For genetic information and genetic counseling referrals: March of Dimes Birth Defects Foundation; National Center for Education in Maternal and Child Health (NCEMCH).

References

Hyperphenylalaninaemia Due to Impaired Dihydrobiopterin Biosynthesis: Leukocyte Function and Effect of Tetrahydrobiopterin Therapy: K. Fukuda, et al.; J. Inherited Metab. Dis., 1985, issue 8(2), pp. 49–52.

Hyperphenylalaninaemia Caused by Defects in Biopterin Metabolism: S. Kaufman; J. Inherited Metab. Dis., 1985, issue 8(suppl. 1), pp. 20-27.

Differential Diagnosis of Tetrahydrobiopterin Deficiency: A. Neiderweiser, et al.; J. Inherited Metab. Dis., 1985, issue 8(suppl. 1), pp. 34–38.

TYROSINEMIA I

Description Tyrosinemia I is a metabolic disorder caused by a lack of the enzyme fumarylacetoacetate hydrolyase, yielding elevated levels of tyrosine and its metabolites. Clinically, acute and chronic forms are seen.

Synonyms
> Tyrosinemia, Hereditary, Hepatorenal Type
> Tyrosyluria

Signs and Symptoms Acute tyrosinemia I is present at birth. Within weeks or months the infant fails to thrive, demonstrating vomiting, diarrhea, and a cabbage-like odor. Other frequent symptoms and signs include hepatomegaly, edema, ascites, melena, and hemorrhagic diathesis. This form, if untreated, is fatal in the first year of life.

The chronic form is milder, with symptoms that include rickets, a mild cirrhosis, renal tubular dysfunction, hypertension, and neurologic abnormalities. Hepatoma may develop.

The diagnosis is established by testing for succinylacetone in the urine and for fumarylacetoacetate hydrolyase in tissues. Prenatal diagnosis of tyrosinemia can be done by identification of amniotic cells that show a reduction in activity of fumarylacetoacetase, or by detection of succinylacetone in amniotic fluid.

Etiology Tyrosinemia is inherited as an autosomal recessive trait. The genetic abnormality results in insufficient levels of the enzyme fumarylacetoacetate hydrolyase.

Epidemiology Tyrosinemia in the acute form affects approximately 1:100,000 newborns in the United States, with both sexes being affected equally. The chronic form of this disorder affects far fewer patients. Both forms may be found in the same family.

Treatment—Standard Treatment is by dietary restriction of phenylalanine, tyrosine, and methionine. Liver transplantation has been helpful for severely affected patients. Other treatment is symptomatic and supportive. Genetic counseling is recommended.

Treatment—Investigational Please contact the agencies listed under Resources, below, for the most current information.

Resources

For more information on hereditary tyrosinemia: National Organization for Rare Disorders (NORD); Research Trust for Metabolic Diseases in Children; National Institute of Diabetes, Digestive & Kidney Diseases Information Clearinghouse; Jess Thoene, M.D., Department of Pediatrics, University of Michigan School of Medicine.

For genetic information and genetic counseling referrals: March of Dimes Birth Defects Foundation; National Center for Education in Maternal and Child Health.

References
The Metabolic Basis of Inherited Disease, 6th ed.: C.R. Scriver, et al., eds.; McGraw-Hill, 1989, pp. 547–559.
Prenatal Diagnosis of Hereditary Tyrosinemia by Determination of Fumarylacetoacetase in Cultured Amniotic Fluid Cells: E.A. Kvittingen, et al.; Pediatr. Res., April 1985, issue 19(4), pp. 334–337.
Neurologic Crises in Hereditary Tyrosinemia: G. Mitchell, et al.; New Eng. J. Med., February 15, 1990, issue 322(7), pp. 432–437.

VALINEMIA

Description Valinemia is a very rare metabolic disorder characterized by elevated levels of the amino acid valine in the blood and urine resulting from a deficiency of valine transaminase.

Synonyms
  Hypervalinemia
  Valine Transaminase Deficiency

Signs and Symptoms Typical findings include poor appetite, frequent vomiting, and failure to thrive. Hypotonia, excessive drowsiness, and hyperactivity may also be seen.

Etiology Valinemia is thought to be inherited as an autosomal recessive trait.

Epidemiology The disorder is very rare. It is present at birth.

Treatment—Standard Valine is restricted in the diet.

Treatment—Investigational Please contact the agencies listed under Resources, below, for the most current information.

Resources
  For more information on valinemia: National Organization for Rare Disorders (NORD); National Digestive Diseases Information Clearinghouse; Research Trust for Metabolic Diseases in Children.
  For genetic information and genetic counseling referrals: March of Dimes Birth Defects Foundation; National Center for Education in Maternal and Child Health (NCEMCH).

References
Mendelian Inheritance in Man, 9th ed.: V.A. McKusick; The Johns Hopkins University Press, 1990, p. 1524.
The Metabolic Basis of Inherited Disease, 6th ed.: C.R. Scriver, et al., eds.; McGraw-Hill, 1989, p. 678.

VITAMIN E DEFICIENCY

Description Vitamin E deficiency, which occurs most often in infants with impaired bile flow, may lead to progressive neuromuscular dysfunction characterized in part by areflexia and loss of balance.

Synonyms
Tocopherol Deficiency

Signs and Symptoms The first sign of vitamin E deficiency is usually areflexia, which may progress to ataxia, loss of balance, and peripheral muscle weakness. There may be difficulties with walking, such as stumbling and staggering (titubation), and abnormal posturing. Ophthalmoplegia and bradykinesia may occur, and sensations of pain, vibration, and position may be impaired.

Vitamin E deficiency in premature and low-birth-weight infants also may cause hemolytic anemia.

Etiology Rarely is vitamin E deficiency caused by dietary deficiency. It usually is associated with an underlying disease such as fat malabsorption, liver disease, or disorders of bile secretion (see *Acanthocytosis; Cholestasis)*. Recent research suggests that vitamin E deficiency with no underlying disease may derive from an inherited defect of vitamin E storage.

Epidemiology Vitamin E deficiency is extremely rare where there is no underlying disorder. It is more common in infants, children, and young adults than in adults. Males and females are affected in equal numbers except when an underlying disorder affects one sex more readily.

Approximately 1:5000 infants have an impairment of their bile flow due to liver diseases such as hepatitis or biliary atresia, and in these infants, the vitamin deficiency causes degenerative progressive neuromuscular disease.

Related Disorders Symptoms of the following disorders can be similar to those of the neurologic complications of vitamin E deficiency. See *Ataxia, Friedreich; Ataxia, Marie; Charcot-Marie-Tooth Disease; Olivopontocerebellar Atrophy.*

Treatment—Standard Any causative underlying disorder must be corrected. Supplementation with vitamin E, alpha tocopherol, alpha tocopheryl acetate, and alpha tocopheryl succinate have not been successful.

Treatment—Investigational Intramuscular injection of an investigational form of vitamin E (*dl*-alpha-tocopherol) has, in some cases, stabilized or reversed the neurologic symptoms caused by vitamin E deficiency. This experimental drug is manufactured by Hoffmann-La Roche.

A water-soluble form of Vitamin E (*d*-alpha tocopheryl polyethylene glycol-1000 succinate, or TPGS), which does not require bile for intestinal absorption, is being investigated under a grant from the National Organization for Rare Disorders (NORD). Preliminary studies indicate that this approach may stabilize or reverse neurologic dysfunction in infants with bile duct obstruction. Participants in this study must be older than 6 months and under 20 years of age, and their vitamin E deficiency must be caused by some form of cholestatic hepatobiliary liver disease. For information, contact Ronald J. Sokol, M.D., Associate Professor of Pediatrics, University of Colorado School of Medicine, Box C228, 4200 East Ninth Avenue, Denver, Colorado 80262; (303) 270-7805.

Please contact the agencies listed under Resources, below, for the most current information.

Resources

For more information on vitamin E deficiency: National Organization for Rare Disorders (NORD); NIH/National Institute of Diabetes, Digestive and Kidney Diseases (NIDDK); American Liver Foundation; The United Liver Foundation; Children's Liver Foundation.

References

Intramuscular Vitamin E Repletion in Children with Chronic Cholestrasis: D.H. Perlmutter, et al.; Am. J. Dis. Child, February 1987, issue 141(2), pp. 170–174.

Vitamin E Deficiency and Neurologic Disease in Adults with Cystic Fibrosis: M.D. Sitrin, et al.; Ann. Intern. Med., July 1987, issue 107(1), p. 51–54.

Vitamin E Deficiency Linked to Liver Disease in Children: C. Pierce; Research Resources Reporter, October 1986; National Institutes of Health, pp. 7–9.

VON GIERKE DISEASE

Description An inborn lack of the enzyme glucose-6-phosphatase is responsible for von Gierke disease, a glycogen storage disease. The enzyme is required for the conversion of glycogen into glucose. A deficiency causes deposits of excess glycogen in liver and kidney cells.

Synonyms

Glycogen Storage Disease I
Glycogenosis Type I
Hepatorenal Glycogenosis

Signs and Symptoms Manifestations of von Gierke disease are usually noticed during the first year of life. Findings include persistent hunger, fatigue, and irritability. Hepatomegaly, weight loss, and a slow growth rate are also seen. Hypoglycemia and lactic acidosis develop if food is withheld, and seizures may occur if the hypoglycemia is severe. The diagnosis can be confirmed with a glucose test and glucagon tolerance test, and by enzymatic assay.

Other findings seen during childhood include easy bruisability and frequent nosebleeds, lipidemia, xanthomas, and hyperuricemia. Microscopic glycogen deposits may be seen in liver cells and throughout the kidneys. Although the disease may be severe at times, symptoms tend to improve with age, and with appropriate dietary control.

Etiology The disease is inherited as an autosomal recessive trait.

Epidemiology This and other glycogen storage diseases together affect about 1:40,000 persons in the United States. Males and females are affected in equal numbers.

Related Disorders See *Forbes Disease; Andersen Disease.*

Treatment—Standard A nearly normal blood glucose level can be maintained through frequent small daily meals of carbohydrates plus a nighttime nasogastric infusion of glucose. An alternative to the nasogastric feeding is the use of uncooked cornstarch in the daily diet. The daily meals should include a high-protein diet. This regimen will promote a normal childhood growth rate.

The uric acid concentration in the blood must be carefully monitored to prevent the development of gouty arthritis during adolescence or adulthood. Allopurinol may be needed if symptoms of gout-like arthritis develop.

Treatment—Investigational Yuan-Tsong Chen, M.D., Ph.D. of Duke University, Durham, North Carolina, was awarded a grant in 1988 for his work using cornstarch as a treatment for von Gierke disease (Type I glycogen storage disease).

Please contact the agencies listed under Resources, below, for the most current information.

Resources

For more information on von Gierke disease: National Organization for Rare Disorders (NORD); Association for Glycogen Storage Diseases; National Institute of Diabetes, Digestive & Kidney Diseases Information Clearinghouse; Research Trust for Metabolic Diseases in Children.

For genetic information and genetic counseling referrals: March of Dimes Birth Defects Foundation; National Center for Education in Maternal and Child Health (NCEMCH).

References

The Metabolic Basis of Inherited Disease, 6th ed.: C.R. Scriver, et al., eds.; McGraw-Hill, 1989, pp. 433–437.

Optimal Rate of Enteral Glucose Administration in Children with Glycogen Storage Disease Type I: W.F. Schwenk, et al.; New Eng. J. of Medicine, March 13, 1986, issue 314(11), pp. 682–685.

Glycogen Storage Disease Type I. Results of Treatment with Frequent Daytime Feeding, Combined with Nocturnal Intragastric Feeding and with Administration of an Alpha-Glucosidase Inhibitor: H. Grube, et al.; European J. of Ped., April 1983, issue 140(2), pp. 102–104.

WILSON DISEASE

Description Wilson disease is a rare genetic disorder characterized by excess copper stored in various body tissues, particularly the liver, brain, and corneas. Eventual developments include hepatic disease and central nervous system dysfunction. Early diagnosis and treatment can prevent serious longterm disability.

Synonyms
Hepatolenticular Degeneration
Lenticular Degeneration, Progressive

Signs and Symptoms The usual presentation of Wilson disease is with hepatic or neurologic disturbances, or both. Symptoms of liver disease usually appear after 6 years of age, and include jaundice and vomiting. Neurologic symptoms are first seen between the ages of 12 and 32 years. Findings include drooling, dysarthria, dysphagia, lack of coordination, tremor, spasticity, muscle rigidity, and double vision. Other presenting signs and symptoms include renal stones, joint disorders, acute hemolytic crisis, and cardiomyopathy.

The Kayser-Fleischer ring, a rusty-brown deposit in the cornea that may not be present in the early stages of Wilson disease, is an important sign that appears in almost all patients and in 100 percent of those with neurologic involvement.

Neurologic signs and symptoms that may appear later in the course include decreased mentation and behavioral disturbances. Joint and bone involvement includes osteoporosis, the appearance of osteophytes at large joints, and reduced spinal and extremity joint spaces. Kidney involvement includes renal tubular damage.

The psychiatric manifestations of Wilson disease vary from patient to patient, and may be confused with psychiatric disorders, ranging from depression to schizophrenia. Accurate diagnosis is crucial; phenothiazines can aggravate the neurologic and psychiatric symptoms of Wilson disease. The side effects of these drugs also may appear similar to symptoms of Wilson disease. Most patients with psychiatric symptoms deriving from Wilson disease also have neurologic disease and Kayser-Fleischer rings in their eyes.

In adolescent females, menstruation may not begin until the disease is treated, because of the general disturbances in metabolism.

Etiology Wilson disease is inherited as a recessive genetic trait located on chromosome 13 at position q14, which prevents the liver from adequately excreting copper in the bile. The resulting gradual accumulation of copper in the body is toxic.

Epidemiology Males and females are affected in equal numbers, and the disease is found in all races and ethnic groups. The incidence is approximately 1:100,000 worldwide, with about 2,000 diagnosed cases in the United States. Many cases are misdiagnosed, however, usually as mental illness, and the true incidence may actually be higher.

Treatment—Standard The standard treatment for Wilson disease is D-penicillamine. Treatment must be lifelong, but some patients cannot tolerate longterm penicillamine therapy. The orphan drug trientine (Syprine, manufactured by Merck Sharp and Dohme) has been found effective for patients who are unable to tolerate penicillamine.

Foods high in copper content, such as chocolate, nuts, and shellfish, should be avoided. Dietary information is available from the Wilson Disease Association.

Physical therapy and speech therapy may be useful for neurologic involvement. In cases of severe liver disease, transplantation has been effective.

Treatment—Investigational The orphan drug zinc acetate is being tested as maintenance therapy for Wilson disease. This is a common nutritional substance, but it must be taken in certain doses at specific times during the day in order to affect copper metabolism. Careful monitoring is therefore necessary. For more information, please contact either George J. Brewer, M.D., University of Michigan Medical School, Medical Science MU708, Box 0618, University of Michigan, Ann Arbor, Michigan 48109-0618; or the manufacturer, Lemmon Company, 650 Carthill Road, Sellersville, Pennsylvania 18960.

Please contact the agencies listed under Resources, below, for the most current information.

Resources

For more information on Wilson Disease: National Organization for Rare Disorders (NORD); Wilson Disease Association; American Liver Foundation; The United Liver Foundation; Children's Liver Foundation; NIH/National Institute of Neurological Disorders & Stroke (NINDS);

For genetic information and genetic counseling referrals: March of Dimes Birth Defects Foundation; National Center for Education in Maternal and Child Health (NCEMCH).

References

The Metabolic Basis of Inherited Disease, 6th ed.: C.R. Scriver, et al., eds.; McGraw-Hill, 1989, pp. 1416–1421.

ZELLWEGER SYNDROME

Description Zellweger syndrome is a rare hereditary disorder characterized by decreased or missing peroxisomes in liver, kidney, and brain cells. Manifestations include facial dysmorphology, ophthalmologic and neurologic abnormalities, hepatomegaly, and unusual problems in prenatal development.

Signs and Symptoms Affected newborns have a typical flat facies, with a high forehead, shallow supraorbital ridges, hypertelorism, and epicanthal folds. The neonate also has profound hypotonia, feeding difficulty, seizures, cardiac defects, hepatomegaly, and vision abnormalities such as clouding of the cornea and cataracts. Jaundice and gastrointestinal bleeding may develop because of a deficient coagulation factor in the blood. Pneumonia or respiratory distress may develop if infections are not prevented and controlled. The syndrome is usually fatal within 6 months.

Etiology Zellweger syndrome is inherited as an autosomal recessive trait. Symptoms result from a deficiency or absence of peroxisomes in brain, liver, and kidney tissues. The cause of the peroxisome deficiency is not known.

Epidemiology An Australian study indicated that the syndrome may occur once in 100,000 live births, but it is possible that some cases have gone undiagnosed.

Related Disorders See *Nemaline Myopathy.*

Infantile muscular atrophy (amyotonia congenital syndrome) is a severe and usually progressive neuromuscular disorder of infants, manifested by a generalized weakness of the muscles in the trunk and extremities. The weakness, seen in other neuromuscular disorders, results from degenerative changes in the central horn cells of the spinal cord.

Treatment—Standard Treatment is symptomatic and supportive. Careful infection prevention and control is crucial. Genetic counseling can be of benefit to families of patients with this disorder.

Treatment—Investigational Use of the antihyperlipidemic agent, clofibrate, has been tried but has not proven effective in treating Zellweger syndrome.Please contact the agencies listed under Resources, below, for the most current information.

Resources

For more information on Zellweger syndrome: National Organization for Rare Disorders (NORD); United Leukodystrophy Foundation; Muscular Dystrophy Association; NIH/National Institute of Neurological Disorders & Stroke (NINDS).

For genetic information and genetic counseling referrals: March of Dimes Birth Defects Foundation; National Center for Education in Maternal and Child Health (NCEMCH).

References

The Metabolic Basis of Inherited Disease, 6th ed.: C.R. Scriver, et al., eds.; McGraw-Hill, 1989, pp. 1486–1494.

Smith's Recognizable Patterns of Human Malformation, 4th ed.: K.L. Jones; W.B. Saunders Company, 1988, pp. 178–179.

Zellweger Syndrome: Diagnostic Assays, Syndrome Delineation, and Potential Therapy: G.N. Wilson, et al.; Am. J. Med. Genet., May 1986, issue 24(1), pp. 69–82.

Unsuccessful Attempts to Induce Peroxisomes in Two Cases of Zellweger Disease by Treatment with Clofibrate: I. Bjorkhem, et al.; Pediatr. Res., June 1985, issue 19(6), pp. 590–593.

3 | NEUROLOGIC AND PSYCHIATRIC DISORDERS
By Melvin H. Van Woert, M.D.

The diagnosis of a neurologic disease requires the anatomical localization of the lesion on the basis of symptomatology, physical signs, and special laboratory and imaging techniques. For example, the loss of normal movement of an extremity could be due to an abnormality in one or several different parts of the central or peripheral nervous system. Some of the regions which regulate motor function and could produce this symptom include the motor cortex; spinal motor neurons; peripheral nerves; vestibular, red, and medullary reticular nuclei; basal ganglia; cerebellum; and accessory motor cortex. Accurate diagnosis requires the identification of the involved areas of the nervous system. A similar complexity in anatomical localization applies to other neurologic symptoms such as visual disturbances, sensory loss, tremor, impairment of balance, and pain. In some cases, the office neurologic examination will identify the abnormal neuronal pathways producing the symptoms. More frequently, special neurologic procedures will be necessary to confirm clinical impressions.

The anatomical localization may suggest the etiological diagnosis immediately. In other cases, medical facts such as age of onset, family history, evolution of symptoms, and sometimes specific laboratory tests will be necessary. Based upon etiology, neurologic diseases are divided into categories such as inflammations; neoplasms; vascular disorders; demyelination; trauma; and degenerative, congenital, and metabolic disorders. Some of these categories, particularly degenerative, congenital, and metabolic disorders, contain a significant number of genetic diseases.

Psychiatric diagnosis relies predominantly upon observation of the patient and critical evaluation of the patient's statements and opinions. There are rarely any objective signs, as in most neurologic disorders. Interpretation of the patient's behavior and response to questions can reveal symptoms such as hallucinations, delusions, or impaired memory, which form the basis for a psychiatric diagnosis. Psychiatric diagnoses have been divided into categories which have been precisely classified in the American Psychiatric Association's *Diagnostic and Statistical Manual of Mental Disorders, 3rd Edition, Revised (DSM-III-R)*: for example, personality disorders, mood disorders, schizophrenia, anxiety disorders, and disorders first evident in infancy, childhood, or adolescence. Formal personality tests, such as the Minnesota Multiphasic Personality Inventory, can be used to obtain scores on conditions such as anxiety, mania, depression, schizophrenia, paranoia, and hypochondriasis. Intelligence tests (Wechsler Adult Intelligence Scale-Revised and Wechsler Intelligence Scale for Children-Revised) and neuropsychological testing for specific cognitive functions such as memory, attention, and fluency of thinking are particularly useful in evaluating organic mental diseases.

Recently, major advances in neuroradiology and genetic studies have resulted in even earlier and more accurate assessment of many pathological processes in the central nervous system. The introduction of computerized tomography **(CT)** and magnetic resonance imaging **(MRI)** has produced dramatic improvements in the diagnosis of neurologic diseases and has greatly diminished the need for risky invasive diagnostic procedures. In addition, CT and MRI have been used in psychiatry to rule out organic diseases, e.g., multi-infarct dementia or subdural hematoma, as causes of symptoms such as memory impairment, personality changes, delusions, or depression. However, as patients with different psychiatric disorders are examined by CT, abnormalities are being detected in some of these mental conditions. For example, schizophrenic patients tend to have an increase in the size of their ventricles compared with normal individuals. This ventricular enlargement in schizophrenia has been confirmed by MRI studies. MRI has also detected decreased temporal lobe size in schizophrenia and cerebellar abnormalities in children with autism.

Older diagnostic procedures like cerebrospinal fluid examinations, electroencephalography and electromyography, and stimulus-induced evoked potential and arteriographic examinations remain very useful, particularly in neurologic disorders.

Position emission tomography **(PET)** offers a new dimension in neuroradiological sophistication by allowing studies of biochemical, physiological, and pharmacological processes to be carried out in patients. Because of the enormous expense and its early stage of development, this procedure is not available to most neurologists and psychiatrists at this time. Abnormal patterns of glucose utilization in the brain, detected by PET studies, have been observed in stroke, Alzheimer disease, seizures, and tumors, and in psychiatric disorders such as schizophrenia, bipolar depression, and obsessive-compulsive disorder. Dementia also is known to occur with progressive supranuclear palsy, and studies of regional glucose metabolism by PET scanning have found a decreased glucose uptake in the prefrontal cortex. Other PET studies can detect neuroreceptor abnormalities in basal ganglia diseases such as Parkinson disease.

Molecular genetic techniques are rapidly being applied to hereditary neurologic and psychiatric diseases to localize abnormal genes. One method is to digest deoxyribonucleic acid **(DNA)** with an enzyme called restriction endonuclease, which splits the DNA at specific sites to form multiple segments known as restriction fragment length polymorphisms **(RFLPs).** The variation in fragment lengths of these segments is a genetic characteristic, and it may be possible to localize an abnormal disease-producing gene within a RFLP in an afflicted family. Lymphocytic DNA from family members is scanned to determine whether a specific variation in restriction fragment length is linked to the disease in family members. This RFLP linkage technique was used to establish that chromosome 4 contains the abnormal gene for Huntington disease; this information led to a diagnostic test for individuals at risk for this condition. The same technique applied to psychiatric disorders showed a close linkage between bipolar illness and the X chromosome marker for color blindness.

There are approximately 1,000 genetic disorders that can impair neurologic or mental function. Specific therapy for these conditions is uncommon. However, dietary treatment has been successful in patients with phenylketonuria, maple syrup urine disease, galactosemia, and Refsum syndrome, by limiting the intake of a precursor which may have a toxic accumulation. In Wilson disease, the toxic accumulation of copper in the body can be prevented by chelation therapy with penicillamine and triethylene tetramine. As the site and product of the abnormal genes present in hereditary diseases of the nervous system are identified, new therapeutic approaches are expected.

Advances in neuroimmunology have greatly improved diagnosis and treatment of diseases such as Guillain-Barré syndrome, myasthenia gravis, and multiple sclerosis.

The identification of multiple neurotransmitters in the brain has led to the association of abnormalities of these chemical messengers with various disease states. Impetus was thus provided for pharmaceutical companies to research and develop drugs that alter neurotransmitter metabolism for the treatment of central nervous system diseases. The development of therapy for Parkinson disease is an excellent example. In the early 1960s, concentration of the neurotransmitter dopamine was found to be markedly depleted in the striatum of the parkinsonian brain because of degeneration of the dopaminergic nigro-striatal neuronal pathway. L-Dopa, which is converted to dopamine in the brain, was observed to produce dramatic clinical improvement. This observation stimulated continued research along the same lines, which led to the marketing of antiparkinsonian dopaminergic agonists (e.g., bromocriptine, pergolide); the monoamine oxidase B inhibitor selegiline (Eldepryl—see the chapter on Orphan Drugs); and, currently, clinical research on fetal dopaminergic neuronal transplants into the caudates of patients with Parkinson disease.

Abnormalities of cholinergic, serotonergic, peptidergic, gabaergic, and noradrenergic systems are being identified in other neurologic and psychiatric diseases. Certain types of myoclonic disorders appear to be due to diminished serotonin metabolism; and the serotonin precursor, L-5-hydroxytryptophan, has been demonstrated to have a beneficial effect. The loss of cholinergic input to the cerebral cortex has been observed in the Alzheimer disease patient's brain, and clinical trials of drugs that increase brain acetylcholine levels are producing some encouraging results. Neuropharmacological manipulation of neurotransmitters in various regions of the brain also has been successfully applied to the development of drugs for the treatment of psychiatric disorders such as anxiety and depression.

References

Principles of Neurology, 4th ed.: R.D. Adams and M. Victor; McGraw-Hill, 1989.

Merritt's Textbook of Neurology, 8th ed.: L.P. Rowland, ed.; Lea & Febiger, 1989.

Diagnostic and Statistical Manual of Mental Disorders, 3rd ed., revised: R.L. Spitzer, et al., eds.; American Psychiatric Association, 1987.

Treatments of Psychiatric Disorders. Task Force Report of the American Psychiatric Association, vols. 1–3: American Psychiatric Association, 1989.

Handbook of Clinical Neurology, vols. 1–58: P.J. Vinken, G.W. Bruyn, and H.L. Klawans, eds.; Elsevier Science Publishers, 1990.

NEUROLOGIC AND PSYCHIATRIC DISORDERS
Listings in This Section

ACOUSTIC NEUROMA

Description An acoustic neuroma is a benign tumor of the 8th cranial nerve. This nerve lies within the internal auditory canal.

Synonyms
>Acoustic Neurilemoma
>Bilateral Acoustic Neuroma
>Cerebellopontine Angle Tumor
>Fibroblastoma, Perineural
>Neurinoma
>Neurofibroma
>Schwannoma

Signs and Symptoms The early manifestations of an acoustic neuroma include tinnitus, hearing loss, or both; these symptoms arise from pressure on the 8th cranial nerve.

Other nerves also may be affected by an acoustic neuroma. Compression of the facial nerve (7th cranial nerve) produces facial muscle weakness. The trigeminal nerve (5th cranial nerve) is responsible for sensation on the skin of the face and the surface of the eye. Tumor involvement of this nerve may lead to facial numbness.

The direction of tumor growth determines symptom development. Tumor growth in the direction of the brain stem may push toward the cerebellum, causing ataxia of the arms and legs. Downward expansion of the tumor can produce numbness in the mouth, dysphagia, and hoarseness.

With increasing intracranial pressure, personality changes and impaired cognition may develop, and as pressure increases on the facial nerve, facial twitching and asymmetry may result. Sudden expansion of the tumor may be caused by hemorrhage or edema.

Etiology The cause of acoustic neuroma is unknown, although there appears to be a hereditary predisposition in a small group of patients with bilateral involvement.

Epidemiology Small, asymptomatic acoustic neuromas have been found on autopsy in 2.4 percent of the general population. Estimates of occurrence of symptomatic acoustic neuroma range from 1:3500 persons to 5:one million, with women being affected more often than men. An unusually large concentration of cases have been found in Humboldt County, California. Most surgical procedures for acoustic neuroma are performed on individuals between 30 and 60 years of age.

Related Disorders See *Neurofibromatosis,* which discusses the acoustic neuromas seen in NF 2.

Treatment—Standard At the present time, the only curative treatment is surgical removal of the tumor. The location and size of the tumor determine whether the approach is suboccipital or translabyrinthine. Postoperative problems can include headache, cerebrospinal fluid leak, meningitis, and decreased mental alertness due to development of a blood clot or obstruction of flow of cerebrospinal fluid. Large acoustic neuromas may have to be resected in stages.

Removal of an acoustic neuroma is a complex and delicate process, and complications relating to the cranial nerves may develop after surgery.

Hearing is often lost, partially or completely, with medium or large tumors, particularly if the tumor protrudes into the brain. It may be possible to preserve hearing, however, with tumors smaller than 0.6 inches. Monitoring of hearing function during surgery may lessen the possibility of hearing loss.

Tinnitus may persist after surgery, and occasionally only begins after surgery.

The facial nerve may be damaged during the procedure, and in some cases, portions of it are removed. Temporary or permanent facial paralysis may result and may lead to eventual dental problems. Nerve regeneration may take up to a year. If the paralysis persists, hypoglossal facial nerve anastomosis may bring improvement.

Ocular complications develop in approximately 50 percent of patients following surgical removal of an acoustic neuroma. Diplopia may occur if there is pressure on the 6th nerve, and there may be impairment of the eyelid muscles. Artificial tears or eye lubricants are often needed by these patients.

Because the vestibular portion of the 8th nerve is often removed during surgery, dizziness and unsteadiness are common until the vestibular apparatus in the normal ear can compensate. Unsteadiness in the dark may be permanent.

Treatment—Investigational Surgical techniques are improving dramatically, and research is continuing on the development of safer and more effective procedures and rehabilitation.

A new type of treatment, developed in Sweden, involves a special form of radiation therapy. The longterm benefits and side effects are not known, however.

The National Institute of Deafness and other Communication Disorders (NIDCD) and a colleague in Cleveland, Ohio are conducting research on hereditary acoustic neuroma.

Please contact the agencies listed under Resources, below, for the most current information.

Resources

For more information on acoustic neuroma: National Organization for Rare Disorders (NORD); Acoustic Neuroma Association; Alexander Graham Bell Association for the Deaf; Deafness Research Foundation; International Association of Parents of the Deaf; National Information Center on Deafness; NIH/National Institute of Deafness & Other Communication Disorders (NIDCD).

For acoustic neuroma associated with neurofibromatosis: National Neurofibromatosis Foundation, Inc.; Neurofibromatosis, Inc.

For genetic information and genetic counseling referrals: March of Dimes Birth Defects Foundation; National Center for Education in Maternal and Child Health (NCEMCH).

References

Cecil Textbook of Medicine, 18th ed.: J.B. Wyngaarden and L.H. Smith, Jr., eds.: W.B. Saunders Company, 1988, p. 2119.

Mendelian Inheritance in Man, 9th ed.: V.A. McKusick; The Johns Hopkins University Press, 1990, pp. 12-13.

AGENESIS OF THE CORPUS CALLOSUM (ACC)

Description Agenesis of the corpus callosum is a rare congenital abnormality involving a partial or complete absence of the transverse fibers that connect the 2 cerebral hemispheres. In some cases mental retardation may result, but other cases may be asymptomatic and intelligence normal. ACC is diagnosed during the first 2 years of life in 90 percent of cases. Affected patients can expect a normal lifespan.

Synonyms
> Agenesis of Commissura Magna Cerebri
> Asymptomatic Callosal Agenesis
> Corpus Callosum, Agenesis

Signs and Symptoms The initial manifestation may be the onset of grand mal or Jacksonian epileptic seizures. This may occur during the first weeks or within the first 2 years of life.

Hydrocephalus and impairment of mental and physical development also occur in some patients in the early stages of ACC. Neurologic evaluation may reveal nonprogressive mental retardation, impaired hand-eye coordination, and visual or auditory memory impairment.

In some mild cases, symptoms may not appear for many years and the disorder is diagnosed when an older patient develops seizures.

Etiology ACC is usually inherited as an X-linked recessive trait, but it may also be caused by an intrauterine infection during pregnancy leading to developmental disturbance in the fetal brain.

Epidemiology ACC is a very rare condition that usually produces symptoms during the first 2 years of life.

Related Disorders See *Aicardi Syndrome; Spina Bifida.*

Andermann syndrome is a genetic disorder characterized by a combination of ACC, mental retardation, and progressive neuropathy. All known cases of this disorder originate from Charlevois County and the Saguenay-Lac St. Jean area of Quebec, Canada. The exact mode of inheritance is unknown.

Treatment—Standard Treatment is symptomatic and supportive, involving anticonvulsive medications, special education, and physical therapy. The pressure of hydrocephalus may be relieved with a surgical shunt. Genetic counseling is recommended for families with this disorder.

Treatment—Investigational Please contact the agencies listed under Resources, below, for the most current information.

Resources
   For more information on ACC: National Organization for Rare Disorders (NORD); NIH/National Institute of Neurological Disorders & Stroke (NINDS).
   For more information on shunts: Association for Brain Tumor Research.
   For genetic information and genetic counseling referrals: March of Dimes Birth Defects Foundation; National Center for Education in Maternal and Child Health (NCEMCH).

References
   Anatomical and Behavioral Study of a Case of Asymptomatic Callosal Agenesis: R. Bruyer, et al.; Cortex, September 1985, issue 21(3), pp. 417–430.
   The Andermann Syndrome: Agenesis of the Corpus Callosum Associated with Mental Retardation and Progressive Sensorimotor Neuronopathy: A. Larbrisseau, et al.; Can. J. Neurol. Sci., May 1984, issue 11(2), pp. 257–261.
   Aicardi's Syndrome: (Agenesis of the Corpus Callosum, Infantile Spasms, and Ocular Anomalies); S. Dinani, et al.; J. Ment. Defic. Res., June 1984, issue 28(Pt.2), pp. 143–149.
   About Shunts: Association for Brain Tumor Research pamphlet.

AICARDI SYNDROME

Description Aicardi syndrome is an extremely rare, congenital disorder in which the corpus callosum has failed to develop. The absence of this structure linking the 2 cerebral hemispheres is associated with frequent seizures, marked abnormalities of the chorionic and retinal layers of the eye, and severe mental retardation.

Synonyms
   Callosal Agenesis
   Chorioretinal Anomalies
   Corpus Callosum Agenesis
   Infantile Spasms
   Spasm in Flexion

Signs and Symptoms Infantile spasms, beginning between birth and 4 months of age, are the first manifestations of the syndrome. The diagnostic sign is the presence of many cream-colored lacunae in the fundus. Subsequent findings include epilepsy, mental retardation, hypotonia, microcephaly, microphthalmia, colobomas, and abnormalities of the ribs and vertebrae. Computed tomographic scans or autopsy reveal that the corpus callosum is missing.
   Patients with this disorder tend to deteriorate with age. Children as old as 4 years may be unable to achieve normal standing posture. Mortality is unusually high, although some patients survive to adulthood.

Etiology The cause of Aicardi syndrome is unknown. A single dominant gene on the X chromosome may be involved.

Epidemiology Aicardi syndrome is extremely rare. Only females are affected; males are thought to die in utero.

Treatment—Standard Drug therapy includes corticosteroids, anticonvulsants, and adrenocorticotropic hormone, and treatment otherwise is symptomatic and supportive.

Treatment—Investigational Please contact the agencies listed under Resources, below, for the most current information.

Resources

For more information on Aicardi syndrome: National Organization for Rare Disorders (NORD); Aicardi Newsletter, NIH/National Institute of Neurological Disorders and Stroke; Richard Allen, M.D., Pediatric Neurology Service, University of Michigan Medical Center.

For genetic information and genetic counseling referrals: March of Dimes Birth Defects Foundation; National Center for Education in Maternal and Child Health (NCEMCH).

References

A New Syndrome: Spasms in Flexion, Callosal Agenesis, Ocular Abnormalities: J. Aicardi, et al.; Electroencephalography and Clinical Neurology, 1965, vol. 19, pp. 609–610.
The Aicardi Syndrome: Report of Four Cases and Review of the Literature: J. Bertoni, et al.; Annals of Neurology, 1979, vol. 5(5), pp. 475–482.

ALEXANDER DISEASE

Description Alexander disease is one of the rarest of the dystrophies, a group of progressive metabolic neurologic disorders, frequently inherited. Histologically the disease is characterized by demyelination and the formation of Rosenthal fibers in the white matter of the brain, especially around blood vessels and on the surface of the brain. Onset typically occurs in infancy and is associated with mental and physical retardation. Juvenile- and adult-onset forms are recognized but occur infrequently.

Synonyms

Dysmyelogenic Leukodystrophy-Megalobarencephaly
Fibrinoid Degeneration of Astrocytes
Leukodystrophy with Rosenthal Fibers
Megalencephaly with Hyaline Inclusion
Megalencephaly with Hyaline Panneuropathy

Signs and Symptoms Early symptoms of Alexander disease in infants include muscle spasticity and mental and physical retardation associated with megalencephaly. With progression of the disease seizures may occur. Juvenile-onset Alexander disease has a long course. In adult-onset cases, Rosenthal fibers may form in the absence of other symptoms. CT scanning can confirm the presence of a leukodystrophy.

Etiology An autosomal recessive inheritance has been postulated. The precise metabolic defect has not been identified.

Epidemiology Males and females are equally affected.

Related Disorders Alexander disease must be distinguished from other leukodystrophies and from brain or metabolic disorders producing similar symptoms. See *Astrocytoma, Malignant; Astrocytoma, Benign; Hydrocephalus; Adrenoleukodystrophy; Leukodystrophy, Canavan; Leukodystrophy, Krabbe; Leukodystrophy, Metachromatic; Pelizaeus-Merzbacher Brain Sclerosis; Refsum Syndrome; Multiple Sclerosis.*

Treatment—Standard Treatment is symptomatic and supportive.

Treatment—Investigational Current research focused on identifying the exact composition of the Rosenthal fibers and the permissive conditions for growth may lead to new methods of diagnosis and, eventually, specific treatment.

Please contact the agencies listed under Resources, below, for the most current information.

Resources

For more information on **Alexander disease:** National Organization for Rare Disorders (NORD); United Leukodystrophy Foundation; NIH/National Institute of Neurological Disorders and Stroke (NINDS); Children's Brain Diseases Foundation.

For **genetic information and genetic counseling referrals:** March of Dimes Birth Defects Foundation; NIH/National Center for Education in Maternal and Child Health (NCEMCH).

References

The Metabolic Basis of Inherited Disease, 6th ed.: Charles R. Scriver, et al., eds.; McGraw-Hill, 1989, pp. 1699–1705.

Merrit's Textbook of Neurology, 8th ed.: L.P. Rowland, ed.; Lea & Febiger, 1989.

Progressive Fibrinoid Degeneration of Fibrillary Astrocytes Associated with Mental Retardation in a Hydrocephalic Infant: W.S. Alexander; Brain, issue 1949(72), pp. 373–381.

ALPERS DISEASE

Description Alpers disease is a progressive neurologic condition affecting infants and children. It is characterized by degeneration of the cerebral gray matter, resulting in motor disturbances, seizures, and dementia. Liver disease is often associated.

Synonyms

Alpers Diffuse Degeneration of Cerebral Gray Matter with Hepatic Cirrhosis

Alpers Progressive Infantile Poliodystrophy

Poliodystrophia Cerebri Progressiva

Progressive Poliodystrophy

Signs and Symptoms Characteristic features include motor retardation, partial paralysis, myoclonus, liver damage, blindness, and growth retardation. Intractable seizures and progressive mental deterioration may also occur. Symptoms of the disease may be intensified by stress or other illnesses.

Etiology The cause is unknown in most cases. A familial form has been identified.

Epidemiology Males and females are affected equally.

Related Disorders See the discussion of myoclonic seizures in *Epilepsy*. See also *Leigh Disease; Batten Disease; Tay-Sachs Disease.*

Treatment—Standard Treatment is symptomatic and supportive.

Treatment—Investigational Please contact the agencies listed under Resources, below, for the most current information.

Resources

For more information on **Alpers disease:** National Organization for Rare Disorders (NORD); Association for Neurometabolic Disorders; Children's Brain Diseases Foundation for Research; NIH/National Institute of Neurological Disorders & Stroke (NINDS).

References
Mendelian Inheritance in Man, 9th ed.: V.A. McKusick; The Johns Hopkins University Press, 1990, p. 1023–1024.
Progressive Infantile Poliodystrophy (Alpers Disease) with a Defect in Citric Acid Cycle Activity in Liver and Fibroblasts: M.J. Prick, et al.; Neuropediatrics, May 1982, vol. 13(2), pp. 108–111.
Progressive Neuronal Degeneration of Childhood with Liver Disease (Alpers Disease): Characteristic Neurophysiological Features: S.G. Boyd, et al.; Neuropediatrics, May 1986, vol. 17(2), pp. 75–80.
Progressive Poliodystrophy (Alpers Disease) with a Defect in Cytochrome aa3 in Muscle; A Report of Two Unrelated Patients: M.J. Prick, et al.; Clin. Neurol. Neurosurg., 1983, vol. 85(1), pp. 57–70.

ALZHEIMER DISEASE

Description Alzheimer disease is a progressive condition of the brain affecting memory, thought, and language. The degenerative changes lead to plaques and neurofibrillary tangles, as well as a loss of cholinergic innervation in the brain.

Synonyms
Presenile Dementia
Senility

Signs and Symptoms The early behavioral changes of Alzheimer disease may be barely noticeable, but with disease progression memory losses increase; and personality, mood, and behavior change. Disturbances of judgment, concentration, and speech occur, along with confusion and restlessness. The type, severity, sequence, and progression of mental changes vary widely. Long periods with little change are common, although in some cases the disease is rapidly progressive.

Persons with Alzheimer disease should be given regular physical examinations to detect other organic disorders that may develop, because these patients may be unable to communicate clearly regarding the development of new or unrelated symptoms.

Etiology At least 10 percent of cases are inherited through a dominant gene. Alzheimer disease frequently occurs in individuals with Down syndrome who live past 35 years of age. Chromosome 21 abnormalities are common to both Down syndrome patients and some of the familial Alzheimer patients.

Some studies suggest that the disease may not be a single illness and that several factors may be involved. Researchers at the UCLA Medical School found that 100 percent of men with early Alzheimer disease (before age 60) had the protein HLA-A2 on the surface of their white blood cells, compared to 30 percent of healthy men under 60, and 40 percent of men with late-onset disease. It is suggested that HLA-A2—positive men under 60 may be at higher risk of early-onset Alzheimer disease.

Researchers at the Johns Hopkins University are studying brain tissue of deceased Alzheimer patients, and have found neuronal degeneration at the nucleus basalis. These neurons are believed to contain the neurotransmitter acetylcholine, and some patients had lost 90 percent of these cells. There appear to be abnormally low levels of acetylcholine in the brains of Alzheimer disease patients.

Other areas of investigation include the role of aluminum, and possible changes in the immune system.

Epidemiology Alzheimer disease occurs in 2 percent to 3 percent of the general population over 60 years of age. Approximately 2.5 million people in the United States are affected. The disease affects females more than males and blacks more than whites.

Related Disorders See *Pick's Disease.*

Treatment—Standard Treatment is symptomatic and supportive. Tranquilizers may decrease agitation, anxiety, and behavior disturbances. Depression accompanying the illness can be treated with various antidepressant drugs. Other helpful general measures include proper diet and fluid intake, and exercise and physical therapy. Alcoholic beverages should be avoided. The daily routine of a patient should be maintained as normally as possible, with continuation of social activities.

Treatment—Investigational Diagnosed Alzheimer disease patients who have one or more relatives (living or deceased) also diagnosed with the disease may participate in a clinical research study being conducted at the National Institute of Neurological and Communicative Disorders and Stroke (NINCDS). Please contact Linda Nee, MSW, or Ronald Polinsky, M.D., NIH/National Institute of Neurological and Communicative Disorders and Stroke, Medical Neurology Branch, Building 10, Room 5N236, Bethesda, Maryland 20892, (301) 496-8350.

Studies of the drug tetrahydroaminoacridine (tacrine) for treatment of Alzheimer disease are presently under way. It is hoped that tacrine may help preserve acetylcholine in the brain. Although this would not stop the progression of the disease, it might help improve symptoms such as memory loss and confusion. For information, please contact Warner-Lambert Co., 2800 Plymouth Road, PO Box 1047, Ann Arbor, Michigan 48106. During October 1987, the Food and Drug Administration temporarily stopped clinical trials of tacrine because one-fifth of the test subjects experienced changes in liver function as a side effect of the drug. Testing was resumed in 1988 using much lower doses than in earlier tests.

The National Institute of Mental Health (NIMH) and the Neuropsychiatric Research Hospital are studying early-onset dementia occurring as a result of Alzheimer disease. This study includes a thorough neuropsychologic evaluation, state-of-the-art brain imaging, and evaluation using newly developed biochemical assay techniques. Participants in this study must be under 45 years of age and should not require special medical care. For information, contact Denise Juliano, MSW, Coordinator of Admissions, Neuropsychiatric Research Hospital, 2700 Martin Luther King Jr. Ave., SE, Washington, DC 20032, (202) 373-6100.

The narcotic antagonist drug naltrexone is being tested for treatment of senile dementia of the Alzheimer type.

For information regarding donation of brain tissue for research on neurologic diseases, please contact Wallace W. Tourtelotte, M.D., Director, Human Neurospecimen Bank, VA Wadsworth Hospital Center, Los Angeles, California 90073; or Edward D. Bird, M.D., Director, Brain Tissue Bank, Mailman Research Center, McLean Hospital, 115 Hill Street, Belmont, Massachusetts 02178.

Please contact the agencies listed under Resources, below, for the most current information.

Resources

For more information on Alzheimer disease: National Organization for Rare Disorders (NORD); Alzheimer Disease and Related Disorders Association, Inc.; NIH/National Institute of Neurological Disorders & Stroke (NINDS); NIH/National Institute on Aging.

References

Cecil Textbook of Medicine, 18th ed.: J.B. Wyngaarden and L.H. Smith, Jr., eds.: W.B. Saunders Company, 1988, pp. 28–29, 2083, 2089–2090.

AMYOTROPHIC LATERAL SCLEROSIS (ALS)

Description ALS is a disease of the motor neurons that innervate skeletal muscles. It generally affects both upper and lower motor neurons and results in progressive wasting and weakness of involved muscles. Several variant forms of ALS exist.

Disease forms and related disease entities include slow motor neuron disease; focal motor neuron disease; spinal muscular atrophy (Kugelberg-Welander disease; juvenile spinal muscular atrophy) progressive bulbar palsy; benign focal amyotrophy; primary lateral sclerosis; infantile spinal muscular atrophy (Werdnig-

Hoffmann disease); Wohlfart-Kugelberg-Welander disease; and floppy infant syndrome.

Synonyms
Aran-Duchenne Muscular Atrophy
Lou Gehrig's Disease
Motor Neuron Disease
Progressive Bulbar Paralysis
Progressive Muscular Atrophy
Pseudobulbar Palsy

Signs and Symptoms Early symptoms include slight, patchy muscular weakness; clumsy hand movements; difficulty in performing fine motor tasks; leg weakness, often resulting in tripping; slowed speech; dysphagia; bulbar symptoms; and nocturnal leg cramps, often in calf or thigh muscles. In weeks or months, the disease involves more muscles. Other signs and symptoms may include muscle fasciculations, leg stiffness, hyperactive deep tendon reflexes, and coughing. Severe weight loss occurs in 5 percent of cases. As mobility impairment progresses, the patient is at increasing risk of respiratory failure and anoxia, aspiration pneumonia, or inadequate nutrition.

Etiology The etiology of ALS is unknown. Allergic, infectious, and viral causes have been proposed. Five to 10 percent of all cases are familial.

Epidemiology Amyotrophic lateral sclerosis is estimated to affect about 2,500 persons in the United States, mainly between the ages of 40 and 70. Sixty percent of cases involve men; 40 percent, women.

Related Disorders It is unclear whether the following disorders are separate disease entities or are variants of ALS.
See *Kugelberg-Welander Syndrome (Spinal Muscular Atrophy; Juvenile Spinal Muscular Atrophy); Primary Lateral Sclerosis; Werdnig-Hoffmann Disease.*
Focal motor neuron disease affects only one area of the body, most commonly the shoulder girdle. The disease progresses over several months, leaving the patient with a fixed deficit. Some patients later develop more extensive motor neuron disease. If focal motor neuron disease is considered as a diagnosis, care should be taken to exclude other causes of focal atrophy.
Progressive bulbar palsy is a variant of ALS characterized by weakness and atrophy of the muscles innervated by the cranial nerves.
Benign focal amyotrophy is a variant in which muscle weakness and atrophy are limited to a single limb. The onset may resemble that of classical ALS.

Treatment—Standard Medical management generally requires a team approach that includes physical therapists, speech pathologists and therapists, pulmonary therapists, medical social workers, and nurses.
Several drugs may be useful in controlling symptoms. Baclofen may reduce spasticity. Patients troubled by leg cramps may benefit from quinine compounds. Fasciculations, which may interfere with sleep, can be treated with agents such as

diazepam.

Maintaining proper nutrition is essential, but vitamin therapy has not been shown to affect the course of ALS. Soft foods should be carefully chosen for patients with dysphagia.

Physical therapy, consisting of daily range-of-motion exercises, is very important. The exercises can help maintain joint flexibility and prevent fixation of muscle contractions.

Communication devices can be useful for patients with dysarthria. Aids to communication include codes involving extraocular movement; artificial speech articulation utilizing small computers; the use of written messages; and other methods that can help to combat feelings of isolation.

Treatment—Investigational Extensive ALS research is directed toward nerve growth factors, axonal transport, androgen receptors in motor neurons, alterations in DNA and RNA, and metabolic studies of the neuromuscular junction.

Thyrotropin-releasing hormone (TRH), an orphan drug developed by Abbott Laboratories, has been investigated for the treatment of ALS, but the drug has not proved effective in clinical trials.

Some evidence suggests that defective metabolism of the amino acid glutamate may be responsible for degeneration of the nerve cells in the muscles of patients with ALS. The effects of branched chain amino acids, particularly L-leucine, L-isoleucine, and L-valine, are being studied to determine whether these substances will prevent the toxic effects of glutamate. Other research focuses on the orphan drug L-threonine, which may increase the inhibitory amino acid glycine, an inhibitory neurotransmitter. L-threonine (Threostat) is manufactured by Tyson & Associates, 1661 Lincoln Blvd., Suite 300, Santa Monica, CA 90404. The longterm safety and effectiveness of these experimental treatments must be assessed before they are recommended for ALS patients.

Please contact the agencies listed under Resources, below, for the most current information.

Resources

For more information on ALS: National Organization for Rare Disorders (NORD); The Amyotrophic Lateral Sclerosis Association; NIH/National Institute of Neurological Disorders & Stroke (NINDS).

For information on the childhood form of motor neuron disease: Families of Spinal Muscular Atrophy.

References

Cecil Textbook of Medicine, 18th ed.: J.B. Wyngaarden and L.H. Smith, Jr., eds.: W.B. Saunders Company, 1988, pp. 2154–2157, 2254.

ANOREXIA NERVOSA

Description Anorexia nervosa is an illness of self-starvation associated with a disturbed sense of body image and extreme anxiety about weight gain.

Synonyms
> Apepsia Hysterica
> Eating Disorder
> Magersucht

Signs and Symptoms Persons suffering from anorexia nervosa have an extreme preoccupation with food and usually consider themselves to be fat when in reality that is not the case. Periods of self-starvation often alternate with periods of binge eating **(bulimia).** A 20- to 25-percent body weight loss is typical. Females with anorexia nervosa usually experience amenorrhea, and hyperactivity combined with depression is seen in many patients.

Etiology Anorexia nervosa is currently considered to be a psychiatric condition, possibly associated with a stressful life situation. Many individuals are described as having been perfectionists and model children. A biological cause has not been established.

Epidemiology Approximately 95 percent of affected persons are female. Onset of the disorder is usually in early to late adolescence. A 1989 study of the disorder's prevalence in South Australia found that the condition affected 1.05 out of 1000 female secondary school students.

Related Disorders See *Bulimia.*

Treatment—Standard Treatment begins with correction of the malnutrition. Psychotherapy is usually essential, and family therapy can be most helpful toward provision of a calm, supportive, stable environment.

Treatment—Investigational Please contact the agencies listed under Resources, below, for the most current information.

Resources
> **For more information on anorexia nervosa:** National Organization for Rare Disorders (NORD); American Anorexia/Bulimia Association (AA/BA); National Anorexic Aid Society, Inc.; Anorexia Nervosa and Associated Disorders, Inc.; Anorexia Nervosa and Related Eating Disorders, Inc.; Bulimia, Anorexia Self-Help; NIH/National Institute of Mental Health; National Mental Health Association.

References
> Diagnostic and Statistical Manual of Mental Disorders, 3rd ed., revised: R.L. Spitzer, et al., eds.; American Psychiatric Association, 1987, pp. 65–67.
> The Prevalence of Anorexia Nervosa: D.I. Ben-Tovim, et al.; Daw Park, South Australia 5041, Repatriation General Hospital; N. Engl. J. Med., March 16, 1989, issue 320(11), pp. 736–737.

ANTISOCIAL PERSONALITY (ASP) DISORDER

Description ASP disorder is a mental illness that is usually observed before the age of 15, characterized by antisocial behavior and a lack of concern for the rights of others.

Signs and Symptoms Signs in early childhood include behavior such as lying, stealing, fighting, truancy, and resisting authority. In adolescence, there may be excessive drinking, drug use, and aggressive sexual behavior. The behavior difficulties usually persist throughout life, with markedly impaired capacity to sustain lasting, responsible relationships with family, friends, or sexual partners. In many cases, individuals with antisocial personality disorder are unable to be consistently self-sufficient, and problems with legal authorities are common. They tend to be irritable and aggressive, which results in physical fights, assaults, and criminality.

Etiology The cause is unknown. There may be association with a single-parent home, absence of parental discipline, extreme poverty, or removal from the home. Lack of educational achievement and the use of drugs may contribute. Predisposing factors may include childhood disturbances such as attention deficit disorder and conduct disorder. (See *Attention Deficit Hyperactivity Disorder.*)

Epidemiology ASP disorder affects approximately 3 percent of American males and 1 percent of American females. Males are affected at a much earlier age than females, with behavioral difficulties beginning in childhood.

Related Disorders See *Attention Deficit Hyperactivity Disorder.*

Substance abuse refers to the maladaptive behavior associated with regular or excessive use of a substance that can modify mood or behavior, such as alcohol or drugs. Social, occupational, psychological, or physical problems may result. Symptoms of addiction must persist for at least 1 month or occur repeatedly over a longer period of time in order to be diagnosed as a substance abuse disorder.

Treatment—Standard Psychological counseling is required for antisocial personality disorder, and in serious cases hospitalization and drug therapy may be necessary. Other treatment is symptomatic and supportive.

Treatment—Investigational Please contact the agencies listed under Resources, below, for the most current information.

Resources

For more information on antisocial personality disorder: National Organization for Rare Disorders (NORD); National Mental Health Association; NIH/National Institute of Mental Health.

References

Diagnostic and Statistical Manual of Mental Disorders, 3rd ed., revised: R.L. Spitzer, et al., eds.; American Psychiatric Association, 1987, pp. 342–346, 165–185.

Genetic and Environmental Factors in Alcohol Abuse and Antisocial Personality: R.J. Cadoret, et al.; J. Stud. Alcohol, January 1987, issue 48(1), pp. 1–8.

The Relationship Between Attention Problems in Childhood and Antisocial Behavior Eight Years Later: J.L. Wallander; J. Child Psychol., Psychiatry, January 1988, issue 29(1), pp. 53–61.

Parental Behavior in the Cycle of Aggression: J. McCord; Psychiatry, February 1988, issue 51(1), pp. 14–23.

APNEA, INFANTILE

Description Apnea ("without breath") denotes the temporary cessation of breathing as a result of neural arrest of respiration and consequent inhibition of air flow through the air passages. Mechanical, neurologic, and traumatic events may contribute in varying degrees to the different subdivisions of apnea. Infantile apnea, defined as apnea occurring in children less than 1 year old, may be related to some cases of infant death syndrome. Episodes of apnea may decrease with age.

Synonyms
> Central Apnea (Diaphragmatic Apnea)
> Mixed Apnea
> Obstructive Apnea (Upper Airway Apnea)
> Sleep Apnea

Signs and Symptoms The clinical picture of apnea includes a temporary cessation of breathing, accompanied by cyanosis and bradycardia. The precise physiologic derangements leading to cessation of breathing vary. In central or diaphragmatic apnea there are no chest movements and no air passes through the mouth or nostrils. When there are diaphragmatic and thoracic movements but no air flow into the lungs, the disorder is known as obstructive apnea. Central apnea followed by or mixed with obstructive apnea is called mixed apnea.

Etiology The cause of infantile apnea is not known.

Epidemiology Infantile apnea by definition occurs in children less than 1 year old.

Related Disorders See *Apnea, Sleep.*

Treatment—Standard Respiratory stimulants such as theophylline or caffeine may be prescribed. Parents and caretakers should be knowledgeable in cardiopulmonary resuscitation. Home monitoring devices may be purchased and used under the advice of a physician.

Treatment—Investigational Please contact the agencies listed under Resources, below, for the most current information.

Resources
  For more information on infantile apnea: National Organization for Rare Disorders (NORD); National Sudden Infant Death Syndrome Clearinghouse; National Sudden Infant Death Syndrome Foundation (NSIDSF); NIH/National Institute of Neurological Disorders and Stroke (NINDS).

References
Neurology in Clinical Practice, Vol II.: The Neurological Disorders: W.G. Bradley et al., eds.: Butterworth-Heinemann, 1991, p. 1493.
Cecil Textbook of Medicine, 18th ed.: J.B. Wyngaarden and L.H. Smith, Jr., eds.; W.B. Saunders Company, 1988, p. 2079.

APNEA, SLEEP

Description Sleep apnea syndrome is characterized by temporary, recurrent interruptions of respiration during sleep. Nocturnal wakefulness, daytime sleepiness, and obesity are typical features. The disorder occurs in 3 forms. **Obstructive sleep apnea (upper airway apnea),** the most common, results from blockage of the respiratory passages. Respiratory drive is normal. In the rarer **central sleep apnea,** there is little brain respiratory activity; breathing stops until the oxygen-starved brain sends impulses that activate the diaphragm and lungs. The **pickwickian syndrome** is a combination of obstructive apnea and obesity.

Signs and Symptoms The most common manifestations of sleep apnea are daytime sleepiness and loud nocturnal snoring. In obstructive apnea the labored breathing is interrupted by airway constriction. The episode ends when the muscles of the diaphragm and the chest build up sufficient pressure to force the airway open. Partial awakening then occurs, as the person gasps for air; sleep is resumed as breathing begins again. This cycle may be repeated several times during the night, and may lead to sleep deprivation if the person is unable to return to sleep quickly.

Complications associated with untreated sleep apnea include hypertension, arrhythmias, abnormal blood levels of oxygen and carbon dioxide, and peripheral edema. Other complications include sleepwalking, blackouts, automatic robotlike behavior, intellectual deterioration, hallucinations, anxiety, irritability, aggressiveness, jealousy, suspiciousness, and irrational behavior. Loss of interest in sex, morning headaches, and bedwetting may also occur with time.

Diagnosis of sleep apnea may require evaluation at a sleep disorder center. The patient fills out a questionnaire or a sleep/wake diary, and overnight examination or daytime sleep tests may be undertaken.

Etiology Several conditions are often associated with obstructive sleep apnea. These include obesity and a short thick neck, and reduction in muscle tone of the soft palate, the uvula, and the pharynx. The upper airway may be narrowed by enlarged tonsils or adenoids, a deviated nasal septum, nasal polyps, or congenital abnormalities. At high altitudes sleep disruption may occur because of low oxygen concentration.

The unstable brain respiratory control in central apnea may be associated with elevated partial pressure carbon dioxide or with decreased metabolic rate during sleep. Central sleep apnea may be produced by lesions of the region of the primary respiratory neurons of the medulla or of the descending pathways in the cervical cord.

Epidemiology About 2.5 million people in the United States suffer from sleep apnea, with males outnumbering premenopausal females 30 to 1. Many affected individuals are at least 20 percent above ideal body weight.

Related Disorders See *Apnea, Infantile; Narcolepsy; Ondine's Curse.*

Treatment—Standard Treatment of mild cases of obstructive sleep apnea usually consists of elevating the head with pillows, sleeping in a recliner chair, or elevating the bed's headposts by 6 to 8 inches. Elevation of the head can keep the tongue from falling backward and blocking the upper airway. In some cases drugs are used, including theophylline, protriptyline, clomipramine, pemoline, thioridazine, or nicotine.

When positional apnea is diagnosed (occurring when the patient sleeps in positions that predispose to breathing obstruction), sewing a bulky object in the back of the sleeping garment can make the supine position so uncomfortable that the person turns over.

Many patients with either central or obstructive sleep apnea have responded well to treatment with continuous positive airway pressure **(CPAP).** The device is effective in approximately 85 percent of obstructive sleep apnea patients.

A surgical technique being used increasingly is uvulo-palato-pharyngoplasty **(UPPP).** Loose tissues are tightened in the back of the mouth and top of the throat, and excess tissues that block the airway in those areas are trimmed away. UPPP has been helpful in about 55 percent of patients with obstructive sleep apnea.

Treatment—Investigational Please contact the agencies listed under Resources, below, for the most current information.

Resources

For more information on sleep apnea: National Organization for Rare Disorders (NORD); American Narcolepsy Association, Inc.; Narcolepsy and Cataplexy Foundation of America; Narcolepsy Network; NIH/National Institute of Neurological Disorders and Stroke (NINDS).

References
Snoring by Night? Snoozing by Day? Sounds Like Sleep Apnea: Harold Hopkins; FDA Consumer, December 1986–January 1987, pp. 29–32.

Nasal CPAP Therapy Upper Airway Muscle Activation, and Obstructive Sleep Apnea: K.P. Strohl, et al.; Am. Rev. Respir. Dis., September 1986, pp. 555–558.

The Effects of Posture on Obstructive Sleep Apnea: R.D. McEvoy, et al.; Am. Rev. Respir. Dis., April 1986, issue 133(4), pp. 662–666.

APRAXIA

Description Apraxia is a disorder of brain function in which a person is unable to carry out familiar movements, even though the desire is there and the physical ability exists.

Synonyms
Wieacker syndrome

Signs and Symptoms When intended movement does occur, it may be clumsy, uncontrolled, and inappropriate. Some patients with apraxia are unable to dress themselves. Movement may also occur unintentionally. Apraxia is sometimes accompanied by aphasia.

Constructional apraxia refers to the inability to draw or construct simple configurations. Persons with **buccofacial apraxia** are not able to lick their lips, whistle, cough, or wink, and those with **oculomotor apraxia** find it difficult to move their eyes, although eye reflex movement can occur.

Etiology The lesion that causes apraxia may be the result of metabolic or structural diseases that involve several different regions of the brain. It may be caused by stroke, with symptoms usually appearing during the acute phase and diminishing within weeks of onset. Head injuries and degenerative dementia may result in apraxia. Some cases are the result of congenital malformations of the central nervous system.

Related Disorders Aphasia is a disturbance in the ability to comprehend or use language, usually resulting from injury to the cerebral cortex. Affected individuals may select the wrong words in conversing and may have difficulties interpreting verbal messages.

Treatment—Standard Treatment involves relearning limb gestures in conjunction with physical and occupational therapy. When apraxia is a symptom of another neurologic disorder, the underlying condition must be treated.

Treatment—Investigational Please contact the agencies listed under Resources, below, for the most current information.

Resources

For more information on apraxia: National Organization for Rare Disorders (NORD); NIH/National Institute of Neurological Disorders and Stroke.

References
Cecil Textbook of Medicine, 18th ed.: J.B. Wyngaarden et al., eds.; W.B. Saunders Company, 1988, pp. 2082, 2087.

Harrison's Principles of Internal Medicine, 12th ed.: J.D. Wilson, et al., eds.; McGraw-Hill, 1991, pp. 159–160.

Apraxia and the Supplementary Motor Area: R.T. Watson, et al.; Arch. Neurol., August 1986, issue 43(8), pp. 787–792.

On the Cerebral Localization of Constructional Apraxia: K. Ruessman et al.; Int. J. Neurosci., September 1988, issue 42(1-2), pp. 59–62.

The Relationship Between Limb Apraxia and the Spontaneous Use of Communicative Gesture in Aphasia: J.C. Borod, et al.; Brain Cogn., May 1989, issue 10(1), pp. 121–131.

ARACHNOIDITIS

Description Arachnoiditis is a progressive inflammatory disorder of the arachnoid membrane, with possible involvement of the brain and spinal cord.

Synonyms
Arachnitis
Cerebral Arachnoiditis
Chronic Adhesive Arachnoiditis

Serous Circumscribed Meningitis
Spinal Arachnoiditis

Signs and Symptoms Cerebral involvement leads to symptoms such as severe headaches, visual disturbances, dizziness, nausea, and vomiting. Spinal involvement may cause pain, weakness, and paralysis. The disorder usually is first noticed with gradual loss of sensations and movement of the legs; as the condition progresses, muscle atrophy, weakness, and involuntary twitching of muscles are seen. In the most severe cases, loss of vision and paralysis may develop. Ossification of the arachnoid membrane also may occur.

Etiology Arachnoiditis can be a complication of meningitis, trauma, or subarachnoid hemorrhage, or may develop following local injections of anesthetic agents or testing dyes. An immune deficiency may also contribute.

Epidemiology Males and females are affected in equal numbers. Individuals who have had spinal surgery or injuries to the spine or head may be at greater risk.

Related Disorders See *Pseudotumor Cerebri.*

Leptomeningitis is characterized by inflammation of the soft membranes surrounding the brain and spinal cord, including the pia mater and arachnoid membrane. This disorder is thought to be a complication of chronic meningitis.

Epiduritis is characterized by inflammation of the dura mater.

Treatment—Standard Treatment consists of a combination of surgery and drug therapy. Surgical removal of adhesions and accumulated fluids may be helpful in some cases, especially if pressure develops. Cyclophosphamide and nitrogen mustard may improve headaches and vision loss, and antiinflammatory drugs may also be used. Other treatment is symptomatic and supportive.

Treatment—Investigational For arachnoiditis caused by a parasitic infection (a rare cause in the United States), the drug praziquinatel has been used with some success.

Please contact the agencies listed under Resources, below, for the most current information.

Resources

For more information on arachnoiditis: National Organization for Rare Disorders (NORD); NIH/National Institute of Neurological Disorders and Stroke (NINDS); American Paraplegia Society; Spinal Cord Society; Spinal Cord Injury Hotline.

References

Spinal Arachnoiditis Due to *Aspergillus* Meningitis in a Previously Healthy Patient: F.A. Van de Wyngaert, et al.; J. Neurol., February 1986, issue 233(1), pp. 41–43.

Pathogenesis of Postmyelographic Arachnoiditis: J.C. Garancis, et al.; Invest. Radiol., January–February 1985, issue 20(1), pp. 85–89.

Spinal Ossifying Arachnoiditis. Case Report: F. Tomasello, et al.; J. Neurosurg. Sci., October–December 1985, issue 29(4), pp. 335–340.

ARNOLD-CHIARI SYNDROME

Description The syndrome is characterized by displacement of the distal brain stem (medulla) through the foramen magnum where it becomes impacted in the upper cervical canal. Infantile Arnold-Chiari syndrome is usually associated with myelomeningocele. Hydrocephalus is commonly present, as well as other malformations of the brain and spinal cord.

Synonyms
> Arnold-Chiari Malformation
> Cerebellomedullary Malformation Syndrome

Signs and Symptoms In infants, vomiting, mental impairment, head and facial muscle weakness, and difficulties with swallowing may be present. The extremities may be paralyzed.

In adults and adolescents the malformation may be asymptomatic until gradual signs and symptoms of cerebellar, lower cranial nerve, and pyramidal dysfunction occur. Downbeat nystagmus is characteristic. Dizziness, headache, vomiting, diplopia, deafness, weakness of the legs, ataxia, and occipital neuralgia may occur.

Symptoms may also simulate those produced by tumors near the foramen magnum or by multiple sclerosis.

Etiology Because of the complexity and associated defects, the cause is uncertain; it appears to be due to a failure of normal development of the brain stem and upper cervical region.

Epidemiology The Arnold-Chiari syndrome is usually found in infants, but may occur in adolescents and adults.

Related Disorders Hydrocephalus is frequently found with this syndrome; the cause is unclear. In addition, myelomeningocele, stenosis of the aqueduct, platybasia, syringobulbia, and syringomyelia are often associated with Arnold-Chiari syndrome. See *Hydrocephalus; Spina Bifida; Syringobulbia; Syringomyelia.*

Treatment—Standard Surgical repair of an existing meningocele and ventricular shunting procedures for relief of hydrocephalus are necessary. Prognosis is poor for infants with extensive defects.

In adults, surgical enlargement of the foramen magnum and decompression of the cervicomedullary junction may prove beneficial.

Treatment—Investigational Please contact the agencies listed under Resources, below, for the most current information.

Resources

For more information on Arnold-Chiari syndrome: National Organization for Rare Disorders (NORD); Arnold-Chiari Family Network; NIH/National Institute of Neurological Disorders & Stroke (NINDS).

For genetic information and genetic counseling referrals: March of Dimes Birth Defects Foundation; National Center for Education in Maternal and

Child Health (NCEMCH).

References
Textbook of Neuropathy: R.L. Davis and D.M. Robertson; Williams and Wilkins, 1985, pp. 202–207.
Cecil Textbook of Medicine, 18th ed.: J.B. Wyngaarden and L.H. Smith, eds.; W.B. Saunders Company, 1988, p. 2258.
Mendelian Inheritance in Man, 9th ed.: V.A. McKusick; The Johns Hopkins University Press, 1990, p. 1043.

ASPERGER SYNDROME

Description Asperger syndrome is a neuropsychiatric disorder whose major manifestation is an inability to understand how to interact socially. Other features include poor verbal and motor skills, singlemindedness, and social withdrawal. The syndrome has similarities to autism.

Signs and Symptoms Symptoms of Asperger syndrome are not usually recognized until a child reaches 30 months of age. The child displays little interest or pleasure in other persons, and imaginative play may be absent or repetitious.

Speech begins at the normal age but is unusual, with the child talking at length on a single subject. Grammar may eventually be understood, but the child has difficulty with pronouns, referring to himself or herself in the 2nd or 3rd person. Speaking usually is monotonous or, contrarily, exaggerated. Many children with Asperger syndrome have excellent rote memory and musical ability.

Nonverbal communication is also affected. The face is usually expressionless unless the child feels strong emotions. Bodily movement may be limited or inappropriate, and walking may be delayed. Lack of coordination results in difficulties with running, ball throwing, and other games, as well as with writing and drawing.

The lack of social and communicative skills results in a feeling of being different and an inability to understand and participate in social interaction, leading to withdrawal from society. These difficulties reach a peak during adolescence. A young man with Asperger syndrome and a strong sex drive, wanting to be normal but with no understanding, may show inappropriate behavior towards the opposite sex.

Etiology The cause is unclear. Some affected children and adults have had a history of pre-, peri-, or postnatal problems. Cerebral damage has been postulated; almost 50 percent of those studied suffered lack of oxygen at birth. An organic deficiency of brain function has also been suggested as a cause. Possible hereditary aspects of Asperger syndrome have not been well investigated.

Epidemiology Males are affected more often than females.

Treatment—Standard Intensive, highly structured, skill-oriented training on a continual basis is most useful for both children and adults with this syndrome. Other treatment is symptomatic and supportive.

Treatment—Investigational Please contact the agencies listed under Resources, below, for the most current information.

Resources

For more information on Asperger syndrome: National Organization for Rare Disorders (NORD); NIH/National Institute of Neurological Disorders & Stroke (NINDS); Association for Children and Adults with Learning Disabilities; NIH/National Society for Children and Adults with Autism (NSAC).

References

Asperger Syndrome: A Clinical Account: L. Wing; Psychol. Med., February 1981, issue 11, pp. 115–129.

Identical Triplets with Asperger Syndrome: E. Bourgoine, et al.; Br. J. Psychiatry, September 1983, issue 143, pp. 261–265.

Asperger Syndrome and Aminoaciduria: A Case Example: S.W. Miles, et al.; Br. J. Psychiatry, March 1987, issue 150, pp. 397–400.

A Possible Case of Asperger Syndrome: A. Munro, et al.; Can. J. Psychiatry, August 1987, issue 32(6), pp. 465–466.

ASTROCYTOMA, BENIGN

Description Benign astrocytomas, tumors composed of glial cells (astrocytes), can occur anywhere in the brain or spinal cord. The subcortical white matter is the most common location in adults, and the optic nerve, cerebellum, and brain stem are the most common locations in children.

Synonyms

Astrocytoma Grade I
Astrocytoma Grade II
Brain Tumor
Intracranial Neoplasm
Intracranial Tumor

Signs and Symptoms Manifestations of a benign astrocytoma depend on its size, location, and rate of growth. Onset may be sudden or gradual.

Recurrent headache, usually resulting from pressure on blood vessels, cranial nerves, or pain-sensitive tissue, is the initial symptom in 50 percent of cases. Seizures are the initial manifestation in 20 percent, and are typically the result of slow-growing astrocytomas.

Gradual-onset symptoms include mental changes such as increased irritability, emotional instability, forgetfulness, reduced mental activity, and loss of initiative or spontaneity. With increased tumor size, symptoms may progress to confusion, lethargy, and stupor.

Other manifestations may include nausea, vomiting, slowed heartbeat, incontinence, astereognosis, paralysis, ataxia, aphasia, nystagmus, and facial pain or numbness.

Etiology The cause is not known; chromosomal abnormalities have been found in malignancies of the glia.

Epidemiology Benign astrocytomas may occur in anyone at any age, but white males between the ages of 40 and 70 are most commonly affected.

Related Disorders See *Astrocytoma, Malignant; Multiple Sclerosis.*

Treatment—Standard Benign astrocytomas are generally detected by computed tomography or magnetic resonance imaging, and biopsy is then performed to determine the optimal treatment approach.

Preoperative treatment attempts to control fluid accumulation with corticosteroids or a shunt; anticonvulsant agents are given to prevent seizures. Surgical removal of the astrocytoma may be successful if the tumor is accessible. Laser microsurgery now can remove local infiltrates with minimal tissue damage. Surgery is usually followed by radiation therapy.

Radiation is used as primary therapy in some instances, followed by chemotherapy.

Treatment—Investigational Various experimental approaches are now being used as treatment for astrocytomas. Brachytherapy involves surgical implantation of radioactive pellets of iodine, iridium, or gold isotopes. This procedure can be used for a tumor that is less than 2.5 inches in diameter and is confined to one side of the brain. Other investigational therapies include use of cell radiosensitizers that can increase the effectiveness of radiation, hyperthermia and photoradiation, intraoperative radiation, and hyperfractionation.

A multitude of new drugs, drug combinations, and drug delivery systems are being tested for effectiveness against astrocytomas. Agents being used to boost the immune system include interferon, levamisole, interleukin-2, thymosine, and bacile Calmette-Guérin.

A new orphan drug and delivery system being tested uses a biodegradable wafer containing a cytotoxic agent that is implanted at the site of the tumor. As the wafer dissolves over a period of many weeks, the drug is slowly released. For more information: Nova Pharmaceutical Corp., 6200 Freeport Centre, Baltimore, Maryland 21224; (301) 522-7000.

Please contact the agencies listed under Resources, below, for the most current information.

Resources

For more information on benign astrocytoma: National Organization for Rare Disorders (NORD); NIH/National Institute of Neurological Disorders and Stroke (NINDS); Association for Brain Tumor Research.

References
Cecil Textbook of Medicine, 18th ed.: J.B. Wyngaarden and L.H. Smith, Jr., eds.; W.B. Saunders Company, 1988, pp. 2229–2235.

Low-Grade Astrocytomas: Treatment with Unconventionally Fractionated External, Beam Stereotactic Radiation Therapy: F. Pozza, et al.; Radiology, May 1989, issue 171(2), pp. 565–569.

Benign Astrocytic and Oligodendrocytic Tumors of the Cerebral Hemispheres in Children: J.F. Hirsch, et al.; J. Neurosurg., April 1989, issue 70(4), pp. 568–572.

Low-Grade Astrocytomas: Treatment Results and Prognostic Variables: C.A. Medbery 3rd, et al.; Int. J. Radiat. Oncol. Biol. Phys., October 1988, issue 15(4), pp. 837–841.
Long-term Follow-up After Surgical Treatment of Cerebellar Astrocytomas in 100 Children: S. Undjian, et al.; Childs. Nerv. Syst., April 1989, issue 5(2), pp. 99–101.

ASTROCYTOMA, MALIGNANT

Description An astrocytoma is a highly malignant, infiltrating primary brain tumor composed of astrocytes. Typical onset is in late middle age. Tentacles from the tumor invade normal tissue, spreading through the white matter of the cerebral hemispheres in a butterfly pattern. Occasionally the dura or ventricles (reached through the spinal fluid) are involved. Familial cases have been identified, and an association with exposure to industrial chemicals is recognized. About one-third of cases are fatal in the first year.

Synonyms

Anaplastic Astrocytoma
Astrocytoma, Grades III and IV
Giant-Cell Glioblastoma
Spongioblastoma Multiforme

Signs and Symptoms The earliest symptom typically is headache, caused by increased intracranial pressure as the growing tumor exceeds the volumetric capacity of the skull. The headache is generalized, worse in the morning, and accompanied by vomiting. Personality changes may accompany or precede the headache.

Other symptoms are referable to the particular area of brain affected. Frontal lobe tumors are associated with memory loss, intellectual impairment, and a flat affect; these symptoms may be accompanied by contralateral convulsions or paralysis. Parietal lobe tumors result in agraphia, paresthesias, loss of proprioception, and occasionally seizures. Symptoms of temporal lobe tumors are less marked initially but eventually include seizures, muscle incoordination, and difficulty in language use and interpretation.

Sixty-five to 70 percent of patients are alive one year after diagnosis; 40 percent survive for 2 years.

Etiology The cause of malignant astrocytoma is unknown. Because of an apparent familial predilection, a hereditary component has been postulated but not proved. A viral etiology has also been postulated. Some cases have been linked to exposure to industrial chemicals such as polyvinyl chloride and agricultural pesticides.

Epidemiology Malignant astrocytoma commonly affects individuals between the ages of 48 and 60 years, although it has also occurred in children. The prevalence is higher in men than in women, especially men with type A blood, and higher in whites than in nonwhites.

Related Disorders See *Glioblastoma Multiforme.*

Treatment—Standard Open surgery or laser microsurgery is the preferred treatment for astrocytomas. Surgery is followed by irradiation of the whole brain to halt microscopic progression, and chemotherapy. For inoperable tumors a subtotal decompressive resection may be performed to reduce the number of tumor cells and increase the effectiveness of radiation therapy and chemotherapy.

Treatment—Investigational Brachytherapy has been tried experimentally, primarily for small recurrences. The mode, fraction schedule, and time of delivery of conventional radiation therapy have been manipulated in various trials. The use of cell radiosensitizers may increase the effectiveness of radiation.

Immunotherapy drugs may be administered to stimulate the body's defenses against the tumor. Techniques under investigation include the intraarterial delivery of various drugs, and disruption of the blood-brain barrier to facilitate drug entry into the brain.

Please contact the agencies listed under Resources, below, for the most current information.

Resources

For more information on malignant astrocytoma: National Organization for Rare Disorders (NORD); Association for Brain Tumor Research; American Cancer Society; NIH/National Institute of Neurological Disorders & Stroke (NINDS); NIH/National Cancer Institute PDQ (Physician Data Query) phoneline.

References
About Glioblastoma Multiforme and Malignant Astrocytoma: D.P. Hesser, et al., eds.; Association for Brain Tumor Research, 1985.

ATAXIA, FRIEDREICH

Description Friedreich ataxia is a progressive, hereditary neuromuscular syndrome that typically manifests in childhood or adolescence. Slow degenerative changes of the spinal cord and brain affect speech and motor coordination, producing numbness or weakness of the arms and legs, secondary lateral scoliosis, and lower limb paralysis. Although the disorder is progressive and treatment is symptomatic only, spontaneous remissions of 5 to 10 years in duration have been reported.

Synonyms
Familial Ataxia
Friedreich Disease
Friedreich Tabes
Hereditary Ataxia
Spinocerebellar Ataxia

Signs and Symptoms Ataxia denotes a failure of muscle coordination that typically results in an unsteady gait. The hallmark of Friedreich ataxia is progressive weakness of the legs, reflected in a staggering, lurching gait, or trembling when the subject is standing still. Partial loss of the sense of touch or sensitivity to pain and temperature may occur. With time, reflexes may remit, and a high-arched foot may develop with hyperextension of the big toe. Involvement of the throat muscles leads to impaired swallowing and choking and may result in difficulty eating. The intellect and emotions are rarely affected. Scoliosis, diabetes mellitus, or cardiomyopathy may occur but are not necessary for a differential diagnosis.

Etiology Friedreich ataxia is usually inherited as a recessive trait. A variant form may be inherited as a dominant trait. Symptoms are caused by degeneration of nerve cells in the dorsal root ganglia, spinal cord, and brain.

Epidemiology Although Friedreich ataxia can be present at birth, symptoms usually first appear between the ages of 8 and 15 years. Estimates of prevalence in the United States range from 2000 to 3000 cases to as many as 20,000. A more precise estimate is difficult to render, as many cases are likely misdiagnosed. The syndrome is the most common of the various forms of hereditary ataxia.

Related Disorders Ataxia is common to several disorders and may take many forms, not all hereditary in origin. See *Ataxia, Marie; Charcot-Marie-Tooth Disease; Ataxia Telangiectasia; Olivopontocerebellar Atrophy.*

Treatment—Standard Treatment is symptomatic and supportive. Therapy includes medication, physiotherapy, orthotic support, and surgery. Propranolol may be effective against the static tremors of Friedreich ataxia and, less often, against intention tremors. Use of these drugs must be monitored in the individual patient to avoid toxicity. Physiotherapy to promote remaining muscle function is frequently helpful, and orthopedic surgery or braces may be prescribed to correct scoliosis and abnormalities of the feet. Vision and hearing problems may be alleviated with corrective devices, drugs, or in some cases surgery.

Continuous medical supervision is necessary to avoid complications involving the heart, lungs, skeleton, and muscles. Preventing pneumonia in advanced stages of Friedreich ataxia is a medical challenge. Medication may be used to treat the cardiomyopathy and diabetes mellitus associated with Friedreich ataxia. These secondary problems may increase the patient's susceptibility to infection, leading to the need for further drug therapy.

Genetic and psychological counseling can assist many patients and families affected by one of the hereditary ataxias. Prenatal diagnosis is available for pregnant women.

Treatment—Investigational Epidural spinal electrostimulation **(ESES)** with the multiprogrammable spinal cord stimulator is currently being evaluated in the treatment of motor dysfunction. The device, which can be implanted surgically over the spine, may provide therapeutic benefit in some types of ataxia when other measures have failed. The goal is to increase the range of mobility and alleviate muscle spasms and pain. For further information on experimental ESES devices: Food and Drug Administration, Office for Orphan Product Development, HF-35 FDA, Room 12-11, 5600 Fishers Lane, Rockville, Maryland 20857.

A genetic marker for Friedreich ataxia has been located on chromosome 9. Once the exact gene has been cloned and the defective protein identified, new treatments may become available that will interrupt progression of the disease, and genetic tests may more readily identify carriers of the gene.

Please contact the agencies listed under Resources, below, for the most current information.

Resources

For more information on Friedreich ataxia: National Organization for Rare Disorders (NORD); National Ataxia Foundation; NIH/National Institute of Neurological Disorders & Stroke (NINDS).

For information on clinical services for persons with Friedreich ataxia, including provision of orthopedic aids, recreation at summer and winter camps, and transportation assistance: The Muscular Dystrophy Association.

For more information on scoliosis: National Scoliosis Foundation, Inc.

For more information on diabetes: American Diabetes Association.

For genetic information and genetic counseling referrals: March of Dimes Birth Defects Foundation; National Center for Education in Maternal and Child Health (NCEMCH).

References

Treatment of Patients with Degenerative Diseases of the Central Nervous System by Electrical Stimulation of the Spinal Cord: D.M. Dooley, et al.; Contin. Neurol., 1981, issue 44(1-3), pp. 71–76.

Epidural Spinal Electrostimulation (ESES) in Patients with Chronic Pain and Central Motor Disturbances (Author's Transl.): D. Klingler, et al.; Wien Klin. Wochenschr., Nov. 27, 1981, issue 93(22), pp. 688–695.

The Inherited Ataxias: D.A. Stampf; Neurol. Clin., February 1985, issue 3(1), pp. 47–57.

Incidence, Natural History, and Treatment of Scoliosis in Friedreich Ataxia: R.B. Cady, et al.; J. Pediatr. Orthop., November, 1984, issue 4(6), pp. 673–676.

ATAXIA, MARIE

Description Marie ataxia is a hereditary cerebellar disorder that affects muscle coordination, producing an early symptom of unsteady gait. Progressive spinal nerve degeneration leads to muscle atrophy in the limbs and head and neck area. The condition appears to have 2 peaks of onset, one in early adulthood and the second in middle age. Persons first affected in middle age are more likely to have mild cases that respond to treatment.

Synonyms

Cerebellar Syndrome
Hereditary Cerebellar Ataxia
Nonne Syndrome
Pierre-Marie Disease

Signs and Symptoms Marie ataxia typically manifests first with lower limb motor deficits that are noticed as the afflicted person walks up or down stairs or over uneven ground. The likelihood of falls increases with progression of the disease. The discoordination and muscle tremors eventually involve the arms and head. When muscles of the head and neck are affected, speech may be difficult to produce, and choking becomes a major concern. Because the ability to clear secretions from the lungs is also affected, patients are more susceptible to pneumonia and other respiratory tract diseases. Extraocular and facial muscle weakness and tongue atrophy may occur. Vision abnormalities are a late development.

A set of manifestations rarely found with other ataxias may occur in Marie ataxia; these include abnormal reflexes, muscle contractions, and diminished perception of pain or touch. The patient usually retains good bladder control and sexual function.

Etiology Marie ataxia is inherited as a dominant trait. Atrophy of the cerebellum and spinal cord is believed responsible for the symptoms.

Epidemiology Some 7000 cases of Marie ataxia have been diagnosed in the United States, although the total may be higher as a result of misdiagnosis and underreporting.

Related Disorders Ataxia, or failure of muscle coordination with a notable early symptom of unsteady gait, occurs in many disorders. There are as well many forms of ataxia, some inherited, others acquired, frequently secondary to another disorder. See *Ataxia, Friedreich; Charcot-Marie-Tooth Disease; Ataxia Telangiectasia; Olivopontocerebellar Atrophy.*

Treatment—Standard Physiotherapy and daily walking, assisted as necessary, will promote remaining muscle function. Surgery, prescription lenses, or drugs may be used to address vision problems. The patient is advised to avoid foods that could precipitate choking spells. Prevention of pneumonia is a challenge that may be met with a combination of antibiotics and postural drainage.

Treatment—Investigational The multiprogrammable spinal cord stimulator, an implantable device that delivers epidural spinal electrostimulation **(ESES),** may aid in the treatment of ataxias and other neuromuscular disorders refractory to medical treatment by improving mobility and alleviating spasticity and pain. For further information on ESES devices: Food and Drug Administration, Office for Orphan Product Development, HF-35 FDA Room 12-11, 5600 Fishers Lane, Rockville, Maryland 20857. For a controlled study of ESES devices: Neuromed, 5000 Oakes Road, Fort Lauderdale, Florida 33314.

The orphan drug physostigmine salicylate (Antilirium) is being studied in the treatment of the inherited ataxias. For additional information: Forest Pharmaceuticals, 2510 Metro Boulevard, St. Louis, Missouri 64043.

Please contact the agencies listed under Resources, below, for the most current information.

Resources

For more information on Marie ataxia: National Organization for Rare Disorders (NORD); National Ataxia Foundation; NIH/National Institute of Neurological Disorders & Stroke (NINDS).

For information on clinical services for persons with ataxia, including provision of orthopedic aids, recreation at summer and winter camps, and transportation assistance: Muscular Dystrophy Association.

For genetic information and genetic counseling referrals: March of Dimes Birth Defects Foundation; National Center for Education in Maternal and Child Health (NCEMCH).

References

Spinocerebellar Ataxia Associated with Localized Amyotrophy of the Hands, Sensorineural Deafness and Spastic Paraparesis in Two Brothers: F. Gemignani; J. Neurogenet., March 1986, issue 3(2), pp. 125–133.

Treatment of Patients with Degenerative Diseases of the Central Nervous System by Electrical Stimulation of the Spinal Cord: D.M. Dooley, et al.; Contin. Neurol., 1981, issue 44(1-3), pp. 71–76.

Otoneurologic Symptomatology in Hereditary Cerebellar Ataxia (Pierre-Marie disease): Ila Kalinovskaia, et al.; Zh. Nevropatol. Psikhiatr., 1980, issue 80(3), pp. 367–372.

ATAXIA TELANGIECTASIA

Description Ataxia telangiectasia is a severe inherited cerebellar ataxia characterized by progressive loss of motor coordination in the limbs and head, vascular oculocutaneous lesions, heightened susceptibility to sinopulmonary disease and neoplasms, and, frequently, premature aging. In some cases the disorder is associated with IgA or IgE immunodeficiency. Mental development may be normal in the early stages of the disease, but progressive dementia can occur during the 2nd decade of life. The clinical presentation may resemble that of Friedreich ataxia; however, the telangiectasia distinguishes ataxia telangiectasia.

Synonyms

Louis-Bar Syndrome
Cerebello-Oculocutaneous Telangiectasia
Immunodeficiency with Ataxia Telangiectasia

Signs and Symptoms The signs and symptoms of ataxia telangiectasia are wide-ranging and affect many distinct systems. Manifestations usually begin in infancy; some may not appear until the child is school age. An early sign is impaired muscle coordination, which usually becomes evident when walking is attempted. Coordination of the head and neck muscles is also impaired, and tremors may occur. Mental development may be delayed or regress as the disorder advances.

At 3 to 6 years the hallmark telangiectasia appears in the eyes, followed by the face and roof of the mouth. Other symptoms, especially those linked to growth and development, become more prominent at this age. Impaired neuromuscular function in the head and neck area leads to abnormal eye movements, faulty speech production, dysphagia, choking, and poor cough reflexes. Abnormal development or nondevelopment of thymus, adenoids, tonsils, and peripheral lymph nodes is a component in some cases of ataxia telangiectasia. A variety of tics, jerks, and other irregular nonvoluntary movements may accompany the disorder. Diminished immune system function and cell-mediated immunity make patients increasingly susceptible to sinopulmonary infections at about 3 years.

Premature aging occurs in 90 percent of cases, typically against a background of growth retardation. Incomplete sexual development and other endocrine abnormalities affect children of both sexes.

Persons with ataxia telangiectasia have a higher-than-normal incidence of carcinoma and lymphoma, first noticeable in adulthood. Exposure to X-irradiation may trigger the development of tumors.

Etiology Ataxia telangiectasia is believed to be inherited as an autosomal recessive trait. Various mechanisms have been postulated to account for the multiplicity of symptoms in this disorder. Neuromuscular symptoms may be due to degenerative central nervous system changes. A thymus gland deficiency has been linked to the immunologic abnormalities. The disorder has also been attributed variously to a defect in early fetal development and to a genetic defect in ability to repair damaged cells.

Epidemiology Ataxia telangiectasia has a familial tendency, frequently affecting more than one sibling. No sex predominance has been discerned. Approximately 1:40,000 newborns in the United States are affected.

Related Disorders See *Ataxia, Friedreich; Ataxia, Marie; Olivopontocerebellar Atrophy.*

Treatment—Standard Medication and physiotherapy are the mainstays of the symptomatic treatment of ataxia telangiectasia. Rigorous medical supervision is necessary to avoid infections or reduce their impact. Antibiotics, gammaglobulin, and postural drainage may be prescribed for respiratory tract infections. The neuromuscular effects such as slurred speech and muscle contractions may improve with diazepam. Reducing exposure to sunlight will help prevent the spread of lesions. Vitamin E has reportedly provided some symptomatic benefit but must be used cautiously to avoid toxic effects. Physiotherapy promotes muscle strength and may delay the onset of limb contractures.

Treatment—Investigational Specific diagnostic and therapeutic efforts directed toward the immunologic and endocrinologic components of ataxia telangiectasia are under way. The drugs under investigation in these research protocols include levamisole, interleukin-2, and interferon, for their immune effects, and various chemotherapeutic agents. The orphan drug physostigmine salicylate (Antilirium) is in clinical trial for the treatment of the inherited ataxias. For more information: Forest Pharmaceuticals, 2510 Metro Boulevard, St. Louis, Missouri 64043.

Please contact the agencies listed under Resources, below, for the most current information.

Resources

For more information on ataxia telangiectasia: National Organization for Rare Disorders (NORD); NIH/National Institute of Neurological Disorders & Stroke (NINDS); National Ataxia Foundation; Ataxia Telangiectasia Research Foundation.

For more information on tumors: American Cancer Society; NIH/National Cancer Institute PDQ (Physician Data Query) phoneline.

For genetic information and genetic counseling referrals: March of Dimes Birth Defects Foundation; National Center for Education in Maternal and Child Health (NCEMCH).

References

Treatment of Patients with Degenerative Diseases of the Central Nervous System by Electrical Stimulation of the Spinal Cord: D.M. Dooley, et al.; Contin. Neurol., 1981, issue 44(1–3), pp. 71–76.

Ataxia-Telangiectasia of Louis-Bar Syndrome: S.L. Conerly, et al.; J. Am. Acad. Dermatol., April 1985, issue 12(4), pp. 681–696.

Vascular Disorders: Amy S. Paller, M.D.; Dermatol. Clin.: The Genodermatoses, February 1987, issue 5(1), pp. 239–250.

ATTENTION DEFICIT HYPERACTIVITY DISORDER (ADHD)

Description Attention deficit hyperactivity disorder is a behavioral disorder of childhood characterized by a short attention span, excessive impulsiveness, and inappropriate hyperactivity.

Synonyms

Attention Deficit Disorder
Hyperactivity
Hyperkinetic Syndrome

Signs and Symptoms ADHD usually is observed before the child reaches 4 years of age, but in some instances is not diagnosed until he or she starts school. Symptoms vary depending on environmental factors, and typically worsen where sustained attention is required. Symptoms usually improve with frequent reinforcement in a structured setting where there are no distractions, and may also improve with maturity.

Characteristic motor overactivity in preschool children is displayed by excessive running, jumping, or climbing; in older children and adolescents, by excessive fidgeting, interrupting, and restlessness. Inattention and impulsiveness are hallmarks at any age. Other features of persons with ADHD include academic underachievement, low self-esteem and frustration tolerance, displays of temper, nonlocalized associated neurologic signs, and poor eye-hand coordination. Specific learning disabilities in reading or math can occur in conjunction with ADHD. Features of the disorder are often seen in children with Tourette syndrome.

Etiology The cause is not known. ADHD is thought to be more common among first-degree relatives. Other disorders that also are found more commonly among family members include developmental disorders, alcohol abuse, conduct disorder, antisocial personality disorder, and learning disabilities. (See ***Antisocial Personality Disorder.***)

Epidemiology Up to 3 percent of children may be affected, and at least 3 times more males than females. Symptoms of ADHD usually continue throughout childhood, and in about one-third of affected children, persist during adulthood.

Related Disorders In **mental retardation,** many features similar to ADHD are seen because of the intellectual development delay. The additional diagnosis of ADHD is made only if hyperactivity and impulsiveness also occur.

Pervasive developmental disorders are characterized by qualitative impairment in the development of social skills, verbal and nonverbal communication skills, and imaginative activity. Activities and interests are restricted, stereotyped, and repetitive. The severity of impairments may vary greatly.

Treatment—Standard Treatment is by counseling and/or the administration of stimulant drugs such as methylphenidate. A structured environment with minimal distractions can also be beneficial.

Treatment—Investigational Please contact the agencies listed under Resources, below, for the most current information.

Resources
For more information on attention deficit hyperactivity disorder: National Organization for Rare Disorders (NORD); C.H.A.D.D., Children with Attention Deficit Disorders; NIH/National Institute of Neurological, Communicative Disorders & Stroke (NINCDS); NIH/National Institute of Mental Health; Association for Children and Adults with Learning Disabilities.

References
Diagnostic and Statistical Manual of Mental Disorders, 3rd ed., revised: R.L. Spitzer, et al., eds.; Am. Psychiat. Assoc., 1987, pp. 50–53.

Sustained Release and Standard Methylphenidate Effects on Cognitive and Social Behavior in Children with Attention Deficit Disorder: W.E. Pelham, Jr., et al.; Pediatrics, October 1987, issue 80(4), pp. 491–501.

Attention Deficit Disorder with Hyperactivity: Differential Effects of Methylphenidate on Impulsivity: M.D. Rapport, et al.; Pediatrics, December 1985, issue 76(6), pp. 938–943.

Fifteen-Year Follow-up of a Behavioral History of Attention Deficit Disorder: D.C. Howell, et al.; Pediatrics, August 1985, issue 76(2), pp. 185–190.

High Rate of Affective Disorders in Probands with Attention Deficit Disorder and in Their Relatives: A Controlled Family Study: J. Biederman, et al.; Am. J. Psychiatry, March 1987, issue 144(3) pp. 330–333.

AUTISM

Description Autism is a lifelong, nonprogressive neurologic disorder characterized by onset usually before age 30 months, language and communication disorders, withdrawal from social contacts, and extreme reactions to changes in the immediate environment. About 75 percent of autistic children have low scores on standardized intelligence tests. The prognosis for independent living may be improved with intensive training but is generally poor. Life span is normal.

Synonyms
Infantile Autism
Kanner Syndrome

Signs and Symptoms Autism generally manifests before age 3. Among the earliest symptoms are lack of response to other persons and a marked preference for passive, solitary activity. The child does not watch others and avoids physical contact. Toddlers tend to form stronger attachments to objects than to people. Slight rearrangement of the objects in the physical environment, such as furniture, may provoke a violent and extreme reaction. Autistic children's response to aural and visual stimuli is unpredictable, ranging from seeming indifference to violent emotion. Hyperactivity is common and may lead to sleeping and eating disorders. Tantrums may occur if the child feels confused or is hindered in the pursuit of some activity. Autistic children may spend hours rocking rhythmically or engaged in some other solitary repetitive activity; the child appears self-absorbed. Motor development is frequently delayed.

Delayed acquisition of language skills is prominent among the communication disorders observed in autistic children. When speech does develop it is characterized by echophrasia and lack of grammar. Voluntary statements are often inappropriate in pitch, rhythm, or inflection. Some children stop speaking for years. Although hearing is intact, autistic children often appear deaf. Proposed deficits in information processing by the brain at the level of synthesis and abstraction may account for the difficulties in acquiring and using language.

Emotional lability and a preference for solitude remain prominent as the autistic child grows up. Play has a strong ritualistic, repetitive component. Unusual mannerisms develop, and bodily posture or limb movements may be contorted. Oral expression may pass into a stage of tooth grinding and muttering in place of speech. Reading and writing are learned with great difficulty. A few children exhibit unusual ability in aspects of music, mathematics, or rote memory.

Clinically, electroencephalographic abnormalities occur in some autistic patients.

Behavior usually improves around school age. Nevertheless, only a small proportion of autistic people ever adjust to independent living, even with intensive social and educational training. Most remain fully dependent and in need of sheltered homes for life.

Etiology Earlier theories proposing a psychogenic basis for autism have been superseded by the theory that the condition is an organic brain disorder. Several of the defects in autism can be traced to a central nervous system incapacity to process and respond to informational input, particularly auditory and visual stimuli. A deficit in information-processing capability could account for the impaired interpretive and conceptualizing skills exhibited by the autistic person.

A familial or genetic cause for some types of autism has been postulated, in part because of the higher incidence of the disorder in siblings. Autism may be inherited through autosomal recessive genes. A genetic component is also suggested by the greater number of boys than girls with infantile autism.

The role of metabolic, infectious, genetic, and environmental influences pre-

and perinatally is under investigation. Defective tryptophan processing has been proposed as a metabolic factor. More research is needed to confirm a genetic origin and to elucidate the contribution of prenatal events to the development of autism.

Epidemiology About 5:10,000 children have the fully expressed syndrome; some 15:10,000 children have 2 or more of the cardinal features of autism. Boys are affected 4 times more frequently than girls.

Related Disorders Other childhood disorders such as epilepsy, metabolic diseases, congenital rubella, and mental retardation of other cause may have an autistic component. The autistic syndrome must be differentiated from other conditions in which impaired language reception and use or schizophrenia are prominent symptoms. See *Epilepsy; Phenylketonuria; Rubella, Congenital.*

Treatment—Standard Treatment is primarily educational. Highly structured programs initiated early in life and providing around-the-clock care and oversight will maximize the child's chances of normal adaptation. Parental education programs and support groups benefit families considerably. Institutionalization is not recommended. Major tranquilizers such as trifluoperazine or haloperidol may be used to control hyperactivity or emotional lability.

Treatment—Investigational Fenfluramine is being studied investigationally as treatment for a subcategory of autistic people. For more information: Edward Ritvo, M.D., University of California, Los Angeles, California; Donald Cohen, M.D., Director, Yale Child Study Center, 333 Cedar Street, New Haven, Connecticut 06510.

Brain opioid levels may be unusually high in autism. Naltrexone, a drug manufactured for the treatment of opioid drug abuse, is being studied as therapy for autism on the theory that it will block brain cell receptors for natural opioids and secondarily decrease the high levels of these neurochemicals in autistic persons.

Please contact the agencies listed under Resources, below, for the most current information.

Resources

For more information on autism: National Organization for Rare Disorders (NORD); The National Society for Children and Adults with Autism (NSAC); NIH/National Institute of Neurological Disorders & Stroke (NINDS); NIH/National Institute of Mental Health.

For genetic information and genetic counseling referrals: March of Dimes Birth Defects Foundation; National Center for Education in Maternal and Child Health (NCEMCH).

References

Mendelian Inheritance in Man, 9th ed.: V.A. McKusick; The Johns Hopkins University Press, 1990, pp. 1058–1059.

BALÓ DISEASE

Description Baló disease is a childhood condition of brain demyelination characterized by progressive spastic paralysis and other neurologic symptoms depending on which parts of the brain are affected. The areas of demyelination can be localized in any part of the brain (e.g., the cerebral hemispheres, the cerebellum, and the brain stem); the lesions consist of irregular patches in concentric circles. The disease may progress rapidly over several weeks, or over 2 to 3 years.

Synonyms
> Concentric Sclerosis
> Encephalitis Periaxialis Concentrica
> Leukoencephalitis Periaxialis Concentrica

Signs and Symptoms The child gradually becomes spastic and paralyzed. Other neurologic, intellectual, and physiologic abnormalities may also develop, depending on the area of the brain affected.

Etiology The cause is unknown. There may be involvement of autoimmune factors or a slow virus.

Epidemiology Baló disease affects children of both sexes.

Related Disorders Schilder disease, a more severe form of brain demyelinization, appears to differ in its progression. The two diseases may be related.

Treatment—Standard There is no specific treatment. Care is supportive and symptomatic.

Treatment—Investigational Please contact the agencies listed under Resources, below, for the most current information.

Resources
> **For more information on Baló disease:** National Organization for Rare Disorders (NORD); NIH/National Institute of Neurological Disorders & Stroke (NINDS).

References
> Cecil Textbook of Medicine, 18th ed.: J.B. Wyngaarden and L.H. Smith, Jr., eds.; W.B. Saunders Company, 1988, p. 1889.

BATTEN DISEASE

Description Batten disease is the juvenile form of a group of inherited progressive neurologic diseases known as **neuronal ceroid lipofuscinoses.** It is characterized by accumulation of lipopigment in the brain and other tissues, leading to rapidly progressive optic atrophy, seizures, and intellectual impairment.
> **Santavuori disease** is the early infantile form; **Jansky-Bielchowsky disease,**

the late infantile form, usually begins before 4 years of age; and **Kufs disease,** the adult-onset form, usually begins in the late teens or early 20s (see *Kufs Disease).*

Synonyms
Batten-Mayou Syndrome
Batten-Spielmeyer-Vogt Disease
Batten-Vogt Syndrome
Neuronal Ceroid Lipofuscinosis
Spielmeyer-Vogt-Batten Syndrome
Spielmeyer-Vogt Disease
Stengel-Batten-Mayou-Spielmeyer-Vogt-Stock Disease
Stengel Syndrome

Signs and Symptoms The major findings are ocular atrophy with pigmentary degeneration, intellectual deterioration, and seizures. Other manifestations include kyphoscoliosis, twitching, spasticity, and ataxia.

The diagnosis of Batten disease requires blood tests and skin or conjunctival punch biopsy for biochemical and ultrastructural studies. Other useful information may be derived from an electroencephalogram, electroretinogram, and visual evoked response test, as well as from magnetic resonance imaging and computed tomography. A biochemical evaluation is also performed to determine the urinary level of dolichol, which is elevated in patients with Batten disease.

Etiology Batten disease is transmitted as an autosomal recessive trait. It is suspected that an enzyme deficiency leads to accumulation of lipopigments in nerves and other tissues.

Epidemiology In the United States, all forms of neuronal ceroid lipofuscinoses occur in approximately 3:100,000 live births. It is seen more commonly in families of Northern European Scandinavian ancestry, particularly the Swedish.

Related Disorders Symptoms of all the neuronal ceroid lipofuscinoses are similar; they are mainly differentiated by age of onset (see Description, above).

Treatment—Standard Treatment is usually symptomatic and supportive. Regular ophthalmic evaluation and services that benefit persons with visual impairment are beneficial. Genetic counseling may be useful.

Treatment—Investigational Clinical, pathological, biochemical, and genetic research on the neuronal ceroid lipofuscinoses began in 1987. Please contact the agencies listed under Resources, below, for the most current information.

The National Institute of Neurological & Communicative Disorders and Stroke and the National Institute of Mental Health support 2 national human brain specimen banks that supply tissue for investigation into neurologic and psychiatric diseases. Prospective donors are asked to contact Wallace W. Tourtellotte, M.D., or Edward D. Bird, M.D. (see the comprehensive Resources list elsewhere in the book).

Resources
For more information on Batten disease: National Organization for Rare

Disorders (NORD); Batten Disease Support & Research Association, National Batten Disease Registry; New York State Institute for Basic Research in Developmental Disabilities; NIH/National Institute of Neurological Disorders & Stroke (NINDS); National Tay-Sachs and Allied Diseases Association; National Lipid Diseases Foundation; Children's Brain Disease Foundation; Research Trust for Metabolic Disease in Children.

For genetic information and genetic counseling referrals: March of Dimes Birth Defects Foundation; National Center for Education in Maternal and Child Health (NCEMCH).

References

Mendelian Inheritance in Man, 9th ed.: V.A. McKusick; The Johns Hopkins University Press, 1990, pp. 1026–1027, 1028, 1382.

BELL'S PALSY

Description Bell's palsy is a nonprogressive facial nerve disorder characterized by sudden onset of facial paralysis. The paralysis results from ischemia and compression of the 7th cranial nerve.

Synonyms
    Facial Nerve Palsy
    Refrigeration Palsy
    Facial Paralysis

Signs and Symptoms Early symptoms include a slight fever, pain behind the ear, a stiff neck, and unilateral facial weakness and stiffness. Onset can be rapid, over several hours, and sometimes follows exposure to cold or a draft. Part or all of the face may be affected.

In most cases, only muscle weakness is involved, and the facial paralysis is temporary. Occasionally, only the upper or lower half of the face is affected. In severe cases, the facial muscles on the affected side are completely paralyzed, causing that side of the face to become smooth, expressionless, and immobile. Often the palpebral fissure is enlarged, remaining open even during sleep, with the result that the eyes cannot be closed. Corneal reflex also may be absent. If the lesion is proximal to the nerve branching, there may be decreased salivation, lacrimation, ipsilateral loss of the sense of taste, and hyperacusis. In some cases, pinprick sensation behind the ear also is decreased.

Recovery depends on the extent and severity of nerve damage. If the facial paralysis is only partial, complete recovery can be expected. The affected muscles usually regain their original function within 1 to 2 months. If, as recovery proceeds, the nerve fibers regrow to muscles other than the ones they originally innervated, there may be synkinesia. Crocodile tears associated with facial muscular contractions occasionally develop in the aftermath of Bell's palsy.

Etiology Ischemia and compression of the facial nerve within the canal occur as the result of nerve swelling and hyperemia of the nerve sheath. Although the cause is unknown, viral and immune diseases often are implicated. There also appears to be an inherited tendency toward developing this disorder.

Related Disorders See *Acoustic Neuroma; Melkersson-Rosenthal Syndrome.*
Other disorders of the 7th cranial nerve and nucleus include mastoid and middle ear infections, Ramsay Hunt syndrome (geniculate ganglion herpes), pontine tumors, and nerve invasion by carcinoma. Supranuclear lesions from stroke or tumor are characterized by weakness only below the eyes. Unilateral myasthenia gravis may present similar clinical findings. See *Myasthenia Gravis.*

Treatment—Standard Prompt decompression of the facial nerve is necessary to minimize permanent nerve damage. Massage and mild electrical stimulation of the paralyzed muscles maintains muscle tone and prevents atrophy. Treatment with oral corticosteroids, such as prednisone, has been more successful than surgical attempts to widen the facial canal. Methylcellulose drops, eyeglasses or goggles, temporary patching, or, in extreme cases, tarsorrhaphy, can help protect the exposed eye. If permanent paralysis has resulted, the peripheral facial nerve can be surgically anastomosed with the spinal accessory or hypoglossal nerves to allow some eventual return of muscle function.

Treatment—Investigational Please contact the agencies listed under Resources, below, for the most current information.

Resources
For more information on Bell's palsy: National Organization for Rare Disorders (NORD); NIH/National Institute of Neurological Disorders & Strokes (NINDS).

References
A Textbook of Neurology, 6th ed.: H.H. Merritt; Lea & Febiger, 1979.

BENIGN ESSENTIAL BLEPHAROSPASM (BEB)

Description BEB is a disorder in which the orbiculares oculi muscles do not function properly, and there is intermittent involuntary contraction or spasm of the musculature around the eyes. Although the eyes themselves are unaffected, the patient may eventually become functionally blind because of inability to open the eyes.

Synonyms
Blepharospasm
Secondary Blepharospasm

Signs and Symptoms In the early stages BEB is characterized by unusually frequent or forceful blinking, as well as occasional short episodes of involuntary eye closure. Over a period of several years, the episodes increase in frequency and duration. Ultimately, the eyes may be closed 75 percent of the time.
Approximately two-thirds of patients also have a general lack of facial muscle

tone, and one-third experience tremor. Episodes may be provoked by bright light, emotional stress, motion (such as riding in a car), and reading.

Etiology The disorder results from dysfunction of the 7th cranial nerve, but the underlying cause is not known. BEB is frequently but incorrectly considered to be a problem of psychological origin.

Epidemiology Females are affected more often than males in an approximate ratio of 3:2. Most patients are older than 50, but onset may be as early as the 2nd decade. All types of blepharospasm together are estimated to affect approximately 150,000 individuals in the United States.

Related Disorders Tetany is a mineral imbalance characterized by spasms of the voluntary muscles.

Tetanus is a bacterial infection characterized by spasms of the voluntary muscles and especially the muscles of the jaw.

See *Meige Syndrome; Tardive Dyskinesia; Wilson Disease; Tourette Syndrome.*

Treatment—Standard Anticholinergic drugs and dopamine depleters have been administered with moderate but often temporary effect.

Two surgical approaches are in use, but also with limited success. Following neurectomy, paralysis of the entire upper face may result, with nerve regeneration after a period of months or years. The second procedure, a protractor myectomy, involves the destruction of the eyelid muscles themselves.

The orphan drug botulinum A toxin (Oculinum) has been approved by the Food and Drug Administration as a treatment for blepharospasm. Small amounts of this agent are injected into the orbicularis oculi, paralyzing these muscles for several months. The procedure must then be repeated. These injections have been very helpful for some, but not all, patients with blepharospasm. The drug is available from Allergan, Inc., Irvine, California, and financial assistance is available.

Treatment—Investigational Please contact the agencies listed under Resources, below, for the most current information.

Resources

For more information on benign essential blepharospasm: National Organization for Rare Disorders (NORD); Benign Essential Blepharospasm Research Foundation, Inc.; NIH/National Institute of Neurological Disorders and Stroke (NINDS); Dystonia Medical Research Foundation.

References

Cranial Dystonia, Blepharospasm and Hemifacial Spasm: Clinical Features and Treatment, Including the Use of Botulinum Toxin: Kraft, S.P., et al.; Can. Med. Assoc. J., Nov. 1, 1988, issue 139(9), pp. 837–844.

Botulinum Toxin in the Management of Blepharospasm: Dutton, J.J., et al.; Arch. Neurol., April 1986, issue 43(4), pp. 380–382.

BENIGN ESSENTIAL TREMOR SYNDROME

Description Benign essential tremor is a disorder of unknown etiology primarily affecting the hands and head. The disease may be slowly progressive, eventually affecting other parts of the body.

Synonyms
> Hereditary Benign Tremor
> Presenile Tremor Syndrome

Signs and Symptoms The primary characteristic is a fine or coarse rhythmic tremor, with a frequency of 4 to 12 times per second when the affected part is in movement or voluntarily held in one position. This is in contrast to Parkinson disease tremors, which usually diminish or disappear entirely with purposeful movement. The tremors mainly affect the upper extremities and are aggravated by stress, anxiety, fatigue, and cold. Speech involvement and hyperhidrosis may be seen.

Etiology The cause is unknown. The disorder may be inherited as an autosomal dominant trait.

Epidemiology Males and females are affected equally. Onset may occur in childhood or old age, but young adults are affected most frequently. The mean age of onset is 45.

Treatment—Standard Tremors may be diminished or controlled by the use of propranolol or primidone. Rest may be helpful. Alcohol can relieve the symptoms but should be used with care because of its potential for abuse.

Treatment—Investigational Please contact the agencies listed under Resources, below, for the most current information.

Resources
 For more information on benign essential tremor syndrome: National Organization for Rare Disorders (NORD); International Tremor Foundation; NIH/National Institute of Neurological Disorders & Stroke (NINDS).
 For genetic information and genetic counseling referrals: March of Dimes Birth Defects Foundation; National Center for Education in Maternal and Child Health (NCEMCH).

References
Cecil Textbook Of Medicine, 18th ed.: J.B. Wyngaarden and L.H. Smith, Jr., eds.; W.B. Saunders Company, 1988, p. 2146.

BENIGN PAROXYSMAL POSITIONAL VERTIGO (BPPV)

Description Benign paroxysmal positional vertigo is characterized by extreme dizziness on certain movements of the head, and by nystagmus.

Synonyms
> Cupulolithiasis
> Postural Vertigo

Signs and Symptoms Episodes of violent dizziness occur without warning, triggered by movements such as turning the head from side to side, by lying on the right or left ear, and by moving to a sitting position. The dizziness (vertigo) is often accompanied by nausea and vomiting, and nystagmus usually also occurs. The symptoms may last only a few weeks or months and may disappear spontaneously.

Etiology Head trauma, ear infection, and ear surgery are among the causes of BPPV. In many cases the cause is unknown.

Epidemiology BPPV primarily affects females during middle or late adulthood.

Related Disorders See *Meniere Disease.*
Vestibular neuronitis of Dix and Hallpike is characterized by dizziness, nausea, and vomiting, and symptoms may worsen with head movement. Hearing is usually not impaired. Onset is abrupt in young adulthood, and the disorder may continue through the 40s. Etiology is unknown, although there is often an association with upper respiratory tract infection and fever.

Treatment—Standard Patients learn to avoid the precipitating positions. Medications can be used to decrease dizziness and to control nausea or vomiting. If bacterial infection is present in the ear, antibiotics are appropriate.

Treatment—Investigational A Jannetta procedure may be helpful in some cases of BPPV. For more information on this type of experimental surgery, contact Margareta Moller, M.D., Presbyterian University Hospital, Room 9402, PUH, 230 Lothrup Street, Pittsburgh, Pennsylvania 15213; (412) 624-3376.

Please contact the agencies listed under Resources, below, for the most current information.

Resources
For more information on benign paroxysmal positional vertigo: National Organization for Rare Disorders (NORD); E.A.R. Foundation; NIH/National Institute of Neurological Disorders & Stroke (NINDS); Dizziness and Balance Disorder Association.

References
Internal Medicine, 3rd ed.: J.H. Stein, ed.-in-chief; Little, Brown and Company, 1990, p. 1929.

BINSWANGER DISEASE

Description Binswanger disease is a form of senile dementia associated with lesions of the deep white matter in the brain due to small vessel arteriosclerotic changes.

Synonyms

Binswanger Encephalopathy
Multi-Infarct Dementia
Ischemic Periventricular Leukoencephalopathy
Subcortical Arteriosclerotic Encephalopathy

Signs and Symptoms Progressive loss of recent memory, difficulty coping with unusual events, self-centeredness, and childish behavior are typical findings. Urinary incontinence, difficulty walking, parkinsonian-type tremors, and depression are also prominent features of the disease.

Diagnosis may be made through the use of such imaging methods as computed tomography and magnetic resonance imaging.

Etiology Binswanger disease is a form of chronic cerebrovascular disease. Hypertension and diabetes may predispose to this condition. A history of repeated small strokes is commonly obtained.

Epidemiology Males are affected more often than females. Disease onset is generally after 60 years of age.

Related Disorders Many neurologic disorders can cause dementia and memory disturbances. See *Alzheimer Disease; Pick Disease; Creutzfeldt-Jakob Disease.*

Treatment—Standard Treatment is symptomatic and supportive, relying on antihypertensive and antidepressant agents.

Treatment—Investigational Please contact the agencies listed under Resources, below, for the most current information.

Resources

For more information on Binswanger disease: National Organization for Rare Disorders (NORD); Alzheimer's Disease and Related Disorders Association, Inc.; NIH/National Institute of Neurological Disorders & Stroke (NINDS); NIH/National Institute on Aging.

References

Senile Dementia of the Binswanger Type. A Vascular Form of Dementia in the Elderly: G.C. Roman; JAMA, October 1987, issue 258(13), pp. 1782–1788.

Subcortical Arteriosclerotic Encephalopathy (Binswanger Disease). Computed Tomographic, Nuclear Magnetic Resonance, and Clinical Correlations: W.R. Kinkel, et al.; Arch. Neurol., October 1985, issue 42(10), pp. 951–959.

White Matter Lucencies on Computed Tomography, Subacute Arteriosclerotic Encephalopathy (Binswanger Disease), and Blood Pressure: B.A. McQuinn, et al.; Stroke, September–October 1987, issue 18(5), pp. 900–905.

Reversible Depression in Binswanger Disease: N. Venna, et al.; J. Clin. Psychiatry, January 1988, issue 49(1), pp. 23–26.

BULIMIA

Description Bulimia is a psychiatric disorder characterized by binge eating followed by self-induced vomiting or purging with laxatives or diuretics.

Signs and Symptoms The alternating binging and purging or fasting typical of the patient with bulimia can lead to significant weight fluctuations. Menstrual irregularities and lymphadenopathy also may be seen. Many patients fear they cannot stop eating voluntarily.

Etiology The cause is unknown.

Epidemiology Approximately 95 percent of bulimic persons are female. Onset is usually during adolescence or early adulthood.

Related Disorders See *Anorexia Nervosa.*

Treatment—Standard Treatment attempts to improve self-image and stabilize eating patterns through provision of a calm, supportive, stable environment and psychotherapy.

Treatment—Investigational Please contact the agencies listed under Resources, below, for the most current information.

Resources

    For more information on bulimia: National Organization for Rare Disorders (NORD); Bulimia, Anorexia Self-Help; American Anorexia/Bulimia Association; Anorexia Nervosa and Associated Disorders, Inc.; Anorexia Nervosa and Related Eating Disorders, Inc.; NIH/National Institute of Mental Health; National Mental Health Association.

References

    Diagnostic and Statistical Manual of Mental Disorders, 3rd ed., revised: R.L. Spitzer, et al., eds.; American Psychiatric Association, 1987, pp. 67–69.

    Cecil Textbook of Medicine, 18th ed.: J.B. Wyngaarden and L.H. Smith, Jr., eds.; W.B. Saunders Company, 1988, pp. 656, 1218–1219.

CARPAL TUNNEL SYNDROME (CTS)

Description Carpal tunnel syndrome, a peripheral nerve entrapment neuropathy, results from compression of the median nerve as it passes through the carpal tunnel at the wrist. Pain, numbness, and paresthesias in the wrist and areas of the hand supplied by the median nerve are characteristic. With timely treatment, the prognosis in most cases is favorable.

Synonyms

    Constrictive Median Neuropathy
    Median Neuritis
    Median Neuropathy

Thenar Amyotrophy of Carpal Origin

Signs and Symptoms Pain and numbness are the most frequent symptoms; paresthesias may also be present. Awakening at night with a burning discomfort that is relieved by vigorously shaking the hand or flexing the wrist and fingers is classic. The thumb, index, middle, and lateral half of the ring finger are most commonly involved. In some cases pain may radiate up the forearm as high as the shoulder. If the thumb is involved, weakness or clumsiness in gripping objects may occur. Symptoms may be aggravated by activities that require wrist flexion or prolonged gripping, e.g., driving for long periods of time.

The CTS can appear as a secondary symptom of various systemic diseases (see under Etiology, below) or may occur as a single primary condition. Left untreated, muscle atrophy may develop in the hand.

Etiology Any narrowing of the carpal canal may cause compression of the median nerve, with nonspecific tenosynovitis being the most common cause. Occupational or sports activities requiring prolonged gripping motion or wrist flexion may increase the risk of occurrence. Trauma or posttraumatic sequelae may initiate the syndrome.

CTS may occur as a result of amyloid neuropathy, the mucopolysaccharidoses, and the mucolipidoses. (See *Amyloidosis; Mucopolysaccharidosis.*) Other inflammatory disorders include rheumatoid arthritis and gout. CTS may develop secondarily to acromegaly, myxedema, diabetes, or lupus erythematosus. Pregnancy, the use of the contraceptive pill, menopause, and renal dialysis are also contributory. Space-occupying lesions may encroach on the carpal.

Epidemiology CTS occurs up to 5 times more frequently in females (usually between 40 and 65 years of age) than in males.

Related Disorders See *Peripheral Neuropathy.*

Ulnar nerve palsy, due to trauma or pressure in the ulnar groove of the elbow, can occur as the result of repeated leaning on the elbow or by abnormal bone growth after a childhood fracture **(tardy ulnar palsy).** Symptoms include pain, numbness, and paresthesias in the 4th and 5th fingers plus weakness and wasting of the thumb and surrounding muscles.

Radial nerve palsy is caused by pressure on the nerve, as can occur when the arm is draped over the back of a chair for long periods of time. Symptoms include weakness of the wrist and hand, wrist drop, and numbness, particularly of the first 2 fingers.

Anterior interosseous nerve syndrome is characterized by pain in the forearm with weakness and loss of dexterity in the hand. The disorder can be caused by injuries or strenuous exercise. Pain is a major symptom; numbness usually does not occur. Some muscle changes may develop in time.

Pronator quadratus syndrome is a median nerve compression syndrome that occurs less frequently than carpal tunnel syndrome, but must be differentiated from it. Pain in the forearm and palm is characteristic. Strenuous exercise often increases the pain. A tingling sensation may be felt when pressure is applied to the affected area.

Cervical degenerative disc disease may cause pain and numbness of the hand. Onset of symptoms usually is abrupt. Nerve root compression may cause gradual loss of reflexes.

Thoracic outlet syndromes involve compression of the subclavian artery and brachial plexus in the interscalene space or costoclavicular space. Symptoms include pain, numbness, and paresthesias along the ulnar side of the forearm and the ulnar portion of the hand.

Treatment—Standard Treatment of carpal tunnel syndrome varies according to severity and type of symptoms. For mild symptoms with no neurologic deficit, conservative treatment is advocated. Immobilization of the wrist, nonsteroidal antiinflammatory agents, and vitamin B6 (pyridoxine) are recommended. Local injection of corticosteroids has given a high percentage of short-term relief. Progressive, persistent symptoms, significant functional impairment, or the presence of neurologic deficit may require surgical decompression. Electromyography is useful for diagnosis before surgery. With prolonged compression, recovery may be incomplete.

Treatment—Investigational Please contact the agencies listed under Resources, below, for the most current information.

Resources

For more information on carpal tunnel syndrome: National Organization for Rare Disorders (NORD); American Carpal Tunnel Syndrome Association; NIH/National Institute of Neurological Disorders & Stroke (NINDS).

References
Nerve Entrapment Syndromes in the Upper Extremity: M.P. Coyle; *in* Principles of Orthopedic Practice, vol. I: Dee, et al., eds.; McGraw-Hill Book Company, 1989, pp. 672–683.

Cecil Textbook of Medicine, 18th ed.: J.B. Wyngaarden and L.A. Smith, eds.; W.B. Saunders Company, 1988, pp. 2267–2268.

Carpal Tunnel Syndrome: D.M. Ditmars, et al.; Hand Clin., August 1986, issue 2(3), pp. 525–532.

Sports-Related Extraarticular Wrist Syndromes: M.B. Wood, et al.; Clin. Orthop., January 1986, issue 202, pp. 93–102.

Acute Carpal Tunnel Syndrome. Complications of Delayed Decompression: D.J. Ford, et al.; J. Bone Joint Surg., November 1986, issue 68(5), pp. 758–759.

CENTRAL CORE DISEASE

Description Central core disease, characterized by muscle weakness beginning in the neonatal period, is one of the diseases contributing to floppy baby syndrome. The legs are usually most severely involved. The disease derives its name from the characteristic biopsy finding of an abnormal core in each muscle fiber.

Synonyms
Muscle Core Disease
Nonprogressive Congenital Myopathy

Signs and Symptoms The muscles of the upper arm are hypotonic and somewhat underdeveloped. Infants find it difficult to learn to sit and to walk. By about 6 years of age, however, most affected children can walk, and as adults, the disease often is experienced only as slight weakness in the legs. Persons with central core disease seem to be unusually susceptible to malignant hyperthermia in response to anesthesia.

Etiology Families with central core disease usually demonstrate dominant gene inheritance. The biochemical abnormality causing muscular weakness and the presence of the core in the muscle fibers is not known. Absence of mitochondria and certain oxidative enzymes is observed in the involved muscle fibers.

Epidemiology Males and females are affected equally.

Related Disorders See *Nemaline Myopathy.*

Treatment—Standard Treatment of central core disease is symptomatic and supportive.

Treatment—Investigational Please contact the agencies listed under Resources, below, for the most current information.

Resources

For more information on central core disease: National Organization for Rare Disorders (NORD); NIH/National Institute of Neurological Disorders & Stroke (NINDS); Muscular Dystrophy Association.

For genetic information and genetic counseling referrals: March of Dimes Birth Defects Foundation; National Center for Education in Maternal and Child Health (NCEMCH).

References

Mendelian Inheritance in Man, 9th ed.: V.A. McKusick; The Johns Hopkins University Press, 1990, pp. 177–178.

CEREBRAL PALSY

Description Cerebral palsy is a neuromuscular disorder resulting from injury to the brain during early development or at birth. Affected individuals typically exhibit a lack of muscle control and coordination. The disorder is not progressive.

Synonyms

Cerebral Diplegia
Infantile Cerebral Paralysis
Little's Disease
Palsy

Signs and Symptoms Infants with cerebral palsy may exhibit developmental delay during the 1st or 2nd year, and may have muscle weakness and abnormal muscle tone.

As the child grows, typical findings include drooling, difficulty gaining bladder or bowel control, convulsive seizures, hand tremors, and the inability to identify objects by touch. Poor vision is found more often in these patients than in the general population. The intellect may be average or above average, or there may be impairment ranging from mild to severe.

Cerebral palsy is classified according to which limbs are affected and to the quality of the movement disturbance. If both legs are affected, the condition is called diplegia; if both arms and legs are affected, quadriplegia.

Spastic cerebral palsy is characterized by involuntary contraction of the muscles and a scissor gait. The lower legs may turn in and cross at the ankle. In some cases, the extensor leg muscles are so tightly contracted that the heels do not touch the floor and the child walks on tiptoe.

Athetoid cerebral palsy is characterized by athetosis that may be accompanied by facial grimacing, abnormal tongue movements, and drooling. Involuntary flailing or jerky motions may also occur.

In **ataxic cerebral palsy,** the principal disturbance in movement is a lack of balance and coordination. The person may sway when standing, have trouble maintaining balance, and may walk with the feet spread wide apart to avoid falling.

Etiology Cerebral palsy is caused by injury to the brain during the early stages of development or at birth. The injury may result from maternal-fetal infection, bleeding into the brain, or lack of oxygen at birth. Premature infants are especially susceptible.

Cerebral palsy also may be acquired postnatally. Head injuries, infections such as meningitis, and other forms of brain damage occurring in the first months or years of life are the main causes.

Epidemiology The United Cerebral Palsy Association estimates that between 1:1000 and 3:1000 infants develop cerebral palsy each year, or about 9000 new cases. Severity can range from mild to very severe.

Treatment—Standard Treatment relies on physical therapy, biofeedback, occupational therapy, and vocational training.

Certain drugs are useful in treating cerebral palsy. Anticonvulsant drugs are usually prescribed to treat associated seizures. Diazepam and other muscle relaxants can sometimes relieve spasticity.

Treatment—Investigational Local electrical stimulation of nerves important for motor coordination and control is under investigation as a possible treatment.

Please contact the agencies listed under Resources, below, for the most current information.

Resources
    For more information on cerebral palsy: National Organization for Rare Disorders (NORD); United Cerebral Palsy Association, Inc.; NIH/National Institute of Neurological Disorders and Stroke (NINDS); The National Easter Seal Society, Inc.
    For genetic information and genetic counseling referrals: March of

Dimes Birth Defects Foundation; National Center for Education in Maternal and Child Health (NCEMCH).

References

Cervical Spinal Cord Stimulation for Spasticity in Cerebral Palsy: H. Hugenholtz et al.; Neurosurgery, April 1988, issue 22(4), pp. 707–714.

Submandibular Gland Resection and Bilateral Parotid Duct Litigation as a Management for Chronic Drooling in Cerebral Palsy: Brundage, et al.; Plast. Reconstr. Surg., March 1989, issue 83(3), pp. 443–446.

CEREBRO-OCULO-FACIO-SKELETAL (COFS) SYNDROME

Description COFS syndrome is a degenerative disorder of the brain and spinal cord characterized by craniofacial and skeletal abnormalities, hypotonia, and diminished or absent reflexes. The white matter of the brain is reduced, with gray mottling.

Synonyms

Pena Shokeir II Syndrome

Signs and Symptoms Craniofacial characteristics include microcephaly and micrognathia; small eyes, cataracts, and blepharophimosis; and large ears and a long philtrum. Kyphosis and osteoporosis may be present. There may be campto-dactyly, flexion contractures, and rocker-bottom feet.

The child fails to thrive and is highly vulnerable to respiratory infections. Death may occur within 5 years.

Etiology COFS syndrome is inherited as an autosomal recessive trait.

Epidemiology The syndrome is present at birth and is seen in infants of diverse ethnic heritage.

Related Disorders Neu-Laxova syndrome is characterized by in utero growth retardation. Multiple abnormalities are present at birth and include microcephaly and anomalies of the placenta, limbs, external genitalia, and skin. Manifestations of both COFS and Neu-Laxova syndromes have been seen in some children.

Treatment—Standard Treatment is symptomatic and supportive. Genetic counseling is recommended for families of affected children.

Treatment—Investigational Please contact the agencies listed under Resources, below, for the most current information.

Resources

For more information on cerebro-oculo-facio-skeletal syndrome: National Organization for Rare Disorders (NORD); NIH/National Institute of Neurological Disorders & Stroke (NINDS); FACES—National Association for the Craniofacially Handicapped; National Craniofacial Foundation; Society for the

Rehabilitation of the Facially Disfigured; About Face.

For genetic information and genetic counseling referrals: March of Dimes Birth Defects Foundation; National Center for Education in Maternal and Child Health (NCEMCH).

References
Smith's Recognizable Patterns of Human Malformation, 4th ed.: K.L. Jones; W.B. Saunders Company, 1988, pp. 146–147.

Chondro-Osseous Changes in Cerebro-Oculo-Facio-Skeletal (COFS) Syndrome: W.S. Hwang, et al.; J. Pathol., September 1982, issue 138(1), pp. 33–40.

Intracranial Calcifications in Cerebro-Oculo-Facio-Skeletal (COFS) Syndrome: S.L. Linna, et al.; Pediatr. Radiol., 1982, issue 12(1), pp. 28–30.

The Neu-Cofs (Cerebro-Oculo-Facio-Skeletal) Syndrome: Report of a Case: M.C. Silengo, et al.; Clin. Genet., February 1984, issue 25(2), pp. 201–204.

CHARCOT-MARIE-TOOTH DISEASE

Description Charcot-Marie-Tooth disease is a progressive, hereditary motor and sensory neuropathy characterized by weakness and atrophy, primarily in the peroneal and distal leg muscles.

Synonyms
Hereditary Sensory Motor Neuropathy
Peroneal Muscular Atrophy

Signs and Symptoms Symptoms of type I Charcot-Marie-Tooth disease manifest in middle childhood or teenage years, with pes cavus and slowly progressive weakness and atrophy of peroneal muscle groups producing a "stork leg" deformity. Eventually, impairment spreads to the upper extremities, with a stocking-glove pattern of decrease in sensitivity to vibration, pain, and temperature. Nerve conduction responses become slower over time, deep tendon reflexes are absent, and enlarged peripheral nerves may be palpable.

Type II Charcot-Marie-Tooth disease symptoms develop later in life and the disorder progresses more slowly. Individuals affected by both types I and II have normal life spans.

Etiology The disease is inherited as an autosomal dominant trait.

Epidemiology Males and females are affected in equal numbers.

Related Disorders See *Dejerine-Sottas Disease;* the age of onset, clinical findings, and prognosis are similar to those of Charcot-Marie-Tooth disease. See also *Refsum Syndrome,* in which peripheral neuropathy is present.

Familial amyloid neuropathy is characterized by accumulation of amyloid in peripheral nerves. This rare disorder is inherited as an autosomal dominant trait.

Hereditary sensory radicular neuropathy manifests initially as pain and decreased sensitivity to temperature in the foot and lower leg. As the disease progresses, weakness and foot ulcers may be accompanied by attacks of sharp pain throughout the body.

Treatment—Standard Bracing to correct foot drop, or orthopedic surgery to stabilize the foot are appropriate therapeutic options. Vocational counseling may also be helpful.

Treatment—Investigational Please contact the agencies listed under Resources, below, for the most current information.

Resources

For more information on Charcot-Marie-Tooth disease: National Organization for Rare Disorders (NORD); Charcot-Marie-Tooth Association; Charcot-Marie-Tooth International; NIH/National Institute of Neurological Disorders & Stroke (NINDS).

For genetic information and genetic counseling referrals: March of Dimes Birth Defects Foundation; National Center for Education in Maternal and Child Health (NCEMCH).

References

Cecil Textbook of Medicine, 18th ed.: J.B. Wyngaarden and L.H. Smith, Jr., eds.: W.B. Saunders Company, 1988, pp. 2264, 2155.

Mendelian Inheritance in Man, 8th ed.: V.A. McKusick; The Johns Hopkins University Press, 1986, pp. 140–143, 860, 1262.

Scientific American MEDICINE: E. Rubinstein and D. Federman, eds.; Scientific American, Inc., 1978–1991, pp. 11:II:1–2.

CHRONIC HICCUPS

Description Hiccups are involuntary spasms of the diaphragm that occur suddenly and repeatedly, usually a few times per minute. Most episodes are transient, lasting only a few minutes. When hiccups persist, the possibility of underlying illness must be investigated.

Synonyms
Singultus

Signs and Symptoms Chronic hiccups may last hours or days, and may recur frequently with only a few hours of relief between spasms. Lack of sleep, exhaustion, and weight loss may result if chronic hiccups are not controlled.

Etiology The characteristic "hic" sound is caused by intake of air into the larynx.

Hiccups develop in response to irritation of afferent or efferent nerves, or of the medullary centers in the brain that control the diaphragm muscle. Chronic hiccups can occur idiopathically, although a persistent form may suggest the presence of such underlying conditions as brain lesions or tumors, pancreatitis, or intestinal, hepatic, or renal disease. Pregnancy, pleurisy of the diaphragm, pneumonia, and alcoholism have also been associated. Surgery or anesthesia can cause hiccups.

Epidemiology Males are affected more frequently than females. The occurrence of ordinary, transient hiccups is common; the occurrence of chronic hiccups is very rare.

Related Disorders Many disorders involving the autonomic nervous system control unconscious activities of the body such as breathing, sweating, heartbeat, hiccups, and coughing.

Treatment—Standard Since ordinary hiccups tend to be self-limited, they do not require treatment.

Chronic hiccups may be controlled with drugs such as chlorpromazine, metoclopramide, anticonvulsants, quinidine, or intramuscular haloperidol. Ephedrine or ketamine are the drugs of choice if hiccups develop during anesthesia and surgery. Hypnosis and acupuncture have been successful in treating some patients. For unresponsive cases, small amounts of procaine solution may be injected into the phrenic nerve to block stimulation of the diaphragm. Surgery to sever the phrenic nerve in the neck has been of limited value and does not cure all cases.

Treatment—Investigational In research at Walter Reed Hospital, nifedipine was found to be successful in stopping chronic hiccuping in 5 of 7 patients treated. The longterm efficacy of nifedipine for this purpose is being evaluated.

Please contact the agencies listed under Resources, below, for the most current information.

Resources

For more information on chronic hiccups: National Organization for Rare Disorders (NORD); NIH/National Heart, Lung and Blood Institute (NHLBI).

References
Treatment of Intractable Hiccups with Intramuscular Haloperidol: T.J. Ives, et al.; Am. J. Psychiatry, November 1985, issue 142(11), pp. 1368–1369.
Chronic Hiccups: M.S. Lipsky; Am. Fam. Physician, November 1986, issue 34(5), pp. 173–177.
Hiccups: Causes and Cures: J.H. Lewis; J. Clin. Gastroenterol., December 1985, issue 7(6), pp. 539–552.
Hiccups and Esophageal Dysfunction: G. Triadafilopoulos; Am. J. Gastroenterol., February 1989, issue 84(2), pp. 164–149.
Sleep Hiccup: J.J. Askenasy; Sleep, April 1988, issue 11(2), pp. 187–194.

CHRONIC SPASMODIC DYSPHONIA (CSD)

Description CSD is a speech disorder that resembles stuttering and is caused by vigorous adduction or abduction of the vocal cords. The voice sounds hoarse, soft, and strained, and the breathing pattern is abnormal.

Synonyms
Abductor Spasmodic Dysphonia
Abductor Spastic Dysphonia
Adductor Spasmodic Dysphonia

Adductor Spastic Dysphonia
Dysphonia Spastica

Signs and Symptoms Chronic spasmodic dysphonia is characterized by uncontrolled vocal spasms, conscious effort in order to speak, tightness in the throat, and intermittent hoarseness.

Symptoms gradually progress over the first 2 years and then generally stabilize. The disorder usually remains chronic without marked changes over a period of years, although symptoms may worsen with stress.

In the most severe form of CSD, patients may experience aphonia. Coughing, laughing, and sometimes singing may be less affected than speaking.

A milder subtype of CSD is characterized by difficulty controlling speech after certain sounds (e.g., "P," "T," and "K").

Diagnosis of chronic spasmodic dysphonia usually includes indirect laryngoscopy to rule out vocal cord structural abnormalities such as nodules, polyps, or tumors.

Etiology The cause is not known. It is possible that the adduction or abduction of the vocal cords may relate to brain stem dysfunction. In about 60 percent of patients, symptoms onset follows a severe upper respiratory tract infection with laryngitis. The disorder may also occur after head injury or prolonged use of phenothiazines. Some patients may have associated movement disorders, such as tardive dyskinesia, oral-facial dystonia, torticollis, or essential tremor.

Epidemiology The disorder occurs most often in those who use their voices a great deal and who have had voice training. Onset usually is between 20 and 60 years of age, and over 70 percent of affected persons are female.

Related Disorders In **chronic stuttering** there is an abnormal speech pattern characterized by repetitions, prolongations, unusual hesitations, and pauses that disrupt rhythmic flow of speech. The disorder usually appears before age 12 and is often familial.

Essential voice tremor is an involuntary movement of the vocal cords produced by rhythmic alternate contractions of opposing laryngeal muscles (see **Benign Essential Tremor Syndrome**).

Vocal cord polyps may be caused by voice abuse, chronic allergies affecting the larynx, or irritation of the vocal cords by industrial fumes or cigarette smoke. Vocal cord polyps typically result in hoarseness and breathiness.

Vocal cord nodules (singer's, teacher's, or screamer's nodules) are concentrations of connective tissue on the vocal cords. These nodules may be due to chronic voice abuse, or unnatural lowering of the voice. Hoarseness and a breathy voice quality result.

Vocal cord paralysis may result from lesions in several locations in the brain, the 10th cranial nerve (nervus vagus), laryngeal nerves, or neck or thoracic lesions; neurotoxins such as lead; infections such as diphtheria; or viral illness. Vocal cord paralysis usually results in loss of vocal cord abduction or adduction, and may affect speech, respiration, and swallowing.

If the vocal cord paralysis is unilateral, the voice is hoarse and breathy. If the paralysis is bilateral, the voice is very soft but of good quality. Breathing difficulty with wheezing may occur on moderate exertion.

Squamous cell carcinoma of the larynx is the most common malignant laryngeal tumor. The earliest symptom is usually hoarseness. Early treatment with radiation or cordectomy usually results in a cure rate of 85 to 95 percent.

Treatment—Standard In 40 percent of cases, the symptoms of chronic spasmodic dysphonia improve with severance of one of the recurrent laryngeal nerves. However, the nerve can grow back 3 to 9 months after surgery, resulting in return of symptoms. Another 40 percent of patients may benefit from treatment with propranolol. Speech therapy also can be helpful.

Treatment—Investigational Researchers at 12 treatment centers including the National Institute of Deafness and Other Communication Disorders are currently treating adults who suffer from chronic spasmodic dysphonia with the orphan drug botulinum A toxin (Oculinum). The drug is injected into the thyroarytenoid cartilage at intervals of several weeks. To date, this procedure has been beneficial in all test cases, with varying degrees of hoarseness and swallowing difficulties as side effects, depending on dosage. Symptoms usually return after 2 to 3 months, and reinjections are required.

Adults over 18 years of age who have had dysphonia for more than 2 years may contact the following persons if they wish to participate in research projects on spasmodic dysphonia: Christy Ludlow, Ph.D., NIH/National Institute of Deafness & Other Communication Disorders (NIDCD), Speech Pathology Unit, Building 10, Room 5N226, 9000 Rockville Pike, Bethesda, Maryland 20892, (301) 496-9365; or Andrew Blitzer, M.D., Professor, Clinical Otolaryngology and Vice-Chairman, College of Physicians and Surgeons, Columbia University, New York, NY 10032.

For information concerning research on spasmodic dysphonia as well as other debilitating communicative disorders: Dr. Sandra Chapman, Callier Center for Communicative Disorders, Dallas Center for Vocal Motor Control, 1966 Inwood Road., Dallas, Texas 75235.

Botulinum toxin is available from Alan Scott, M.D., Smith-Kettlewell Eye Research Foundation, 2232 Webster Street, San Francisco, California 94115, (415) 567-0667.

For information on an epidemiologic study on spastic dysphonia, contact Clarence T. Sasaki, M.D., Yale University School of Medicine, 333 Cedar St., New Haven, Connecticut 06510.

Please also check with the agencies listed under Resources, below, for further information.

Resources

For more information on chronic spasmodic dysphonia: National Organization for Rare Disorders (NORD); Spastic Dysphonia Support Group; VOCAL (Voluntary Organization for Communication and Language).

CLUSTER HEADACHE

Description Cluster headaches are a rare disabling neuralgia characterized by profound unilateral, nonthrobbing pain, and accompanied by rhinorrhea and lacrimation. Attacks usually last 15 to 30 minutes and may recur several times daily. Onset occurs during sleep. Cyclic and chronic forms of cluster headache are recognized.

Synonyms
> Histamine Cephalalgia
> Vasogenic Facial Pain

Signs and Symptoms The patient with cluster headaches may awake from sleep with deep, nonthrobbing pain in the face, eye, temple, or forehead. When the pain passes the patient falls into a deep sleep, only to be aroused again by another attack in the same site. The eyelid over an affected eye may droop, and an involved eye or nostril may water copiously.

Attacks occur in groups of 1 to 4 headaches, daily or more often, and may continue for weeks to months. The cyclic variant is characterized by a headache-free period of variable duration; a remission for several years may be followed by a new onslaught of cluster headaches. When the headaches recur regularly without intervening headache-free periods, the condition is considered chronic. Alcohol ingestion appears to trigger the attacks in some patients.

Etiology The cause of cluster headaches is unknown. The condition has been speculatively linked to hormonal imbalances, spasms, edema, and carotid artery inflammation.

Epidemiology Cluster headaches have a strong male sex predominance. Young to middle-aged males can be affected, but incidence is most common in the 5th, 6th, or 7th decade of life. Women are rarely affected.

Related Disorders Severe headache is a feature of many disorders, particularly neuralgias, cerebrovascular syndromes, and brain tumors. Like cluster headaches, **migraine headaches** typically are unilateral. The headaches may be accompanied by gastrointestinal upset (nausea, vomiting, constipation, or diarrhea), irritability, and visual problems such as photosensitivity or double vision. Affected individuals appear to have a genetic predisposition. Migraine headache has been attributed to constriction of the cranial arteries, but the cause of the constriction is unknown.

See *Tolosa-Hunt Syndrome; Trigeminal Neuralgia; Arteritis, Giant-Cell.*

Treatment—Standard Inhalation of ergotamine and oxygen may speed recovery from an attack. Methysergide, lithium carbonate, prednisone, verapamil, and nifedipine may be prescribed to help prevent recurrences. Alcohol ingestion should be avoided.

Treatment—Investigational Various surgical procedures have been proposed for extreme cases of cluster headache unresponsive to medication. Sphenopalatine ganglion neurectomy has been tried experimentally to relieve pain when medical treatment has failed. The safety and efficacy of this procedure are unknown. Please contact the agencies listed under Resources, below, for the most current information.

Resources

For more information on cluster headache: National Organization for Rare Disorders (NORD); NIH/National Institute of Neurological Disorders and Stroke; National Migraine Foundation.

References

Internal Medicine, 2nd ed.: J.H. Stein, ed.-in-chief; Little, Brown and Company, 1987, pp. 2180–2185.

Vasogenic Facial Pain (Cluster Headache): L.R. Eversole, et al.; Int. J. Oral Maxillofac. Surg., February 1987; issue 16(1), pp. 25–35.

Cluster Headaches: J.P. McKenna; Am. Fam. Physician, April 1988; issue 37(4), pp. 173–178.

Cluster Headache Pain vs. Other Vascular Headache Pain. Differences Revealed with Two Approaches to the McGill Pain Questionnaire: A. Jerome, et al.; Pain, July 1988, issue 34(1), pp. 35–42.

Unilateral Impairment of Pupillary Response to Trigeminal Nerve Stimulation in Cluster Headache: M. Fanciullacci, et al.; Pain, February 1989, issue 36(2), pp. 185–191.

CONVERSION DISORDER

Description Conversion disorder is a psychological, neurotic condition involving physical symptoms that develop out of emotional conflicts or needs, without any physiological basis and without any intention for effect. The physical symptoms usually appear suddenly during times of extreme psychological stress. Conversion disorder can be distinguished from other physiological disorders by the associated inappropriate lack of concern over debilitating symptoms (la belle indifférence).

Synonyms

Hysterical Neurosis, Conversion Type

Signs and Symptoms Common symptoms of conversion disorder, which often resemble neurologic diseases, include paralysis, seizures, aphonia, dyskinesia, and temporary blindness. Patients usually exhibit only one symptom, and an episode tends to appear and disappear suddenly. With recurrent episodes, the symptom may appear in a different location or with varying severity.

The conversion symptoms are thought to be symbolic resolutions to psychological conflicts, i.e., vomiting may represent revulsion and disgust, or blindness portray an inability to accept witnessing a traumatic event. Physiological disease must be ruled out before establishing a diagnosis of conversion disorder.

Etiology The source of this disorder is an inner conflict that creates extreme psychological stress. Conversion symptoms arise as a means to partially resolve the inner conflict. For example, a soldier who subconsciously wishes to avoid firing a gun may develop a paralyzed hand.

Epidemiology Onset is usually in the teens and 20s, but can be later in life. Individuals with previous physical disorders and individuals who are exposed to persons with real physical symptoms are susceptible to developing this disorder. A large number of the known cases of conversion disorder have appeared in military settings, particularly during wartime. One particular symptom, globus hystericus, is more common in females.

Related Disorders Physical disorders with vague somatic symptoms may initially be misdiagnosed as conversion disorder; these include multiple sclerosis, Wilson disease, demyelinating polyneuropathy.

Treatment—Standard Treatment is individualized and can include psychoanalysis, family therapy, or specific life changes. Antidepressant and antipsychotic drugs can be helpful in reducing some symptoms. Although hypnosis may eliminate certain specific symptoms, often a substitute symptom arises. Temporary paralysis may be treated by electromyographic biofeedback.

Treatment—Investigational Please contact the agencies listed under Resources, below, for the most current information.

Resources

For more information on conversion disorder: National Organization for Rare Disorders (NORD); National Mental Health Association; NIH/National Institute of Mental Health (NIMH).

References

Diagnostic and Statistical Manual of Mental Disorders, 3rd ed., revised: R.L. Spitzer, et al., eds.; Am. Psychiat. Assoc., 1987, pp. 257–259.

Globus Hystericus Syndrome Responsiveness to Antidepressants: I.H. Bangash, et al.; Am. J. Psychiatry, July 1986, issue 143(7), pp. 917–918.

The Utility of Electromyographic Biofeedback in the Treatment of Conversion Paralysis: D.A. Fishbain, et al.; Am. J. Psychiatry, December 1988, issue 145(12), pp. 1572–1575.

CREUTZFELDT-JAKOB DISEASE

Description Creutzfeldt-Jakob disease is a rare, fatal, transmissable spongiform encephalopathy, occurring in middle life, and characterized by progressive degeneration of the central nervous system and by neuromuscular disturbances.

Synonyms

Corticostriatal-Spinal Degeneration
Jakob-Creutzfeldt Disease
Spastic Pseudosclerosis
Subacute Spongiform Encephalopathy

Signs and Symptoms The early stages are marked by memory failures, behavioral changes, difficulty in concentration and coordination, or visual disturbances. Myoclonus, extensor plantar reflexes, and hyperreflexia may be seen. The illness progresses to pronounced mental deterioration, hemiparesis, sensory disturbances, and progressive muscular atrophy, and mutism, akinesia, seizures, and semicoma may ensue. Death generally occurs within a year, and may take place after only a few months.

The disease can produce characteristic changes in the electroencephalograph (EEG). CT scan can demonstrate atrophy of the brain.

Etiology The etiologic agent in Creutzfeldt-Jakob disease is believed to be a small infectious particle called a prion. The mode of transmission is not completely understood. About 10 percent of reported cases are familial.

Epidemiology Creutzfeldt-Jakob disease affects both males and females, with peak incidence of the disorder occurring in the late 50s.

Related Disorders See *Alzheimer Disease.*

Treatment—Standard Although there is no specific therapy for Creutzfeldt-Jakob disease, there is some evidence that vidarabine and amantidine may be helpful in some patients.

Treatment—Investigational The following investigators have expressed an interest in receiving biopsy and autopsy tissue, blood, and cerebrospinal fluid from patients with Creutzfeldt-Jakob and related diseases:

Stephen DeArmone, M.D., and Stanley Prusiner, M.D., Department of Pathology/Neuropathology Unit, HSW 430, University of California, San Francisco, California 94143, (415) 476-5236;

Clarence J. Gibbs, M.D., and D. Carleton Gajdusek, M.D., NIH/National Institute of Neurological Disorders and Stroke Laboratory of Central Nervous System Studies, Building 36, Room 4A-15, 9000 Rockville Pike, Bethesda, Maryland 20892, (301) 496-4821 (call collect);

Elias Manuelidis, M.D., Yale University School of Medicine, Section of Neuropathology, 333 Cedar Street, New Haven, Connecticut 06510, (203) 785-4442.

A study of early-onset dementia occurring as a result of Creutzfeldt-Jakob disease is being conducted by the National Institute of Mental Health (NIMH) and the Neuropsychiatric Research Hospital. Participants in this study must be under 45 years of age and not require special medical care. Please contact Denise Juliano, MSW, Coordinator of Admissions, Neuropsychiatric Research Hospital, 2700 Martin Luther King Jr. Avenue, SE, Washington DC 20032, (202) 373-6100.

Please contact the agencies listed under Resources, below, for the most current information.

Resources
For more information on Creutzfeldt-Jakob disease: National Organization for Rare Disorders (NORD); Alzheimers Disease and Related Disorders Association; NIH/National Institute of Neurological Disorders & Stroke (NINDS).

For more information on longterm care facilities: National Hospice Organization.

References
NIH Publication No. 86-2760, May 1986.

Scientific American MEDICINE: E. Rubinstein and D. Federman, eds.; Scientific American, Inc., 1978–1991, pp. 7:XXXII:1–3.

DANDY-WALKER SYNDROME

Description Dandy-Walker syndrome is characterized by congenital hydrocephalus resulting from obstruction of the foramina of Magendie and Luschka.

Synonyms
> Dandy-Walker Cysts
> Dandy-Walker Deformity
> Internal Hydrocephalus
> Noncommunicating Hydrocephalus
> Obstructive Hydrocephalus

Signs and Symptoms Hydrocephalus is accompanied by headache, transient visual disturbances, and papilledema in affected infants.

Etiology The syndrome is inherited as an autosomal recessive trait. The disorder is caused by a developmental malformation in which the 4th ventricle of the brain is cystic.

Epidemiology Dandy-Walker syndrome is very rare. Males appear to be affected more often than females.

Related Disorders See *Arnold-Chiari Syndrome; Hydrocephalus.*

Treatment—Standard Dandy-Walker syndrome may be treated with a ventriculoperitoneal shunt procedure.

Treatment—Investigational Please contact the agencies listed under Resources, below, for the most current information.

Resources

For more information on Dandy-Walker syndrome: National Organization for Rare Disorders (NORD); Hydrocephalus Parent Support Group; National Hydrocephalus Foundation; NIH/National Institute of Neurological Disorders & Stroke (NINDS).

For genetic information and genetic counseling referrals: March of Dimes Birth Defects Foundation; National Center for Education in Maternal and Child Health (NCEMCH).

References
Problems of Diagnosis and Treatment in the Dandy-Walker Syndrome: H.E. James, et al.; Childs Brain, 1979, issue 5, pp. 24–30.
Scientific American MEDICINE: E. Rubinstein and D. Federman, eds.; Scientific American, Inc., 1978–1991, p. 11:III:1.

DEJERINE-SOTTAS DISEASE

Description Dejerine-Sottas disease is an irregularly progressive, hereditary hypertrophic neuropathy that affects motor function of the legs and, in later stages, muscle strength and coordination in the hands and forearms. Enlargement of the peripheral nerves, accompanied by recurrent loss of myelin, is the cause of the muscle weakness.

Synonyms
Hereditary Motor Sensory Neuropathy Type III
Hypertrophic Interstitial Neuritis
Hypertrophic Interstitial Neuropathy
Hypertrophic Interstitial Radiculoneuropathy
Onion-Bulb Neuropathy

Signs and Symptoms The patient with Dejerine-Sottas disease first notices a tingling or burning sensation, followed by weakness in the back of the leg that then spreads to the front of the leg. Walking becomes difficult and painful; eventually the leg muscles atrophy. Reflexes and heat sensitivity may be lost. As the disease progresses, the hands and forearms are affected. Mild vision problems may be associated. Dejerine-Sottas disease is only partially disabling; affected persons may remain active and can expect a normal lifespan.

Etiology Dejerine-Sottas disease is a hereditary condition that is transmitted as a recessive trait. The cause of the recurrent loss of myelin is not known.

Epidemiology Onset usually occurs between ages 10 and 30 years. Males and females are believed to be equally affected.

Related Disorders See *Charcot-Marie-Tooth Disease.*
Dejerine-Sottas disease must be distinguished from hereditary sensory radicular neuropathy, in which the early symptoms are pain and loss of thermal sensitivity in the foot and lower leg, followed by muscle weakness and ulcerations on the toes.

Treatment—Standard The cornerstones of treatment are physiotherapy, which promotes remaining muscle function, and orthopedic supports, which help stabilize involved joints. Surgery may be necessary. Patients and their families may benefit from genetic and occupational counseling.

Treatment—Investigational Please contact the agencies listed under Resources, below, for the most current information.

Resources
For more information on Dejerine-Sottas disease: National Organization for Rare Disorders (NORD); Muscular Dystrophy Association; NIH/National Institute of Neurological Disorders & Stroke (NINDS).

For genetic information and genetic counseling referrals: March of Dimes Birth Defects Foundation; National Center for Education in Maternal and Child Health (NCEMCH).

References
Abnormal Auditory Evoked Potentials in Dejerine-Sottas Disease. Report of Two Cases with Central Acoustic and Vestibular Impairment: F. Baiocco, et al.; J. Neurol., 1984, issue 231(1), pp. 46–49.

The Importance of Quantitative Electron Microscopy in Studying Hypertrophic Neuropathies.

A Comparison Between a Case of Dejerine Sottas Disease (HMSN III) and a Case of the Hypertrophic Form of Charcot-Marie-Tooth disease (HMSN I): G. Tredici, et al.; Int. J. Tissue React., 1984, issue 6(3), pp. 267–274.

DEPERSONALIZATION DISORDER

Description Depersonalization disorder is marked by persistent or recurring episodes of loss of the sense of self or reality.

Synonyms
Depersonalization Neurosis

Signs and Symptoms During an episode of depersonalization disorder, a person's perception of self is altered, so that there is a feeling of detachment from and lack of control over his or her own reality, i.e., actions, thoughts, and physical self. Symptoms may be aggravated by mild anxiety or depression.

The condition usually begins during adolescence or early adulthood, and is chronic with periods of remissions and exacerbations.

Etiology The specific cause of depersonalization disorder is unknown, although attacks may be precipitated by severely stressful situations, anxiety, or depression. Psychoactive drug use also is associated with the disorder.

Epidemiology The prevalence and sex distribution of depersonalization disorder are unknown. Brief periods involving feelings of depersonalization may be fairly common during adolescence.

Related Disorders See *Panic-Anxiety Syndrome.*

Agoraphobia is an intense fear of finding oneself alone or among other persons in public areas where one might have an attack of panic and be humiliated, or be unable to get to a safe place. The anxiety associated with attacks causes many individuals with agoraphobia to be unwilling to leave their homes.

Treatment—Standard Treatment of depersonalization disorder involves psychotherapy. The antidepressant drug desipramine may be beneficial. Other treatment is symptomatic and supportive.

Treatment—Investigational Please contact the agencies listed under Resources, below, for the most current information.

Resources
For more information on depersonalization disorder: National Organization for Rare Disorders (NORD); NIH/National Institute of Mental Health; National Mental Health Association.

References

Diagnostic and Statistical Manual of Mental Disorders, 3rd ed., revised: R.L. Spitzer, et al., eds.; Am. Psychiat. Asso., 1987, pp. 275–277.

Desipramine: A Possible Treatment for Depersonalization Disorder: R. Noyes, Jr., et al.; Can. J. Psychiatry, December 1987, issue 32(9), pp. 782–784.

Depersonalization in a Nonclinical Population: D. Trueman; J. Psychol., January 1984, issue 116(1st half), pp. 107–112.

Depersonalization and Agoraphobia Associated with Marijuana Use: C. Moran; Br. J. Med. Psychol., June 1986, issue 59(pt. 2), pp. 187–196.

DEVIC DISEASE

Description Devic disease is a rare nerve condition characterized by demyelination of the optic nerve and the nerves in the spinal cord.

Synonyms

> Neuromyelitis Optica
> Ophthalmoneuromyelitis
> Optic Neuroencephalomyelopathy
> Optic Neuromyelitis
> Opticomyelitis
> Retrobulbar Neuropathy

Signs and Symptoms The initial symptoms are slight fever, sore throat, or head cold. The inflammation and demyelination of the optic nerve lead to swelling and pain within the eye and eventual loss of clear vision. The ocular findings initially may be unilateral, but may become bilateral. Spinal cord abnormalities associated with mild paraparesis of the lower limbs and loss of bowel and bladder control develop later. Deep tendon reflexes are diminished or absent, and variable sensory loss occurs. With time there may be improvement of both paraparesis and ocular symptoms; but this may be followed by worsening.

Etiology The cause is not known. Some research indicates that Devic disease may be an autoimmune or genetic disorder. The disease may occur spontaneously, usually following a fever, or in conjunction with multiple sclerosis or systemic lupus erythematosus.

Epidemiology Males and females are affected in equal numbers.

Related Disorders See *Guillain-Barré Syndrome.* Also see *Multiple Sclerosis* and *Systemic Lupus Erythematosus,* disorders which may precede the development of Devic disease.

Acute disseminated encephalomyelitis (postinfectious encephalitis), a central nervous system disorder characterized by inflammation of the brain and spinal cord caused by damage to the myelin sheath, can occur spontaneously but more commonly follows a viral infection or inoculation, e.g., of a bacterial or viral vaccine.

Treatment—Standard Early treatment using adrenocorticotropic hormone or corticosteroid drugs may successfully control inflammation of the optic nerve and spinal cord. Other treatment is symptomatic and supportive.

Treatment—Investigational Lymphocytaplasmapheresis is being investigated as a possible treatment for patients with Devic disease.

Please contact the agencies listed under Resources, below, for the most current information.

Resources

For more information on Devic disease: National Organization for Rare Disorders (NORD); NIH/National Eye Institute; NIH/National Institute of Neurological Disorders & Stroke (NINDS).

References

Lymphocytaplasmapheresis in Devic's Syndrome: A.J. Aguilera, et al.; Transfusion, January–February 1985, issue 25(1), pp. 54–56.

Devic's Syndrome and Systemic Lupus Erythematosus: A Case Report with Necropsy: E.L. Kinney, et al.; Arch. Neurol., October 1979, issue 36(10), pp. 643–644.

DYSLEXIA

Description Dyslexia is the inability to interpret written language by a person with normal vision and hearing and no mental impairment or cultural deprivation. The condition is usually noted in childhood.

Synonyms

Congenital Word Blindness
Developmental Reading Disorder
Primary Reading Disability
Specific Reading Disability

Signs and Symptoms The perceptual confusion of letters may lead to difficulties in other areas of symbolic processing such as arithmetic; however, spelling is not necessarily impaired. The child may not be able to tell right from left. Sensory perception and gross neurologic status are usually normal. Facility with mirror reading or mirror writing is common.

When asked to read, a dyslexic child may make up a story to fit a picture in the text, or may substitute other words for those that are not understood. Reading is hesitant and slow. The inevitable frustration with classroom performance may lead to behavioral problems such as delinquency, aggression, and poor social relations with parents and peers.

To forestall or interrupt development of a pattern of failure, early diagnosis is important. Audiometric and vision testing as well as psychological and neurologic examinations are advised.

Etiology An autosomal dominant inheritance has been suggested for some cases. There may be a central nervous system defect in the ability to organize graphic symbols. Dyslexia can also result from injury to the cerebral cortex.

Epidemiology Dyslexia is usually noticed between ages 6 and 9 years. Prevalence among school children appears to be between 2 and 8 percent.

Related Disorders Inability to understand written language may follow injury to the language-processing centers in the cerebral cortex **(alexia).**

Treatment—Standard The treatment of dyslexia entails remedial education for children and various self-checking strategies for adults.

Treatment—Investigational Please contact the agencies listed under Resources, below, for the most current information.

Resources
    For more information on dyslexia: National Organization for Rare Disorders (NORD); NIH/National Institute of Neurological Disorders & Stroke (NINDS); Orton Dyslexia Society; Association for Children and Adults with Learning Disabilities; National Network of Learning–Disabled Adults, Inc.; HEATH Resource Center (Higher Education and the Handicapped).
    For genetic information and genetic counseling referrals: March of Dimes Birth Defects Foundation; National Center for Education in Maternal and Child Health (NCEMCH).

References
Mendelian Inheritance in Man, 9th ed.: V.A. McKusick; The Johns Hopkins University Press, 1990, pp. 275–276.
Diagnostic and Statistical Manual of Mental Disorders, 3rd ed., revised: R.L. Spitzer, et al., eds.; Am. Psychiat. Asso., 1987, pp. 43–44.

EMPTY SELLA SYNDROME

Description Empty sella syndrome is a rare brain disorder in which the sella turcica appears as an extension of the subarachnoid space and is filled with cerebrospinal fluid. This results from a defect in the diaphragma sellae. Alternatively, the syndrome may be primary or secondary to a pituitary tumor or irradiation or surgery on the pituitary gland.

Synonyms
    Empty Sella Turcica

Signs and Symptoms The clinical picture is dominated by headaches, impaired vision, and obesity. In some cases these findings are accompanied by hypertension and cold intolerance. Sex-specific differences may be seen: hirsutism in women, and gynecomastia and reduced libido in men.
    Computed tomography may show a vestigial diaphragma sellae and an apparently empty pituitary fossa. Other diagnostic studies include hormone assays and neurologic examination.

Etiology The primary form of empty sella syndrome is inherited as an autosomal dominant trait. Secondary cases develop as a result of birth defects, pituitary adenomas, and irradiation or surgery on the pituitary gland.

Epidemiology Empty sella syndrome predominantly develops in obese middle-aged women, although men and, rarely, children may also be affected.

Related Disorders The syndrome must be distinguished from tumors of the brain or optic nerve, especially in the setting of diabetes and visual deficits. Thus, the entity must be distinguished from Achard-Thiers syndrome, characterized by diabetes and adrenal overproduction of androgens, resulting in virilization in postmenopausal women; from craniopharyngiomas, fast-growing cystic tumors derived from Rathke's pouch that may invade the hypothalamus, sella turcica, 3rd ventricle, and optic nerve, producing hydrocephalus and visual deficits in children and young adults; from meningiomas, benign slow-growing tumors of the meninges; and from optic glioma, a slow-growing optic nerve tumor that occasionally extends to the 3rd ventricle. See *Meningioma.*

Treatment—Standard Treatment is symptomatic and supportive.

Treatment—Investigational Please contact the agencies listed under Resources, below, for the most current information.

Resources

For more information on empty sella syndrome: National Organization for Rare Disorders (NORD); NIH/National Institute of Neurological Disorders & Stroke (NINDS).

For genetic information and genetic counseling referrals: March of Dimes Birth Defects Foundation; National Center for Education in Maternal and Child Health (NCEMCH).

References

The "Empty Sella" in Childhood: D.C. Costigan, et al.; Clin. Pediatr., August 1984, issue 23(8), pp. 437–440.

Subarachnoid Hemorrhage with Normal Cerebral Angiography: A Prospective Study on Sellar Abnormalities and Pituitary Function: P. Bjerre, et al.; Neurosurgery, December 1986, issue 19(6), pp. 1012–1015.

MRI and CT of Sellar and Parasellar Disorders: M.H. Naheedy, et al.; Radiol. Clin. North Am., July 1987, issue 25(4), pp. 819–847.

Mendelian Inheritance in Man, 8th ed.: V.A. McKusick; The Johns Hopkins University Press, 1988, p. 226.

EPILEPSY

Description Epilepsy, a disorder of the central nervous system, is characterized by recurrent paroxysmal electrical disturbances in the brain. Manifestations include loss of consciousness, convulsions, spasms, sensory confusion, and disturbances in the autonomic nervous system. Attacks are frequently preceded by an "aura," a feeling of unease or sensory discomfort; the aura marks the beginning of the seizure in the brain. If the electrical disturbances or symptoms respond to medication, the patient can expect an otherwise normal life.

Epilepsy may take a number of different forms. Some of the types are grand mal epilepsy (major epilepsy, status epilepticus); Jacksonian epilepsy (focal epilepsy); myoclonic progressive familial epilepsy (Unverricht syndrome, Lundborg-Unverricht disease, Lafora disease, Unverricht-Lundborg-Laf disease); petit mal epilepsy (minor epilepsy, pyknoepilepsy, akinetic seizure, myoclonic seizure); myoclonic astatic petit mal epilepsy (Lennox-Gastaut syndrome, petit mal variant); febrile seizures; and psychomotor epilepsy (temporal lobe epilepsy, psychomotor equivalent, psychomotor convulsion with epilepsia procursiva, abdominal epilepsy).

Synonyms

Convulsions

Seizures

Signs and Symptoms There are no established precipitants of an epileptic seizure that are common to all patients. However, visual phenomena such as flickering lights or sunbursts are frequently cited as precipitants. In predisposed patients, the likelihood of a seizure increases with stress, fatigue, insufficient food intake, or failure to take prescribed medications.

Of the various ways to subdivide epileptic seizures, general and partial seizures will be considered here.

GENERALIZED SEIZURES. EEG changes occur simultaneously in both hemispheres of the brain, and the patient typically develops impaired consciousness. Subjective symptoms shortly preceding the attack may include abdominal and chest discomfort, nausea, dizziness, palpitations, headache, aphasia, dyspnea, throat constriction, and numbness in the hands, lips, and tongue. Some patients report experiencing visions or hallucinations, or find themselves in a dreamlike state. Auditory and olfactory distortions may be present. Prodromal symptoms that may precede the attack by hours to weeks include irritability and odd mannerisms, such as smacking the lips repeatedly.

Grand mal (tonic-clonic) seizures follow sudden electrical disruptions in both hemispheres of the brain. Seizures of this type may occur repeatedly or only once per episode. In **status epilepticus,** a severe form of grand mal seizure, a series of convulsions takes place while the patient is unconscious. The condition is life-threatening and requires immediate hospitalization.

There are 3 stages to tonic-clonic seizures. In the first stage, which lasts about 30 seconds, the patient loses consciousness and falls, and may emit a loud cry. Tonic contraction of the muscles results in bodily rigidity; this is followed by violent clonic spasms in the muscles of the face, head, and limbs; rolling eyes; and gnashing teeth. Breathing may cease temporarily. These features may be accompanied by a discharge of saliva, cyanosis, and loss of bladder and bowel control. This stage may continue for several minutes. In the 3rd or postictal stage, consciousness returns. Recovery may take seconds to hours and is often followed by an extended period of confusion, drowsiness, fatigue, or excitement.

The onset of **petit mal seizures** usually occurs between the ages of 4 and 12, very infrequently after age 20. Seizures are brief, may occur daily, and consist of loss of consciousness, eye fluttering, and cessation of motor activity. Interpretation of these symptoms as "behavior disorder" or "daydreaming" will delay the diagnosis.

Infantile spasms ("jackknife" or "salaam" seizures) are generalized seizures that occur in children 3 months to 2 years old. The head and torso curve forward as the knees are drawn up toward the chest in the characteristic posture. The spasms last only a few seconds but may occur repeatedly throughout the day.

Myoclonic (bilateral massive epileptic) seizures are sudden, brief spasms of the limbs or entire body. The myoclonic jerks may recur rapidly or may be limited to one episode only.

PARTIAL SEIZURES. Simple partial seizures with elementary symptomatology are characterized by clinical symptoms referable to the involved area of the cortex. The seizure is brief and the patient does not lose consciousness. **Jacksonian (rolandic) seizures** begin with twitching in a digit or extremity that then progresses to adjoining muscles. Symptoms are unilateral and the patient does not lose consciousness. **Partial seizures with mixed symptomatology** (complex partial seizures, temporal lobe or psychomotor seizures) may be characterized by unprovoked aggressive behavior and other abnormal behaviors with impairment of consciousness. The electrical storm usually occurs in the temporal lobes.

Etiology The exact cause of epilepsy is unknown, although hereditary factors have been implicated in essential epilepsy. Some types of epilepsy occur in conjunction with or following other disorders or accidents. Common causes of recurring seizures in infants are genetic inborn errors of metabolism, other metabolic disorders, developmental brain defects, perinatal injuries, and hypoxia. In children, new-onset epileptic seizures can be caused by meningitis, encephalitis or brain abscesses, tumors, exposure to toxins, vascular diseases, degenerative diseases, and head trauma. Febrile seizures usually do not recur. In adults, the onset of seizures can be temporally linked to brain tumor, head trauma, stroke, cerebrovascular disease, and degenerative brain disease.

Epidemiology No sex prevalence is apparent. Three-fourths of patients exhibit symptoms before age 20 years, but onset can occur at any age. An estimated 150,000 persons develop epilepsy each year.

Related Disorders See *Myoclonus; Wilson Disease.*

Kok disease is a rare hereditary neurologic disorder characterized by myoclonic jerks, hypertonia, hyperreflexia, arching of the head, unstable gait, or excessive startle reactions that include falling stiffly to the ground without loss of consciousness.

Treatment—Standard The anticonvulsant drugs used to prevent and control seizures include phenytoin, valproic acid, carbamazepine, phenobarbital, clonazepam, ethosuximide, primidone, corticotropin, and corticosteroids. Surgery may be effective for seizures stemming from tumors or drug-resistant temporal lobe epilepsy but is not performed until other treatment methods have failed.

Self-injury during a seizure is a major danger of epilepsy. The patient should be turned on the side to prevent aspiration, and the head protected by a soft surface. Restraint is inadvisable. Artificial respiration should only be attempted if breathing does not resume by the end of the seizure.

Treatment—Investigational Experimental anticonvulsant drugs include nimodipine, praziquantel, clomiphene, and lorazepam. More research is necessary to determine their longterm safety and efficacy.

Please contact the agencies listed under Resources, below, for the most current information.

Resources

For more information on epilepsy: National Organization for Rare Disorders (NORD); The Epilepsy Foundation of America; NIH/National Institute of Neurological Disorders and Stroke (NINDS).

References

Internal Medicine, 2nd ed.: J.H. Stein, ed.-in-chief; Little, Brown & Company, 1987, p. 2145.
Sublingual Lorazepam in Childhood Serial Seizures: J. Yager, et al.; Am. J. Dis. Child., September 1988, issue 142(9), pp. 931–932.
Seizure Control with Clomiphene Therapy. A Case Report: A. Herzog; Arch. Neurol., February 1988, issue 45(2), pp. 209–210.
Disseminated Cysticerosis. New Observations, Including CT Scan Findings and Experience with Treatment by Praziquantel: N. Wadia, et al.; Brain, June 1988, issue 111(3), pp. 597–614.
Control of Epilepsy Partialis Continuans with Intravenous Nimodipine. Report of Two Cases: L. Brandt, et al.; J. Neurosurg., December 1988, issue 69(6), pp. 949–950.

ERB PALSY

Description Erb palsy is a disorder in newborns or infants of the peripheral nervous system resulting from an injury to one or more nerves of the upper brachial plexus. Paralysis of the shoulder and upper extremity is characteristic.

Synonyms

Erb/Duchenne Palsy
Erb Paralysis

Signs and Symptoms Following an injury to the upper brachial plexus, adduction and internal turning of the shoulder occurs, with pronation of the forearm and hand. The shoulder and upper extremity may become paralyzed. There also may be paralysis of the diaphragm on the affected side, with associated loss of feeling and muscle atrophy. Feeling and function in the wrist and hand usually are not affected.

Etiology The cause of this disorder is an injury to the nerve roots and surrounding nerves of the upper brachial plexus. The injury may involve abnormal stretching of the shoulder during a difficult labor, breech delivery, or excessive sideways movement of the neck during delivery.

Epidemiology Males and females are affected equally.

Related Disorders See *Parsonnage-Turner Syndrome; Peripheral Neuropathy.*

Treatment—Standard Patients usually respond promptly to the standard treatment of physical therapy and splinting of the affected area. Surgery may be necessary to repair damaged nerves when injury has been extensive. Other treatment is symptomatic and supportive.

Treatment—Investigational Please contact the agencies listed under Resources, below, for the most current information.

Resources

For more information on Erb palsy: National Organization for Rare Disorders (NORD); NIH/National Institute on Arthritis, Musculoskeletal and Skin Diseases (NIAMS) Information Clearinghouse.

References

Erb/Duchenne Palsy: A Consequence of Fetal Macrosomia and Method of Delivery: L. McFarland, et al.; Obstet. Gynecol., December 1986, issue 68(6), pp. 784–788.

Brachial Plexus Palsy in the Newborn: S. Jackson, et al.; J. Bone Joint Surg. [Am], September 1988, issue 70(8), pp. 1217–1220.

Early Microsurgical Reconstruction in Birth Palsy: H. Kawabata, et al.; Clin. Orthop., February 1987, pp. 233–242.

Duchenne-Erb Palsy. Experience with Direct Surgery: J. Comtet, et al.; Clin. Orthop., December 1988, issue 237, pp. 17–23.

Preliminary Experience with Brachial Plexus Exploration in Children: Birth Injury and Vehicular Trauma: J. Piatt Jr., et al.; Neurosurgery, April 1988, issue 22(4), pp. 715–723.

FAHR DISEASE

Description Fahr disease is a rare neurologic condition characterized by abnormal deposition of calcium in certain areas of the brain. The clinical picture is one of progressive deterioration in mental and motor function, mental retardation, spastic paralysis, and athetosis. Parkinson disease may be secondarily associated.

Synonyms

Cerebrovascular Ferrocalcinosis
Intracranial Calcification
Nonarteriosclerotic Cerebral Calcification
Striopallidodentate Calcinosis

Signs and Symptoms Abnormal calcium deposits accrue in the basal ganglia, cerebral cortex, dentate nucleus, subthalamus, and red nucleus areas of the brain, attended by loss of brain cells. Calcium may also be deposited in areas of demyelination and in lipid deposits.

The head often appears round and smaller than normal. Dementia and loss of previously attained motor function are characteristic and accompanied by spastic paralysis and occasionally athetosis.

Features of Parkinson disease that may be found in Fahr disease include tremors and rigidity, a masklike facies, shuffling walk, and a "pill rolling" motion of the fingers. Dystonia, chorea, and seizures are occasionally reported. A parkinsonian component is not necessary for the differential diagnosis.

Etiology An autosomal recessive inheritance of Fahr disease has been postulated. Some cases occur sporadically, perhaps reflecting fetal infection rather than a genetic origin.

Epidemiology Fahr disease is a very rare disorder. Males and females are equally affected.

Related Disorders See *Parkinson Disease.*

Treatment—Standard Some psychotic symptoms may be ameliorated with lithium carbonate. Other treatment is symptomatic and supportive. Genetic counseling may be beneficial for patients and families with the hereditary form of the disease.

Treatment—Investigational A Fahr disease registry has been developed. Cases may be registered with Bala V. Manyam, M.D., Fahr Disease Registry, Parkinson's Disease and Movement Disorders Clinic, Southern Illinois University School of Medicine, P.O. Box 19230, Springfield, Illinois 62794-9230.

Please contact the agencies listed under Resources, below, for the most current information.

Resources

For more information on Fahr disease: National Organization for Rare Disorders (NORD); NIH/National Institute of Neurological Disorders & Stroke (NINDS); Fahr Disease Registry.

For genetic information and genetic counseling referrals: March of Dimes Birth Defects Foundation; NIH/National Center for Education in Maternal and Child Health (NCEMCH).

References

Mendelian Inheritance in Man, 9th ed.: V.A. McKusick; The Johns Hopkins University Press, 1990, pp. 1084–1085.

Idiopathic Nonarteriosclerotic Cerebral Calcification (Fahr's Disease): An Electron Microscopic Study: S. Kobayashi, et al.; Acta Neuropathol. (Berl.), 1987, issue 73(1), pp. 62–66.

The Treatment of Psychotic Symptoms in Fahr's Disease with Lithium Carbonate: K.M. Munir; J. Clin. Psychopharmacol., February 1986, issue 6(1), pp. 36–38.

FAMILIAL DYSAUTONOMIA

Description Familial dysautonomia is a rare genetic disorder of the autonomic nervous system **(ANS)** associated with pain, loss of sensation, and unsteadiness.

Two types of the disorder (I and II) are recognized. Type II is better known as congenital sensory neuropathy with anhidrosis. There may be a 3rd type with adult onset of impaired ANS functioning.

Synonyms

Congenital Sensory Neuropathy with Anhidrosis (Type II Familial
Dysautonomia)
Hereditary Sensory and Autonomic Neuropathy
Riley-Day Syndrome

Signs and Symptoms Types I and II familial dysautonomia for the most part have
similar symptoms. Differential diagnosis can be made by biopsy.

An infant born with this disorder has poor sucking and swallowing reflexes, low
ocular fluid pressure, and hypothermia.

There is typically a decreased perception of pain and temperature, which can
lead to cutaneous trauma. A lack of tears and insensitivity of the eye to pain from
foreign objects can lead to corneal inflammation and ulceration.

Other findings include unstable blood pressure, an absence of sense of taste,
impaired speech, drooling, attacks of vomiting, and skin blotching. There may be
episodes of pneumonia, absence of tendon reflexes, skeletal defects, and stunted
height.

By adolescence, 95 percent of patients have evidence of spinal curvature, and
may experience increased sweating and an accelerated heart rate. Other adolescent symptoms include weakness; leg cramping; difficulty concentrating; and personality changes characterized by depression, irritability, insomnia, and nega-
tivism. Kidney insufficiency develops in 20 percent of patients over 20 years of
age. Neurologic deterioration also progresses, and unsteadiness in walking
becomes more apparent at this age.

Patients with type II familial dysautonomia also may have anhidrosis and mental
retardation.

There may be an adult-onset type of familial dysautonomia, the genetic defect
expressed later than in the childhood forms.

Etiology Type I familial dysautonomia has a dominant inheritance; type II, a recessive inheritance.

Epidemiology Type I familial dysautonomia primarily affects individuals of Ashkenazi Jewish ancestry; the genetic carrier rate is estimated to be 1:30. Both males
and females are affected. Type II is not limited to a specific group.

Related Disorders Many conditions characterized by the symptom of dysautonomia should not be confused with this specific hereditary disorder.

Biemond congenital and familial analgesia symptoms are similar to those of
familial dysautonomia, and include insensitivity to pain, a diminished sense of
temperature and touch, and absence of tendon reflexes.

Treatment—Standard Drugs used to relieve the symptoms of familial dysautonomia are diazepam, metoclopramide, bethanechol, metaproterenol, chloral hydrate,
and chlorpromazine. Artificial tears may be needed for the eyes. Physical therapy,
chest physiotherapy, occupational therapy, feeding facilitation, and speech therapy
may be needed. Patients may also benefit from a variety of orthopedic and ocular
aids.

Treatment—Investigational Please contact the agencies listed under Resources, below, for the most current information.

Resources
  For more information on familial dysautonomia: National Organization for Rare Disorders (NORD); Dysautonomia Foundation, Inc.; National Foundation for Jewish Genetic Diseases; NIH/National Institute of Neurological Disorders and Stroke (NINDS).
  For genetic information and genetic counseling referrals: March of Dimes Birth Defects Foundation; NIH/National Center for Education in Maternal and Child Health (NCEMCH).

References
  Cecil Textbook of Medicine, 18th ed.: J.B. Wyngaarden and L.H. Smith, Jr., eds.; W.B. Saunders Company, 1988, pp. 2264–2265.
  Mendelian Inheritance in Man, 9th ed.: V.A. McKusick; The Johns Hopkins University Press, 1990, pp. 1382–1383.
  Adult Onset Autonomic Dysfunction Coexistent with Familial Dysautonomia in a Consanguineous Family: A.E. Rubenstein and M.D. Yahr; Neurology (Minneap.), February 1977, issue 27(2), pp. 168–170.
  Congenital Sensory Neuropathy with Anhydrosis: N. Ishii, et al.; Arch. Dermatol., April 1988, issue 124(4), pp. 564–566.
  Neonatal Recognition of Familial Dysautonomia: F.B. Axelrod, et al.; J. Pediatr., June 1987, issue 110(6), pp. 946–948.

FIBER TYPE DISPROPORTION, CONGENITAL (CFTD)

Description Congenital fiber type disproportion is a rare hereditary disease affecting the growth of type I muscle fibers. The clinical picture is dominated by hypotonia and weakness, various skeletal deformities, and short stature; however, none of these findings is pathognomonic. The disorder can usually be diagnosed at birth. Function tends to improve as the patient ages.

Synonyms
  Atrophy of Type I Fibers
  Myopathy, Congenital, with Fiber Type Disproportion
  Myopathy of Congenital Fiber Type Disproportion

Signs and Symptoms The muscles of a newborn infant with CFTD are unusually weak and hypotonic. The nonprogressive hypotonia may be accompanied by failure to grow and by developmental skeletal anomalies such as scoliosis, dislocated hip joints, foot deformities, and a high arched palate. Mental retardation may occur in some cases. The clinical findings may occur singly or in combination, but the diagnosis rests on muscle biopsy, which shows type I muscle fibers smaller than type II fibers.

Etiology CFTD is inherited as an autosomal recessive trait.

Epidemiology CFTD is usually present at birth. Males and females are affected equally.

Related Disorders Various neuromuscular disorders, especially the dystrophies, can produce symptoms resembling those of CFTD. **Emery-Dreifuss muscular dystrophy** is commonly diagnosed from the early symptom of toe-walking in a 4- or 5-year-old child. As the muscle weakness progresses the child assumes a waddling gait. Eventually shoulder, neck, and spinal muscles may be involved. Cardiac problems are a frequent, serious accompaniment of the disease.

Leyden-Moebius muscular dystrophy (limb-girdle muscular dystrophy) is a slowly progressive disorder with onset in childhood. Most frequently the pelvic muscles in the pelvic girdle become weak and atrophy; the shoulder girdle and facial muscles may also be involved. Persons of either sex may be affected.

Gowers muscular dystrophy (late distal hereditary myopathy) is a hereditary disorder with an early symptom of mild weakness in the small muscles of the hands and feet, spreading proximally to involve neighboring muscles. The disorder is transmitted as an autosomal dominant trait and is rare. Onset usually occurs in middle age or later, and symptoms typically remain mild to moderate.

See *Muscular Dystrophy, Batten Turner; Muscular Dystrophy, Becker; Muscular Dystrophy, Duchenne; Myotonic Dystrophy.*

Treatment—Standard Physiotherapy with active and passive exercise is recommended to promote muscle function in CFTD. The effects of the disorder usually diminish as the patient ages. Genetic counseling may be helpful.

Treatment—Investigational Please contact the agencies listed under Resources, below, for the most current information.

Resources
For more information on congenital fiber type disproportion: National Organization for Rare Disorders (NORD); NIH/National Institute of Neurological Disorders & Stroke (NINDS); Muscular Dystrophy Association.

For genetic information and genetic counseling referrals: March of Dimes Birth Defects Foundation; NIH/National Center for Education in Maternal and Child Health (NCEMCH).

References
Mendelian Inheritance in Man, 8th ed.: V.A. McKusick; The Johns Hopkins University Press, 1986, p. 1094.

Clinical Variability in Congenital Fiber Type Disproportion: R.R. Clancy, et al.; J. Neurol. Sci., June 1980, issue 46(3), pp. 257–266.

Congenital Fiber Disproportion. Atrophy of Type I Fibers. Report of 11 Cases: J.A. Levy, et al.; Arq. Neuropsiquiatr., June 1987, issue 45(2), pp. 153–158.

Muscle Fiber Type Transformation in Nemaline Myopathy and Congenital Fiber Type Disproportion: T. Miike, et al.; Brain Dev., 1986, issue 8(5), pp. 526–632.

FREY SYNDROME

Description Frey syndrome results from injury to the facial nerve near the parotid glands and is characterized by flushing or sweating on one side of the face when certain foods are consumed. The symptoms usually are mild and well tolerated by most patients, although symptomatic treatment is necessary in some cases.

Synonyms
> Auriculotemporal Syndrome
> Baillarger Syndrome
> Dupuy Syndrome
> Salivosudoriparous Syndrome
> Sweating-Gustatory Syndrome

Signs and Symptoms Sweating is the predominant symptom in men; women typically experience flushing symptoms. Eating hot, spicy, or very acidic food causes sweating and flushing on the cheek and ear on one side of the face.

Etiology Frey syndrome usually develops after injury or surgery on the parotid glands resulting in damage to the facial nerve. The sweating and flushing are due to abnormal regeneration of parasympathetic, rather than sympathetic, nerve fibers following injury. These aberrant parasympathetic nerves are stimulated by eating the offending foods.

Related Disorders See *Hyperhidrosis.*

Treatment—Standard Treatment is symptomatic and directed toward relieving excessive discomfort. Scopolamine cream may be applied to the skin. In more severe cases, nerve projections near the ear and cheek may be modified surgically.

Treatment—Investigational An orphan drug, glycopurrolate, is being developed by Robins Corporation for treatment of Frey syndrome.

Please contact the agencies listed under Resources, below, for the most current information.

Resources
For more information on Frey syndrome: National Organization for Rare Disorders (NORD); Association for Glycogen Storage Diseases; The National Arthritis and Musculoskeletal and Skin Diseases Information Clearinghouse.

GUILLAIN-BARRÉ SYNDROME

Description Guillain-Barré syndrome (acute idiopathic polyneuritis) is a rare, rapidly progressive form of ascending polyneuropathy. Although the precise etiology is unknown, a viral enteric or respiratory infection precedes the onset of the syndrome in about half of cases, which has led to postulation of an autoimmune mechanism. Damage to the myelin and nerve axons through immune system mechanisms results in delayed nervous signal transmission, with a corresponding weakness in the muscles innervated by those nerves. With proper treatment, more than half of patients recover completely with no residual neurologic signs. The syndrome is fatal in 2 to 5 percent of cases.

The following subdivisions are recognized: Miller-Fischer syndrome (Fischer syndrome, acute disseminated encephalomyeloradiculopathy); chronic Guillain-Barré syndrome (chronic idiopathic polyneuritis); relapsing Guillain-Barré syndrome; chronic inflammatory demyelinating polyradiculoneuropathy; chronic relapsing polyneuropathy; polyneuropathy; and polyradiculoneuropathy.

Synonyms
Acute Idiopathic Polyneuritis
Ascending Paralysis
Kussmaul-Landry Paralysis (Landry Paralysis)
Landry Ascending Paralysis
Postinfective Polyneuritis

Signs and Symptoms In the typical pattern in this ascending polyneuritis, paresthesias begin in the feet, followed by weakness and flaccid paralysis of the legs. Eventually the torso, upper limbs, and face are affected. Symptoms progress over hours to weeks. Deep tendon reflexes may be lost; among the first to go is the ankle jerk. The paralysis may be accompanied by fever, bulbar palsy, and an increase in cerebrospinal fluid protein levels.

Specific symptoms are bilateral and reflect the portion of the nervous system involved. Sensory nerve damage produces numbness and tingling in the feet, hands, gums, and face. The face may appear pouchy and lopsided, and the patient may have difficulty breathing or swallowing food without choking. Involvement of the autonomic nervous system may cause sinus tachycardia or bradycardia, hypertension, postural hypotension, and changes in body temperature, vision, bladder function, and blood chemistries.

Fischer syndrome is a rare form of Guillain-Barré syndrome that commonly follows an upper respiratory tract infection. Men are predominantly affected. A generalized weakness occurs that is particularly severe in the ocular muscles, resulting in vision problems. Involvement of facial and neck musculature leads to impaired speech production and a sagging face. Deep tendon reflexes may be lost, and an awkward, unsteady (ataxic) gait is common.

Chronic idiopathic polyneuritis produces symptoms indistinguishable from those of Guillain-Barré syndrome except that the eyes and face are involved in only 15 percent of cases. The course is unpredictable; however, symptoms tend to progress over 6 to 12 months, then remit for a variable period before recurring.

Etiology An autoimmune mechanism triggered by a preceding viral infection has been postulated as the cause of Guillain-Barré syndrome. The viral infections incriminated have ranged from a common cold to viral hepatitis and mononucleosis. Cases have also occurred following surgery, an insect sting, a swine flu injection, or porphyria.

Epidemiology Guillain-Barré syndrome is extremely rare, with a reported incidence of 1 or 2 cases per 100,000 persons.

Treatment—Standard The clinical course is highly variable. Paralysis generally peaks in less than 10 days, although it may continue to progress for months. Recovery begins after the condition has stabilized and may take 6 months to 2 years. The prognosis generally correlates with the speed of recovery.

Although no cure for Guillain-Barré syndrome is available, various forms of treatment have proved effective. Physiotherapy is helpful for restoring muscle strength as innervation returns. Strength is usually recovered in the upper body first. Respiratory assistance may be needed by hospitalized patients. Corticosteroids (for chronic Guillain-Barré syndrome) and plasmapheresis may be prescribed. Plasmapheresis appears most beneficial in younger patients with severe locomotor disability at the time of the first plasma exchange. Other therapy is customized to the particular deficit or complication present.

Treatment—Investigational For information on plasmapheresis, physicians may contact The Johns Hopkins University Hospital, Plasmapheresis Center, 601 North Broadway, Baltimore, Maryland 20205.

A pilot study published in 1988 suggested that high-dose intravenous gammaglobulin may be therapeutic in severe cases of Guillain-Barré syndrome; this finding awaits confirmation. In the August, 1986, issue of "Research Currents," The National Institute of Neurological Disorders and Stroke reviewed the use of plasmapheresis and steroids, finding no clear benefit for the latter.

Please contact the agencies listed under Resources, below, for the most current information.

Resources
For more information on Guillain-Barré syndrome: National Organization for Rare Disorders (NORD); Guillain-Barré Syndrome Support Group International; NIH/National Institute of Neurological Disorders & Stroke (NINDS).

References
Cecil Textbook of Medicine, 18th ed.: J.B. Wyngaarden and L.H. Smith, Jr., eds.; W.B. Saunders Company, 1988, pp. 2198, 2259, 2261–2262, 489–490.

HALLERVORDEN-SPATZ DISEASE

Description Hallervorden-Spatz disease affects movement. It is associated with degeneration of the nervous system. A variety of symptoms can develop, including dystonia, muscular rigidity, spasticity, and dementia. Onset typically occurs during childhood, although occasionally the disease onset may be in adulthood.

Synonyms
Progressive Pallid Degeneration Syndrome

Signs and Symptoms The most common symptoms are dystonia, muscular rigidity, and dementia. Spasticity develops in one-third of cases. Dysarthria, mental retardation, facial grimacing, dysphasia, and visual loss due to optic atrophy are reported less frequently. Symptoms tend to vary among individuals. The clinical syndrome may resemble parkinsonism in some cases.

Etiology Hallervorden-Spatz disease is thought to be inherited as an autosomal recessive trait. More than one child in a family may be affected. In such cases, siblings are likely to experience similar symptoms.

Related Disorders Other movement disorders such as static encephalopathy, Sandifer syndrome, benign paroxysmal torticollis, and infections and tumors of the spine and soft tissues of the neck may also cause dystonic symptoms or uncontrolled muscle contractions.

Treatment—Standard Treatment is symptomatic and supportive.

Treatment—Investigational Please contact the agencies listed under Resources, below, for the most current information.

Resources
For more information on Hallervorden-Spatz disease: National Organization for Rare Disorders (NORD); United Leukodystrophy Foundation; NIH/National Institute of Neurological Disorders & Stroke (NINDS); Research Trust for Metabolic Diseases in Children.

For genetic information and genetic counseling referrals: March of Dimes Birth Defects Foundation; NIH/National Center for Education in Maternal and Child Health (NCEMCH).

References
Mendelian Inheritance in Man, 8th ed.: V.A. McKusick; Johns Hopkins University Press, 1986, p. 976.

HUNTINGTON DISEASE

Description Huntington disease (Huntington chorea) is an inherited, progressively degenerative neurologic condition that produces chorea and dementia.

Synonyms
Chronic Progressive Chorea
Degenerative Chorea
Hereditary Chorea
Hereditary Chronic Progressive Chorea
Huntington Chorea
Woody Guthrie's Disease

Signs and Symptoms Huntington disease runs a 10- to 25-year progressive course. Initial characteristics include mild choreiform movements and personality changes. In time, speech and memory become impaired, and the choreiform movements become severe. With further progression the chorea may subside and akinesia develop, and dementia gradually ensues. Patients with advanced disease are at high risk of pneumonia, the result of being bedridden and emaciated. Death occurs, on the average, about 14 years after onset.

Magnetic resonance imaging and computerized tomography, electroen-cephalography, neuropsychologic testing, and recently a DNA marker test can be utilized in making the diagnosis. The gene for Huntington disease is located on the tip of chromosome 4. DNA linkage analysis, which is 99 percent accurate when enough family members are tested, is now being widely used at genetic clinics.

Etiology The mode of inheritance is autosomal dominant.

Epidemiology Huntington disease affects approximately 1:10,000 persons in the United States, with another 150,000 at risk. The disease occurs in both sexes equally, and is most common in whites. Symptoms usually appear between 30 and 50 years of age, although onset may be as late as the 7th or 8th decade. A rarer childhood form of the disease, accounting for 10 percent of cases, can occur in children as young as age 2 years.

Treatment—Standard Therapy is symptomatic and supportive. Phenothiazine and other neuroleptics are only marginally effective.

Treatment—Investigational Paul F. Consroe, Ph.D., has been awarded a grant from the Office of Orphan Products Development, Food and Drug Administration, for studies involving clinical trials of the orphan drug cannabidiol in the treatment of Huntington disease. For more information, contact Paul F. Consroe, Ph.D., Department of Pharmacology & Toxicology, College of Pharmacology, University of Arizona, Tucson, Arizona 85721.

Another experimental drug, MK-801, is being tested to determine whether it can block the effects of quinolinic acid, thought to damage brain neurons in persons with Huntington disease. The drug idebenone is being used in Japan to treat patients with cognitive problems resulting from strokes, but it also appears to prevent brain cell degeneration. It is reported to be well tolerated, with few side effects. Idebenone has been approved by the FDA for a clinical trial in Huntington disease patients to determine the drug's effectiveness in preventing brain cell degeneration. For more information, contact The Drug Study Project at the Johns Hopkins University School of Medicine, Baltimore; (301) 955-2398.

Please also contact the agencies listed under Resources, below, for the most current information.

Resources

For more information on Huntington disease: National Organization for Rare Disorders (NORD); Huntington Disease Society of America; NIH/National Institute of Neurological Disorders & Stroke (NINDS); The Hereditary Disease Foundation; Huntington Society of Canada.

For genetic information and genetic counseling referrals: March of Dimes Birth Defects Foundation; National Center for Education in Maternal and Child Health (NCEMCH).

References
Cecil Textbook of Medicine, 18th ed.: J.B. Wyngaarden and L.H. Smith, Jr., eds.; W.B. Saunders Company, 1988, pp. 148, 2090–2091, 2147–2148.

HYDRANENCEPHALY

Description In hydranencephaly, portions of the cerebral hemispheres may be missing, replaced by fluid within the cranium. The disorder is a very rare form of porencephaly (see Related Disorders, below).

Synonyms
Hydroanencephaly

Signs and Symptoms At birth, irritability and spasticity of the arms and legs are common. A neurologic examination may be inconclusive. Other symptoms may include inadequate body temperature regulation, visual impairment, mental retardation, seizures, myoclonus, and respiratory failure. There is usually nothing specific about the neurologic findings.

Etiology Most cases are due to acquired distinctive processes in utero such as from vascular lesions, hypoxia, intraventricular hemorrhage, viral infections, and, possibly, genetic factors.

Epidemiology Hydranencephaly is present at birth. Males and females are affected equally.

Related Disorders See *Hydrocephalus.*

Porencephaly is a central nervous system disorder in which cysts develop in cortical brain tissue. Accumulated fluid can be drained by means of a surgical shunt. Some patients may be only mildly affected neurologicly, and have normal intelligence; for others, the disablement may be severe.

Treatment—Standard Treatment is symptomatic and supportive. Increased intracranial pressure often is relieved with a shunt, which must be monitored carefully for potential infection and blockage.

Treatment—Investigational Please contact the agencies listed under Resources, below, for the most current information.

Resources
For more information on hydranencephaly: National Organization for Rare Disorders (NORD); NIH/National Institute of Neurological Disorders & Stroke (NINDS); The Children's Brain Diseases Foundation For Research.
For information on shunts: Association for Brain Tumor Research.
For genetic information and genetic counseling referrals: March of Dimes Birth Defects Foundation; NIH/National Center for Education in Maternal and Child Health (NCEMCH).

References

Hydranencephaly: Prenatal and Neonatal Ultrasonographic Appearance: D.J. Coady, et al.; Am. J. Perinatol., July 1985, issue 2(3), pp. 228–230.

Ultrasonographic Prenatal Diagnosis of Hydranencephaly. A Case Report: H.A. Hadi, et al.; J. Reprod. Med., April 1986, issue 31(4).

HYDROCEPHALUS

Description Hydrocephalus is a condition in which dilated cerebral ventricles inhibit normal flow of cerebrospinal fluid **(CSF)**. The CSF accumulates in the skull and puts pressure on the brain tissue. An enlarged head in infants and increased CSF pressure are frequent findings but are not necessary for the diagnosis. The following forms are recognized: communicating hydrocephalus, noncommunicating or obstructive hydrocephalus, internal hydrocephalus, normal-pressure hydrocephalus, and benign hydrocephalus.

Synonyms

Hydrocephaly

Signs and Symptoms Characteristic features of hydrocephalus in children include cephalomegaly, a thin, transparent scalp, a bulging forehead with prominent fontanelles, and a downward gaze. Other clinical findings include convulsions, abnormal reflexes, a slowed heartbeat and respiratory rate, headache, vomiting, irritability, weakness, and problems with vision. Blindness and continuing mental deterioration from brain atrophy can result if treatment is not instituted.

In adolescent- or adult-onset hydrocephalus the physiognomic abnormalities are less evident than in children with congenital or early-onset hydrocephalus. Many of the other mental and physiologic manifestations are the same, with the added loss of previously acquired motor coordination. Acquired hydrocephalus in children and adolescents is often associated with symptoms of hypopituitarism such as delayed growth and obesity, and generalized weakness.

Hydrocephalus is subdivided according to the ventricular defect and the CSF pressure, high or normal. In **communicating hydrocephalus** there is no obstruction in the ventricular system; the CSF flows readily into the subarachnoid space but is insufficiently absorbed, or perhaps produced in too great a quantity to be absorbed. In **noncommunicating (obstructing) hydrocephalus,** a ventricular block to CSF flow causes dilation of the pathways upstream of the block, leading to increased CSF pressure in the skull. **Normal-pressure hydrocephalus,** which affects middle-aged and older persons, is characterized by dilated ventricles but normal lumbar CSF pressure. The hydrocephalus may be detected by pneumoencephalography. Other symptoms of normal-pressure hydrocephalus include dementia, ataxia, and urinary incontinence.

Etiology The cause of hydrocephalus is unknown. Some cases are caused by a birth defect; others follow hemorrhage, viral infection, or meningitis. A genetic predisposition has been proposed, with transmission through autosomal recessive or X-linked genes.

Epidemiology Most cases of hydrocephalus are diagnosed in the first 2 years of life, but onset may occur at any age, depending on the etiology. No particular sex prevalence has been identified.

Related Disorders Among the disorders that can occur in conjunction with hydrocephalus are spina bifida, Arnold-Chiari syndrome, epilepsy, and meningitis. See *Spina Bifida; Arnold-Chiari Syndrome; Epilepsy.*

Treatment—Standard Standard treatment entails placement of a ventriculoperitoneal shunt to drain the excess CSF. Periodic lengthening of the shunt is necessary to accommodate growth in children. A clogged or nonfunctioning shunt may have to be replaced.

Treatment—Investigational Please contact the agencies listed under Resources, below, for the most current information.

Resources

    For more information on hydrocephalus: National Organization for Rare Disorders (NORD); Hydrocephalus Parent Support Group; National Hydrocephalus Foundation; NIH/National Institute of Neurological Disorders and Stroke (NINDS); Association for Retarded Citizens.

    For genetic information and genetic counseling referrals: March of Dimes Birth Defects Foundation; NIH/National Center for Education in Maternal and Child Health (NCEMCH).

References

Mendelian Inheritance in Man, 8th ed.: V.A. McKusick; The Johns Hopkins University Press, 1986, pp. 991, 1313.

Internal Medicine, 2nd ed.: J.H. Stein, ed.-in-chief; Little, Brown and Company, 1987, p. 2213.

JOSEPH DISEASE

Description Joseph disease is a derangement of the central nervous system producing a cerebellar deficit and peripheral sensory loss. There are 3 forms: types I, II, III.

Synonyms

    Stiatonigral Degeneration

Signs and Symptoms Type I Joseph disease is identified by a lurching, unsteady gait which may be accompanied by dysarthria, muscle rigidity, dystonia, athetosis, and irregular eye movements. Mental alertness and intellect usually remain unaffected.

Type II symptoms are similar to those of type I but progress less rapidly. The distinctive characteristic of type II is increased cerebellar dysfunction marked by difficulty in walking and coordinating movement of the extremities, and spasticity.

Type III (Machado disease) typically presents with ataxia and is distinguished from the other 2 forms by a loss of muscle mass that is due to motor polyneuropathy. Impaired sensation and diminished ability to move the extremities are common, as is diabetes.

Etiology Joseph disease is inherited as an autosomal dominant trait. Currently, it is unknown whether 3 different gene abnormalities are responsible for each form of the disease, or whether all 3 forms result from the expression of a single gene.

Epidemiology Individuals of Portuguese ancestry are most susceptible to Joseph disease. Onset of type I usually occurs around age 20 years; type II typically begins about 30 years of age; and type III usually is not evident until after age 40 years.

Treatment—Standard Treatment is symptomatic and supportive. Pharmacotherapy with L-dopa and baclofen may help relieve muscle rigidity and spasticity. Genetic testing is recommended for families in which at least one member has been diagnosed with the disease.

Treatment—Investigational Please contact the agencies listed under Resources, below, for the most current information.

Resources
   For more information on Joseph disease: National Organization for Rare Disorders (NORD); International Joseph Disease Foundation, Inc.; NIH/National Institute of Neurological Disorders & Stroke (NINDS); Roger N. Rosenberg, M.D., University of Texas Southwestern Medical School.
   For genetic information and genetic counseling referrals: March of Dimes Birth Defects Foundation; NIH/National Center for Education in Maternal and Child Health (NCEMCH).

References
   Mendelian Inheritance in Man, 8th ed.: V.A. McKusick; The Johns Hopkins University Press, 1986, p. 88.

JOUBERT SYNDROME

Description Joubert syndrome is a rare neurologic disorder involving malformation of the area of the brain that controls balance and coordination. Psychomotor retardation, abnormal eye movements, and respiratory irregularities are characteristic.

Synonyms
   Cerebellar Hypoplasia
   Cerebellar Vermis Aplasia
   Cerebellarparenchymal Disorder IV
   Familial Cerebellar Vermis Agenesis
   Vermis Cerebellar Agenesis

Signs and Symptoms Sleep apnea and periods of deep, abnormal breathing are common in infants and may be triggered by emotional stimulation, e.g., crying. Unusually deep inhalations occasionally may occur. These respiratory irregularities usually decrease with age.

Abnormal eye movements such as irregular jerking and eye rolling or crossing may be present. Ataxia, dysmetria, hypermetria, and tremors also may be observed. Weakness of the skeletal muscles may be accompanied by clumsy or rapid alternating movements. Mental retardation also may occur.

Etiology The cause is not known; the disorder may be inherited as an autosomal recessive trait.

Epidemiology Onset is usually in infancy. The syndrome is extremely rare; only 10 cases were reported in the medical literature in 1981. Both males and females can be affected, and the disorder can occur more than once in the same family.

Related Disorders See *Dandy-Walker Syndrome.*

Treatment—Standard Treatment is symptomatic and supportive. Genetic counseling, special education services, and physical therapy may benefit patients and their families.

Treatment—Investigational Please contact the agencies listed under Resources, below, for the most current information.

Resources

For more information on **Joubert syndrome:** National Organization for Rare Disorders (NORD); NIH/National Institute of Neurological Disorders & Stroke (NINDS); Children's Brain Diseases Foundation; David B. Flannery, M.D., Medical College of Georgia.

For **genetic information and genetic counseling referrals:** March of Dimes Birth Defects Foundation; NIH/National Center for Education in Maternal and Child Health (NCEMCH).

References

Mendelian Inheritance in Man, 6th ed.: V.A. McKusick; The Johns Hopkins University Press, 1983, p. 640.

JUMPING FRENCHMEN OF MAINE

Description "Jumping Frenchmen" is an appellation for an unusually extreme startle reaction that occurs in selected populations. The symptoms are elicited by sudden, unexpected noise or movement but greatly exceed, in range and severity, the normal startle reaction.

Synonyms

Jumping Frenchmen
Latah (observed in Malaysia)
Myriachit (observed in Siberia)

Signs and Symptoms The symptoms of "jumping Frenchmen" usually become apparent in adolescence and tend to remit with age. The extreme startle reaction response includes jumping, raising the arms, hitting, yelling, echolalia, obeying sudden orders, and echopraxia. The reaction may include violence, and the intensity of the response increases with fatigue and stress. An unexpected event is necessary to elicit the reaction, and affected individuals may become the subjects of practical jokes designed to provoke the reaction.

Etiology The cause is unknown.

Epidemiology The disorder was originally described in French Canadian lumberjacks in the Moosehead Lake region of Maine in the late 19th and early 20th centuries. Similar behaviors have been observed in specific populations in Southeast Asia, Siberia, India, Somalia, and Yemen. Males appear to be affected more often than females.

Related Disorders Several syndromes or reactive behaviors have features in common with "jumping Frenchmen" but are unrelated to it. See *Tourette Syndrome*, which is similarly characterized by echolalia or echopraxia. **Hyperexplexia**, thought to be a hereditary disorder, lacks the echolalia, echopraxia, and the forced obedience response characteristic of "jumping Frenchmen." The brief, predominantly unilateral muscle contractions of **startle epilepsy** are not as complex and directed as the startle reaction in "jumping Frenchmen," and affected subjects have other seizure manifestations. Individuals with **Kok disease,** a rare hereditary neurologic disorder, have an excessive startle reaction to sudden, unexpected noise, movement, or touch, but also exhibit specific seizure activity.

Treatment—Standard Anticipation of a sudden noise or movement can help the patient avoid the startle response. As the response appears to be reinforced by repetition, elimination of teasing or provocative behavior from others will also help to end episodes.

Treatment—Investigational Please contact the agencies listed under Resources, below, for the most current information.

Resources
 For more information on **Jumping Frenchmen of Maine:** National Organization for Rare Disorders (NORD); NIH/National Institute of Neurological Disorders & Stroke (NINDS).

References
 Jumping Frenchmen of Maine: M. Sainte-Hilaire, et al.; Neurology, September 1986, issue 36(9), pp. 1269–1271.

KEARNS-SAYRE SYNDROME

Description Kearns-Sayre syndrome is a rare myopathy associated with mitochondrial dysfunction, cardiomyopathy, neuropathy, and ophthalmoplegia and retinal disease.

Synonyms

Oculocraniosomatic Neuromuscular Disease

Signs and Symptoms The cardiac wall becomes inflamed and the heart may be enlarged. Cardiac arrhythmias may develop. Eye muscles become progressively weaker, causing ophthalmoplegia and ptosis. Associated retinal degeneration can result in impaired vision. Muscle function in the arms and legs also may be diminished, and growth may be retarded. Dementia, epilepsy, and ataxia may occur.

Etiology The cause is unknown.

Epidemiology Males and females may be affected equally. Onset typically occurs before age 20 years.

Treatment—Standard Treatment of reduced muscle function is symptomatic and supportive. Associated heartbeat irregularities may be treated with various antiarrhythmic drugs or the use of a pacemaker.

Treatment—Investigational Coenzyme Q10, a new compound being investigated, appears to improve the release of energy by muscle mitochondria. This treatment also may improve heart, vision, and neurologic symptoms. The longterm safety and effectiveness of Coenzyme Q10 is yet to be determined.

Please contact the agencies listed under Resources, below, for the most current information.

Resources

For more information on Kearns-Sayre syndrome: National Organization for Rare Disorders (NORD); American Heart Association; Retinitis Pigmentosa Foundation Fighting Blindness; NIH/National Eye Institute; The National Arthritis and Musculoskeletal and Skin Diseases Information Clearinghouse.

References

Heart Involvement in Progressive External Ophthalmoplegia (Kearns-Sayre Syndrome): Electrophysiologic, Hemodynamic and Morphologic Findings: B. Schwartzkopff, et al.; Z. Kardiol., March 1986, issue 75(3), pp. 161–169.

Treatment of Kearns-Sayre Syndrome with Coenzyme Q10: S. Ogasahara, et al.; Neurology, January 1986, issue 36(1), pp. 45–53.

The Fine Structure of the Intramitochondrial Crystalloids in Mitochondrial Myopathy: T.M. Mukherjee, et al.; J. Submicrosc. Cytol., July 1986, issue 18(3), pp. 595–604.

KERNICTERUS

Description Kernicterus is a condition in infants characterized by high levels of bilirubin in the blood. The bilirubin accumulates in the brain stem and basal ganglia. The condition exists in utero and is most prevalent in premature or very sick neonates. It is associated with severe neural symptoms in the form of mental retardation and neuromuscular disorders.

Synonyms

Bilirubin Encephalopathy
Nuclear Jaundice
Posticteric Encephalopathy

Signs and Symptoms Early general symptoms of kernicterus in full-term infants include lethargy, poor feeding, and vomiting; neuromuscular symptoms reflecting degenerative changes include opisthotonos, upward deviation of the eyes, convulsions, and rigidity. Children who survive the initial period may develop the complete neurologic syndrome, with bilateral choreoathetosis, sensorineural hearing loss, extrapyramidal signs, seizures, and loss of upward gaze. In mild cases the dysfunction may be limited to perceptual-motor handicaps and learning disorders.

Etiology Historically, kernicterus was a common sequela of severe hemolytic jaundice of the newborn. Today kernicterus commonly results from severe erythroblastosis fetalis, a hemolytic anemia of newborn infants that is caused by transplacental transmission of maternally formed antibody, evoked by maternal-fetal blood group incompatibility. With the availability of specific treatments for jaundice, kernicterus now develops only in premature or very low birth weight infants with hyperbilirubinemia. Factors predisposing to the development of kernicterus include hypoxemia, acidosis, infections, hypoalbuminemia, and hypothermia.

Epidemiology Newborn infants of either sex may be affected.

Related Disorders Hepatic diseases and hemolytic anemias are among the disorders producing jaundice.

Treatment—Standard Various measures can be implemented to avoid or treat kernicterus in neonates. Early frequent feedings increase the frequency of stools, mobilizing the bowel and reducing the levels of bilirubin in the liver and intestines. Infants with high bilirubin levels may be given exchange blood transfusions through a catheter placed in the umbilical vein. Phototherapy is widely used to treat hyperbilirubinemia in infants, although the longterm effects on mental development are unknown.

Treatment—Investigational The orphan drug Zixoryn (flumecinol) has been used in the investigational treatment of hyperbilirubinemia in newborns unresponsive to phototherapy.

Please contact the agencies listed under Resources, below, for the most current information.

Resources

For more information on kernicterus: National Organization for Rare Disorders (NORD); American Liver Foundation; The United Liver Foundation; Children's Liver Foundation; NIH/National Institute of Child Health and Human Development.

For genetic information and genetic counseling referrals: March of Dimes Birth Defects Foundation; National Center for Education in Maternal and Child Health (NCEMCH).

References
Nelson Textbook of Pediatrics, 13th ed.: R.E. Behrman and V.C. Vaughan, III, eds.; W.B. Saunders Company, 1987, pp. 407–409.
Cecil Textbook of Medicine, 18th ed.: J.B. Wyngaarden and L.H. Smith, Jr., eds.; W.B. Saunders Company, 1988, pp. 812, 1076.

KUFS DISEASE

Description The cerebral lipofuscinoses are a group of inherited disorders marked by excess accumulation of lipofuscin in the brain. The various diseases in this group are differentiated according to age at onset; Kufs disease is a late adolescent or adult form. Symptoms are predominantly neurologic, resembling those of mental disorders, and dermatologic, resembling ichthyosis. Deposits of lipofuscin are found throughout the central nervous system **(CNS)**. The disorder is usually slowly progressive and may be fatal.

Synonyms
> Amaurotic Familial Idiocy, Adult
> Ceroid Lipofuscinosis, Adult Form
> Ceroidosis, Adult-Onset
> Lipofuscinosis, Generalized
> Neuronal Ceroid Lipofuscinosis

Signs and Symptoms Manifestations of Kufs disease first appear in the late teens or early 20s. The early symptoms of muscle weakness and incoordination increase in severity and may be replaced by seizures and chorea as the disease progresses. Excessive amounts of keratin in the skin lead to ichthyosis vulgaris. Neurologic manifestations begin with confusion and behavioral changes reminiscent of psychosis. Convulsions and more severe mental disturbances resembling mental illness may ensue. The neurologic deficits result from excess accumulation of lipofuscin in the brains of affected individuals.

Etiology Kufs disease may be inherited as a dominant or recessive trait. The dominant form produces milder symptoms than the recessive form. An inborn defect in lipid metabolism is responsible for the accumulation of lipofuscins in the CNS.

Epidemiology Kufs disease, the adult-onset form of cerebral sphingolipidosis, begins between the ages of 15 and 26 years. It is an extremely rare condition, affecting perhaps a few hundred people in the United States. There is no racial predilection.

Related Disorders Jansky-Bielschowsky disease is the late infantile form of cerebral sphingolipidosis, with onset occurring between 3 and 4 years of age; **Batten disease** is the juvenile form, and begins between the ages of 5 and 7 years. Both are inherited as recessive traits and are hereditary disorders of lipid metabolism or storage. The cardinal features of Jansky-Bielschowsky disease are rapid neurologic deterioration, retinal pigment changes, and optic atrophy leading to blindness. It is a rare disease that appears to occur predominantly in persons of Scandinavian ancestry. Batten disease is a rare condition diagnosed from the finding of ceroid lipofuscin pigments and the characteristic "salt-and-pepper" retinal appearance.

Of the 14 known lipid storage diseases, **Gaucher disease** is the most common. Gaucher disease is the comprehensive term for a number of disorders characterized by the defective production or metabolism of glucocerebrosidase and diagnosed from the presence of Gaucher cells in the marrow and other organs. Infantile, juvenile, and adult forms are recognized. See *Batten Disease; Gaucher Disease; Niemann-Pick Disease; Sandhoff Disease; Tay-Sachs Disease.*

Treatment—Standard Treatment of Kufs disease is symptomatic and supportive. Patients and their families may benefit from genetic counseling and services for the mentally disabled.

Treatment—Investigational Specific treatments for lipid storage disease may be available in the near future. Gene replacement therapy may eventually prove useful.

Please contact the agencies listed under Resources, below, for the most current information.

Resources

For more information on Kufs disease: National Organization for Rare Disorders (NORD); National Lipid Diseases Foundation; NIH/National Institute of Neurological Disorders & Stroke (NINDS); The Children's Brain Diseases Foundation for Research; National Tay-Sachs/Allied Diseases Association.

For genetic information and genetic counseling referrals: March of Dimes Birth Defects Foundation; National Center for Education in Maternal and Child Health (NCEMCH).

References

Adult Ceroid-Lipofuscinosis. Diagnostic Value of Biopsies and of Neurophysiological Investigations: A. Vercruyssen, et al.; J. Neurol. Neurosurg. Psychiatry, November 1982, issue 45(11), pp. 1056–1059.

Familial Occurrence of Adult-Type Neuronal Ceroid Lipofuscinosis: M. Tobo, et al.; Arch. Neurol., October 1984, issue 41(10), pp. 1091–1094.

Autofluorescence Emission Spectra of Neuronal Lipopigment in a Case of Adult-Onset Ceroidosis (Kufs Disease): J.H. Dowson, Acta Neuropathol. (Berl.), 1983, issue 59(4), pp. 241–245.

KUGELBERG-WELANDER SYNDROME

Description Kugelberg-Welander syndrome is a rare inherited disorder in which degeneration of motor neurons causes progressive weakness and muscle atrophy, notably in the legs, accompanied by loss of reflexes. An early symptom is uncoordinated gait.

Synonyms

Juvenile Spinal Muscular Atrophy
Spinal Muscular Atrophy

Signs and Symptoms The clinical picture of Kugelberg-Welander syndrome is dominated by muscle atrophy in the limbs and trunk, producing a slumped-forward posture and impaired motor control. Patients with this condition describe difficulty walking, climbing stairs, and getting out of bed. They may lose bowel control, and reflexes may be slowed. Involvement of the ocular muscles leads to profound myopia and impaired vision. Rhythm irregularities may occur when the heart muscle is affected.

Etiology Kugelberg-Welander syndrome is attributed to degeneration of the motor neurons in the spinal cord. It is commonly inherited as an autosomal recessive trait. An autosomal dominant or X-linked recessive transmission has been postulated for some cases.

Epidemiology More males than females have Kugelberg-Welander syndrome, and those women who are affected tend to have less severe symptoms. Onset generally occurs between 2 and 17 years of age.

Related Disorders See *Werdnig-Hoffmann Disease.*

Treatment—Standard Treatment of Kugelberg-Welander syndrome is symptomatic and supportive. The mainstays of treatment are physiotherapy and orthotic supports. An implanted pacemaker may be necessary to correct cardiac irregularities. Genetic counseling may be offered to patients and their families.

Treatment—Investigational Lithium carbonate is being used experimentally in the treatment of Kugelberg-Welander syndrome.

Please contact the agencies listed under Resources, below, for the most current information.

Resources

For more information on Kugelberg-Welander syndrome: National Organization for Rare Disorders (NORD); Families of Spinal Muscular Atrophy; National Institute of Neurological Disorders & Stroke (NINDS).

For genetic information and genetic counseling referrals: March of Dimes Birth Defects Foundation; National Center for Education in Maternal and Child Health (NCEMCH).

References

Mendelian Inheritance in Man, 9th ed.: V.A. McKusick; The Johns Hopkins University Press, 1990, p. 1355.

Late Onset Spinal Muscle Atrophy. A Sex Linked Variant of Kugelberg-Welander: G.W. Paulson, et al.; Acta Neurol. Scand., January 1980, issue 61(1), pp. 49–55.

Chronic Proximal Spinal Muscular Atrophy of Childhood and Adolescence. Sex Influence: I. Hausmanowa-Petrusewicz, et al.; J. Med. Genet., December 1984, issue 21(6), pp. 447–450.

Is Kugelberg-Welander Spinal Muscular Atrophy a Fetal Defect?: I. Hausmanowa-Petrusewicz, et al.; Muscle Nerve, September–October 1980, issue 3(5), pp. 389–402.

LANDAU-KLEFFNER SYNDROME

Description Landau-Kleffner syndrome is a neurologic disorder characterized by aphasia and occasionally epileptic seizures and auditory agnosia. The electroencephalogram **(EEG)** is abnormal.

Synonyms
Infantile Acquired Aphasia

Signs and Symptoms Symptoms develop slowly and include aphasia, paroxysmal abnormalities in the EEG, and occasionally epileptic seizures and auditory agnosia. The aphasia varies among patients and is related to the location and extent of dysfunction in the brain. Some patients improve spontaneously. In general, the prognosis is poorer for those who develop symptoms at an early age. Diagnosis is aided by neuroradiological examination.

Etiology The cause is unknown.

Epidemiology Children only are affected. The disorder was first identified in 1957; as of 1982 only 80 cases had been reported.

Related Disorders See *Epilepsy.*

Treatment—Standard Treatment is generally symptomatic and supportive. Antiepileptic drugs have had varying effectiveness. Some patients may benefit from speech therapy or sign language.

Treatment—Investigational A new type of surgery is being investigated for children suffering from Landau-Kleffner syndrome. Subpial transection may restore hearing and speech and eliminate seizures. For more information: Rush Presbyterian, St. Luke's Medical Center, 1753 West Congress Parkway, Chicago, Illinois 60612; (312) 942-5000 or (312) 942-5939.

Please contact the agencies listed under Resources, below, for the most current information.

Resources
For more information on Landau-Kleffner syndrome: National Organization for Rare Disorders (NORD); C.A.N.D.L.E. (Childhood Aphasia, Neurological Disorders, Landau-Kleffner Syndrome, and Epilepsy); NIH/National Institute of Deafness & Other Communication Disorders (NIDCD); American Speech-Language-Hearing Association.

References
Age of Onset and Outcome in "Acquired Aphasia with Convulsive Disorder" (Landau-Kleffner Syndrome): D.V. Bishop; Dev. Med. Child Neurol., December 1985, issue 27(6), pp. 705–712.

LEUKODYSTROPHY, CANAVAN

Description Canavan leukodystrophy is a rare inherited disorder in which spongy degeneration of the central nervous system leads to progressive mental deterioration accompanied by increased muscle tone, poor head control, megalocephaly, and blindness. The disorder is caused by a chemical imbalance in the brain. Symptoms appear in early infancy and progress rapidly, resulting in early death.

Synonyms
> Canavan-Van Bogaert-Bertrand Disease
> Familial Idiocy with Spongy Degeneration of Neuraxis
> Spongy Degeneration of the Brain
> Van Bogaert-Bertrand Syndrome

Signs and Symptoms Canavan leukodystrophy is usually noticed by 6 months of age as mental and physical regression occurs. Early symptoms include apathy, floppiness, and loss of previously acquired mental and motor skills. Disease progression is characterized by limb spasticity, atonicity of the neck muscles, and megalocephaly as the brain swells and the bones of the skull fail to fuse normally. Paralysis may ensue. With diminished chest muscle function, the infant is susceptible to respiratory tract disease. Progressive atrophy of the optic muscles results in blindness in many cases; less often, hearing is also impaired. Death typically occurs before the age of 4 years.

Neurologic and radiological studies aid in the diagnosis. Computed tomography is helpful in distinguishing Canavan leukodystrophy from hydrocephaly; the scans show severe, widespread white matter changes, predominantly demyelination and vacuolation.

Etiology Canavan leukodystrophy is transmitted as an autosomal recessive trait. The degenerative brain changes are attributed to insufficient production of aspartoacylase, the enzyme that breaks down N-acetylaspartic acid, which occurs in high levels in the brain. Breakdown of this acid may act to trigger chemical reactions requisite to proper brain function, or the excessively high levels may be damaging per se.

Epidemiology Patients with Canavan dystrophy are usually of Eastern European Jewish ancestry. Both sexes are affected. A familial tendency has been recognized.

Related Disorders See *Adrenoleukodystrophy; Alexander Disease.*

Treatment—Standard Treatment is symptomatic and supportive.

Treatment—Investigational With the identification of the enzyme defect causing Canavan leukodystrophy, prenatal testing and specific therapies may become available in the future. Basic pathologic (tissue and fluid) research, not intended to provide counseling or devise treatment, is being conducted on various peroxisomal diseases, including Canavan leukodystrophy. For more information: Anne B. Johnson, M.D., Department of Pathology—K427, Albert Einstein College of Medicine, 1300 Morris Park Ave., Bronx, NY 10461.

Please contact the agencies listed under Resources, below, for the most current information.

Resources

For more information on Canavan leukodystrophy: National Organization for Rare Disorders (NORD); United Leukodystrophy Foundation; NIH/National Institute of Neurological Disorders & Stroke (NINDS); National Foundation for Jewish Genetic Diseases; National Tay-Sachs/Allied Diseases Association, Inc.

For genetic information and genetic counseling referrals: March of Dimes Birth Defects Foundation; National Center for Education in Maternal and Child Health (NCEMCH).

References

The Cecil Textbook of Medicine, 18th ed.: J.B. Wyngaarden and L.H. Smith, Jr., eds.; W.B. Saunders Company, 1988, p. 2216.

LEUKODYSTROPHY, KRABBE

Description Krabbe leukodystrophy is a rare familial metabolic disorder in which the sphingolipid ceramide galactoside accumulates in the white matter of the brain, owing to a deficiency of the enzyme galactoside beta-galactosidase (galactosylceramidase). The resulting demyelination leads to brain degeneration and progressive neurologic dysfunction. The clinical picture includes mental retardation, paralysis, blindness, deafness, and pseudobulbar palsy.

Synonyms

Galactocerebrosidase Deficiency
Galactoside Beta-Galactosidase Deficiency
Galactosyl Ceramide Lipidosis
Galactosylceramidase Deficiency
Globoid Leukodystrophy
Krabbe Disease
Leukodystrophy, Globoid Cell
Sphingolipidosis

Signs and Symptoms The infantile form of Krabbe leukodystrophy, which accounts for 90 percent of cases, manifests between 3 and 5 months of age. A late-onset form has been identified with onset at age 6 to 18 months. Apathy, irritability, and fretfulness are among the first symptoms to appear; vomiting and episodes of partial unconsciousness may also occur. These early symptoms are followed by seizures, spastic contractions of the lower extremities, dysphagia, and mental deterioration. With progressive brain degeneration, paraplegia and blindness may occur. Lesions in specific areas of the brain produce decerebrate rigidity. Sensitivity to sounds is a component of the disorder in some cases.

The diagnosis is established by galactocerebrosidase assays performed on fibroblast cells from an infant or fetus. Pathologic examination shows extensive demyelination and characteristic globoid cells filled with unmetabolized cerebroside.

Etiology Krabbe leukodystrophy is inherited as a recessive trait. The disorder is caused by a deficiency of galactoside beta-galactosidase, an enzyme that aids in the metabolism of galactocerebroside, a component of myelin. The neurologic symptoms are due to demyelination of the brain and brain stem.

Epidemiology Krabbe leukodystrophy affects 1:40,000 newborns in the United States. The sex distribution is equal.

Related Disorders See *Adrenoleukodystrophy; Alexander Disease; Leukodystrophy, Canavan; Leukodystrophy, Metachromatic.*

Treatment—Standard Treatment for Krabbe leukodystrophy is symptomatic and supportive. Prenatal diagnosis is available.

Treatment—Investigational Bone marrow transplantation is being studied as possible therapy for mild, early cases of Krabbe leukodystrophy. Other research focuses on defining the gene abnormality that causes leukodystrophy.

Please contact the agencies listed under Resources, below, for the most current information.

Resources

For more information on Krabbe leukodystrophy: National Organization for Rare Disorders (NORD); National Lipid Diseases Foundation; United Leukodystrophy Foundation; Adrenoleukodystrophy Project; NIH/National Institute of Neurological Disorders and Stroke (NINDS); Research Trust for Metabolic Diseases in Children.

For genetic information and genetic counseling referrals: March of Dimes Birth Defects Foundation; National Center for Education in Maternal and Child Health (NCEMCH).

References

A Correlative Synopsis of the Leukodystrophies: P. Morell; Neuropediatrics, September 1984, Suppl. 15, pp. 62–65.

Prenatal Diagnosis of Krabbe Disease Using a Fluorescent Derivative of Galactosylceramide: M. Zeigler, et al.; Clin. Chim. Acta, October 15, 1984, issue 142(3), pp. 313–318.

LEUKODYSTROPHY, METACHROMATIC (MLD)

Description Metachromatic leukodystrophy is a form of leukoencephalopathy in which sulfatide, a sphingolipid, accumulates in neural and nonneural tissues, producing blindness, convulsions, motor disturbances progressing to paralysis, and dementia. Myelin is lost from the central nervous system (**CNS**). The disorder is inherited as an autosomal recessive trait. Infantile, juvenile, and adult forms are recognized.

Synonyms

Arylsulfatase A Deficiency

Cerebroside Sulfatase Deficiency
Diffuse Cerebral Sclerosis
Greenfield Disease
Leukoencephalopathy
Metachromatic Form of Diffuse Cerebral Sclerosis
Metachromatic Leukoencephalopathy
Sulfatide Lipidosis
Sulfatidosis

Signs and Symptoms The early signs and symptoms of MLD may be vague and gradual in onset, and therefore difficult to diagnose correctly. A subtle change in mentation, memory, or posture may be the first symptom observed. In occasional cases the earliest symptom is a disturbance in vision, or numbness somewhere in the body.

Infantile MLD usually is detected in the 2nd year of life, commonly before 30 months of age. Clinical features include blindness, motor disturbances, rigidity, mental deterioration, and occasionally convulsions. A juvenile form has an onset between ages 4 and 10 years. Adult MLD begins after 16 years of age and is characterized by psychiatric disturbances evolving to dementia; truncal ataxia, and intention tremor develop later in this form of MLD.

Etiology MLD is caused by a deficiency in arylsulfatase A, an enzyme that acts on the sulfatide of the myelin of nerve cells in the white matter of the CNS. An autosomal recessive inheritance has been identified.

Epidemiology Persons of all nationalities and both sexes may be affected by MLD.

Related Disorders See *Adrenoleukodystrophy; Alexander Disease; Leukodystrophy, Canavan; Leukodystrophy, Krabbe.*
See also *Tay-Sachs Disease; Sandhoff Disease.*

Treatment—Standard Treatment for MLD is symptomatic and supportive.

Treatment—Investigational Bone marrow transplantation has been used experimentally for children with mild forms of MLD. The safety and efficacy of the procedure in this setting are not known. Laboratory research is directed toward identifying the abnormal gene responsible for MLD.

Please contact the agencies listed under Resources, below, for the most current information.

Resources
For more information on metachromatic leukodystrophy: National Organization for Rare Disorders (NORD); United Leukodystrophy Foundation, Inc.; National Tay-Sachs/Allied Diseases Association; NIH/National Institute of Neurological Disorders & Stroke (NINDS).

For genetic information and genetic counseling referrals: March of Dimes Birth Defects Foundation; National Center for Education in Maternal and Child Health (NCEMCH).

References
Cecil Textbook of Medicine, 18th ed.: J.B. Wyngaarden and L.H. Smith, Jr., eds.; W.B. Saunders Company, 1988, pp. 2215–2216.

LISSENCEPHALY

Description Lissencephaly ("smooth brain"), also called agyria ("without rings"), is a rare brain formation disorder characterized by lack of normal development of convolutions in the cerebral cortex and a small brain. Persons with this disorder have a small head and characteristic facies; developmental anomalies of the renal, cardiovascular, and gastrointestinal systems may be present as well. The developmental abnormalities begin before birth, perhaps with interruption of normal brain development in the 4th month of gestation. An autosomal recessive inheritance has been postulated.

Synonyms
Agyria
Lissencephaly Syndrome

Signs and Symptoms Lissencephaly can be diagnosed at or soon after birth. In addition to the small head and unusual facies, young infants suffer from failure to thrive, in part due to difficulty in feeding. The newborn is cyanotic and floppy, has a feeble cry, and may have respiratory difficulties, especially while sleeping. Some are jaundiced and have hepatomegaly or splenomegaly. Hair may cover large areas of the body, and the digits may be malformed. As the infant grows, lack of response to stimuli may be noted, with intermittent bouts of hyperactivity. The initial poor muscle tone may be replaced by seizures and pronounced muscle spasms. Psychomotor retardation is prominent. Other developmental anomalies that may be noted early include undescended testicles, hernias, congenital heart disease, solitary kidney, and duodenal atresia.

Of the 8 possible variants of lissencephaly, 2 occur most frequently: Miller-Dieker syndrome and Norman-Roberts syndrome. The facial features of patients with **Miller-Dieker** syndrome include a high, narrow, wrinkled forehead and a wide, flat lip span ("carp mouth"). Skeletal abnormalities show up as a poorly developed jaw and a prominent posterior aspect to the skull. The corneas may be clouded and the ears may have an unusual shape. By contrast, the physiognomy in **Norman-Roberts syndrome** is characterized by a low sloping forehead and a prominent bridge of the nose.

Etiology Lissencephaly is thought to be inherited as an autosomal recessive trait. Specific chromosomal abnormalities have been identified in some cases and speculatively linked to the Miller-Dieker variant. The Norman-Roberts variant is not known to be associated with a chromosomal abnormality.

Epidemiology Lissencephaly is a very rare disorder. No particular sex prevalence has been identified.

Related Disorders Lissencephaly may occur as part of a suite of disorders, particularly in the triad of hydrocephalus, agyria (lissencephaly), and retinal dysplasia (**HARD**). This triad is known variously as Warburg syndrome, Chemke syndrome, Pagon syndrome, Walker-Warburg syndrome, and cerebro-ocular dysgenesis. When encephalocele is also present, the mnemonic is **HARD + E.** Lissencephaly may also occur as part of the **Neu-Laxova syndrome,** an intrauterine growth disorder characterized by multiple developmental anomalies, including microcephaly, lissencephaly, and abnormalities of the limbs, skin, and external genitalia. The placenta is abnormal in Neu-Laxova syndrome.

Treatment—Standard Treatment of lissencephaly is symptomatic and supportive. Patients and families may benefit from genetic counseling.

Treatment—Investigational Please contact the agencies listed under Resources, below, for the most current information.

Resources
For more information on lissencephaly: National Organization for Rare Disorders (NORD); Support Network for Pachygyria, Agyria, Lissencephaly; NIH/National Institute of Neurological Disorders & Stroke (NINDS); The Children's Brain Diseases Foundation for Research.
For genetic information and genetic counseling referrals: March of Dimes Birth Defects Foundation; National Center for Education in Maternal and Child Health (NCEMCH).

References
Miller-Dieker Syndrome. Lissencephaly and Monosomy 17P: W.B. Dobyns, et al.; J. Pediatr., April 1983, issue 102(4), pp. 552–558.

Syndromes with Lissencephaly. I. Miller-Dieker and Norman-Roberts Syndromes and Isolated Lissencephaly: W.B. Dobyns, et al.; Am. J. Med. Genet., July 1984, issue 18(3), pp. 509–526.

LOCKED-IN SYNDROME

Description Locked-in syndrome is a very rare neuromuscular disorder characterized by complete paralysis of voluntary muscles, with the exception of the muscles that control voluntary eye movements. Paralysis can result from lesions in motor nerve centers, or from a blood clot that interferes with oxygen flow to the brain stem, particularly the ventral pons.

Synonyms
Cerebromedullospinal Disconnection
Deefferented State
Pseudocoma

Signs and Symptoms Complete paralysis of all voluntary muscles occurs. The only muscles that remain unaffected are those that control eye movements. Consciousness is maintained but individuals are unable to speak. Communication is limited to the use of an eye blink code.

Etiology Lesions across the corticospinal and corticobulbar nerve tracts separate all motor nerves except those to the eye muscles. In some cases, the circulation to the brain stem may be blocked by a blood clot. Reduced blood flow and oxygen supply to the internal capsule of the brain can cause tissue death on both sides of the body. If circulation can be restored, the patient's condition may improve.

Epidemiology Males and females are affected equally.

Related Disorders In **akinetic mutism,** patients' eyes are open and they seem to be awake, but they cannot communicate. The disorder is a result of bilateral frontal lobe damage or destruction of the brain's reticular activating system. Muscle response to painful stimuli is poor.

Treatment—Standard Several devices to facilitate communication are available for people who cannot speak. Other treatment is symptomatic and supportive.

Treatment—Investigational Please contact the agencies listed under Resources, below, for the most current information.

Resources

For more information on **locked-in syndrome:** National Organization for Rare Disorders (NORD); NIH/National Institute of Neurological Disorders & Stroke (NINDS).

References

Adaptive Equipment for C6 Quadriplegia: An Approach to Effective, Simple, and Inexpensive Devices: J.R. Basford, et al.; Arch. Phys. Med. Rehabil., December 1985, issue 66(12), pp. 829–831.

Recovery from Locked-in Syndrome After Posttraumatic Bilateral Distal Vertebral Artery Occlusion: J.M. Cabezudo, et al.; Surg. Neurol., February 1986, issue 25(2), pp. 185–190.

MEDULLOBLASTOMA

Description A medulloblastoma is a cerebellar tumor consisting of undifferentiated glial cells. About half of medulloblastomas invade the pons and medulla, with subsequent extension or metastasis. Headache and vomiting are early symptoms; however, the full spectrum of symptoms varies with the precise location of the tumor.

Signs and Symptoms The signs and symptoms of medulloblastoma fall into 2 general categories, those due to increased intracranial pressure (**ICP**) and those due to the tumor's effects on brain tissue. Increased ICP may result from tumor growth in the nonexpansile skull, with subsequent displacement of normal brain tissue. Other tumor mass effects include brain tissue edema and obstruction of cerebrospinal fluid (**CSF**) flow.

The first sign of a medulloblastoma in infants may be cephalomegaly without other apparent symptoms. Older children experience early-morning vomiting, with or without nausea. The vomiting is attributed to increased ICP but may also result from some other disturbance of the brain tissue without ICP changes. Because the child may feel transiently well after vomiting, the diagnosis may be delayed until growth of the tumor produces other symptoms. As the ICP continues to increase, the child may become irritable and lethargic, with personality changes and attention deficit. Vomiting is more frequent as the tumor grows.

Signs of tumor impingement on normal cerebellar tissue include loss of skilled muscle activity controlled by the cerebellum, such as walking and speech. Ataxia and ataxic gait are other early manifestations of cerebellar disorder.

The precise location of the tumor determines which of the many other symptoms will occur in a given case. Symptoms commonly observed include muscle weakness, spasticity, hypotonicity, reflex changes, stiff neck muscles, strabismus, and nystagmus.

Etiology The cause of medulloblastoma is unknown.

Epidemiology Medulloblastomas have been found in persons of all ages, from neonates to people in the 8th decade of life. The greatest prevalence (80 percent) is in children, in whom 3 peaks of onset have been noticed: at 3 years, at 5½ years, and at 7 to 9 years. Twice as many boys as girls are affected, but the sex distinction diminishes with increasing age at onset. In adults, peak onset occurs at 20 to 24 years.

Treatment—Standard Treatment of medulloblastoma entails some combination of surgery, radiation therapy, and chemotherapy. Because the tumor frequently obstructs normal CSF flow, a shunt may be inserted to drain the excess fluid and decrease ICP before surgical excision of the tumor is attempted. Posterior fossa craniectomy is the preferred procedure to debulk the tumor and to promote the efficacy of subsequent chemotherapy or radiation therapy.

Medulloblastoma is a highly radiation-sensitive tumor. Radiation therapy is usually begun 7 to 10 days after surgery. Because medulloblastoma may spread extensively throughout the neural axis, the entire central nervous system must be irradiated, with a booster dose to the posterior fossa. Five-year survival rates of 60 to 70 percent have been reported following total excision of the tumor and irradiation.

Treatment is complex in young children, especially those with extensive initial involvement or in whom the tumor cannot be completely excised. Chemotherapy is usually prescribed in these cases to delay recurrence.

Treatment—Investigational Please contact the agencies listed under Resources, below, for the most current information.

Resources

For more information on medulloblastoma: National Organization for Rare Disorders (NORD); Association for Brain Tumor Research; American Cancer Society; NIH/National Cancer Institute PDQ (Physician Data Query) phoneline.

References
About Medulloblastoma: W. Kretzmer, et al.; Association for Brain Tumor Research, 1985.

MEIGE SYNDROME

Description Meige syndrome is a neurologic movement disorder characterized by blepharospasm, dystonia, and occasionally spasms in the facial musculature. Persons in late middle age and older are affected.

Synonyms
Blepharospasm Oromandibular Dystonic Syndrome
Bruegel Syndrome

Signs and Symptoms The clinical picture of Meige syndrome is dominated by the gradual onset of dyskinesia and dystonia of the facial muscles in middle-aged or older persons. Intermittent involuntary eyelid closure may result from spasms of the muscles around the eye. Spasms of the tongue, throat, and respiratory tract may also occur, leading to breathing difficulties. Occasionally the neuromuscular involvement extends to the trunk and extremities.

Etiology The cause is unknown.

Epidemiology Meige syndrome typically affects persons of either sex 50 years of age or older, although it can occur at younger ages.

Related Disorders See *Benign Essential Blepharospasm.*

Treatment—Standard Various drugs may be used to treat the symptoms, particularly the blepharospasm, of Meige syndrome. These drugs include diazepam, levodopa, methyldopa, trihexyphenidyl, lithium, baclofen, and clonazepam.

The orphan drug botulinum A toxin (Oculinum) when injected intramuscularly causes temporary paralysis and for this reason has been used to treat the spasms of Meige syndrome. After a few months the spasms return and treatment must be repeated.

Treatment—Investigational Please contact the agencies listed under Resources, below, for the most current information.

Resources
For more information on **Meige syndrome:** National Organization for Rare Disorders (NORD); NIH/National Institute of Neurological Disorders & Stroke (NINDS); Dystonia Medical Research Foundation; Benign Essential Blepharospasm Research Foundation, Inc. (BEBRF, Inc.).

References
The Cecil Textbook of Medicine, 18th ed.: J.B. Wyngaarden and L.H. Smith, Jr., eds.; W.B. Saunders Company, 1988, pp. 2150–2151.

MELKERSSON-ROSENTHAL SYNDROME

Description Melkersson-Rosenthal syndrome is a rare hereditary neurologic condition characterized by chronic noninflammatory facial edema, predominantly of the lips, accompanied by paresis and occasionally lingua plicata (scrotal tongue). Symptoms typically begin before adulthood.

Synonyms
>   Cheilitis Granulomatosa
>   Melkersson Syndrome

Signs and Symptoms The chronic facial edema in Melkersson-Rosenthal syndrome is most noticeable in the lips, although sometimes only one lip is involved. Affected tissue sites may permanently increase in size with the buildup of fibrous tissue. Peripheral facial paralysis, unilateral or bilateral, is another diagnostic feature but does not necessarily co-occur with the edema. Lingua plicata occurs in some cases and may be associated with sensory defects on the anterior two-thirds of the tongue. Symptomatic episodes may follow long symptom-free periods.

Etiology The cause is not known.

Epidemiology Melkersson-Rosenthal syndrome was first identified in European populations. Onset typically occurs during childhood or adolescence, and more girls than boys have been diagnosed with the syndrome.

Related Disorders See *Bell's Palsy,* which should be included in the differential diagnosis of facial paralysis.

Treatment—Standard Specific treatment of Melkersson-Rosenthal syndrome involves surgery, to decompress the facial nerve and reduce the amount of fibrous tissue in the lips, and triamcinolone injections, for treatment of swelling and fibrosis.

Treatment—Investigational Clofazimine, a drug used in the treatment of leprosy, is undergoing trial in the treatment of Melkersson-Rosenthal syndrome.

Please contact the agencies listed under Resources, below, for the most current information.

Resources
    For more information on Melkersson-Rosenthal syndrome: National Organization for Rare Disorders (NORD); NIH/National Institute of Neurological Disorders & Stroke (NINDS).

References
Internal Medicine, 2nd ed.: J.H. Stein, ed.-in-chief; Little, Brown and Company, 1987, p. 486.
Melkersson-Rosenthal Syndrome: M.W. Minor, et al.; J. Allergy Clin. Immunol., July 1987, issue 80(1), pp. 64–67.
Intralesional T Lymphocyte Phenotypes and HLA-DR Expression in Melkersson-Rosenthal Syndrome: L. Ronnblom, et al.; Int. J. Oral Maxillofac. Surg., October 1986, issue 15(5), pp. 614–619.
Total Facial Nerve Decompression in Recurrent Facial Paralysis and the Melkersson-Rosenthal Syndrome. A Preliminary Report: M.D. Graham, et al.; Am. J. Otol., January 1986, issue 7(1), pp. 34–37.
The Melkersson-Rosenthal Syndrome: W.B. Wadlington, et al.; Pediatrics, April 1984, issue 73(4), pp. 502–560.

MENIERE DISEASE

Description Meniere disease is associated with endolymphatic hydrops and is characterized by vertigo, fluctuating hearing loss, and tinnitus.

Synonyms
    Endolymphatic Hydrops
    Labyrinthine Hydrops
    Labyrinthine Syndrome
    Lermoyez Syndrome

Signs and Symptoms The attacks of vertigo usually are sudden in onset, persist for hours, and slowly decrease. Nausea and vomiting may accompany the vertigo. The tinnitus characteristic of Meniere disease may be ever-present or recurrent, and there may be an intermittent hearing loss. Symptoms are unilateral in 85 to 90 percent of cases.

The Lermoyez variant of Meniere disease is distinguished by initial tinnitus and hearing loss and later onset of vertigo, from months to years. In another variant, vertigo is not present and the endolymphatic distention is limited to the cochlea.

Etiology The cause of Meniere disease is not known. It is thought that the membrane between the inner and middle ear may become more porous, causing an alteration in the labyrinthine osmotic pressure. Other possible factors include disturbance of the autonomic regulation of the endolymphatic system, local allergy of the inner ear, and vascular disturbance of the stria vascularis. Stress and emotional disturbances can precipitate attacks.

Epidemiology A recent study suggests that 0.4 percent of the population in the United States may be affected with Meniere disease. Males are affected more commonly than females, and onset is usually during the 5th decade of life.

Treatment—Standard Anticholinergic agents may relieve the tinnitus and gastrointestinal disturbances. Antihistamines and diazepam may also be helpful. Barbiturates such as phenobarbital also are used for general sedation during severe episodes.

Treatment—Investigational When recurring attacks of vertigo become more frequent and severe and intensive medical therapy has failed to control them, the patient becomes a candidate for conservative or destructive surgery.

Conservative approaches are used if residual hearing is good or adequate with a hearing aid. These procedures are the endolymphatic shunt, middle cranial fossa vestibular neurectomy, and retrolabyrinthine vestibular neurectomy.

Destructive approaches are used if residual hearing is poor and cannot be helped with amplification. The 3 such procedures in use today are the oval window labyrinthectomy, postauricular labyrinthectomy, and translabyrinthine vestibular neurectomy.

For further information on experimental surgery, contact Margareta Moller, M.D., Presbyterian University Hospital, Room 9402, PUH, 230 Lothrup Street,

Pittsburgh, Pennsylvania 15213, (412) 624-3376; and the Ear Research Foundation, Department P, 1921 Floyd St., Sarasota, Florida 34239.

Please contact the agencies listed under Resources, below, for the most current information.

Resources
   For more information on Meniere disease: National Organization for Rare Disorders (NORD); The E.A.R. Foundation; Vestibular Disorders Association; American Tinnitus Association; NIH/National Institute of Deafness & Other Communication Disorders (NIDCD).

MENINGIOMA

Description Meningiomas are benign, slow-growing tumors of the meninges that occasionally cause thickening or thinning of adjoining skull bones. Meningiomas are characterized as frontal, temporal, and parietal.

Synonyms
   Arachnoidal Fibroblastoma
   Dural Endothelioma
   Leptomeningioma
   Meningeal Fibroblastoma

Signs and Symptoms The symptoms of meningioma vary according to the size and location of the tumor. Many, but not all, brain tumors cause headaches.

   With **frontal tumors,** progressive weakness develops on one side of the body or in a localized area (e.g., a leg). Focal or generalized seizures and mental changes such as drowsiness, listlessness, dullness, or personality changes may occur. If the tumor is in the dominant hemisphere, aphasia may result. Frontal lobe tumors can also produce anosmia, diplopia, and incontinence.

   Temporal tumors, particularly in the nondominant hemisphere, usually cause no symptoms other than seizures. Some patients experience anomia if the tumor is in the dominant hemisphere.

   Parietal tumors, meningiomas over the parietal lobe, may produce either generalized or focal sensory seizures. Astereognosis is also seen.

Etiology The cause is unknown. These tumors usually develop from cell clusters associated with arachnoidal villi.

Epidemiology Meningiomas most frequently are found in middle-aged persons, and are rare in children. The ratio of affected women to affected men is 3:2. American blacks are seldom affected.

Treatment—Standard Many meningiomas can be completely removed surgically. If complete removal is impossible because of the risk of damaging an artery or other local tissue, even partial removal may alleviate symptoms. Because meningiomas grow so slowly, further surgery may not be necessary for many years. Radiation and chemotherapy are usually not used as treatment for meningiomas.

If the patient experiences muscle weakness, coordination problems, or speech impairment, physical, occupational, or speech therapy may be helpful.

Treatment—Investigational Please contact the agencies listed under Resources, below, for the most current information.

Resources

For more information on meningioma: National Organization for Rare Disorders (NORD); American Cancer Society; NIH/National Cancer Institute PDQ (Physician Data Query) phoneline; Association for Brain Tumor Research.

References

About Meningiomas: B. Fine, et al.; Association for Brain Tumor Research, 1982.

MOYAMOYA DISEASE

Description Moyamoya disease affects the cerebrovascular circulation by increasingly narrowing and in some cases eventually occluding the terminal portion of the internal carotid artery.

Synonyms

Cerebrovascular Moyamoya Disease

Signs and Symptoms The age at onset appears to dictate the manifestations. For example, children may experience seizures or involuntary movements and even exhibit signs of mental retardation. In young patients, moyamoya disease is usually associated with headaches; speech difficulties; paralytic episodes involving the feet, legs, or upper extremities; hemorrhage; and anemia. In adults, disturbance of consciousness or subarachnoid hemorrhage is prominent.

The patient may have syncopal episodes. In addition, these visual abnormalities may occur alone or in combination: hemianopia, diplopia, bilaterally diminished visual acuity, and the inability to recognize objects; papilledema may indicate subarachnoid or cerebral hemorrhage.

Etiology Moyamoya disease is idiopathic. In a few patients, it has been attributed to an autosomal recessive trait. Studies have implicated oral contraceptives in a small number of female patients, but this has not been substantiated. Pregnancy also may be a factor.

Epidemiology Although onset can be at any age, moyamoya disease often affects females under age 20, especially Japanese girls. In one Japanese study, 7 percent of the cases were familial, and similar cases, including those involving identical twins, have been recognized in Europe.

Related Disorders Symptoms of cerebrovascular accidents and malformations can be similar to those of moyamoya disease.

Treatment—Standard Arteriography and magnetic resonance imaging (**MRI**) are diagnostic in moyamoya disease. The disease may plateau in some patients in whom it has been advancing, but it has not responded to therapy in the past. Today, however, both surgical treatment and drug therapy offer hope. Current drug therapy consists of IV verapamil, a calcium-channel blocker. The effectiveness of the complicated surgical procedures in use varies among patients.

Other treatment is symptomatic and supportive.

Treatment—Investigational The potential roles of calcium-channel blockers and anticoagulants are being investigated.

Please contact the agencies listed under Resources, below, for the most current information.

Resources

For more information on moyamoya disease: National Organization for Rare Disorders (NORD); National Institute of Neurological Disorders & Stroke (NINDS); The Children's Brain Diseases Foundation for Research.

For genetic information and genetic counseling referrals: March of Dimes Birth Defects Foundation; National Center for Education in Maternal and Child Health (NCEMCH).

References

Mendelian Inheritance in Man, 9th ed.: V.A. McKusick; The Johns Hopkins University Press, 1990, p. 1338.

Nelson Textbook of Pediatrics, 13th ed.: R.E. Behrman and V.C. Vaughan, III, eds.; W.B. Saunders Company, 1987, pp. 1324–1325.

Cerebral Infarction Due to Moyamoya Disease in Young Adults: A. Bruno, et al.; Stroke, July 1988, issue 19(7), pp. 826–833.

Ocular Symptoms of Moyamoya Disease: S. Noda, et al.; Am. J. Ophthalmol., June 15, 1987, issue 103(6), pp. 812–816.

Pitfalls in the Surgical Treatment of Moyamoya Disease. Operative Techniques for Refractory Cases: S. Miyamoto, et al.; J. Neurosurg. April 1988, issue 68(4), pp. 537–543.

Treatment of Acute Deficits of Moyamoya Disease with Verapamil: M.J. McLean, et al.; Ann. Acad. Med. Singapore, January 1985, issue 14(1), pp. 65–70.

MULTIPLE SCLEROSIS (MS)

Description The course of MS, a chronic demyelinating central nervous system **(CNS)** disorder, is variable; it may advance, relapse, remit, or stabilize. Demyelinating plaques scattered throughout the CNS interfere with neurotransmission and cause a range of neurologic symptoms.

Synonyms

Disseminated Sclerosis

Insular Sclerosis

Signs and Symptoms Symptoms can range from visual impairment, including blind spots, diplopia, and nystagmus, to impairment of speech, paresthesias or numbness, difficult ambulation, and dysfunction of the bladder and bowel. MS is rarely fatal; the average life expectancy is 93 percent that of the general population. One in 5 MS patients experiences but one attack, followed by little or no advance in the disorder. Two-thirds of patients are independently ambulatory 25 years post diagnosis. Approximately 50 percent of those pursue most of the activities they engaged in prior to onset of the disease. In some, however, paralysis of varying severity necessitates the use of canes, crutches, and other ambulatory aids. In a small minority of patients the disease accelerates quickly and may result in life-threatening complications.

Etiology Multiple sclerosis is idiopathic. An autoimmune association, possibly in a viral or an environmental setting, has been suggested. The human T-lymphotropic virus (HTLV-I), a retrovirus that has been associated with other CNS disorders and certain blood malignancies, has been implicated. A hereditary predisposition has been suggested, but a precipitating factor must also be present.

Studies have shown that siblings of a patient with MS are at a 10 to 15 percent higher risk of developing MS than the general population, whose risk is 0.1 percent. A Canadian study indicated that daughters of mothers with MS have a 5 percent risk. Certain histocompatibility antigens may be involved.

A 1989 Australian study implicated a feline virus. Approximately 7 percent of domestic cats have been shown to have a demyelinating disease that closely resembles MS. Both infected cats and patients with MS have yielded a morbillivirus. Confirmatory studies are yet to come.

Epidemiology In the United States, MS affects approximately 58:100,000 persons in the United States, numbering approximately 130,000 individuals. The disease may appear at any age, but diagnosis is most often made between the ages of 20 and 40. MS is more common in whites than in American blacks and Orientals. In a few ethnic societies (Eskimos, Bantus, American Indians), MS is rare or absent, which may hint at a genetic link. MS seems to occur more often in temperate regions of the world.

Treatment—Standard MS has evaded both cure and prevention. Routinely, ACTH, prednisone, or another corticosteroid is given to alleviate attacks, but these drugs have no effect on the progression of the disorder. Several classes of drugs bring symptomatic relief, including muscle relaxants to reduce muscle spasms, and antidepressants, aspirin, or acetaminophen to lessen pain. Physical therapy and exercise, particularly aquatic programs, may be beneficial.

Treatment—Investigational Research regarding MS is vigorous. Among the drugs and modalities under investigation are the following.

Cyclophosphamide. Some patients in studies have had temporary improvement. The goal of current treatment protocols, in which maintenance booster injections are given, is sustaining the effects of the drug.

Beta-interferon. Intrathecal injections appear to halve the rate of exacerbations in some patients.

Copolymer 1. This orphan drug, a synthetic polypeptide developed in Israel and manufactured by Lemmon Pharmaceuticals, has had a 2-year trial, the results of which have been announced by Dr. Murray Bornstein of Albert Einstein College of Medicine. The subjects were 50 patients with relapsing-remitting MS, some of whom received copolymer I and some a placebo. The average number of attacks per patient was markedly lower in the copolymer group. Currently an international trial of several hundred patients is ongoing.

4-Aminopyridine. Intravenous injections of this drug, which can increase conduction in demyelinated pathways, resulted in varying degrees of improvement of vision, eye movement, coordination, and walking in 10 of the 12 subjects. Investigators at the Rush Medical College in Chicago reported that the improvements lasted about 4 hours, and a current study is evaluating the effects of longterm treatment with 4-aminopyridine.

Hyperbaric oxygen. This method of therapy has been disappointing.

Monoclonal antibodies. Researchers are exploring the potential of monoclonal antibodies in preventing MS progression; these antibodies may interrupt the autoimmune process. Initial trials have shown the treatment to be without adverse effects. A prime candidate is an antibody to the immune response antigen, an antibody that may disrupt the physiology of MS but not interfere with the immune system.

Immunosuppressive drugs. The immunosuppressive drugs are under investigation for use in MS. Recent research involving one immunosuppressive drug, cyclosporine, however, found that the therapeutic dose required in MS is so high that it would entail unacceptable side effects.

Betaseron. This orphan drug, a type of beta-interferon, is manufactured by Triton Biosciences. Patients currently being treated are those with a relapsing and remitting form of MS.

Baclofen. Intrathecal infusion of baclofen through a surgically implanted pump is under study for its effect on spasticity. Infusion into the spinal space, rather than the oral route, seems to afford better reduction in spasticity and improvement of muscle tone for longer periods. Also, a lower dose seems to be required when the drug is infused. Research on baclofen for spasticity is supported by an orphan drug grant from the FDA.

Alpha-interferon. This antiviral compound has been given experimentally to patients with MS. Early findings indicate that alpha-interferon may delay attacks, thereby reducing their number.

Irradiation. This modality is in experimental use to reduce T-cell—producing tissue in patients with MS. Lymphoid irradiation focuses on the spleen and the lymph nodes.

Other therapies undergoing study are plasmapheresis and regimens of amantadine and colchicine.

Please contact the agencies listed under Resources, below, for the most current information.

Resources

For more information on multiple sclerosis: National Organization for Rare Disorders (NORD); NIH/National Institute of Neurological Disorders & Stroke (NINDS); National Multiple Sclerosis Society, National Headquarters. (The National Multiple Sclerosis Society maintains over 120 chapters throughout the United States. These chapters provide direct services to people with MS and their families, including occupational and physical therapy, support groups, clinics, and professional and public education. Information about chapters can be obtained from the national office.)

For genetic information and genetic counseling: March of Dimes Birth Defects Foundation; National Center for Education in Maternal and Child Health (NCEMCH).

References
Intrathecal Baclofen for Severe Spasticity: R.D. Penn, et al.; N. Engl. J. Med., June 8, 1989, issue 320(23), pp. 1517–1521.

MUSCULAR DYSTROPHY, BATTEN TURNER

Description Batten Turner syndrome is a benign congenital form of muscular dystrophy.

Synonyms
Benign Congenital Muscular Dystrophy Syndrome

Signs and Symptoms The initial sign in an infant may be floppiness. Later a mild muscular weakness and hypotonia make the child prone to falling and stumbling. Early motor development and milestone achievements may be minimally retarded. Especially susceptible to weakness and hypotonia are the pelvic girdle, neck, and shoulder girdle. As a rule, walking becomes normal later in life, but physical activities may be hampered. Fractures and paralysis are not part of the symptom complex.

Etiology Batten Turner muscular dystrophy is idiopathic.

Epidemiology Infants and young children of either sex are affected.

Treatment—Standard Exercise and avoidance of obesity are important for patients with Batten Turner muscular dystrophy. The outlook for minimal muscular deficiency is excellent. Many patients have no major physical handicaps.

Treatment—Investigational Please contact the agencies listed under Resources, below, for the most current information.

Resources
For more information on Batten Turner muscular dystrophy: National Organization for Rare Disorders (NORD); Muscular Dystrophy Association; Muscular Dystrophy Group of Great Britain and Northern Ireland; Society for Muscular Dystrophy International; NIH/National Institute of Neurological Disorders & Stroke (NINDS).

References
Mendelian Inheritance in Man, 9th ed.: V.A. McKusick; The Johns Hopkins University Press, 1990, p. 1367.

Cecil Textbook of Medicine, 18th ed.: J.B. Wyngaarden and L.H. Smith, Jr., eds.: W.B. Saunders Company, 1988, pp. 2272–2275.

MUSCULAR DYSTROPHY, BECKER (BMD)

Description Becker muscular dystrophy is a slowly progressive wasting myopathy that affects particularly the hip and shoulder muscles.

Synonyms
> Benign Juvenile Muscular Dystrophy
> Progressive Tardive Muscular Dystrophy

Signs and Symptoms Onset of BMD is usually during the patient's 2nd or 3rd decade. On palpation, the muscles have a firm, rubbery feel. Deep tendon reflexes may be absent early in the disorder. Walking is impaired. Eventually, joint contractures, scoliosis, and restrictive lung disease may appear. Cardiac complications are rare. The patient may have mild mental retardation.

It is possible to test for muscular dystrophy in utero and postnatally. The prenatal genetic test identifies the fetus as a carrier of the gene associated with muscular dystrophy. The postnatal test uses antidystrophin antibodies to check for the protein dystrophin in muscle tissue. A deficiency or an abnormality of dystrophin is responsible for the symptoms in BMD.

Etiology The disorder is inherited as an X-linked recessive trait. However, approximately 30 percent of patients with any type of muscular dystrophy have no familial history. Diagnosis in these cases is facilitated by the ability to test for dystrophin.

Epidemiology BMD is almost exclusively limited to males, with an incidence of about 1:30,000 live births. Females may be carriers; usually they remain asymptomatic but in most carriers the serum creatine phosphokinase (CPK) is high.

Related Disorders Onset of **Leyden-Moebius muscular dystrophy (limb-girdle muscular dystrophy)** is before adolescence. Progressive weakness and muscle deterioration occur most severely in the pelvic girdle, but muscles of the face, shoulders, and arms are also affected.

Gower muscular dystrophy, usually with onset in adulthood, begins in the hands and feet, slowly progressing to proximal body areas. Only moderate weakness occurs.

Treatment—Standard Treatment consists of exercise, physical therapy, and the use of orthoses. Genetic counseling may be helpful.

Treatment—Investigational Please contact the agencies listed under Resources, below, for the most current information.

Resources
For more information on Becker muscular dystrophy: National Organization for Rare Disorders (NORD); Muscular Dystrophy Association; NIH/National

Institute of Neurological Disorders & Stroke (NINDS); Muscular Dystrophy Group of Great Britain and Northern Ireland; Society for Muscular Dystrophy International.

For genetic information and genetic counseling referrals: March of Dimes Birth Defects Foundation; NIH/National Center for Education in Maternal and Child Health (NCEMCH).

References

Mendelian Inheritance in Man, 9th ed.: V.A. McKusick; The Johns Hopkins University Press, 1990, pp. 1679–1688.

Evaluation of Carrier Detection Rates for Duchenne and Becker Muscular Dystrophies Using Serum Creatine-Kinase (CK) and Pyruvate-Kinase (PK) through Discriminant Analysis: M. Zatz, et al.; Am. J. Med. Genet., October 1986, issue 25(2), pp. 219–230.

Preferential Deletion of Exons in Duchenne and Becker Muscular Dystrophies: S.M. Forrest, et al.; Nature, October 15–21, 1987, issue 329(6140), pp. 638–640.

MUSCULAR DYSTROPHY, DUCHENNE (DMD)

Description DMD is one of the most frequently encountered types of muscular dystrophy. It is also the fastest in its spread of muscle degeneration. Almost all affected children are boys.

Synonyms

Childhood Muscular Dystrophy

Pseudohypertrophic Muscular Dystrophy

Signs and Symptoms The weakness associated with DMD usually does not manifest before age 2 to 5 years. Initially, muscle wasting is confined to the pelvic and shoulder girdle muscles. Infiltration of fat and connective tissue produces hypertrophy of the calf muscles. Within several years the disorder affects the musculature of the upper trunk and arms, and finally all major muscles. DMD runs a consistent and consequently a predictable course.

The affected child's symptoms include falls, waddling gait, and awkwardness in raising himself from the floor; these are often attributed to clumsiness. By age 3 to 5 years, however, weakness becomes apparent. The parents may be falsely encouraged by a seeming improvement between ages 3 and 7, but it is due to natural growth and development. Weakness progresses rapidly after age 8 or 9, resulting in inability to walk or stand alone. Leg braces may make walking possible for a year or two, but the patient will need a wheelchair by early adolescence, or before.

As a rule, the next stage produces a marked increase in contractures and scoliosis. Lung capacity may be diminished, increasing susceptibility to respiratory infections.

Tests are available to detect muscular dystrophy either before or after birth. The prenatal examination determines whether the fetus is carrying the DMD gene. The postnatal test employs antidystrophin antibodies to locate dystrophin in muscle tissue. Individuals with DMD lack dystrophin; those with Becker muscular dystrophy have a normal amount of dystrophin in the tissue, but the molecule is abnormal.

Etiology DMD is inherited as an X-linked trait; the responsible gene has been identified. Approximately 30 percent of patients are without a familial history, however, in which case the disorder is diagnosed by finding a deficiency of dystrophin in the muscles.

Epidemiology DMD is almost exclusively limited to boys. The estimated incidence is 1:4,000 male neonates.

Treatment—Standard Treatment consists only of supportive measures. Physical therapy and orthopedic devices can lessen some of the crippling associated with the disease.

Treatment—Investigational The gene appears to serve as the blueprint for the manufacture of dystrophin in muscle tissue. Symptoms occur when dystrophin is completely absent from the body. Investigation involving replacement of dystrophin is under way in individuals with DMD. Other studies involve prednisone, which appears to improve muscle strength in affected patients.

Please contact the agencies listed under Resources, below, for the most current information.

Resources

For more information on DMD: National Organization for Rare Disorders (NORD); Muscular Dystrophy Association; NIH/National Institute of Neurological Disorders & Stroke (NINDS); Muscular Dystrophy Group of Great Britain and Northern Ireland; Society for Muscular Dystrophy International.

For genetic information and genetic counseling referrals: March of Dimes Birth Defects Foundation; National Center for Education in Maternal and Child Health (NCEMCH).

References

Mendelian Inheritance in Man, 9th ed.: V.A. McKusick; The Johns Hopkins University Press, 1990, pp. 1679–1688.
Randomized, Double-blind Six-month Trial of Prednisone in Duchenne's Muscular Dystrophy: J.R. Mendell, et al; New Engl. J. Med., June 15, 1989, issue 320(24), pp. 1592–1597.

MUSCULAR DYSTROPHY, EMERY-DREIFUSS

Description Emery-Dreifuss muscular dystrophy attacks the musculature of the arms, legs, face, neck, spine, and heart. Encroachment is frequently slow.

Synonyms
Dreifuss-Emery Type Muscular Dystrophy with Contractures
Rigid Spine Syndrome
Tardive Muscular Dystrophy

Signs and Symptoms As a rule, the first sign of Emery-Dreifuss muscular dystrophy is toe-walking in a child age 4 to 5 years. This initial manifestation of slowly advancing muscle weakness in the legs may later be followed by waddling that is due to pelvic girdle weakness, and significant weakness of the shoulder muscles. Eventually the disorder may affect the nuchal muscles. Flexion contractures of the elbows and ankles may occur. The effect on the heart muscle is of major concern; the potential for severe cardiac complications is high.

Etiology Emery-Dreifuss is inherited as an X-linked trait. The recent appearance in females of a disorder with symptoms resembling those of Emery-Dreifuss raises the possibility of an additional route of inheritance, however.

Epidemiology Emery-Dreifuss is almost exclusively limited to males.

Related Disorders See *Muscular Dystrophy, Duchenne; Myotonic Dystrophy.*

Treatment—Standard Treatment is supportive, consisting of physical therapy and active and passive exercise. Agencies that provide services to handicapped people and their families may be helpful, as may genetic counseling.

Patients with cardiac complications are usually candidates for a pacemaker; antiarrhythmic drugs may be indicated.

Treatment—Investigational Heart transplantation has been attempted in patients with severe cardiac complications.

Please contact the agencies listed under Resources, below, for the most current information.

Resources

For more information on **Emery-Dreifuss muscular dystrophy:** National Organization for Rare Disorders (NORD); Muscular Dystrophy Association; Muscular Dystrophy Group of Great Britain and Northern Ireland; Society for Muscular Dystrophy International; NIH/National Institute of Neurological Disorders and Stroke (NINDS).

For **genetic information and genetic counseling referrals:** March of Dimes Birth Defects Foundation; NIH/National Center for Education in Maternal and Child Health (NCEMCH).

References

Mendelian Inheritance in Man, 9th ed.: V.A. McKusick; The Johns Hopkins University Press, 1990, pp. 1688–1690.

Cardiologic Evaluation in a Family with Emery-Dreifuss Muscular Dystrophy: G. Pinelli, et al.; G. Ital. Cardiol., July 1987, issue 17(7), pp. 589–593.

Lethal Cardiac Conduction Defects in Emery-Dreifuss Muscular Dystrophy: A.H. Oswald, et al.; S. Afr. Med. J., October 1987, issue 72(8), pp. 567–570.

X-Linked Muscular Dystrophy with Early Contractures and Cardiomyopathy (Emery-Dreifuss type): A.E. Emery; Clin. Genet. November 1987, issue 32(5), pp. 360–367.

MUTISM, ELECTIVE

Description Elective mutism is a rare pediatric psychiatric disorder in which a child chooses not to speak in a social setting. Comprehension and vocal ability are usually intact.

Signs and Symptoms The child may be overly shy, anxious, depressed, and manipulative. Usually mute in school—which he or she may refuse to attend—the child often talks normally at home. Some children, however, remain mute in almost every social setting, substituting gestures, nodding, sound, or words of one syllable for speech. Temper tantrums may occur, and the patient may respond negatively when given a chore. With strangers the child typically is compliant, reticent, and almost rigid. Progress in school and social life may be adversely affected. Usually elective mutism continues for only a few weeks or months, but a few cases on record have endured for several years.

Etiology Precipitating factors in elective mutism are recent immigration, hospitalization or trauma at a young age, social isolation, a language or speech disorder, and mental retardation. In addition, the child's family may be innately overly shy and reserved. When immigration is a factor, the diagnosis can only be made after the child has learned the new language.

Epidemiology While the onset of elective mutism is usually before age 5 years, it may not be apparent until the child starts school. The disorder occurs slightly more often in females than in males.

Related Disorders See *Autism.*

Delayed speech and language development may indicate a disorder of the nervous system, a cognitive impairment, or a degree of deafness. Or, delayed development may reflect an emotional, social, family, or behavioral problem. It is important to rule out tracheal and laryngeal dysfunction and an abnormality in oral-motor development.

In **aphasia,** trauma to the area in the brain that controls language adversely affects comprehension or oral expression. The highest incidence of aphasia is in individuals who have had a stroke or head trauma, but in children it may be congenital. The severity of cerebral trauma dictates the severity of the deficit. Severe damage may result in lack of comprehension of information given orally. Minor injuries may result in selective language impairment.

Pervasive developmental disorders are a group of uncommon psychiatric disorders with the common denominators of deficient social skills, impaired development of verbal and nonverbal communication, and an inability to participate in activities requiring imagination. The child may be slow in developing intellect, language and speech, and motor activity, including posture. The degree and form of these deficiencies vary widely among afflicted children. The most well-known pervasive developmental disorder is autism.

Developmental expressive language disorder is infrequently encountered. The child starts speaking late, and expansion of the words used is slow to evolve. When severe, the disorder is generally apparent before age 3; milder forms may go unnoticed until early adolescence.

Treatment—Standard The initial step is a workup, including hearing tests, to confirm elective mutism by exclusion. Upon confirmation, psychotherapy and behavior management constitute treatment. One method used is reinforcement conditioning, in which the patient is rewarded for compliance with an assigned task. A 2nd technique is counterconditioning, which entails substituting new behaviors for the unacceptable previous behaviors. The 3rd approach is shaping, a means of developing complex behaviors through increasing reinforcement of simple behaviors; the goal is that the child in time will adopt the desired complex behavior. Paramount in sustaining the positive changes is resolution of any attendant family problems.

Treatment—Investigational Please contact the agencies listed under Resources, below, for the most current information.

Resources

For more information on elective mutism: National Organization for Rare Disorders (NORD); NIH/National Institute of Mental Health; National Mental Health Association.

References

Diagnostic and Statistical Manual of Mental Disorders, 3rd ed., revised: R.L. Spitzer, et al., eds.; American Psychiatric Association, 1987, pp. 32–33, 38–39, 45–47, 88–89.

A Comparison of Elective Mutism and Emotional Disorders in Children: R. Wilkins; Br. J. Psychiatry, February 1985, issue 146, pp. 198–203.

Speech and Language Disorders in Children: D.C. Van Dyke, et al.; Am. Fam. Physician, May 1984, issue 29(5), pp. 257–268.

Stranger Reaction and Elective Mutism in Young Children: M. Lesser-Katz; Am. J. Orthopsychiatry, July 1986, issue 56(3), pp. 458–469.

MYASTHENIA GRAVIS (MG)

Description MG is a chronic neuromuscular disease marked by weakness and easy fatigability of the musculature, particularly of the bulbar-innervated muscles. MG is responsive to rest. Any muscle may be involved, but the extraocular muscles and those used in swallowing are most frequently affected.

Synonyms

Goldflam Disease

Signs and Symptoms The disorder may be so insidious in its initial stage that it is unrecognized. On the other hand, the onset of severe generalized weakness may be sudden. Symptoms correlate with the weakened muscles. Early symptoms reflect fatigue in the muscles employed in speech, swallowing, and chewing. The voice is nasal and tends to fade. Dysphagia poses the threat of food lodging in the trachea. Weakness of the extraocular musculature leads to 2 early signs, ptosis and diplopia, which worsen as the day goes on and improve with rest. Weakness of the limbs is often present and is most intense after exercise and in the evening.

In most patients, intervals of improved strength intersperse those of greater weakness. Many events, such as infection, overdoing physical activity, emotional upset, menstruation, and pregnancy can trigger short-term intensity of symptoms. At its worst, the sudden escalation of MG may lead to **myasthenia gravis crisis**. In that case, the patient experiences sudden, severe muscle weakness, particularly in the muscles used in respiration. The symptoms resemble those of cholinergic crisis, the cause of which is excessive dosage of anticholinesterase agents.

Rarely, patients have become asymptomatic spontaneously.

Maternal MG may result in the infant having a transient form of the disorder. Weakness is apparent at birth and persists for 18 to 50 days, after which function becomes normal.

Etiology Evidence indicates that MG is an autoimmune disorder in which antibodies bind to the acetylcholine receptor on muscles, thus interrupting neuromuscular transmission. This interference causes weakening of the muscles upon repeated use.

Epidemiology Approximately 100,000 individuals in the United States have MG. Onset is at any age; in females, it is usually at ages 15 to 35 and in males at ages 40 to 70. Younger females tend to have generalized MG, while males are more likely to have localized symptoms in the extraocular muscles. Any type may strike at any age in either sex, however.

Treatment—Standard For many years the agents of choice for symptomatic relief have been the anticholinesterase drugs, especially pyridostigmine and neostigmine. Edrophonium is used to diagnose MG. ACTH is indicated for severely ill patients.

Physicians at the National Institute of Neurological and Disorders and Stroke are trying a new drug regimen for MG: a longterm course of alternate-day prednisone in a single high dose. This treatment has been effective over long periods in most of the patients treated, with patients over age 40, especially males, showing the best response.

Thymectomy has been therapeutic in a number of patients, many of whom had advanced disease. Recent studies have led a number of physicians to consider that thymectomy should be done in most patients with MG.

Certain drugs can aggravate symptoms in MG. Contraindicated are curare, quinidine, quinine, and some antibiotics; tonic water is a source of quinine.

Treatment—Investigational The National Institute of Neurological Disorders and Stroke (NINDS) has studied plasmapheresis as a treatment for MG. The procedure has been effective in strengthening patients before and after thymectomy. It is also useful in reducing symptoms during treatment with immunosuppressive drugs and in MG crisis.

Cyclosporine, an immunosuppressive drug, is undergoing trials as a treatment for MG. Some patients have shown increased strength after using the drug.

Studies are being conducted to evaluate the use of sandoglobulin in MG.

Please contact the agencies listed under Resources, below, for the most current information.

Resources

For more information on MG: National Organization for Rare Disorders (NORD); Myasthenia Gravis Foundation, Inc.; NIH/National Institute of Neurological Disorders & Stroke (NINDS); Muscular Dystrophy Association.

For genetic information and genetic counseling referrals: March of Dimes Birth Defects Foundation; National Center for Education in Maternal and Child Health (NCEMCH).

References

Cecil Textbook of Medicine, 18th ed.: J.B. Wyngaarden and L.H. Smith, Jr., eds.: W.B. Saunders Company, 1988, pp. 2285–2287.

MYELITIS

Description Myelitis refers to inflammation of segments of the spinal cord. The disease may be acute or chronic and has many subdivisions: acute transverse myelitis; ascending myelitis; Brown-Séquard syndrome; concussion myelitis; Foix-Alajouanine myelitis (subacute necrotizing myelitis); funicular myelitis; systemic myelitis; transverse myelitis.

Signs and Symptoms Local back pain is a common presenting symptom. Frequently present are muscle spasms, malaise, headache, anorexia, and numbness or paresthesias of the legs. Sensorimotor paralysis below the level of the lesion may cause urinary retention, sexual dysfunction, and fecal incontinence. Below the spinal lesion tendon reflexes may be absent. Frequently the thoracic area is affected, resulting in abdominal muscle paralysis. Symptoms may abate minimally in time, but this is cause-dependent.

In **acute transverse myelitis,** there may be congested or obstructed blood vessels, edema, cellular infiltration or loss, and demyelination.

In **ascending myelitis,** loss of sensation becomes more extensive with time.

Brown-Séquard syndrome is a disorder in which spinal cord compression and lesions affect one half of the spinal cord. Inflammation, trauma, foreign bodies, or meningovascular syphilis may be causative.

In **disseminated myelitis** there is more than one spinal cord segment lesion.

Etiology Although myelitis is often idiopathic, a viral infection, trauma to the spinal cord, an immune reaction, or a circulatory deficiency in the cord per se may be the cause. Furthermore, the disorder may be a complication of demyelination, a reaction to rubella or varicella vaccines, or a symptom of neurovascular syphilis or acute encephalomyelitis.

Epidemiology Onset may be at any age. Males and females are affected in equal numbers.

Related Disorders See *Spinal Stenosis.*

Cervical spondylitis is the result of nerve root compression and a narrowed spinal canal. The precipitating factors are collapse of disc spaces, thickening of ligaments, and bony overdevelopment. Pain, initially in the nuchal area, may eventually extend to the shoulders and arms and possibly affect motion.

Treatment—Standard Treatment is symptomatic and supportive.

Treatment—Investigational Electrical stimulation is under study as therapy in some cases of myelitis. The multiprogrammable spinal cord stimulator, which is being assessed for its ability to control motor dysfunction, produces epidural spinal electrostimulation (**ESES**). When implanted in the spine, it may improve the range of motion and reduce muscle spasms and pain in some types of myelitis or myelopathy as well as in other neuromuscular disorders that are refractory to more conventional modalities.

Please contact the agencies listed under Resources, below, for the most current information.

Resources

For more information on myelitis: National Organization for Rare Disorders (NORD); American Paraplegia Society; American Spinal Injury Association; Spinal Cord Society; Spinal Cord Injury Hotline; NIH/National Institute of Neurological Disorders & Stroke (NINDS); NIH/National Institute of Allergy and Infectious Diseases (NIAID).

References

Acute Transverse Myelopathy in Childhood: K. Dunne, et al.; Dev. Med. Child. Neurol., April 1986, issue 28(2), pp. 198–204.

Evoked Potentials in Acute Transverse Myelopathy: C.H. Wulff; Dan. Med. Bull., October 1985, issue 32(5), pp. 282–286.

Recurrent Transverse Myelitis Associated with Collagen Disease: M. Yamamato; J. Neurol., June 1986, issue 233(3), pp. 185–187.

MYOCLONUS

Description Myoclonus is a movement disorder in which a skeletal muscle undergoes sudden, involuntary contractions. Clinically, there are 3 types of myoclonus—intention, rhythmical, and arrhythmic; the following are some examples of these types.

Intention myoclonus (action myoclonus): postanoxic; postencephalitic.

Arrhythmic myoclonus (stimulus-sensitive myoclonus): hereditary essential myoclonus (paramyoclonus multiplex); hyperexplexia (essential startle disease); opsoclonus (infantile myoclonic encephalopathy, polymyoclonia familial arrhythmic myoclonus); progressive myoclonic epilepsy; Ramsay Hunt syndrome (dyssynergia cerebellaris myoclonia).

Rhythmical myoclonus (segmental myoclonus): nocturnal myoclonus; palatal myoclonus; respiratory myoclonus.

Signs and Symptoms Intention myoclonus is marked by episodes triggered by voluntary movements, such as a purposeful action.

In **arrhythmic myoclonus,** muscle jerks are arrhythmic and unforeseeable.

The jerking may be confined to a single muscle or involve the whole skeletal musculature. Severity, simultaneity, and symmetry of muscle contractions differ in the individual patient as well as among patients. The stimulus may be visual, auditory, or tactile, or it may be physical fatigue, stress, or anxiety. In women, myoclonus is often more intense premenstrually.

In **hyperexplexia,** the patient's startle reaction is extreme; muscle jerks come and go. **Opsoclonus** is localized; both eyes jerk simultaneously and irregularly. When opsoclonus occurs in infants with generalized myoclonus, the infant is said to have **infantile myoclonic encephalopathy** or **polymyoclonia familial. Progressive myoclonic epilepsy,** which is potentially disabling, combines severe epilepsy with significant stimulus-sensitive myoclonus. In advanced disease, dementia may appear. **Ramsay Hunt syndrome** comprises many disorders: epilepsy, myoclonus, and marked spinocerebellar degeneration as well as other nonstable neurologic abnormalities.

Rhythmical (segmental) myoclonus has a distinctive hallmark: the muscles jerk at a frequency of 10 to 180 jerks/minute. The affected muscles are generally those innervated by one or more contiguous spinal cord segments. In contrast to arrhythmic myoclonus, this type is not relieved by sleep or coma and is not triggered by sudden stimuli or voluntary movements. In **nocturnal myoclonus** there is frequent jerking of the body or extremities, particularly the legs, 2 to 3 times a minute when falling asleep, sleeping, or during deep relaxation during the day. Insomnia frequently accompanies these attacks. In **palatal myoclonus** there are quick rhythmical contractions of the soft palate and sometimes other muscles including those of the pharynx, larynx, eyes, face, and diaphragm occur. **Respiratory myoclonus** causes rapid rhythmic muscular contractions of the diaphragm, sometimes leading to dyspnea.

Etiology Several types of arrhythmic myoclonus are hereditary: hereditary essential myoclonus (autosomal dominant), progressive myoclonic epilepsy (usually autosomal recessive, whether alone or in conjunction with a hereditary disease such as Tay-Sachs or Kufs), and Ramsay Hunt syndrome (autosomal dominant).

Myoclonus is believed in the majority of patients to be due to excessive neuronal discharge. In rhythmical or segmental myoclonus, local trauma to the spinal motor neurons is usually responsible. Hyperexcitability of foci in the medullary reticular formation or cerebral cortical pathways is the cause of arrhythmic myoclonus. Some types of intention myoclonus, essential myoclonus, and progressive myoclonus epilepsy may be associated with a drop in the activity in the brain of the neurotransmitter, serotonin.

Viral, vascular, neoplastic, or traumatic lesions to the central nervous system may precede either rhythmical or arrythymic myoclonus. Cerebral oxygen deprivation due to cardiac or respiratory failure can cause myoclonus. Also implicated are certain toxins, including some therapeutic drugs in high doses, and metabolic disorders.

Related Disorders The differential diagnosis of myoclonus includes fasciculations, tics, chorea, athetosis, dystonia, and hemiballismus. It is important to rule out tremor, particularly that associated with cerebellar disease.

Treatment—Standard Certain drugs are indicated for treating the various types of arrhythmic myoclonus. For example, the benzodiazepine derivatives, especially clonazepam, are given in most forms of arrhythmic myoclonus, including progressive myoclonus epilepsy, Ramsay Hunt syndrome, myoclonus associated with idiopathic epilepsy, infantile spasms, and postencephalitic and postanoxic intention myoclonus. Diazepam is also used in these disorders. The patient may become tolerant to these drugs after a course of several months. Meanwhile, side effects, such as sleepiness, ataxia, lethargy, and aberrant behavior may appear. Anticonvulsant drugs with antimyoclonic activity may also be useful.

Valproic acid is most therapeutic in the longterm treatment of progressive myoclonus epilepsy; it is less effective in some other forms of the disorder. The drug is not without side effects, however, which may be transient: nausea, vomiting, diarrhea, abdominal pain, and possibly hepatic damage.

ACTH or prednisone is indicated in a few types of myoclonus. These include infantile spasms, infantile myoclonic encephalopathy, and opsoclonus accompanying neuroblastoma.

Rhythmical myoclonus is more refractory. Among the drugs that have recently shown therapeutic potential in the disorder are clonazepam, tetrabenazine, and haloperidol.

Treatment—Investigational An antimyoclonic drug, L-5 hydroxytryptophan (L-5HTP) is still undergoing study. This serotonin precursor, in combination with carbidopa, which prevents the conversion of L-5HTP to serotonin outside the central nervous system, is being investigated for its efficacy in postanoxic intention myoclonus, progressive myoclonus epilepsy, essential myoclonus, and palatal myoclonus. The gastrointestinal side effects of diarrhea and nausea are kept to a minimum by correct proportions of carbidopa. Combinations of clonazepam, valproic acid, and L-5HTP with carbidopa may in some patients be the therapy of choice. L-5HTP is being developed by Bolar Pharmaceutical Co., Inc., 130 Lincoln Street, Copiague, New York 11726.

The Food and Drug Administration (FDA) has awarded a research grant to Lawrence Scrima, Ph.D., University of Arkansas for Medical Science, Little Rock, Arkansas, for studies on gamma-hydroxybutyrate as a treatment for nocturnal myoclonus.

Please contact the agencies listed under Resources, below, for the most current information.

Resources

For more information on myoclonus: National Organization for Rare Disorders (NORD); National Myoclonus Foundation; NIH/National Institute of Neurological Disorders & Stroke (NINDS); Epilepsy Foundation of America.

References

Myoclonus: M.H. Van Woert and H.E. Chung; in Handbook of Clinical Neurology, vol. 38: P.J. Vinken and G.W. Bruyn, eds.; North Holland Publishing Co., 1979, pp. 575–593.

Myoclonus. What Causes It, What Controls It: M.H. Van Woert and H.E. Chung; in Consultant, April 1982, pp. 263–273.

Treatment of Myoclonus: M.H. Van Woert and H.E. Chung; *in* Current Status of Modern Therapy, vol. 8: A. Barbeau, ed.; MTP Press, 1980.

MYOSITIS, INCLUSION BODY (IBM)

Description IBM is a slowly progressive inflammatory disease of the skeletal muscles associated with microtubular filament inclusions in muscle cells.

Signs and Symptoms As a rule, the disorder is not accompanied by skin rash, malignancy, or collagen vascular disease, although one or more of these have been present in certain patients with IBM. The absence of fever, headache, and joint and muscle pain differentiates IBM from polymyositis and dermatomyositis; the histopathology of IBM does, however, include macrophages (also associated with polymyositis). Distal muscle weakness and atrophy are prominent. Serum creatine kinase is only slightly elevated. Muscle biopsy and electromyography are useful for making a diagnosis.

Etiology Inclusion body myositis seems to be a distinct type of inflammatory muscle disease. Its cause is unknown.

Epidemiology In general, IBM is a disease of the elderly, most often male. On the average, onset occurs at age 53, but it has been reported in patients in their teens.

Related Disorders See *Polymyositis/Dermatomyositis; Mixed Connective Tissue Disease.*

Distal myopathy primarily attacks the small muscles of the extremities. As a rule, a patient is over age 40 when he experiences the first symptoms—weakness of the hands. The disorder is considered to be hereditary; the trait is autosomal dominant.

Generally, **oculopharyngeal muscular dystrophy** appears in adulthood with involvement of the extraocular muscles and those employed in swallowing. The characteristic facies, particularly ptosis, is similar to that of myasthenia gravis. The inheritance pattern is frequently autosomal dominant, but at times the disorder may be sporadic or autosomal recessive.

Treatment—Standard Inclusion body myositis is unresponsive to corticosteroids and other immunosuppressive drugs. To date, therapy is only symptomatic and supportive.

Treatment—Investigational Please contact the agencies listed under Resources, below, for the most current information.

Resources

For more information on inclusion body myositis: National Organization for Rare Disorders (NORD); The National Arthritis and Musculoskeletal and Skin Diseases Information Clearinghouse; Muscular Dystrophy Association.

References

Inclusion Body Myositis: A Chronic Persistent Mumps Myositis?: S.M. Chou; Hum. Pathol., August, 1986, issue 17(8), pp. 765–777.

Inclusion Body Myositis and Systemic Lupus Erythematosus: R.A. Yood, et al.; J. Rheumatol., June 1985, issue 12(3), pp. 568–570.

Mendelian Inheritance in Man, 8th ed.: V.A. McKusick; The Johns Hopkins University Press, 1986, p. 427.

Monoclonal Antibody Analysis of Mononuclear Cells in Myopathies. V: Identification and Quantitation of T8+ Cytotoxic and T8+ Suppressor Cells: K. Arahata, et al.; Ann. Neurol., May, 1988, issue 23(5), pp. 493–499.

MYOSITIS OSSIFICANS

Description Myositis ossificans is a progressive disorder characterized by calcifications in the skeletal musculature.

Synonyms

Fibrodysplasia Ossificans Progressiva (FOP)
Fibrosis Ossificans Progressiva
Guy-Patin Syndrome
Muenchmeyer Syndrome
Patin Syndrome
Stone Man

Signs and Symptoms The muscles invaded by calcification increasingly weaken and become rigid. Related tissue—that linking muscle to muscle and tendon to muscle—and the tendons themselves may be similarly affected. Upon muscular contraction, the patient usually experiences pain and tenderness. Some patients have bruise-like swelling of the skin over the site of the calcifications. In addition, shortened digits may be present. On rare occasions, deafness, baldness, or mental retardation may accompany the disorder. In the later stages of the disease, it may be impossible to predict its course. For example, scoliosis may or may not occur. In the most severely afflicted patients, ambulation may be impaired.

Etiology It is thought that myositis ossificans is inherited as an autosomal dominant trait. Muscle injuries that cause calcifications can, however, mimic hereditary myositis ossificans.

Epidemiology The medical literature has reported approximately 350 cases of myositis ossificans in this century. The disorder affects males and females in equal numbers; onset is commonly before age 10.

Related Disorders In **a variant of myositis ossificans,** calcifications are due to muscle injury. This form is not hereditary.

Pseudohypoparathyroidism is hereditary and X-linked. Normal quantities of the parathyroid hormone are present, but response to the hormone is insufficient, adversely affecting bone growth. Headaches, weakness, easy fatigability, lethargy, and blurred vision or photophobia may be present. Paresthesias, stiffness, or cramps in arms or legs; palpitations; and abdominal pain may occur. A round face, thick short stature, shortened digits, and mental deficiencies are also part of the pattern. The prognosis is favorable in most cases. Hormonal and calcium replacement therapy is often beneficial, but the stunting of growth may continue.

Calcinosis universalis is a skin disorder in which calcium deposits produce tenderness. Onset of this progressive disorder may be at any age. Calcium deposits around joints or in muscles may cause weakness and edema. Deposits may also settle in the kidneys, stomach, or lungs. The outlook depends on the extent of the disorder and treatment of associated infections.

Treatment—Standard Surgery or biopsy of calcifications may sometimes aggravate symptoms; surgery is reserved for the most seriously afflicted patients. Intramuscular injections, muscle trauma, puncture of a vein, or dental surgery may also worsen calcifications.

Corticosteroids and lidocaine may lessen inflammation and muscle stiffness. Prompt treatment of infections is essential. Otherwise, treatment is symptomatic and supportive. Agencies and programs for the handicapped may benefit patients and their families. Genetic counseling can help families with the hereditary form of myositis ossificans.

Treatment—Investigational Sonography, x-ray, and scintigraphy are being evaluated for their ability to locate and monitor the growth and size of calcifications in muscles.

Please contact the agencies listed under Resources, below, for the most current information.

Resources

For more information on myositis ossificans: National Organization for Rare Disorders (NORD); The National Arthritis and Musculoskeletal and Skin Diseases Information Clearinghouse; Muscular Dystrophy Association; International FOP Organization.

For information about scoliosis: National Scoliosis Foundation, Inc.

For genetic information and genetic counseling referrals: March of Dimes Birth Defects Foundation; National Center for Education in Maternal and Child Health (NCEMCH).

References

Diagnostic and Therapeutic Aspects of Myositis Ossificans (Author Transl.): P. Jenny, et al.; Z. Kinderchir., March 1982, issue 35(3), pp. 86–87.

Fibrodysplasia Ossificans Progressiva. The Clinical Features and Natural History of 34 Patients: J.M. Connor, et al.; J. Bone Joint Surg. [Br.], 1982, issue 64(1), pp. 76–83.

Treatment of Traumatic Myositis Ossificans Circumscripta; Use of Aspiration and Steroids: J.C. Molloy, et al.; J. Trauma, November 1976, issue 16(11), pp. 851–857.

MYOTONIC DYSTROPHY

Description Myotonic dystrophy is a rare, slowly progressive, inherited condition in which the relaxing power of the muscles is decreased and muscle atrophy occurs, especially in the muscles of the face and neck. Ocular muscles, the endocrine system, and the cardiovascular system may also be affected. Myotonic dystrophy may be mild or severe. If the latter, mentation may be affected. Onset typically occurs in late adolescence or young adulthood.

Synonyms
Curschmann-Batten-Steinert Syndrome
Myotonia Atrophica
Steinert Disease

Signs and Symptoms Early symptoms of myotonic dystrophy are the inability to relax muscles after they have been contracted, and muscle weakness. Depending on the muscles involved, manifestations may include drooping eyelids, a continually furrowed forehead, weakness in lifting, tongue weakness, and inability to relax the hand after shaking hands. The patient may trip or fall easily. Muscles of the face and neck are principally affected, but limb dystrophy is also common. Eventually generalized weakness ensues. Speech, finger grasp, and cardiac muscles are affected.

Myotonic dystrophy may be accompanied by mental deterioration or retardation and endocrine abnormalities such as low testosterone levels, amenorrhea, menstrual irregularities, infertility, and glucose intolerance.

Etiology Myotonic dystrophy is inherited as a dominant trait with incomplete penetrance. The responsible gene has been localized to chromosome 9. A genetic test is available with a 90 percent predictive accuracy.

Epidemiology Equal numbers of males and females are affected. New cases are primarily seen in young adults.

Related Disorders See **_Thomsen Disease (myotonia congenita)_,** in which there is a similar problem of muscle inability to relax after contraction, but in which the muscles themselves are well-developed and even large.

Treatment—Standard Treatment is symptomatic and supportive. Physiotherapy may be helpful in promoting remaining muscle strength. Genetic testing is available.

Treatment—Investigational Drugs under investigation for the treatment of myotonic dystrophy include tocainide (Xylotocan) and nifedipine. In addition, it is thought that selenium and vitamin E may increase muscle strength and alleviate some symptoms. Administration of these substances must be supervised to prevent toxic overdose.

Please contact the agencies listed under Resources, below, for the most current information.

Resources
For more information on myotonic dystrophy: National Organization for Rare Disorders (NORD); Muscular Dystrophy Association; NIH/National Institute of Neurological Disorders & Stroke (NINDS); The National Arthritis and Musculoskeletal and Skin Diseases Information Clearinghouse.

For genetic information and genetic counseling referrals: March of Dimes Birth Defects Foundation; National Center for Education in Maternal and Child Health (NCEMCH).

References

The Problem of Diagnosis and Therapy of Myotonic Dystrophy: F. Reisecker; Wien Med. Wochenschr., June 30, 1983, issue 133(12), pp. 319–321.

Nifedipine in the Treatment of Myotonia in Myotonic Dystrophy: R. Grant, et al.; J. Neurol. Neurosurg. Psychiatry, February 1987, issue 50(2), pp. 199–206.

Myotonic Dystrophy Treated with Selenium and Vitamin E: G. Orndahl, et al.; Acta Med. Scand., 1986, issue 219(4), pp. 407–414.

Antimyotonic Therapy with Tocainide Under ECG Control in the Myotonic Dystrophy of Curschmann-Steinert: U. Mielke, et al.; J. Neurol., 1985, issue 232(5), pp. 271–274.

NARCOLEPSY

Description Narcolepsy is marked by unnatural drowsiness during the day, cataplexy, hallucinations, sleep paralysis, and disrupted sleep during the night.

Synonyms
Gélineau Syndrome
Paroxysmal Sleep
Sleep Epilepsy

Signs and Symptoms Onset of narcolepsy is generally between ages 10 and 20. The development and the degree of symptoms vary greatly among patients. The various symptoms usually appear singly. Each onset may be separated by years from another, and there is variability in symptoms sequence. As a rule, the patient is an adolescent whose initial manifestations are mild. These intensify over the years, sometimes without change for months or years; at other times, changes can be rapid.

Exaggerated daytime drowsiness is usually the initial symptom, and may be described by the patient as sleepiness, tiredness, lack of energy, a sleep attack, or an inability to resist sleep. This unending susceptibility to drowsiness or falling asleep occurs daily, but the severity varies throughout each day. Total sleep time in each 24 hours is generally normal.

Cataplexy is a sudden loss of voluntary muscle tone. The usual background of an attack is anger, elation, or surprise. The episode may be a short period of partial muscle weakness, or almost complete loss of muscle control that persists for several minutes and climaxes in postural collapse. During the attack, the cataplectic patient cannot move or speak despite consciousness and at least partial awareness of surrounding activities.

Hypnagogic hallucinations are startling occurrences during the beginning or end of a sleep period. The hallucinations may pertain to any or all of the senses and be almost indistinguishable from reality.

In **sleep paralysis,** the patient wants to move but cannot do so and feels panic. The timing of this symptom coincides with falling asleep or waking up.

Many awakenings are typical in **disrupted nighttime sleep.** Nightmares, the urge to urinate, or sleep apnea (common in narcolepsy) may awaken the patient. At times there is no apparent reason for awakening, and frequently this type of awakening is associated with a craving for food, especially something sweet.

Etiology The cause is unknown. The disorder is known to be familial, and HLA associations have been reported.

Epidemiology The American Narcolepsy Association estimates the incidence of narcolepsy to be approximately 200,000 individuals in the United States. Approximately 5 percent of patients are symptomatic by age 10; 25 percent after age 20; and 18 percent after age 30. Onset after age 40 is unlikely. Narcolepsy tends to remain a lifelong condition.

Related Disorders Symptoms resembling those of narcolepsy may occur secondary to intracranial tumors, head trauma, cerebral arteriosclerosis, psychosis, and uremia. Cataplexy can be differentiated from familial periodic paralysis; in the latter, episodes are longer lasting and the metabolism of potassium is faulty.

Treatment—Standard Specific treatment for narcolepsy is lacking, but there are several drugs that may bring symptomatic relief. The treatment selected relates to the symptoms and prior response to therapy. In some patients, the disorder has more of an element of cataplexy, and in others, sleep attacks predominate. Those who are not seriously hampered by sleep attacks, sleepiness, or cataplexy may not require drug therapy.

Drugs indicated in sleep attacks and sleepiness include methamphetamines and amphetamines, although their side effects are potentially harmful. The most frequently encountered side effects are personality changes (particularly tenseness and irritability) and depression. These manifest during the late afternoon and evening as the drugs wear off, or on weekends if the patient has a tendency to reduce the dose during that period. Methylphenidate is the analeptic drug of choice in sleep attacks and drowsiness.

Treatment of cataplexy includes imipramine, desimipramine, and chlorimipramine. There is even less knowledge of the effects of lifelong use of these drugs than there is concerning those of the amphetamines. Two recognized side effects are sleepiness and impotence. Chlorimipramine is currently the most effective of these compounds.

Tolerance and the need for too-high dosage or the necessity to assess the symptom status may make withdrawal of drug therapy necessary. Sudden cessation of analeptic medications may result in exaggerated drowsiness and often a severe depression. Sudden withdrawal from imipraminic compounds may result in a marked acceleration of the cataplectic symptoms.

Sleep habits are an essential part of therapy. Assuring regular bedtimes and prevention of interruptions are important. Intervals of naps during the day may avert the hard-to-control continual need for daytime sleep. A physician-directed program can set the most beneficial sleep pattern.

Treatment—Investigational Two of the National Institutes of Health—the

National Institute of Mental Health and the National Institute of Neurological, Communicative Disorders and Stroke—support research in sleep disorders, including narcolepsy. Gamma-hydroxybutyrate (GHB), an orphan drug, is on trial for cataplexy in sleep disorder centers and is currently regarded favorably in the treatment of narcolepsy and cataplexy. Fewer episodes of sleep paralysis and hypnagogic hallucinations have also been recorded, and some patients have been able to stop or reduce their use of stimulants while taking GHB. Controlled studies of this drug, sponsored by an FDA Orphan Drug research grant, began in 1985. GHB is produced by Biocraft Laboratories, P.O. Box CN0200, Elmwood Park, New Jersey 07407.

Vitoxazine hydrochloride is also under study, especially in the control of cataplectic symptoms. For further information contact Stuart Pharmaceuticals, Division of ICI Americas, Inc., Wilmington, Delaware 19897.

Studies have begun in regard to human brain tissue in narcolepsy. Preliminary supposition is that narcoleptic patients may have an excess of dopamine receptors in the amygdala, the area that controls emotions. This abnormality of dopamine receptors may be associated with the emotional aspect that precipitates cataplexy.

Please contact the agencies listed under Resources, below, for the most current information.

Resources

For more information on narcolepsy: National Organization for Rare Disorders (NORD); American Narcolepsy Association, Inc.; Narcolepsy and Cataplexy Foundation of America; Narcolepsy Network; NIH/National Institute of Neurological Disorders & Stroke (NINDS).

For genetic information and genetic counseling referrals: March of Dimes Birth Defects Foundation; National Center for Education in Maternal and Child Health (NCEMCH).

References

Mendelian Inheritance in Man, 9th ed.: V.A. McKusick; The Johns Hopkins University Press, 1990, p. 645.

Genetic Markers in Narcolepsy: N. Langdon, et al.; Lancet, November 24, 1984, issue 8413(2), pp. 1178–1180.

Importance of Mazindol in the Treatment of Narcolepsy: H. Vespignani, et al.; Sleep, July 1986, issue 3(7), pp. 274–275.

Problems & Strategies Identified by Narcoleptic Patients: A.E. Rogers; Neurosurg. Nurs., December 1984, issue 6(16), pp. 326–336.

NEMALINE MYOPATHY

Description Nemaline myopathy is a congenital disease of the skeletal muscles. Under the microscope, nemaline rods—fine threads—are seen in the muscle fibers.

Synonyms

Congenital Rod Disease

Rod Myopathy

Signs and Symptoms Skeletal muscle floppiness may be apparent in the newborn. The musculature of the thin thighs and upper arms is very weak, as are the trunk muscles; posture may be affected. Neurologic examination of the infant may reveal absence of the deep tendon reflexes, impaired muscle tone, and soft muscles. Involvement of the muscles used in respiration or swallowing may be life-threatening. Aside from this complication, the prognosis is unpredictable. The disease progresses during childhood, but increase in muscle mass during the growing years may offset the progression and the child may show general improvement. The facial muscles can be markedly affected. High arched palate, thin face, prominent jaw, and pectus carinatum are sometimes seen. In the adult-onset cases, varying degrees of weakness of shoulder and pelvic girdle muscles are seen.

Etiology Nemaline myopathy is inherited as an autosomal dominant trait; a recessive inheritance has been reported. The biochemical defect involved is not known.

Epidemiology The age of onset varies from early childhood to middle life.

Related Disorders See *Central Core Disease.*

Treatment—Standard Treatment is symptomatic and supportive.

Treatment—Investigational Please contact the agencies listed under Resources, below, for the most current information.

Resources

For more information on nemaline myopathy: National Organization for Rare Disorders (NORD); NIH/National Institute of Neurological Disorders & Stroke (NINDS).

For genetic information and genetic counseling referrals: March of Dimes Birth Defects Foundation; National Center for Education in Maternal and Child Health (NCEMCH).

References
Mendelian Inheritance in Man, 9th ed.: V.A. McKusick; The Johns Hopkins University Press, 1990, pp. 646–647.
Harrison's Principles of Internal Medicine, 12th ed.: J.D. Wilson, et al., eds.; McGraw-Hill, 1991, p. 2114.

OBSESSIVE-COMPULSIVE DISORDER

Description Obsessive-compulsive disorder is a neurotic condition in which persistently recurrent ideas and fantasies and specific repetitive actions and impulses cause marked distress and interfere with the person's normal routine. Inner conflict, anxiety, and depression are common associated characteristics.

Synonyms
Obsessive-Compulsive Neurosis

Signs and Symptoms Common obsessions range from worrying over whether one has locked a door or been contaminated by contact with another person or thing, to repeated impulses toward violence. The individual usually recognizes that these ideas, images, or impulses are intrinsic to himself and attempts to suppress them. Compulsive behaviors include repetitive hand-washing, verifying, and touching. The individual may resist such impulses, but acting on them relieves tension. The course of the disorder is variable and chronic, with mild, moderate, or severe symptomatic episodes followed by intermittent periods of remission.

Etiology The cause of obsessive-compulsive disorder is not known.

Epidemiology Symptoms are commonly first seen in the teen and early adult years, although childhood onset is possible. Males and females are affected in equal numbers. The mild form of this disorder may be quite common; only a small percentage of affected persons are impaired significantly enough to warrant treatment.

Related Disorders The disorder may be differentiated from **obsessive-compulsive personality disorder,** whose characteristics are perfectionism and inflexibility, exemplified by such behaviors as avoidance of decision-making; preoccupation with details, rules, and efficiency; and inability to express affection.

Treatment—Standard Appropriate treatment options for obsessive-compulsive disorder include insight psychotherapy, supportive therapy, behavioral techniques, or pharmacologic therapy with tricyclic antidepressants and monoamine oxidase inhibitors.

Treatment—Investigational Clinical trials of the drug fluoxetine for obsessive-compulsive disorder are under way. For more information: Eli Lilly & Company, Lilly Corporate Center, Indianapolis Indiana 46285; (201) 261-2000.

Please contact the agencies listed under Resources, below, for the most current information.

Resources

For more information on obsessive-compulsive disorder: National Organization for Rare Disorders (NORD); Obsessive-Compulsive Disorder Foundation, Inc.; NIH/National Institute of Mental Health (NIMH); National Mental Health Association.

References
Diagnostic and Statistical Manual of Mental Disorders, 3rd ed., revised: R.L. Spitzer, et al., eds.; Am. Psychiat. Asso., 1987, pp. 245–247, 354–356.

Intravenous Chlorimipramine in the Treatment of Obsessional Disorder in Adolescence: Case Report: L.B. Warneke; J. Clin. Psychiatry, March 1985, issue 46(3), pp. 100–103.

Psychotherapeutic Management of Obsessive-Compulsive Patients: L. Salzman; Am. J. Psychother., July 1985, issue 39(3), pp. 323–330.

Successful Treatment of Obsessive-Compulsive Disorder with ECT: L.A. Melman, et al.; Am. J. Psychiatry, April 1984, issue 141(4), pp. 596–597.

Biological Factors in Obsessive-Compulsive Disorders: S.M. Turner, et al.; Psychol. Bull., 1985, issue 97(3), pp. 430–450.

Evidence for a Biological Hypothesis of Obsessive-Compulsive Disorder: J.Lieberman; Neuropsychobiology, 1984, issue 11, pp. 14–21.

OLIVOPONTOCEREBELLAR ATROPHY

Description Olivopontocerebellar atrophy describes 5 inherited forms of ataxia characterized by wasting or diminution of the cerebellar cortex, the middle peduncles, and the inferior olivary bodies: type I (Menzel type); type II (Fickler-Winkler type; Dejerine-Thomas type); type III (with retinal degeneration); type IV (Schut-Haymaker type); type V (with dementia and extrapyramidal signs).

Synonyms
　　Multiple Systems Atrophy

Signs and Symptoms Manifestations vary, and include ataxia, spasticity, and extrapyramidal rigidity. Optic atrophy, retinitis pigmentosa, ophthalmoplegia, dysphagia, and dementia may also be present. As discussed above, 5 clinical types of olivopontocerebellar atrophy have been described.

Olivopontocerebellar atrophy I (Menzel type) is characterized by cerebellar degeneration, speech disturbances, and chorea. Average age at onset of symptoms is 30 years.

Olivopontocerebellar atrophy II (Fickler-Winkler or Dejerine-Thomas type) is not well understood; the disorder appears to manifest at around age 50 years.

Olivopontocerebellar atrophy III (with retinal degeneration) is characterized by blindness, tremor, weakness, and ataxia.

Olivopontocerebellar atrophy IV (Schut-Haymaker type) is accompanied by abnormalities of the spinal cord and cranial nerves. Spastic paraplegia and other symptoms manifest during the middle 20s.

Olivopontocerebellar atrophy V (with dementia and extrapyramidal signs) manifests as cerebellar atrophy, tremor, ataxia, rigidity, and mental deterioration in affected adults.

Etiology Types I and III through V are inherited as autosomal dominant traits. Olivopontocerebellar atrophy type II is inherited as an autosomal recessive trait.

Epidemiology The 5 forms of the disorder appear to affect males and females in equal numbers.

Related Disorders See *Ataxia, Friedreich; Ataxia, Marie; Charcot-Marie-Tooth Disease.*

Treatment—Standard Treatment of olivopontocerebellar atrophy is symptomatic and supportive. Pharmacologic therapy with propranolol or dantrolene sodium may be beneficial in the management of static tremors and muscle spasms, respectively. Physical therapy may be helpful; genetic counseling is recommended.

Treatment—Investigational Please contact the agencies listed under Resources, below, for the most current information.

Resources

For more information on olivopontocerebellar atrophy: National Organization for Rare Disorders (NORD); National Ataxia Foundation; NIH/National Institute of Neurological Disorders & Stroke (NINDS).

For genetic information and genetic counseling referrals: March of Dimes Birth Defects Foundation; National Center for Education in Maternal and Child Health (NCEMCH).

References

Mendelian Inheritance in Man, 9th ed.: V.A. McKusick; The Johns Hopkins University Press, 1990, pp. 671–674, 1392.

Olivopontocerebellar Atrophy with Dementia, Blindness, and Chorea. Response to Baclofen: D.A. Trauner; Arch. Neural., August 1985, issue 42(8), pp. 757–758.

Olivopontocerebellar Atrophy. A Review of 117 Cases: J. Berciano; J. Neurol. Sci., February 1982, issue 53(2), pp. 253–272.

An Apology and an Introduction to the Olivopontocerebellar Atrophies: R.C. Duvoisin; Adv. Neurol., 1984, issue 41, pp. 5–12.

ONDINE'S CURSE

Description Congenital central hypoventilation syndrome is characterized by dysfunction of the central regulation of respiration. The disorder typically affects infants. Insufficient aeration of the lungs due to shallow breathing may cause brain damage and death.

Synonyms

Congenital Central Hypoventilation Syndrome (CCHS)
Primary Central Hypoventilation Syndrome

Signs and Symptoms The clinical picture is dominated by nocturnal hypoventilation, resulting in hypoxemia, hypercapnia, and acidosis. Severity of the symptoms in infants may decrease with age.

Etiology The cause is not known.

Epidemiology Congenital central hypoventilation syndrome begins in infancy. Rarely, trauma (surgical or accidental) may precipitate the syndrome in adolescents and adults. Very few cases have been reported.

Related Disorders Congenital central hypoventilation syndrome must be distinguished from infantile apnea, characterized by intermittent cessation of breathing, and from chronic obstructive lung disease, characterized by dyspnea, coughing, and an onset coinciding with bronchiolitis. See *Apnea, Infantile.*

Treatment—Standard Monitoring of sleep patterns is recommended.

Respiratory stimulants such as almitrine and dimefline may be prescribed to deepen nocturnal respiration and improve blood gas values. Tracheostomy and cribral cannulation have been used for surgical correction.

Treatment—Investigational Radiofrequency electrophrenic respiration (diaphragmatic pacing) lowers pulmonary artery pressure and improves alveolar respiration; its use is still experimental but promising. Low-flow oxygen with a body respirator 2 nights a week has also been used successfully.

Please contact the agencies listed under Resources, below, for the most current information.

Resources
For more information on Ondine's curse: National Organization for Rare Disorders (NORD); NIH/National Institute of Neurological Disorders & Stroke (NINDS); NIH/National Institute of Child Health and Human Development (NICHHD).

References
Cecil Textbook of Medicine, 18th ed.: J.B. Wyngaarden and L.H. Smith, Jr., eds.; W.B. Saunders Company, 1988, p. 111.

ORGANIC PERSONALITY SYNDROME

Description Organic personality syndrome is a neuropsychiatric disorder caused by structural brain damage or impaired cerebral function. Persistent psychiatric and neurotic symptoms may involve mood, perception, attention, intellectual functioning (including cognition and memory), and personality. The duration and degree of significant personality changes depend upon the organic cause.

Synonyms
Organic Brain Syndrome

Signs and Symptoms Typical character traits may be more pronounced, or the individual's usual behavior may change. Symptoms are related to the nature and location of the brain dysfunction. Marked apathy, emotional instability, impaired judgment, and belligerence are common characteristics.

Etiology The most frequent cause of organic personality syndrome is structural brain damage from neoplasms, head trauma, or cerebrovascular disease. Endocrine disorders such as thyroid and adrenocortical disease, vitamin B12 deficiency, and the use of psychoactive drugs (including drug and alcohol abuse) are associated less often with this syndrome.

Epidemiology Males and females of all ages are equally affected. Organic personality syndrome frequently is a sign of an underlying disease or condition (see Related Disorders).

Related Disorders Huntington disease or dementia often is a primary underlying cause of organic personality syndrome. (See *Huntington Disease.)*

Symptoms of the following disorders can be similar to those of organic personality syndrome: schizophrenia; antisocial personality disorder; attention deficit hyperactivity disorder. (See *Antisocial Personality Disorder; Attention Deficit*

Hyperactivity Disorder.) Since personality changes can occur in many disorders not due to an organic cause, a psychiatric and/or neurologic evaluation should be performed to establish a differential diagnosis and to determine the cause of any extreme or persistent change in behavior.

Treatment—Standard Treatment depends upon the cause. Personality changes due to medications or drug abuse often can be reversed when the offending agent has been eliminated or reduced. Appropriate treatment of an underlying neurologic disorder can help eliminate symptoms of organic personality syndrome. When the syndrome arises from neoplasms in the brain, prognosis depends upon the tumor type, the patient's age, and the tumor location. Surgery may be effective in some cases, causing little or no permanent change in intellectual ability and quality of life.

Treatment—Investigational Please contact the agencies listed under Resources, below, for the most current information.

Resources

For more information on organic personality syndrome: National Organization for Rare Disorders (NORD); National Mental Health Association; NIH/National Institute of Mental Health (NIMH).

References
Diagnostic and Statistical Manual of Mental Disorders, 3rd ed., revised: R.L. Spitzer, et al., eds.; Am. Psychiat. Asso., 1987, pp. 114–116.

Cognitive Outcome and Quality of Life One Year After Subarachnoid Haemorrhage: P. McKenna, et al.; Neurosurgery, March 1989, issue 24(3), pp. 361–367.

National Survey of Patterns of Care for Brain-Tumor Patients: M.S. Mahaley, Jr, et al.; J. Neurosurgery, December 1989, issue 71(6), pp. 826–836.

Nonpsychotic Involutional Inhibited Depressions and Psycho-Organic Deteriorations: Treatment with Viloxazine and Piracetam: A. Borromei, et al.; Minerva Med., May 1989, issue 80(5), pp. 475–482.

Partial Section of the Corpus Callosum: Focal Signs and Their Recovery: A. Castro-Caldas, et al.; Neurosurgery, September 1989, issue 25(3), pp. 442–447.

PANIC-ANXIETY SYNDROME

Description Panic-anxiety syndrome is a psychiatric disorder characterized by acute attacks of anxiety or panic with no apparent cause. These attacks tend to be unpredictable and recurrent.

Synonyms
Anxiety Neurosis
Anxiety State
Panic Disorder

Signs and Symptoms The primary feature is acute anxiety, or panic, that initially develops abruptly for no evident reason and interferes temporarily with rational thoughts and behavior. Later, the patient may relate certain events with his feelings of anxiety or panic. Psychological symptoms may include intense apprehension, unreasonable fear of impending doom, such as fear of dying or becoming insane, or dread of losing self-control. Cardiorespiratory symptoms are the most common physical manifestations, such as dyspnea, tachycardia, palpitations, sweating, trembling, and dizziness or faintness. Patients also may experience chest pain, feelings of unreality, unusual sensations (burning or pricking), or hot and cold flashes. Attacks occur suddenly, typically last only a few minutes to an hour, and follow a chronic course.

Secondary complications may develop. Fear of losing control may result in **agoraphobia,** the fear of being in places or situations which are difficult to escape from or in which help might not be available. Fear of future attacks may cause patients to experience nervousness, muscle tension, and increased blood pressure and heart rate between attacks. Attempts to alleviate the constant nervousness can lead to abuse of alcohol or antianxiety medications. Depressive disorders also can develop as an associated complication.

Etiology Although the specific cause of panic-anxiety disorder is unknown, disruption of important interpersonal relationships may predispose to the development of the condition. Excessive secretion of the hormone norepinephrine, which stimulates the autonomic nervous system, is one possible effect of panic-anxiety disorders which may produce some of the symptoms, such as tachycardia. Hypersensitivity to lactates, which usually accumulate during physical exertion, also may be a contributing factor. Studies with caffeine suggest a potential relationship between panic-anxiety syndrome and abnormalities in the neural systems involving adenosine.

Researchers have been able to trigger panic attacks by exposing patients to carbon dioxide or some other substances. A brain chemical, cholecystokinin, has been found to provoke panic attacks 20 seconds after injection. The significance of this finding is unclear.

Epidemiology Females tend to be affected more frequently than males in panic disorder with agoraphobia, but panic disorder without agoraphobia is equally common in males and females. The average age of onset is usually in the late 20s.

Related Disorders Phobias can cause physical symptoms that resemble panic-anxiety syndrome; however, these symptoms occur only in response to specific stimuli. Panic-anxiety syndrome may be differentiated by the unpredictability of the anxiety attacks.

Withdrawal from barbiturates and substance intoxications (caffeine, alcohol, or amphetamines) also may produce symptoms of panic attacks.

The chronic anxiety characteristic of **generalized anxiety disorder** often resembles the anxiety that can develop between attacks in panic-anxiety syndrome. However, the typical recurrent fits of panic associated with the latter are not evident in generalized anxiety disorder.

Panic attacks can occur with such other psychiatric disorders as **major depression** or **somatization disorder.**

Treatment—Standard Alprazolam and imipramine hydrochloride are the main therapeutic agents used to treat panic-anxiety syndrome.

Treatment—Investigational Please contact the agencies listed under Resources, below, for the most current information.

Resources

For more information on panic-anxiety syndrome: National Organization for Rare Disorders (NORD); Anxiety Disorder Association of America; Mental Health Association; NIH/National Institute of Mental Health (NIMH).

References

Diagnostic and Statistical Manual of Psychiatric Illness, 3rd ed., revised: R.L. Spitzer, et al., eds.; Am. Psychiat. Asso., 1987, pp. 235–241.

Neuroendocrine Correlates of Lactate-Induced Anxiety and Their Response to Chronic Alprazolam Therapy: D.B. Carr, et al.; Am. J. Psychiatry, April 1986, issue 4(143), pp. 483–494.

Noradrenergic Function and the Mechanism of Action of Antianxiety Treatment: D.S. Charney and G.R. Heninger; Arch. Gen. Psychiatry, May 1985, issue 5(42), pp. 473–481.

Increased Anxiogenic Effects of Caffeine in Panic Disorders: D.S. Charney, et al.; Arch. Gen. Psychiatry, March 1985, issue 3(42), pp. 233–243.

PARAPLEGIA, HEREDITARY SPASTIC

Description Hereditary spastic paraplegia is characterized by slow, progressive degeneration of the corticospinal tract. Manifestations of the disorder vary in accordance with the extent of neurologic damage and the mode of genetic inheritance, but they generally include muscle spasticity, weakness, and paralysis.

Synonyms

Familial Spastic Paraplegia
Spasmodic Infantile Paraplegia
Spastic Congenital Paraplegia
Spastic Spinal Familial Paralysis
Strümpell Familial Paraplegia
Strümpell-Lorrain Familial Spasmodic Paraplegia

Signs and Symptoms Symptoms may first appear in early childhood, or later in life. Weakness, stiffness, and spasticity of leg muscles may progress to muscle groups in other parts of the body. Increased tendon reflexes, generalized weakness, and urinary disturbances develop as the disorder progresses.

Etiology The disorder may be inherited as an autosomal dominant or recessive trait.

Related Disorders See *Arteriovenous Malformation; Werdnig-Hoffmann Disease.*

Treatment—Standard Treatment of hereditary spastic paraplegia is symptomatic and supportive. Foot bracing and physical therapy may be beneficial. Genetic counseling is recommended.

Treatment—Investigational The Food and Drug Administration (**FDA**) has awarded an orphan drug research grant to John H. Growdon, M.D., Massachusetts General Hospital, Boston, for studies on the experimental drug L-threonine for hereditary spastic paraplegia.

Infusion of the drug baclofen by a surgically implanted pump is being studied for spasticity, under an FDA orphan drug grant. Infusion of the drug directly into the spinal space, rather than oral administration, seems to provide patients with better relief of spasticity and improve muscle tone for longer periods of time. Less baclofen seems to be needed when administered in this way.

Please contact the agencies listed under Resources, below, for the most current information.

Resources

For more information on hereditary spastic paraplegia: National Organization for Rare Disorders (NORD); NIH/National Institute of Neurological Disorders & Stroke (NINDS).

For genetic information and genetic counseling referrals: March of Dimes Birth Defects Foundation; National Center for Education in Maternal and Child Health (NCEMCH).

References

Hereditary "Pure" Spastic Paraplegia: A Clinical and Genetic Study of 22 Families: A.E. Harding; J. Neurol. Neurosurg. Psychiatry, October 1981, issue 44(10), pp. 871–883.

Familial Spastic Paraplegia, Mental Retardation, and Precocious Puberty: M.I. Raphaelson, et al.; Arch. Neurol., December 1983, issue 40(13), pp. 809–810.

The Spinal Canal in Familial Spastic Paraplegia: D. Vassilopoulos, et al.; Eur. Neurol., 1981, issue 20(2), pp. 110–114.

Intrathecal Baclofen for Severe Spasticity: R.D. Penn, et al.; New Engl. J. Med., June 8, 1989, issue 320(23), pp. 1517–1521.

PARENCHYMATOUS CORTICAL DEGENERATION OF THE CEREBELLUM

Description Deterioration of the superficial layer of the cerebellum occurs in parenchymatous cortical degeneration of the cerebellum. Disability increases as the disease progresses.

Synonyms

Parenchymatous Cerebellar Disease

Signs and Symptoms Deterioration of the cerebellum gradually leads to slurring of speech, tremor of the lower extremities, and incoordination of the upper extremities.

Microscopic examination reveals the loss of certain cells and fibers of the cerebellar cortex, such as Purkinje cells, granular cells, and olivocerebellar fibers.

Etiology Parenchymatous cortical degeneration of the cerebellum may be inherited, or may be associated with underlying disease, especially cancer or alcoholism.

Epidemiology Symptom onset is usually during adulthood, although it may occur at any time.

Treatment—Standard Treatment is symptomatic and supportive.

Treatment—Investigational Please contact the agencies listed under Resources, below, for the most current information.

Resources

For more information on parenchymatous cortical degeneration of the cerebellum: National Organization for Rare Disorders (NORD); NIH/National Institute of Neurological Disorders & Stroke (NINDS); NIH/National Institute on Aging (NIA).

For genetic information and genetic counseling referrals: March of Dimes Birth Defects Foundation; National Center for Education in Maternal and Child Health (NCEMCH).

Parkinson Disease

Description Parkinson disease is a slowly progressive neurologic condition marked by tremor, muscular rigidity, slowness of movement, and difficulty initiating voluntary movements. Degenerative changes occur in the substantia nigra and other pigmented regions of the brain, accompanied by a decrease in dopamine levels in the brain. Parkinsonian symptoms occasionally develop secondary to hydrocephalus, cerebral trauma, encephalitis, infarcts or tumors near the basal ganglia, or exposure to certain drugs and toxins. The disease may not become incapacitating for many years.

Synonyms

    Juvenile Parkinsonism of Hunt (Hunt Corpus Striatum Syndrome; Pallidopyramidal Syndrome)

    Parkinsonism (Paralysis Agitans; Shaking Palsy; Secondary Parkinsonism; Symptomatic Parkinsonism; Postencephalitic Parkinsonism; Drug-Induced Parkinsonism; Parkinsonism Dementia Complex)

Signs and Symptoms Onset is insidious and often marked by a slight tremor, especially in the hands. Initially, the tremor occurs at rest, then becomes more pronounced with fatigue and emotional stress, diminishing during voluntary movements. The tremor may be limited to the arms or extend to the neck, jaw, and legs. Voluntary movements such as walking become increasingly difficult, and gait becomes slow, stiff, and shuffling. Cognition and sensation generally remain normal, although some patients experience mild to severe dementia. The depression that commonly develops may be part of the disease or a reactive response.

As the disease advances, a stooped posture and an immobile, unblinking facial expression with frequent drooling develops. Seborrhea may arise on the face and scalp.

Etiology In most cases, the cause of Parkinson disease is unknown. A few cases result from carbon monoxide or manganese poisoning. Drug-induced parkinsonian symptoms can develop from dopamine-receptor antagonistic drugs used to treat psychiatric disorders. These symptoms usually disappear when the drugs are withdrawn or the dosage is decreased, or with time during treatment.

Epidemiology Although 10 to 20 percent of all cases are diagnosed in individuals under age 40 years, Parkinson disease occurs primarily in the middle-aged and elderly populations. Between 300,000 and 500,000 cases of classic Parkinson disease are found in the United States. The National Institute of Neurological Disorders and Stroke reported recently that from a study of the prevalence of major neurologic disorders in a biracial population, the incidence of Parkinson disease demonstrates no gender or racial differences.

Juvenile parkinsonism of Hunt is an extremely rare hereditary syndrome with onset in teens, 20s, or early 30s. **Parkinsonism dementia complex** is associated with motor neuron disease or amyotrophic lateral sclerosis. This rare form has been found in western Pacific Islands and has been determined to be caused by consumption of a locally grown toxic bean.

A **drug-induced parkinsonism** was identified in young heroin addicts who abused a "designer drug" originally in a fairly localized community in California. Primates given the same toxic substance are considered a model for this disorder.

Treatment—Standard Some patients can enjoy a normal life span with drug treatment that provides varying degrees of symptomatic relief. A combination of levodopa and carbidopa is the treatment of choice, although this drug combination tends to become less effective over time.

Other useful drugs include anticholinergics and amantadine, a dopamine-releasing agent that works with levodopa. Anticholinergic agents, such as trihexyphenidyl, benztropine mesylate, biperiden, and diphenhydramine help control tremors and rigidity. Amantadine hydrochloride helps reduce tremors and rigidity and improves spontaneous movements. Bromocriptine and pergolide, which are dopamine agonists, may be useful in some cases, particularly in conjunction with the levodopa/carbidopa combination.

An orphan drug, deprenyl, is a monoamine-oxidase inhibitor that was approved by the FDA for use in the United States in 1989. This drug has been used in late-stage Parkinson disease to enhance the levodopa/carbidopa combination. Recent research suggests that the progression of more advanced symptoms may be delayed significantly by using deprenyl in the early stages of Parkinson disease.

Physical therapy involves exercises that may improve walking and speaking. Exercise does not stop the progression of the disease, but tends to reduce disability and improve emotional wellbeing.

Treatment—Investigational Dopamine agonists are a class of drugs being investigated for the treatment of Parkinson disease. A surgical treatment procedure in the very early stages of experimentation involves implanting cells from the patient's adrenal gland or from fetal tissue into the brain to increase the amount of dopamine available to the affected structures. Ongoing animal studies will help determine whether this procedure can be improved so that it will be more effective in humans.

Please contact the agencies listed under Resources, below, for the most current information.

Resources

For more information on Parkinson disease: National Organization for Rare Disorders (NORD); Parkinson Disease Foundation; United Parkinson Foundation; NIH/National Institute of Neurological Disorders & Stroke (NINDS).

References

Cecil Textbook of Medicine, 18th ed.: J.B. Wyngaarden and L.H. Smith, Jr., eds.; W.B. Saunders Company, 1988, pp. 2143–2147.

PARSONNAGE-TURNER SYNDROME

Description Parsonnage-Turner syndrome is characterized by neuritis of the brachial plexus.

Synonyms

Brachial Neuritis
Brachial Plexus Neuritis
Idiopathic Brachial Plexus Neuropathy
Neuralgic Amyotrophy

Signs and Symptoms The chief symptom is severe, sharp, lancinating pain in the shoulder, scapular region, and upper arm. The pain may be accompanied by unilateral or bilateral muscle weakness, atrophy, and hyperesthesia. Persons with this disorder generally recover within a few months, although symptoms may persist for several years.

Etiology The etiology is unknown. The syndrome may develop after immunization, viral infection, surgery, or Lyme disease. An autoimmune association is suspected.

Epidemiology Parsonnage-Turner syndrome occurs most often in young males, but anyone can be affected.

Related Disorders See *Peripheral Neuropathy.*

Rheumatoid arthritis is distinguished by morning stiffness, pain or tenderness, and swelling of one or more joints, chiefly in the hands, knees, feet, jaw, and spine. It is thought to be an autoimmune disorder.

Treatment—Standard Most patients with Parsonnage-Turner syndrome recover without treatment. Physical therapy may be helpful. Other measures are symptomatic and supportive.

Treatment—Investigational Please contact the agencies listed under Resources, below, for the most current information.

Resources
  For more information on Parsonnage-Turner syndrome: National Organization for Rare Disorders (NORD); The National Arthritis and Musculoskeletal and Skin Diseases (NIAMS) Information Clearinghouse.

References
Postpartum Idiopathic Brachial Neuritis: D. Dimitru, et al.; Obstet. Gynecol., March 1989, vol. 73(3), pp. 473–475.
Hypertrophic Brachial Plexus Neuritis: A Pathological Study of Two Cases: M. Cusiamano, et al.; Ann. Neurol., November 1988, vol. 24(5), pp. 615–622.
Brachial Neuritis Involving the Bilateral Phrenic Nerves: N. Walsh, et al.; Arch. Phys. Med. Rehabil., January 1987, vol. 68(1), pp. 46–48.
Injury to the Brachial Plexus During Putti-Platt and Bristow Procedures. A Report of Eight Cases: R. Richards, et al.; Am. J. Sports Med., July–August 1987, vol. 15(4), pp. 374–380.
Surgery for Lesions of the Brachial Plexus: D. Kline, et al.; Arch. Neurol., February 1986, vol. 43(2), pp. 170–181.
Brachial Neuritis: L. Dillin, et al.; J. Bone Joint Surg. [Am], July 1985, vol. 67(6), pp. 878–883.

PELIZAEUS-MERZBACHER BRAIN SCLEROSIS

Description Pelizaeus-Merzbacher brain sclerosis is a progressive disease of the central nervous system associated with deterioration of the white matter of the brain. The pathologic changes in the brain consist of destruction of the myelin sheath surrounding nerve cell axons with accumulation of the breakdown products of myelin. Affected areas include the subcortical cerebrum, cerebellum, and brain stem.

Coordination, motor abilities, and intellectual function deteriorate, and disease progression is usually rapid.

Synonyms
  Aplasia Axialis Extracorticalis Congenita
  Diffuse Familial Brain Sclerosis
  Pelizaeus-Merzbacher Disease
  Sudanophilic Leukodystrophy

Signs and Symptoms The first manifestations usually appear in early infancy, although onset is later in one form of the disease. The child grows slowly and fails to develop normal control of the head and eyes. Tremor, spasticity, grimacing, unsteadiness, muscle contractures, weakness, optic atrophy, and ocular nystagmus eventually develop. Skeletal deformations and convulsions also are sometimes seen.

Etiology Pelizaeus-Merzbacher brain sclerosis is hereditary, with infantile forms being either autosomal recessive or X-linked. A form with adult onset is autosomal dominant. The reasons for the degeneration of the white matter of the brain are not understood.

Epidemiology The infantile form affects males, while other forms may affect either sex.

Related Disorders Pelizaeus-Merzbacher brain sclerosis belongs to a group of degenerative brain diseases known as leukodystrophies, which are characterized by destruction of the white matter of the brain. See *Adrenoleukodystrophy; Alexander Disease; Leukodystrophy, Canavan; Leukodystrophy, Krabbe; Leukodystrophy, Metachromatic; Refsum Syndrome.*

Treatment—Standard Treatment for Pelizaeus-Merzbacher brain sclerosis is symptomatic. Supportive care, including emotional support for family members, is recommended as needed.

Treatment—Investigational Current research is directed toward the identification of the gene that causes Pelizaeus-Merzbacher brain sclerosis.

Please contact the agencies listed under Resources, below, for the most current information.

Resources

For more information on Pelizaeus-Merzbacher brain sclerosis: National Organization for Rare Disorders (NORD); United Leukodystrophy Foundation; NIH/National Institute of Neurological Disorders & Stroke (NINDS); Research Trust for Metabolic Diseases in Children.

References
Cecil Textbook of Medicine, 18th ed.: J.B. Wyngaarden and L.H. Smith, Jr., eds.: W.B. Saunders Company, 1988, p. 2216.

PERIPHERAL NEUROPATHY

Description Peripheral neuropathy produces sensory, motor, and autonomic symptoms. These can appear alone or in combination.

Synonyms
>
> Mononeuritis
> Mononeuritis Multiplex
> Mononeuropathy
> Multiple Peripheral Neuritis
> Peripheral Neuritis
> Polyneuritis
> Polyneuropathy

Signs and Symptoms Symptoms reflect disease of a single nerve (mononeuropathy, mononeuritis), several nerves in asymmetric areas of the body (mononeuritis multiplex), or symmetric involvement (polyneuropathy, polyneuritis, multiple peripheral neuritis). As a rule, lesions are degenerative; their sites are the nerve roots or the peripheral nerves. Tinel sign is helpful in locating the site of damage in some neuropathies, but electrical nerve conduction studies are the sine qua non.

Involvement of a single nerve produces mononeuropathy (mononeuritis), as in the compression and entrapment syndromes. Symptoms include weakness, pain, and paresthesias. In mononeuritis multiplex the nerves destined to be ultimately affected may all be diseased at onset or they may become involved as the disorder advances. The symptoms of multineural disease frequently mimic those of polyneuropathy.

Polyneuropathy is usually bilaterally symmetric, with a diverse spectrum of symptoms due to the variability of nerve involvement and the range of etiologies, including malnutrition, poisoning, diseases such as diabetes mellitus, and metabolic disorders. Development may take months or years, commonly starting with sensory disorders in the legs such as peripheral tingling, numbness, or burning pain. When the sensory loss is major, nontender ulcers on the digits or Charcot joints may be evident. A neurologic examination will show absence or weakening of the Achilles and other deep tendon reflexes. Weakness and atrophy of distal limb muscles and flaccid tone signal that the motor nerve fibers are affected.

Etiology Peripheral neuropathy has many different causes:

Mechanical pressure (e.g., compression, direct trauma, penetrating injuries, contusions, fracture, or dislocated bones), which can result in mononeuritis and sometimes mononeuritis multiplex.

Another type of mechanically induced neuritis may be due to heavy muscular activity and forced overextension of a nerve, as in certain construction or craft activities.

Neuropathy due to pressure, which commonly involves the superficial nerves (ulnar, radial, or peroneal) and may result from prolonged use of crutches, or staying in one position for too long. A tumor may exert such pressure, and nerves in narrow canals such as in the entrapment syndromes may be similarly affected.

Intraneural hemorrhage or **exposure to cold or to radiation.**

Vascular or collagen disorders such as polyarteritis nodosa, atherosclerosis, systemic lupus erythematosus, scleroderma, sarcoidosis, and rheumatoid arthritis, which can result in mononeuritis multiplex.

Related Disorders See *Guillain-Barré Syndrome; Carpal Tunnel Syndrome.*

Treatment—Standard Depending upon the type of peripheral neuropathy, the patient may recover without residual effects or partially recover and have sensory, motor, or vasomotor deficits and, if severely afflicted, chronic muscular atrophy.

Therapy is cause-oriented, e.g., control of diabetes, nutritional needs, changing recreational or work habits, or surgery to remove a tumor or repair a ruptured intervertebral disc. In entrapment or compression neuropathy, splinting or surgical decompression of the ulnar or median nerves is frequently curative. Peroneal and radial compression neuropathies require avoidance of pressure. Recovery is frequently slow; physical therapy and/or splints may be useful in preventing contractures.

Treatment—Investigational Please contact the agencies listed under Resources, below, for the most current information.

Resources

For more information on peripheral neuropathy: National Organization for Rare Disorders (NORD); NIH/National Institute of Neurological Disorders & Stroke (NINDS).

References

Cecil Textbook of Medicine, 18th ed.: J.B. Wyngaarden and L.H. Smith, Jr., eds.; W.B. Saunders Company, 1988, p. 507.

PICK'S DISEASE

Description Pick's disease is a degenerative neurologic disease affecting the frontal and temporal lobes of the brain. It is characterized by progressive dementia.

Synonyms

> Diffuse Degenerative Cerebral Disease
> Lobar Atrophy

Signs and Symptoms Clinically, Pick's disease closely resembles Alzheimer disease. In the early stages, memory is usually intact, and disorientation may be less pronounced than in Alzheimer disease. In later stages, however, there is loss of motor control and language functions, and severe dementia.

The disease is characterized by uneven atrophy of the brain, with marked changes in the frontal and temporal lobes, and other areas apparently intact. Brain tissue from persons with Pick's disease does not exhibit the neurofibrillary tangles and senile plaques characteristic of Alzheimer disease. Pick's argentophilic inclusion bodies are found in certain nerve cells of the brain.

Diagnosis of Pick's disease is usually made after a careful history and physical examination, including thorough neurologic evaluation, psychometric studies, magnetic resonance imaging and computed tomography, and electroencephalographic testing.

Etiology The cause is unknown, although some cases have been reported with dominant inheritance.

Epidemiology Females are affected more often than males. The disease usually begins in the 5th or 6th decade, but onset may be as early as age 30. The reported incidence in the United States is much lower than that of Alzheimer disease. Investigators in Michigan have reported 12 cases of Pick's disease in 35 years; in Minnesota, however, Pick's disease accounts for about 4 percent of dementias.

Related Disorders See *Alzheimer Disease; Huntington Disease.*

Dementia can be a symptom of many disorders, mimicking Alzheimer and Pick's diseases.

Treatment—Standard Treatment is symptomatic and supportive. Patients with progressive dementia often experience frustration, anxiety, and depression resulting from their inability to function at their previous level. These problems can be minimized by maintaining a stable home environment and a structured routine that does not place excessive demands on the patient. Sedatives should generally be avoided.

Treatment—Investigational Please contact the agencies listed under Resources, below, for the most current information.

Resources

For more information on Pick's disease: National Organization for Rare Disorders (NORD); NIH/National Institute of Neurological Disorders & Stroke (NINDS); NIH/National Institute on Aging; Alzheimers Disease and Related Disorders Association, Inc.

References

Harrison's Principles of Internal Medicine, 12th ed.: J.D. Wilson, et al., eds.; McGraw-Hill, 1991, p. 2062.

Mendelian Inheritance in Man, 9th ed.: V.A. McKusick; The Johns Hopkins University Press, 1990, p. 748.

POST-POLIO SYNDROME

Description Post-polio syndrome is characterized by progressive muscle weakness and deterioration of function in the previously affected muscles of an individual who had poliomyelitis at least 10 years earlier. Partial or complete recovery from the initial episode of polio is common, followed years later by a gradual recurrence of muscle weakness for which there is no other apparent cause.

Synonyms

Polio, Late Effects
Post-Polio Muscular Atrophy
Post-Polio Sequelae

Signs and Symptoms Muscle function gradually decreases and muscle weakness develops, usually in the limbs that previously had been most affected by the polio virus. Occasionally muscles are affected that are fully recovered or never had been involved in the initial polio episode. This latent polio syndrome may involve the muscles necessary for respiration, and cause other symptoms such as fatigue, muscle pain, and fasciculations.

Etiology The exact cause of post-polio syndrome remains unknown. Research has failed to prove early theories of reactivation of the dormant polio virus and a more rapid aging in certain parts of the nervous system of post-polio patients than their unaffected peers. Scientists recently determined that post-polio syndrome is not a form of amyotropic lateral sclerosis.

In a 1987 study of patients with post-polio syndrome, it was found that nerve cells in affected muscles may grow many small sprouts from the axons of healthy nerve cells during the recovery phase. These sprouts acquire the function of the polio-damaged neurons. After years of functioning beyond capacity, the healthy nerve cells can weaken and lose the ability to maintain the sprouts. The muscle becomes weaker as the sprouts begin to shrink. This discovery may be helpful in development of an experimental treatment to improve the sprouting of axons.

Other research being conducted to determine the cause of post-polio syndrome includes investigating the presence of abnormal proteins in cerebrospinal fluid, and examining the effect of the polio virus on nerve cells in muscle fibers of post-polio patients.

Epidemiology Approximately 20 percent of persons who recovered from poliomyelitis more than 10 years earlier may be affected by post-polio syndrome. Symptoms of this syndrome can appear 30 or more years after the initial polio episode.

Related Disorders Symptoms of poliomyelitis (infantile paralysis) are similar to those of post-polio syndrome.

Treatment—Standard Persons who had polio before the vaccine was developed should be evaluated for post-polio syndrome, including a complete physical examination and comprehensive muscle testing and gait analysis. Rehabilitation in the form of physical and occupational therapy may be helpful. Exercise, not exceeding 5 to 20 minutes' duration, and regular rest periods may be advised. Swimming is a particularly good form of exercise for post-polio patients. Changes in braces and medication and diet modification may be recommended. Excess weight is very disabling for weakened muscles. Occasionally a respirator is prescribed, such as a mouth intermittent positive pressure ventilation system, if breathing has been affected.

Treatment—Investigational Please contact the agencies listed under Resources, below, for the most current information.

Resources

For more information on post-polio syndrome: National Organization for Rare Disorders (NORD); Post-Polio National, Inc. (Post-Polio League for Information and Outreach); Polio Information Center; British Polio Fellowship; Centers for Disease Control.

For rehabilitation services: National Easter Seal Society for Crippled Children and Adults.

References
Mouth Intermittent Positive Pressure Ventilation in the Management of PostPolio Respiratory Insufficiency: J.R. Bach, et al.; Chest, June 1987, issue 91(6), pp. 859–864.

Handbook of the Late Effects of Poliomyelitis for Physicians and Survivors: G. Laurie, et al., eds.; G.I.N.I., 1984.

Late Effects of Poliomyelitis: L. Halstead, et al., eds.; Symposia Foundation, 1984.

PRIMARY LATERAL SCLEROSIS

Description Primary lateral sclerosis is an adult neurologic disease that affects the upper motor neurons (corticospinal tract). It is characterized by progressive muscle weakness in the facial area and the extremities, associated with spasticity and hyperactive deep tendon reflexes.

Synonyms
> Central Motor Neuron Disease
> Motor Neuron Disease

Signs and Symptoms Initially there are few symptoms, and neurologic dysfunction progresses slowly. Spasticity in the hands, feet, or legs produces slowness and stiffness of movement. Dragging of the feet is followed by inability to walk. Facial involvement may result in dysarthria. Sensory function and intellectual function remain intact. The disease may progress gradually over a number of years, with wasting and weakening of the affected muscles.

Etiology The etiology is unknown.

Epidemiology Males and females are affected equally. The average age of onset is about 32 years.

Related Disorders See *Amyotrophic Lateral Sclerosis.*

Multifocal motor neuropathy is clinically similar to ALS. However, lower motor neurons are mainly affected. The disease is characterized by slowly progressive muscle wasting and weakness without spasticity and stiffness. Immunosuppressive drugs have produced improvement in some cases.

Treatment—Standard Symptomatic treatment includes the use of baclofen and diazepam for spasticity and quinine to control cramps. Other measures may include physical therapy to prevent joint immobility and speech therapy for patients with dysarthria.

Treatment—Investigational Current research on motor neuron diseases involves nerve growth factors, axonal transport, androgen receptor in motor neurons, and DNA/RNA changes.

Please contact the agencies listed under Resources, below, for the most current information.

Resources

For more information on primary lateral sclerosis: National Organization for Rare Disorders; NIH/National Institute of Neurological and Disorders & Stroke (NINDS); The Amyotrophic Lateral Sclerosis Association.

References
Harrison's Principles of Internal Medicine, 12th ed.: J.D. Wilson, et al., eds.; McGraw-Hill, 1991, p. 2074.

Chronic Progressive Spinobulbar Spasticity. A Rare Form of Primary Lateral Sclerosis: J.L. Gastaut, et al.; Arch. Neurol., May 1988, vol. 45(5), pp. 509–513.

Clinical and Electrophysiological Studies in Primary Lateral Sclerosis: L.S. Russo, Jr.; Arch. Neurol., October 1982, vol. 39(10), pp. 662–664.

Primary Lateral Sclerosis; A Case Report: M.F. Beal, et al.; Arch. Neurol., October 1981, vol. 38(10), pp. 630–633.

Primary Lateral Sclerosis, a Debated Entity: K.A. Sotaniemi, et al.; Acta Neurol. Scand., April 1985, vol. 71(4), pp. 334–336.

PROGRESSIVE SUPRANUCLEAR PALSY (PSP)

Description PSP is characterized by impaired motor control, abnormal eye movements, and dementia.

Synonyms

    Nuchal Dystonia Dementia Syndrome

    Steele-Richardson-Olszewski Syndrome

Signs and Symptoms Onset of symptoms occurs from ages 50 to 70 years, and includes bradykinesia, visual impairment, and falling. Loss of voluntary (but preservation of reflexive) eye movements, particularly of vertical gaze, is accompanied by spastic weakness of the pharyngeal musculature, and signs of parkinsonism. The face is expressionless, and speech is forced and slurred. Apathy and dementia develop late in the course of the disorder, which progresses over a 6- to 8-year period. Degenerative changes occur in the basal ganglia, brain stem, and cerebellum.

Etiology The cause of PSP is unknown.

Epidemiology Males are affected twice as often as females.

Related Disorders See *Parkinson Disease.*

    Lacunar state is characterized by a progression of neurologic symptoms similar to that found in cases of stroke.

    Pseudobulbar palsy is characterized by symptoms similar to those of PSP; however, eye movements in affected individuals are normal.

Treatment—Standard Medical treatment of PSP is generally disappointing. Tricyclic antidepressant drugs such as amitryptiline and imipramine may bring symptomatic relief in some cases. Agents such as carbidopa/levodopa, bromocriptine, trihexyphenidyl, amantadine, and benztropine may relieve extrapyramidal symptoms early in the course. Pergolide has been helpful in some cases.

    Walking aids, such as a walker weighted in front, and wearing shoes with built-up heels, may help prevent patients from falling backwards.

Treatment—Investigational The National Institute of Neurological Disorders and Stroke (NINDS) is seeking certain individuals affected by progressive supranuclear palsy for participation in a clinical research study. For complete information, contact Irene Litvan, M.D., NINCDS Experimental Therapeutics Branch, Building 10, Room 5C106, Bethesda, Maryland 20892; (301) 496-7993.

Please contact the agencies listed under Resources, below, for the most current information.

Resources

For more information on progressive supranuclear palsy: National Organization for Rare Disorders (NORD); NIH/National Institute of Neurological Disorders & Stroke (NINDS); International Tremor Foundation; Society for Progressive Supranuclear Palsy (SPSP); Progressive Supranuclear Palsy Research Fund.

References

Progressive Supranuclear Palsy: H.L. Klawans; United Parkinson Foundation, 1981.

Scientific American MEDICINE: E. Rubinstein and D. Federman, eds.; Scientific American, Inc., 1978–1991, pp. 11:IV:8–9.

PSEUDOTUMOR CEREBRI

Description Pseudotumor cerebri is a syndrome of increased intracranial pressure. Although symptoms can mimic those of a brain tumor, no tumor is present.

Synonyms

Benign Intracranial Hypertension

Signs and Symptoms Symptoms include headache that typically is mild and resistant to analgesics. Features seen occasionally include papilledema with progressive visual loss, memory impairment, dizziness, and asthenia.

Spinal fluid pressure is elevated. Electroencephalogram findings usually are normal.

Etiology In most cases no specific cause can be identified. Possible causes include increased intracranial pressure secondary to chronic carbon dioxide retention and hypoxia, a parathyroid or adrenal gland disorder, iron deficiency anemia, and venous sinus thrombosis. Agents that have been implicated include corticosteroids, sex hormones, tetracycline, and nalidixic acid, and vitamin A in excessive amounts.

Epidemiology The female-to-male ratio is 8:1, and prevalence is highest among overweight females between the ages of 15 and 50. The general public appears to be affected at a rate of 0.9:100,000 persons, but this incidence increases to 13 to 15:100,000 persons among those who are 10 percent overweight, and to 19.3:100,000 persons among those who are 20 percent or more over their ideal weight.

Related Disorders See *Arachnoiditis.*

Epiduritis is characterized by inflammation of the dura mater. Symptoms can be similar to pseudotumor cerebri.

Treatment—Standard The cause determines treatment. Implicated medications should be discontinued. Lumbar punctures, performed daily at first, may lower pressure and relieve some of the symptoms. Occasionally a lumbar-peritoneal shunt may be required. Diuretics may be used.

Treatment—Investigational Please contact the agencies listed under Resources, below, for the most current information.

Resources

For more information on pseudotumor cerebri: National Organization for Rare Disorders (NORD); NIH/National Institute of Neurological Disorders and Stroke (NINDS).

References

Internal Medicine, 3rd ed.: J.H. Stein, ed.-in-chief; Little, Brown and Company, 1990, p. 2023.

Optic Nerve Head Drusen and Pseudotumor Cerebri: B. Katz, et al.; Arch. Neurol., January 1988, issue 45(1), pp. 45–47.

The Incidence of Pseudotumor Cerebri. Population Studies in Iowa and Louisiana: F.J. Durcan, et al.; Arch. Neurol., August 1988, issue 45(1), pp. 875–877.

Clinical Course and Prognosis of Pseudotumor Cerebri. A Prospective Study of 24 Patients: P.S. Sorenson, et al.; Acta Neurol. Scand., February 1988, issue 77(2), pp. 164–172.

Pseudotumor Cerebri in Men: K.B. Digre, et al.; Arch. Neurol., August 1988, issue 45(8), pp. 866–872.

REFLEX SYMPATHETIC DYSTROPHY SYNDROME (RSDS)

Description The wide variety of disorders encompassed in this syndrome are all characterized by chronic, severe pain that occurs with posttraumatic vasomotor changes. RSDS is easily misdiagnosed as just a painful nerve injury.

Synonyms

Algodystrophy
Algoneurodystrophy
Causalgia Syndrome
Posttraumatic Dystrophy
Reflex Neurovascular Dystrophy
Shoulder-Hand Syndrome
Steinbrocker Syndrome

Signs and Symptoms The usual presenting symptom is burning pain and stiffness in an arm or leg (although any area of the body may be affected) at the site of a previous injury but extending beyond the area of the earlier injury. Pain severity may be worse than the original injury. In the early stages, there may also be erythema, tenderness, and swelling. Hyperhidrosis may be present, and heat may intensify the discomfort. Range of motion may be decreased.

In some patients the condition progresses. Pain worsens, range of motion is further restricted, and motor weakness may be present. The skin may appear pale, pitted, or cyanotic.

A further stage may be associated with a decrease in pain, although more commonly pain becomes intractable and only mild relief can be obtained with treatment. Severe tendon contractures and muscle atrophy may accompany loss of strength. At this late stage, changes may become permanent. Osteoporosis and grooved nails may be present.

Etiology The cause is unclear, but a number of factors may contribute, particularly changes in autonomic nervous system function.

RSDS may be associated with infections, burns, radiation therapy, hemiparesis, and myocardial infarction. Spinal disorders such as cervical osteoarthritis also may be associated with the syndrome. No cause is found, however, in approximately 30 percent of cases.

Epidemiology RSDS appears to be more common among women than men, and among individuals over 50 years of age. It has also been seen among children and young adults.

Related Disorders See *Carpal Tunnel Syndrome; Erythromelalgia.*

Treatment—Standard Although no standard treatment for RSDS has been developed, prevention and early treatment of symptoms are recommended. Daily physical therapy should begin as soon as the diagnosis is confirmed. Whirlpool and paraffin wax baths are sometimes beneficial. Ice or heat applications should be avoided in most cases because they seem to cause overstimulation of nerve endings, resulting in increased discomfort.

Transcutaneous electrical nerve stimulation **(TENS)** may be used in the early stages of RSDS or added to an existing therapy program. Local or systemic glucocorticosteroids can be effective but must be used cautiously. Side effects are rarely seen with the lower doses recommended for RSDS, but weight gain, moon facies, and digestive upsets have been reported. Nonsteroidal antiinflammatory medications, other analgesics, and muscle relaxants are sometimes helpful. Other agents that have been used include guanethidine, propranolol, nifedipine, phenytoin, and tricyclic antidepressants.

Sympathetic blockade can be helpful for the intractable pain of the later stage of the disorder. A stellate ganglion block is used for upper extremity pain, and a lumbar sympathetic block is performed for lower extremity pain. Surgical or chemical sympathectomy may be undertaken if blockade is inadequate.

Treatment—Investigational Preliminary investigation of dorsal column stimulation, which involves a spinal implant device, shows promise. A similar device, the implanted morphine pump, is being used to deliver morphine directly to the spinal fluid.

Guanethidine monosulfate is being used experimentally as a treatment. For additional information, contact Ciba-Geigy Corporation, 556 Morris Ave., Summit, New Jersey 07901.

Please contact the agencies listed under Resources, below, for the most current information.

Resources
For more information on RSDS: National Organization for Rare Disorders

(NORD); Reflex Sympathetic Dystrophy Syndrome Association (RSDSA); The Arthritis Foundation; The National Arthritis and Musculoskeletal and Skin Diseases Information Clearinghouse.

References
Reflex Sympathetic Dystrophy Syndrome: Diagnosis and Treatment: R.W. Rothrock and D. Weiss, D.O.; Osteopathic Medical News, February 1987, pp. 20–25.

RESTLESS LEGS SYNDROME

Description Restless legs syndrome is a neurologic disorder in which aching and crawling sensations occur in the legs, usually at night. Patients attempt to relieve these irritating sensations by constantly moving their feet and legs. This syndrome can be hereditary, or it can develop as a complication of alcoholism, iron deficiency anemia, pregnancy, or diabetes.

Synonyms
Anxietas Tibialis
Ekbom Syndrome
Hereditary Acromelalgia

Signs and Symptoms Attacks commonly begin at times when the legs are resting, such as when going to bed or sitting still. Intense discomfort involving aching sensations and paresthesias occurs between the knee and ankle. These often intolerable sensations precipitate movement of the legs and feet, and interfere with the ability to fall asleep and maintain sleep. Myoclonic leg jerks just prior to the onset of sleep are reported more frequently in persons with restless legs syndrome, even when awake, than in the normal adult population. Psychological stress typically exacerbates symptoms.

Etiology Restless legs syndrome is inherited as an autosomal dominant trait in about one-third of all cases. Some research suggests that restless legs syndrome may be related to a slight defect in the way sleep is organized in the brain.

Epidemiology Males and females are equally affected. Onset usually occurs during adolescence, and the course is chronic. Alcoholism, anemia, diabetes, and pregnancy increase the risk of developing this disorder.

Related Disorders See *Myoclonus.*

Treatment—Standard Treatment is symptomatic. The application of cold compresses sometimes helps relieve aching sensations in the legs. Drug therapy with clonazepam, carbamazepine, and low doses of a combination of L-dopa and carbidopa has been reported to be effective. Patients with an inherited form of this disorder may benefit from genetic counseling.

Treatment—Investigational Please contact the agencies listed under Resources, below, for the most current information.

Resources
For more information on restless legs syndrome: National Organization for Rare Disorders (NORD); NIH/National Institute of Neurological Disorders & Stroke (NINDS).
For genetic information and genetic counseling referrals: March of Dimes Birth Defects Foundation; National Center for Education in Maternal and Child Health (NCEMCH).

References
Mendelian Inheritance in Man, 9th ed: V.A. McKusick; The Johns Hopkins University Press, 1990, p. 16.
Restless Legs Syndrome: Harvard Medical School Health Letter; August 1987, issue 10(12), pp. 2–3.

RETT SYNDROME

Description Rett syndrome, a degenerative disease with progressive encephalopathy, is behaviorally similar to autism and characterized by developmental regression or loss of previously acquired skills.

Synonyms
Cerebroatrophic Hyperammonemia

Signs and Symptoms Rett syndrome manifests after the first 7 to 18 months of the female infant's life. Rapid deterioration occurs for the next 18 months and leads to mental and physical retardation. Patients develop severe dementia, lose purposeful movements of hands, and appear autistic. Walking, if acquired at all, is characterized by a broad-based gait. Microcephaly develops with increasing age. Episodes of apnea followed by hyperventilation are common. Later, seizures, gait apraxia, and truncal ataxia are prominent. There is continued deterioration often resulting in death before 40 years of age.

Etiology Rett syndrome is an X-linked dominant genetic disorder.

Epidemiology Thus far, Rett syndrome has only been diagnosed in females. As of October 1986, 1100 cases had been reported worldwide; however, based on studies conducted in Sweden and Scotland, the disorder may be as prevalent as 1:12,000 live female births.

Related Disorders See *Autism; Cerebral Palsy.*

Treatment—Standard Physical therapy may help prevent stiffening and encourage mobility. Braces and splints are sometimes used to treat toe-walking, scoliosis, and clenched hands. Hydrotherapy or underwater jet massage may also be helpful. Seizures associated with Rett syndrome are treated with anticonvulsive medications. Music therapy has been helpful in achieving communication with some patients. Special education and related services in school are recommended.

Treatment—Investigational The drug naltretone is under investigation but has not been approved by the Food and Drug Administration for general use. Please contact the agencies listed under Resources, below, for the most current information.

Resources
    For more information on Rett syndrome: National Organization for Rare Disorders (NORD); International Rett's Syndrome Association; NIH/National Institute of Neurological Disorders & Stroke (NINDS).
    For genetic information and genetic counseling referrals: March of Dimes Birth Defects Foundation; National Center for Education in Maternal and Child Health (NCEMCH).

References
    Mendelian Inheritance in Man, 9th ed.: V.A. McKusick; The Johns Hopkins University Press, 1990, pp. 1715–1716.

SCAPULOPERONEAL MYOPATHY

Description Scapuloperoneal myopathy is a hereditary condition in which muscle wasting and consequent weakness of the scapular and peroneal musculature are hallmarks. It can be a single entity, but it may accompany several other disorders.

Synonyms
        Myogenic (Facio)-Scapulo-Peroneal Syndrome
        Scapuloperoneal Muscular Dystrophy
        Scapuloperoneal Syndrome, Myopathic Type

Signs and Symptoms Onset of muscle wasting and weakness may occur during the childhood years, but these features may have their onset in adulthood as well. The patient's initial complaint is likely to be one of weakness in the legs; symptoms involving the peroneal muscles usually precede those of the shoulder muscles. A few patients have wasting of the facial muscles. Both the rate of progression and the degree of weakness vary among patients.

Etiology Scapuloperoneal myopathy is hereditary; the trait is autosomal dominant.

Epidemiology Males and females are affected in equal numbers.

Related Disorders Davidenkov's syndrome (Kaeser syndrome; neurogenic scapuloperoneal amyotrophy) is marked by peroneal muscle weakness and atrophy with pedal abnormalities and an unusual gait. These signs and symptoms precede involvement of the shoulder muscles. Unlike scapuloperoneal myopathy, in this syndrome the nerve impulses may become significantly delayed. Pain, paresthesias in the legs, cardiac complications, and muscle contractures may also occur.

Treatment—Standard Treatment of scapuloperoneal myopathy consists of programmed therapeutic exercise and physical therapy interspersed with rest. Genetic counseling is advisable for patients and their families. Other treatment is symptomatic and supportive.

Treatment—Investigational Please contact the agencies listed under Resources, below, for the most current information.

Resources

For more information on scapuloperoneal myopathy: National Organization for Rare Disorders (NORD); The National Arthritis and Musculoskeletal and Skin Diseases Information Clearinghouse.

For genetic information and genetic counseling referrals: March of Dimes Birth Defects Foundation; National Center for Education in Maternal and Child Health (NCEMCH).

References

Scapuloperoneal Myopathy: D.H. Todman, et al.; Clin. Exp. Neurol., 1984, issue 20, pp. 169–174.

Scapuloperoneal Syndrome with Cardiomyopathy: Report of a Family with Autosomal Dominant Inheritance and Unusual Features: A. Chakrabarti, et al.; J. Neurol. Neurosurg. Psychiatry, December 1981, issue 44(12), pp. 1146–1152.

SEITELBERGER DISEASE

Description Seitelberger disease is an inherited central nervous system condition in which progressive muscular and coordination difficulties, speech and vision deficits, and impaired cerebral function develop.

Synonyms

Infantile Neuroaxonal Dystrophy

Signs and Symptoms Features of Seitelberger disease include impaired ability to speak or walk, hypotonia and loss of coordination, spasticity, loss of reflexes, and deafness. In later stages of the disease, there may be progressively impaired vision and involuntary rapid eye movements, dementia, and seizures. Most affected children die before age 6 years.

Etiology The disease is inherited as an autosomal recessive trait. There is some indication that it is the infantile form of Hallervorden-Spatz syndrome.

Epidemiology There is a slight predilection for females, with onset usually before the age of 2 years.

Related Disorders See *Hallervorden-Spatz Disease; Leukodystrophy, Metachromatic.*

Primary optic atrophy, which causes diminished visual acuity and decreased ability to see light, can be a symptom of Seitelberger disease. Symptoms may be caused by degeneration, shrinkage, or disappearance of nerve fibers.

Treatment—Standard Treatment is symptomatic and supportive, and services for visually and physically impaired persons can provide assistance. Genetic counseling may benefit families of affected patients.

Treatment—Investigational Please contact the agencies listed under Resources, below, for the most current information.

Resources

For more information on Seitelberger disease: National Organization for Rare Disorders (NORD); The Children's Brain Diseases Foundation For Research; NIH/National Institute of Neurological Disorders & Stroke (NINDS); United Leukodystrophy Foundation; National Ataxia Foundation.

For genetic information and genetic counseling referrals: March of Dimes Birth Defects Foundation; National Center for Education in Maternal and Child Health (NCEMCH).

References

Neuroaxonal Dystrophy in Childhood. Report of Two Second Cousins with Hallervorden-Spatz Disease, and a Case of Seitelberger Disease: K. Kristensson, et al.; Acta Paediatr. Scand., November 1982, issue 71(6), pp. 1045–1049.

Histological and Ultrastructural Features of Dystrophic Isocortical Axons in Infantile Neuroaxonal Dystrophy (Seitelberger Disease): M.H. Mitchell, et al.; Acta Neuropathol. (Berl), 1985, issue 66(2), pp. 89–97.

SHY-DRAGER SYNDROME

Description Shy-Drager syndrome is a progressive disorder of unknown cause marked by autonomic insufficiency associated with degeneration of cell bodies of preganglionic sympathetic nerves in the intermediolateral column of the spinal cord. Degeneration in other parts of the central nervous system can produce olivopontocerebellar and parkinsonian syndromes.

Synonyms

Orthostatic Hypotension in Neurologic Disease
Postural Hypotension
Progressive Autonomic Failure

Signs and Symptoms Onset of symptoms occurs at ages 40 to 75 years. The hallmark of the disorder is orthostatic hypotension. Urinary and bowel dysfunction, sexual impotence, and anhidrosis occur, followed by parkinsonlike neurologic disturbances, cerebellar incoordination, muscle wasting and fasciculations, and coarse tremors of the legs. The disease progresses over a course of 7 to 8 years, with fatal outcome.

Etiology The cause is not known, although environmental or genetic factors have been suggested. Symptoms result from an impairment of the autonomic nervous system.

Epidemiology Males are more commonly afflicted than females.

Related Disorders See *Parkinson Disease.*

Treatment—Standard Therapy should include counterpressure, as in the use of elastic stockings. Antiparkinson medication must be used cautiously because it may lower blood pressure. Dietary increases of salt used with flurohydrocortisone to increase intravascular pressure also should be used with care.

Treatment—Investigational The orphan drug midodrine is being investigated as a treatment for Shy-Drager syndrome. For more information, contact Roberts Pharmaceuticals, Meridian Center III, 6 Industrial Way West, Eatontown, New Jersey 07724; (201) 389-1182.

The National Institute of Neurological Disorders and Stroke (NINDS) is seeking certain individuals affected by Shy-Drager syndrome for participation in a clinical research project. For information, contact Ms. Linda Nee, M.S.W., or Ronald Polinsky, M.D., NINCDS Medical Neurology Branch, Building 10, Room 5N236, Bethesda Maryland 20892; (301) 496-8850.

Please contact the agencies listed under Resources, below, for the most current information.

Resources
For more information on Shy-Drager syndrome: National Organization for Rare Disorders (NORD); Shy-Drager Syndrome Support Group; International Tremor Foundation; NIH/National Institute of Neurological Disorders & Stroke (NINDS).

References
Cecil Textbook of Medicine, 18th ed.: J.B. Wyngaarden and L.H. Smith, Jr., eds.; W.B. Saunders Company, 1988, pp. 1466, 2106–2107, 2153.
Scientific American MEDICINE: E. Rubinstein and D. Federman, eds.; Scientific American, Inc., 1978–1991, p. 11:IV:8.

SPASMODIC TORTICOLLIS

Description Spasmodic torticollis is characterized by repetitive or continuous spasm of the cervical muscles, resulting in twisting of the neck and an unusual head posture.

Synonyms
Spasmodic Wryneck

Signs and Symptoms The onset may be gradual, with the head tending to rotate to one side when the patient attempts to hold it straight or is experiencing stress. One shoulder may be higher than the other. The symptoms may slowly progress, often reaching a plateau after 2 to 5 years.

In some cases pain is present, usually unilateral and in one site, often at the side of the neck, the back, or the shoulder. The severity of pain varies from person to person. After a night's sleep, for a period of 10 minutes to 4 hours, spasmodic torticollis may be relieved or subside completely. Lying supine also may relieve the spasms.

Approximately 5 percent of patients recover spontaneously, most often within 5 years. Recovery seems to be more common in milder cases and in those with onset before age 40. The disorder may recur after apparent remission.

Etiology In most cases, etiology is unknown. Occasionally, basal ganglia disease, central nervous system infection, or tumors in the neck have been thought to be the underlying cause.

Epidemiology Onset is generally in the 4th or 5th decade of life but may occur at any age. Females are affected slightly more often than males.

Related Disorders See *Torsion Dystonia.*

Treatment—Standard No treatment is effective in every case. Medications reported to be useful for some patients include clonazepam and diazepam; trihexyphenidyl and procyclidine; baclofen; carbamazepine; amitriptyline; amantadine; reserpine; bromocriptine; perphenazine/amitriptyline; and lithium.

Physical therapy may reduce pain associated with spasms. Cervical collars or orthopedic devices are generally not effective. Although surgery is not usually beneficial, it may be helpful in severe cases. Transcutaneous electrical nerve stimulation **(TENS),** biofeedback, nerve blocks, and relaxation techniques may also relieve pain. Supportive counseling is often of benefit. An occupational therapist may be able to help patients increase their comfort and improve mobility.

Treatment—Investigational The use of electronic spinal implants to improve motor function is being studied. A double-blind controlled study involving 300 patients using an electronic orphan device is being conducted by Neuromed, Inc. Contact William F. Jackson, Clinical Affairs Manager, Neuromed, Inc., 5000 Oakes Road, Fort Lauderdale, Florida 33314; (800) 327-9910.

Clinical trials of the orphan drug botulinum toxin for treating spasmodic torticollis are in progress. For additional information, contact Alan B. Scott, M.D., 2232 Webster St., San Francisco, California 94115. The NIH is giving botulinum injections to persons who qualify for the program. For additional information, contact Mark Hallet, M.D., National Institutes of Health, Building 10, Room 5N226, Bethesda, Maryland 20892; (301) 496-1561.

Please contact the agencies listed under Resources, below, for the most current information.

Resources

For more information on spasmodic torticollis: National Organization for Rare Disorders (NORD); National Spasmodic Torticollis Association, Inc.; Dystonia Medical Research Foundation; NIH/National Institute of Neurological Disorders & Stroke (NINDS).

References

Cecil Textbook of Medicine, 18th ed.: J.B. Wyngaarden and L.H. Smith, Jr., eds.; W.B. Saunders Company, 1988, p. 2150.

SPINA BIFIDA

Description A closure defect of the posterior portion of the neural tube produces spina bifida; part of the contents of the spinal canal protrude through this opening. In the most severe form, **rachischisis,** the opening is extensive.

Synonyms
Rachischisis Posterior

Signs and Symptoms Physical findings in spina bifida can range from mild to severe. The mildest form of the condition, spina bifida occulta, causes few if any symptoms, and may go undetected. The lack of closure affects only a small area of the spine. Spina bifida occulta is sometimes found on x-ray, and is occasionally suspected because of a dimple or tuft of hair overlying the affected area. Impaired bladder control is a common finding, even with relatively mild forms of the condition.

In the more severe forms of spina bifida, a meningocele or meningomyelocele protrudes from the lower back. This sac, which may be as large as a grapefruit, may be covered with skin, or the nerve tissue may be exposed, and it may contain spinal fluid.

The malformation of the lower spinal cord causes abnormalities of the lower trunk and extremities of varying severity. If the condition is mild, the person may only experience muscle weakness and impaired skin sensations. In more severe cases, the legs may be paralyzed and without sensation. In patients with meningocele, fluid may accumulate in cavities in the brain, leading to hydrocephalus.

Although spina bifida is usually present at birth, it occasionally is first seen during adolescence, when rapid growth stretches shortened nerves and causes progressive weakness.

Etiology The cause of spina bifida is not known. Hereditary and other prenatal factors may contribute.

Epidemiology In the United States, it is estimated that spina bifida occurs in approximately 1:2000 live births. The condition is more frequent in Ireland and Wales and less common in Israel and among Jews in general. Spina bifida is also 3 to 4 times more common among lower socioeconomic groups of all cultures.

Treatment—Standard The mildest forms of spina bifida generally require no treatment, but in moderate to severe conditions, surgery may be considered, as early as a few hours after birth. Special surgical considerations include imminent breakage of the sac, and placement of a shunt to drain the fluid of hydrocephalus. A coiled catheter may be implanted, which will expand as the child grows.

Leg paralysis may lead to contractures, and physical therapy, further surgery, orthopedic devices, and range of motion exercises may help the patient minimize the disability.

Treatment—Investigational Various aspects of the causes of spina bifida, hydrocephalus, and related defects are being investigated, including the effects of drugs, chemicals, viruses, and other agents on nervous system development. Another area of research is nonsurgical drainage of hydrocephalus and prevention of the associated brain damage.

The National Institute of Neurological Disorders and Stroke is sponsoring a nationwide project involving 55,000 affected individuals, to collect and analyze information about spina bifida and related conditions.

Please contact the agencies listed under Resources, below, for the most current information.

Resources

For more information on spina bifida: National Organization for Rare Disorders (NORD); Spina Bifida Association of America; The National Easter Seal Society for Crippled Children and Adults; NIH/National Institute of Neurological Disorders & Stroke (NINDS); Spina Bifida Association of Canada.

For genetic information and genetic counseling referrals: March of Dimes Birth Defects Foundation; National Center for Education in Maternal and Child Health (NCEMCH).

References
Cecil Textbook of Medicine, 18th ed.: J.B. Wyngaarden and L.H. Smith, Jr., eds.: W.B. Saunders Company, 1988, p. 170.

SPINAL STENOSIS

Description Spinal stenosis is characterized by measurable constriction or compression of the space within the spinal canal, nerve root canals, or vertebrae.

Synonyms
Cervical Spinal Stenosis
Degenerative Lumbar Spinal Stenosis
Familial Lumbar Stenosis
Lumbar Canal Stenosis
Lumbar Spinal Stenosis
Lumbosacral Spinal Stenosis
Stenosis of the Lumbar Vertebral Canal
Tandem Spinal Stenosis
Thoracic Spinal Canal Stenosis

Signs and Symptoms The nerve and blood vessel compression associated with spinal stenosis can lead to intermittent limping and other difficulties with walking, urinary incontinence, temporary paralysis of the legs, and pain or burning sensations in the lower back and legs. Progressive ataxia may also occur.

Diagnosis relies on imaging procedures such as magnetic resonance imaging, computed tomography, myelography, and intraoperative spinal sonography.

Etiology Symptoms may be associated with spinal injury or surgery or abnormal bone growth or deterioration, as in osteoarthritis or Paget's disease of bone. The constriction is sometimes progressive. Spinal stenosis may be inherited, at least in some cases, as an autosomal dominant trait.

Epidemiology Spinal stenosis tends to affect males more often than females, and is usually found among middle-aged or elderly persons, although it can be present at birth. Persons engaging in extremely rough contact sports may have a greater incidence of the condition than the general population.

Related Disorders See *Achondroplasia,* which may precede the development of spinal stenosis; and *Paget's Disease of Bone.*

Sciatica is characterized by pain that travels along the route of the sciatic nerve. The cause can be peripheral nerve root compression from spinal disc abnormalities, tumors, or, rarely, from infection.

Cauda equina syndrome is characterized by dull pain in the upper sacral region with loss of sensation in the buttocks, genitalia, or thighs, and disturbance of bowel and bladder function. The condition is caused by compression of the cauda equina below the first lumbar vertebra. Symptoms are sometimes successfully managed with surgical decompression.

A **herniated intervertebral lumbar disc** (or "slipped" disc) refers to an abnormal protrusion of the fibrous tissue into the spinal canal, causing local compression and nerve injury. This painful condition is common, and may require surgical intervention.

Treatment—Standard Surgery to decompress the affected areas of the spinal canal may be helpful; other treatment is symptomatic and supportive.

Treatment—Investigational Internal spinal fixation devices are being evaluated to alleviate pressure on nerves or blood vessels in the spinal canal, by mechanically altering the position of the bony vertebrae.

Please contact the agencies listed under Resources, below, for the most current information.

Resources

For more information on spinal stenosis: National Organization for Rare Disorders (NORD); National Scoliosis Foundation, Inc.; NIH/National Institute of Arthritis, Musculoskeletal & Skin Diseases (NIAMS) Information Clearinghouse.

References

Surgical Management of Lumbar Spinal Stenosis: R.J. Nasca; Spine, October 1987, issue 12(8), pp. 809–816.

Lumbar Herniated Disc Disease and Canal Stenosis: Prospective Evaluation by Surface Coil MR, CT, and Myelography: M.T. Modic, et al.; Am. J. Roentgenol., October 1986, issue 147(4), pp. 757–765.

Tandem Lumbar and Cervical Spinal Stenosis. Natural History, Prognostic Indices, and Results after Surgical Decompression: T.F. Dagi, et al.; J. Neurosurg., June 1987, issue 66(6), pp. 842–849.

Cauda Equina Syndrome: A Complication of Lumbar Discectomy: A.C. McLaren, et al.; Clin. Orthop., March 1986, issue 204, pp. 143–149.

Thoracic Spinal Canal Stenosis: G.H. Barnett, et al.; J. Neurosurg., March 1987, issue 66(3), pp. 338–344.

Interpeduncular Segmental Fixation: E. Luque; Clin. Orthop., February 1986, issue 203, pp. 54–57.

STIFF-MAN SYNDROME

Description Stiff-man syndrome is a very rare neurologic disorder characterized by diffuse hypertonia that includes the voluntary muscles of the neck, trunk, shoulders, and proximal extremities, and painful muscle spasms.

Synonyms
Moersch-Woltmann Syndrome

Signs and Symptoms Onset is gradual. Initial symptoms include aching and tightness of the involved muscles, possibly bilaterally. As muscular rigidity progresses, pain may increase, and patients may have difficulty making sudden movements. In severe cases bone fractures may result from the extreme twisting and contracting of the muscles. Hyperhidrosis and tachycardia may accompany muscle spasms. Contractions usually are relieved by sleep.

The course of this disorder is progressive, with eventual involvement of the muscles of the back and abdomen. As stiffness increases, patients may develop kyphosis or lordosis.

Etiology The cause of stiff-man syndrome is unknown. Genetic factors have not been established clearly, although the disorder appears to be familial.

An autoimmune association has been postulated. External factors such as sudden noise and emotional stimuli can precipitate muscle spasms.

Related Disorders See *Torsion Dystonia.*

Treatment—Standard Diazepam may provide dramatic relief of muscle rigidity and spasms.

Treatment—Investigational Pietro DeCamilli, M.D., and Michele Solemana, M.D., at Yale University theorize that stiff-man syndrome may be an autoimmune disorder and are studying the use of plasma exchange combined with steroid drugs as a potential treatment. The effectiveness and side effects of this therapy currently are being investigated.

Please contact the agencies listed under Resources, below, for the most current information.

Resources
For more information on stiff-man syndrome: National Organization for Rare Disorders (NORD); Mark Hallet, M.D., NIH/National Institute of Neurological Disorders & Stroke (NINDS).

References
Mendelian Inheritance in Man, 9th ed: V.A. McKusick; The Johns Hopkins University Press, 1990, pp. 553, 880.

SYDENHAM CHOREA

Description Sydenham chorea is an acute, usually self-limited, disorder of early life that occurs in about 5 to 10 percent of cases of rheumatic fever, beginning several months after the polyarthritis has subsided.

Synonyms
Chorea Minor
Infectious Chorea
Rheumatic Chorea
St. Vitus Dance

Signs and Symptoms Affected individuals develop rapid, involuntary, nonrepetitive movements that gradually become severe, affecting gait, arm movements, and speech. Fatigue and restlessness may precede the onset of chorea. Clumsiness and facial grimacing are common. The disorder is bilateral in 75 percent of cases. Choreic movements disappear with sleep. Occasionally the patient may require sedation to avoid self-injury. The disorder subsides in 3 to 6 months with no neurologic residua.

Etiology Sydenham chorea is a complication of streptococcal infection.

Epidemiology Onset of choreic symptoms may occur up to 6 months after the streptococcal infection has been cleared. Girls are affected more often than boys, usually between the ages of 5 and 15 years.

Related Disorders See *Cerebral Palsy; Huntington Disease; Tourette Syndrome; Wilson Disease.*

Scarlet fever and rheumatic fever may precede the development of Sydenham chorea. See *Rheumatic Fever.*

Treatment—Standard No medication is consistently effective in the treatment of Sydenham chorea. Tranquilizers, barbiturates, salicylates, or corticosteroids may be helpful in some patients. The condition should be regarded as transitory.

Treatment—Investigational Please contact the agencies listed under Resources, below, for the most current information.

Resources
For more information on Sydenham chorea: National Organization for Rare Disorders (NORD); NIH/National Institute of Neurological Disorders and Stroke (NINDS); Center for Disease Control (CDC).

References
Harrison's Principles of Internal Medicine, 12th ed.: J.D. Wilson, et al., eds.; McGraw-Hill, 1991, p. 935.

Carbamazepine: An Alternative Drug for the Treatment of Nonhereditary Chorea: M. Roig, et al.; Pediatrics, September 1988, issue 82(pt. 2), pp. 492–495.

Tetrabenazine Therapy of Dystonia, Chorea, Tics and Other Dyskinesias: J. Jankovic, et al.; Neurology, March 1988, issue 38(3), pp. 391–394.

Scientific American MEDICINE: E. Rubinstein and D. Federman, eds.; Scientific American, Inc., 1978–1991, p. 15:VII:2.

SYRINGOBULBIA

Description Syringobulbia is a slowly progressive neurologic disorder in which cavitation occurs in the brain stem. The cavity (syrinx) in **syringomyelia** is usually in the central portion of the spinal cord, but may extend from the cervical to the lumbar regions (see *Syringomyelia*). In **syringobulbia,** the syrinx is in the lower brain stem.

Syringobulbia is often associated with craniovertebral anomalies, including Arnold-Chiari syndrome.

Signs and Symptoms Features of syringobulbia may include vocal cord paralysis, atrophy and fibrillation of the tongue muscle, dysarthria, vertigo, and nystagmus. There also may be anhidrosis and flushing on the affected side of the face (Horner syndrome).

Etiology The defect may be congenital but does not increase in size and cause symptoms until later in life (e.g., early adulthood). Brain stem injury from trauma, tumors, or compression may also cause syringobulbia.

Epidemiology Syringobulbia can affect persons of either sex. Onset usually occurs before 30 years of age.

Related Disorders See *Syringomyelia; Arnold-Chiari Syndrome.*

The symptoms in some forms of amyloid neuropathy are similar to those of syringobulbia (see *Amyloidosis).*

Neoplasms and vascular malformations in the brain stem may cause neurologic symptoms similar to those of syringobulbia.

Treatment—Standard Surgical drainage may be indicated in some cases. Nonsurgical treatment of syringobulbia is symptomatic and supportive. Radiation therapy has not been beneficial.

Treatment—Investigational Please contact the agencies listed under Resources, below, for the most current information.

Resources

For more information on syringobulbia: National Organization for Rare Disorders (NORD); NIH/National Institute of Neurological Disorders & Stroke (NINDS); Spinal Cord Injury; American Spinal Injury Association; National Spinal Cord Injury Association.

References
Harrison's Principles of Internal Medicine, 12th ed.: J.D. Wilson, et al., eds.; McGraw-Hill, 1991, p. 2086.
Infantile Hypoventilation Syndrome, Neurenteric Cyst, and Syringobulbia: H.D. Chung, et al.; Neurology (NY), April 1982, issue 32(4), pp. 441–444.

SYRINGOMYELIA

Description Syringomyelia is a slowly progressive neurologic disorder in which cavitation occurs in the spinal cord. The cavity (syrinx) is usually paramedian and may extend up into the medulla oblongata (see *Syringobulbia)* or down as far as the lumbar region.

Syringomyelia is often associated with craniovertebral anomalies, including Arnold-Chiari syndrome.

Synonyms
Morvan Disease
Myelosyringosis

Signs and Symptoms If the syrinx is located in the cervical or thoracic areas of the spine, the initial symptoms may include loss of pain and temperature perception in the upper extremities and chest, spreading to the shoulders and back. Reflexes may be absent. The sense of touch is not affected, however.

When the lumbar and sacral segments of the spine are affected, typical findings include spasticity, muscle weakness, and ataxia in the lower extremities as well as paralysis of the bladder.

Syringomyelia is a slowly progressive disorder. Erosion of the bony spinal canal, osteoporosis, joint contractures, and progressive scoliosis may occur.

Diagnosis relies on imaging techniques such as delayed computed tomographic metrizamide myelography or magnetic resonance imaging.

Morvan disease is a severe form of syringomyelia accompanied by ulceration of fingers and toes.

Etiology Autosomal dominant inheritance for some cases has been suggested. Syringomyelia may also be caused by injury of the spinal cord from trauma, tumors, or compression.

Epidemiology Usually, males and females under age 30 years are affected. About 1000 cases are identified in the United States each year.

Related Disorders See *Syringobulbia; Arnold-Chiari Syndrome.*

The symptoms in some forms of amyloid neuropathy are similar to those of syringomyelia (see *Amyloidosis).*

Neoplasms and vascular malformations in the spinal cord may also cause neurologic symptoms similar to those of syringomyelia.

Treatment—Standard Syringoperitoneal shunting to drain the fluid has been effective in reversing or arresting neurologic deterioration in some patients. Radiation therapy has not been beneficial.

Intraoperative sonography (**IOS**) has been used during surgery to evaluate the effectiveness of the procedure as it is being performed.

Treatment—Investigational Please contact the agencies listed under Resources, below, for the most current information.

Resources

For more information on syringomyelia: National Organization for Rare Disorders (NORD); American Syringomyelia Alliance Project, Inc.; NIH/National Institute of Neurological Disorders & Stroke (NINDS).

References
Mendelian Inheritance in Man, 9th ed.: V.A. McKusick; The Johns Hopkins University Press, 1990, pp. 890–891, 1490.

Harrison's Principles of Internal Medicine, 12th ed.: J.D. Wilson, et al., eds.; McGraw-Hill, 1991, p. 2086.

Surgical Treatment of Syringomyelia. Favorable Results with Syringoperitoneal Shunting: N.M. Barbaro, et al.; J. Neurosurg., September 1984, issue 61(3), pp. 531–538.

Posttraumatic Syringomyelia: G.E. Dworkin, et al.; Arch. Phys. Med. Rehabil., May 1985, issue 66(5), pp. 329–331.

TARDIVE DYSKINESIA

Description Tardive dyskinesia is a neurologic syndrome associated with the longterm use of neuroleptic drugs, producing symptoms that mimic certain neurologic diseases but which are neurotoxic side effects of the drugs. The syndrome usually appears late in the course of drug therapy and may persist indefinitely after discontinuation of the medication.

Synonyms
Tardive Dystonia
Oral-Facial Dyskinesia

Signs and Symptoms Typical involuntary and abnormal facial movements include grimacing, sticking out the tongue, and sucking and smacking of the lips. Involuntary, rapid movements of the arms and legs (chorea and athetosis) also may occur. These symptoms often remain long after the neuroleptic drugs have been discontinued, although some may disappear with time.

Etiology Tardive dyskinesia results from longterm use (3 months to years) of neuroleptic drugs, prescribed not only for the treatment of psychoses but also for certain gastrointestinal and neurologic disorders.

Epidemiology Prevalence in patients being treated with neuroleptics is 15 to 40 percent. The risk is higher for women and with advancing age.

Related Disorders See *Huntington Disease; Cerebral Palsy; Tourette Syndrome*—the symptoms of which tardive dyskinesia may mimic.

Treatment—Standard Prevention is important because most symptomatic treatment is unsatisfactory and potentially dangerous. The neuroleptic drug must be discontinued as soon as any involuntary facial movements are observed. Psychiatric disorders treated with neuroleptic drugs may go into remissions, at which time the drugs should be reduced and discontinued when possible to prevent tardive dyskinesia.

Treatment—Investigational The use of vitamin E is being evaluated for the possible treatment of tardive dyskinesia. Patients involved in this study have persistent, moderate-to-severe symptoms of tardive dyskinesia, and are between the ages of 18 and 70 years. Information about this research project can be obtained from Denise Juliano, MSW, Coordinator of Admissions, Neuropsychiatric Research Hospital, 2700 Martin Luther King Jr. Avenue, SE, Washington, DC 20032; (202) 373-6100.

Please contact the agencies listed under Resources, below, for the most current information.

Resources
 For more information on tardive dyskinesia: National Organization for Rare Disorders (NORD); Tardive Dyskinesia/Tardive Dystonia National Association; NIH/National Institute of Mental Health (NIMH); National Mental Health Association.

References
Internal Medicine, 3rd ed.: J.H. Stein, ed.-in-chief; Little, Brown and Company, 1990, pp. 1955, 2003.
Suppression of Tardive Dyskinesia with Amoxapine: Case Report: D.A. D'Mello, et al.; J. Clin. Psychiatry, March 1986, issue 47(3), p. 148.
Facial Dyskinesia: J. Janovic, et al.; Adv. Neurol., 1988, p. 49.

TARSAL TUNNEL SYNDROME

Description Tarsal tunnel syndrome is a compression neuropathy of the posterior tibial nerve at the ankle.

Synonyms
 Posterior Tibial Nerve Neuralgia

Signs and Symptoms Symptoms typically are painful burning, tingling, or numbness in the foot. Pain is often more intense at night, and is relieved by moving the foot.

Etiology The posterior tibial nerve may become compressed where it enters a confined compartment or tunnel inferior to the medial malleolus of the tibia at the ankle. An old fracture, hypertrophied adjacent muscles, or vascular compression may be responsible for the compression; but in some cases no abnormality can be demonstrated.

Epidemiology Onset can be at any age. Males and females appear to be affected in equal numbers. The disorder is most common among individuals who stand for long periods.

Related Disorders See *Erythromelalgia; Peripheral Neuropathy.*

Burning feet syndrome (Gopalan syndrome) is thought to be caused by deficiency of a B vitamin. Symptoms include severe burning, aching, cramping, and pins-and-needles sensations in the soles of the feet. In some cases the palms of the hands are affected.

Treatment—Standard Tension on the affected nerve should be alleviated by immobilization of the foot or adaptation of the shoe. Antiinflammatory drugs and local corticosteroid injection are the usual treatment. Surgery should be reserved for cases that do not respond to conservative treatment.

Treatment—Investigational Please contact the agencies listed under Resources, below, for the most current information.

Resources

For more information on tarsal tunnel syndrome: National Organization for Rare Disorders (NORD); The National Arthritis and Musculoskeletal and Skin Diseases Information Clearinghouse.

References

Tarsal Tunnel Syndrome: E.L. Radin; Clin. Orthop., December 1983, issue 181, pp. 167–170.

Tarsal Tunnel Syndrome. A Case Report and Review of the Literature: G.M. O'Malley, et al.; Orthopedics, June 1985, issue 8(6), pp. 758–760.

THOMSEN DISEASE

Description Thomsen disease is a rare nonprogressive, inherited neuromuscular condition, usually beginning in infancy, that is characterized by muscle stiffness on first attempting movement and also by muscle inability to relax following movement. If all the body muscles are involved, the entire body may become stiff.

Synonyms

Myotonia Congenita
Myotonia Hereditaria
Thomsen-Becker Myotonia

Signs and Symptoms When movement is attempted after rest, muscles become rigid. Contraction may continue for 30 seconds or more after mechanical stimulation, but the stiffness subsides as the same movement is repeated a few times. Slowness in chewing, swallowing, talking, and walking are typical, and muscles are often large and well-developed for the child's age. The symptoms may improve as the child grows older.

Etiology Thomsen disease is inherited as an autosomal dominant trait.

Epidemiology Thomsen disease usually begins at birth or shortly after, although, rarely, it appears at puberty. Males seem to be affected more often than females.

Related Disorders See *Myotonic Dystrophy*, in which there is a similar problem of muscle inability to relax after contraction. Differentiation can be made, however, by the muscular weakness and atrophy seen in myotonic dystrophy.

Schwartz-Jampel syndrome (chondrodystrophic myotonia) is characterized by failure of muscle development to keep pace with overall growth. The condition begins in early infancy.

Treatment—Standard The antiarrhythmic drug tocainide is used as a treatment for Thomsen disease. Careful monitoring of dosage and heart function is important. Procainamide, phenytoin, and quinine also have been effective.

There is usually a poor response to physical therapy in Thomsen disease, but active and passive exercises may be helpful in some instances. Agencies that provide services to handicapped persons and their families may be of benefit. Genetic counseling also may be useful.

Treatment—Investigational The experimental antimyotonic drug mexiletine may improve muscle weakness in some patients, but this treatment is still under investigation.

Please contact the agencies listed under Resources, below, for the most current information.

Resources

For more information on Thomsen disease: National Organization for Rare Disorders (NORD); NIH/National Institute of Neurological Disorders & Stroke (NINDS); The National Arthritis and Musculoskeletal and Skin Diseases Information Clearinghouse; Muscular Dystrophy Association.

For genetic information and genetic counseling referrals: March of Dimes Birth Defects Foundation; National Center for Education in Maternal and Child Health (NCEMCH).

References

Mendelian Inheritance in Man, 9th ed.: V.A. McKusick; The Johns Hopkins University Press, 1990, p. 638.

Nelson Textbook of Pediatrics, 13th ed.: R.E. Behrman and V.C. Vaughan, III, eds.; W.B. Saunders Company, 1987, p. 1339.

Successful Treatment with Tocainide of Recessive Generalized Congenital Myotonia: E.W. Streib; Ann. Neurol., May 1986, issue 19(5), pp. 501–504.

Value of Mexiletine in the Treatment of Thomsen-Becker Myotonia: F. Himon, et al.; Arch. Fr. Pediatr., January 1986, issue 43(1), pp. 49–50.

TINNITUS

Description Tinnitus is a person's subjective experience of sound that does not exist in the environment.

Signs and Symptoms The sounds of tinnitus have variously been described as clicking, buzzing, whistling, ringing, roaring, etc. They may always be present, or may be intermittent. There frequently is an associated hearing loss.

Etiology Many ear disorders are associated with tinnitus, including infection, obstruction, and tumors. Certain medications and environmental toxins may be implicated, as may head injuries and alcohol abuse.

Related Disorders Bruits, heard in auscultation by the examiner, can sometimes be heard by the patient and may be mistaken for tinnitus.

Internal (though imaginary) sounds are a feature of some mental illnesses such as schizophrenia.

Treatment—Standard Treatment of any underlying disease may cure the tinnitus. Otherwise, relief may be obtained through the use of pleasant background noise, e.g., music or other sounds attractive to the patient such as ocean surf.

Treatment—Investigational Please contact the agencies listed under Resources, below, for the most current information.

Resources

For more information on tinnitus: National Organization for Rare Disorders (NORD); American Tinnitus Association; NIH/National Institute of Deafness & Other Communication Disorders (NIDCD).

References

Harrison's Principles of Internal Medicine, 12th ed.: J.D. Wilson, et al., eds.; McGraw-Hill, 1991, p. 156.

TORSION DYSTONIA

Description Torsion dystonia is a neurologic disorder characterized by involuntary contortions of muscles in the neck, torso, and extremities. Occasionally only one or a few muscles are involved. The disorder is most noticeable on walking, when involvement of several muscle groups may produce a sideways gait, with the body twisting as if writhing.

Synonyms

        Dystonia Lenticularis
        Dystonia Musculorum Deformans
        Segawa Dystonia
        Ziehen-Oppenheim Disease

Signs and Symptoms In the early stages, the symptoms may be mild and sporadic, occurring only after prolonged activity or stress. As the disease progresses the contortions begin to occur during any physical activity, particularly walking; in advanced disease they also occur during rest. Not all cases are progressive, however, and the dystonia may plateau at a mild level.

Secondary symptoms include foot drag, cramps in the hands and feet, difficulty in grasping objects, and unclear speech. The contractured tendons and buildup of connective tissue in muscle may cause permanent physical deformities.

Etiology Torsion dystonia may be inherited as a recessive, dominant, or X-linked trait, or may be acquired. A chromosome marker for hereditary forms of dystonia, identified in 1989, indicates that the gene is located on the long arm of chromosome 9.

In the autosomal recessive form, muscle contractions of the feet and hands typically appear in childhood or adolescence. Symptoms spread quickly to involve the trunk and extremities, but progression slows after adolescence. This form is more severe than the autosomal dominant form.

In the autosomal dominant form, muscles in the torso and neck are affected first. Symptoms progress slowly, but new muscle groups may be initially involved well beyond adolescence.

An X-linked form of torsion dystonia has been described in which the initial symptom is spasmodic eye blinking.

Torsion dystonia acquired as a result of brain injury due to infection, trauma, birth injury, or stroke is frequently unilateral and nonprogressive.

Epidemiology The autosomal recessive form usually becomes apparent by puberty and primarily affects Ashkenazic Jews. The defective gene is carried by 1:100 Ashkenazic Jews in the United States. Males and females are affected in equal numbers.

Onset of the rarer autosomal dominant form is in late adolescence or early adulthood.

The average age at onset for the X-linked form seems to be about 38 years.

Related Disorders Torsion dystonia must be differentiated from other conditions associated with involuntary contortions. See *Ataxia, Marie; Cerebral Palsy; Glutaricaciduria I; Spasmodic Torticollis; Tardive Dyskinesia.*

Treatment—Standard Drugs used to treat dystonia include trihexyphenidyl, benztropine, diazepam, clonazepam, baclofen, carbamazepine, levodopa, bromocriptine, chlorpromazine, thiopropazate, haloperidol, pimozide, tetrabenazine, and amantadine.

Treatment—Investigational Surgical techniques in development for the treatment of torsion dystonia include the implantation of electrical devices to stimulate nerve impulse transmission. Other surgical procedures are ablative. A high-risk procedure involves destruction of the cells of the basal ganglia that are transmitting incorrect instructions. In severe cases, the nerves connecting with the contracting muscles may be severed.

Botulinum toxin, an orphan drug approved by the FDA in 1989, is being tested in connection with certain forms of dystonia. The drug is manufactured by Oculinum, Inc.

Sinemet, being tested at the National Institute of Neurological Disorders and Stroke in Bethesda, Maryland, for treatment of Segawa dystonia, has dramatically alleviated symptoms in patients with this inherited disorder, which is often misdiagnosed as cerebral palsy. Sinemet's property of stimulating the production of dopamine is useful in this case, since children with Segawa dystonia are deficient in dopamine. For more information, contact John K. Fink, M.D., NINDS Developmental and Metabolic Neurology Branch, NIH, Building 10, Room 3D03, Bethesda, Maryland 20892.

Please contact the agencies listed under Resources, below, for the most current information.

Resources

For more information on torsion dystonia: National Organization for Rare Disorders, Inc. (NORD); NIH/National Institute of Neurological Disorders and Stroke (NINDS); Dystonia Medical Research Foundation; National Foundation for Jewish Genetic Diseases.

For genetic information and genetic counseling referrals: March of Dimes Birth Defects Foundation; NIH/National Center for Education in Maternal and Child Health (NCEMCH).

References

Mendelian Inheritance in Man, 9th ed.: V.A. McKusick; The Johns Hopkins University Press, 1990, pp. 277–278, 1155–1156, 1731.

Brain Neurotransmitters in Dystonia Musculorum Deformans: Hornykiewicz; N. Engl. J. Med., August 7, 1986, issue 315(6), pp. 347–353.

Clinical Course of Idiopathic Torsion Dystonia Among Jews in Israel: R. Inzelberg, et al.; Adv. Neurol., 1988, issue 50, pp. 93–100.

Autosomal Dominant Torsion Dystonia in a Swedish Family: L. Forsgren, et al.; Adv. Neurol., 1988, issue 50, pp. 83–92.

TOURETTE SYNDROME

Description Tourette syndrome is a neurologic disorder characterized by motor and vocal tics, manifested as involuntary muscle movements of the extremities, shoulder, face, and the voluntary muscles, and uncontrollable, inarticulate sounds and sometimes inappropriate words. Tourette syndrome is not a progressive or degenerative disorder; rather, symptoms tend to be variable and follow a chronic waxing and waning course throughout an otherwise normal life span.

Synonyms

Brissaud II
Chronic Multiple Tics
Coprolalia-Generalized Tic Disorder
Gilles de la Tourette Syndrome
Guinon Myospasia Impulsiva
Maladie de Tics
Tics

Signs and Symptoms Onset usually occurs in childhood with a tic in a facial muscle, causing excessive blinking, nose twitching, or grimacing. Other gestures include involuntary head shaking, shoulder jerking, arm flapping, foot stamping, and the uncontrollable imitation of another person's movements. Some patients may have self-mutilating symptoms.

The sounds produced can be inarticulate and incoherent, such as grunts, barks, screams, or sniffing, or they can include words. **Coprolalia** occurs in approximately 30 percent of all patients. Involuntary repetition of a word or sentence spoken by the patient or another person (**palilalia** or **echolalia**) also is common.

Tics may subside when the patient is concentrating on a particular task, but intensify during stress. Over periods of months to years some symptoms may disappear and be replaced by new tics; or new symptoms may be added to old ones.

Etiology Seventy percent of all cases appear to be genetic, inherited as an autosomal dominant trait, although an X-linked Tourette modifier gene has been described. Research suggests that there may be a biochemical dysfunction that affects neurotransmitter systems in the brain.

The effect of gene penetrance is suggested by the high prevalence of first-degree relatives with mild tic conditions in families with Tourette syndrome. Some relatives may have chronic tics, while others may not display any tics but exhibit obsessive-compulsive behaviors, which recent research indicates are frequently associated with Tourette syndrome.

Genetic studies suggest that only about 10 percent of affected relatives have symptoms severe enough to interfere with normal, daily living. The chance of an affected parent having a child with Tourette symptoms has been estimated to be approximately 40 to 50 percent. In many cases, however, the child will have a mild form of the syndrome, although severity of symptoms currently cannot be predicted.

Epidemiology A childhood onset between the ages of 2 and 16 years is most typical, although there are rare cases with later onset as well as symptoms appearing at one year. The male:female ratio is 3:1. Tourette syndrome occurs in all nationalities and across all economic groups.

Related Disorders Transient tics of childhood are common among children. These motor or vocal tics usually disappear within one year.

Chronic tics begin in childhood, or after age 40. Usually either motor or vocal tics are present, not both, and are more limited than in Tourette syndrome.

Treatment—Standard Haloperidol in low doses helps suppress symptoms in many patients, but side effects often limit its use.

Clonidine appears to improve motor, vocal, and behavioral symptoms in approximately 50 percent of patients, according to some reports.

Pimozide, an approved orphan drug with dopaminergic blocking action, appears to be as effective as haloperidol with fewer side effects for some Tourette patients. Other dopamine-blocking drugs (e.g., fluphenazine) also are useful for reducing Tourette symptoms.

Supportive psychotherapy can help patients adjust to this chronic, often socially crippling disorder.

Treatment—Investigational Drugs that treat the obsessive-compulsive symptoms of Tourette syndrome are being studied; these drugs include clomipramine (Anafranil) and fluoxetine (Prozac).

Geneticists also are studying several large families with many members affected by Tourette syndrome to help identify a causative gene.

Research also is ongoing in the area of neurotransmitters.

Please contact the agencies listed under Resources, below, for the most current information.

Resources

For more information on Tourette syndrome: National Organization for Rare Disorders (NORD); Tourette Syndrome Association; NIH/National Institute of Neurological Disorders & Stroke (NINDS).

For genetic information and genetic counseling referrals: March of Dimes Birth Defects Foundation; NIH/National Center for Education in Maternal and Child Health (NCEMCH).

References

Mendelian Inheritance in Man, 9th ed.: V.A. McKusick; The Johns Hopkins University Press, 1990, pp. 351–352, 1675.

Diagnostic and Statistical Manual of Mental Disorders, 3rd ed., revised: R.L. Spitzer, et al., eds.; Am. Psychiat. Asso., 1987, pp. 79–82.

Cecil Textbook of Medicine, 18th ed.: J.B. Wyngaarden and L.H. Smith, Jr., eds.; W.B. Saunders Company, 1988, pp. 2151–2152.

TRIGEMINAL NEURALGIA

Description Trigeminal neuralgia is characterized by excruciating episodic pain in the areas supplied by the trigeminal nerve.

Synonyms
Fothergill Disease
Tic Douloureux

Signs and Symptoms Brief (seconds to minutes) but intense bursts of pain occur along the maxillary and mandibular nerves, usually in adults over age 50 years. Pain may be triggered by talking, brushing teeth, touching the face, chewing, or swallowing. No other clinical or pathologic signs are present. During any one attack the pain is usually limited to one side of the face.

Etiology The cause is unknown. Vascular compression of the root entry zone of the trigeminal nerve, as well as toxic, nutritional, and infectious factors have been discussed.

Epidemiology Trigeminal neuralgia usually affects older adults of both sexes. It is more common in women than in men.

Related Disorders Glossopharyngeal neuralgia is characterized by severe paroxysmal pain originating on the side of the throat and radiating to the ear. The petrosal and jugular ganglia of the glossopharyngeal nerve are involved.

Sphenopalatine ganglion neuralgia (Sluder neuralgia) is characterized by burning and boring pain in the area of the superior maxilla. Pain radiates to the neck and shoulder.

Postherpetic pain may also occur in the face.

Treatment—Standard Carbamazepine, phenytoin, and baclofen have been reported to be effective in treating trigeminal neuralgia. Surgical therapy includes radiofrequency coagulation of the gasserian ganglion and the Jannetta procedure, involving removal of vascular structures pressing on the trigeminal ganglion.

Treatment—Investigational Tinzanidine, used experimentally as a treatment in trigeminal neuralgia, has been approved for study in the United States by the Food and Drug Administration. Although this orphan drug is available experimentally in the United States, conclusive results have not yet been reported.

Please contact the agencies listed under Resources, below, for the most current information.

Resources

For more information on trigeminal neuralgia: National Organization for Rare Disorders (NORD); Trigeminal Neuralgia Support Group; NIH/National Institute of Dental Research, Clinical Pain Division; NIH/National Institute of Neurological Disorders & Stroke (NINDS).

References

Trigeminal Neuralgia: Treatment by Microvascular Decompression: P.J. Jannetta; *in* Neurosurgery: Wilkins, et al., eds.; McGraw-Hill, 1984.
Scientific American MEDICINE: E. Rubinstein and D. Federman, eds.; Scientific American, Inc., 1978–1991, p. 11:II:7.

TUBEROUS SCLEROSIS (TS)

Description Tuberous sclerosis is characterized by seizures, mental retardation, developmental delay, and skin and ocular lesions. The disorder's manifestations and severity vary.

Synonyms

Bourneville Pringle Syndrome
Epiloia
Phakomatosis

Signs and Symptoms Seizures, often the first symptoms of tuberous sclerosis, occur in about 90 percent of patients. They may include myoclonic jerks and hypsarrhythmia. Two-thirds of patients are mildly to severely mentally retarded.

Prenatal benign brain tumors may be detected with a CT scan; they may calcify within the first years after birth.

Between 60 and 90 percent of infants have hypomelanotic macules at birth. Adenoma sebaceum appears between the ages of 3 and 5 years and proliferates during puberty. Collagen accumulates in skin of the lower back and nape of the neck and appears as slightly elevated, yellowish-brown patches with an orange peel texture. Periungual or subungual fibromas may develop, and café-au-lait spots and nodules appear on the skin. About 90 percent of patients develop retinal astrocytic hamartomas or phakomas.

Delayed speech, slow motor development, and learning disabilities may be associated. Typical behavior patterns include manifestations resembling childhood autism; episodes of screaming, crying, and rage; and catatonic rigidity.

Etiology Tuberous sclerosis is believed to be an autosomal dominant inherited disorder traced to the long arm of chromosome 9. Instances of presumed spontaneous mutation may represent mildly affected parents.

Epidemiology TS occurs in approximately 1:20,000 births and affects 10,000 individuals in the United States. Males and females are affected equally.

Treatment—Standard Although mental impairment does not always occur, its severity has a direct correlation to early onset and duration or severity of the seizures. Early diagnosis and seizure control are important. Treatment is limited to abolishing or minimizing symptoms and includes anticonvulsants. Conventional anticonvulsants include closely monitored use of phenobarbital, phenytoin, clonazepam, valproic acid, carbamazepine, ethosuximide, or acetazolamide. Some "infantile spasms" can be treated with prednisone or adrenocorticotropic hormone (ACTH). Immunizations, such as DPT and rubella, can prompt seizures in children.

Dermabrasion or laser therapy is used to eliminate facial angiofibromas. Surgery may be required for rapidly growing tumors.

Intracranial hypertension caused by a benign tumor may require a shunting procedure or surgical removal of the tumor. Some rhabdomyomas require surgery. Large cystic lesions of the kidneys may require surgical decompression or excision, possibly leading to removal of a kidney.

Treatment—Investigational Investigators are attempting to isolate the genetic marker, which could lead to the development of both prenatal testing and a diagnostic blood test. Blood and skin cells from TS individuals have been banked at the Camden Cell Repository, New Jersey, and are available for worldwide research.

Please contact the agencies listed under Resources, below, for the most current information.

Resources

For more information on tuberous sclerosis: National Organization for Rare Disorders (NORD); National Tuberous Sclerosis Association, Inc.; American Tuberous Sclerosis Association; NIH/National Institute of Neurological Disorders & Stroke (NINDS).

For information about seizures: Epilepsy Foundation of America.

For genetic information and genetic counseling referrals: March of Dimes Birth Defects Foundation; National Center for Education in Maternal and Child Health (NCEMCH).

References
Cecil Textbook of Medicine, 18th ed.: J.B. Wyngaarden and Lloyd H. Smith, Jr., eds.; W.B. Saunders Company, 1988, pp. 2158–2159, 2344–2345.

VASCULAR MALFORMATIONS OF THE BRAIN

Description Vascular malformations of the brain include arteriovenous malformations, cavernous angiomas (or hemangiomas), venous malformations, and telangiectasia.

Synonyms
Intracranial Vascular Malformations
Occult Intracranial Vascular Malformations

Signs and Symptoms Manifestations of cerebrovascular malformations vary according to the type and severity of the disorder.

Arteriovenous malformations (AVMs) are congenital. These anomalous shunts can produce neurologic symptoms as they enlarge and compress neural tissue, or in response to hemorrhage. Parenchymal (or subarachnoid) hemorrhage, focal epilepsy, and progressive focal sensory-motor deficits may occur.

Cavernous angiomas (or hemangiomas) may be congenital or appear shortly after birth. These raised red or purplish lesions may contain mature vasculature and lymphatics. They rarely involute spontaneously.

Venous malformations vary in size and may cause headaches, seizures, strokes, or hemorrhage.

Telangiectasia can occur on the face, eyes, meninges, and mucous membranes.

Etiology Vascular malformation of the brain may be congenital (inherited as an autosomal dominant trait with variable expression and incomplete penetrance) or acquired, the result of an injury or trauma.

Epidemiology Vascular malformations of the brain generally affect males and females in equal numbers, although AVMs occur more frequently in males. A hereditary form of cavernous malformations may be found more frequently in Mexican-Americans.

Related Disorders See *Moyamoya Disease.*

Embolic, hemorrhagic, and thrombotic strokes should be considered in the differential diagnosis of cerebrovascular malformations.

Treatment—Standard AVMs may be treated with anticonvulsants; surgical excision may be required. Intravascular thrombosing via intraarterial catheters and coagulation with focused proton beams may also be effective.

Cavernous angiomas may resolve in response to systemic administration of prednisone, but electrocoagulation or surgical excision may be required.

Treatment—Investigational Several types of surgery are being investigated for treatment of vascular malformations of the brain: charged-particle radiosurgery, interventriculostomy, and catheter placement.

Please contact the agencies listed under Resources, below, for the most current information.

Resources

For more information on vascular malformations of the brain: National Organization for Rare Disorders (NORD); NIH/National Institute of Neurological Disorders and Stroke (NINDS).

For genetic information and genetic counseling referrals: March of Dimes Birth Defects Foundation; NIH/National Center for Education in Maternal and Child Health (NCEMCH).

References

Vascular Malformations of the Brain: B.M. Stein & J.P. Mohr; New Engl. J. Med., August 11, 1988, issue 319(6), pp. 368–370.

Cerebral Cavernous Malformations: Incidence and Familial Occurrence: D. Rigamonti, et al.; New Engl. J. Med., August 11, 1988, issue 319(6), pp. 343–347.

Clinical, Radiological, and Pathological Spectrum of Angiographically Occult Intracranial Vascular Malformations. Analysis of 21 Cases and Review of the Literature: R.D. Lobato, et al.; J. Neurosurg., April 1988, issue 68(4), pp. 518–531.

WERDNIG-HOFFMANN DISEASE

Description Werdnig-Hoffmann disease is an inherited neuromuscular condition of infants. It is characterized by degenerative changes in the ventral horn cells of the spinal cord, resulting in progressive atrophy and weakness of the muscles of the trunk and extremities.

Synonyms

Infantile Spinal Muscular Atrophy

Werdnig-Hoffmann Paralysis

Signs and Symptoms Onset occurs before age 2 years and may be in utero. The earlier the onset, the graver the prognosis. Initial signs include hypotonia and weakness of the skeletal musculature, with hypermobility of joints; absent tendon reflexes; fasciculations of the tongue; and a froglike position, with hips abducted and knees flexed. Mental development is normal. Typically, the child never gains head control, does not turn over, and never sits or stands.

The rate of progression varies. In the form that begins in utero, generalized muscle atrophy and weakness progress rapidly. Within a few months, respiratory and excretory difficulties develop, and the infant is unable to swallow. Death occurs because of respiratory failure or aspiration of food. The form that begins during the first few months of life may have a more slowly progressive course, even extending into adult life. In rare cases, the disease may become arrested.

Etiology Werdnig-Hoffmann disease is an autosomal recessive disorder. In rare instances there appears to be autosomal dominant inheritance.

Epidemiology Males and females are affected equally. There may be no known family history of the disease, since the genetic defect is recessive. The estimated incidence is 1:1,000,000 live births per year.

Treatment—Standard Medical management is symptomatic. Physical therapy, respiratory care, and aggressive treatment of respiratory infections are used. Orthopedic devices may be helpful when the condition is relatively static.

Treatment—Investigational The Muscular Dystrophy Association (MDA) supports basic and applied studies in nerve and muscle metabolism in the hope that these will identify the biologic processes that give rise to muscular dystrophy and related neuromuscular diseases, such as Werdnig-Hoffmann disease.

Please contact the agencies listed under Resources, below, for the most current information.

Resources

For more information on **Werdnig-Hoffmann disease:** National Organization for Rare Disorders (NORD); Muscular Dystrophy Association; NIH/National Institute of Neurological Disorders & Stroke (NINDS); Families of Spinal Muscular Atrophy; Muscular Dystrophy Group of Great Britain and Northern Ireland.

For genetic information and genetic counseling referrals: March of Dimes Birth Defects Foundation; National Center for Education in Maternal and Child Health (NCEMCH).

References
Mendelian Inheritance in Man, 9th ed.: V.A. McKusick; The Johns Hopkins University Press, 1990, p. 1354.

Nelson Textbook of Pediatrics, 13th ed.: R.E. Behrman and V.C. Vaughan, III, eds.; W.B. Saunders Company, 1987, pp. 1331–1332.

Cecil Textbook of Medicine, 18th ed.: J.B. Wyngaarden and L.H. Smith, Jr., eds.; W.B. Saunders Company, 1988, p. 2155.

4 CARDIOVASCULAR AND RESPIRATORY DISEASES
By Amnon Rosenthal, M.D.

In this brief introduction, I have outlined an approach to the recognition and detection of rare cardiovascular and respiratory diseases in the infant, child, and young adult. Only a broad classification and generalizations are provided. In general, cardiovascular diseases in childhood are congenital, acquired, or associated with other hereditary conditions. The rarity of any of these is relative to the population examined, methods used in detection, and the training and subspecialty expertise of the physician. For example, ventricular septal defect, which is a congenital cardiac malformation, is seen frequently by the pediatric cardiologist, less often by the pediatrician or general practitioner, and rarely by an internist. Since many of these defects close spontaneously with advancing age, they occur more frequently in the infant than in the child and are truly rare in adults. Many of the rare diseases described are specific to infancy with few survivors into adulthood (e.g., hypoplastic left heart syndrome), while others may be silent in childhood and are more frequently observed in adults (e.g., mitral valve prolapse syndrome). Some diseases are rare at any age (e.g., primary pulmonary artery hypertension or Romano-Ward syndrome).

In more than 90 percent of infants and children with cardiovascular disease, the condition is congenital and not acquired. The prevalence of congenital heart disease is approximately 8:1,000 to 10:1,000 live births. The clinician should have a high index of suspicion for the possible presence of congenital heart disease in the following circumstances.

(1) A history of prematurity or being small for gestational age.

(2) An identifiable syndrome with or without associated chromosomal abnormality. For example, heart disease is very common in children with Down syndrome. Nearly 50 percent have an atrioventricular septal defect, ventricular septal defect, or patent ductus arteriosus. Turner syndrome is frequently associated with left heart lesions, especially coarctation of the aorta; and Noonan syndrome with right heart lesions such as pulmonary stenosis or atrial septal defect.

(3) The presence of other noncardiac congenital malformations. Nearly a quarter of all children with congenital cardiac disease have associated cardiac anomalies. The presence of congenital heart disease should be especially suspected in those infants and children with anomalies in the musculoskeletal system, central nervous system, and gastrointestinal system.

(4) Delayed height and weight maturation during infancy.

(5) Recurrent respiratory infections or episodes of bronchospasm.

The history and physical examination are particularly useful in eliciting symptoms and signs which may clearly point to involvement of the cardiovascular system. The assessment should include evaluation of growth and development, blood pressure measurement, and auscultation for abnormal heart sounds and murmurs. The possible presence of congestive heart failure or a chronic shunt hypoxemia (cyanosis) is almost invariably indicative of cardiac disease. Other symptoms and signs which point to the possible presence of cardiac disease include syncope (e.g., orthostatic hypotension, congenital complete heart block); dyspnea (e.g., fibrosing alveolitis) or wheezing (e.g., cor triatriatum); easy fatigability (e.g., pulmonary artery hypertension); chest pain (e.g., mitral valve prolapse); palpitations (e.g., Wolff-Parkinson-White syndrome); a cerebrovascular accident (e.g., arteriovenous malformation); seizures or abortive sudden death (e.g., Romano-Ward syndrome). If pulmonary disease is present, evidence of cor pulmonale should be sought.

Primary physicians should employ commonly used studies which they themselves can interpret. The most useful are the chest x-ray, electrocardiogram, and performance of systemic arterial oxygen saturation by pulse volume oximeter. These, in addition to the history and physical examination, will usually lead to the strong suspicion or identification of cardiac disease. Performance of more extensive studies such as echocardiograms, radionuclide imaging, exercise testing, or holter monitoring should be at the discretion of the cardiologist. Adequate performance of an echocardiogram requires great skill, knowledge of the pediatric cardiac disease searched for, and in infants and young children, adequate sedation. It is also rather expensive.

In addition to referral to a cardiologist, multiple consultations are often necessary in the management of patients with hereditary, metabolic, or acquired diseases. These consultations may include the geneticist (e.g., for Marfan syndrome); pulmonologist (e.g., fibrosing alveolitis); endocrinologist (e.g., Turner syndrome); rheumatologist (e.g., collagen diseases); or an expert in metabolic diseases (e.g., Pompe disease).

A pediatric cardiologist should be consulted when an infant exhibits one or more of the following: (a) central cyanosis; (b) persistent tachypnea; (c) congestive heart failure; (d) absent or weak femoral pulses; (e) loud murmur; (f) a heart rate greater than 200 or slower than 80 beats per minute; (g) chest x-ray with cardiomegaly, increased or decreased pulmonary vascularity; and (h) an abnormal electrocardiogram. In children and adolescents, consultation should be obtained when the following are present: (a) loud systolic murmur (grade 3/6 or greater); (b) any diastolic murmur; (c) cyanosis or clubbing; (d) chest pain suggestive of angina; (e) systemic hypertension with or without decreased femoral pulses; (f) palpitations, syncope, or exercise intolerance; (g) an abnormal rhythm; (h) an ECG with ventricular hypertrophy; and (i) cardiomegaly or pulmonary congestion on chest x-ray.

General principles in the management of children with any cardiac disease include appropriate dietary and nutritional recommendations, activity recommendations, the need for antimicrobial prophylaxis in the prevention of infective endocarditis at times of predictable risk, and appropriate therapy of intercurrent infections. Also important is attention to the psychosocial aspects of the cardiac disease, genetic counseling, advice with respect to travel, insurance, or employability, and sometimes the need for home therapy including oxygen, intravenous administration, or other devices. Special considerations may be required for both cardiac and noncardiac surgery, as well as the anesthetic used.

References

Fetal, Neonatal, and Infant Cardiac Disease: J.H. Moller and W.A. Neal, eds.; Appleton and Lange, 1989.

Smith's Recognizable Patterns of Human Malformations, 4th ed.: K.L. Jones; W.B. Saunders Company, 1988.

Moss' Heart Disease in Infants, Children and Adolescents, 4th ed.: F.H. Adams, G.C. Emmanouilides, and T.A. Riemenschneider, eds.; Williams and Wilkins, 1989.

CARDIOVASCULAR AND RESPIRATORY DISEASES
Listings in This Section

ALVEOLITIS, EXTRINSIC ALLERGIC

Description Extrinsic allergic alveolitis is a lung disease usually associated with certain occupations that provide the possibility of recurrent organic dust inhalation. Acute respiratory symptoms and fever may begin several hours after exposure. Chronic disease, marked by gradual changes in lung tissue, is associated with repeated episodes or longterm exposure (over years) to a specific organic dust.

Associated forms of the disease include bird breeder disease, bathtub refinisher's lung, mushroom picker disease, mushroom worker's lung, laboratory technician's lung, pituitary snuff-taker's lung, plastic worker's lung, epoxy resin lung, maltworker's lung, maple bark stripper disease, sequoiosis, suberosis, bagassosis, wheat weevil disease, farmer's lung, ventilation pneumonitis, and cheese-worker's lung.

Synonyms
Allergic Interstitial Pneumonitis
Extrinsic Allergic Pneumonia
Hypersensitivity Pneumonitis

Signs and Symptoms Symptoms generally include dyspnea, wheezing, and dry coughs that seem to shake the entire body. Additional symptoms may include chills, sweating, aching, and fatigue. Most cases involve typical episodes that are mild and short and may be misdiagnosed. The chronic disease that develops with prolonged exposure to the irritant may be characterized by fever, rales, cyanosis, and, possibly, expectoration of blood.

Etiology Repeated exposure to organic substances, often associated with a specific occupation, is linked to the disorder. The irritants may include avian dust, a paint catalyst used in bath tub refinishing, mushroom compost, rat or gerbil urine residue, snuff, plastic residue, heated epoxy residue, and a variety of molds, including moldy barley, maple bark dust, redwood bark dust (sequoiosis), cork dust (suberosis), sugar cane dust (bagasse), moldy wheat and hay dust, moldy water from heating and cooling systems, and cheese mold.

Epidemiology Males and females are both affected, depending on occupations and individual allergic reactions.

Related Disorders See *Alveolitis, Fibrosing.*
Asthma is often associated with allergies.

Desquamative interstitial pneumonia is a chronic pneumonia of unknown etiology characterized by dyspnea and a harsh cough that does not seem to clear the obstruction. Symptoms are caused by desquamation in the lungs and thickening of the air passage walls.

Treatment—Standard Identification and, if possible, avoidance of the irritant are the initial concerns of treatment. In an occupational setting, improved ventilation and air filtering masks are recommended for mild symptoms. If permanent lung changes have not occurred, corticosteroids and avoidance measures often reduce

466 | CARDIOVASCULAR AND RESPIRATORY DISEASES

severity and may resolve acute symptoms. Corticosteroids may also be tried in persistent cases. Change of occupation may be necessary.

Treatment—Investigational Please contact the agencies listed under Resources, below, for the most current information.

Resources

For more information on extrinsic allergic alveolitis: National Organization for Rare Disorders (NORD); American Lung Association; NIH/National Institute of Allergy and Infectious Diseases (NIAID); National Institute of Environmental Health Sciences.

References

Extrinsic Allergic Alveolitis in Children. Apropos of 4 Cases: M. Bost, et al.; Pediatrie, June 1984, 39(4), pp. 253–260.
Allergic Alveolitis (Pathogenesis and Diagnosis): K.C. Bergman; A. Gesamte Inn. Med., January 1980, 35(2), pp. 77–80.
Diagnostic Approach to New or Unrecognized Risks in Hypersensitivity Pneumopathies: C. Molina; Rev. Fr. Mal. Respir., 1983, 11(4), pp. 427–438.

ALVEOLITIS, FIBROSING

Description Fibrosing alveolitis is an inflammatory lung disorder characterized by abnormal formation of fibrous tissue between alveoli.

Synonyms

Alveolocapillary Block
Cryptogenic Fibrosing Alveolitis
Diffuse Fibrosing Alveolitis
Hamman-Rich Syndrome
Interstitial Diffuse Pulmonary Fibrosis
Pulmonary Fibrosis, Idiopathic

Signs and Symptoms Manifestations include progressive dyspnea and coughing that may not ease bronchial irritation. Rapid, shallow breathing and coughing occur with moderate exercise. The skin may appear cyanotic, and fingers or toes may become clubbed. Loss of appetite and weight, fatigue, fever, weakness, and vague chest pains are common. Infections occur easily, and untreated individuals develop complications that include emphysema, pulmonary infections, or cardiac disease. Imaging techniques monitor progressive lung changes.

Etiology The cause is unknown. Scleroderma, a blood factor associated with rheumatoid arthritis, or an autoimmune factor may be involved.

Epidemiology The disease affects males and females equally, primarily during middle age.

Related Disorders See *Alveolitis, Extrinsic Allergic.*

Treatment—Standard Early treatment with systemic corticosteroids (high doses followed by a lower maintenance dosage) may prevent widespread or permanent lung morbidity. Azathioprine may be effective in cases resistant to steroids. Other treatments include oxygen administered in high concentrations if blood oxygen is diminished, antibiotics for bacterial infections, and digitalis or diuretics for heart problems. Other treatment is symptomatic and supportive.

Treatment—Investigational Lung transplantation is under investigation as a possible treatment.

Please contact the agencies listed under Resources, below, for the most current information.

Resources

For more information on fibrosing alveolitis: National Organization for Rare Disorders (NORD); American Lung Association; NIH/National Heart, Lung, and Blood Institute (NHLBI).

References

Effect of Intermittent High Dose Parenteral Corticosteroids on the Alveolitis of Idiopathic Pulmonary Fibrosis: B.A. Keogh, et al.; Am. Rev. Respir. Dis., January 1983, 127(1), pp. 18–22.

Bronchoalveolar Lavage Fluid Neutrophils Increase after Corticosteroid Therapy in Smokers with Idiopathic Pulmonary Fibrosis: K.L. Christopher, et al.; Am. Rev. Respir. Dis., January 1986, 133(1), pp. 104–109.

Concentration, Biosynthesis and Degradation of Collagen in Idiopathic Pulmonary Fibrosis: M. Selman, et al.; Thorax, May 1986, 41(5), pp. 355–359.

ARTERIOVENOUS MALFORMATION (AVM)

Description AVM is a congenital disorder involving abnormal vascular communication between arteries and veins. AVM may occur in the central nervous system, spine, liver, or limbs.

Signs and Symptoms Spinal AVM is characterized by back pain associated with sensory loss and leg weakness, and, infrequently, acute hemorrhage. Urination is impaired early. Rarely, a murmur at auscultation can be heard over the spine, or a skin angioma may be seen. An x-ray of the spine may reveal the distinctive worm-like impression of tangled vessels.

There are 3 types of lesions. Type I, the most common, occurs in adults. It is a single coiled feeding vessel, usually with a single feeding artery arising from another artery between the ribs or a lumbar segmental artery. Located dorsally, Type I AVM is often surgically accessible.

Type II is less common, occurs in adults, and also has a single feeding vessel. A glomus-type anomaly, Type II presents delayed opacification after contrast medium injection prior to x-ray.

Type III typically occurs in the neck area in children, and has the poorest overall prognosis. There are multiple feeding vessels with a large malformation that often appears to fill the entire spinal canal, demonstrating rapid flow with marked arteriovenous shunting. The multiple arterial feeders and the location inside the spinal canal usually prohibit surgery, and bleeding occurs more frequently.

Large **cranial AVM** in infants result in congestive heart failure within 24 hours of delivery. Forty percent of older patients with cranial AVM initially have focal or generalized seizures. Headaches may occur with or without bleeding. A ruptured AVM causes bleeding in the subarachnoid space under the inner membrane of the brain or inside the brain itself. Clinical symptoms are similar to those of ruptured cerebral aneurysms. A steal syndrome occurs as blood is shunted away from normal brain tissue toward the AVM, causing focal neurologic deficits secondary to ischemia. Bleeding to the affected brain area, AVM size, and individual response to treatment affect outcome.

A CT scan of spinal cord AVM may be useful for both screening and follow-up. Digital intravenous computerized angiography may eventually replace common angiography as a diagnostic tool.

Etiology AVMs are congenital defects of unknown etiology.

Epidemiology Onset of symptoms is from early childhood to the 9th decade, affecting males slightly more often than females.

Treatment—Standard If spinal cord function is threatened, spinal AVM surgery using specialized microtechniques is indicated.

Treatment of cranial AVM includes anticonvulsants. Embolization or surgical removal may be attempted. If all the arterial feeders can be identified and embolized or ligated, the condition may be successfully treated (see below). In most instances, however, the location and size of the lesions preclude satisfactory therapy.

Treatment—Investigational Occlusion of feeder arteries by embolization (collapsing of the veins by shooting plastic pellets into them through a catheter) is being evaluated as a treatment for spinal AVM.

Cranial AVM patients are being treated experimentally with stereotactic Bragg-peak proton-beam therapy. This therapy is designed to induce subendothelial deposits of a collagen and hyaline substance that will narrow small vessel lumens and thicken the malformation's walls during the first 12 to 24 months following this procedure.

Please contact the agencies listed under Resources, below, for the most current information.

Resources

For more information on arteriovenous malformations: National Organization for Rare Disorders (NORD); NIH/National Institute of Neurological Disorders & Stroke (NINDS).

References
Harrison's Principles of Internal Medicine, 12th ed.: J.D. Wilson, et al., eds.; McGraw-Hill, 1991, pp. 2000–2001.

ATRIAL SEPTAL DEFECTS

Description A small opening (foramen ovale) is present in all normal infants at birth, but closes in the majority with advancing age. If the septum separating the 2 atria is incompletely and abnormally formed before birth, a large opening may persist. The defect leads to an increased workload on the right heart, and excessive blood flow to the lung. Symptoms tend to be absent or mild at first, so that the defect is often not recognized until school age or adulthood. In adults, various cardiorespiratory problems and heart failure begin to develop. Atrial defects can take several forms, including the most common, secundum defect, the less frequent ostium primum defect, and sinus venosus defect, or coronary sinus defect.

Signs and Symptoms In the **ostium secundum defect** the middle portion of the atrial septum, in the region of the foramen ovale, fails to close during fetal development. Although superficially similar to patent foramen ovale, the ostium secundum defect develops differently and has a different course.

In **ostium primum defects,** which may be associated with Down syndrome, the lower part of the atrial septum fails to develop normally. Often, the valves separating the atrium from the ventricle on each side (tricuspid valve—right side; mitral valve—left side) are also malformed, and the ventricular septum may be deficient.

Sinus venosus occurs high in the atrial septum and is often associated with anomalous entry of the right pulmonary veins into the right atrium or superior vena cave.

Many children are asymptomatic. A few have mild growth retardation and an unusual susceptibility to respiratory infections. At approximately 40 years of age (and earlier at high altitudes where there is more constriction of the pulmonary arteries), patients may begin to have difficulties because of the gradually developing hypertension in the pulmonary circulation, changing the direction in which the blood is shunted through the defect.

Clinical consequences of right-to-left shunts include cyanosis, clubbing of the fingertips, and polycythemia. Patients are predisposed to brain abscesses. Severe cases may result in heart failure, with edema and breathlessness. Arrhythmias, including atrial fibrillation, may occur in the disease's later stages. Patients are also predisposed to paradoxical embolism, especially during pregnancy. Death may result without surgical repair of the defect.

Etiology The causes of the arrest in embryonic development resulting in atrial septal defects are poorly understood. The defects may occur in association with a variety of other congenital cardiac defects, or in infants small for gestational age. Ostium primum defects often occur in individuals with Down syndrome.

Epidemiology Approximately one percent of live births have some type of congenital heart defect; of these, about 10 percent are atrial septal defects. Females are affected more often than males.

Related Disorders See *Atrioventricular Septal Defect.*

Treatment—Standard The definitive treatment is surgery, suturing shut the hole in the septum, or patching it with a graft. The success rate is high for this procedure. For ostium primum (endocardial cushion) defects, which may require repairing or replacing of the atrioventricular valves, the success rate is considerably lower. Surgery is optimally performed between the ages of 3 and 6.

Digitalis can be used as a preoperative, palliative treatment for arrhythmias, tachycardias, and heart failure. Sodium restriction, diuretics, and rest are also effective in treating congestive heart failure. Respiratory infections are treated vigorously and early. Because of the risk of bacterial endocarditis, patients should be given antibiotics prophylactically with surgery and procedures such as tooth extractions.

Treatment—Investigational Please contact the agencies listed under Resources, below, for the most current information.

Resources

For more information on atrial septal defects: National Organization for Rare Disorders (NORD); American Heart Association; American Lung Association; NIH/National Heart, Lung and Blood Institute (NHLBI).

References

Harrison's Principles of Internal Medicine, 12th ed.: J.D. Wilson, et al., eds.; McGraw-Hill, 1991, pp. 927–928.

ATRIOVENTRICULAR SEPTAL DEFECT

Description This form of congenital heart defect is characterized by improperly developed atrial and ventricular septa and atrioventricular valves. Symptoms and prognosis depend on the severity of the malformation. There is an incomplete form (atrial septal defect primum), transitional form (atrial septal defect and small ventricular septal defect), or complete form (large atrial and ventricular defects). In addition, the extent of leakage of the valves between the atria and ventricles and size of the ventricles influence symptoms and prognosis.

Synonyms

Cor Biloculare (Complete Atrioventricular Septal Defect)

Signs and Symptoms In the complete form, congestive heart failure usually develops during infancy, with congestion of the lungs and other tissues, and dyspnea. Initial indications include poor feeding, tachypnea, excessive sweating, and tachycardia. Mild cyanosis is often present. Pneumonias and bronchitis may occur frequently and precipitate heart failure. Pulmonary artery hypertension is present and leads to the development of permanent pulmonary vascular disease before one year of age. Older patients are also at risk for embolisms or thrombosis, brain abscesses, and bacterial endocarditis. Diagnosis can be suspected by electrocardiogram and made by echocardiography or cardiac catheterization and angiography.

Etiology The etiology of atrioventricular septal defects in unknown. The malformation occurs frequently in Down syndrome.

Epidemiology Children with Down syndrome constitute the majority of all cases.

Related Disorders Related disorders include **cor triloculare biatriatum,** in which there are 3 heart chambers (2 atria and 1 ventricle), and **cor triloculare biventricularis** (2 ventricles and 1 large atrium). See *Atrial Septal Defects; Cor Triatriatum; Ventricular Septal Defects.*

Treatment—Standard Surgical repair before 6 to 12 months of age is recommended, whenever feasible. Prior to surgery, congestive heart failure must be managed by digoxin and diuretics. Oxygen therapy and adequate nutrition may also prove beneficial. Some patients may survive into adulthood without surgery, and develop the Eisenmenger syndrome.

Because they are susceptible to bacterial endocarditis, patients should be given appropriate antimicrobial prophylaxis at times of predictable risk (e.g., dental work). Similarly, respiratory infections are treated vigorously and early.

Treatment—Investigational Please contact the agencies listed under Resources, below, for the most current information.

Resources

For more information on atrioventricular septal defect: National Organization for Rare Disorders (NORD); American Heart Association; NIH/National Heart, Lung and Blood Institute (NHLBI); American Lung Association; National Down Syndrome Society; National Down Syndrome Congress.

For genetic information and genetic counseling referrals: March of Dimes Birth Defects Foundation; National Center for Education in Maternal and Child Health (NCEMCH).

BROAD BETA DISEASE

Description This hereditary lipid transport disorder is marked by the presence of xanthomas under certain skin areas. The patient is predisposed to obesity, atherosclerosis, and occlusion of blood vessels.

Synonyms
>Familial Broad Beta Disease
>Familial Dysbetalipoproteinemia
>Hyperlipoproteinemia, Type III
>Xanthoma Tuberosum

Signs and Symptoms Xanthomas appear in adults on the palms of the hands, fingers (occasionally), knees, elbows, arms, legs, and buttocks, and within the Achilles tendon. The cornea may also be affected (arcus lipidus corneae).

The primary complications are cardiovascular. An imbalance of cholesterol-transporting protein-lipid molecules and other fats leads to elevated cholesterol and triglyceride blood levels. The patient's obesity resulting from this disorder increases the risk of cardiovascular disease.

Etiology Broad beta disease is believed to be an inherited autosomal dominant trait. It has been associated rarely with diabetes or hypothyroidism.

Epidemiology Adults of both sexes may be affected.

Related Disorders Broad beta disease is one of several forms of hyperlipoproteinemia.

Treatment—Standard Reducing the amounts of cholesterol and fats in the patient's diet may prevent xanthomas and hyperlipidemia. Xanthomas can sometimes be removed surgically. Treatment of cardiovascular disease is symptomatic.

Treatment—Investigational Please contact the agencies listed under Resources, below, for the most current information.

Resources
   For more information on broad beta disease: National Organization for Rare Disorders (NORD); National Lipid Diseases Foundation; American Heart Association; NIH/National Heart, Lung and Blood Institute (NHLBI).
   For genetic information and genetic counseling referrals: March of Dimes Birth Defects Foundation; National Center for Education in Maternal and Child Health (NCEMCH).

CHURG-STRAUSS SYNDROME

Description Churg-Strauss syndrome is a lung disorder which often occurs as a complication of other conditions. Angiitis or vasculitis is accompanied by granulomas.

Synonyms
   Allergic Angiitis and Granulomatosis
   Allergic Granulomatosis and Angiitis
   Allergic Granulomatous Angiitis
   System Vasculitis with Asthma and Eosinophilia

Signs and Symptoms An allergic reaction or asthma may precede the syndrome's development by several years. Asthma tends to subside as vasculitis occurs. Lung tissue infiltrations (short term or persistent), fever, and weight loss are often initial signs. Interstitial lung disease, ophthalmic lesions, and seizures may develop.
   Granulomas may infiltrate tissue and cause deterioration; they may be accompanied by eosinophils, which can unite with the granulomas to form larger lesions. Histiocytes and a variable number of giant cells may invade tissues, especially in the lungs. Vascular growths can bring about both deterioration and infiltrating inflammation. Lesions can heal with or without scar formation.
   Malaise, skin rash, kidney inflammation, peripheral neuropathy, asymmetric

polyarthralgia, or arthritis may occur.

Etiology Although the exact etiology is unknown, the disease may be associated with an autoimmune disorder, possibly involving antibodies to thyroglobulin, parietal cells, adrenal cells, or thyroid.

Epidemiology Onset may occur from 15 to 70 years of age. The disease affects both males and females.

Related Disorders See *Polyarteritis Nodosa; Wegener Granulomatosis.*

Treatment—Standard Corticosteroids and/or cyclophosphamide are used for inflammation and kidney problems. Intravenous methylprednisolone may be effective in severe cases. Other treatment is symptomatic and supportive.

Treatment—Investigational Plasma exchange in conjunction with corticosteroids and cyclophosphamide is being evaluated.

Please contact the agencies listed under Resources, below, for the most current information.

Resources

For more information on Churg-Strauss syndrome: National Organization for Rare Disorders (NORD); American Lung Association; NIH/National Heart, Lung and Blood Institute (NHLBI).

References

Internal Medicine, 2nd ed.: J.H. Stein, ed.-in-chief; Little, Brown and Company, 1987, pp. 1285–1286.

Allergic Angiitis of Churg-Strauss Syndrome. Response to Pulse Methylprednisolone: R. MacFadyen, et al.; Chest, April 1987, 91(4), pp. 629–631.

Systemic Vasculitis with Asthma and Eosinophilia. A Clinical Approach to the Churg-Strauss Syndrome: J.G. Lanham, et al.; Medicine (Baltimore), March 1984, 63(2), pp. 65–81.

Conjunctival Involvement in Churg-Strauss Syndrome: C.L. Shields, et al.; Am. J. Ophthalmol., November 1986, 102(5), pp. 601–605.

COR TRIATRIATUM

Description Cor triatriatum is a rare congenital heart defect characterized by a small extra chamber above the left atrium into which the pulmonary veins drain. As a result, the passage of blood to the left atrium and ventricle is slowed, simulating obstruction of the mitral valve.

Synonyms
Triatrial Heart

Signs and Symptoms Depending on the size of the opening between the extra chamber and the left atrium proper, when the opening is small symptoms develop early in infancy. Symptoms include tachypnea, wheezing, coughing, and pulmonary congestion. Progressive enlargement of the heart occurs, often resulting in the development of high pulmonary artery pressure and right heart congestive failure. Heart murmurs may be present. In older patients, generalized edema, extreme dyspnea, poor oxygenation of the tissues, and tachycardia occur. Frequent pneumonias and bronchitis are likely, in turn precipitating heart failure. Patients are also at risk for bacterial endocarditis. Diagnosis can be made through echocardiography, magnetic resonance imaging, or heart catheterization and angiography.

Etiology The cause of cor triatriatum is unknown.

Related Disorders The condition simulates **mitral valve stenosis.**

Epidemiology Infants of both sexes may be affected.

Treatment—Standard Most patients will require surgery, which should be performed at a young age. Prior to surgery, congestive heart failure should be managed by diuretics and, if necessary, fluid and salt restriction. Digitalis should also be administered to increase the strength and decrease the rate of the heart contractions. Oxygen therapy may also prove beneficial. Respiratory infections are treated vigorously and early.

Treatment—Investigational Please contact the agencies listed under Resources, below, for the most current information.

Resources

For more information on cor triatriatum: National Organization for Rare Disorders (NORD); American Heart Association; American Lung Association; NIH/National Heart, Lung and Blood Institute (NHLBI).

For genetic information and genetic counseling referrals: March of Dimes Birth Defects Foundation; National Center for Education in Maternal and Child Health (NCEMCH).

References

Moss' Heart Disease in Infants, Children, and Adolescents, 4th ed.: F.H. Adams, G.C. Emmanouilides, and T.A. Riemenschneider, eds.; Williams and Wilkins, 1989.

DEXTROCARDIA WITH SITUS INVERSUS

Description The condition is characterized by a right-sided positioning of the heart, with reversal of its chambers and the abdominal viscera.

Synonyms

Heterotaxy Syndrome
Mirror-Image Dextrocardia
Situs Inversus Totalis

Signs and Symptoms The cardiac silhouette is positioned on the right side of the chest with the apex pointing to the right; the position of the chambers and of the abdominal organs is reversed. Heart sounds emanating more clearly from the right chest provide physical evidence of the condition. Chest roentgenography reveals malpositioning of the heart. The electrocardiogram shows inversion of electrical waves. Most patients live a normal life without associated symptoms or disability. However, about 20 percent of patients have Kartagener syndrome, or the triad of situs inversus, sinusitis, and bronchiectasis. While situs inversus totalis is rarely associated with congenital heart disease, situs inversus of the abdominal organs and a normally positioned heart are commonly associated with heart defects. Similarly, a heart in the right chest with normal or ambiguous abdominal situs is often associated with severe heart defects.

Etiology The disorder, present at birth, is transmitted by autosomal recessive genes.

Epidemiology The incidence of dextrocardia with complete situs inversus is about 2:10,000 live births. Males and females are affected in equal numbers.

Related Disorders See *Kartagener Syndrome.*

Treatment—Standard Treatment is symptomatic and supportive. If the condition is associated with other more serious heart malformations, the prognosis and treatment will vary. Genetic counseling may be helpful.

Treatment—Investigational Please contact the agencies listed under Resources, below, for the most current information.

Resources

  For more information on dextrocardia with situs inversus: National Organization for Rare Disorders (NORD); American Heart Association; NIH/National Heart, Lung and Blood Institute (NHLBI).

  For genetic information and genetic counseling referrals: March of Dimes Birth Defects Foundation; National Center for Education in Maternal and Child Health (NCEMCH).

References

Congenitally Corrected Transposition in the Adult. Detection by Radionuclide Angiocardiography: G.L. Guit, et al.; Radiology, November 1985, issue 157(2), pp. 521–527.
A Possible Increase in the Incidence of Congenital Heart Defects Among the Offspring of Affected Parents: V. Rose, et al.; J. Am. Coll. Cardiol., August 1985, issue 6(2), pp. 376–382.
Internal Medicine, 2nd ed.: J.H. Stein, ed.-in-chief; Little, Brown and Company, 1987, pp. 525.
The Heart, Arteries and Veins, 7th ed.: J.W. Hurst, et al., eds.; McGraw-Hill, 1990, pp. 255, 757–758.

DILATATION OF THE PULMONARY ARTERY, IDIOPATHIC (IDPA)

Description IDPA is a rare congenital defect in which the main pulmonary artery is dilated in the absence of any apparent anatomic or physiologic cause.

Signs and Symptoms IDPA generally produces no symptoms because there is no circulation abnormality. The minimal clinical signs consist of a pulmonary ejection sound that disappears on inhalation, a soft pulmonary ejection systolic murmur, and splitting of the 2nd sound on inhalation. The disorder does not cause pulmonary valve disease, nor does bacterial endocarditis occur. The electrocardiogram is normal, and diagnosis is made when chest x-ray films reveal a dilated main pulmonary artery without cardiac chamber enlargement. An echocardiogram confirms the diagnosis.

Etiology The cause is unknown; however, a defect in the normal development of pulmonary artery elastic tissue before or after birth has been postulated. The dilatation also may be a consequence of a generalized connective tissue disease, because it is occasionally found in Marfan syndrome or Ehlers-Danlos syndrome (see *Marfan Syndrome; Ehlers-Danlos Syndrome*).

Treatment—Standard Treatment is not required. Affected persons have a normal life expectancy provided there are no cardiac lesions.

Treatment—Investigational Please contact the agencies listed under Resources, below, for the most current information.

Resources
For more information on idiopathic dilatation of the pulmonary artery: National Organization for Rare Disorders (NORD); NIH/National Heart, Lung and Blood Institute (NHLBI); American Lung Association.

EISENMENGER SYNDROME

Description The syndrome is characterized by a congenital ventricular septal defect. Pulmonary vascular resistance **(PVR)** increases as the child matures, resulting in high pulmonary artery pressure. The term Eisenmenger syndrome has also been applied to the association of other congenital heart defects with advanced pulmonary vascular disease.

The patient has dyspnea, cyanosis, and polycythemia. Some patients do not deteriorate until age 40 or 50.

Signs and Symptoms Onset of noticeable symptoms usually occurs between ages 5 and 15. Cyanosis develops, especially during exertion, and a heart murmur may be detected. In persistent ductus arteriosus (without a ventricular septal defect), the feet will appear more bluish than the hands. Swelling due to soft-tissue proliferation at the fingertips and toes (clubbing) may also occur. Dyspnea and easy fatigability are common, and angina and syncope may occur.

Older patients have an abnormally high blood pressure, and atrial fibrillation may present in the later stages.

An enlarged right ventricle, and loud pulmonary valve closure, may be evident on medical examination. Signs of pulmonary hypertension may be identified by a heaving parasternal cardiac impulse; a loud pulmonary second sound transmitted to the apex of the heart, by high diastolic pressure closing the valve forcibly; a pulmonary ejection click; a high-frequency decrescendo murmur during diastole down the left edge of the sternum; and a pansystolic murmur caused by incomplete closure of the tricuspid valve.

Failure of the right cardiac ventricle is characterized by dyspnea and fluid retention, often resulting in edema.

Hemoptysis may occur in advanced stages. Chest x-rays may show enlarged pulmonary arteries close to the lungs and ischemia in the periphery of the lungs. An enlarged atrium and tissue death due to pulmonary infarction may occur during late stages.

Etiology The cause of the defective development of the fetal heart and pulmonary vasculature are not known.

Epidemiology Male and female infants are affected in equal numbers.

Related Disorders See *Pulmonary Hypertension, Primary; Ventricular Septal Defects.*

Treatment—Standard Treatment is symptomatic and supportive. Anticoagulants should be avoided because of the risk of hemorrhaging in the lungs.

Treatment—Investigational Repair of the cardiac defect with single lung transplantation or combined heart and lung transplantation has been performed with a reasonable success rate.

Please contact the agencies listed under Resources, below, for the most current information.

Resources

For more information on Eisenmenger syndrome: National Organization for Rare Disorders (NORD); NIH/National Heart, Lung and Blood Institute (NHLBI).

For genetic information and genetic counseling referrals: March of Dimes Birth Defects Foundation; National Center for Education in Maternal and Child Health (NCEMCH).

References

Abnormal Architecture of the Ventricles in Hearts with an Overriding Aortic Valve and a Perimembranous Ventricular Septal Defect ("Eisenmenger VSD"): A. Oppenheimer-Dekker, et al.; Int'l. J. Cardiol., November 1985, 9(3), pp. 341–355.

Combined Heart and Lung Transplantation: S.W. Jamieson, et al.; Lancet, May 1983, 1(8334), pp. 1130–1132.

Eisenmenger's Syndrome and Pregnancy: S. Lieber, et al.; Acta Cardiol. (Brux.), 1985, 40(4), pp. 421–424.

Endocardial Fibroelastosis (EFE)

Description EFE, a serious and rare heart disorder affecting infants and children, is characterized by a thickened endocardium that shows an increase in collagenous and elastic tissue. These lesions cause cardiac hypertrophy and congestive heart failure. Two forms are recognized: the rare restrictive cardiomyopathy and the more common congestive cardiomyopathy.

Synonyms
Endocardial Dysplasia
Endocardial Sclerosis
Fetal Endomyocardial Fibrosis
Subendocardial Sclerosis

Signs and Symptoms Elastic tissue proliferates in the subendocardium, causing a diffuse, milky-white thickening of the endocardium and subendocardium. The onset of symptoms, which generally occurs between 4 and 12 months of age, is rapid and most commonly features dyspnea, grunting respirations, cough, irritability, weakness, and pallor. The physical examination may reveal respiratory distress; intercostal retractions; fine, moist rales; and a gallop rhythm of the heart. The chest film shows an enlarged heart.

Left ventricular hypertrophy suggests the diagnosis. The earliest signs of myocardial damage are shown in subtle S-T segment and T-wave changes on the electrocardiogram **(ECG).** Serial ECGs reveal progression or regression of the disorder. Ventricular failure may also be encountered with tachycardia and atrial and ventricular arrhythmias. Severe mitral regurgitation is common.

Etiology The cause is not known. EFE may be hereditary.

Epidemiology EFE affects less than 1 percent of infants and children with congenital heart disease. Infants and children of both sexes between the ages of 4 months and 2 years are affected. A few adult cases have been reported.

Related Disorders Idiopathic cardiomyopathy, a disorder of unknown origin, is characterized by cardiac hypertrophy and dilatation. **Viral myocarditis** is marked by severe dyspnea, an enlarged heart, tachycardia, arrhythmias, and generalized edema.

Treatment—Standard Response to treatment is most favorable when the damage is noted early. Bed rest may facilitate healing of the myocardial lesions while the myocardium is working at a reduced load. Further therapy is directed at control of congestive heart failure, with agents such as afterload reduction digitalis and diuretics. Associated arrhythmias require appropriate antiarrhythmic therapy. Anticoagulation may be necessary. Prognosis is guarded despite therapy. Cardiac transplantation is effective surgical treatment.

Treatment—Investigational Please contact the agencies listed under Resources, below, for the most current information.

Resources
For more information on endocardial fibroelastosis: National Organization for Rare Disorders (NORD); American Heart Association; NIH/National Heart, Lung and Blood Institute (NHLBI).

References
Cecil Textbook of Medicine, 18th ed.: J.B. Wyngaarden and L.H. Smith, Jr., eds.; W.B. Saunders Company, 1988, p. 351.

The Heart, Arteries and Veins, 17th ed.: J.S. Hurst, et al., eds.; McGraw-Hill, 1990, pp. 725–726, 1312–1313.

ENDOMYOCARDIAL FIBROSIS (EMF)

Description A heart disease of unknown etiology, EMF is commonly characterized by a gross fibrosis of the endocardium lining of one or both ventricles, which progresses toward ventricular cavities constriction and involvement of the chordae tendineae and atrioventricular valves. EMF may be progressive **Loeffler disease,** a heart and small-arteries disease of unknown origin characterized by eosinophilia, gross fibrosis of the endocardium, small-vessel arteritis, and infiltration of other organs.

Synonyms
Davies Disease
Fibroelastic Endocarditis

Pathophysiology, Signs, and Symptoms Fibrotic lesions may be over 1 cm thick, project into the myocardium, and frequently affect the heart asymmetrically. The left ventricle may be involved at its base, or on its posterior left wall, including the chordae tendineae. The right ventricle may be involved at its apex and along the inflow tract, encasing the tricuspid valve's papillary muscles and chordae tendineae. Thrombosis often develops on the surface of the fibrotic lesions, and calcification may occur.

Left ventricular fibrosis is characterized by restricted left ventricle filling with diminished diastolic compliance. Mitral valve incompetence is frequent, resulting in mitral regurgitation, left atrial dilatation, pulmonary venous hypertension, left ventricular enlargement, and first-degree arteriovenous block. Atrial fibrillation is common. A chest x-ray may reveal a normal or mildly enlarged heart except for left atrial enlargement and signs of pulmonary venous hypertension. The electrocardiogram **(ECG)** shows a low QRS voltage and a nonspecific S-T segment with T-wave changes.

Right ventricular fibrosis is characterized by restricted filling of the right ventricle and poor ventricular compliance. It is often associated with tricuspid valve incompetence. Tricuspid regurgitation, right atrial dilatation, and systemic venous hypertension result. Ascites, hepatosplenomegaly, and jugular vein distention with facial edema may be present. Findings similar to left ventricular fibrosis are seen on ECG. Chest x-rays show an enlarged right atrium.

Biventricular fibrosis is a combination of right and left ventricular fibrosis.

The extracardiac manifestations of **Loeffler disease** include stroke, petechial hemorrhages, and hepatomegaly.

Etiology Suggested causes have included filariasis and diet. An immunologic mechanism is currently suspected.

Epidemiology EMF is endemic in the tropics but rare in Europe and North America. All races can be affected, mostly children and young adults. The disease has occurred in a few patients over age 60.

Treatment—Standard Open-heart surgery is the only effective treatment. The procedure involves endomyocardiectomy to allow normal diastolic ventricular filling; repair or replacement of the mitral or tricuspid valve (or both) to ensure valvular competence; and leaving a portion of fibrous endocardium on the left ventricular septum to prevent postoperative heart block. Cardiac transplantation may also be an option.

Treatment—Investigational Please contact the agencies listed under Resources, below, for the most current information.

Resources

For more information on endomyocardial fibrosis: National Organization for Rare Disorders (NORD); American Heart Association; NIH/National Heart, Lung and Blood Institute (NHLBI); Centers for Disease Control (CDC).

References
Cecil Textbook of Medicine, 18th ed.: J.B. Wyngaarden and L.H. Smith, Jr., eds.; W.B. Saunders Company, 1988, pp. 361–362.

GOODPASTURE SYNDROME

Description Goodpasture syndrome is a rare disease that causes inflammation of pulmonary and renal membranes. It is classified into 3 groups according to its etiology: autoimmune or antibody-induced disease, systemic vasculitis, and idiopathic Goodpasture. When the disease is antibody-induced, the antibodies that cause inflammation appear to be deposited in capillary membranes of the lungs and kidneys.

Synonyms
Pneumorenal Syndrome

Signs and Symptoms Lung hemorrhage and renal dysfunction are the major features of Goodpasture syndrome. Symptoms include hemoptysis, rhonchi, and dyspnea, and, less commonly, coughing, chills, hypertension, fatigue, and weakness. Fibrous tissue may form in the lungs.

Glomerulonephritis may progress rapidly to renal failure. Anemia and pallor give evidence of renal dysfunction, and hematuria and proteinuria may be present.

Although symptoms may recur during therapy, continued treatment is effective for many patients.

Etiology The known causes of Goodpasture syndrome are toxins, such as hydrocarbon chemical exposure, and infections, such as influenza. Even simple infections can cause Goodpasture syndrome in some patients. Antiglomerular basement membrane (**anti-GBM**) antibodies appear to circulate throughout the blood and damage pneumorenal membranes.

Epidemiology Goodpasture syndrome occurs worldwide and at any age, and seems to be more frequent in males.

Related Disorders See *Wegener Granulomatosis.*

A lung disorder similar to Goodpasture syndrome that occurs mostly in young children is **idiopathic pulmonary hemosiderosis.** This disorder is marked by chronic secondary anemia; however, it does not produce the antibody reaction found in Goodpasture syndrome.

A lung and kidney disorder that also has some clinical similarities to Goodpasture syndrome is **bacterial endocarditis.** This disease also affects the heart and can cause heart murmurs and embolism. Other symptoms are skin lesions, splenomegaly, and intermittent high fever.

Treatment—Standard The use of plasmapheresis combined with immunosuppressive drugs to treat Goodpasture syndrome has been successful in most patients. Corticosteroids alone or in combination with azathioprine or mercaptopurine may be of benefit in some cases. In some patients hemodialysis and/or renal transplantation seem to be the best treatment options; transplantation must await decrease in levels of circulating anti-GBM antibody.

Goodpasture syndrome has been considered a highly fatal disease, but recent studies have shown that the mortality rate for the syndrome dropped from 86 percent in 1955 to 13 percent in 1982 as a result of improved therapy. These studies have also shown that as many as 51 percent of patients no longer require renal dialysis.

Treatment—Investigational Researchers are investigating the benefits of selective methods of plasmapheresis over nonspecific methods in the treatment of Goodpasture syndrome as well as many other autoimmune disorders. Cascade filtration, cryofiltration, immunoabsorption, enzymatic degradation, and continuous electrophoresis are among the procedures under investigation.

Please contact the agencies listed under Resources, below, for the most current information.

Resources

For more information on Goodpasture syndrome: National Organization for Rare Disorders (NORD); Immune Deficiency Foundation; The National Kidney Foundation; American Lung Association; National Kidney and Urologic Diseases Information Clearinghouse.

References
Immunomodulation with Apheresis Technics: A. Liebert, et al.; Allerg. Immunol. (Leipz.), 1986, issue 32(1), pp. 5–18.

Goodpasture's Syndrome: Development of its Prognosis from 1955 to 1982: J. Marcandoro, et al.; Presse Med., May 28, 1985, issue 12(23), pp. 1483–1487.

The Clinical Spectrum of Acute Glomerulonephritis and Lung Haemorrhage (Goodpasture's Syndrome): S. Holdsworth, et al.; Q. J. Med., April 1985, issue 55(216), pp. 75–86.

HEART BLOCK, CONGENITAL

Description This rare congenital heart disease involves the conduction system of the heart, and results in a slow heart rate. There are 3 forms of congenital heart block: first, second, and third degree.

Synonyms
>Atrioventricular (AV) Block

Signs and Symptoms First-degree atrioventricular **(AV)** block is characterized by slowed conduction of electrical impulses within the AV node and is detectable only by electrocardiogram. The condition is benign and not associated with symptoms. Second-degree AV block may be associated with symptoms. In third-degree (complete) AV block, no atrial impulses are conducted to the ventricles. There is independent beating of the atria and ventricles. Some patients may be asymptomatic, but others develop fatigue with exertion, lightheadedness, syncope, or sudden death.

Etiology The etiology is unknown. Some cases may be caused during pregnancy by an intrauterine infection or by the presence of an autoimmune disorder, such as systemic lupus erythematosus, in the mother.

Epidemiology Males and females are affected equally.

Related Disorders Mobitz type I (Wenkebach) AV block is characterized by progressive slowing of AV conduction of atrial impulses. It is usually transient. **Mobitz type II AV block** has an acute onset and generally indicates organic heart disease.

>**Bundle branch block** is due to a lesion in a bundle branch. It is occasionally congenital and usually indicates prior cardiac surgery or cardiovascular disease. Right bundle branch block, characterized by a slowing of conduction in the bundle branches, may occur in patients with no clinical evidence of cardiovascular disease.

Treatment—Standard Atropine increases AV conduction. Complete heart block often requires a pacemaker.

Treatment—Investigational For pregnant women affected with connective tissue disease, especially systemic lupus erythematosus, plasmapheresis may be useful. Dexamethasone is under investigation for this situation.

>Please contact the agencies listed under Resources, below, for the most current information.

Resources
>**For more information on congenital heart block:** National Organization for Rare Disorders (NORD); American Heart Association; NIH/National Heart, Lung and Blood Institute (NHLBI); International Bundle Branch Block Association.
>**For genetic information and genetic counseling referrals:** March of

Dimes Birth Defects Foundation; National Center for Education in Maternal and Child Health (NCEMCH).

References

Internal Medicine, 2nd ed.: J.H. Stein, ed.-in-chief; Little, Brown and Company, 1987, pp. 301–570.

Delayed Maternal Lupus after Delivery of Offspring with Congenital Heart Block: B.S. Kasinath, et al.; Arch. Intern. Med., December 1982, 142(13), p. 2317.

Connective Tissue Disease, Antibodies to Ribonucleoprotein, and Congenital Heart Block: J.S. Scott, et al.; N. Engl. J. Med., July 1983, 28(309), pp. 209–212.

Maternal Antibodies Against Fetal Cardiac Antigens in Congenital Complete Heart Block: P.V. Taylor, et al.; N. Engl. J. Med., September 1986, 315(11), pp. 667–672.

HYPOPLASTIC LEFT HEART SYNDROME

Description Hypoplastic left heart syndrome is a congenital heart defect characterized by an underdeveloped left atrium and ventricle and narrowed valves connecting the chambers to each other (mitral valve) and to an abnormally formed aorta (aortic valve).

Synonyms

Aortic Atresia, Mitral Atresia

Signs and Symptoms Underdevelopment of the left side of the heart impairs blood flow from the lungs to the systemic circulation. There is poor systemic perfusion, metabolic acidosis, and shock. Blood also accumulates in the lungs, and congestive heart failure develops. Without surgical intervention, death usually occurs in the newborn period with very few patients surviving infancy.

Etiology The causes of the arrest in embryonic development of the left heart are poorly understood. Less than 10 percent of the cases appear to be familial.

Epidemiology Hypoplastic left heart syndrome may affect infants of both sexes.

Treatment—Standard Emergency medical treatment is directed to maintenance of adequate systemic perfusion by infusion of prostaglandin E-1 (PGE-1), which keeps the ductus arteriosus patent. Digoxin and diuretics are also useful. More definitive surgical therapy is available and includes the Norwood procedure followed by a bidirectional Glenn or Fontan procedure. Another surgical option is cardiac transplantation.

Treatment—Investigational Please contact the agencies listed under Resources, below, for the most current information.

Resources

For more information on hypoplastic left heart syndrome: National Organization for Rare Disorders (NORD); American Heart Association; NIH/National Heart, Lung and Blood Institute (NHLBI).

References
Fetal, Neonatal and Infant Cardiac Disease: J.H. Moller and W.A. Neal, eds.; Appleton and Lange, 1989.

LYMPHOMATOID GRANULOMATOSIS

Description Lymphomatoid granulomatosis is a vascular disease that is rare and progressive and characterized by nodular lesions that infiltrate and destroy veins and arteries, especially in the lungs. The condition can be benign or malignant.

Synonyms
Benign Lymphangiitis and Granulomatosis
Malignant Lymphangiitis and Granulomatosis
Pulmonary Angiitis
Pulmonary Wegener Granulomatosis

Signs and Symptoms The destructive lesions can occur in the lungs, kidneys, central nervous system, or skin. The patient may have a cough with or without hemoptysis, dyspnea, chest pain, malaise, fever, weight loss, diarrhea, arthralgia, and myalgia. Macules, nodules, and sometimes ulcerations appear when the skin is affected.

Respiratory distress and eventually failure of the respiratory system can result. In severe cases, the lesions sometimes take on the characteristics of **malignant lymphoma**. Lung biopsy may be necessary for diagnosis.

Etiology While the exact cause is unknown, some cases are thought to result from an allergic reaction to an unknown antigen. Others appear to be autoimmune-related.

Epidemiology Although lymphomatoid granulomatosis can affect individuals of any age, it occurs more often in persons over 40 years, and it is slightly more common in males than females.

Related Disorders See *Wegener Granulomatosis; Churg-Strauss Syndrome.*

Treatment—Standard The administration of corticosteroid drugs or cyclophosphamide or both in combination is standard treatment. Other therapy depends on symptoms.

Treatment—Investigational The orphan drug prednimustine is being tested as a treatment for malignant lymphomatoid granulomatosis. For more information, please contact Smith Kline & French Laboratories, 1500 Spring Garden Street, Philadelphia, Pennsylvania 19101.

Please contact the agencies listed under Resources, below, for the most current information.

Resources
For more information on lymphomatoid granulomatosis: National Organization for Rare Disorders (NORD); American Lung Association; American Can-

cer Society; NIH/National Cancer Institute Physicians Data Query (PDQ) phone-line; Cancer Information Service (CIS); NIH/National Heart, Lung and Blood Institute (NHLBI).

References

Internal Medicine, 2nd ed.: J.H. Stein, ed.-in-chief; Little, Brown and Company, 1987, p. 665.

Pulmonary Diseases and Disorders, vol. 2, 2nd ed.: A.P. Fishman, ed.; McGraw-Hill, 1980, p. 1127.

Benign Lymphocytic Angiitis and Granulomatosis: H. Tukianen, et al.; Thorax, August 1988, issue 43(8), pp. 649–650.

Lymphomatoid Granulomatosis: A Review of 12 Cases: J. Prenovault, et al.; Can. Assoc. Radiol. J., December 1988, issue 39(4), pp. 263–266.

Necrotizing Vasculitis with Granulomatosis: I. Yevich; Int. J. Dermatol., October 1988, issue 27(8), pp. 540–546.

MITRAL VALVE PROLAPSE SYNDROME (MVPS)

Description MVPS is a cardiac disorder that may occur alone or be associated with other disorders, such as **connective tissue disease** or **muscular dystrophy**. Mitral regurgitation may cause other complications.

Synonyms

Ballooning Posterior Leaflet Syndrome
Barlow Syndrome
Billowing Posterior Mitral Leaflet Syndrome
Click-Murmur Syndrome
Mitral Click-Murmur Syndrome
Mitral Leaflet Syndrome

Signs and Symptoms Most patients have no noticeable symptoms. When these occur, they may initially include fatigue, weakness, palpitations, and dizzy spells. Other persons experience atypical chest pain or have a history of heart murmur. In some severe cases, patients demonstrate an inability to breathe except when sitting upright. Arrhythmia may develop. Examination may reveal a single or multiple midsystolic click. Mitral regurgitation does not occur in all cases and may be minor, slowly progressive, or sudden and severe. Rare cases may result in endocarditis, transient ischemic episodes, stroke, congestive heart failure, or sudden death.

Diagnostic tests include chest x-ray, stationary and ambulatory electrocardiogram recordings, echocardiography, cardiac catheterization and angiography, radionuclide studies, and exercise testing. The diagnosis is usually established by physical examination and is confirmed by echocardiography.

Etiology The syndrome can be inherited as an autosomal dominant trait. Some cases result from neuroendocrine or autonomic nerve dysfunction. Mitral valve leaflets may be myxomatous or redundant; and chordae tendineae may become elongated, causing prolapse of the mitral valve into the left atrium. Abnormally contracting left ventricular wall segments may also be a cause, as may rheumatic fever.

Epidemiology The syndrome affects both males and females and often appears in women of childbearing age.

Related Disorders See *Marfan Syndrome; Rheumatic Fever.*

Treatment—Standard Patients should receive antibiotics prior to surgery. Oral contraceptives for women with mitral valve prolapse are contraindicated, since serious complications may occur. Surgical replacement of the affected valve is indicated with severe mitral regurgitation.

Treatment—Investigational Beta blockers and moricizine may alleviate arrhythmias and tachycardia, as well as palpitations, dizziness, and syncope.

Please contact the agencies listed under Resources, below, for the most current information.

Resources

For more information on mitral valve prolapse: National Organization for Rare Disorders (NORD); American Heart Association; NIH/National Heart, Lung & Blood Institute (NHLBI).

For genetic information and genetic counseling referrals: March of Dimes Birth Defects Foundation; NIH/National Center for Education in Maternal and Child Health (NCEMCH).

References

Internal Medicine, 2nd ed.: J.H. Stein, ed.-in-chief; Little, Brown and Company, 1987, pp. 475–482.

Mitral Valve Prolapse Syndrome. Evidence of Hyperadrenergic State: H. Boudoulas, et al.; Postgrad. Med., February 1988, pp. 152–162.

Complex Ventricular Arrhythmias Associated with the Mitral Valve Prolapse Syndrome. Effectiveness of Moricizine (Ethmozine) in Patients Resistant to Conventional Antiarrhythmics: C.M. Pratt, et al.; Am. J. Med., April 1986, 80(4), pp. 626–632.

Mitral Valve Prolapse in Women with Oral Contraceptive-Related Cerebrovascular Insufficiency. Associated Persistent Hypercoagulable State: M.B. Elam, et al.; Arch. Intern. Med., January 1986, 146(1), pp. 73–77.

ORTHOSTATIC HYPOTENSION

Description Orthostatic hypotension is an extreme and rapid drop in blood pressure occurring when a person suddenly stands. A defect in the baroreceptors is often involved.

Synonyms

Low Blood Pressure
Postural Hypotension

Signs and Symptoms Symptoms, which usually appear after sudden standing, may include dizziness, lightheadedness, blurred vision, and syncope.

Etiology Hypovolemia—resulting from excessive use of diuretics or vasodilators, or prolonged bed rest—is a common cause. Other types of drugs that can cause orthostatic hypotension include phenothiazines, tricyclic antidepressants, the monoamine oxidase inhibitors, and alpha-adrenergic blocking agents. Specific drugs include alcohol, vincristine, barbiturates, L-dopa, and quinidine.

Conditions associated with orthostatic hypotension include the prolonged bed rest mentioned above, Addison disease, arteriosclerosis, diabetes, and certain neurologic disorders. Tilt table study may be helpful in establishing the diagnosis.

Epidemiology The disorder affects both men and women and is more common in the elderly.

Related Disorders See *Shy-Drager Syndrome.*

In **vasovagal syncope,** blood circulation in the brain is temporarily impaired, possibly from emotional stress, pain, mild shock, fasting, fever, anemia, mild heart disease, and prolonged bed rest. Symptoms, which include orthostatic hypotension, fainting, and pale, cold extremities, may occur at irregular intervals and last from minutes to hours.

Symptoms of **idiopathic orthostatic hypotension** include lowered blood pressure, hypohidrosis, decreased salivation, and impotence. Idiopathic damage to the autonomic nervous system is implicated.

Treatment—Standard When due to hypovolemia because of medications, the condition is easily and rapidly reversed by correcting dosage or discontinuing the medication. When due to extended bed rest, the condition may be improved by allowing the patient to sit up each day with increasing frequency. Oral ephedrine may be given. In some cases, salt intake is increased or salt-retaining drugs prescribed. Beta-blockers may also be useful. In some extreme cases, physical counterpressure is required; e.g., the use of elastic hose, or whole-body inflatable suits.

Treatment—Investigational A grant was awarded in 1988 by the FDA Orphan Products Division, to Roy L. Freeman, M.D., Ph.D., of New England Deaconess Hospital, Boston, Massachusetts, for his work on using the drug DL-*threo*-3, 4-dihydroxyphenylserine in treating orthostatic hypotension.

Other drugs under investigation for treating this disorder are phenylpropanolamine, midodrine, oral ergotamine tartrate or subcutaneous dihydroergotamine, and caffeine. Subcutaneous somatostatin appears to help certain individuals with postprandial hypotension.

Please contact the agencies listed under Resources, below, for the most current information.

Resources

For more information on orthostatic hypotension: National Organization for Rare Disorders (NORD); NIH/National Institute of Neurological Disorders and Stroke (NINDS); David Robertson, M.D., Director of Clinical Research Center, Vanderbilt University.

References
Postural Hypotension: Its Meaning and Management in the Elderly: M.J. Rosenthal, et al.; Geriatrics, December 1988, 43(12), pp. 31–34, 39–42.
Orthostatic Hypotension: J. Susman; Am. Fam. Physician, June 1988, 37(6), pp. 115–118.

Treatment of Orthostatic Hypotension: Interaction of Pressor Drugs and Tilt Table Conditioning: R.D. Hoeldtke, et al.; Arch. Phys. Med. Rehabil., October 1988, 69(10), pp. 895–898.

PERNIOSIS

Description Perniosis, a vascular disorder caused by prolonged exposure to cold damp weather, is characterized by skin lesions on the lower legs, hands, toes, feet, ears, and face.

Synonyms
Chilblains
Cold-Induced Vascular Disease
Erythema, Pernio
Pernio

Signs and Symptoms The disorder usually occurs in cold weather with high humidity and generally lasts several weeks, with some cases persisting into warmer weather. It is characterized by a bluish-red skin discoloration that can cause pain, intense itching, burning, and swelling of the skin, especially as the body becomes warmer. Lesions usually occur on the fingers, toes, lower legs, heels, ears, or nose, and acrocyanosis may be seen on fingertips or extremities. Bullae that ulcerate if rubbed or irritated may appear in severe cases.

Thigh perniosis commonly affects individuals who wear tight-fitting slacks. It is characterized by red or bluish plaques on the outside thighs that cause swelling, burning, itching, and occasionally ulceration. Symptoms can be relieved or avoided by exposure to a warm temperature and looser-fitting thermal insulated clothing.

Etiology The cause is not known. The disease may result from an allergic reaction or hypersensitivity to the cold. Prolonged exposure, insufficient protective clothing, and circulatory or cardiovascular disease may be causative factors.

Epidemiology Females are affected more often than males; children, adults with poor circulation, and smokers are affected most often. The disorder is rarely seen in the United States.

Related Disorders See *Raynaud's Disease; Urticaria, Cold; Vasculitis.*

Treatment—Standard Affected areas should be warmed slowly, and patients should refrain from scratching or rubbing affected skin. Symptoms may be relieved with nifedipine, and corticosteroid creams may relieve itching. Other treatment is symptomatic and supportive.

Treatment—Investigational Please contact the agencies listed under Resources, below, for the most current information.

Resources
For more information on perniosis: National Organization for Rare Disor-

ders (NORD); NIH/National Heart, Lung and Blood Institute (NHLBI).

References

The Treatment of Chilblains with Nifedipine. The Results of a Pilot Study, a Double-Blind Placebo-Controlled Randomized Study and a Long-Term Open Trial: M. Rustin, et al.; Br. J. Dermatol., February 1989, 120(2), p. 267.

Chronic Pernio. A Historical Perspective of Cold-Induced Vascular Disease: J. Jacob, et al.; Arch. Intern. Med., August 1986, 146(8), pp. 1589–1592.

PULMONARY ALVEOLAR PROTEINOSIS

Description Pulmonary alveolar proteinosis is a rare chronic lung disorder in which the alveoli fill with a protein/phospholipid material that interferes with ventilation. Individual cases vary from mild to severe.

Synonyms
  Phospholipidosis

Signs and Symptoms Although some patients are asymptomatic, most cases are characterized by progressively severe dyspnea, especially following exertion. The disorder may remain stable and confined, spread throughout the lungs, or spontaneously clear. Commonly affected regions include the lower and posterior lung; occasionally the disease is restricted to the anterior segments.

Etiology Although the exact etiology is unknown, exposure to aluminum dust or an impaired immune system have been associated with rare cases.

Epidemiology The disease affects males more often than females, usually between ages 20 and 50.

Related Disorders Symptoms of **pneumonia** may be similar.

Treatment—Standard Mild cases may go into spontaneous remission. Lavage (performed once or several times as needed) under general anesthesia is indicated in more severe cases. The clinician should promptly identify and treat secondary lung infections.

Treatment—Investigational Please contact the agencies listed under Resources, below, for the most current information.

Resources
  For more information on pulmonary alveolar proteinosis: National Organization for Rare Disorders (NORD); American Lung Association; NIH/National Heart, Lung and Blood Institute (NHLBI); Info-Line.

References

Bronchopulmonary Lavage in Pulmonary Alveolar Proteinosis: Chest Radiogr. Observations: M.E. Gale, et al.; AJR, May 1986, 146(5), pp. 981–985.

Total Lung Lavage for Pulmonary Alveolar Proteinosis in an Infant Without the Use of Cardiopulmonary Bypass: F. Moazam, et al.; J. Pediatr. Surg., August 1985, 20(4), pp. 398–401.

Morphologic Diagnosis of Idiopathic Pulmonary Alveolar Lipoproteinosis Revisited: I. Rubinstein, et al.; Arch. Int. Med., April 1988, 148(4), pp. 813–816.

PULMONARY HYPERTENSION, PRIMARY (PPH)

Description PPH is a rare and progressive vascular disease characterized by pulmonary artery hypertension and widespread multiple lesions that affect the pulmonary arterioles leading to the capillaries. The pumping ability of the right ventricle eventually diminishes.

Synonyms
Primary Obliterative Pulmonary Vascular Disease

Signs and Symptoms Symptoms include dyspnea (with or without exertion), excessive fatigue, weakness, angina, and syncope. Facial puffiness and eyelid swelling may be present. Cyanosis, coughing, hemoptysis, hypotension, and cardio- and hepatomegaly also may occur. Heart failure may ensue. Cardiac catheterization and pulmonary angiography may be necessary for diagnosis if routine laboratory tests prove inconclusive.

PPH can occur in full-term newborns with no underlying structural heart disease, or in association with meconium aspiration. Infants will have severe hypoxemia and acidosis because of diminished pulmonary blood flow and large right-to-left shunt at a persistent patent ductus arteriosus and/or patent foramen ovale.

Etiology The etiology is unknown, but a genetic predisposition to the disorder may exist through autosomal dominant or recessive genes. In infants, the disorder is believed to be caused by perinatal hypoxemia immediately before, during, or after birth.

Epidemiology Although it can occur in the newborn, the condition appears more frequently in females between age 20 and 50. In males, it usually occurs later in life. The disorder also occurs more frequently at higher altitudes.

Related Disorders See *Pulmonary Hypertension, Secondary.*

Cor pulmonale is associated with enlargement of the right ventricle of the heart, occurring as a result of severe pulmonary disease. Symptoms usually include dyspnea, exertional syncope, and substernal angina pain.

Interstitial pneumonia is characterized by exertional dyspnea, coughing, and anorexia; the symptoms may range from mild to severe, depending on the extent of involvement. Fever usually is not present, nor is there an overproduction of mucus.

Pulmonary veno-occlusive disease is characterized by obstruction in the pulmonary venules leading to pulmonary hypertension and a radiographic picture of pulmonary edema.

Treatment—Standard Treatment is supportive. Physical activity and exercise should be limited. The disorder has been treated with nifedipine, isoproterenol, phentolamine, phenoxybenzamine, and prazosin. Prostacyclin may be used to dilate the pulmonary blood vessels. Vasodilator drugs, alpha-adrenergic blocking agents, beta agonists, and prostaglandins may also be used. However, drugs cannot cure or halt the progression of the disease. Genetic counseling may be beneficial.

Treatment—Investigational Epoprostenol is under investigation. Heart/lung transplantation can be used in severe cases unresponsive to other therapies.

Please contact the agencies listed under Resources, below, for the most current information.

Resources

For more information on primary pulmonary hypertension: National Organization for Rare Disorders (NORD); American Society of Hypertension; American Heart Association; American Lung Association; NIH/National Heart, Lung and Blood Institute (NHLBI).

For genetic information and genetic counseling referrals: March of Dimes Birth Defects Foundation; NIH/National Center for Education in Maternal and Child Health (NCEMCH).

References

Pulmonary Diseases and Disorders, 2nd ed.: A.P. Fishman; McGraw-Hill, 1988, pp. 999–1025.
Familial Pulmonary Capillary Hemangiomatosis Resulting in Primary Pulmonary Hypertension: D. Langleben, et al.; Ann. Intern. Med., July 1988, 109(2), pp. 106–109.
Current Approach to Treatment of Primary Pulmonary Hypertension: B.M. Groves, et al.; Chest, March 1988, 93(suppl.), pp. 175S–178S.

PULMONARY HYPERTENSION, SECONDARY (SPH)

Description SPH affects the blood vessels in the lungs and is usually associated with other lung diseases, such as interstitial pneumonia, or related diseases in other organs.

Synonyms

Pulmonary Arterial Hypertension

Signs and Symptoms Dyspnea (especially after exertion), anxiety, tachypnea, angina, and, in extreme cases, heart failure can occur. In 98 percent of patients, diagnosis can be made by diameter measurements of the right and left descending pulmonary arteries. A right pulmonary artery diameter greater than 16.7 mm and a left pulmonary artery diameter greater than 16.9 mm indicate excessively high pulmonary hypertension. Right-sided cardiac catheterization or echocardiography are used in diagnosis.

Etiology There are a number of causes, including lung disease, congenital heart disease, pulmonary artery embolism or thrombosis, pulmonary vasoconstriction, and the CREST syndrome. High altitudes, thickening of the blood, and portal hypertension may be implicated. SPH may also occur for unknown reasons.

Epidemiology The disease affects both males and females.

Related Disorders See *Pulmonary Hypertension, Primary.*

Treatment—Standard Physical activity should be restricted and underlying causes treated. Vasodilators, such as epoprostenol, hydralazine, and nifedipine, may be used.

Treatment—Investigational Heart/lung transplantation is performed in severe cases.

Please contact the agencies listed under Resources, below, for the most current information.

Resources

For more information on secondary pulmonary hypertension: National Organization for Rare Disorders (NORD); American Heart Association; American Lung Association; NIH/National Heart, Lung and Blood Institute (NHLBI).

References

Pulmonary Diseases and Disorders, 2nd ed.: A.P. Fishman; McGraw-Hill, 1988, pp. 999–1025.

Current Approach to Treatment of Primary Pulmonary Hypertension: B.M. Groves, et al.; Chest, March 1988, 93(3), pp. 175S–178S.

Functional Tricuspid Regurgitation and Right Ventricular Dysfunction in Pulmonary Hypertension: D.A. Morrison, et al.; Am. J. Cardiol., July 1988, 62(1), pp. 108–112.

Prediction of Favourable Responses to Long-Term Vasodilator Treatment of Pulmonary Hypertension by Short-Term Administration of Epoprostenol CC (Prostacyclin) or Nifedipine: A. Rozkovec, et al.; Br. Heart J., June 1988, 59(6), pp. 696–705.

RESPIRATORY DISTRESS SYNDROME, ADULT (ARDS)

Description ARDS, a life-threatening pulmonary disorder, is precipitated by a variety of direct lung injuries or acute illnesses that damage the microvasculature of the lungs. Major symptoms include dyspnea, tachypnea, hyperventilation, and hypoxemia.

Synonyms

Acute Respiratory Distress Syndrome
Pump Lung
Shock Lung
Wet Lung

Signs and Symptoms The onset of ARDS is often within 24 to 48 hours after the pulmonary insult. Dyspnea with intercostal retractions and use of the accessory muscles of respiration are often the first signs. A few fine inspiratory crackles also may be evident in the physical examination. The chest film usually reveals diffuse, bilateral infiltrates. Early analysis of arterial blood gases shows a reduced arterial oxygen tension despite an increased inspired oxygen fraction and an increased carbon dioxide tension.

Complications include pulmonary emboli and barotrauma, secondary infection, stress ulceration and hemorrhage, renal insufficiency, arrhythmias, and anemia. Chronic lung disease, multiple-organ failure, and irreversible respiratory dysfunction may also develop. Death is most often the result of multiple organ failure.

Etiology ARDS is caused by injuries and illnesses such as shock, sepsis or pneumonia, trauma, aspiration of gastric contents, inhalation injury, drug overdose, metabolic disorders (including pancreatitis and uremia), and hematologic disorders (including intravascular coagulation and massive blood transfusion). The major cause of ARDS appears to be the sepsis syndrome.

Epidemiology The syndrome affects males and females of any age who suffer acute injury or illness to the lungs.

Related Disorders Symptoms of bronchial asthma, pneumonia, and emphysema can be similar to ARDS. See also *Respiratory Distress Syndrome, Infant.*

Treatment—Standard Supportive therapies include mechanical ventilation, fluid management, and pharmacologic agents. Mechanical ventilation usually necessitates nasal or endotracheal intubation and the use of positive end-expiratory pressure. Packed red blood cells can correct anemia, and crystalloids can correct hypovolemia. Treatment of secondary infections includes use of antibiotics and surgical drainage of closed space infections. Infection is the most serious complication because it frequently leads to sepsis. Infection control measures are recommended. Other agents that have been suggested include dopamine to augment cardiac output and diuretics to reduce preload and hydrostatic forces. Treatment is considered to be successful when the patient no longer needs mechanical assistance to breathe.

Treatment—Investigational Extracorporeal membrane oxygenator (ECMO) has been utilized successfully in treating ARDS.

Ketoconazole (antifungal) and prostaglandin E-1 are being investigated for preventing secondary infections. The ability of monoclonal antibodies to endotoxin to decrease the progression of sepsis syndrome to ARDS is being studied. Replacing surfactant, which becomes depleted in ARDS, is also under investigation.

Please contact the agencies listed under Resources, below, for the most current information.

Resources

For more information on ARDS: National Organization for Rare Disorders (NORD); American Lung Association; NIH/National Heart, Lung and Blood Institute (NHLBI).

References
Internal Medicine, 2nd Ed.: J.H. Stein, ed.-in-chief; Little, Brown and Company, 1987, pp. 612, 614, 618, 1537.
Ketoconazole Prevents Acute Respiratory Failure in Critically Ill Surgical Patients: G.J. Slotman, et al.; J. Trauma, May 1988, issue 28(5), pp. 648–654.
Adult Respiratory Distress Syndrome in Pediatric Patients. II Management: J. Royall, et al.; J. Pediatr., March 1988, issue 112(3), pp. 335–347.
Pulmonary Extraction and Pharmacokinetics of Prostaglandin E1 During Continuous Intravenous Infusion in Patients with Adult Respiratory Distress Syndrome: J.W. Cox, et al., Am. Rev. Respir. Dis., January 1988, issue 137(1), pp. 5–12.
Adult Respiratory Distress Syndrome: Update for 1984: M. Iannuzzi and T.L. Petty; J. Respir. Dis., February 1984, issue 2, pp. 118–125.
Trends in Respiratory Medicine: Adult Pulmonary Diseases: Roundtable discussion; J. Respir. Dis., October 1989, issue 10, pp. 39–51.

RESPIRATORY DISTRESS SYNDROME, INFANT (IRDS)

Description IRDS is an acute respiratory disorder that affects premature infants who have a deficiency of alveolar surfactant. Clinical manifestations include breathing difficulty and atelectasis.

Synonyms
Infantile Respiratory Distress Syndrome
Hyaline Membrane Disease

Signs and Symptoms IRDS is characterized by rapid respirations with an expiratory grunt, cyanosis, and chest retractions, which generally develop within the first hours of life. Chest film findings include diffuse reticulogranular densities, air bronchograms, and underinflation. Arterial blood gas analysis often shows hypoxemia and hypercapnia.

Etiology IRDS is caused by the absence of surfactant in the lungs of premature infants. The type II alveolar cells that synthesize surfactant are not completely differentiated until 32 weeks of gestation, explaining why RDS is seen in premature infants. Because surfactant acts to decrease surface tension in the alveoli, surfactant-deficient infants have progressive alveolar collapse.

Epidemiology Male and female premature infants of less than 37 weeks' gestation are affected in equal numbers. The risk of IRDS is higher in infants of diabetic mothers.

Related Disorders Bronchopulmonary dysplasia may result from use of mechanical ventilation in infants with RDS. Barotrauma, high inspired oxygen concentrations, and endotracheal intubation may precipitate the condition. Gradual weaning from mechanical ventilation is important along with nutritional support and diuretic therapy.
    Transient tachypnea of the newborn often resembles mild RDS and is

caused by delayed absorption of fetal pulmonary fluid. Predisposing conditions include premature birth (but close to term), cesarean section, precipitous delivery, breech delivery, and maternal diabetes. Mechanical ventilation is rarely needed, and recovery is usually within 2 to 3 days.

Treatment—Standard Conventional treatment in IRDS involves mechanical ventilation using positive end-expiratory pressure and fluid and nutritional support. The recently available synthetic lung surfactant colfosceril palmitate/cetyl alcohol/tyloxapol (Exosurf, Burroughs Wellcome Co., Research Triangle Park, North Carolina 27709) is being used in IRDS. The treatment is administered after birth to high-risk infants through the ventilator tube.

Treatment—Investigational Survanta, a surfactant developed by Abbott Laboratories, is not yet approved by the Food and Drug Administration. Human Surf is being developed by Dr. T. Allen Merritt of the University of California Medical Center, in San Diego.

Please contact the agencies listed under Resources, below, for the most current information.

Resources
For more information on IRDS: National Organization for Rare Disorders (NORD); American Lung Association; NIH/National Heart, Lung and Blood Institute (NHLBI).

References
Internal Medicine, 2nd ed.: J.H. Stein, ed.-in-chief; Little, Brown and Company, 1987, pp. 576.

Changes in Pulmonary Mechanics After the Administration of Surfactant to Infants with Respiratory Distress Syndrome: J.M. Davis, et al.; N. Engl. J. Med., August 1988, issue 319(8), pp. 476–479.

Pulmonary Surfactant Replacement in Respiratory Distress Syndrome: D. Vidyasagar, et al.; Clin. Perinatol., December 1987, issue 14(4), pp. 991–1015.

Randomized Controlled Trial of Exogenous Surfactant for the Treatment of Hyaline Membrane Disease: J.D. Gitlin, et al.; Pediatrics, January 1987, issue 79(1), pp. 31–37.

ROMANO-WARD SYNDROME

Description This genetic heart disorder is characterized primarily by symptoms occurring during infancy or early childhood, with adult onset possible. Recurrent symptoms include syncope, convulsive seizures, and/or arrhythmias with angina.

Synonyms
Q-T Prolongation with Extracellular Hypokalemia
Q-T Prolongation without Congenital Deafness

Signs and Symptoms Initial symptoms include recurring, unexpected partial or total loss of consciousness accompanied by arrhythmias with long Q-T intervals. Overexertion, excitement, or stress may trigger recurrent symptoms, which can also appear without any precipitating factors. The severity of attacks and types of symptoms may vary: e.g., a prolonged Q-T interval may occur with mild angina and without loss of consciousness; or loss of consciousness or grand mal seizures may occur followed by temporary disorientation. Lowered blood potassium levels may be symptomatic and linked to arrhythmias.

Etiology The syndrome is thought to be an inherited autosomal dominant trait with variable penetrance.

Epidemiology Approximately 155 cases, affecting both sexes equally, have been reported in the 20th century.

Related Disorders Jervell and Lange-Nielsen syndrome, inherited as an autosomal recessive trait, is characterized by congenital deafness (unlike in Romano-Ward syndrome) and heartbeat irregularities that lead to loss of consciousness, seizures, and even death.

Treatment—Standard Propranolol is the suggested treatment. Therapies for arrhythmias include surgical removal of certain afferent cardiac nerves or a combination of surgical and pharmaceutical intervention. Raising potassium levels may improve some symptoms, and genetic counseling may be beneficial. First-degree relatives should be investigated. Other treatment is symptomatic and supportive.

Treatment—Investigational Treatment with an implantable automatic cardioverter-defibrillator is being investigated in conjunction with antiarrhythmic drug therapy. The implantable Q-T–sensitive cybernetic pacemaker is also under investigation.

Please contact the agencies listed under Resources, below, for the most current information.

Resources

For more information on Romano-Ward syndrome: National Organization for Rare Disorders (NORD); American Heart Association; NIH/National Heart, Lung and Blood Institute (NHLBI).

For genetic information and genetic counseling referrals: March of Dimes Birth Defects Foundation; National Center for Education in Maternal and Child Health (NCEMCH).

References

Prolonged Q-T Syndrome (Romano-Ward Syndrome). Description of a Case Diagnosed in Infancy: V. Meschi, et al.: Pediatr. Med. Chir., January–February 1985, 7(1), pp. 131–136.

Management of the Prolonged Q-T Syndrome and Recurrent Ventricular Fibrillation with an Implantable Automatic Cardioverterdefibrillator: E.V. Platia, et al.; Clin. Cardiol., September 1985, 8(9), pp. 490–493.

The Q-T–Sensitive Cybernetic Pacemaker: A New Role for an Old Parameter? P.E. Puddu, et al.; Pace, January 1986, 9(1 pt. 1), pp. 108–123.

TETRALOGY OF FALLOT

Description Tetralogy of Fallot is the most prevalent form of cyanotic congenital heart disease. It consists of 4 defects: a ventricular septal defect; subpulmonary stenosis; overriding aorta; and right ventricular hypertrophy. Untreated cases become progressively more severe. There is further diminution in pulmonary blood flow and increasing cyanosis with its associated complications.

Synonyms

Pink Tetralogy of Fallot (Acyanotic Tetralogy of Fallot)
Pseudotruncus Arteriosus

Signs and Symptoms Symptoms can appear at birth or within the first year. The most common symptom is cyanosis at rest or with crying. Excessive fatigue may adversely affect the infant's appetite, resulting in slow weight gain and impeded growth. Exertion can bring about severe, life-threatening attacks of hyperpnea and hypoxia. A characteristic squatting posture is sometimes assumed to aid with difficult breathing. Other symptoms of inadequate tissue oxygenation are cyanosis, clubbing of the fingertips, and polycythemia.

Various complications can occur, such as relative anemia in infancy, polycythemia in children and adults, coagulation defects, infective endocarditis, embolisms in the systemic circulation, cerebral infarctions, infectious sinusitis, and brain abscesses. Congestive heart failure is rare except with endocarditis or arrhythmias. Severe right ventricle obstructions with pulmonary atresia are known as **pseudotruncus arteriosus** (or pulmonary atresia with ventricular septal defect).

The physical examination, electrocardiography, echocardiography, and cardiac catheterization data aid in diagnosis and therapy. X-rays usually reveal a characteristic shape of the heart. Periodic measurements of systemic blood oxygen saturation and hemoglobin are advisable.

Etiology No specific etiologic agent has been identified. Approximately 25 percent of patients have an associated extracardiac congenital abnormality.

Epidemiology About one percent of newborns have congenital heart defects. Of these, about 10 percent have tetralogy of Fallot, which occurs more often in males than females.

Related Disorders Other congenital heart defects include atrial and isolated ventricular septal defects, pulmonary valve stenosis, malformations of the aorta and pulmonary artery, and anomalous positions of the heart. See *Atrial Septal Defects; Ventricular Septal Defects.*

Treatment—Standard Surgical correction of the malformation is best accomplished during infancy. When repair is not feasible, palliative measures taken in infancy or early childhood include construction of a shunt between the aorta and the pulmonary artery. Presurgical, palliative medical treatment includes maintenance of adequate hydration and appropriate hemoglobin, and avoidance of strenuous exercise. Medications may also be needed to treat arrhythmias. Because they are susceptible to bacterial endocarditis, patients should be given antibiotics at times of predictable risk (e.g., tooth extractions and surgery). Similarly, respiratory infections are treated vigorously and early. Severe hypoxic spells may require the administration of oxygen, morphine, sodium bicarbonate, and other drugs to improve oxygen concentration.

Treatment—Investigational Please contact the agencies listed under Resources, below, for the most current information.

Resources
   For more information on tetralogy of Fallot: National Organization for Rare Disorders (NORD); American Heart Association; NIH/National Heart, Lung and Blood Institute (NHLBI); American Lung Association.
   For genetic information and genetic counseling referrals: March of Dimes Birth Defects Foundation; National Center for Education in Maternal and Child Health (NCEMCH).

References
   Moss' Heart Disease in Infants, Children and Adolescents, 4th ed.: F.H. Adams, G.C. Emmanouilides, and T.A. Riemenschneider; Williams and Wilkins, 1989.

TRUNCUS ARTERIOSUS, PERSISTENT

Description Persistent truncus arteriosus is a serious congenital heart defect with a high mortality rate. The truncus arteriosus is a fetal structure which later is divided into the aorta and pulmonary artery by the development of the bulbar septum. The disorder is nearly always accompanied by a ventricular septal defect. Persistence beyond the fetal stage causes blood from both ventricles to mix, affecting the pulmonary and systemic circulation. If the infant survives congestive heart failure in infancy, extreme hypertension in the lungs eventually causes pulmonary vascular obstructive disease.

Signs and Symptoms Similar to those of a severe ventricular septal defect, the symptoms and signs are those related to unrelenting congestive heart failure, an enlarged heart, pulmonary plethora, and gradual development of pulmonary vascular obstructive disease. There may be associated truncal valve stenosis or regurgitation. The infant's appetite is adversely affected, resulting in slow weight gain and impeded growth. Diagnosis is established by echocardiography or heart catheterization. In the absence of surgical correction, nearly 90 percent of infants die by 6 months of age.

Etiology The causes of the arrest in embryonic development resulting in congenital heart disease are poorly understood. About 35 percent of patients with truncus arteriosus have DiGeorge syndrome.

Epidemiology Persistent truncus arteriosus may affect infants of both sexes. It is usually fatal during early infancy.

Related Disorders See *Tetralogy of Fallot; Ventricular Septal Defects.* Other related disorders are interrupted aortic arch and pseudotruncus arteriosus.

Treatment—Standard In addition to surgical intervention, standard medical therapeutic measures for heart failure are used.

Treatment—Investigational Please contact the agencies listed under Resources, below, for the most current information.

Resources

For more information on persistent truncus arteriosus: National Organization for Rare Disorders (NORD); American Heart Association; NIH/National Heart, Lung and Blood Institute (NHLBI).

For genetic information and genetic counseling referrals: March of Dimes Birth Defects Foundation; National Center for Education in Maternal and Child Health (NCEMCH).

References

Fetal, Neonatal and Infant Cardiac Disease: J.H. Moller and W.A. Neal, eds.; Appleton and Lange, 1989.

Moss' Heart Disease in Infants, Children, and Adolescents, 4th ed.: F.H. Adams, G.C. Emmanouilides, and T.A. Riemenschneider, eds.; Williams and Wilkins, 1989.

VENTRICULAR SEPTAL DEFECTS

Description Ventricular septal defects, a relatively common form of congenital heart disease, may occur at any part of the interventricular septum but are generally membranous. The size of the defect determines clinical severity; large defects can result in infant mortality. Ventricular septal defects may close spontaneously (more common with small defects) or become relatively less significant as the heart matures and grows. The disease can result in congestive heart failure, characterized by tachypnea, wheezing, tachycardia, hepatomegaly, and failure to thrive. In addition, persistent high pulmonary artery blood pressure can permanently damage the lungs.

Synonyms

Common Ventricle (Cor Triloculare Biatriatum)
Eisenmenger Syndrome
Roger Disease (Maladie de Roger)

Signs and Symptoms Small defects may be asymptomatic, as may be the case in patients with **Roger disease.** With moderate defects, signs of congestive heart failure may appear, such as fatigue or breathing difficulty during activity or feeding. In infants, poor feeding due to fatigue, cold grayish extremities, and rapid shallow breathing may indicate heart disease. Ventricular septal defects of moderate size are also characterized by cardiomegaly, characteristic heart murmurs, and an abnormal electrocardiogram.

A very large opening causes severe symptoms. If the septum is entirely absent, the 2 ventricles constitute a single chamber, a condition known as **common ventricle** or **cor triloculare biatriatum.** In infants and children, large defects generally cause growth retardation, heart failure, mild cyanosis, and pulmonary artery hypertension. In older children and adults, dyspnea after physical exertion, chest pain, episodes of fainting, hemoptysis, and hypoxia (including cyanosis, clubbing of the fingers, and polycythemia) may occur as a result of pulmonary vascular obstructive disease **(Eisenmenger syndrome).**

Infective endocarditis is associated more with small- or moderate-sized septal defects.

The patterns and quality of the heart sounds, electrocardiography, echocardiography, and cardiac catheterization data help determine the exact anatomic defect and differentiate ventricular septal defects from other similar conditions.

Etiology The causes of the arrest in embryonic development resulting in congenital heart disease are poorly understood. In most infants, ventricular septal defects occur as the only malformation. However, many malformation syndromes are associated with ventricular septal defects, including maternal alcoholism, trisomy syndromes, maternal ingestion of phenylhydantoin, postrubella infection, and maternal phenylketonuria.

Epidemiology Approximately one percent of newborns have a congenital heart defect; 25 to 30 percent of these are ventricular septal defects. Females are affected more often than males.

Related Disorders Other associated or related congenital heart defects include atrioventricular septal defects, atrial septal defects, valve defects of various kinds, malformation of the aorta and pulmonary artery, and anomalous positions of the heart in the chest. See *Tetralogy of Fallot; Atrial Septal Defects; Eisenmenger Syndrome.*

Treatment—Standard Surgery is not indicated for small ventricular septal defects. Medical management includes treatment of congestive heart failure with digoxin, diuretics, and rest. Nutritional considerations are paramount in infants. Because they are susceptible to bacterial endocarditis, patients should be given appropriate antibiotics at times of predictable risk (e.g., dental work and surgery). Similarly, respiratory infections are treated vigorously and early.

Indications for surgical repair in infancy are intractable congestive heart failure, poor weight gain, and significant pulmonary artery hypertension. The development of pulmonary vascular obstructive disease may be prevented if surgical closure of the defect is undertaken in the first 2 years of life. In older children, persistent large left-to-right shunt and cardiomegaly are also treated surgically.

If symptoms persist after conservative treatment, surgery is recommended, especially since it is successful even in infants, and because pulmonary vascular disease may be prevented in the first 2 years of life.

Treatment—Investigational Please contact the agencies listed under Resources, below, for the most current information.

Resources
   For more information on ventricular septal defects: National Organization for Rare Disorders (NORD); American Heart Association; NIH/National Heart, Lung, and Blood Institute (NHLBI).

For genetic information and genetic counseling referrals: March of Dimes Birth Defects Foundation; National Center for Education in Maternal and Child Health (NCEMCH).

References
Fetal, Neonatal and Infant Cardiac Disease: J.H. Moller and W.A. Neal, eds.; Appleton and Lange, 1989.

Moss' Heart Disease in Infants, Children, and Adolescents, 4th ed.: F.H. Adams, G.C. Emmanouilides, and T.A. Riemenschneider, eds.; Williams and Wilkins, 1989.

WOLFF-PARKINSON-WHITE (WPW) SYNDROME

Description WPW syndrome is a genetic disorder resulting in cardiac arrhythmias. An extra conduction pathway in the heart (bundle of Kent) pre-excites the ventricles. Palpitations, weakness, and dyspnea may occur.

Synonyms
Preexcitation Syndrome
Accessory Atrioventricular Pathways

Signs and Symptoms Symptoms include arrhythmias, such as atrial flutter, atrial fibrillation, or paroxysmal supraventricular tachycardia (**PSVT**). In atrial flutter, atria of the heart contract very fast, often more than the ventricles; atrial fibrillation is a "twitching" of the atria instead of regular contractions, which causes the ventricles to respond irregularly. Symptoms associated with atrial flutter may include irregular pulse, tachycardia, pallor, nausea, weakness, dyspnea, syncope, and fatigue. PSVT is a condition in which the heart rate suddenly increases to 100 to 200 beats per minute. A sudden, rapid, regular fluttering sensation and tightness in the chest may occur. These patients may also experience weakness, syncope, palpitations, and dyspnea. Angina may occur in older patients. Diagnosis may be made with electrocardiogram and electrophysiologic study.

Etiology WPW syndrome is inherited as an autosomal dominant trait characterized by an additional conduction pathway, the bundle of Kent, which sends extra electrical impulses from the atria to the ventricles.

Epidemiology This rare congenital disorder affects males and females, and symptoms can occur at any age.

Related Disorders Lown-Ganong-Levine (LGL) syndrome is a genetic disorder involving cardiac arrhythmias that are slightly different from WPW syndrome. The ventricles receive part or all of their electrical impulses from an irregular conduction pathway instead of from the bundle of His. If LGL patients have atrial flutter, atrial fibrillation, or paroxysmal atrial arrhythmias, then palpitations, faintness, weakness, and nausea may occur as they do in WPW syndrome.

Sinus tachycardia is a cardiac arrhythmia that causes the heartbeat to gradually increase to over 100 beats per minute. The disorder may be caused by emotional stress, exercise, infection, and certain drugs.

Sick sinus syndrome is characterized by irregular atrial activity. Bradycardia and tachycardia usually occur. Gradual supraventricular tachycardia, atrial flutter, and atrial fibrillation may also develop. Palpitations, weakness, faintness, and nausea are common symptoms.

Atrial ectopic tachycardia usually occurs gradually. It is the result of premature electrical impulses located within the atrial myocardium. Rapid, regular fluttering sensations and tightness in the chest may occur, as may palpitations, weakness, faintness, shortness of breath, and polyuria.

Treatment—Standard Initial PSVT treatment may involve lying down, stimulation of gagging or vomiting, the Valsalva maneuver, or carotid sinus massage. Quinidine and procainamide may help control atrial flutter, fibrillation, and PSVT. Localization and ablation of the accessory connection can usually be achieved by catheter. Ablating of the accessory pathway by catheter has largely replaced operative surgical division or cryoablation. Implantation of a pacemaker may control tachycardia.Genetic counseling may be beneficial. Other treatment is symptomatic and supportive.

Treatment—Investigational Edrophonium may be helpful for PSVT in WPW patients, but it has not yet been approved by the Food and Drug Administration. Flecainide is also being studied to treat PSVT. Propranolol is under investigation for preventing atrial flutter, fibrillation, and PSVT. Adenosine triphosphate (ATP) is being investigated as a treatment for PSVT and to prevent extra stimulation of the ventricles by the bundle of Kent.

Please contact the agencies listed under Resources, below, for the most current information.

Resources

For more information on Wolff-Parkinson-White syndrome: National Organization for Rare Disorders (NORD); American Heart Association; NIH/National Heart, Blood & Lung Institute.

For genetic information and genetic counseling referrals: March of Dimes Birth Defects Foundation; NIH/National Institute of Maternal & Child Health (NCEMCH).

References

Mendelian Inheritance in Man, 9th ed.: V.A. McKusick; The Johns Hopkins University Press, 1990, p. 985.

Internal Medicine, 3rd ed.: J.H. Stein, ed.-in-chief; Little, Brown and Company, 1990, pp. 77–78.

Comparative Quantitative Electrophysiologic Effects of Adenosine Triphosphate on the Sinus Node and Atrioventricular Node: A.D. Sharma and G.J. Klein; Am. J. Cardiol., February 1, 1988, vol. 61(4), pp. 330–335.

5 HEMATOLOGIC/ONCOLOGIC DISORDERS
By Laurence A. Boxer, M.D.

Clinical Disorders of Anemia and Erythrocytosis

The classification of anemia can be based on physiologic, morphologic, or etiologic factors. The prospective approach to any individual patient requires integration of history, physical findings, blood counts, red cell indices, reticulocyte count, red blood cell morphology, specific tests such as hemoglobin electrophoresis and Coombs' test, and, finally, a search to determine the underlying disease or process. The approach to the diagnosis of anemia in patients takes into consideration the following broad categories: 1) decreased production of red blood cells or blood loss; 2) red blood cell size: normocytic, macrocytic, or microcytic; 3) knowledge of the relative frequency of the causes of anemia at various ages; and 4) appreciation that the diagnosis of anemia depends on normal values corresponding to the patient's age, sex, and cardiopulmonary status (see Figure 5.1).

The history can help focus on a diagnosis, but physical examination is more often nonspecific. In children, signs of anemia include pallor, color of mucous membranes, jaundice, tachycardia, palpitation, fatigue, dyspnea, poor feeding, and weight gain or other evidence of cardiac decompensation. Bruising, petechial and overt bleeding, splenomegaly, and other abdominal organomegaly or lymphadenopathy might suggest an underlying process causing the anemia. In children it is important to be alert to specific dysmorphic features of

Figure 5.1. A Diagnostic Approach To Anemia

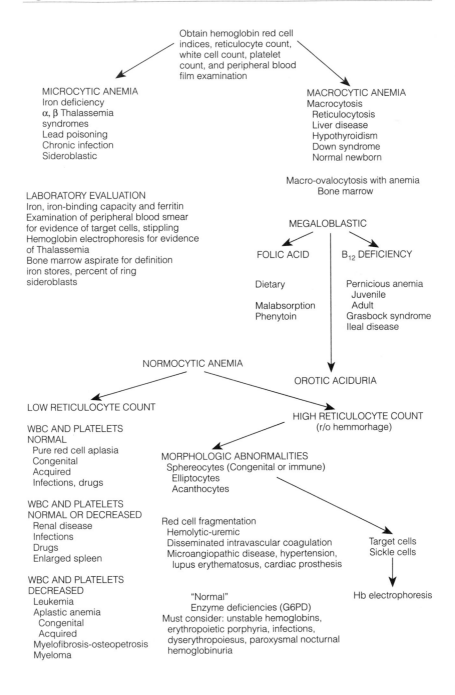

Obtain hemoglobin red cell indices, reticulocyte count, white cell count, platelet count, and peripheral blood film examination

MICROCYTIC ANEMIA
Iron deficiency
α, β Thalassemia syndromes
Lead poisoning
Chronic infection
Sideroblastic

MACROCYTIC ANEMIA
Macrocytosis
Reticulocytosis
Liver disease
Hypothyroidism
Down syndrome
Normal newborn

Macro-ovalocytosis with anemia
Bone marrow

LABORATORY EVALUATION
Iron, iron-binding capacity and ferritin
Examination of peripheral blood smear for evidence of target cells, stippling
Hemoglobin electrophoresis for evidence of Thalassemia
Bone marrow aspirate for definition iron stores, percent of ring sideroblasts

MEGALOBLASTIC

FOLIC ACID

Dietary

Malabsorption
Phenytoin

B_{12} DEFICIENCY

Pernicious anemia
Juvenile
Adult
Grasbock syndrome
Ileal disease

NORMOCYTIC ANEMIA

OROTIC ACIDURIA

LOW RETICULOCYTE COUNT

HIGH RETICULOCYTE COUNT
(r/o hemmorhage)

WBC AND PLATELETS NORMAL
 Pure red cell aplasia
 Congenital
 Acquired
 Infections, drugs

MORPHOLOGIC ABNORMALITIES
 Sphereocytes (Congenital or immune)
 Elliptocytes
 Acanthocytes

WBC AND PLATELETS NORMAL OR DECREASED
 Renal disease
 Infections
 Drugs
 Enlarged spleen

Red cell fragmentation
 Hemolytic-uremic
 Disseminated intravascular coagulation
 Microangiopathic disease, hypertension,
 lupus erythematosus, cardiac prosthesis

Target cells
Sickle cells

WBC AND PLATELETS DECREASED
 Leukemia
 Aplastic anemia
 Congenital
 Acquired
 Myelofibrosis-osteopetrosis
 Myeloma

"Normal"
 Enzyme deficiencies (G6PD)
Must consider: unstable hemoglobins,
 erythropoietic porphyria, infections,
 dyserythropoiesus, paroxysmal nocturnal
 hemoglobinuria

Hb electrophoresis

Diamond-Blackfan and Fanconi anemias, vascular and skin changes of sickle cell anemia, and sickle C disease and the facies of beta-thalassemia major, since these congenital defects usually become symptomatic early in life. A history of chronic diarrhea and cerebellar ataxia may suggest congenital acanthocytosis.

The basic laboratory evaluation for anemia, including accurate interpretation of the blood smear, often confirms the underlying process or suggests other tests that need to be done. Microcytosis out of proportion to the reduction in hemoglobin concentrations suggests a thalassemia trait, which can be established by hemoglobin electrophoresis. Careful examination of the peripheral smear often reveals abnormalities pointing to a specific diagnosis or underlying abnormalities. Perhaps the most difficult group of patients are those with hemolytic anemia and red cell aplasia. Under these circumstances, as well as in hemoglobinopathies, critical information is obtainable by examining the hemogram and peripheral blood smears. For these patients the reticulocyte count corrected as the reticulocyte index (reticulocyte count × hematocrit ÷ by age-appropriate hematocrit) × ½ is an important guide to further evaluation.

The hemolytic anemias are a complex group of disorders associated with an elevated reticulocyte index. The correct diagnosis for an individual patient may be apparent after a history, physical examination, and routine blood study. The smear may allow the crucial distinction to be made between immune and nonimmune hemolysis; this determination will then guide further evaluation. Spherocytes and microspherocytes are classic markers of immune hemolytic anemia; fragmented red blood cells are markers of intravascular nonimmune myelocytic anemia. Since extravascular hemolysis within the spleen does not result in hemoglobinemia, hemoglobinuria, or hemosiderinuria, detection of any of these implies an intravascular hemolytic process. Acute severe intravascular hemolysis may cause detectable hemoglobinemia, which can be seen on visual inspection of the patient's plasma. Hemoglobinuria may be detected with recent intravascular hemolysis. Chronic intravascular hemolysis can be detected by assays for urinary hemosiderin. Frequently, however, additional tests including hemoglobin electrophoresis, haptoglobin determination, red cells' osmotic fragility, specific assays of red blood cell enzymes, acid hemolysis tests, sugar water test, and tests for unstable hemoglobin must be performed to identify the basis for the anemia.

Examination of the bone marrow is important in the diagnosis in relatively few causes of anemia. These include megaloblastic, sideroblastic, aplastic, and dyserythropoietic anemias; acute leukemia; neuroblastoma; lipid storage diseases; and myeloma.

Similarly, when erythrocytosis has been identified, the physician has two goals in dealing with the patient: identification of the correctable cause and reduction of the red cell mass. Polycythemia vera is a form of myeloproliferative syndrome in which the granulocyte, monocyte, and platelet counts as well as the red cell count are usually elevated. This disorder appears to represent occupancy of the bone marrow by the progeny of a neoplastic clone of stem cells, which proliferate with an appropriate exuberance for any given level of external stimulants. Elevation of the counts in all three major cell lineages, red blood cells, white blood cells, and platelets, and the presence of splenomegaly should lead one to suspect this diagnosis strongly as a cause of erythrocytosis. Erythropoietin levels are normal in polycythemia vera, which distinguishes it from the secondary causes of red cell elevation.

Clinical Disorders of Granulopoiesis

Neutropenia is defined as an absolute decrease in the number of circulating, terminally differentiated neutrophils. For whites over one year of age, the lower limit of the normal range for the peripheral blood neutrophil count is 1,500 cells/mm^3 of blood. For white infants under one year, the lower limit of normal is generally considered to be 1,000 cells/mm^3 of blood. Blacks have slightly lower values on average.

Neutropenia appears secondary to or in association with a number of pathophysiologic conditions, including viral and severe bacterial infections; exposure to drugs such as certain antibiotics and anticonvulsants; autoimmune processes such as those seen with systemic lupus erythematosus; marrow infiltrative processes such as leukemia, metastatic tumor, and myelofibrosis; and inborn errors of metabolism such as propionic acidemia and isovaleric acidemia. Finally, some chronic primary neutropenic disorders occur with a well-defined genetic basis (e.g., cyclic neutropenia); and some occur in association with disorders of immune function. Neutropenia can also occur as a consequence of extramedullary physiologic processes.

To establish a diagnosis of cyclic neutropenia, serial blood counts with white blood cell differential counts are essential (see Table 5.1). Usually these should be obtained twice weekly for 6 to 8 weeks in order to confirm the neutrophil cycling at 21-day intervals. Bone marrow aspirate or biopsy or both is particularly important for ruling out the possibility of malignant marrow disorders such as leukemia or metastatic tumor. Other tests that may be useful in ruling out alternative diagnoses include an antineutrophil antibody assay, antinuclear antibody assay, and antimicrobial serologic assays when specific infections such as hepatitis or cytomegalic disease or the infections caused by Epstein-Barr or human immunodeficiency virus are suspected.

Table 5.1: Laboratory Evaluation of Neutropenia

Complete blood count, including platelet count

Serial absolute neutrophil counts: 2x/week for 6 weeks

Serologic studies
    Antineutrophil antibody assay
    Antinuclear antibody assay
    Immunoglobulins (IgG, IgA, IgM)
    Antiviral antibody studies

Cultures to screen for infections

Radiography of long bones (for Schwachman syndrome and Fanconi anemia)

Screening for nutritional deficiency states
    Serum copper, folate, and vitamin B12 levels

Lymphocyte quantitation and function
    T- and B-cell numbers
    Skin test reactivity

Colony-forming unit (CFU) and colony-stimulating activity (CSA) assays

Hydrocortisone stimulation test

Special studies
    Chromosome analysis (for preleukemia states and Fanconi anemia)
    Plasma and urinary amino acid screening (for metabolic acidemias)
    Sucrose hemolysis/Ham tests (for paroxysmal nocturnal hemoglobinuria)
    Pancreatic enzyme determination in duodenal fluid (for Schwachman syndrome)
    Electron microscopic evaluation of neutrophils

Blood cultures, and cultures of other apparent sites of infection may document the presence of an organism causing neutropenia. A bone marrow test with corticosteroids may prove useful in assessing marrow reserve, which is normal in patients with chronic benign neutropenia. Other conditions that may be associated with chronic idiopathic neutropenia include Schwachman syndrome, X-linked agammaglobulinemia, dysgammaglobulinemia, and depressed cellular immunity. Other rare disorders associated with neutropenia but with distinctive features permitting separation from idiopathic neutropenia include cartilage-hair hypoplasia syndrome, dyskeratosis congenita, and Fanconi anemia.

Recurrent Infections

The differential diagnosis for a patient who presents with recurrent infection is formidable, given the complexity of the immune response. The similarities in the clinical presentation of many of the phagocyte disorders can further complicate attempts to establish the diagnosis. Even when appropriate phagocyte function tests are performed, the results can be difficult to interpret in light of the intrinsic variability of these tests from day to day and from laboratory to laboratory. With these caveats in mind, however, the clinician can approach the patient with recurrent infection in an orderly manner and often establish a diagnosis if in fact a phagocytic defect is responsible. A useful algorithm for approaching these patients is presented in Figure 5.2.

When considering the history, one must take into account the frequency of infections, the patient's age, and the associated medical conditions. For example, recurrent otitis media in a two-year-old boy is far less worrisome than a similar history in a 40-year-old. Another consideration is that the more unusual or severe the infection, the less frequently it has to occur before a phagocyte evaluation is indicated. Infections in unexpected anatomical locations should also alert the physician to a possible underlying immune disorder. Hepatic, pulmonary, and rectal abscesses as well as disseminated systemic infections may be indicative of an underlying phagocytic defect. Finally, the identification of certain pathogens such as the catalase-positive organisms including *Serratia marcescens, Aspergillus, Nocardia,* and *Pseudomonas cepacia* in children and young adults should suggest an eval-

Figure 5.2. Algorithm for the workup of a patient with recurrent infection.

Modified from J.T. Curnutte and L.A. Boxer; Disorders of granulopoiesis and granulocyte function: *in* Hematology of Infancy and Childhood, 3rd ed.: D.G. Nathan and F.A. Oski, eds.; W.B. Saunders Company, 1987, p. 835. Used with permission.

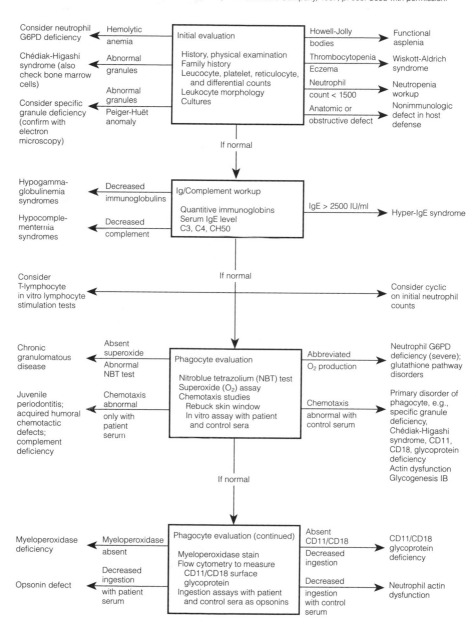

Table 5.2. Classification of Hemorrhagic Disorders

Disorders due to abnormalities of platelet-vessel interaction
Hereditary hemorrhagic telangiectasia
Secondary vasculitis
    Systematic lupus erythematosus
    Sepsis
Scurvy
Henoch-Schoenlein syndrome (anaphylactoid purpura)

Thrombocytopenias
Increased destruction of trapping
    Idiopathic thrombocytopenic purpura
    Immunologic drug purpura
    Splenomegaly
    Acute infection and inflammatory disorders
    Hemolytic-uremic syndrome
    Thrombotic thrombocytopenic purpura
    Giant hemangioma
    Cyanotic congenital heart disease
    Intravascular coagulation
    Isoimmune thrombocytopenias
    Wiskott-Aldrich syndrome
Decreased production
    Leukemia and other malignancies
    Aplastic anemias
    Drugs and toxins
    Hereditary thrombocytopenias
    Thrombopoietin deficiency

Disorders of platelet function
Thromboasthenia or Glanzmann disease
Bernard-Soulier giant platelet syndrome
Platelet release abnormality
    Storage pool disease
    Abnormal release mechanism
von Willebrand disease
Acquired disorders

Disorders of coagulation system
Congenital deficiencies
    Factor VIII (classic hemophilia A) and von Willebrand disease
    Factor IX (Christmas disease)
    Factor XI
    Factor XIII (fibrin-stabilizing factor deficiency)
    Factor I (afibrinogenemia, dysfibrinogenemia)
    Factor II (hypoprothrombinemia, dysprothrombinemias)
    Factor V
    Factor VII
    Factor X
    Alpha-2-antiplasmin deficiency

Acquired deficiencies due to decreased production
    Vitamin K-dependent coagulation factors
    Liver disease
    Altered bowel flora
    Malabsorption
    Coumadin treatment
  Hypothyroidism
Acquired deficiencies due to increased destruction
    Disseminated intravascular coagulation
    Purpura fulminans
    Necrotizing enterocolitis
    Localized venous and arterial thrombosis
  Pathologic anticoagulants

---

uation for chronic granulomatous disease. Certain unusual findings can be helpful in determining which patients warrant further testing. For example, an infant with a history of delayed separation of the umbilical cord who has had several bouts of pneumonia and is noted to have neutrophilia should be evaluated for leukocyte adhesion deficiency; and the child with nystagmus, fair skin, and recurrent staphylococccal infections should be evaluated for Chédiak-Higashi syndrome.

Bleeding Tendency

The history and physical findings are important in classifying a patient with a bleeding tendency. A carefully constructed family pedigree may indicate the hereditary nature of the bleeding manifestation (X-linked inheritance with factor VIII and IX deficiencies; autosomal dominant inheritance (although not solely) with von Willebrand disease; recessive inheritance with factor V and factor VII deficiencies). Characteristic of the hemophilias are bleeding at circumcision (but not invariably), and deep hematoma and hemarthrosis if the disorder is severe. In contrast, thrombocytopenia and abnormalities of platelet function and of von Willebrand factor are frequently manifested by epistaxis, bruising, and petechiae. Patients with factor XIII deficiency characteristically have umbilical cord bleeding in the newborn. Prolonged hemorrhage after a tooth extraction or after nasopharyngeal surgery such as tonsillectomy is a reliable symptom of an abnormal bleeding tendency. Negative personal and family histories are rare in a child with hereditary hemorrhagic disease unless the child is very young or the disease is quite mild. Nevertheless, mild hemophilia may result in bleeding with only severe trauma or major surgery. Hemorrhagic disorders are classified in Table 5.2.

Patients with a positive family history of bleeding or significant hemorrhagic episodes in the past or those who are scheduled for major surgery should have certain laboratory tests performed to determine and classify a potential bleeding diathesis. (See Table 5.3.) These include platelet count or estimation of the platelet number on blood smear; bleeding time by the template method, which is a measure of platelet-vessel interaction; partial thromboplastin time, which measures thrombin generation in the intrinsic pathway and is a function of all the coagulation factors except factor VII; the prothrombin time, which measures thrombin generation in the extrinsic pathway and is a function of factors II, V, VII, and X activity and the fibrinogen level; and thrombin time, which estimates the amount and function of fibrinogen as particular sensitivity to the presence of fibrin degradation products or heparin.

Oncology

Adequate tissue must be obtained from the tumor to establish the specific diagnosis and subtype of cancer. Rare exceptions are those

Table 5.3. Use of screening tests for classifying hemorrhagic disorders

Disorder	Platelet Count	BT	PTT	PT	TT
Afribrinogenemia	N	Mild Abn	No clot	No clot	No clot
Dysfibrinogenemia	N	N	N	Mild Abn	Abn
II, V, X deficiencies	N	N	Abn	Abn	N
VII deficiency	N	N	N	Abn	N
VIII, IX, XI, XII deficiencies	N	N	Abn	N	N
XIII deficiency	N	N	N	N	N
von Willebrand disease	N	Abn	Abn	N	N
Platelet function defects	N or low	Abn	N	N	Abn

BT=bleeding time; PTT=partial thromboplastin time; PT=prothrombin time; TT=thrombin time; N=normal for age; Abn=abnormal prolongation of clotting test time.

incidences in which a biopsy might be life-threatening and the location is virtually pathognomonic of a specific histology. Brain tumors and anterior mediastinal tumors that compress the trachea and blood vessels are two notable examples. In the latter situation, which usually involves a lymphoma, steroids may reduce the tumor size and relieve symptoms before biopsy is attempted. More often, an adequate sample must be obtained before definitive therapy unless complete surgical excision is definitively diagnostic and therapeutic. The specific diagnosis is seldom a problem in the leukemias, since bone marrow aspiration usually affords a ready answer. The solid tumors present the greatest difficulty.

A second diagnostic principle is to establish the extent of the disease. In the leukemias this can be readily accomplished by physical examination, routine laboratory tests, chest x-ray, and examination of the cerebral spinal fluid.

With solid tumors, determining the extent of the disease often involves major surgery and an extensive examination using diagnostic imaging techniques. A coordinated approach involving the surgeon and pathologist is crucial for planning treatment and for judging its success. In addition, modern oncology demands an extensive biological classification of leukemias and solid tumors, often requiring sophisticated scientific approaches using cytogenetics, molecular biology, and immunophenotyping as well as light and electron microscopy with special stains to determine the presence of glycogen, enzymes, or other substances that help classify a variety of tumors.

HEMATOLOGIC/ONCOLOGIC DISORDERS
Listings in This Section

ACANTHOCYTOSIS

Description Acanthocytosis is an inherited blood disorder characterized by the presence of malformed erythrocytes (acanthocytes) in the circulating blood and the absence of chylomicrons and very low density lipoproteins (**VLDL**) in plasma. The disorder leads to ataxia, retinitis pigmentosa, and malabsorption of fat in the alimentary tract that results in steatorrhea.

Synonyms
> Abetalipoproteinemia
> Bassen-Kornzweig Syndrome
> Low-Density Beta-Lipoprotein Deficiency

Signs and Symptoms With onset usually beginning in the first year of life, symptoms of this disorder can occur in the alimentary, neuromuscular, skeletal, and ocular systems.

Some of the symptoms related to the alimentary tract are loss of appetite, copious loose stools, vomiting, and reduced ability to absorb nutrients from food. Although patients tend to have very high levels of fat in the mucous membrane cells of the intestine, they do not metabolize fats well and excrete only 15 to 20 percent of the fat they ingest. They also have trouble absorbing fat-soluble vitamins A, E, and K; vitamin K deficiency then causes reduced levels of coagulation factor in the blood.

During the first 10 years of life, fully one-third of the patients have neuromuscular problems. Slow growth is a common symptom, as is loss of stretch reflexes. Patients generally have ataxia before they turn 20 and are usually unable to stand without assistance by the time they reach 40 because of spinocerebellar degeneration resulting in loss of position and vibration sense. Patients may also have retrospinal demyelination and some loss of sensation to touch, pain, and temperature. Muscle weakness and atrophy sometimes occur and, rarely, cardiac problems. Approximately one-third of patients become mentally retarded.

The symptoms related to the skeletal system, which include kyphoscoliosis, lordosis, pes cavus, and clubfoot, are probably due to muscle imbalances that develop at key stages of bone growth.

Retinitis pigmentosa, loss of clear vision, nystagmus, and ophthalmoplegia are some of the common symptoms related to the eyes. Retinitis pigmentosa usually begins about the time the patient reaches age 10. Loss of clear vision, which can lead to blindness, begins between the ages of 7 and 30.

Laboratory studies reveal the characteristic spiny cytoplasmic projections of acanthocytes, low levels of plasma cholesterol, and an absence or deficiency of VLDLs or **LDLs** (low density lipoproteins). The patient is unable to form chylomicrons in the lymph vessels. Diagnosis of this disorder is based on the demonstration of large intracellular fat particles in biopsy specimens of the jejunum, on the patient's failure to form chylomicrons following a meal, and on the absence of apolipoprotein B in plasma as determined by immunochemical means.

Etiology A genetically transmitted autosomal recessive disorder, acanthocytosis often occurs in patients with consanguineous parentage.

Epidemiology This extremely rare disorder affects equal numbers of males and females.

Related Disorders See *Tangier Disease (Alphalipoproteinemia)*.

Treatment—Standard Restriction of triglycerides in the patient's diet has been successful in helping to relieve symptoms in the gastrointestinal tract. Vitamin E administered in large doses has been shown to improve neuromuscular symptoms and prevent retinopathy in some patients, but it cannot stop the disease from progressing. Other treatments depend on symptoms. A mentally retarded or blind child may benefit from programs offered by social service agencies. The patient's family should receive genetic counseling.

Treatment—Investigational Please contact the agencies listed under Resources, below, for the most current information.

Resources
For more information on acanthocytosis: National Organization for Rare Disorders (NORD); National Lipid Diseases Foundation; National Diabetes, Digestive and Kidney Diseases Information Clearinghouse; National Tay-Sachs/Allied Diseases Association; National Retinitis Pigmentosa Foundation Fighting Blindness; Research Trust for Metabolic Diseases in Children.

For genetic information and genetic counseling referrals: March of Dimes Birth Defects Foundation; National Center for Education in Maternal and Child Health (NCEMCH).

References
The Metabolic Basis of Inherited Disease, 6th ed.: C.R. Scriver, et al., eds.; McGraw-Hill, 1989, pp. 1145–1151.

Agammaglobulinemias, Primary

Description Primary agammaglobulinemias are genetic antibody deficiency disorders characterized by abnormal B lymphocyte development and function in the presence of basically normal T lymphocytes, although T-cell–mediated immune deficits may occur secondary to the disorder. Primary agammaglobulinemias are categorized into 3 types: X-linked agammaglobulinemia **(XLA)**, X-linked agammaglobulinemia with growth hormone deficiency, and autosomal recessive agammaglobulinemia.

Synonyms
>Antibody Deficiency
>Gammaglobulin Deficiency
>Immunoglobulin Deficiency

Signs and Symptoms Bacterial infections, the most frequent symptoms of these antibody deficiencies, result from failures in specific immune responses that are triggered by defects in T and B lymphocytes, which make antibodies. Autoimmune disorders also occur more frequently than normal in patients with some of these diseases. *Giardia lamblia* is a frequent cause of chronic intestinal inflammation and diarrhea in patients with all forms of agammaglobulinemia. Infections begin to occur in boys with X-linked agammaglobulinemia (also known as Bruton agammaglobulinemia) late in the first year of life, only after maternal IgG antibodies have been catabolized. Subsequently these patients suffer recurrent pyogenic infections in the skin, middle ear, and upper and lower respiratory tracts. Most of the infections in XLA patients are bacterial, but persistent viral and parasitic infections can occur as well. Infection by enteroviruses and the poliomyelitis virus results in unusually severe illness. Echovirus infections can cause a syndrome that resembles dermatomyositis. Infections caused by mycoplasma bacteria can lead to severe arthritis. *Hemophilus influenzae* is the most common pyogen found in XLA patients, but they also have recurrent infections with pneumococci, streptococci, and staphylococci, and to a lesser degree with pseudomonas.

XLA patients have abnormally low levels of IgA, IgG, and IgM antibodies in their blood. Their neutrophils are compromised in terms of their ability to engulf microbes that require antibodies for opsonization. Transient, persistent, or cyclical neutropenia may occur. The number of B cells and their plasma cell progeny are reduced consistently by 100-fold or more. XLA patients are virtually devoid of tonsils, which are made up mostly of B lymphocytes.

A single family has been described to have X-linked agammaglobulinemia with growth hormone deficiency. The boys in the family have reduced or undetectable numbers of B cells and may also have panhypogammaglobulinemia and substantial amounts of IgA and IgM. Researchers are unable to explain why growth hormone coexists with XLA. The patients' T cells appear normal.

Familial agammaglobulinemia also occurs in girls, suggesting that one form of the disorder is inherited as an autosomal trait. Because autosomal recessive agammaglobulinemia is rare, researchers have not yet been able to document the exact mode of transmission or the B cell defect.

Etiology XLA is inherited as an X-linked trait that is believed to be intrinsic to the B lymphocyte lineage. Obligate heterozygous carriers have normal immune systems. As noted above, one very rare form is autosomal recessive. The disease has been shown to occur in brothers and in males whose sisters later had male children with XLA.

Epidemiology These rare inherited disorders occur almost exclusively in males.

Related Disorders See *Acquired Immune Deficiency Syndrome (AIDS); Ataxia Telangiectasia; DiGeorge Syndrome; Nezelof Syndrome; Severe Combined Immunodeficiency; Wiskott-Aldrich Syndrome.*

IgA deficiency is a related antibody deficiency disorder characterized by low levels of IgA in the blood in the presence of normal or increased levels of IgG and IgM. It is the most common primary immunodeficiency. Other deficiencies of immunoglobulin isotopes are **IgM deficiency** and **IgG subclass deficiencies**.

Treatment—Standard Intravenous administration of gammaglobulin therapy is the standard treatment. The optimal dose for each XLA patient should be determined empirically but is at least 300 mg/kg every month. Bacterial infections can be controlled with antibiotics. Patients should avoid exposure to infectious diseases, immunizations, corticosteroids, and immunosuppressive drugs.

Treatment—Investigational Please contact the agencies listed under Resources, below, for the most current information.

Resources
   For more information on primary agammaglobulinemias: National Organization for Rare Disorders (NORD); NIH/National Institute of Allergy and Infectious Disease; Immune Deficiency Foundation; Centers for Disease Control (CDC).
   For genetic information and genetic counseling referrals: March of Dimes Birth Defects Foundation; National Center for Education in Maternal and Child Health (NCEMCH).

References
Fundamental Immunology, 2nd ed.: W.E. Paul, ed.; Raven Press, 1989, pp. 1039–1057.
Genetic Deficiencies in Specific Immune Responses: F.S. Rosen; Seminars in Hematology, October 1990, issue 27(4), pp. 333–341.
Immunodeficiency: R.H. Buckley; J. Allergy Clin. Immunol., December 1983, issue 72(6), pp. 627–641.

AGRANULOCYTOSIS, ACQUIRED

Description Acquired agranulocytosis is a blood disorder characterized by a pronounced reduction in the number of granular leukocytes in the circulating blood (often fewer than 500 granulocytes per mm^3) due to an impairment in granulocyte production in bone marrow. Patients are susceptible to bacterial infections that cause ulcers in mucous membranes.

Synonyms
   Agranulocytic Angina
   Malignant Neutropenia
   Primary Granulocytopenia

Signs and Symptoms The first symptoms of bacterial infection may be weakness, chills, fever, or extreme exhaustion. The onset of acute granulocytopenia is marked by infected ulcers in the mucous membranes of the cheek, throat, and intestinal tract. The patient may have difficulty swallowing. Resulting granulocytopenia causes a decrease in the number of neutrophils. If left untreated, the patient could quickly progress into bacterial shock.
   Chronic granulocytopenia generally progresses slowly beginning with many different infections in the patient's bronchopulmonary system, skin, and perirectal region. Canker sores and chronic gingivitis may be a recurrent feature in the mouth, and other infections may recur regularly.

Etiology This disorder is usually drug-induced and dose-related. The most common causes of granulocyte destruction or impairment are chemotherapeutic antineoplastic agents. Other chemical or pathogenic agents that are less commonly involved include chemotherapeutic antimetabolites, alkylating agents, antithyroid drugs, dibenzepin compounds, phenothiazine derivatives, anticonvulsants, antihistamines, sulfonamides, synthetic penicillins, benzene, arsenic, chloramphenicol, and nitrous oxide.

Granulocyte production can also be impaired by drugs regardless of the dosage. The drugs implicated in acute idiosyncratic forms of this disorder include indomethacin, cinchona alkaloids, phenylbutazone, thiazides, procainamide, and nitrofurantoin. The drugs implicated in chronic forms include gold salts, chloramphenicol, and phenylbutazone.

A number of drugs destroy granulocyte precursors in bone marrow and produce granulocytopenia. They include phenytoin, pyrimethamine, methotrexate, and cytarabine. In rare instances, acute agranulocytosis results from the destructive action of leukocyte antibodies that are induced by such drugs as phenylbutazone, gold salts, sulfapyridine, aminopyrine, meralluride, and dipyrine.

Granulocytopenia associated with this disease most often results from stepped-up destruction of neutrophils caused by macrophage destruction of leukocytes, whole-body infections, some form of hypersplenism such as Felty syndrome, an intrinsic granulocyte defect such as in Chédiak-Higashi syndrome, congestive splenomegaly associated with collagen disease, and in rare instances, leukocyte isoantibodies. Acute reversible neutropenia mediated by complement can occasionally occur in hemodialysis.

Aside from antineoplastic chemotherapeutic agents, the drugs that induce granulocytopenia most frequently are phenylbutazone, which carries the highest relative risk, sulfonamides, antithyroid compounds, and phenothiazines.

Treatment—Standard The drugs or other agents that induce this disorder must be identified and eliminated from the patient's regimen. Broad-spectrum antibacterial therapy can be beneficial if the patient has a fever over 38.3°C (100.94°F), is in shock, or has a positive blood culture or significant local infection. In adults initially, the antimicrobial therapy should be combined with gentamicin or tobramycin plus cephalothin, oxacillin, or carbenicillin. The antibiotics should be administered for 7 to 10 days after the fever abates, but no longer or the patient will be exposed to superinfections and renal complications. When granulocyte levels return to 500 mm^3, fever and infections will generally abate.

Corticosteroids are sometimes used to treat shock induced by bacteria, but they should not be used for acute granulocytopenia because they can impede the movement of granulocytes into tissue by masking bacterial infections. Patients with hypogammaglobulinemia should be given human gammaglobulin. Patients with severe neutropenia and sepsis that is resistant to antibiotics have been shown to benefit from massive infusions of leukocytes from matched donors, but the procedure is risky and costly and should not be used routinely.

Mouth and throat ulcers can be soothed with gargles of salt or hydrogen peroxide or with anesthetic lozenges. Mouth washes containing nystatin are used for oral thrush. Patients may have to go on a semisolid or liquid diet when mucous membranes are acutely inflamed.

Patients with chronic granulocytopenia need to be hospitalized during acute episodes and so should be instructed to recognize symptoms early. Chronic patients must be monitored for bacteria resistant to antibiotics and for opportunistic infections.

Treatment—Investigational In recent years, recombinant DNA technology has been able to clone molecularly the genes of granulocyte-colony stimulating factor **(G-CSF)** and granulocyte macrophage-CSF **(GM-CSF)** from various species to produce recombinant human **(rh)** factors. These rhG-CSF and rhGM-CSF glycoproteins stimulate the proliferation and differentiation of hematopoietic progenitors and ultimately increase the number of granulocytes and macrophages and improve their function. This technology is currently under investigation and may prove to be effective in the treatment of agranulocytosis and granulocytopenia in the future.

Please contact the agencies listed under Resources, below, for the most current information.

Resources

For more information on acquired agranulocytosis: National Organization for Rare Disorders (NORD); NIH/National Heart, Lung and Blood Institute.

References
Cecil Textbook of Medicine, 18th ed.: J.B. Wyngaarden and L.H. Smith, Jr., eds.; W.B. Saunders Company, 1988, pp. 1325, 1699.

GM-CSF Treatment in Aplasia after Cytotoxic Therapy: C. Gattringer, et al.; Onkologie, February 1989, issue 12(1), pp. 16–18.

Various Human Hematopoietic Growth Factors (Interleukin-3, GM-CSF, G-CSF) Stimulate Clonal Growth of Nonhematopoietic Tumor Cells: W.E. Berdel, et al.; Blood, January 1989, issue 73(1), pp. 80–83.

ANEMIA, APLASTIC

Description In aplastic anemia, suppression of the bone marrow can cause pancytopenia. In some cases, however, the disorder may be discriminatory and affect only the red blood cells, the white cells, or the platelets.

Synonyms
Aregenerative Anemia
Erythroblastophthisis
Hypoplastic Anemia
Panmyelopathy
Panmyelophthisis
Progressive Hypoerythemia
Refractory Anemia
Toxic Paralytic Anemia

Signs and Symptoms Onset of aplastic anemia may be sudden, but as a rule it is gradual. Weeks or months may pass before the effect of the causative toxin becomes apparent.

The initial symptoms may be increasing weakness, fatigue, and lethargy. Exertion may be followed by headache and respiratory problems. The patient may have bacterial infections more often and be sicker than is usual. While the manifestations depend upon the extent of the pancytopenia, the usual symptoms of anemia are exaggerated.

The typical patient's skin is pale and waxy, but that of a patient with the chronic form of the disorder may show significant brown pigmentation. If marked thrombocytopenia is present, bleeding into the epidermis and the mucous membranes may become apparent. Petechiae also may be noted, and trauma may produce purpura. Other signs may be mucosal ulceration, tachycardia, and systolic murmur.

Etiology Aplastic anemia results from failure of the bone marrow cells to mature. About 50 percent of cases are idiopathic; in most of these, the patients are in their teens and 20s.

Acquired aplastic anemia may be due to exposure to chemicals such as benzene, urethane, and those in some solvents and insecticides. Other causative agents are inorganic arsenic and radiation, and drugs such as phenylbutazone, chloramphenicol, antibiotics, antiinflammatory agents, and anticonvulsants.

The exact mechanism involved in the adverse reaction is not known. An inborn hypersensitivity may be the explanation.

Related Disorders Bone marrow failure may also occur in renal failure, hepatic disease, endocrine abnormalities, late-stage malignancies (particularly with metastasis to the bone marrow), chronic infections, and certain hereditary diseases.

Treatment—Standard In chemical-, radiation-, or drug-related aplastic anemia, the offender must be removed.

A bone marrow transplant offers maximum effectiveness; the marrow of a sibling is compatible in about 30 percent of cases. Repeated blood transfusions lower the chances of a successful transplant and should be avoided if at all possible. Antilymphocyte globulin is the treatment of choice for patients who do not have an HLA-compatible sibling. Androgenic steroids (e.g., oxymetholone) may also trigger bone marrow production in less severe aplastic anemia.

When an immunologic cause has been identified, immunosuppressive drugs such as prednisone, cyclosporin A, and cyclophosphamide may be effective.

The outcome is poor in severe aplastic anemia, with only 20 percent of patients surviving 2 years with supportive therapy alone. Marrow production may resume once removal of the causative toxin is accomplished. The idiopathic form of the disorder may have a longer course with a less optimistic prognosis, but remission may occur. Transfusions may lead to an overall increase in tissue iron stores without trauma to the tissue. Infections (e.g., septicemia) may also intervene.

Treatment—Investigational A new biotechnology product is undergoing study. Recombinant human granulocyte macrophage—colony stimulating factor (rhGM—CSF) is being given in extremely severe refractory cases. It leads to transient but not sustained rises of the neutrophils.

Please contact the agencies listed under Resources, below, for the most current information.

Resources

For more information on aplastic anemia: National Organization for Rare Disorders (NORD); Aplastic Anemia Foundation of America; NIH/National Cancer Institute PDQ (Physician Data Query) phoneline.

References

Cecil Textbook of Medicine, 18th ed.: J.B. Wyngaarden and L.H. Smith, Jr., eds.; W.B. Saunders Company, 1988, pp. 885–889.

ANEMIA, DIAMOND-BLACKFAN

Description Diamond-Blackfan anemia is a hereditary congenital autoimmune blood disorder.

Synonyms

Blackfan-Diamond Anemia
Constitutional Erythroid Hypoplasia

Signs and Symptoms The infant with Diamond-Blackfan anemia has a moderate-to-severe deficiency of red blood cells. About age 1 month, the infant may appear unusually weak, pale, and sluggish. Normal growth may not occur, and facial characteristics such as a snub nose, widely spaced eyes, and a prominent upper lip may be apparent. Vertebral fusion may produce a webbed or shortened and rigid neck. The shoulder blades may protrude, and the hand may be deformed. Spontaneous remissions are possible, but usually drug therapy is responsible for improvement.

Etiology Diamond-Blackfan anemia may be either autosomal dominant or recessive, and is autoimmune-related. Patients have an erythroid-precursor antibody.

Epidemiology Males and females are affected in equal numbers. Since its discovery in 1938, about 150 verified cases of Diamond-Blackfan anemia have been reported in the United States.

Related Disorders See *Anemia, Aplastic; Anemia, Fanconi.*

Treatment—Standard Corticosteroid therapy is begun as soon as possible. Blood transfusions may also be necessary, but when multiple they carry the risk of complications: cardiac and hepatic disorders and iron overload. Prevention of infections is essential since they can aggravate the blood disorder. When treatment is effective, the patient's future health is usually unaffected. Genetic counseling may be helpful. Other treatment is symptomatic and supportive.

Treatment—Investigational Experimental bone marrow transplants are reserved for the gravest cases. Interleukin-III shows promise in raising the red cell count in patients refractory to corticosteroids.

Please contact the agencies listed under Resources, below, for the most current information.

Resources

For more information on Diamond-Blackfan anemia: National Organization for Rare Disorders (NORD); Diamond-Blackfan Anemia Support Group; NIH/National Heart, Lung and Blood Institute (NHLBI); Aplastic Anemia Foundation of America.

For genetic information and genetic counseling referrals: March of Dimes Birth Defects Foundation; National Center for Education in Maternal and Child Health (NCEMCH).

References

Defective Erythroid Progenitor Differentiation System in Congenital Hypoplastic (Diamond-Blackfan) Anemia: J.M. Lipton, et al.; Blood, April 1986, issue 67(4), pp. 962–968.

Diamond-Blackfan Syndrome in Adult Patients: E.P. Balaban, et al.; Am. J. Med., March 1985, issue 78(3), pp. 533–538.

ANEMIA, FANCONI

Description Fanconi anemia is a hereditary aplastic anemia encountered mainly in children and associated with cardiac, renal, and skeletal congenital anomalies as well as changes in skin pigmentation.

Synonyms

Aplastic Anemia with Congenital Anomalies
Congenital Pancytopenia
Constitutional Aplastic Anemia
Fanconi Panmyelopathy

Signs and Symptoms The first signs may be easy bruising and unprovoked epistaxis. Tests reveal inadequate production of red blood cells, white blood cells, and platelets. Diagnosis is generally made before age 9, usually between ages 2 and 6, by which time aplastic anemia per se is present.

The child's growth may be retarded, or may stop. Microcephaly, hypogenitalism, hyperreflexia, and patchy hyperpigmentation may be evident. The upper extremities are likely to reflect the impact of the disorder on the skeleton, such as aplasia of the thumbs and radii. Examination usually reveals a spleen too small for the child's age. Renal abnormalities, and strabismus and microphthalmia may also be present.

Monitoring is essential because patients with Fanconi anemia are cancer-prone, especially to leukemia.

Etiology Fanconi anemia is inherited as an autosomal recessive trait, perhaps precipitated by an environmental factor. Cell hypersensitivity to environmental carcinogens has been implicated.

Epidemiology Males are affected more often than females. Incidence is approximately 1:120,000 individuals.

Treatment—Standard Treatment usually includes methyltestosterone, methyltestosterone plus prednisone, and blood transfusions. Another therapeutic approach is to give cyclophosphamide, alone or in combination with procarbazine and antithymocyte globulin, followed by thoraco-abdominal irradiation to prepare the patient for allogeneic bone marrow transplantation.

Treatment—Investigational An experimental method of lessening the likelihood of rejection of a bone marrow transplant is the use of cyclosporin A to remove donor T lymphocytes. The longterm outcome is not yet known.

Under a grant from the National Organization for Rare Disorders, Blanche Alter, M.D., is studying several possible treatments. For tissue donation contact Dr. Alter at Mount Sinai School of Medicine, 5th Ave. & 100th St., New York, NY 10029.

Please contact the agencies listed under Resources, below, for the most current information.

Resources

For more information on Fanconi anemia: National Organization for Rare Disorders (NORD); Fanconi Anemia Support Group; International Fanconi Registry; Aplastic Anemia Foundation of America; NIH/National Heart, Lung and Blood Institute (NHLBI).

For genetic information and genetic counseling referrals: March of Dimes Birth Defects Foundation; National Center for Education in Maternal and Child Health (NCEMCH).

References
Mendelian Inheritance in Man, 9th ed.: V.A. McKusick; The Johns Hopkins University Press, 1990, pp. 1174–1177.
Fanconi Anemia Study May Give Cancer Insight: Dermatology News, July–August, 1986.

ANEMIA, HEMOLYTIC, COLD-ANTIBODY

Description Cold-antibody hemolytic anemia develops when a temperature of 30°C (86°F) or below causes agglutination and consequent complement fixation when IgM antibodies and erythrocytes bind. As a result, changes in the surface membranes of the red blood cells lead to their removal from the circulating macrophages.

Synonyms
Anemia, Autoimmune Hemolytic
Cold Agglutinin Disease
Cold-Antibody Disease

Signs and Symptoms It is thought that IgM antibody–erythrocyte binding occurs distally. Temperatures can drop to 32 to 28 C (89.6°F to 82.4°F) in the ear lobes, fingertips, the tip of the nose, and the cheeks for lengthy periods.

Patients with cold-antibody hemolytic anemia may have weakness, dizziness, headache, tinnitus, spots before the eyes, fatigue, or sleepiness; they may behave oddly or be irritable. Gastrointestinal upsets and amenorrhea may occur, as may jaundice and splenomegaly, and, less often, hemoglobinuria. Cardiac failure or shock may develop.

Etiology Cold-antibody hemolytic anemia is idiopathic.

Epidemiology Usually the elderly are involved, particularly those whom infectious mononucleosis, lymphoproliferative disease, or mycoplasma pneumonia has rendered susceptible.

Related Disorders See *Hemoglobinuria, Paroxysmal Cold.*

Treatment—Standard Avoidance of cold may be beneficial. Immunosuppressive drugs such as chlorambucil or cyclophosphamide may sometimes lower the cold agglutinin concentration in severely afflicted patients.

When blood transfusions are necessary, certain precautions are essential. Cross-matching to assure compatibility should be carried out at 37°C (98.6°F), and the blood should be heated by an on-line warmer to prevent binding of the new erythrocytes with antibodies.

Treatment—Investigational Plasmapheresis may be effective in some patients, but the side effects and efficacy are still being studied. It is currently reserved for the gravest cases.

Sandoglobulin is also undergoing investigation as a treatment for cold-antibody hemolytic anemia.

Please contact the agencies listed under Resources, below, for the most current information.

Resources

For more information on cold-antibody hemolytic anemia: National Organization for Rare Disorders (NORD); NIH/National Heart, Lung and Blood Institute (NHLBI).

References
Benefit of a 37 Degree Extracorporeal Circuit in Plasma Exchange Therapy for Selected Cases with Cold Agglutinin Disease: C. Andrzejewski Jr., et al.; J. Clin. Apheresis, 1988, issue 4(1), pp. 13–17.
Internal Medicine, 2nd ed.: J.H. Stein, ed.-in-chief; Little, Brown and Co., 1987, pp. 1058–1059.
Isolation of a Peptide Associated with Autoimmune Haemolytic Anaemia from Red Cell Membranes: E. Kajii, et al.; Clin. Exp. Immunol., September 1988, issue 73(3), pp. 406–409.
Patients with Red Cell Autoantibodies: Selection of Blood for Transfusion: R.J. Sokol, et al.; Clin. Lab. Haematol., 1988, issue 10(3), pp. 257–264.

ANEMIA, HEMOLYTIC, HEREDITARY NONSPHEROCYTIC

Description Hereditary nonspherocytic hemolytic anemia is a term used to describe a heterogeneous group of genetic blood disorders characterized by defective erythrocytes that are not spherocytes. The disorders are thought to be caused by deficiencies in hereditary enzymes, such as glucose-6-phosphate dehydrogenase (**G6PD**), which will be discussed here.

G6PD deficiency is recognized as the most common inherited enzyme abnormality in humans. There are close to 300 distinct variants that have been classified into 5 main groups according to their erythrocyte enzymatic activity and the presence of hemolysis. In general terms, patients with hereditary nonspherocytic hemolytic anemia who have a G6PD deficiency have inherited an uncommon variant that has severely decreased enzyme activity, extremely abnormal kinetics, and reduced heat stability, factors that could account for its defective function.

Signs and Symptoms The signs and symptoms of moderate anemia, recurrent jaundice, and splenomegaly or hepatomegaly usually occur in childhood, but some newborns are jaundiced at birth. If the newborn's erythrocytes contain Heinz bodies, a diagnosis of nonspherocytic hemolytic anemia can be made. In some instances a marked decrease in hemoglobin level may be present.

Etiology G6PD deficiency is inherited as a partially dominant X-linked trait. The hemolysis characteristic of these disorders may result from oxidant stress and in turn leads to the symptoms described above. Fava beans and certain drugs, such as some sulfonamides, antimalarial drugs, and phenacetin, can precipitate hemolytic crises.

Epidemiology Males, as hemizygotes with respect to the enzyme, are more likely to be seen clinically.

Treatment—Standard Any precipitating agent for the hemolysis should be discontinued. Patients with this disease may occasionally need blood transfusions. If the need for transfusions becomes chronic, then iron chelation therapy (deferoxamine) is given when indicated. Splenectomy is not beneficial for nonspherocytic hemolytic anemia.

Treatment—Investigational Sandoglobulin is under investigation for the treatment of these disorders, but its safety and effectiveness have not yet been determined.

Please contact the agencies listed under Resources, below, for the most current information.

Resources

For more information on hereditary nonspherocytic hemolytic anemia: National Organization for Rare Disorders (NORD); National Heart, Lung and Blood Institute (NHLBI).

For genetic information and genetic counseling referrals: March of

Dimes Birth Defects Foundation; National Center for Education in Maternal and Child Health (NCEMCH).

References

The Metabolic Basis of Inherited Disease, 6th ed.: C.R. Scriver et al., eds.; McGraw-Hill, 1989, pp. 2247–2249.

Cecil Textbook of Medicine, 18th ed.: J.B. Wyngaarden and L.H. Smith, Jr., eds.; W.B. Saunders Company, 1988, p. 880.

Chronic Nonspherocytic Hemolytic Anemia (CNSHA) and Glucose 6 Phosphate Dehydrogenase (G6PD) Deficiency in a Patient with Familial Amyloidotic Polyneuropathy (FAP): L. Vives-Corrons, et al.; Human Genetics, January 1989, issue 81(2), pp. 161–164.

ANEMIA, HEMOLYTIC, HEREDITARY SPHEROCYTIC

Description Hereditary spherocytic hemolytic anemia is an intracorpuscular abnormality in which defects within the red blood cell shorten its survival. The membrane of the cell is abnormal in lipid content and surface area, both of which are smaller than normal. The red blood cells are sphere-shaped; it is difficult for them to course through the splenic circulation, and when they cannot do so they are lost. The spheroid shape is the hallmark of hereditary spherocytic hemolytic anemia, and it is the result of the inherent metabolic defect.

Synonyms

Acholuric Jaundice (Chronic Acholuric Jaundice)
Chronic Familial Icterus
Congenital Hemolytic Anemia
Congenital Hemolytic Jaundice
Hereditary Spherocytosis

Signs and Symptoms Hereditary spherocytic hemolytic anemia may be present at birth or may not be apparent for years. The nature of the disorder varies significantly among patients. In many patients, the symptoms are mild enough to go unrecognized. Tiredness and moderate persistent jaundice may be present. Onset of puberty may be late. Splenomegaly is commonly found, and it may sometimes manifest in abdominal discomfort.

An infection is the most common trigger of an aplastic crisis, which signals temporary deficiency of red blood cell production. Trauma or pregnancy may intensify the crisis. The patient may complain of fever, headache, abdominal pain, anorexia, vomiting, and lethargy. Children may have epistaxis.

Occasionally hepatomegaly, cholelithiasis, or leg ulcers may develop. Congenital deformities, perhaps polydactylism or a tower-shaped skull, may be present.

Etiology Hemolytic anemias have 2 distinct findings: (1) a reduction in the life span of the erythrocytes, and (2) the retention of iron within the body, mainly in the reticuloendothelial system. In all hemolytic anemias, there is overdestruction of red blood cells.

The abnormality of the red blood cell membrane in spherocytic hemolytic anemia is usually inherited as an autosomal dominant metabolic trait, but severe forms are inherited in an autosomal recessive manner. Usually there is a familial history of anemia, jaundice, or splenomegaly. At times, the disorder may skip one or more generations. No familial history can be traced in some cases.

Epidemiology The greatest incidence of hereditary spherocytic hemolytic anemia is in Northern Europeans.

Related Disorders Spherocytes may be present in hemoglobin C disease, autoimmune hemolytic anemia, drug-induced hemolytic anemia, alcoholism, and individuals with burns.

Treatment—Standard Hereditary spherocytosis usually has a lengthy chronic course. The only currently recognized specific treatment is splenectomy, which is carried out in a patient under age 45 who has had jaundice and biliary colic or aplastic crises. Splenectomy should be avoided in children under age 5 years because of the risk of overwhelming bacterial infection. Following the surgery the patient becomes asymptomatic.

During an aplastic crisis, transfusions may be indicated to avert cardiovascular collapse. If the crisis was triggered by an intercurrent infection, antibiotic treatment may be warranted.

Treatment—Investigational Studies are ongoing in the use of sandoglobulin as a treatment for hereditary spherocytic hemolytic anemia.

Please contact the agencies listed under Resources, below, for the most current information.

Resources
    For more information on hereditary spherocytic hemolytic anemia: National Organization for Rare Disorders (NORD); NIH/National Heart, Lung and Blood Institute (NHLBI); NIH/National Cancer Institute PDQ (Physicians Data Query) phoneline; American Cancer Society.
    For genetic information and genetic counseling referrals: March of Dimes Birth Defects Foundation; National Center for Education in Maternal and Child Health (NCEMCH).

References
    Cecil Textbook of Medicine, 18th ed.: J.B. Wyngaarden and L.H. Smith, Jr., eds.; W.B. Saunders Company, 1988, p. 880.

ANEMIA, HEMOLYTIC, WARM-ANTIBODY

Description Warm-antibody hemolytic anemia is an autoimmune disorder in which IgM antibodies bind with erythrocytes, removing them from circulation and aborting their normal life span of 120 days. Bone marrow production of new cells cannot replace their numbers. The extent of the anemia depends on the duration of the survival of the coated red cells and the ability of the marrow to maintain manufacture of red cells.

Immune hemolytic anemias are classified by the temperature at which erythrocyte removal occurs. Warm-antibody hemolytic anemia is associated with temperatures of 37°C (98.6°F) or higher, while cold-antibody hemolytic anemia generally has its onset at lower temperatures.

Synonyms
> Autoimmune Hemolytic Anemias
> Warm-Reacting Antibody Disease

Signs and Symptoms The degree of the symptoms depends upon the speed of onset and that of the annihilation of red blood cells, and whether an underlying disorder is present; symptoms vary from patient to patient. The manifestations of sudden onset are often paleness, tiredness, exertion-produced breathing problems, dizziness, and palpitations. The slower the onset the less marked the anemia, and a patient may be asymptomatic. Jaundice and splenomegaly are usually part of the complex.

Etiology Approximately 25 percent of reported cases of this disorder are idiopathic; an estimated 65 percent have a precipitating disorder such as chronic lymphocytic leukemia or other disease of the lymph system. Other associated disorders are systemic lupus erythematosus (**SLE**), rheumatoid arthritis, and ulcerative colitis. Another 10 to 15 percent of cases are considered to be reactions to drugs, e.g., methyldopa.

Epidemiology Warm-antibody hemolytic anemia may affect anyone. Individuals with diseases that alter the immune system are at higher risk. Chronic lymphatic leukemia, lymphoma, and SLE may precede the development of warm-antibody hemolytic anemia.

Related Disorders See *Hodgkin Disease; Systemic Lupus Erythematosus.*

Chronic lymphatic leukemia is marked by an oversupply of white blood cells in the bone marrow, spleen, liver, and blood. As the disease advances, the leukemic cells invade other areas including the intestinal tract, kidneys, lungs, gonads, and lymph nodes. The patient may experience tiredness, weakness, itchiness, night sweats, abdominal discomfort, or weight loss. Splenomegaly is generally present.

Treatment—Standard Corticosteroids are the drugs of choice in warm-antibody hemolytic anemia. For the few patients who are refractory, immunosuppressive drugs are indicated. Advanced disease may require splenectomy. In those with an underlying disorder, treatment of that disorder usually significantly improves the anemia. In drug-induced anemia, symptoms generally abate when the medication is discontinued.

Treatment—Investigational Sandoglobulin is being investigated as a potential therapy.

Please contact the agencies listed under Resources, below, for the most current information.

Resources

For more information on warm-antibody hemolytic anemia: National Organization for Rare Disorders (NORD); NIH/National Heart, Lung and Blood Institute (NHLBI).

References

Cecil Textbook of Medicine, 18th ed.: J.B. Wyngaarden and L.H. Smith, Jr., eds.; W.B. Saunders Company, 1988, pp. 917–920.

Incomplete Warm Hemolysins. II. Corresponding Antigens and Pathogenic Mechanisms in Autoimmune Hemolytic Anemias Induced by Incomplete Warm Hemolysins: M.W. Wolf, et al.; Clin. Immunopathol., April 1989, issue 51(1), pp. 68–76.

Internal Medicine, 2nd ed.: J.H. Stein, ed.-in-chief; Little, Brown and Company, 1987, pp. 1057–1059.

Production of Human Warm-Reacting Red Cell Monoclonal Antoantibodies by Epstein-Barr Virus Transformation: C. Andrzejewski, et al.; Transfusion, March–April 1989, issue 29(3), pp. 196–200.

ANEMIA, MEGALOBLASTIC

Description Megaloblasts in the marrow and hypersegmented polymorphonuclear leukocytes are hallmarks of megaloblastic anemia. Leukopenia and thrombocytopenia may also be present.

Synonyms

Megaloblastic Anemia of Pregnancy

Signs and Symptoms As a rule, onset is slow. The initial symptoms may be diarrhea, vomiting, anorexia, and weight loss. Malabsorption may result. Hepatomegaly and splenomegaly may occur. The patient may be jaundiced or pale, and weakness, palpitations, breathing problems, aching limbs, and feeling inappropriately hot or cold may be complaints. Oral infection, neurologic lesions, and irritability also may occur.

Etiology Megaloblastic anemia is due to a deficiency of either vitamin B12 or folic acid. Any of a number of factors may cause these deficiencies: inadequate diet, malabsorption, certain diseases or parasites, or immunosuppressive drugs. In addition, during pregnancy the fetal blood requirement may result in maternal megaloblastic anemia.

Related Disorders Folic acid deficiency causes megaloblastic anemia and other blood findings. Folic acid is available from many plants and from animal tissues, but long cooking destroys it. Infertility, gastrointestinal problems, certain skin diseases, obstetric disorders, neuropathy, and, perhaps, psychiatric disorders may be associated with the deficiency.

See also *Anemia, Pernicious.*

Treatment—Standard Treatment includes intramuscular injections of vitamin B12 or oral iron supplements. A lifetime maintenance dose of vitamin B12 is essential. Folic acid deficiency is treated by oral administration of folate.

Treatment—Investigational Please contact the agencies listed under Resources, below, for the most current information.

Resources

For more information on megaloblastic anemia: National Organization for Rare Disorders (NORD); NIH/National Heart, Lung and Blood Institute (NHLBI).

References

Bone Marrow Status of Anaemic Pregnant Women on Supplemental Iron and Folic Acid in a Nigerian Community: L.A. Okafor, et al.; Angiology, August 1985, issue 36(8), pp. 500–503.

Homocystinuria and Megaloblastic Anemia Responsive to Vitamin B-12 Therapy: S. Schuh, et al.; New Eng. J. of Med., March 15, 1984, issue 310(11), pp. 686–690.

Megaloblastic Anemia due to Vitamin B12 Deficiency Caused by Small Intestinal Bacterial Overgrowth: Possible Role of Vitamin B12 Analogues: M.F. Murphy, et al.; Brit. J. Haematol., January 1986, issue 62(1), pp. 7–12.

ANEMIA, PERNICIOUS

Description Pernicious anemia is characterized by a deficiency of vitamin B12 that is generally due to a failure of the gastric mucosa to secrete intrinsic factor, which is needed to absorb vitamin B12 from the diet. In some cases, intestinal abnormalities prevent absorption of the vitamin.

Synonyms

Addisonian Pernicious Anemia (Addison Anemia)
Addison-Biermer Anemia
Biermer Anemia
Cytogenic Anemia
Malignant Anemia
Primary Anemia

Signs and Symptoms Because the human liver stores enough vitamin B12 to last 3 to 5 years, pernicious anemia progresses slowly as the hepatic reserves of B12 are used. Once symptoms appear, however, they must be treated or the disease could be fatal. Symptoms and signs include weakness, easy fatigability, dyspnea, tachycardia, and angina. Patients may also have gastrointestinal problems, such as anorexia, abdominal pain, indigestion, belching, and possibly intermittent constipation and diarrhea. Weight loss is common. In some cases there is genitourinary involvement as well as hepato- or splenomegaly.

Neurologic involvement can occur, most often in the peripheral nerves but also in the spinal cord. Early neurologic symptoms and signs include paresthesias and loss in the extremities of vibration and position awareness. Ataxia, a positive Babinski sign, and hyperactive reflexes are among the characteristics that may develop. Patients may be depressed and irritable, and experience the paranoia known as megaloblastic madness.

Etiology Pernicious anemia is known to be familial, and a predisposition to the disease may be inherited as an autosomal dominant trait. The most common cause of B12 deficiency is the failure of the gastric mucosa to secrete intrinsic factor, but other causes may be involved, including gastrectomy, malabsorption syndromes, congenital absence of absorptive sites for vitamin B12 in the ileum, absence of absorptive sites due to regional enteritis or surgical resection of the small intestine, chronic atrophic gastritis, chronic pancreatitis, myxedema, blind loop syndrome, and fish tapeworm infestation.

Epidemiology Pernicious anemia primarily affects adults and rarely occurs before the patient reaches the age of 35. It is most common in the moderate climates of North America and Europe among people of Scandinavian, English, and Irish extraction. It is extremely rare in Orientals. A juvenile version of pernicious anemia afflicts infants, children, and adolescents and resembles the adult version in all respects except for certain biochemical reactions.

Related Disorders See *Anemia, Megaloblastic.*

Treatment—Standard Intramuscular injection of vitamin B12 is the standard therapy. A physician must closely monitor the amount given. Patients generally continue to receive maintenance doses of vitamin B12 for life.

Treatment—Investigational Please contact the agencies listed under Resources, below, for the most current information.

Resources
    For more information on pernicious anemia: National Organization for Rare Disorders (NORD); NIH/National Heart, Lung and Blood Institute (NHLBI).
    For genetic information and genetic counseling referrals: March of Dimes Birth Defects Foundation; National Center for Education in Maternal and Child Health (NCEMCH).

References
    Cecil Textbook of Medicine, 18th ed.: J.B. Wyngaarden and Lloyd H. Smith, Jr., eds.; W.B. Saunders Co., 1988, pp. 904–905.

ANEMIA, SIDEROBLASTIC

Description Sideroblastic anemias are disorders in which synthesis of hemoglobin is abnormal because of insufficient or ineffective use of intracellular iron, which may be in abundant supply.

Synonyms
        Idiopathic Refractory Sideroblastic Anemia
        Iron Overload Anemia
        Sideroblastosis

Signs and Symptoms The patient experiences general weakness, fatigue, and difficulty in breathing. Exertion may cause chest pains resembling angina.

In contrast to most other forms of anemia, the blood serum has unusually high levels of iron and iron-containing substances; it also contains sideroblasts. The mucous membranes and the skin of hands and arms may be pale, often with a lemon-yellow cast. Upon occasion, subcutaneous bleeding may produce a brownish-red effect. Splenomegaly or hepatomegaly may be present. A complication in a late stage of sideroblastic anemia is acute leukemia, which occurs in approximately 10 percent of the cases.

Etiology Hereditary sideroblastic anemia is generally inherited as an X-linked trait, but may in rare cases be autosomal recessive. Autosomal dominant inheritance of sideroblastic anemia with erythrocyte dimorphism has been reported.

Acquired forms are most often idiopathic, but in some cases can be attributed to such factors as alcohol abuse and certain drugs (e.g., anti-tuberculosis agents or chloramphenicol). The disorder also may be a symptom of a granulomatous disease, a tumor, rheumatoid arthritis, or myelodysplasia.

Epidemiology Inherited forms usually develop in childhood. The idiopathic acquired disease occurs most often in the elderly. Incidence of other acquired forms depends on the precipitating condition.

Related Disorders Idiopathic hemochromatosis is a hereditary disorder of iron metabolism marked by an overload of iron in the tissues, particularly in the liver, pancreas, and heart, and a bronze cast to the skin. Cirrhosis of the liver, diabetes mellitus, and associated bone and joint changes may also be present.

See ***Thalassemia Major; Thalassemia Minor.***

Treatment—Standard Hereditary sideroblastic anemia often improves with the use of pyridoxine. There is presently no specific therapy for idiopathic sideroblastic anemia. When a precipitating agent has been determined, its use should be discontinued. Pyridoxine has not proved generally effective in cases of acquired sideroblastic anemia. Supportive treatment, including transfusion, may be beneficial in all cases of sideroblastic anemia.

To remove an overload of iron in sideroblastic anemia, deferoxamine is infused subcutaneously or intramuscularly, and has frequently been effective; however, a combination of deferoxamine with ascorbate has been even more effective in many cases.

Treatment—Investigational Please contact the agencies listed under Resources, below, for the most current information.

Resources

For more information on sideroblastic anemia: National Organization for Rare Disorders (NORD); NIH/National Heart, Lung and Blood Institute (NHLBI); Leukemia Society of America.

For genetic information and genetic counseling referrals: March of Dimes Birth Defects Foundation; National Center for Education in Maternal and Child Health (NCEMCH).

536 | HEMATOLOGIC AND ONCOLOGIC DISORDERS

References

Mendelian Inheritance in Man, 9th ed.: V.A. McKusick; The Johns Hopkins University Press, 1990, pp. 858, 1476, 1563–1564.

Harrison's Principles of Internal Medicine, 12th ed.: J.D. Wilson, et al., eds.; McGraw-Hill, 1991, p. 1522.

Effect of Dose, Time and Ascorbate on Iron Excretion after Subcutaneous Desferrioxamine: M.A. Hussein, et al.; Lancet, May 7, 1977, issue 1(8019), pp. 977–979.

Idiopathic Refractory Sideroblastic Anemia, Incidence and Risk Factors for Leukemia Transformation: D.S. Chang, et al.; Cancer, August 1979, issue 44(2), pp. 724–731.

ANGIOEDEMA, HEREDITARY

Description In hereditary angioedema, circumscribed obstruction of lymphatic vessels or the veins causes temporary edema in areas of the skin, mucous membranes, and, sometimes, the internal organs.

Synonyms
Complement-Mediated Urticaria Angioedema
Hereditary Angioneurotic Edema

Signs and Symptoms Most commonly edema affects the backs of the hands or feet, the eyelids, lips, and genitalia. Edema in the mucous membrane lining of the respiratory and gastrointestinal tracts is more usual in hereditary angiodema than in other forms of angiodema. Also, the patient with the hereditary type complains of firm and painful rather than pruritic swellings. Urticaria rarely is present.

Transient attacks recur, becoming more severe. Injury or severe pain, surgery, dental procedures, viral illness, and stress can trigger or worsen the episodes.

Clues to edema in the gastrointestinal tract include nausea, vomiting, acute abdominal pain, and perhaps signs of obstruction. An edematous pharynx or larynx can be life-threatening.

Etiology Hereditary angioedema is autosomal dominant. Either one of 2 defects is present: more commonly, a deficiency of complement component C1 esterase inhibitor; less commonly, synthesis of an abnormal form of this protein.

Epidemiology Males and females are affected equally.

Related Disorders Acute, nonhereditary angioedema affects the skin and mucous membranes and commonly clears spontaneously in 1 to 2 days. Any number of allergens may be responsible, including drugs, insect stings and bites, and certain foods, especially eggs, shellfish, nuts, and fruits.

Chronic nonhereditary angioedema may be due to constant exposure to an allergen, or to stress. Angioedema may also appear during certain illnesses, including systemic lupus erythematosus and chronic sinus or dental infection.

Treatment—Standard Hereditary angioedema is refractory to the routine therapies for acute or chronic angioedema, but several drugs can be preventive. Prophylactic drugs that yield longterm protection include androgens, such as danazol, and oxymetholone. For women, androgens with few masculinizing effects should be prescribed, and the minimal effective dosage should be used.

To avert episodes associated with surgery, dental work, and similar stresses, short-term treatment prior to the expected period of stress is indicated. Fresh frozen plasma, or preparations of the missing enzyme partially purified from whole blood, are effective in these situations.

In acute attacks that threaten airway obstruction, it is essential to maintain or create an airway. A tracheotomy may be indicated and oxygen needed. Epinephrine and antihistamine may be given, but their value is uncertain in this setting.

Treatment—Investigational An effective drug that is still only in experimental use is epsilon-aminocaproic acid.

The orphan drug tranexamic acid is used prophylactically in patients with hereditary angioneurotic edema and those with other congenital coagulopathies who are undergoing surgical procedures such as dental extractions. This drug has been approved for marketing for these procedures only. For additional information contact Kabi Vitrum, Inc., 1311 Harbor Bay Parkway, Alameda, California 94501.

Please contact the agencies listed under Resources, below, for the most current information.

Resources

For more information on hereditary angioedema: National Organization for Rare Disorders (NORD); NIH/National Heart, Lung and Blood Institute (NHLBI).

For genetic information and genetic counseling referrals: March of Dimes Birth Defects Foundation; National Center for Education in Maternal and Child Health (NCEMCH).

References

Cecil Textbook of Medicine, 18th ed.: J.B. Wyngaarden and L.H. Smith, Jr., eds.; W.B. Saunders Company, 1988, pp. 148, 1940.

ANTITHROMBIN III (AT III) DEFICIENCY, CONGENITAL

Description Since antithrombin III limits blood coagulation, congenital antithrombin III deficiency is characterized by a marked tendency toward venous or arterial thrombosis. There are 3 recognized forms of the disorder: classical AT III deficiency and 2 variants, AT III-Ia and AT III-Ib.

Signs and Symptoms Patients usually suffer the first episode of thrombosis between the ages of 10 and 35. Precipitating events include surgery, pregnancy, childbirth, trauma, or use of oral contraceptives. Because pregnancy and estrogen use are significant risk factors, women tend to develop thrombosis at an earlier age than men.

About 40 percent of patients with congenital AT III deficiency develop pulmonary embolisms. Embolisms also commonly occur in the veins deep in the legs and pelvic region, the more superficial veins in the legs, and the mesenteric veins. Edema is common in affected legs and pelvic areas. Clots that form in the heart may result in thromboembolism to other organs, such as the brain or kidneys.

Etiology Congenital AT III deficiency is inherited as an autosomal dominant gene. In the classical form of the disorder, an insufficient amount of antithrombin is produced in the liver. In the variant forms, AT III-Ia and -Ib, both normal and abnormal AT III are produced but interact so that the result is inhibition of normal antithrombin.

Epidemiology The disease is thought to occur in about one in every 3,000 to 5,000 individuals.

Related Disorders Acquired antithrombin III deficiency occurs when AT III levels fall below 75 percent of normal, increasing the risk of thromboembolism. This condition develops after major trauma calling for sustained or large-scale blood coagulation; if there is urinary loss of antithrombin III during failure of renal filtration; or if AT III is destroyed when proteins are broken down, as in starvation. Other causal conditions include liver failure, severe blood loss, late pregnancy, and estrogen use. Acquired antithrombin III deficiency can usually be reversed.

Treatment—Standard The goal of treatment is to prevent thrombosis, primarily through the use of oral anticoagulants, such as coumadin drugs, heparin, and intravenous concentrated AT III. When the risk of thrombosis is high, as during pregnancy or with surgery, AT III replacement therapy is particularly important. Antithrombin III should also be replaced to help dissolve blood clots after thrombosis has occurred.

Heparin and AT III replacement can cause bleeding, so the amount of therapy must be carefully monitored. AT III can also increase the patient's risk of developing hepatitis.

Women who are prone to this disorder should refrain from taking estrogen. Patients who have any of the following characteristics should be screened for AT III deficiency: a family history of thrombosis, a thrombosis before age 35, recurrence of thrombosis even with heparin therapy, deep vein thrombosis early in pregnancy, or loss of large amounts of protein in the urine.

A drug known as AT nativ has received FDA approval as a treatment for congenital antithrombin III deficiency. It is manufactured by Kabivitrum, Inc., 160 Industrial Drive, Franklin, Ohio 45005.

Treatment—Investigational AT III replacement is under development by the following pharmaceutical companies: Miles Inc., 400 Morgan Lane, West Haven, CT 06516, (800) 468-0894; Kabivitrum, Inc., 160 Industrial Drive, Franklin, OH 45005, (800) 447-3846; Hoechst-Roussel Pharmaceuticals, Inc., Route 202-206 North, Somerville, NJ 00876, (800) 445-4774.

Human antithrombin III is under clinical investigation in preventing or arresting episodes of thrombosis in patients with congenital antithrombin III deficiency, especially those who have suffered trauma or are about to undergo surgery or childbirth. For additional information on human antithrombin III: The American National Red Cross National Headquarters, 17th and E Streets, NW, Washington, DC 20006.

Please contact the agencies listed under Resources, below, for the most current information.

Resources

For more information on congenital antithrombin III deficiency: National Organization for Rare Disorders (NORD); NIH/National Heart, Lung and Blood Institute (NHLBI); American Liver Foundation; The United Liver Foundation; Children's Liver Foundation.

References

Substitution of AT III: H.K. Breddin, et al.; Wiener Klinische Wochenschrift, December 21, 1984 (in English), issue 96(24), pp. 875–878.

Antithrombin III Deficiency and Thromboembolism: E. Thaler, et al.; Clinics in Haematology, June 1981, issue 10(2), pp. 369–390.

BANTI SYNDROME

Description Banti syndrome is a chronic splenic disease characterized by splenomegaly that results from thrombosis of the splenic or portal veins, cirrhosis of the liver, narrowing of splenic or portal veins, or birth abnormalities.

Synonyms

Hypersplenism

Signs and Symptoms In the early stages of the disease, patients have splenomegaly, anemia, fatigue, and weakness. In later stages the anemia worsens and esophageal hemorrhaging may occur, which causes bloody vomitus and dark stools. Hepatomegaly may eventually develop. The course of the disease is similar to that of cirrhosis of the liver except that splenomegaly is the major symptom.

Etiology Banti syndrome is the result of chronic hypertension in the vein that transports blood from the spleen; the hypertension is caused by liver cirrhosis, thrombosis or constriction of the splenic or portal veins, or birth abnormalities. The accumulation of trapped blood then causes splenomegaly.

Related Disorders See *Primary Biliary Cirrhosis; Gaucher Disease; Felty's Syndrome.*

Treatment—Standard Treatment varies with the cause of the syndrome. If thrombosis or narrowing of a vein is the cause, a surgical shunt can be used to reroute the blood and bypass the obstruction. If cirrhosis is the cause, treatment is appropriate to the type and underlying cause of cirrhosis. Ethamolin, an orphan drug, has been approved by the U.S. Food and Drug Administration for use in the treatment of bleeding esophageal varices; its manufacturer is Glaxo Pharmaceuticals.

Treatment—Investigational Please contact the agencies listed under Resources, below, for the most current information.

Resources

For more information on Banti syndrome: National Organization for Rare Disorders (NORD); National Institute of Diabetes, Digestive & Kidney Diseases Information Clearinghouse.

References

Evaluation of Splenic Embolization in Patients with Portal Hypertension and Hypersplenism: A. Alwmark, et al.; Ann. Surg., November 1982, issue 196(5), pp. 518–245.

BERNARD-SOULIER SYNDROME

Description Bernard-Soulier syndrome is an inherited coagulation disorder characterized by abnormalities of blood platelets. Patients have a tendency to bleed excessively and bruise easily. There are 2 forms of the disease, which differ according to the way they are inherited: autosomal recessive (thrombasthenia–thrombocytopenia) and autosomal dominant (thrombopathic thrombocytopenia).

Synonyms

Hereditary Giant Platelet Syndrome

Signs and Symptoms From the time of birth and throughout life, patients tend to bleed excessively from cuts and other injuries and commonly have nosebleeds and unusually heavy menstrual flow. They also bruise easily and the bruises tend to linger. Subcutaneous bleeding causes purpura in both small spots and large areas. Thrombopathic thrombocytopenia, the autosomal dominant form of this disorder, has been linked with monoclonal gammopathy, hereditary kidney disease, and deafness.

Laboratory studies show that platelets are reduced in number, larger than normal, and abnormally shaped; they also exhibit unusual biochemical reactions and have a shortened lifespan.

Etiology Bernard-Soulier syndrome is inherited either through an autosomal recessive or an autosomal dominant gene. Thrombocytopenia, the autosomal recessive form, is thought to be caused by a defect in the membrane around the platelets.

Related Disorders See *Thrombasthenia; May-Hegglin Anomaly; Chédiak-Higashi Syndrome*.

Treatment—Standard The standard therapy for this disorder consists of transfusion of normal blood or platelets when the patient's bleeding poses a danger. The patient should not be given aspirin and related drugs for arthritis because of their effect on platelet aggregation.

Treatment—Investigational Please contact the agencies listed under Resources, below, for the most current information.

Resources

For more information on Bernard-Soulier syndrome: National Organization for Rare Disorders (NORD); NIH/National Heart, Lung and Blood Institute (NHLBI).

For genetic information and genetic counseling referrals: March of Dimes Birth Defects Foundation; National Center for Education in Maternal and Child Health (NCEMCH).

References

Cecil Textbook of Medicine, 18th ed.: J.B. Wyngaarden and L.H. Smith, Jr., eds.; W.B. Saunders Company, 1988, pp. 1055–1057.

CASTLEMAN DISEASE

Description Castleman disease is a rare lymph system disorder marked by benign neoplasms in lymph node tissue throughout the body but especially in the neck, base of the head, chest, or stomach.

Synonyms

Angiofollicular Lymph Node Hyperplasia
Angiomatous Lymphoid
Castleman Tumor
Giant Benign Lymphoma
Hamartoma

Signs and Symptoms The neoplasms are single, solid, and contained and are usually surrounded by normal nodes. Occasionally, neoplasms grow in the veins and mimic an aneurysm. The major symptoms are tumors, respiratory tract infections, dyspnea, coughing, bloody sputum, pain or pressure in the chest or back, fever, and lethargy. Other features include microcyte anemia, hypergammaglobulinemia, and growth retardation.

Etiology Although the exact cause is unknown, the disease is thought to reflect the effect of increased IL-6 production.

Epidemiology Castleman disease affects equal numbers of males and females of any age.

Related Disorders See *Hodgkin Disease.*

Another related disease, **malignant lymphoma,** is marked by circumscribed solid tumors made up of cells that most often appear in lymphatic sites, such as lymph nodes and the spleen. Symptoms may mimic Hodgkin disease or leukemia.

Treatment—Standard Surgical excision of the neoplasm is the usual treatment.

Treatment—Investigational Please contact the agencies listed under Resources,

below, for the most current information.

Resources
For more information on Castleman disease: National Organization for Rare Disorders (NORD); American Cancer Society; NIH/National Cancer Institute PDQ (Physician Data Query) phoneline.

References
Castleman Disease: An Unusual Retroperitoneal Mass: D.P. Bartkowski, et al.; J. Urol., January 1988, issue 139(1), pp. 118–120.
Computerized Tomography of Castleman Disease Simulating a False Renal Artery Aneurysm: A Case Report: L. Friedman, et al.; J. Urol., July 1987, issue 138(1), pp. 123–124.
Castleman Disease in Children: R.W. Powell, et al.; J. Pediatr. Surg., August 1986, issue 21(8), pp. 678–682.

CHÉDIAK-HIGASHI SYNDROME

Description A form of albinism, Chédiak-Higashi syndrome is a hereditary disorder characterized by decreased pigmentation, ocular problems, leukocyte anomalies, and increased susceptibility to infections and certain cancers.

Synonyms
Begnez-Cesar Syndrome
Chédiak-Steinbrinck-Higashi Syndrome
Leukocytic Anomaly Albinism
Oculocutaneous Albinism

Signs and Symptoms Because patients have partial albinism, Chédiak-Higashi syndrome can be diagnosed in early infancy when strong light causes ocular discomfort and nystagmus. The number of the patient's leukocytes and platelets is reduced and neutrophils and lymphocytes contain characteristic inclusions. The patient suffers frequent infections accompanied by high fever and has a tendency to bleed excessively on injury and to bruise easily. The patient's defective blood cells can infiltrate other organs, including the lungs, brain, kidneys, adrenal glands, and liver.

Children who have Chédiak-Higashi syndrome are weak, grow poorly, have splenomegaly, hepatomegaly, and enlarged lymph nodes, and are highly susceptible to leukemias and lymphomas.

Etiology Chédiak-Higashi syndrome is transmitted as an autosomal recessive trait. The patient's defective cells are unable to release enzymes into intracellular compartments to destroy foreign material, such as bacteria; they are also unable to produce normal amounts of melanin.

Related Disorders See *May-Hegglin Anomaly.*

Treatment—Standard The disorder is difficult to treat, and treatment varies according to symptoms. Infections must be kept in check with vigorous antibiotic therapy. Transfusions of leukocytes may also be useful in treating infections.

Whole blood transfusions may be necessary if bleeding becomes excessive after injury or surgery. Any cancers must be treated with accepted cancer therapy. The patient should avoid exposure to sunlight as much as possible and use sunscreens and sunglasses.

Treatment—Investigational Please contact the agencies listed under Resources, below, for the most current information.

Resources

For more information on Chédiak-Higashi syndrome: National Organization for Rare Disorders (NORD); National Organization for Albinism and Hypopigmentation; NIH/National Institute of Allergy and Infectious Diseases.

For genetic information and genetic counseling referrals: March of Dimes Birth Defects Foundation; National Center for Education in Maternal and Child Health (NCEMCH).

References

Cecil Textbook of Medicine, 18th ed.: J.B. Wyngaarden and L.H. Smith, Jr., eds.; W.B. Saunders Company, 1988, pp. 958–959, 1057, 1113, 1534–1536.

Smith's Recognizable Patterns of Human Malformation, 4th ed.: K.L. Jones; W.B. Saunders Company, 1988, p. 542.

CYCLIC NEUTROPENIA

Description A rare blood disorder, cyclic neutropenia is marked by an abnormally severe decrease in the number of circulating neutrophils and other blood components. The decrease occurs at regular intervals, with resulting infections and fever.

Synonyms

Cyclic Hematopoiesis
Periodic Neutropenia

Signs and Symptoms Patients have a dramatic drop in neutrophil levels below $500/mm^3$ for 6 to 8 days every 21 days in a constant and consistent cycle that may also affect reticulocytes and platelets. At the same time, levels of eosinophils and monocytes may rise abnormally.

The change in neutrophil levels is usually accompanied by infections and sometimes by aphthous stomatitis. Patients commonly have fatigue, weakness, and fever, and sometimes skin infections, dental problems, and cervical adenopathy. Over the long term, cyclic neutropenia may cause the parotid gland to become inflamed. If the disorder occurs in infancy or childhood, patients tend to improve as they grow older.

Etiology When the disease occurs in infants and children, it may be inherited as an autosomal dominant trait. When it occurs in adults, it is believed to be an acquired disease of unknown etiology. Studies suggest that the cyclic nature of the disorder is caused by leukocytes not properly maturing in the patient's bone marrow.

Epidemiology Cyclic neutropenia occurs all over the world in equal numbers of males and females. About a quarter of the patients have a family history of the disease.

Treatment—Standard Antibiotics are given to treat infections. Granulocyte-colony stimulating factor has been used to increase neutrophil production. Patients require careful oral and dental care. Persons with inherited forms of the disease should receive genetic counseling. Other treatments depend on symptoms.

Treatment—Investigational Please contact the agencies listed under Resources, below, for the most current information.

Resources

For more information on cyclic neutropenia: National Organization for Rare Disorders (NORD); NIH/National Heart, Lung and Blood Institute (NHLBI).

For genetic information and genetic counseling referrals: March of Dimes Birth Defects Foundation; National Center for Education in Maternal and Child Health (NCEMCH).

References

Mendelian Inheritance in Man, 9th ed.: V.A. McKusick; The Johns Hopkins University Press, 1990, pp. 660–661.

Treatment of Cyclic Neutropenia with Granulocyte-Colony Stimulating Factor: W.B. Hammond, et al.; New Eng. J. Med., May 18, 1989, issue 320, pp. 1306–1311.

Human Cyclic Neutropenia: Clinical Review and Long-Term Follow-Up of Patients: D.G. Wright, et al.; Medicine (Baltimore), January 1981, issue 60(1), pp. 1–13.

Cyclic Hematopoiesis: Human Cyclic Neutropenia: R.D. Lange; Exp. Hematol., July 1983, issue 11(6), pp. 435–451.

Adult-Onset Cyclic Neutropenia is a Benign Neoplasm Associated with Clonal Proliferation of Large Granular Lymphocytes: T.P. Loughran, Jr., and W.P. Hammond, 4th; J. Exp. Med., December 1, 1986, issue 164(6), pp. 2089–94.

EWING SARCOMA

Description Ewing sarcoma is an inherited malignant neoplastic disease characterized by round-cell tumors that usually occur in the extremities. It occurs most frequently in young persons aged 10 to 20.

Synonyms

Endothelioma, Diffuse, of Bones

Myeloma, Endothelial

Signs and Symptoms Tumors that are painful to touch (but not always visible) develop usually in the bones of the arms and legs, but can occur in any bone. The tumor tends to involve wide areas of the long bones, sometimes as much as the entire shaft. The femur and humerus are most commonly affected; however, tumors sometimes occur in the pelvis as well. The pain of the tumor worsens with time, and intermittent pain often gets worse at night. Tenderness and swelling are usually present in the area around the tumor; the skin over the tumor may be warm; and blood vessels may be evident on the surface of the skin. The patient may develop anemia and fever. The tumor can spread to lymph nodes, lungs, or the skull if the disease is left untreated.

Etiology Ewing sarcoma is generally transmitted as an autosomal dominant genetic trait.

Epidemiology Ewing sarcoma occurs most frequently in young men 10 and 20 years of age.

Related Disorders The most common primary bone tumor is **osteosarcoma,** which is a painful and highly malignant neoplasm that usually occurs in the knee area, although it can occur in any bone, and commonly metastasizes to the lungs. Patients are usually in the 10-to-20-year age range, but osteosarcoma can occur in persons of any age.

Malignant lymphoma of the bone is characterized by a small round-cell tumor that may occur in any bone and can spread to soft tissue or other bones. It most commonly affects individuals in their 40s and 50s. Pain and swelling are common. The standard treatment is a combination of radiation therapy and chemotherapy.

Another malignant bone tumor is **chondrosarcoma,** which affects cartilage. If the disease is severe, the tumors grow rapidly and metastasize. Chondrosarcomas can also seed themselves in surrounding soft tissue. Surgery is the usual treatment.

The most commonly occurring benign bone tumor is **osteochondroma,** which may be a single or multiple neoplasm that occurs most frequently in young persons aged 10 to 20. Researchers have discovered a strong tendency among family members to develop these tumors.

Treatment—Standard Combinations of surgery, radiation therapy, and chemotherapy are used to treat Ewing sarcoma. The 5-year survival rate is approximately 50 percent.

Treatment—Investigational Please contact the agencies listed under Resources, below, for the most current information.

Resources

For more information on Ewing sarcoma: National Organization for Rare Disorders (NORD); American Cancer Society; NIH/National Cancer Institute PDQ (Physician Data Query) phoneline.

References

Mendelian Inheritance in Man, 9th ed.: V.A. McKusick; The Johns Hopkins University Press, 1990, p. 315.

Immunohistological Characterization of a Ewing's Sarcoma Case: S. Lizard-Nacol, et al.; Cancer Detect. Prev., 1988, issue 12(1-6), pp. 297–302.

Long-Term Results in 144 Localized Ewing's Sarcoma Patients Treated with Combined Therapy: G. Bacci, et al.; Cancer, April 15, 1989, issue 63(8), pp. 1477–1486.

FACTOR IX DEFICIENCY

Description Factor IX deficiency is an inherited coagulation disorder characterized by severe and prolonged hemorrhaging and, in extreme cases, articular pain and bone deformities. The disorder mimics classic hemophilia A, but occurs only 20 percent as often. The mostly male patients have a deficiency of factor IX, which is a component of thromboplastin, at birth; however, the severity of the deficiency varies from family to family. Rarely, a mild form of the disorder is found in female carriers.

Synonyms
> Christmas Disease
> Hemophilia B
> Plasma Thromboplastin Component Deficiency

Signs and Symptoms Patients have prolonged episodes of hemorrhaging that are either spontaneous or related to injury and that occur at or near the surface of the skin or internally. In mild cases, patients hemorrhage only after surgery or tooth extractions. In more severe cases, hemorrhage can occur in any part of the body, including the central nervous system and the gastrointestinal tract. In extreme cases, internal hemorrhaging in muscle, joints, and bone builds up and can cause pain and deformity. Ultimately, the tips of long bones are eroded and chronic problems develop, such as cell necrosis, periosteal pain, and the formation of pseudocysts. Patients who receive transfusions over a long period sometimes develop substances in their blood that inhibit factor IX activity.

Etiology Factor IX deficiency is an X-linked recessive genetic trait whose penetrance is incomplete. Patients have diminished amounts of thromboplastin in their blood as a result of the deficient factor IX.

Epidemiology While factor IX deficiency most commonly affects males, researchers have documented some occurrence in female carriers of the genetic trait.

Related Disorders See *Hemophilia; von Willebrand Disease.*

Treatment—Standard Patients are transfused with fresh-frozen plasma for minor hemorrhaging, or prothrombin complex concentrates rich in factor IX for severe episodes. Patients risk getting hepatitis or AIDS if they receive infected prothrombin concentrates that have not been properly screened. An increased load of factor IX might result in coagulation in veins.

Pseudocysts in bones, muscles, or joints that result in pain and disability can be surgically removed, but patients need to be carefully monitored during any type of surgery, including dental surgery. Patients and their families should receive genetic counseling. Other therapies depend on symptoms.

Treatment—Investigational Plasmapheresis has been used experimentally in extreme cases when conventional procedures have failed to control hemorrhaging, but more research is needed concerning its side effects and efficacy. Monoclonal factor IX has been developed for use in factor IX replacement therapy and to treat complications of hemorrhaging. The manufacturer is Armour Pharmaceutical Co., 920A Harvest Drive, Suite 200, Blue Bell, Pennsylvania 19422.

Please contact the agencies listed under Resources, below, for the most current information.

Resources

For more information on factor IX deficiency: National Organization for Rare Disorders (NORD); National Hemophilia Foundation; Canadian Hemophilia Society; World Federation of Hemophilia; The Haemophilia Society; NIH/National Heart, Lung and Blood Institute (NHLBI).

For genetic information and genetic counseling referrals: March of Dimes Birth Defects Foundation; National Center for Education in Maternal and Child Health (NCEMCH).

References

The Metabolic Basis of Inherited Disease, 6th ed.: C.R. Scriver, et al., eds.; McGraw-Hill, 1989, pp. 2116–2119.

Internal Medicine, 2nd ed.: J.H. Stein, ed.-in-chief; Little, Brown and Company, 1987, p. 1014.

Introduction of Split Tolerance and Clinical Cure in High-Responding Hemophiliacs with Factor IX Antibodies: I.M. Nilsson, et al.; Proc. Natl. Acad. Sci., December 1986, issue 83(23), pp. 9169–9173.

Repair of Ventricular Septal Defect and Aortic Regurgitation Associated with Severe Hemophilia B: A. Mazzucco, et al.; Ann. Thorac. Surg., July 1986, issue 42(1), pp. 97–99.

FACTOR XIII DEFICIENCY

Description Factor XIII deficiency is an extremely rare inherited disorder that prevents the patient's blood from clotting normally and can result in slow internal bleeding. Two forms of the disease are acquired factor XIII deficiency and congenital factor XIII deficiency.

Synonyms

Fibrinase Deficiency
Fibrinoligase Deficiency
Fibrin Stabilizing Factor Deficiency
Laki-Lorand Factor Deficiency
Plasma Transglutaminase Deficiency

Signs and Symptoms Internal bleeding may seep into surrounding soft tissue several days after trauma, even mild trauma such as a bump or bruise. Pain and swelling may precede the bleeding. If the bleeding persists, large cysts can form in the surrounding tissue spaces, destroy surrounding bone, and cause peripheral nerve damage, usually in the thigh and buttocks areas. At birth, the patient may bleed from the umbilical cord, a phenomenon that rarely occurs in other blood disorders. The most serious hemorrhaging occurs in the central nervous system following mild head trauma. Hemorrhaging may stop spontaneously without treatment.

Women with this condition who become pregnant usually have miscarriages. Men may be sterile or have extremely low sperm counts. Replacing factor XIII does not correct sterility. Some of the less frequently seen signs of this disorder are poor wound healing, excessive bleeding from wounds, retroperitoneal hematomas, and blood in the urine.

The following symptoms are seldom or never seen, helping to differentiate factor XIII deficiency from other bleeding disorders: excessive blood loss during menstruation, ocular hemorrhage, gastrointestinal bleeding, arthritis caused by an accumulation of blood in the joints, postoperative hemorrhage, mucous membrane bleeding, and petechiae.

The condition is not generally a threat to patients who need surgery because even small amounts of factor XIII present in blood transfusions will prevent postoperative hemorrhaging. Excessive bleeding from wounds, abrasions, or even spontaneous abortions is not common unless the patient uses aspirin or similar medications.

Etiology Although the exact cause of this disorder is unknown, it is believed to be inherited through autosomal recessive genes. People who inherit only one gene for factor XIII deficiency have reduced levels of factor XIII in their blood but are usually symptomless.

Epidemiology Factor XIII deficiency occurs equally in men and women. The disorder has been seen in pregnant women at term, in newborns, in persons who have undergone major surgery, in those who have sickle cell disease, and in many children with Schoenlein-Henoch purpura.

The disorder sometimes occurs secondary to hepatic carcinoma and cirrhosis. In such cases, levels of factor XIII can be returned to normal when the underlying liver disease is treated. Patients previously treated with isoniazid or who have chronic kidney failure may develop anticoagulation antibodies.

Related Disorders See *von Willebrand Disease; Factor IX Deficiency; Hemophilia; Purpura, Schoenlein-Henoch.*

Treatment—Standard Since normal plasma contains just 10 percent of factor XIII, patients who receive small infusions of fresh or frozen plasma, cryoprecipitate, or factor XIII concentrates every 3 to 4 weeks can have a normal response to trauma. Because some patients have a high incidence of intracranial bleeding, preventive treatment is necessary. Pregnant women can be given exogenous factor XIII to help prevent spontaneous abortion. Patients and their families may need genetic counseling. Other treatments depend on symptoms.

Treatment—Investigational Isolated factor XIII preparations are under development as a potential treatment, as is the orphan drug fibrogammin. For more information on fibrogammin: Hoechst-Roussel Pharmaceuticals, Inc.; Route 202-206 North; Somerville, NJ 08876.

Please contact the agencies listed under Resources, below, for the most current information.

Resources

For more information on factor XIII deficiency: National Organization for Rare Disorders (NORD); National Hemophilia Foundation; World Federation of Hemophilia; NIH/National Heart, Lung and Blood Institute (NHLBI).

For genetic information and genetic counseling referrals: March of Dimes Birth Defects Foundation; National Center for Education in Maternal and Child Health (NCEMCH).

References

Internal Medicine, 2nd ed.: J.H. Stein, ed.; Little, Brown and Company, 1987, p. 1017.

GASTRIC LYMPHOMA, NON-HODGKIN TYPE

Description Non-Hodgkin gastric lymphoma is an extremely rare malignant stomach neoplasm that is characterized by a bulky mass, abdominal pain, and anemia.

Synonyms

Stomach Lymphoma, Non-Hodgkin Type

Signs and Symptoms X-rays reveal a bulky mass in the stomach that is often associated with hemorrhagic gastritis, stress ulcer, or monilial gastritis. Endoscopic biopsy and brushing cytology are also used to diagnose this disease.

Etiology The cause is not known.

Epidemiology Only about 5 percent of the total of all primary malignant stomach neoplasms are non-Hodgkin gastric lymphoma. The disease occurs about 10 years earlier than stomach carcinoma and is most common in persons of Japanese, Thai, and Finnish heritage and those who live in the mountain regions of Colombia. Males are affected more often than females.

Related Disorders See *Zollinger-Ellison Syndrome; Familial Polyposis; Peutz-Jeghers Syndrome.*

Gastric carcinoma, the 3rd most commonly occurring gastrointestinal cancer in the U.S., is characterized by a distended stomach, enlarged gastric folds, obstructing lesions, and an ulcerated mass in the stomach. It generally affects men over 50 and persons who consume foods high in salt and nitrates rather than a diet high in vegetables and fresh fruits.

Treatment—Standard Stomach surgery, multiagent chemotherapy, radiation therapy, or combined radiation therapy and chemotherapy are used to treat this cancer. A chemotherapeutic regimen of cyclophosphamide, nitrogen mustard, Oncovin (vincristine), procarbazine, and prednisone (C-MOPP) is currently being used with success. Also in use is a combination of cyclophosphamide, Oncovin (vincristine), doxorubicin, and prednisone (CHOP) administered along with radiation and other chemicals.

Treatment—Investigational Please contact the agencies listed under Resources,

below, for the most current information.

Resources

  For more information on non-Hodgkin gastric lymphoma: National Organization for Rare Disorders (NORD); American Cancer Society; NIH/National Cancer Institute PDQ (Physician Data Query) phoneline; Cancer Information Service.

References

Internal Medicine, 3rd ed.: J.H. Stein, ed.-in-chief; Little, Brown and Company, 1990, p. 347.

Recent Results of Multimodal Therapy of Gastric Lymphoma: M.H. Shiu, et al.; Cancer, October 1, 1986, issue 54(10), pp. 594–597.

The Role of Brushing Cytology in the Diagnosis of Gastric Malignancy: I. Cook, et al.; Acta Cytol., July–August, 1988, issue 32(4), pp. 461–464.

GLIOBLASTOMA MULTIFORME

Description Glioblastoma multiforme is a highly malignant primary brain tumor that grows rapidly and has the ability to invade surrounding tissue by spreading in a butterfly pattern through the white matter of the cerebral hemispheres. The tumor may invade the dura mater or spread to the ventricles of the brain via cerebrospinal fluid. It rarely metastasizes outside the brain and spinal cord.

Synonyms
  Giant Cell Glioblastoma
  Spongioblastoma Multiforme

Signs and Symptoms Due to glioblastoma multiforme's rapid growth pattern, an increase in cranial pressure is usually the first symptom of this tumor. Pressure builds because the cranium is unable to expand to accommodate the growing tumor. The patient may complain of a generalized headache that is more painful in the morning, accompanied by vomiting but rarely nausea. These symptoms may be preceded by subtle personality changes.

  Glioblastoma multiforme most commonly occurs in the frontal, temporal, and parietal lobes of the cerebral hemispheres, although it may occur in other areas of the hemispheres as well.

  Glioblastomas in the frontal lobe usually cause memory impairment or other intellectual disabilities. Patients may show little or no emotions and may suffer convulsions and hemiplegia of the side of the body opposite the tumor.

  Tumors in the temporal lobe can cause seizures, poor coordination of body parts or other motor disturbances, and interference with the ability to interpret language.

  The symptoms of parietal lobe tumors are agraphia, paresthesia or similar sensory changes, spatial disorientation or loss of position awareness of body parts, and seizures.

Etiology While the cause of glioblastoma multiforme, like most brain tumors, is unknown, tumors have been reported in family members. However, researchers have not proven heredity as a means of transmission.

Certain chemicals in the work place have been associated with some tumors, including vinyl chloride, chemicals used in rubber manufacturing, and chemical sprays used by farmers. Some studies suggest that children exposed to lead or barbiturates may be at a slightly higher risk of developing this tumor. Other studies indicate that a rare virus may cause glioblastomas, but the research is inconclusive.

Epidemiology Men are twice as likely as women to get glioblastoma multiforme, and the tumor occurs more frequently in whites than in non-whites and most often in people between the ages of 48 and 60, although it has been seen in preteens as well. Men with blood type A appear to be at a higher risk.

Related Disorders See *Astrocytoma, Malignant.*

Treatment—Standard Surgery with or without radiation therapy and chemotherapy is the standard treatment for accessible glioblastomas. If the tumor is not accessible, a biopsy may be done to determine if the tumor is amenable to other treatments, and steroid medications given to control swelling. To ameliorate symptoms and increase the effectiveness of other therapies, subtotal decompressive resection may be performed. If the tumor has invaded the brain extensively, either biopsy or partial resection may be used primarily to relieve symptoms.

Aggressive surgery or total resection, often done with the use of an operating microscope, attempts to remove all identifiable tumor. A laser or ultrasonic aspirator can be used in some cases. Surgeons use lasers to vaporize tissue beyond the tumor's border and try to remove tumor infiltrates with a minimal amount of damage to normal tissue. Because glioblastomas infiltrate so extensively, even aggressive resection cannot totally remove the tumor, and follow-up radiation therapy and chemotherapy are needed. If the tumor recurs, a 2nd or even 3rd operation may be performed. External irradiation to both the tumor and the entire brain usually follows surgery almost immediately.

Either during or after radiation therapy, cytotoxic drugs are given in an attempt to destroy any remaining tumor cells. However, since cytotoxins are not completely cell-specific, they may also cause damage to normal tissue. Carmustine (BCNU) and lomustine (CCNU) are the most commonly used drugs.

Treatment—Investigational Brachytherapy is an experimental treatment for glioblastoma multiforme that surgically implants radioactive pellets, such as iodine, iridium, or gold isotopes, directly into the tumor. It is used primarily when a recurrent tumor is confined to one side of the brain and measures less than 2½ inches.

Other therapies under investigation are the use of cell radiosensitizers to increase the effectiveness of radiation; the use of different types of radiation, such as neutrons, hyperthermia, and photoradiation; intraoperative radiation; and hyperfractionation.

Immunotherapy with such drugs as interferon, levamisole, interleukin-2, thymosine, and BCG (bacille Calmette-Guérin), is also being tried. Clinical trials are under way of the orphan drug sodium monomercaptoundecahydro-closo-dodecaborate (Boralife), used as an alternative to conventional photon therapy.

Please contact the agencies listed under Resources, below, for the most current information.

Resources
For more information on glioblastoma multiforme: National Organization for Rare Disorders (NORD); NIH/National Institute of Neurological Disorders & Stroke (NINDS); Association for Brain Tumor Research; American Cancer Society; NIH/National Cancer Institute PDQ (Physician Data Query) phoneline.

References
About Glioblastoma Multiforme and Malignant Astrocytoma: D.P. Hesser et al., eds.; Association for Brain Tumor Research (1985).

GLUCOSE-6-PHOSPHATE DEHYDROGENASE (G6PD) DEFICIENCY

Description G6PD deficiency is a genetically determined enzyme abnormality that usually has no symptoms but can lead to serious medical consequences, such as hemolytic anemia or favism. G6PD is an enzyme present in all cells that is essential to glucose metabolism and provides erythrocytes with a defense against the destructive effects of certain drugs.

Signs and Symptoms Most patients are asymptomatic; however, the symptoms that do occur range in intensity from mild and chronic to life-threatening, and they usually mimic those of acute hemolytic anemia, i.e., shock, fever, chills, pain in the abdomen and back, and sometimes hemoglobinuria and renal failure. Drugs implicated in causing hemolytic anemia include acetanilid, methylene blue, nalidixic acid, naphthalene, niridazole, nitrofurantoin, pamaquine, pentaquine, phenylhydrazine, primaquine, sulfacetamide, sulfamethoxazole, sulfanilamide, sulfapyridine, thiacolesulfone, toluidine blue, and trinitrotoluene. Aspirin, certain derivatives of vitamin K, fava beans, diabetes acidosis, and acute viral or bacterial infections can also cause acute hemolytic anemia in G6PD-deficient patients.

Etiology Glucose-6-phosphate dehydrogenase deficiency is an X-linked genetically transmitted trait.

Epidemiology G6PD deficiency is the most common genetically determined enzyme deficiency in humans, affecting an estimated 400 million people in the world. It occurs most frequently in tropical and subtropical Asia, tropical Africa, areas of the Mediterranean, the Middle East, and New Guinea. Scientists have identified more than 300 different varieties of this deficiency, all of which result from G6PD gene mutations. Some variations are more common among black American males. The condition is difficult to diagnose because serious symptoms do not occur until the patient is exposed to certain drugs.

Related Disorders Favism occurs when individuals with G6PD deficiency consume fava beans or inhale fava pollen. Researchers believe that 2 chemicals present in high concentrations in fava beans, divicine and isouramil, are responsible for the reactions, which include jaundice, severe anemia, possible coma, fever, pallor, tachycardia, weakness, pain in the abdomen or back, and dark red urine. Onset is sudden, occurring within 5 to 24 hours after the person ingests fava beans or only minutes after he or she inhales the pollen.

Treatment—Standard Preventive measures should be taken, such as screening patients for G6PD deficiency before they are given antimalarial drugs or any of the drugs listed in the Signs and Symptoms section above. If hemolysis occurs after any of these drugs are administered, the drug should be discontinued and hydration should be maintained. People found to have G6PD deficiency should avoid fava beans and areas where they are grown. Patients and their families should receive genetic counseling. Other treatments depend on symptoms.

Treatment—Investigational Please contact the agencies listed under Resources, below, for the most current information.

Resources
For more information on G6PD deficiency: National Organization for Rare Disorders (NORD); NIH/National Institute of Diabetes, Digestive and Kidney Diseases; Research Trust for Metabolic Disease in Children.

For genetic information and genetic counseling referrals: March of Dimes Birth Defects Foundation; NIH/National Center for Education in Maternal and Child Health (NCEMCH).

References
Mendelian Inheritance in Man, 9th ed.: V.A. McKusick; The Johns Hopkins University Press, 1990, pp. 357–358, 1213–1215, 1595–1611.

Internal Medicine, 2nd ed.: J.H. Stein, ed.-in-chief; Little, Brown and Company, 1987, pp. 1052–1054.

The Suitability of Saliva for Detection of Glucose-6–Phosphate Dehydrogenase Deficiency: A.H. Beaumont, et al.; Mol. Biol. Rep., 1988, issue 13(2), pp. 73–78.

Chronic Nonspherocytic Hemolytic Anemia (CNSHA) and Glucose–6-Phosphate Dehydrogenase (G6PD) Deficiency in a Patient with Familial Amyloidotic Polyneuropathy (FAP). Molecular Study of a New Variant (G6PD Clinic) with Markedly Acidic PH Optimum: J.L. Vives-Corrons, et al.; Hum. Genet., January 1989, issue 81(2), pp. 161–164.

Tolerability of Tiaprofenic Acid in Patients with Glucose–6-Phosphate Dehydrogenase (G6PD) Deficiency: Q. Mela, et al.; Drugs, 1988, issue 35 (suppl. 1), pp. 107–110.

Diverse Point Mutations in the Human Glucose-6-Phosphate Dehydrogenase Gene Cause Enzyme Deficiency and Mild or Severe Hemolytic Anemia: T.J. Vulliamy, et al.; Proc. Natl. Acad. Sci. USA, July 1988, issue 85(14), pp. 5171–5175.

GRANULOMATOUS DISEASE, CHRONIC (CGD)

Description Chronic granulomatous disease is a very rare blood disorder that affects neutrophils and is characterized by widespread granulomatous lesions. The affected patient is unable to resist infections.

Synonyms
Chronic Dysphagocytosis
Granulomatosis, Chronic, Familial
Granulomatosis, Septic, Progressive

Signs and Symptoms Patients suffer repeated infections that include suppurative lymphadenitis, liver abscesses, pneumonia, and osteomyelitis. Chronic infections may be evident in the liver, gastrointestinal tract, eyes, and brain. Hypergammaglobulinemia, anemia, leukocytosis, and hepatomegaly are characteristic. Dermatitis, diarrhea, perianal abscesses, and rhinitis may also be present. The widespread granulomatous lesions may occur in any organ, and commonly cause obstruction of the gastrointestinal tract.

Etiology The cause of the X-linked form of CGD is a lack of cytochrome b, a component of the NADPH oxidase enzyme responsible for making H_2O_2. The gene for the X-linked form of CGD has been located in the middle of the short arm of the X-chromosome, but autosomal variants of the disorder may involve other genes in females and males coding for other protein components which are necessary for NADPH oxidase.

Epidemiology The disorder affects only one in a million persons, males more often than females. Symptoms usually occur during childhood but may be delayed to early teens and rarely into adulthood.

Related Disorders See *Wegener Granulomatosis; Churg-Strauss Syndrome; Polyarteritis Nodosa.*

Treatment—Standard The standard treatment is antibiotic therapy with such agents as trimethoprim and sulfamethoxazole; corticosteroid drugs are also beneficial. Patients and their families may require genetic counseling. Any other therapy should be based on symptoms and designed to help the patient's body resist infection. The orphan drug interferon-gamma attenuates the number of infections.

Treatment—Investigational Bone marrow transplants can be successful when the procedure is performed on a young patient.

Please contact the agencies listed under Resources, below, for the most current information.

Resources
For more information on chronic granulomatous disease: National Organization for Rare Disorders (NORD); NIH/National Institute of Allergy and Infectious Diseases (NIAID).

For genetic information and genetic counseling referrals: March of Dimes Birth Defects Foundation; National Center for Education in Maternal and Child Health (NCEMCH).

References
Mendelian Inheritance in Man, 8th ed.: V.A. McKusick; The Johns Hopkins University Press, 1986, p. 973.

Internal Medicine, 2nd ed.: J.H. Stein, ed.-in-chief; Little, Brown and Company, 1987, pp. 1286–1288.

Research Highlights: J.E. Smith, Ph.D.; NIH Research Resources Reporter, March 1989.

Corticosteroids in Treatment of Obstructive Lesions of Chronic Granulomatous Disease: T.W. Chin, et al.; J. Pediatrics, September 1987, issue 111(3), pp. 512–518.

Clinical Features and Current Management of Chronic Granulomatous Disease: C.B. Forrest, et al.; Hematol. Oncol. Clin. North Am., June 1988, issue 2(2), pp. 253–266.

Detection of Carriers of the Autosomal Form of Chronic Granulomatous Disease: A.J. Verhoeven, et al.; Blood, February 1988, issue 71(2), pp. 505–507.

Recombinant Human Interferon-Gamma Reconstitutes Defective Phagocyte Function in Patients with Chronic Granulomatous Disease in Childhood: J.M. Sechler, et al.; Proc. Natl. Acad. Sci. USA, July 1988, issue 85(13), pp. 4874–4878.

HAGEMAN FACTOR DEFICIENCY

Description Hageman factor deficiency is a genetic blood disorder caused by a lack of blood factor XII (the Hageman factor), a single-chain glycoprotein necessary for blood clotting. Because other blood-clotting factors tend to compensate for factor XII, there are usually no symptoms and the disorder is only accidentally discovered through preoperative blood tests.

Signs and Symptoms Although it happens rarely, Hageman factor deficiency can lead to blood clots at an early age that inhibit circulation and might cause myocardial infarction or thrombophlebitis.

Patients are not prone to unusual bleeding, and petechiae and ecchymoses are absent. However, the blood of affected patients takes an abnormally long time to clot and serum prothrombin and thromboplastin time are usually abnormal. The blood level of Hageman factor tends to vary greatly in affected patients.

Diagnosis is made if blood from a person suspected to have the disorder does not correct the deficiency in blood from a person known to have the disorder.

Etiology Although the exact mechanism is not well understood, Hageman factor deficiency is genetically transmitted through autosomal recessive genes believed to be defective on either chromosome 6 or 7.

Epidemiology Men and women are affected in equal numbers. Orientals inherit Hageman factor deficiency more often than those of European descent. The patients' parents are closely related in about 10 percent of cases.

Related Disorders See *Factor IX Deficiency; Factor XIII Deficiency.*

Treatment—Standard Because bleeding caused by this disorder is usually mild, Hageman factor deficiency is generally not treated.

Treatment—Investigational Please contact the agencies listed under Resources, below, for the most current information.

Resources

For more information on Hageman factor deficiency: National Organization for Rare Disorders (NORD); National Hemophilia Foundation; NIH/National Heart, Lung and Blood Institute (NHLBI).

References

The Metabolic Basis of Inherited Disease, 5th ed.: J.B. Stanbury, et al., eds.; McGraw-Hill, 1983, pp. 1548–1549.

Mendelian Inheritance in Man, 7th ed.: V.A. McKusick; The Johns Hopkins University Press, 1986, pp. 1015–1016.

The Contact Activation System: Biochemistry and Interactions of These Surface-Mediated Defense Reactions: R.W. Colman, et al.; Crc. Crit. Rev. Oncol. Hematol., 1986, issue 5(1), pp. 57–85.

Immunoblotting Studies of Coagulation Factor XII, Plasma Prekallikrein, and High Molecular Weight Kininogen: B. Lammle, et al.; Semin. Thromb. Hemost., January 1987, issue 13(1), pp. 106–114.

HEMOCHROMATOSIS, HEREDITARY

Description Hereditary hemochromatosis is a metabolic disorder characterized by excessive absorption of iron in the gastrointestinal tract. The accumulation of iron eventually damages numerous organs. Involvement of the liver, pancreas, or heart may lead to serious consequences, particularly in elderly patients. Joints and skin may also become diseased.

Synonyms

Bronze Diabetes
Familial Hemochromatosis
Iron Overload Disease
Primary Hemochromatosis
Troisier-Hanot-Chauffard Syndrome

Signs and Symptoms Symptoms develop usually in men between ages 40 and 60 years, and later in women. The symptoms vary according to the organs involved. Early symptoms are nonspecific and include weakness, weight loss, apathy, loss of libido, and pain in the extremities. Muscle tenderness and cramps in the legs may develop.

Later stages of the disease are characterized by cirrhosis of the liver, diabetes, gradual darkening of the skin, and congestive heart failure. Enlargement of the liver may begin years before it becomes impaired. Eventually, this organ becomes firm and smooth, with iron deposits in the parenchymal cells. Cancer of the liver is more prevalent in patients with hemochromatosis than in unaffected individuals.

When the heart muscle is involved, cardiac enlargement, arrhythmias, and congestive heart failure may result. Involvement of the pituitary gland can cause secondary dysfunction of the various endocrine glands it regulates: thyroid dysfunction may lead to increased sensitivity to cold; secondary adrenocortical insufficiency, to weakness and lack of resistance to stress; and secondary gonadal dysfunction, to testicular atrophy, loss of libido, and amenorrhea.

Etiology Hemochromatosis is inherited as an autosomal recessive trait. The exact enzymatic deficiency is unknown. Relatives of an individual who is homozygous for the mutant gene can be identified by tissue typing; however, the test is expensive and impractical for mass screening. Researchers have measured the degree of saturation of transferrin in the serum to screen for the disease. This test is inexpensive and can detect the disorder before organs become damaged.

Epidemiology Hemochromatosis affects an estimated 600,000 to 1.6 million Americans, with carriers ranging from 24 million to 32 million. The disorder is diagnosed rarely, however; fewer than 250,000 cases have been identified in the United States.

Hemochromatosis is expressed fully in homozygotes only. Heterozygotes may develop it if they have diabetes or are alcoholic. Symptoms occur more often in men than in women because women lose blood during menstruation and pregnancy.

Treatment—Standard After hemochromatosis has been diagnosed, damage to organs can be prevented by repeated phlebotomies to remove iron. Beginning this treatment early in the course will improve the prognosis. In those cases where multiple phlebotomies cause anemia, injections of deferoxamine may reduce levels of iron without producing anemia. Secondary disorders are treated symptomatically.

Treatment—Investigational Gary M. Brittenham, M.D., has been awarded a grant from the Office of Orphan Products Development, Food and Drug Administration, for his research work on chelation therapy with oral iron chelators. For more information: Gary M. Brittenham, M.D.; 2040 Adelbert Road; Case Western Reserve University School of Medicine; Cleveland, Ohio 44106

Please contact the agencies listed under Resources, below, for the most current information.

Resources

For more information on hereditary hemochromatosis: National Organization for Rare Disorders (NORD); Hereditary Hemochromatosis Research Foundation; NIH/National Institute of Diabetes, Digestive & Kidney Diseases Information Clearinghouse; Iron Overload Diseases Association.

For genetic information and genetic counseling referrals: March of Dimes Birth Defects Foundation; National Center for Education in Maternal and Child Health (NCEMCH).

References

Mendelian Inheritance in Man, 9th ed.: V.A. McKusick; The Johns Hopkins University Press, 1990, pp. 1235–1238.

Cecil Textbook of Medicine, 18th ed.: J.B. Wyngaarden and L.H. Smith, Jr., eds.; W.B. Saunders Company, 1988, pp. 1189–1192.

HEMOGLOBINURIA, PAROXYSMAL COLD (PCH)

Description PCH is an extremely rare autoimmune hemolytic disorder. Healthy erythrocytes are destroyed prematurely and suddenly after exposure to temperatures of 15°C (59°F) or lower.

Synonyms
> Donath-Landsteiner Hemolytic Anemia
> Donath-Landsteiner Syndrome

Signs and Symptoms Attacks of PCH can occur within minutes or up to 8 hours after exposure to cold. Symptoms and signs may include fever, malaise, anorexia, pain in the flanks and in the back and legs, headache, vomiting, diarrhea, mild anemia, and hemoglobinuria. Jaundice may follow attacks. Liver and spleen may be enlarged.

Etiology Most cases occur after a viral infection (such as chickenpox or mumps) or in conjunction with congenital or acquired syphilis. Hemolysis is mediated by a complement-fixing IgG antibody. The disease may also affect individuals with no histories of other disorders. Localized exposure to cold water (by hand washing or drinking) may also trigger an attack in some severe cases.

Epidemiology Anyone may acquire PCH. An individual with a viral infection (such as chickenpox or mumps) or with syphilis is at higher risk of contracting the disorder.

Related Disorders See *Anemia, Hemolytic, Cold-Antibody; Hemoglobinuria, Paroxysmal Nocturnal.*

Treatment—Standard Treatment of the accompanying viral infection by supportive therapy, bed rest, and protection of the affected individual from cold temperatures is usually effective. If the disorder is chronic, it may respond to treatment with glucocorticoids or immunosuppressive drugs (such as cyclophosphamide). The following guidelines must be met when blood transfusions are needed: blood should be cross-matched at 37°C to find compatible units, and the blood should be warmed by an on-line warmer to prevent new erythrocytes from being coated with antibodies and destroyed.

Treatment—Investigational Please contact the agencies listed under Resources, below, for the most current information.

Resources
> **For more information on paroxysmal cold hemoglobinuria:** National Organization for Rare Disorders (NORD); NIH/National Heart, Lung and Blood Institute (NHLBI).

References
> Cecil Textbook of Medicine, 18th ed.: J.B. Wyngaarden and L.H. Smith, Jr., eds; W.B. Saunders Company, 1988, p. 921.
> Internal Medicine, 2nd ed.: J.H. Stein, ed.-in-chief; Little, Brown and Company, 1987, p. 1059.

Donath-Landsteiner Hemolytic Anemia due to an Anti-Pr-Like Biphasic Hemolysin: W.J. Judd, et al.; Transfusion, September–October, 1986, issue 26(5), pp. 423–425.

An Unusual Donath-Landsteiner Antibody Detectable at 37 Degrees C by the Antiglobulin Test: S. Lindgren, et al.; March–April, 1985: issue 25(2), pp. 142–144.

HEMOGLOBINURIA, PAROXYSMAL NOCTURNAL (PNH)

Description PNH is an anemia caused by a defect in the membrane of erythrocytes. The breakdown of red blood cells causes hemoglobinuria and hemoglobinemia, which occur at night in classical PNH but in fact may occur more often throughout the day or intermittently.

Synonyms
Marchiafava-Micheli Syndrome

Signs and Symptoms Severe abdominal or back pain may occur during hemolysis. Hemoglobinuria, paleness, and jaundice may be present. Venous thrombosis may occur, usually in the spleen, liver, and inferior vena cava. The spleen and the liver may be enlarged. Patients usually experience mild anemia for several years before the major symptoms of hemoglobinuria become apparent.

Etiology PNH appears to result from a defect in the membrane of erythrocytes that leads to complement-mediated intravascular hemolysis. Aplastic anemia may develop in 20 to 30 percent of cases. An infection, the administration of iron or of a vaccine, or menstruation may precipitate hemolysis that results in hemoglobinemia and hemoglobinuria.

Epidemiology PNH may occur at any age but is most common between 20 and 45 years of age. No racial predominance has been noted.

Related Disorders See *Hemoglobinuria, Paroxysmal Cold.*

Treatment—Standard Androgens may be administered in some cases. Packed red blood cells may be transfused during crises. Used cautiously, anticoagulants such as heparin appear useful in treating thrombi. Iron supplements may be prescribed. Normal bone marrow has been transplanted in some patients. Other treatment may be symptomatic.

Treatment—Investigational Please contact the agencies listed under Resources, below, for the most current information.

Resources
For more information on paroxysmal nocturnal hemoglobinuria: National Organization for Rare Disorders (NORD); NIH/National Heart, Lung and Blood Institute (NHLBI).

References
Internal Medicine, 3rd ed.: J.H. Stein, ed.-in-chief; Little, Brown and Company, 1990, pp. 1113–1114.
Thrombolytic Therapy for Inferior Vena Cava Thrombosis in Paroxysmal Nocturnal Hemoglobinuria: P.W. Sholar, et al.; Ann. Intern. Med., October 1985, issue 103(4), pp. 539–541.

HEMOPHILIA

Description Hemophilia is an inherited blood-coagulation disorder caused by inactive or deficient blood proteins, usually factor VIII. It is found in males almost exclusively and can be classified as mild, moderate, or severe. The level of severity is determined by the percentage of active clotting factor in the blood (normal percentage ranges from 50 to 150 percent). People who have severe hemophilia have less than 1 percent in their blood.

There are 3 major types of hemophilia: hemophilia A (also known as classical hemophilia or factor VIII deficiency or antihemophilic globulin **[AHG]** deficiency); hemophilia B (Christmas disease or factor IX deficiency); and hemophilia C (factor XI deficiency). Von Willebrand disease and other rare clotting disorders have similar symptoms but are not usually called hemophilia.

Synonyms
Antihemophilic Globulin (AHG) Deficiency
Christmas Disease
Classical Hemophilia
Factor VIII Deficiency
Factor IX Deficiency
Factor XI Deficiency
Von Willebrand Disease (Vascular Hemophilia)

Signs and Symptoms The most serious symptom of hemophilia is uncontrolled internal bleeding that begins spontaneously without an apparent cause and, over time, can cause permanent damage to joints and muscles. A hemophiliac bleeds for a longer period of time than normal. External bleeding can usually be controlled and minor cuts can be treated as normal.

Etiology Hemophilia is a recessive genetic condition linked to the X chromosome. Although most patients have a family history of the disease, as many as one-third of new cases are found in persons without a family history of the disease. A hemophiliac male cannot pass the disease on to his sons, but all of his daughters will be genetic carriers capable of passing the disease on to succeeding generations.

Epidemiology An estimated 20,000 males in the United States have hemophilia, not including the many mild cases that remain undiagnosed until they are discovered following major trauma or surgery. Hemophilia occurs in one out of every 4,000 male newborns. Medical advances have enabled hemophiliacs to reach a near-normal life expectancy.

Related Disorders See *von Willebrand Disease.*

Treatment—Standard While there is no cure for hemophilia, the disorder can be controlled through infusions of a blood-clotting factor, generally factor VIII. The clotting factor remains active in the hemophiliac's blood for only a short time; new infusions are required each time internal bleeding occurs to avoid permanent damage. This therapy is necessary for the life of the patient.

The Food and Drug Administration has approved the drug desmopressin (Stimate) for treatment of moderately severe cases of hemophilia. The FDA has also approved the orphan drug tranexamic acid (Cyclokapron) for short-term use (2 to 8 days) in hemophiliacs before and after such minor surgery as a tooth extraction. This drug reduces the need for blood transfusions after surgery.

Treatment—Investigational The National Hemophilia Foundation has funded AIDS-related research in collaboration with the federal Centers for Disease Control and commercial research into the preparation of factor VIII by recombinant gene technology.

Researchers at the National Institute of Diabetes, Digestive & Kidney Diseases have developed a method for culturing endothelial cells and a cell line that produces factor VIII:C, the clotting factor missing from the blood of persons with hemophilia A.

Dr. Harvey Pollard, Chief of the Laboratory of Cell Biology and Genetics, and his colleagues have cultured endothelial cells from the adrenal glands of cows that produce large amounts of factor VIII:C. Hemophiliacs frequently develop antibodies against factor VIII:C obtained from blood donors and therefore must use factor VIII:C from animal or other nonhuman sources. Factor VIII:C obtained from human sources might also expose hemophiliacs to hepatitis and AIDS. Large-scale production of endothelial-produced Factor VIII:C may provide a viable alternative to current therapies.

Shirley I. Miekka, Ph.D., at the American Red Cross in Washington, D.C., is studying coagulation factor X as a treatment for hemophilia under an FDA grant.

A new orphan drug known as monoclonal factor IX is being used as a treatment for hemophilia B. It is manufactured by Armour Pharmaceutical Co., 920A Harvest Dr., Suite 200, Blue Bell, Pennsylvania 19422. Another orphan drug, recombinant antihemophilic factor, is under investigation for treatment of hemorrhage in individuals with hemophilia A. It is manufactured by Miles, Inc., Cutter Biological, 400 Morgan Lane, West Haven, Connecticut 06516. E(rGM-CSF) is another drug being tested for hemophilia. The drug is manufactured by Schering Corp., 2000 Galloping Hill Road., Kenilworth, New Jersey 07033.

Please contact the agencies listed under Resources, below, for the most current information.

Resources

For more information on hemophilia: National Organization for Rare Disorders (NORD); National Hemophilia Foundation; World Federation of Hemophilia; Canadian Hemophilia Society; The Haemophilia Society;

NIH/National Heart, Lung, and Blood Institute (NHLBI).

For genetic information and genetic counseling referrals: March of Dimes Birth Defects Foundation; National Center for Education in Maternal and Child Health (NCEMCH).

References
Cecil Textbook of Medicine, 18th ed.: J.B. Wyngaarden and L.H. Smith, Jr., eds.; W.B. Saunders Company, 1988, p. 1045.

HEMORRHAGIC TELANGIECTASIA, HEREDITARY

Description Hereditary hemorrhagic telangiectasia is an inherited disorder characterized by capillary lesions on the skin, mucous membranes, and many internal organs. Patients often suffer anemia caused by hemorrhaging telangiectases.

Synonyms
Osler-Weber-Rendu Syndrome
Rendu-Osler-Weber Syndrome

Signs and Symptoms Lesions that are red to violet in color develop chiefly on the patient's cheeks, ears, lips, and tongue and in the nasal mucosa. The lesions may also occur in the gastrointestinal tract, lungs, brain, spinal cord, and liver. Hemorrhaging occurs either spontaneously or as a result of injury. Epistaxis and gastrointestinal hemorrhaging become more severe with age and can cause chronic anemia. Arteriovenous fistulae are formed that can cause cyanosis, polycythemia, clubbed fingers, and possibly stroke. The mortality from hereditary hemorrhagic telangiectasia is less than 10 percent, but this disorder can lead to many complications because it is often misdiagnosed or undiagnosed.

Etiology Hereditary hemorrhagic telangiectasia is transmitted as an autosomal dominant characteristic. Telangiectases in the lungs, brain, and liver are thought to be caused by arteriovenous fistulae that form to replace the capillaries that normally connect venules and arterioles. When the capillaries are missing, the lesions bleed profusely.

Epidemiology Hereditary hemorrhagic telangiectasia affects both sexes and all ages. In Europe, the incidence of the disease has been reported to be 1:50,000. However, because the disorder is often misdiagnosed, this estimate may be inaccurate.

Related Disorders See *von Willebrand Disease; Scleroderma; Raynaud's Disease and Phenomenon.* Other related disorders are **Calcinosis-Raynaud-Sclerodactyly-Telangiectasia (CRST); multiple phlebectasia; spider nevi;** and **cherry angiomas (senile hemangiomas; DeMorgan** or **ruby spots).** CRST is characterized by calcium salt deposits in focal nodules in various body tissues other than the parenchymatous viscera. Multiple phlebectasias are enlarged veins. Spider nevi are small, visible, abnormally enlarged arteries that have radiating branches resembling spider legs. Cherry angiomas are red papules caused by a weakening of the capillary wall.

Treatment—Standard Treatment is designed to stop the hemorrhaging and remove or block exceptionally large lesions or arteriovenous fistulae. Cauterization of telangiectases in the nasal mucosa stops the growth of new lesions and thus offers temporary benefit. Surgical excision of arteriovenous fistulae has been accomplished, and balloon embolotherapy has been found effective in occluding pulmonary arteriovenous fistulae. Application of a compress saturated with vaso-constrictors, such as phenylephrine, has been used to control epistaxis. Anemia can be treated by blood transfusions or iron replacement therapy using iron dex-tran administered either orally or intravenously. Surgery may be necessary for gas-trointestinal lesions that produce severe hemorrhaging.

Treatment—Investigational Estrogen and progesterone therapy to prevent hem-orrhaging has been investigated. Estrogen has not been effective, but proges-terone holds some promise.

Please contact the agencies listed under Resources, below, for the most current information.

Resources
For more information on hereditary hemorrhagic telangiectasia: Nation-al Organization for Rare Disorders (NORD); Hereditary Hemorrhagic Telangiec-tasis Registry; NIH/National Heart, Lung and Blood Institute (NHLBI); NIH/National Institute of Child Health and Human Development (NICHHD).

For genetic information and genetic counseling referrals: March of Dimes Birth Defects Foundation; National Center for Education in Maternal and Child Health (NCEMCH).

References
Harrison's Principles of Internal Medicine, 12th ed.: J.D. Wilson, et al., eds.; McGraw-Hill, 1991, p. 326.

HISTIOCYTOSIS X

Description Histiocytosis X is an older term for Langerhans cell histiocytosis **(LCH),** a name given to a group of childhood blood disorders characterized by an abnormal proliferation of histiocytes throughout the body but especially in the skin, bones, brain, lungs, spleen, and liver. The child develops nonmalignant growths that represent accumulations of histiocytes. The clinical course of these disorders is aggressive, and treatment depends on the extent of damage to the affected organ, which varies according to the extent and location of the growths.

Synonyms
Eosinophilic Granuloma
Hand-Schüller-Christian Syndrome
Langerhans Cell Granulomatosis
Langerhans Cell Histiocytosis

Letterer-Siwe Disease

Signs and Symptoms Symptoms vary widely from child to child and according to the organ affected. Patients with acute forms of this disease have splenomegaly, bone marrow damage, and abnormal blood counts due to blood cell deficiencies. Platelet deficiencies may cause excessive hemorrhaging; erythrocyte loss can cause anemia; and leukocyte deficiencies may cause infection.

Secondary lung infection or histiocytic infiltration may result in breathing difficulties. When bone is affected, the patient will have pain at the site. The patient's skin may have lesions containing small sacs of pus, scaly or greasy rashes, purplish red spots, hemorrhaging beneath the skin, knots visible under the skin, and small, hard, red elevations on the surface of the skin.

Diabetes insipidus occurs if the hypothalamus and pituitary are affected. Pituitary damage can cause growth problems, thyroid deficiencies, and sex hormone abnormalities. In chronic cases, healing and scarring may be difficult to differentiate from histiocyte growth, particularly in the lungs and liver. Effects in the mouth include gingival swelling, tooth loss, and premature tooth eruption. The patient's eyeballs may protrude, and clear vision may be lost.

Rarely, in patients who have had no signs of the disease for many years, neurologic damage leads to difficulty in walking and controlling the body. Some limited short-term symptoms may heal spontaneously and permanently, but more widespread symptoms may continue for years.

Etiology Researchers are unable to explain what causes histiocytes to grow and spread abnormally. Some theories suggest that infections or immune system deficiencies are involved, since Langerhans cells respond to immune system stimuli.

Epidemiology While a few cases of this disease have occurred in family members, most are nonfamilial. The disease occurs most frequently in children, although onset can begin in adulthood as well. Children under 2 years of age are the most severely affected.

Related Disorders Hemophagocytic lymphohistiocytosis (hemophagocytic reticulosis), a genetic blood disorder with onset in infancy, is characterized by blood cell abnormalities, splenomegaly, hepatomegaly, fever, liver damage, neurologic damage, easy hemorrhaging, and fever. **Infection-associated hemophagocytic syndrome** is characterized by hepatic lesions and lesions in the central nervous system that are associated with infectious agents or a family history of the disease.

Treatment—Standard Although the histiocytic growths resulting from this disorder are not malignant, some therapies are similar to those used in cancer patients. Chemotherapy is routinely used to treat chronic and aggressive forms of histiocytosis X that are widespread. Radiotherapy and steroid injections are used to treat local lesions, depending on where they are, whether or not pain is severe, and if function might be diminished. Longterm therapy with corticosteroids or radiation may be used for adults with lung involvement only. Other therapies depend on symptoms. Some forms of this disorder may require no treatment at all once a confirmed diagnosis has been made.

Treatment—Investigational Experimental research is under way in the United States, Germany, Austria, and Italy into the use of bone marrow transplants, immune system modulators, and other procedures to treat this disorder. Definitive results have not yet been achieved.

Please contact the agencies listed under Resources, below, for the most current information.

Resources

For more information on histiocytosis X: National Organization for Rare Disorders (NORD); Histiocytosis-X Association; NIH/National Heart, Lung and Blood Institute (NHLBI); Diane Komp, M.D., Yale University School of Medicine; Izaak Walton Killam Hospital for Children.

References

Point of View: Histiocytosis Syndromes in Children: B. Favara, et al.; Lancet, January 24, 1987, pp. 208–209.

Editorial: Langerhans Cell Histiocytosis: D. Komp; New Eng. J. of Med., issue 316(12), pp. 747–748.

HODGKIN DISEASE

Description Hodgkin disease is a form of malignant lymphoma. Its characteristics include lymph node, lymphoid tissue, and spleen enlargement and the presence of Reed Sternberg cells.

Synonyms

Hodgkin Lymphoma

Signs and Symptoms Initially, lymph nodes begin to swell, most frequently in the neck (two-thirds of the time) but also in the chest, armpits, abdomen, and groin. Eventually, the tissue around the nodes may be affected, as well as the patient's lungs, liver, spleen, and bone marrow. Patients may or may not have night sweats, weight loss, and fever. In rare cases bone pain is present. Reed-Sternberg cells are found in the affected lymph nodes. Since enlarged lymph nodes are symptoms of other cancers and infectious diseases, diagnosis can be difficult.

Etiology The cause is unknown. A viral agent may be involved.

Epidemiology Symptoms usually occur in patients between the ages of 15 and 40 years, although in rare instances Hodgkin disease affects persons over 50; it also may occur in children. Four distinct types of malignant cells have been recognized. The most common type affects young women primarily. Two other less common types affect male teenagers and older men predominantly, and the rarest form affects older men and women. Clusters of this disease have appeared in certain geographic areas and occasionally in families, but these are rare.

Related Disorders A group of cancers known as **non-Hodgkin lymphomas** is also characterized by enlarged lymph nodes that begin in the neck or groin and usually spread. Patients can be affected at any age and may have leukemia, anemia, and night sweats.

Burkitt lymphoma is another lymphatic cancer that is possibly infectious and affects not only the lymph nodes but also bone marrow, the central nervous system, kidneys, and gonads. It occurs in Central Africa but rarely in the United States.

Treatment—Standard The stage of the disease determines the appropriate treatment, which depends on the number of tumors and their location and whether or not the patient has fever, night sweats, and weight loss. Staging is generally done according to the Ann Arbor classification system.

Radiation therapy is used to shrink affected lymph nodes and destroy diseased lymphocytes. Chemotherapeutic regimens are also used, including such combinations as MOPP (nitrogen mustard, Oncovin [vincristine], prednisone, and procarbazine); ABVD (Adriamycin [doxorubicin], bleomycin, vinblastine, and dacarbazine); MOP-BAP (nitrogen mustard, Oncovin, procarbazine, bleomycin, Adriamycin, and prednisone); and ChlVPP (chlorambucil, vinblastine, prednisone, and procarbazine). MOPP and ABVD can be used together but alternated every month. Other treatments depend on symptoms.

Treatment—Investigational Fournier, a French pharmaceutical company, has developed an experimental drug, LF1695, for use in children with immune system damage due to Hodgkin disease, Chagas disease, and Schwachman syndrome. For information, contact Fournier Laboratories, BP90, Daix, 21121 Fontaine, Les Dijon, France. Please contact the agencies listed under Resources, below, for the most current information, especially the National Cancer Institute, which may be conducting clinical trials on new drugs for Hodgkin disease and other cancers (1-800-4-CANCER).

Resources

For more information on Hodgkin disease: National Organization for Rare Disorders (NORD); American Cancer Society; NIH/National Cancer Institute PDQ (Physician Data Query) phoneline.

References

Internal Medicine, 3rd Ed.: J.H. Stein, ed.-in-chief; Little, Brown and Company, 1987, pp. 1136–1141.

Winning the Battle Against Hodgkin's Disease: K. Consalvo and M. Gallagher; RN, December 1986, pp. 20–25.

Treatment Strategies for Hodgkin's Disease: G. Bonadonna; Semin. Hematol., April 1988, issue 25(2, suppl. 2), pp. 51–57.

IDIOPATHIC EDEMA

Description Idiopathic edema is a common disorder characterized by episodic or persistent swelling due to salt and water retention that is not caused by cardiac, hepatic, or splenic disease. It occurs in women almost exclusively and usually affects the face, abdomen, and extremities.

Synonyms
    Cyclic Edema
    Distress Edema
    Periodic Edema
    Periodic Swelling
    Stress Edema

Signs and Symptoms Swelling occurs either occasionally or chronically and develops rapidly, especially in the feet, hands, and face. Significant pitting edema in the lower extremities occurs after standing for a long time. Patients may also have a bloated abdomen and gain weight, sometimes as much as 10 to 12 pounds in a 24-hour period. Other signs and symptoms are a drop in urine output, irritability, depression, fatigue, headache, and tension. Idiopathic edema is often associated with the menstrual cycle.

Etiology The cause is unknown; an imbalance of estrogens or progesterone is suspected. The patients' abnormal aldosterone response to standing upright apparently plays a role in their retention of sodium and water.

Epidemiology Almost all patients are women who are middle-aged or younger.

Related Disorders See *Angioedema, Hereditary.*

Treatment—Standard The drugs captopril and spironolactone have been found to be successful in restoring normal aldosterone response and reversing the edema.

Treatment—Investigational Please contact the agencies listed under Resources, below, for the most current information.

Resources
    For more information on idiopathic edema: National Organization for Rare Disorders (NORD); National Institute of Diabetes, Digestive & Kidney Diseases Information Clearinghouse.

References
Long-Term Furosemide Treatment in Idiopathic Edema: M. Shichiri, et al.; Arch. Intern. Med., November 1984, issue 144(11), pp. 2161–2164.
Idiopathic Edema in a Male: I. Weinberger, et al.; American J. Med. Sci., July–August 1984, issue 288(1), pp. 27–31.
Therapeutic Response of Idiopathic Edema to Captopril: D. Docci, et al.; Nephron, 1983, issue 34(3), pp. 198–200.

LEUKEMIA, CHRONIC MYELOGENOUS

Description Chronic myelogenous leukemia is characterized by excessive numbers of leukocytes in the blood, bone marrow, liver, and spleen that infiltrate the lungs, kidneys, intestinal tract, lymph nodes, and gonads. In the first or chronic phase of the disease, leukocytes are overproduced in the bone marrow. In the advanced or acute phase, known as the blast crisis, immature blast cells or promelocytes make up more than 50 percent of the cells in the bone marrow, and the disease becomes extremely aggressive and unresponsive to therapy. The majority of patients (approximately 85 percent) enter the advanced phase.

Synonyms
> Chronic Granulocytic Leukemia
> Chronic Myelocytic Leukemia
> Chronic Myeloid Leukemia

Signs and Symptoms Patients generally present with nonspecific symptoms, such as weakness, fatigue, night sweats, splenomegaly, weight loss, abdominal discomfort, or itchiness. Routine blood tests may reveal the underlying problem. In the acute phase, patients have hepatosplenomegaly, pain in bones, extreme weight loss, high fever, excessive calcium in the blood, arthralgia, and hemorrhagic purplish patches in the epidermis and mucous membranes.

Etiology While the precise cause is unknown, researchers have implicated excessive radiation exposure as a high-risk factor. Patients have a proliferation of abnormal and useless neoplastic cells in their blood, 90 percent of which have a consistent rearrangement of chromosomes that results from the transfer of genetic material from chromosome 9 to chromosome 22, or vice versa. Known as the Philadelphia chromosome, chromosome 22 becomes shorter than normal and is suspected of playing a role in the onset or development of the disease.

Epidemiology Chronic myelogenous leukemia occurs slightly more often in men than in women, and patients are usually in their 40s or 50s, although the disease can occur at any age.

Related Disorders See *Polycythemia Vera.*

Treatment—Standard Chemotherapy and radiation therapy are used to reduce the number of leukocytes and the size of the spleen in an attempt to induce remission. Busulfan and hydroxyurea are commonly prescribed. Other chemotherapeutic agents, splenectomy, and bone marrow transplantation are sometimes tried to keep patients from entering the acute phase. Marrow transplants are the most successful, and the best results are achieved in patients under 40 who have not entered the acute phase. Once the acute phase begins, transplants are not very successful.

Some patients in the acute phase appear to improve temporarily with prednisone and vincristine therapy, but because the acute phase of this disease proceeds aggressively and rapidly, a second remission is less likely.

Treatment—Investigational The orphan drug recombinant interferon alpha-2a (Roferon-A) is under investigation as a treatment for chronic myelogenous leukemia. Its manufacturer is Hoffman-LaRoche, Inc., 340 Kingsland St., Nutley, New Jersey 07110.

Please contact the agencies listed under Resources, below, for the most current

information.

Resources
For more information on chronic myelogenous leukemia: National Organization for Rare Disorders (NORD); Leukemia Society of America; American Cancer Society; NIH/National Cancer Institute PDQ (Physician Data Query) phoneline.

References
Internal Medicine, 3rd ed.: J.H. Stein, ed.-in-chief; Little, Brown and Company, 1990, pp. 1561–1563.

Blast Crisis of Philadelphia Chromosome-Positive Chronic Myelocytic Leukemia (CML): B. Anger, et al.; Blut, September 1988, issue 57(3), pp. 131–137.

Bone Marrow Transplantation for Chronic Myelogenous Leukemia in Chronic Phase: J.M. Goldman, et al.; Ann. Intern. Med., June 1988, issue 108(6), pp. 806–814.

LEUKEMIA, HAIRY CELL

Description Hairy cell leukemia is a neoplastic disease characterized by the presence in the blood of abnormal mononuclear cells (hairy cells) and pancytopenia.

Synonyms
Leukemic Reticuloendotheliosis

Signs and Symptoms Symptoms generally occur gradually and include vague abdominal pain, a feeling of fullness in the stomach, weakness, malaise, fatigue, weight loss, and easy bruising. Hairy cells heavily infiltrate the splenic pulp and sinuses, bone marrow, lymph nodes, and the liver. In chronic cases, splenectomy provides longterm survival. However, in acute cases, the prognosis is not as good.

Etiology The cause is not known.

Epidemiology Approximately 2,000 to 3,000 people in the United States are affected every year.

Related Disorders Letterer-Siwe disease (Abt-Letterer-Siwe disease; systemic aleukemic reticuloendotheliosis) is an inherited autosomal recessive hereditary disorder characterized by swollen lymph nodes, hepatomegaly, splenomegaly, and a persistent, spiking, low-grade fever. Other symptoms are pallor and discrete yellowish-brown maculopapular lesions that are sometimes ulcerated.

Treatment—Standard Until recently, splenectomy was the standard treatment. Methotrexate was also used, along with leucovorin as an antidote against its toxic effects, as were glucocorticoids for vasculitic symptoms, and alkylation agents.

Within recent years, the Food and Drug Administration has approved the orphan drug alpha-interferon, manufactured by Hoffman-LaRoche, Inc. and Schering Corporation, as a treatment for hairy cell leukemia. Clinical trials of this drug showed that 92 to 94 percent of treated patients were alive 2 years after treatment was begun, compared with fewer than 50 percent of patients who were treated by conventional therapies. In 75 to 90 percent of treated patients, the disease went into remission. Alpha-interferon may be injected daily for up to 6 months, followed by maintenance injections 3 times a week. Flulike side effects diminish over time.

Treatment—Investigational Under investigation is the use of interleukin-2 to restore the patient's natural killer cell activity.

Clinical trials are also being conducted on the drug deoxycoformycin. For information, contact The Comprehensive Cancer Center (Dr. Eric Kraut), Ohio State University, Columbus, Ohio, or the Investigational Drug Branch of the National Cancer Institute in Bethesda, Maryland.

Please contact the agencies listed under Resources, below, for the most current information.

Resources

For more information on hairy cell leukemia: National Organization for Rare Disorders (NORD); Hairy Cell Leukemia Foundation; Leukemia Society of America; American Cancer Society; NIH/National Cancer Institute PDQ (Physician Data Query) phoneline.

References
Recombinant Alpha-2 Interferon in the Treatment of Hairy Cell Leukemia: J.A. Thompson, et al.; Cancer Treatment Rep., July–August 1985, issue 69(7-8), pp. 791–793.

Splenectomy for Hairy Cell Leukemia; A Clinical Review of 63 Patients: A.S. Van Norman, et al.; Cancer, February 1, 1986, issue 57(3), pp. 644–648.

Therapeutic Options in Hairy Cell Leukemia: J.E. Groopman; Seminars in Oncology, December 1985, issue 12(4 suppl. 5), pp. 30–34.

LYMPHADENOPATHY, ANGIOIMMUNOBLASTIC WITH DYSPROTEINEMIA (AILD)

Description A progressive immune disorder that affects people over 50, AILD is characterized by an abnormal proliferation of immunoblasts, capillaries, and plasma cells in lymph nodes that leaves the patient vulnerable to life-threatening infections. It is believed to be caused by chronic stimulation of the immune system resulting from drug therapy given for another condition, by viral infections, or by other stimuli.

Synonyms
    Immunoblastic Lymphadenopathy

Signs and Symptoms The major symptoms of AILD are enlarged lymph nodes, acute infections, anemia, hypergammaglobulinemia, hepatosplenomegaly, chills, acute fever, sweating, weight loss, general discomfort, and sometimes a skin rash. In some cases, acute lymphoma develops.

Etiology AILD is believed to be an overreaction to immune system stimuli, such as drug therapy, viral infections, insect bites, or immunizations; or it could be an early form of a lymphoproliferative disorder.

Epidemiology AILD usually affects men and women over 50 in equal numbers.

Related Disorders See *Acquired Immune Deficiency Syndrome (AIDS)*.

Dermatopathic lymphadenopathy (lipomelanic reticulosis) is a skin condition marked by enlarged lymph nodes and abnormal proliferation of histiocytes and macrophages that contain fat and melanin. Other skin conditions that involve exfoliation or pruritus are thought to be the cause.

Treatment—Standard Corticosteroids and cyclophosphamides, which reduce swollen lymph nodes and diminish blood cell deficiencies, are the standard treatment for this disorder. The patient must be carefully shielded against infections. Other therapies depend upon symptoms.

Treatment—Investigational Please contact the agencies listed under Resources, below, for the most current information.

Resources

For more information on **AILD:** National Organization for Rare Disorders (NORD); Immune Deficiency Foundation; NIH/National Cancer Institute PDQ (Physician Data Query) phoneline; NIH/National Institute of Allergy and Infectious Diseases (NIAID).

References

Effect of Cyclophosphamide Therapy On Oncogene Expression in Angioimmunoblastic Lymphadenopathy: D.M. Klinman, et al.; Lancet, November 8, 1986, issue 2(8515), pp. 1055–1058.

Angioimmunoblastic Lymphadenopathy: W.P. Su; Dermatol. Clin., October 1985, issue 3(4), pp. 759–768.

Modulation of C-MYB Transcription in Autoimmune Disease by Cyclophosphamide: J.D. Mountz, et al.; J. Immunol., October 1985, issue 135(4), pp. 2417–2422.

LYMPHANGIOMA, CAVERNOUS

Description Cavernous lymphangioma is a congenital lymphatic disorder characterized by dilated lymph vessels and benign lesions under the skin that are made up of lymphoid tissue. Usually present at birth, lymphangioma may also develop later in life.

Synonyms

Chylangioma

Signs and Symptoms Deep-seated, benign lesions that are gray, pink, or yellow in color appear around the patient's neck and on the upper extremities, as well as in the mouth, on the tongue, around the eyes and eyelids, and on the lower extremities. These soft tumors of the lymph vessels vary in shape and size. If the lymphangiomas are punctured or cut, prolonged draining of lymph fluid results.

Etiology The cause is unknown.

Epidemiology Cavernous lymphangioma affects males and females in equal numbers, usually at birth.

Related Disorders See *Lymphedema, Hereditary.*

Treatment—Standard Surgery is used to remove the involved tissue. Other treatment depends on symptoms.

Treatment—Investigational Please contact the agencies listed under Resources, below, for the most current information.

Resources

For more information on cavernous lymphangioma: National Organization for Rare Disorders (NORD); American Cancer Society; NIH/National Cancer Institute PDQ (Physician Data Query) phoneline.

References

Cavernous Lymphangioma of the Duodenum: Case Report and Review of the Literature: M. Davis, et al.; Gastrointest. Radiol., 1987, issue 12(1), pp. 10–12.

Cavernous Lymphangioma of the Lip: Report of a Case: B.L. Eppley, et al.; J. Am. Dent. Assoc., April 1985, issue 110(4), pp. 503–504.

LYMPHANGIOMYOMATOSIS

Description A progressive disorder that primarily affects the lungs of women of childbearing age, lymphangiomyomatosis is characterized by abnormal growth of smooth muscle cells into spindle shapes. The irregularly shaped cells block airways over time and cause breathing difficulties. The disorder may also affect the smooth muscle tissue of the thoracic duct, lymph nodes, and the liver, and can lead to weight loss despite a proper diet. Injections of chorionic gonadotropin and other hormones have been shown to trigger this disorder in some rare cases.

Synonyms

Lymphangioleiomatosis

Pulmonary Lymphangiomyomatosis

Signs and Symptoms The patient usually develops shortness of breath first and then excess fluid or air in the pleurae. Hemorrhaging may eventually occur in the lungs, followed by bloody expectorations. When lymphangiomyomatosis occurs in the lymphatic vessels of the intestines and liver, causing vessel rupture or blockage, chyle and other fluids collect in the walls of the abdominal or thoracic cavity. Excessive urinary fat cell loss turns the urine milky and may cause weight loss. Symptoms and signs become more severe with hormone injections or a pregnancy. In very rare cases, manifestations are confined to lymphatic vessels in the patient's legs.

Etiology While the exact cause of this disorder is not known, the fact that it occurs only in women leads researchers to believe that it may be transmitted as a sex-linked trait or genetic disposition. Hormone therapy given to the patient to combat some other malady has also been implicated.

Epidemiology Lymphangiomyomatosis occurs only in women and usually in their childbearing years.

Treatment—Standard Treatment depends on symptoms. Shunts or tubes are used to drain pleural fluid, and bronchodilators can relieve breathing problems. Oophorectomy has been beneficial for some patients. Tamoxifen has been shown to be successful in arresting the progression of the disease. Pleurodesis of tetracycline diminishes accumulations of fluid. A fat replacement diet may or may not be beneficial. In extreme cases, excision of abnormal lung tissue may benefit the patient.

Treatment—Investigational Scientists are investigating the role of hormone therapy in the development of lymphangiomyomatosis and whether or not a genetic disposition is a prerequisite to the disorder. Also under investigation is the therapeutic value of progestin for lymphangiomyomatosis; however, more research is needed.

Please contact the agencies listed under Resources, below, for the most current information.

Resources

For more information on lymphangiomyomatosis: National Organization for Rare Disorders (NORD); American Lung Association; NIH/National Heart, Lung and Blood Institute (NHLBI).

For genetic information and genetic counseling referrals: March of Dimes Birth Defects Foundation; National Center for Education in Maternal and Child Health (NCEMCH).

References

Successful Treatment of Pulmonary Lymphangiomyomatosis with Oophorectomy and Progesterone: D. Adamson, et al.; Am. Rev. Respir. Dis., October 1985, issue 132(4), pp. 916–921.

Pulmonary Lymphangiomyomatosis Associated with Tuberous Sclerosis. Treatment with Tamoxifen and Tetracycline-Pleurodesis: C.M. Luna, et al.; Chest, September 1985, issue 88(3), pp. 473–475.

Lymphangiomyomatosis with Chylous Ascites: Treatment with Dietary Fat Restriction and Medium Chain Triglycerides: P.R. Calabrese, et al.; Cancer, August 1977, issue 40(2), pp. 895–897.

LYMPHEDEMA, HEREDITARY

Description Hereditary lymphedema is an inherited lymph-system disorder characterized by swelling of subcutaneous tissue caused by obstruction of lymphatic vessels and resulting edema of lymph fluid.

There are 3 forms of hereditary lymphedema: congenital (Milroy disease;

Nonne-Milroy-Meige syndrome); lymphedema praecox (Meige disease); and lymphedema tarda.

Signs and Symptoms The edema generally occurs below the waist, but may also be present in the face, larynx, and upper extremities. Patients with an edematous leg may feel uncomfortable but there is usually no pain. The swelling may begin in the foot and move upwards.

Patients with **Milroy disease** have nonulcerating lymphedema from birth. **Meige disease** usually occurs in the 1st or 2nd decade of the patient's life and can cause severe lymphedema in areas below the waist. Initially the patient presents with redness, swelling, pain, and inflammation. Related abnormalities can also occur, such as distichiasis, extradural cysts, vertebral abnormalities, cerebrovascular malformation, pleural effusion, cleft palate, hearing loss, and yellowing of nails.

Onset of **lymphedema tarda** usually occurs after age 35.

Etiology Hereditary lymphedema is transmitted as an autosomal dominant trait; less commonly, autosomal or sex-linked recessive.

Epidemiology Women are affected more often than men.

Related Disorders See *Angioedema, Hereditary.*

Traumatic lymphedema results from an injury to the lymphatic system, such as a bruise, that blocks the lymph vessels.

Treatment—Standard The leg should be elevated to reduce swelling. Other measures include use of support hose and, in some instances, pneumatic compression. Foot and skin hygiene is necessary to prevent lymphangitis and drying of the skin. Microsurgical anastomosis procedures have recently been used with some success.

Treatment of other symptoms and signs is symptomatic and supportive. Genetic counseling may benefit patients and their families.

Treatment—Investigational Please contact the agencies listed under Resources, below, for the most current information.

Resources

For more information on hereditary lymphedema: National Organization for Rare Disorders (NORD); National Lymphedema Network; National Lymphatic & Venous Diseases Foundation, Inc.; NIH/National Heart, Lung and Blood Institute.

For genetic information and genetic counseling referrals: March of Dimes Birth Defects Foundation; National Center for Education in Maternal and Child Health (NCEMCH).

References
Harrison's Principles of Internal Medicine, 12th ed.: J.D. Wilson, et al., eds.; McGraw-Hill, 1991, pp. 1025–1026.

Mendelian Inheritance in Man, 9th ed.: V.A. McKusick; Johns Hopkins University Press, 1990, p. 584.

Pulmonary Diseases and Disorders, 2nd ed.: A.P. Fishman; McGraw-Hill, 1988, p. 2134.

Familial Lymphedema Praecox: Meige's Disease: E.S. Wheeler, et al; Plast. Reconstr. Surg., May 1981, issue 67(3), pp. 362–364.

LYMPHOCYTIC INFILTRATE OF JESSNER

Description In lymphocytic infiltrate of Jessner, benign solid lesions composed of accumulated lymphocytes appear on the epidermis of the neck, face, or back. They may disappear spontaneously without leaving scars after remaining unchanged for several years.

Synonyms

Benign Lymphocytic Infiltrate of the Skin
Jessner-Kanof Lymphocytic Infiltration of the Skin

Signs and Symptoms The lesions typically are smooth and pink or red, have no hair follicles, and are sometimes clear in the center. They most commonly appear on the cheeks, eyelids, and upper face but may also occur on the back and neck. The surrounding skin is usually pruritic and erythematous. Rarely, lesions are sensitive to sunlight. After several years, the lesions generally disappear.

Etiology The exact reason for the abnormal lymphocytic accumulation in the skin is not known.

Epidemiology Males and females are affected in equal numbers.

Related Disorders See *Leprosy; Systemic Lupus Erythematosus; Mycosis Fungoides.*

Lymphocytoma cutis is a related disorder marked by skin nodules composed of accumulated lymphocytes and histiocytes. These lesions may be widespread or limited to a small area, are purple to yellow-brown in color, often form glistening spherical masses, and have a narrow noninfiltrating layer that separates them from the epidermis.

Treatment—Standard Chloroquine or other antimalarial drugs are usually administered for periods ranging from 6 weeks to 3 months. Superficial radiation may also be given in small doses to eliminate the lesions. Other therapy depends on symptoms.

Treatment—Investigational Thalidomide has been used experimentally when the lesions caused by lymphocytic infiltrate of Jessner resist other treatment; however, this drug has been shown to result in birth defects when taken by pregnant women, and it has been disapproved for use in the United States.

Please contact the agencies listed under Resources, below, for the most current information.

Resources

For more information on lymphocytic infiltrate of Jessner: National Organization for Rare Disorders (NORD); The National Arthritis and Musculoskeletal and Skin Diseases Information Clearinghouse.

References

Lymphocytic Infiltration of the Skin (Jessner and Kanof): W. Kenneth Blaylock; *in* Clinical Dermatology: Demis, et al.; Harper & Row, 1982.

Treatment of Jessner-Kanof Disease with Thalidomide: G. Moulin, et al.; Ann. Dermatol. Venereol., 1983, issue 110(8), pp. 611–614.

Lymphocytic Infiltration of the Skin (Jessner). A T-Cell Lymphoproliferative Disease: R. Willemze, et al.; Br. J. Dermatol., May 1984, issue 110(5), pp. 523–529.

MALIGNANT MELANOMA

Description Malignant melanoma is a skin neoplasm derived from epidermal or nevose melanin cells. The neoplastic cells eventually invade the dermis and adjacent tissue and frequently metastasize widely. Subtypes of this neoplasm are known as juvenile melanoma, malignant lentigo melanoma, and acral lentiginous melanoma.

Signs and Symptoms The early stages of this disease are usually asymptomatic, but later, a lesion appears that does not heal, or a mole begins to change in color or size.

Juvenile melanoma is marked by a benign pink-to-purplish-red papule on the face (usually the cheeks) that has a slightly scaly surface. It generally occurs before the juvenile reaches puberty and is often mistaken for the malignant form of the disease.

A malignant lentigo melanoma is a brown or black precancerous spot on the epidermis (usually of the face) that is irregular in shape and resembles a freckle. It most often occurs in older persons.

An acral lentiginous melanoma is a malignant neoplasm that occurs on areas of the epidermis that have no hair follicles and have not been overly exposed to the sun.

Etiology While the exact cause of this disease is unknown, research indicates that individuals who allow their skin to be exposed to the sun excessively, particularly before puberty, and who live in sunny climates are at greater risk of developing malignant melanoma. Studies have also found that some persons may have a genetic predisposition to the disease that is inherited as an autosomal dominant trait.

Epidemiology In recent years, malignant melanoma has increased in incidence at a much greater rate than any other malignant neoplastic disease. It affects equal numbers of males and females, although blue-eyed and fair-complected Caucasians are at greater risk than other populations.

Related Disorders See *Squamous Cell Carcinoma, Cutaneous.*

Basal cell carcinoma is a common skin cancer characterized by hard and shiny nodules, hardened scarlike patches that hemorrhage, or ulcerated and encrusted lesions. A biopsy is necessary to distinguish it from localized dermatitis or psoriasis.

Kaposi's sarcoma is a malignant neoplasm associated with acquired immunodeficiency syndrome (**AIDS**) and characterized by small tumors, plaques, papules, nodules, or ulcers that are tan to purple in color. The neoplasms occur in the oropharyngeal and gastrointestinal tracts and infiltrate the lungs, liver, and bone. Before AIDS was first recognized, Kaposi's sarcoma was usually found only in elderly Jewish or Mediterranean men and in persons with compromised immune systems. Today about 30 percent of AIDS patients have Kaposi's sarcoma.

The lesions of **seborrheic keratosis** can resemble those of the early stages of malignant melanoma.

Treatment—Standard Treatment varies with the stage of disease and the location of the lesion. In stage 1, the lesion is surgically excised along with a 5-cm margin around the lesion. Smaller margins are excised in certain areas, such as the face. In stage 2, which involves the lymph nodes, a lymphadenectomy is performed. Once the disease has metastasized, chemotherapy is administered. Dacarbazine has been shown to be effective in some patients. High-dose combinations of cisplatin, cyclophosphamide, and carmustine have also been beneficial for some patients.

Treatment—Investigational Interferon is under investigation as a treatment for this disease, either alone or in combination with other agents. Autologous bone marrow transplantation is also being used on an experimental basis.

Please contact the agencies listed under Resources, below, for the most current information.

Resources

For more information on malignant melanoma: National Organization for Rare Disorders (NORD); The Skin Cancer Foundation; American Cancer Society; NIH/National Cancer Institute PDQ (Physician Data Query) phoneline.

References
Internal Medicine, 3rd ed.: J.H. Stein, ed.-in-chief; Little, Brown and Company, 1990, pp. 1154–1156.

Malignant Melanoma. Treatment with High Dose Combination Alkylating Agent Chemotherapy and Autologous Bone Marrow Support: T.C. Shea; Arch. Dermatol., June 1988, issue 124(6), pp. 878–884.

Changing Trends in Melanoma: C.M. Balch, M.D., ed.-in-chief; Mel. Let., 1987, Vol. 5, No. 1.

Immunotherapy for Malignant Melanoma, Vaccines: J.C. Bystryn; Mel. Let., 1986, Vol. 4, No. 2.

MASTOCYTOSIS

Description Mastocytosis is an inherited blood disorder marked by abnormal mast cell infiltration of skin, bone, bone marrow, lungs, liver, spleen, and occasionally the meninges. In adults, the solid organs are affected more than the skin, whereas in children, the reverse is true (see *Urticaria Pigmentosa*). **Mast cell leukemia** is one form of mastocytosis.

Synonyms

Cutaneous Mastocytosis
Systemic Mast Cell Disease

Signs and Symptoms Patients with mastocytosis initially feel a vague sense of discomfort or poor health, accompanied by weight loss, diarrhea, nausea, vomiting, weakness, and irregular heart beat. In children, the skin is primarily affected and not other organs. The skin is marked with dilated blood vessels, thick and discolored spots that run together, patches resulting from a proliferation of leukocytes, and chronic skin growths that are flat and patterned. The affected skin may show minimal discoloration, but gentle rubbing or stroking can produce swelling and redness.

Adults tend to have greater involvement of internal organs, including mucous membranes in the nose, mouth, and rectum. Lymph nodes, spleen, and liver become swollen and bone softens and deteriorates, although new bone may grow as the hard outer layer or the spongy inner substance of bone thickens. Patients rarely may have duodenal ulcers that are associated with hemorrhaging or pain in the upper abdomen.

Etiology The precise method of genetic transmission of this disorder is not known. Histamine seems to be overproduced and released from mast cells that infiltrate various organs.

Epidemiology Mastocytosis most commonly affects adult men and women in equal numbers, although it can also begin in childhood.

Related Disorders See *Urticaria Pigmentosa.*

Treatment—Standard A combination of the antihistamines chlorpheniramine and cimetidine is used to control the growth of mast cells and block the effects of histamine release. More recently, oral cromolyn sodium (Gastrocrom R) has been developed; it not only relieves symptoms but prevents recurrence. The drug's manufacturer has established a patient assistance program to provide free Gastrocrom R for needy patients. Contact Fisons Corp., Gastrocrom Patient Assistance Program, Box 1776, Rochester, New York 14603 or call 1-800-727-6100.

Surgical excision of mast cells may be necessary to improve organ function in advanced stages of the disorder.

Treatment—Investigational Please contact the agencies listed under Resources, below, for the most current information.

Resources

For more information on mastocytosis: National Organization for Rare Disorders (NORD); The National Arthritis and Musculoskeletal and Skin Diseases Information Clearinghouse; NIH/National Cancer Institute PDQ (Physician Data Query) phoneline.

References

Mastocytosis: A Review: D.H. Stein; Pediatr. Dermatol., November 1986, issue 3(5), pp. 365–375.

MAY-HEGGLIN ANOMALY

Description May-Hegglin anomaly is a sometimes symptomless hereditary condition characterized by abnormalities of blood platelets and certain leukocytes. Treatment is usually not necessary; prognosis is good.

Synonyms
>Döhle Bodies-Myelopathy
>Hegglin Disease
>Leukocytic Inclusions with Platelet Abnormality

Signs and Symptoms Some patients with May-Hegglin anomaly may show symptoms from birth but others remain asymptomatic for life. The symptoms that do occur include purpura, epistaxis, excessive bleeding from the mouth during dental work, headaches, and muscular weakness on one side of the body due to intracranial bleeding. Excessive bleeding may be brought about when steroid therapy used to treat some other disorder is discontinued.

Laboratory results show giant, oddly shaped platelets and characteristic inclusions in the polymorphonuclear leukocytes. There also might be slightly fewer platelets than normal.

Etiology May-Hegglin anomaly is an inherited blood disorder transmitted by an autosomal dominant gene.

Epidemiology This anomaly occurs primarily in persons of Greek or Italian descent.

Related Disorders Related disorders of abnormal platelet function are Bernard-Soulier syndrome, thrombasthenia, Chédiak-Higashi syndrome, the gray platelet syndrome, and various defects related to collagen-induced platelet aggregation. See **Bernard-Soulier Syndrome; Thrombasthenia; Chédiak-Higashi Syndrome.** Platelet disorders have also been linked with such congenital conditions as Wiskott-Aldrich syndrome, Down syndrome, thrombocytopenia with absent radius syndrome, and von Willebrand disease.

Treatment—Standard May-Hegglin anomaly generally does not require therapy.

Treatment—Investigational Please contact the agencies listed under Resources, below, for the most current information.

Resources
  For more information on May-Hegglin anomaly: National Organization for Rare Disorders (NORD); NIH/National Heart, Lung, and Blood Institute (NHLBI).

  For genetic information and genetic counseling referrals: March of Dimes Birth Defects Foundation; National Center for Education in Maternal and Child Health (NCEMCH).

References
   Cecil Textbook of Medicine, 18th ed.: J.B. Wyngaarden and L.H. Smith, Jr., eds.; W.B. Saunders
   Company, 1988, p. 1048.

MULTIPLE MYELOMA

Description Multiple myeloma is a rare malignant neoplasm that develops in bone marrow and is characterized by neoplastic proliferation of plasma cells in the marrow of various bones, especially the skull, spine, rib cage, pelvis, and legs. Subdivisions of the disease are known as plasma cell leukemia, nonsecretory myeloma, osteosclerotic myeloma, smoldering myeloma, extramedullary plasmacytoma, and solitary plasmacytoma of bone (see under Related Disorders, below).

Synonyms
   Kahler Disease
   Myelomatosis
   Plasma Cell Myeloma

Signs and Symptoms The features most often seen in multiple myeloma are bone pain, anemia, and renal insufficiency. Body movements trigger pain in the bones of the chest or back, which may be followed by pallor, anemia, fatigue, weakness, complications in the kidneys, hepatosplenomegaly, compressed nerves in the spinal column, and greater susceptibility to bacterial infections (especially pneumonia). Results of blood studies show increased levels of suppressor T cells and decreased levels of helper T cells.

Etiology While the precise etiology of this cancer is not known, scientists have implicated a number of possible causes, including such environmental factors as exposure to asbestos, radiation, and toxic chemicals used in agriculture and industry, as well as viruses and a genetic disposition to the disease.

Epidemiology Twice as many men as women are affected by multiple myeloma, and symptoms usually occur between the ages of 40 and 70. This cancer makes up one percent of all cancers and fully 10 percent of all malignant blood disorders.

Related Disorders See *Amyloidosis; Waldenström Macroglobulinemia.*
   A group of disorders known as **heavy chain diseases** are related to multiple myeloma in that they are characterized by an excessive number of plasma cells or lymphocytes that look like plasma cells, in the lymph nodes and bone marrow. These proliferative disorders are of 3 types: **alpha, gamma,** and **mu heavy chain diseases.** In the alpha form, patients have progressive weight loss, malabsorption of nutrients, steatorrhea, and diarrhea. In the gamma form, patients have anemia, amino acid deficiencies, hepatosplenomegaly, and lymphadenoma. In the mu form, patients have chronic lymphocytic leukemia or lymph gland neoplasms and gammaglobulinemia.
   In addition, a number of disorders are secondary to multiple myeloma and considered subdivisions of the disease. However, they do not have to be present for differential diagnosis of multiple myeloma.

The first is **plasma cell leukemia,** which is marked by plasma cell hyperplasia in the blood. Thirty percent of these patients have documented multiple myeloma, although initially patients present with signs of leukemia.

The second is **nonsecretory myeloma,** in which multiple myeloma patients fail to produce M protein in their blood or urine.

The third is **osteosclerotic myeloma,** which is a chronic inflammatory disease marked by very low numbers of plasma cells (5 percent or less of normal), osteosclerotic lesions, and sometimes lytic lesions. It causes motor deficiencies, poor motor nerve conduction, high levels of protein in spinal fluid, club fingers, fluid retention, hepatosplenomegaly, and skin discoloration.

The fourth is **smoldering myeloma,** in which atypical plasma cells are present in bone marrow in unusually high numbers but without signs of disease. However, protein is present in the urine of many patients.

The fifth is **extramedullary plasmacytoma,** which is marked by the presence of plasma cell neoplasms in places other than bone marrow, most notably in the upper respiratory tract but also in almost every other organ of the body.

Finally, the last is **solitary plasmacytoma of bone,** which is marked by the presence of only one bone lesion and no evidence of multiple myeloma in the marrow.

Treatment—Standard Analgesic drugs and chemotherapy are usually given to relieve pain. Interferon is sometimes administered along with chemotherapy. Fluid administration may be necessary if the kidneys are affected. Radiation therapy may be given to shrink any bone masses that develop.

Treatment—Investigational Plasmapheresis has been used experimentally and has potential benefit; however, more research is needed. Sandoglobulin is also under investigation as a treatment, but its safety and efficacy have not yet been determined.

Please contact the agencies listed under Resources, below, for the most current information.

Resources

For more information on multiple myeloma: National Organization for Rare Disorders (NORD); American Cancer Society; NIH/National Cancer Institute PDQ (Physician Data Query) phoneline; National Kidney Foundation.

References

Internal Medicine, 3rd ed.: J.H. Stein, ed.-in-chief; Little, Brown and Company, 1990, pp. 1146–1149.

Effects of Plasmapheresis on the Plasma Concentration of Proteins Used to Monitor the Disease Process in Multiple Myeloma: A. Wahlin, et al.; Acta Med. Scand., 1988, issue 223(3), pp. 263–267.

Interferon in the Treatment of Multiple Myeloma: M.R. Cooper, et al.; Cancer, February 1987, issue 59(3 suppl.), pp. 594–600.

The Use of Interferon in the Treatment of Multiple Myeloma: J.J. Costanzi, et al.; Semin. Oncol., June 1987, issue 14(2, suppl. 2), pp. 24–28.

MYCOSIS FUNGOIDES

Description Mycosis fungoides is a chronic lymphocyte disorder that arises in the skin and is characterized by progressive infiltration by malignant lymph cells. In the late stages, the patient may have lymph-node infiltrations and ulcerated tumors that resemble mushrooms. In addition to skin, the malignant cells may infiltrate other parts of the body, such as the brain, spleen, liver, and gastrointestinal tract. One type of this disorder is called Vidal-Brocq mycosis fungoides.

Synonyms
   Granuloma Fungoides

Signs and Symptoms Stage I: The first signs of mycosis fungoides usually resemble eczema or other skin disorders, such as psoriasis and lichen planus, and are marked by pruritus and pain in the dermal area affected. The patient has scattered erythematous patches on the skin of his trunk and extremities. He or she may also suffer insomnia.

Stage II: Lymphoid cells infiltrate the skin, and bluish-red elevated plaques develop that are initially tiny but eventually grow larger and run together to look like exfoliative dermatitis. At this stage, lipomelanotic reticulosis may develop in lymph nodes, and lymphadenitis can occur.

Stage III: Lobulated tumors develop that resemble mushrooms. They are bluish or red-brown ulcerated lesions measuring 1 to 15 cm in diameter. The dermis may thicken and atypical lymphoid cells may infiltrate the upper dermis in bands and the clear spaces of the lower dermis, causing necrosis.

Stage IV: The final stage is marked by generalized spread of diseased lymphocytes throughout the body, accompanied by anemia, weight loss, fever, gastrointestinal tract involvement with or without intestinal ulceration, and hepatosplenomegaly. Cardiac muscle may also be involved, and dysphagia and coughing may occur. When the brain is affected, the patient may lose clear vision and experience eye pain.

Etiology While the precise cause of this disorder is unknown, researchers believe the cause is probably a lymphoma arising in the skin or reticulum.

Epidemiology Mycosis fungoides generally occurs in patients over 40 years, and twice as often in men as in women.

Related Disorders See *Leprosy; Lymphocytic Infiltrate of Jessner.*

Chronic lymphocytic leukemia is a related disorder characterized by an abnormal buildup of lymph cells that infiltrate bone marrow and cause deficiencies in blood cell development.

In **Sézary syndrome (Sézary reticulosis syndrome; Sézary erythroderma),** reticular cells infiltrate the skin, causing patches to fall off in scales. Patients have intense pruritus, hair loss, hyperkeratosis, and swelling.

Treatment—Standard The standard treatments for mycosis fungoides are electron beam radiation and local administration of the drugs psoralen and mechlorethamine, followed by exposure to long wavelength ultraviolet light or sunlight.

Treatment—Investigational Clinical trials of intramuscular injections of high-dose recombinant leukocyte alpha-interferon for advanced stages of the disease are under way with positive initial results. Lowering the dosage can reduce side effects, but more research into safety and effectiveness is needed.

While cyclosporine has potential benefit in the treatment of mycosis fungoides and a number of other dermatologic disorders, its side effects can be life-threatening and its use must be limited. It remains an experimental drug for even the most extreme cases, and its longterm effects are not known.

Please contact the agencies listed under Resources, below, for the most current information.

Resources

For more information on mycosis fungoides: National Organization for Rare Disorders (NORD); American Cancer Society; The Skin Cancer Foundation; NIH/National Cancer Institute PDQ (Physician Data Query) phoneline.

References

Alpha-Interferon Treatment of Cutaneous T-Cell Lymphoma and Chronic Lymphocytic Leukemia: K.A. Foon, et al.; Semin. Oncol., December 1986, issue 13(4 suppl. 5), pp. 35–39.

Combined Total Body Electron Beam Irradiation and Chemotherapy for Mycosis Fungoides: I.M. Braverman, et al.; J. Am. Acad. Dermatol., January 1987, issue 16(1, pt. 1), pp. 45–60.

Cutaneous Malignancies and Metastatic Squamous Cell Carcinoma Following Topical Therapies for Mycosis Fungoides: E.A. Abel, et al.; J. Am. Acad. Dermatol., June 1986, issue 14(6), pp. 1029–1038.

MYELOFIBROSIS-OSTEOSCLEROSIS (MOS)

Description Myelofibrosis-osteosclerosis is a bone marrow condition characterized by proliferation of fibrous tissue to repair or replace damaged bone marrow, and generalized anemia and splenomegaly.

Synonyms

Agnogenic Myeloid Metaplasia
Myelofibrosis
Myelofibrosis and Myeloid Metaplasia
Osteosclerosis

Signs and Symptoms About 30 percent of patients are asymptomatic. The rest experience the signs and symptoms of anemia, such as pallor, weakness, fatigue, dizziness, and headache. Splenomegaly occurs in almost all patients, and hepatomegaly in about 50 percent. Other features include drowsiness, irritability, sweating, gastrointestinal complaints, jaundice, weight loss, and amenorrhea. The patient usually suffers bouts of severe pain in the abdomen, bones, and joints.

Etiology Myelofibrosis-osteosclerosis is thought to be a connective tissue reaction to several different types of injury that destroy bone marrow tissue. One cause of MOS is metastasis to bone marrow of primary tumors in the breast, prostate, kidney, lung, or adrenal or thyroid glands. A rare cause of MOS in children is osteopetrosis. Tuberculosis and exposure to such toxic substances as benzene, fluoride, or phosphorus are often associated with secondary MOS.

Epidemiology MOS occurs in both sexes, usually during mid-life, and rarely in children. The disorder is seen in about 2:100,000 persons, slightly more often in whites.

Treatment—Standard If the cause of MOS is known, therapy involves treating the underlying cause. If the cause is not known, therapy involves treating the symptoms. If anemia produces cardiovascular symptoms, blood transfusions are effective. Moderate success has been achieved in treating primary MOS with androgens or corticosteroids or both to increase erythrocyte production and decrease their destruction.

Treatment—Investigational Please contact the agencies listed under Resources, below, for the most current information.

Resources
    For more information on myelofibrosis-osteosclerosis: National Organization for Rare Disorders (NORD); American Cancer Society; NIH/National Cancer Institute PDQ (Physician Data Query) phoneline; NIH/National Heart, Lung and Blood Institute (NHLBI).

References
Internal Medicine, 3rd ed.: J.H. Stein, ed.-in-chief; Little, Brown and Company, 1990, pp. 1126–1128.

NEVOID BASAL CELL CARCINOMA SYNDROME

Description Nevoid basal cell carcinoma syndrome is a malignant neoplastic disease marked by lesions in the epidermis or mucous membranes of the patient's mouth, as well as bony formations and multiple cysts on the head and face. The syndrome may also involve the nervous and vascular systems and connective tissue. The epidermal lesions do not usually have external causes and are limited in size but unlimited in number.

Synonyms
    Basal Cell Nevus Syndrome
    Gorlin-Goltz Syndrome
    Herzberg-Wiskemann Phakomatosis
    Nevus, Epitheliomatosis Multiplex with Jaw Cysts

Signs and Symptoms Multiple lesions appear on the patient's face, neck, chest, and back; they increase in number with age. Onset usually occurs after puberty.

Multiple cysts can cause mandibular swelling and frontal bossing. Other manifestations include mental retardation, cataracts, coloboma of the choroid and optic nerve, vertebral defects, scoliosis, bifid ribs, calcification of the falx cerebri, and late eruption of teeth in children.

Etiology While the precise cause of nevoid basal cell carcinoma is not known, it is believed that patients may have a genetic predisposition to the disease, which is inherited as an autosomal dominant trait.

Epidemiology Equal numbers of males and females are affected by this disorder.

Related Disorders See *Malignant Melanoma; Squamous Cell Carcinoma, Cutaneous.*

Basal cell carcinoma is a common skin cancer characterized by hard and shiny nodules, hardened scarlike patches that hemorrhage, or ulcerated and encrusted lesions.

Treatment—Standard The lesions are usually removed surgically, although their numbers and locations make this difficult. If the lesions cannot be completely removed by surgery, chemotherapy is also given. Many patients benefit from the chemotherapeutic drug etretinate, which has been shown to destroy the lesions and prevent the formation of new tumors. Patients and their families should receive genetic counseling. Other treatments depend on symptoms.

Treatment—Investigational Oral isotretinoin is under investigation as a treatment for this disease, but more research is needed to determine its longterm safety and efficacy.

Please contact the agencies listed under Resources, below, for the most current information.

Resources

For more information on nevoid basal cell carcinoma: National Organization for Rare Disorders (NORD); The Skin Cancer Foundation; American Cancer Society; NIH/National Cancer Institute PDQ (Physician Data Query) phoneline.

References

Mendelian Inheritance in Man, 9th ed.: V.A. McKusick; The Johns Hopkins University Press, 1990, pp. 120–122.

Long Term Retinoid Therapy is Needed for Maintenance of Cancer Chemopreventative Effect: G.L. Peck; Dermatologica, 1987, issue 175(suppl. 1), pp. 138–144.

Etretinate Treatment of the Nevoid Basal Cell Carcinoma Syndrome. Therapeutic and Chemopreventive Effect: E. Hodak, Int. J. Dermatol., November 1987, issue 26(9), pp. 606–609.

Aromatic Retinoid in the Chemoprevention of the Progression of Nevoid Basal-Cell Carcinoma Syndrome: M. Cristofolini; J. Dermatol. Surg. Oncol., October 1984, issue 10(10), pp. 778–781.

NEZELOF SYNDROME

Description Nezelof syndrome is an immune deficiency disorder that impairs cellular immunity against infections, especially opportunistic infections. The syndrome also includes some abnormalities in humoral immunity. In a subgroup of about 12 patients, immune deficiency appears to be due to a lack of purine nucleoside phosphorylase (**PNP**).

Synonyms
Cellular Immunodeficiency with Abnormal Immunoglobulin Synthesis

Signs and Symptoms Patients suffer frequent and severe infections from birth, including oral candidiasis, diarrhea, skin infections, septicemia, urinary tract infections, measles, pulmonary infections, and vaccinia. *Pneumocystis carinii* pneumonia and chronic diarrhea are characteristic of the syndrome. Cytomegalovirus, rubeola, *Pseudomonas,* and mycobacterial infections may also occur. The patient's growth is retarded and general wasting is evident.

Impairment of cellular immunity results in delayed cutaneous anergy, an inability to reject foreign tissue grafts, potentially fatal reactions to vaccination, and a high incidence of malignant tumors. Patients are susceptible to graft-versus-host disease, which causes fever, skin reactions, hepatitis, and gastrointestinal disturbances, such as diarrhea, vomiting, intestinal obstruction, and malabsorption. Patients with PNP deficiency show progressive neurologic deterioration characterized by spastic paralysis of all limbs, autoimmune hemolytic anemia, and thrombocytopenic purpura.

Low T cell counts and lymphopenia are common laboratory findings in Nezelof syndrome patients. Leukocytes may show a reduced number of neutrophils and high concentrations of eosinophils. Lymph glands shrink in size. The patient's thymus gland is small and histologically abnormal. All classes of antibodies are present, often in normal concentrations, and the patient sometimes has a selective IgA deficiency and substantial elevations of IgE and/or IgD antibodies. Patients with PNP deficiency have very low uric acid levels in the blood and urine.

Etiology While the means of transmission and pathophysiology are not clear, Nezelof syndrome is thought to be hereditary, either through an autosomal or a sex-linked gene. A dysfunction of the thymus gland is suspected in most cases. In patients with PNP deficiency, researchers think that the PNP substrate accumulates because of enzyme deficiency and is then preferentially taken up by T lymphocytes. High concentrations of the substrate molecule inhibit DNA synthesis and impair cell function.

Epidemiology This extremely rare syndrome affects both males and females.

Related Disorders See *Acquired Immune Deficiency Syndrome; Severe Combined Immunodeficiency; DiGeorge Syndrome; Wiskott-Aldrich Syndrome; Ataxia Telangiectasia.*

Treatment—Standard Each infection must be treated vigorously according to symptoms, with antifungal, antibiotic, and supportive measures. In several cases, bone marrow transplants taken from immunologically compatible siblings have been successful in treating the disease.

Pneumocystis carinii pneumonia is particularly resistant to treatment. Trimethoprim-sulfamethoxazole and the orphan drug pentamidine isethionate are usually used. Idoxuridine, floxuridine, or cytarabine are preferred in the treatment of cytomegalovirus and generalized herpes simplex infections. Amphotericin B therapy has been successful in treating severe infections from *Candida* and related fungi.

For patients with PNP deficiency, researchers have tried to replace the missing enzyme or at least dilute the excess purine bases by giving blood transfusions, but with little success. Also unsuccessful has been deoxycytidine therapy. Patients have to be protected from exposure to infectious agents, including live viral vaccines. They should not be given corticosteroids or immunosuppressant drugs, nor should they undergo splenectomy. If blood transfusions become necessary, the blood must be irradiated to avoid graft-versus-host disease. The prognosis for survival beyond childhood is poor unless matched sibling bone marrow transplants are successful.

Treatment—Investigational Please contact the agencies listed under Resources, below, for the most current information.

Resources

For more information on Nezelof syndrome: National Organization for Rare Disorders (NORD); NIH/National Institute of Allergy and Infectious Diseases; Immune Deficiency Foundation; NIH/National Cancer Institute PDQ (Physician Data Query) phoneline; American Cancer Society.

For genetic information and genetic counseling referrals: March of Dimes Birth Defects Foundation; National Center for Education in Maternal and Child Health (NCEMCH).

References

Immunodeficiency: R.H. Buckley; J. Allergy Clin. Immunol., December 1983, issue 72(6), pp. 627–641.

Combined Immunodeficiency and Thymic Abnormalities: R.D. Webster; J. Clin. Pathol. (suppl.), 1979, issue 13, pp. 10–14.

Metabolic Defects in Immunodeficiency Diseases: R.D. Webster; Clin. Exp. Immunol., July 1982, issue 49(1), pp. 1–10.

PHEOCHROMOCYTOMA

Description Pheochromocytoma is a rare neoplastic disorder marked by usually benign chromaffinoma derived from tumors in the adrenal medullary tissue and characterized by hypertension that does not respond to usual treatment.

Synonyms

Adrenal Tumor

Chromaffin Cell Tumor

Signs and Symptoms The patient's hypertension may be associated with heart palpitations, angina, rapid breathing, profuse sweating, headache, pallor, cold and clammy skin, nausea, stomach pain, vomiting, constipation, tingling sensations, and visual disturbances.

Diagnosis is by urine testing, magnetic resonance imaging, and lack of response to hypertension medication.

Etiology Pheochromocytoma results from tumors growing in adrenal glands and possibly along certain nerve pathways as well. In some cases, it has been shown to appear without an apparent cause, while in other cases it has been linked to an autosomal dominant gene whose penetrance is incomplete.

Epidemiology Symptoms usually appear before the patient reaches age 50, but pheochromocytoma can strike at any age. Equal numbers of women and men are affected.

Related Disorders See *Neurofibromatosis; von Hippel-Lindau Disease.*

Sipple syndrome is a related disorder marked by adrenal tumors associated with other endocrine gland tumors.

Treatment—Standard The standard treatment is removal of the neoplasm by surgery. Other treatments depend on symptoms. When pheochromocytoma is shown to occur in families, genetic counseling is recommended.

Treatment—Investigational Please contact the agencies listed under Resources, below, for the most current information.

Resources

For more information on pheochromocytoma: National Organization for Rare Disorders (NORD); American Cancer Society; NIH/National Cancer Institute PDQ (Physician Data Query) phoneline.

For genetic information and genetic counseling referrals: March of Dimes Birth Defects Foundation; National Center for Education in Maternal and Child Health (NCEMCH).

References

Localization of Ectopic Pheochromocytomas by Magnetic Resonance Imaging: J.E. Schmedt, et al.; Am. J. Med., October 1987, issue 83(4), pp. 770–772.

Clinically Unsuspected Pheochromocytomas. Experience at Henry Ford Hospital and a Review of the Literature: N.K. Krane; Arch. Intern. Med., January 1986, issue 146(1), pp. 54–57.

Diagnosis and Management of Pheochromocytoma: G.W. Gifford, et al.; Cardiology, 1985, issue 72(suppl. 1), pp. 126–130.

POLYCYTHEMIA VERA

Description A chronic proliferative disorder involving bone marrow, polycythemia vera is characterized by an increase in the number of erythrocytes and a rise in the concentration of hemoglobin in the blood.

Synonyms
Erythremia

Signs and Symptoms Patients experience fatigue, malaise, difficulty in concentrating, headache, drowsiness, dizziness, and forgetfulness. Pruritis occurs in about 50 percent of cases, especially after a hot bath. The patient's skin is sometimes erythematous, or it may be normal in color and have only dusky redness in the mucous membranes. Retinal veins may be dark red, full, and tortuous, and the spleen is generally palpable. Osteonecrosis may occur. Some patients are symptomless.

Etiology The cause is unknown.

Related Disorders Leukemia is a related disorder.

Treatment—Standard Phlebotomy is the most common treatment. From 3 to 6 phlebotomies are usually required to return the number of erythrocytes in the blood to normal by reducing the hematocrit level to less than 50 percent. However, repeated phlebotomy usually causes iron-deficiency anemia, and the treatment is not as effective in patients with high iron absorption rates or greatly elevated platelet counts. It is not convenient in patients with poor veins. If the patient is elderly and has advanced arteriosclerosis or a heart condition, less blood should be removed with each phlebotomy.

The patient should not be given supplemental iron when phlebotomy is the only therapy because the iron tends to accelerate hemoglobin production. Neither should the patient eat foods rich in iron, such as clams, oysters, liver, and legumes.

Almost all patients treated by phlebotomy followed by radiophosphorus (32_P) therapy experience clinical and hematologic remission that usually lasts 18 months but can vary from 6 months to several years. Most patients so treated usually have no immediate side effects, but approximately 10 percent of patients treated with 32_P develop acute leukemia that usually occurs after more than 10 years of treatment. Chemotherapy for polycythemia vera increases the risk of acute leukemia.

Patients suffer hyperuricemia that requires treatment with allopurinol. Acute gouty arthritis can develop; it should be treated with colchicine or nonsteroidal antiinflammatory drugs. Although corticosteroids can produce rapid and complete remission in some patients, they are generally used only when other drugs are not effective.

Treatment—Investigational The Food and Drug Administration has approved the experimental use of the orphan drug Anagrelide, manufactured by Bristol-Myers, for polycythemia vera.

Please contact the agencies listed under Resources, below, for the most current information.

Resources
For more information on polycythemia vera: National Organization for Rare Disorders (NORD); Myeloproliferative Disease Foundation; NIH/National

Heart, Lung and Blood Institute (NHLBI).

References
Cecil Textbook of Medicine, 18th ed.: J.B. Wyngaarden and L.H. Smith, Jr., eds.; W.B. Saunders Company, 1988, pp. 973, 980–984.

PURE RED CELL APLASIA

Description A rare blood disorder that affects only erythrocytes, pure red cell aplasia is marked by a sudden decline in the number of red blood cells produced by the bone marrow.

Signs and Symptoms Pallor, weakness, and lethargy are seen, with the course determined by the degree of aplasia. Patients have a deficient number of erythroblasts despite elevated levels of erythropoietin.

Etiology Believed to be an autoimmune disorder, pure red cell aplasia is one of a group of syndromes related to bone marrow failure. The possible causes of this disorder are viral infection, a neoplasm in the thymus gland, or certain drugs, such as the sulfonylureas, anesthetic halothane, gold used in the treatment of arthritis, and antiepileptic drugs, e.g., phenobarbital, phenytoin, and penicillin.

Epidemiology This rare disorder affects equal numbers of adult males and females.

Related Disorders See *Anemia, Aplastic.*

Treatment—Standard When drugs are the cause of pure red cell aplasia and those drugs are discontinued, the disorder usually goes into remission.

The antiinflammatory drugs prednisone and antithymocyte globulin are used to treat patients under 30, while older patients are treated with cytotoxic immunosuppressants (e.g., azathioprine, cyclophosphamide, and 6-mercaptopurine). Anti-human thymocyte gammaglobulin is used for patients resistant to conventional immunosuppressive agents. All patients may require blood transfusions periodically until the drugs take effect. If the drugs lead to remission, they are discontinued.

Surgical removal of the thymus gland often results in remission.

Treatment—Investigational Please contact the agencies listed under Resources, below, for the most current information.

Resources
For more information on pure red cell aplasia: National Organization for Rare Disorders (NORD); NIH/National Heart, Lung and Blood Institute (NHLBI); Aplastic Anemia Foundation of America.

References
Pure Red Cell Aplasia Characterized by Erythropoietic Maturation Arrest. Response to Anti-Thymocyte Globulin: A.D. Jacobs, et al.; Amer. J. Med., March 1985, issue 78(3), pp. 515–517.

New Therapies for Aplastic Anemia: S.B. Krantz; Amer. J. Med. Sciences, 1986, issue 291, pp. 371–379.

Diphenylhydantoin-Induced Pure Red Cell Aplasia: E.N. Dessypris, et al.; Blood, 1985, issue 65, pp. 789–794.

PURPURA, IDIOPATHIC THROMBOCYTOPENIC (ITP)

Description ITP is a platelet disorder characterized by abnormal hemorrhaging into the skin and mucous membranes without an apparent cause or underlying disease. Anemia may result.

Synonyms
> Purpura Hemorrhagica
> Werlhof Disease

Signs and Symptoms The signs of hemorrhaging from the mucous membranes are epistaxis, and gastrointestinal, genitourinary, and vaginal bleeding. Hemarthrosis and bleeding into the central nervous system are less common features. Anemia produces weakness, fatigue, or signs of congestive heart failure. Fever and splenomegaly may also occur.

Etiology Although the cause of ITP is not known, symptoms are sometimes preceded by an acute viral infection. There is evidence to support an immunologic basis for the disorder, since antiplatelet antibodies have been identified in most patients. Bone-marrow samples show the presence of a large number of inactive or nonproductive megakaryocytes.

Epidemiology ITP affects children and young adults most frequently, and occurs in females more often than males. Pregnant women who have systemic lupus erythematosus are particularly vulnerable to ITP.

Related Disorders Allergic purpura is acute or chronic vasculitis that involves the skin, joints, and gastrointestinal and renal systems.

Treatment—Standard Corticosteroids (hydrocortisone or prednisone) are effective in about 15 percent of ITP patients. About one-half of those who do not respond to steroid therapy or who have recurrence when steroids are discontinued respond well to splenectomy. Immunosuppressive drugs, such as cyclophosphamide and azathioprine, have been effective in some patients who did not respond to steroids or splenectomy. The antineoplastic drug vincristine has sometimes been therapeutic.

While platelet concentrates can be transfused to control hemorrhaging until more specific therapy has time to be effective, the short survival time of platelets limits the usefulness of this treatment. Patients also risk an immune reaction to repeated platelet transfusions.

The Food and Drug Administration has approved the use of intravenous immunoglobulin for short periods in patients (especially children) who have an acute form of ITP. Chronic ITP may require monthly injections of immunoglobulin.

Treatment—Investigational The orphan drug defibrotide is under investigation as a treatment for ITP. Crinos International in Italy makes the drug available on an experimental basis.

Please contact the agencies listed under Resources, below, for the most current information.

Resources
For more information on idiopathic thrombocytopenic purpura: National Organization for Rare Disorders (NORD); NIH/National Heart, Blood and Lung Institute (NHBLI).

References
Cecil Textbook of Medicine, 18th ed.: J.B. Wyngaarden and L.H. Smith, Jr., eds.; W.B. Saunders Company, 1988, pp. 1050–1051.

PURPURA, SCHOENLEIN-HENOCH

Description Schoenlein-Henoch purpura is a capillary disorder characterized by purpural skin lesions and internal hemorrhaging. The disorder can also affect the joints, gastrointestinal tract, kidneys, and, rarely, the central nervous system.

If the skin and joints are affected, but not the gastrointestinal tract, the disorder is termed **Schoenlein purpura.** If the patient has skin purpura and acute abdominal problems without joint disease, he or she has **Henoch purpura.**

Synonyms
Anaphylactoid Purpura
Allergic Purpura
Hemorrhagic Capillary Toxicosis
Henoch-Schoenlein Purpura
Nonthrombocytopenic Idiopathic Purpura
Peliosis Rheumatica
Rheumatic Purpura

Signs and Symptoms Initially, the patient's skin reddens, swells, and develops hives, which are associated with capillary inflammation or hemorrhaging beneath the skin that produces a reddish-brown or reddish-purple appearance. In most patients, hives appear on the buttocks and lower extremities first and may then spread or worsen.

Patients may also experience fever and a general feeling of discomfort or weakness. Acute local pain can result if blood and plasma accumulate in the joints or abdomen. Gastrointestinal hemorrhaging may cause iron-deficiency anemia and other gastrointestinal disturbances, such as vomiting or blood in the stool.

Approximately 10 percent of patients have kidney inflammation or lesions that can appear at any time and signify a more severe form of the disorder. When the central nervous system is affected, the patient may suffer headaches, perceptual changes, and seizures.

Etiology Although the cause is not known, it is suggested that the disorder may be an extreme allergic reaction to certain foods, such as chocolate, milk, eggs, or beans; various drugs; or insect bites. Upper respiratory tract infection or rubella sometimes precedes the disease, but a causal link to viral infections has not been proved.

Epidemiology While Schoenlein-Henoch purpura can occur at any age, it most commonly occurs in childhood. Males are apparently affected slightly more often than females; one study showed a ratio of 35 males to 25 females.

Related Disorders Common purpura is the most prevalent type of purpura, occurring most often in women over age 50. Where there has been no injury, purpural lesions occur more often than subcutaneous bleeding. However, following surgery or even minor injury, blood vessel fragility results in excessive bleeding. The bleeding may be reduced by short-term corticosteroid therapy and, in postmenopausal women, estrogen.

Scurvy, a type of purpura, results from a deficiency of vitamin C in the diet. Patients suffer weakness, anemia, spongy gums, and a tendency to subcutaneous and mucous membrane hemorrhaging.

Gardener-Diamond syndrome, sometimes called painful bruising syndrome, is also a type of purpura which chiefly occurs in young women. An autoimmune association has been suggested.

Treatment—Standard If the cause of the disorder is found to be an allergic reaction, the patient should avoid the precipitant. Other therapy depends on symptoms. Mild childhood cases tend to improve spontaneously with age. Hemodialysis has been found to benefit some patients with renal failure. In most patients, the disease has a limited course and the prognosis is good.

Treatment—Investigational Adults with severe cases of this disorder have been experimentally treated with combination therapy of anticoagulants (heparin and acenocoumarol), corticosteroids, and immunosuppressants. Cyclophosphamide has been successfully used alone in a few patients. Plasmapheresis has been tried, but more research is needed.

Please contact the agencies listed under Resources, below, for the most current information.

Resources

For more information on Schoenlein-Henoch purpura: National Organization for Rare Disorders (NORD); National Kidney Foundation; NIH/National Institute of Allergy and Infectious Diseases (NIAID); NIH/National Heart, Lung and Blood Institute (NHLBI).

References

Schoenlein-Henoch Syndrome in Adults: D.A. Roth, et al.; Q. J. Med., May 1985, issue 55(217), pp. 145–152.

Clinical Aspects of the Nephropathy in Schoenlein-Henoch Syndrome: E. Verrina, et al.; Pediatr. Med. Chir., May–June 1986, issue 8(3), pp. 317–320.

Neurological Manifestations of Schoenlein-Henoch Purpura: Report of Three Cases and Review of the Literature: A.L. Belman, et al.; Pediatrics, April 1985, issue 75(4), pp. 687–692.

Purpura, Thrombotic Thrombocytopenic (TTP)

Description TTP is a rare blood disease characterized by an abnormally small number of platelets in the blood, abnormal destruction of erythrocytes, kidney dysfunction, nervous system disturbances, fever, and the presence of purpura in the skin and mucous membranes.

Synonyms
Moschowitz Disease

Signs and Symptoms Onset is often sudden, severe, and persistent. Normal blood flow may be blocked by platelets clotting the blood vessels of many of the patient's organs. Headaches, arthralgias, slight or partial paresis, changes in the patient's mental condition, seizures, and coma may also occur, as well as proteinuria, hematuria, and fever. Hemorrhaging in mucous membranes and skin causes purpura. Pallor, fatigue, weakness, nausea, vomiting, and abdominal pain are further signs and symptoms. Increased levels of creatinine are found in the blood of 50 percent of these patients.

Ten percent of patients suffer acute kidney failure. Urine flow decreases to a very low level, followed by shortness of breath, swelling of feet, fever, and headache. High blood pressure, heart and lung congestion, and brain metabolism alterations result from retention of salt and water in the blood. Irregular heartbeat can result from hyperkalemia.

Retinal abnormalities sometimes occur in women patients who take oral contraceptives, but clarity of vision is generally not affected. Female TTP patients may also have severe complications while they are pregnant.

Etiology While the precise cause is not known, studies have implicated some kind of autoimmune reaction or infectious agent. It has also been shown that the disease may be inherited in some cases, with TTP occurring in members of the same family many years apart. Other studies have shown a hormonal influence on the disease and that oral contraceptives and the menstrual cycle (**cyclic TTP**) may affect relapses. **AIDS** (acquired immunodeficiency syndrome), **ARC** (the AIDS-related complex), and **HIV** infection (human immunodeficiency virus) have also been shown to be causative factors.

Epidemiology TTP literally affects one in a million persons every year, two-thirds of them women who are mostly between the ages of 20 and 50. Individuals with HIV infection are more often affected. Pregnant women and persons with collagen-vascular diseases may occasionally develop TTP.

Related Disorders See *Hemolytic-Uremic Syndrome (HUS); Purpura, Idiopathic Thrombocytopenic (ITP); Purpura, Schoenlein-Henoch; Thrombocytopenia, Essential.*

The combination of TTP and hemolytic-uremic syndrome has been called **thrombotic microangiopathy** or **TTP-HUS complex.** Some researchers suggest that the two are really variations of the same disease.

Treatment—Standard Immediate diagnosis and treatment are important to the outcome. Prednisone is used as an antiinflammatory and immunosuppressant. Treatment also includes plasmapheresis or infusions of fresh-frozen plasma.

Patients and families genetically affected by this disorder should receive genetic counseling. Other treatments depend on symptoms.

Treatment—Investigational Whole blood exchange and splenectomy are being investigated as therapies. The immunosuppressive drug vincristine has been used for patients who do not respond to other therapy, as have the vasodilator dipyridamole and aspirin. Antiplatelet drugs have shown some promise, but their safety and efficacy are not yet known. An Italian pharmaceutical company has developed the orphan drug defibrotide for experimental use. For information, contact Crinos International, Via Belvedere 1, 22079 Villa Guardia, Como, Italy.

Please contact the agencies listed under Resources, below, for the most current information.

Resources

For more information on TTP: National Organization for Rare Disorders (NORD); NIH/National Heart, Lung and Blood Institute (NHLBI).

For genetic information and genetic counseling referrals: March of Dimes Birth Defects Foundation; National Center for Education in Maternal and Child Health (NCEMCH).

References

Internal Medicine, 3rd ed.: J.H. Stein, ed.-in-chief; Little, Brown and Company, 1990, pp. 1046–1047, 897.

Thrombotic Thrombocytopenic Purpura. A Review: S.J. Sierakow and E.J. Kucharz; Cor. Vasa., 1988, issue 30(1), pp. 60–72.

Thrombotic Thrombocytopenic Purpura in Patients with the Acquired Immunodeficiency Syndrome (AIDS)-Related Complex. A Report of Two Cases: J.M. Nair, et al.; Ann. Intern. Med., August 1, 1988, issue 109(3), pp. 209–212.

SCHWACHMAN SYNDROME

Description Schwachman syndrome is a digestive and respiratory disorder characterized by insufficient digestive enzymes and abnormally low leukocyte counts. Onset is usually in infancy or early childhood. Because the infant does not digest nutrients properly, short stature and other problems with bone growth, and chronic diarrhea may result. The patient usually suffers persistent respiratory and skin infections as well.

Synonyms

Burke Syndrome
Metaphyseal Dysostosis (Type B IV)
Neutropenia-Pancreatic Insufficiency
Schwachman-Diamond Syndrome

Signs and Symptoms The initial symptom of this syndrome is usually diarrhea. Affected infants frequently have respiratory and skin infections and tend to bleed easily. Some infants may fail to thrive or suffer anemia because of insufficient absorption of nutrients. One-third of patients are short of stature. Bone deformities that can impair walking occur in some.

Etiology While the exact cause of the spectrum of this disease is not known, studies have shown that the digestive and respiratory effects are due to insufficient amounts of digestive enzymes and leukocytes.

Epidemiology The syndrome begins to manifest itself in infancy or early childhood. Males and females appear to be equally affected.

Related Disorders See *Agranulocytosis, Acquired.*

The respiratory and digestive symptoms of Schwachman syndrome may mimic those of cystic fibrosis.

Treatment—Standard Antibiotics are used to treat infections, pancreatic enzymes are administered to correct enzyme deficiencies, and the patient is fed a diet high in protein, calories, and vitamins. Other therapy depends on symptoms.

Treatment—Investigational The severe chronic neutropenia which may develop responds to treatment with granulocyte-colony stimulating factor.

Please contact the agencies listed under Resources, below, for the most current information.

Resources

For more information on Schwachman syndrome: National Organization for Rare Disorders (NORD); NIH/National Institute of Diabetes, Digestive & Kidney Diseases Information Clearinghouse; Cystic Fibrosis Foundation; American Lung Association.

References

Pancreatic Lipomatosis in the Schwachman-Diamond Syndrome. Identification by Sonography and CT-Scan: E. Robberecht, et al.; Pediatr. Radiol., 1985, issue 15(5), pp. 348–349.

Cystic Fibrosis "Factor(s)": Present Also in Sera of Schwachman's Pancreatic Insufficiency: G. Banchini, et al.; Pediatr. Res., July 1981, issue 15(7), pp. 1073–1075.

Chronic Diarrhea and Neutropenia Not Associated with Pancreatic Insufficiency: A Non-Schwachman-Diamond Entity: L.R. Marino, et al.; J. Pediatr. Gastroenterol. Nutr., 1983, issue 2(3), pp. 559–562.

SICKLE CELL DISEASE

Description Any disease that results from the presence of sickle- or crescent-shaped erythrocytes in the peripheral blood is known as sickle cell disease. These abnormally shaped red blood cells become rigid and lodge in capillaries, preventing the flow of oxygen to tissue and organs and causing anemia. This disorder takes a number of forms, including sickle cell anemia, sickle cell-hemoglobin C disease, and sickle cell-thalassemia disease.

Synonyms

Hemolytic Anemia
Sickle Cell Anemia
Sickle Cell Trait
Thalassemia

Signs and Symptoms The features of sickle cell anemia, which is the most prevalent of the sickle cell diseases, are hemolytic anemia, acute attacks of pain, sickle cell dactylitis, lingering upper respiratory infection, pallor of tongue and lips, irritability, crying, poor eating habits, splenomegaly, hepatosplenomegaly, jaundice, stroke, scleral icterus, and hemic murmurs.

Onset in most patients is in the first 3 years of life. In patients ages 3 to 5, the signs of the disease are pain in the chest, abdomen, limbs, and joints that usually follows exposure to cold, overexertion, infection, or dehydration and is not accompanied by swelling; slow growth; and nosebleeds.

In adolescents and young adults, the signs include severe pain, delayed puberty, progressive anemia, leg ulcers, nosebleeds, dental disease, renal disease, aseptic necrosis of the femoral head, retinal lesions, and cardiac effects.

Individuals 20 and over experience painful episodes that may become less frequent with advancing age; leg ulcers; retinitis; and often gallbladder disease.

Both sickle cell-thalassemia disease and sickle cell-hemoglobin C disease are milder forms of sickle cell disease, and hemoglobin C disease is late in onset. Sickle cell trait occurs when an individual only inherits one sickle cell gene. Individuals who inherit one sickle cell gene are said to have sickle cell trait and are generally symptomless carriers of sickle cell disease.

Etiology Sickle cell disease is inherited through a recessive gene. Offspring of affected patients may or may not have the disease.

Epidemiology Of the estimated 50,000 persons in the United States who have sickle cell disease, most are Afro-Americans, although Asiatic Indians and Italians, Greeks, and others of Mediterranean ancestry are also afflicted. Sickle cell anemia affects 0.6 percent of the black population in the United States. Sickle cell trait is present in as much as 40 percent of the population in some areas of Africa. The incidence of sickle cell trait in those of African descent in the United States is 9 percent.

Treatment—Standard Specific treatment depends on symptoms. Patients are required to get regular checkups, avoid chills, dress warmly, eat balanced meals, get ample sleep, avoid standing in the cold without exercising, and practice deep breathing for 5 minutes before sleep. Vaccines against pneumococcal infections may be given to children over the age of 2. Cord blood screening is used to detect sickle cell disease in newborns, and hemoglobin electrophoresis can detect the major varieties of sickle cell disease.

Treatment—Investigational A number of treatments are being tested in an effort to raise levels of fetal hemoglobin in patients with sickle cell disease. One is hydroxyurea, an antineoplastic agent normally used against leukemia; another is erythropoietin, a protein that enhances erythropoiesis. Researchers are also investigating danazol, a gonadotropin inhibitor that may enable sickle cell erythrocytes to flow through very small capillaries. This drug is being tested by Dr. William Harrington of the University of Miami School of Medicine.

An orphan drug called poloxamer 188, N.F. (RheothRx Copolymer) is being tried as a treatment for acute episodes of pain from sickle cell anemia. It is manufactured by CytRx Corp., 150 Technology Parkway, Technology Park/Atlanta, Norcross, GA 30092. Studies are also being conducted on sandoglobulin as a treatment for sickle cell disease. The longterm effects and effectiveness of these treatments are not yet known.

Please contact the agencies listed under Resources, below, for the most current information.

Resources

For more information on sickle cell disease: National Organization for Rare Disorders (NORD); National Association for Sickle Cell Disease, Inc.; NIH/National Heart, Lung and Blood Institute (NHLBI); Cooley's Anemia Foundation, Inc.; The Canadian Sickle Cell Society.

For genetic information and genetic counseling referrals: March of Dimes Birth Defects Foundation; National Center for Education in Maternal and Child Health (NCEMCH).

References

Cecil Textbook of Medicine, 18th ed.: J.B. Wyngaarden and L.H. Smith, Jr., eds.; W.B. Saunders Company, 1988, pp. 149, 152, 936–942.

SQUAMOUS CELL CARCINOMA, CUTANEOUS

Description Squamous cell carcinoma is a common epithelial neoplasm that often occurs in sun-exposed skin. The carcinoma may also develop in mucous membranes and in fact anywhere on the body.

Signs and Symptoms Cutaneous squamous cell carcinoma is a red, scaly, sharply outlined keratosis that may develop on normal tissue or on precancerous leukoplakia. There may be satellite nodules. The tumor can reach to the lower reticular dermis.

Etiology The most common cause of cutaneous squamous cell carcinoma is exposure to the sun. The cancer may also arise on the site of preexisting lesions such as a scar from a burn or from trauma, or a lesion of systemic lupus erythematosus.

Epidemiology Males and females appear to be affected equally in cutaneous squamous cell carcinoma. Persons with fair complexions are the most vulnerable.

Related Disorders See *Malignant Melanoma; Bowen Disease.*

Basal cell carcinoma is a common skin cancer characterized by hard and shiny nodules, hardened scarlike patches that hemorrhage, or ulcerated and encrusted lesions.

Treatment—Standard Biopsy must be done to diagnose the tumor type.
Cutaneous squamous cell carcinoma is treated with excision or Moh's surgery.

Treatment—Investigational Please contact the agencies listed under Resources, below, for the most current information.

Resources
For more information on cutaneous squamous cell carcinoma: National Organization for Rare Disorders (NORD); NIH/National Cancer Institute PDQ (Physician Data Query) phoneline; The Skin Cancer Foundation; American Cancer Society.

References
Harrison's Principles of Internal Medicine, 12th ed.: J.D. Wilson, et al., eds.; McGraw-Hill, 1991, pp. 245–247, 1249, 1102–1109, 1211, 1633–1634.

Histologic Tumor Regression Grades in Squamous Cell Carcinoma of the Head and Neck after Preoperative Radiochemotherapy: O.M. Braun, et al.; Cancer, March 15, 1989, issue 63(6), pp. 1097–1100.

Ultrastructural Effects of Irradiation on Squamous Cell Carcinoma of the Head and Neck: P. Kellokumou-Lehtinen, et al.; Cancer, March 15, 1989, issue 63(6), pp. 1108–1118.

Treatment of Recurrent Squamous Cell Carcinoma of the Head and Neck with Low Doses of Interleukin-2 Injected Perilymphatically: G. Cortesina, et al.; Cancer, December 15, 1989, issue 62(12), pp. 2482–2485.

THALASSEMIA MAJOR

Description Characterized by a marked increase in F hemoglobin and decreased synthesis of the beta polypeptide chains in the hemoglobin molecule, thalassemia major is the most severe form of chronic familial hemolytic anemias found originally in persons living in the Mediterranean basin. Patients also have a decreased number of erythrocytes.

Synonyms
Beta Thalassemia Major
Cooley Anemia
Erythroblastotic Anemia of Childhood
Hemolytic Anemia
Hereditary Leptocytosis

Mediterranean Anemia
Target Cell Anemia
Thalassemia

Signs and Symptoms Symptoms, which occur insidiously and generally in infancy or early childhood, include generalized weakness, malaise, dyspepsia, and palpitations. Patients may be jaundiced and suffer from leg ulcers, hepatomegaly, splenomegaly, cholelithiasis, and an enlarged abdomen. Hyperactive bone marrow growth may result in thickened cranial bones and prominent cheek bones. Osteoporosis may occur in the long bones, and pathologic fractures are common. Patients may be underdeveloped and short in stature for their age. Iron deposits in the cardiac muscle can cause cardiac dysfunction and eventual cardiac failure. Patients may show mental deterioration. Intercurrent infections may cause additional complications.

Etiology Thalassemia major is a congenital disorder inherited as an autosomal recessive trait. Homozygotic individuals are more severely afflicted than heterozygotic ones. The disorder is more prevalent among those families who intermarry and in those whose parents both have genes for thalassemia minor.

Epidemiology Thalassemia major most commonly occurs in individuals of Mediterranean ancestry, especially Italians and Greeks, and in an area that extends from northern Africa and southern Europe to Thailand, including Iran, Iraq, Indonesia, and southern China.

Treatment—Standard Patients are treated for severe anemia; chronic blood transfusions are necessary to maintain the hemoglobin above 10 gm percent and to allow for normal growth. Splenectomy may help patients with splenomegaly by reducing the number of blood transfusions required. To avoid iron overload, children should be given daily administration of deferoxamine.

Treatment—Investigational Several iron chelating compounds are being clinically investigated for thalassemia major therapy. Bone marrow transplantation is also under investigation.

Please contact the agencies listed under Resources, below, for the most current information.

Resources

For more information on thalassemia major: National Organization for Rare Disorders (NORD); National Association for Sickle Cell Disease Inc.; Cooley's Anemia Foundation, Inc.; NIH/National Heart, Lung, and Blood Institute.

For genetic information and genetic counseling referrals: March of Dimes Birth Defects Foundation; National Center for Education in Maternal and Child Health (NCEMCH).

References
Cecil Textbook of Medicine, 18th ed.: J.B. Wyngaarden and L.H. Smith, Jr., eds.; W.B. Saunders Company, 1988, pp. 149, 930–936.

THALASSEMIA MINOR

Description A relatively mild form of anemia that is both congenital and familial, thalassemia minor is the heterozygous state of a thalassemia gene.

Synonyms
> Beta Thalassemia Minor
> Hereditary Leptocytosis
> Heterozygous Beta Thalassemia
> Thalassemia

Signs and Symptoms Persistent fatigue may be the only sign of this disorder. However, if anemia becomes severe, the patient may have slight splenomegaly and pallor, and occasionally complain of pain in the left upper quadrant of the abdomen. The life span of patients is normal. The disease may be exacerbated when the patient is under stress, suffers infections or malnutrition, or is pregnant.

Etiology Thalassemia minor is inherited as an autosomal recessive trait.

Epidemiology The disorder most commonly occurs in persons of Mediterranean or southern Chinese descent. The occurrence rate in some Italian populations is as high as 20 percent.

Related Disorders See *Thalassemia Major.*

Treatment—Standard Treatment is generally not necessary. Iron therapy is ineffective and might be detrimental; prolonged administration of parenteral iron could result in excess iron storage. Pregnant women might require blood transfusions during pregnancy to maintain hemoglobin levels.

Treatment—Investigational Please contact the agencies listed under Resources, below, for the most current information.

Resources
   For more information on thalassemia minor: National Organization for Rare Disorders (NORD); National Association for Sickle Cell Disease Inc.; Cooley's Anemia Foundation, Inc.; NIH/National Heart, Lung and Blood Institute.
   For genetic information and genetic counseling referrals: March of Dimes Birth Defects Foundation; National Center for Education in Maternal and Child Health (NCEMCH).

References
   Cecil Textbook of Medicine, 18th ed.: J.B. Wyngaarden and L.H. Smith, Jr., eds.; W.B. Saunders Company, 1988, pp. 147, 930–936, 1038.

THROMBASTHENIA

Description Thrombasthenia is an inherited coagulation disorder that causes hemorrhage due to abnormal functioning of platelets. A variety of genetic abnormalities may cause the disease. The condition is not progressive and seems to improve with age. However, if prolonged hemorrhaging is not treated successfully, the patient's life may be endangered.

Synonyms
Diacyclothrombopathia
Glanzmann Disease
Glanzmann-Naegeli Syndrome

Signs and Symptoms Beginning at birth or shortly thereafter, thrombasthenia patients tend to bleed easily and profusely, particularly after injury and during surgery, and are susceptible to developing bruises and large purplish spots on the skin that are caused by subcutaneous bleeding. They may also suffer nosebleeds, unusually heavy menstrual flow, and irregular uterine bleeding with varying degrees of severity. Laboratory results show that platelets are abnormal in appearance, fail to aggregate normally, and evidence unusual retraction of clots.

Etiology Thrombasthenia is a congenital disorder transmitted either through autosomal dominant or recessive genes. Researchers have found 4 different genetic abnormalities that they associate with thrombasthenia.

Related Disorders Related disorders of abnormal platelet function are Bernard-Soulier syndrome, May-Hegglin anomaly, Chédiak-Higashi syndrome, the gray platelet syndrome, and various defects related to collagen-induced platelet aggregation. See ***Bernard-Soulier Syndrome; May-Hegglin Anomaly; Chédiak-Higashi Syndrome.*** Platelet disorders have also been linked with such congenital conditions as Wiskott-Aldrich syndrome, Down syndrome, thrombocytopenia with absent radius syndrome, and von Willebrand disease.

Treatment—Standard When hemorrhaging is severe, the standard therapy is transfusion of platelets from a normal donor.

Treatment—Investigational Please contact the agencies listed under Resources, below, for the most current information.

Resources
For more information on thrombasthenia: National Organization for Rare Disorders (NORD); NIH/National Heart, Lung and Blood Institute (NHLBI).

For genetic information and genetic counseling referrals: March of Dimes Birth Defects Foundation; National Center for Education in Maternal and Child Health (NCEMCH).

References
Cecil Textbook of Medicine, 18th ed.: J.B. Wyngaarden and L.H. Smith, Jr., eds.; W.B. Saunders Company, 1988, pp. 1056–1057.

THROMBOCYTHEMIA, ESSENTIAL

Description Essential thrombocythemia is a rare blood platelet disorder characterized by abnormally increased circulating platelets and associated thrombosis, hemorrhaging, and splenomegaly.

Synonyms
    Essential Hemorrhagic Thrombocythemia
    Essential Thrombocytosis
    Idiopathic Thrombocythemia
    Primary Thrombocythemia

Signs and Symptoms Bleeding occurs in two-thirds of patients, as a result of abnormal platelet function. These patients may experience epistaxis, easy bruising, or bleeding in the gastrointestinal tract. Thrombosis may produce peripheral vascular ischemia such as pulmonary emboli and deep vein thrombosis as well as digital ischemia, or central nervous system ischemia that includes transient ischemic attacks (TIAs), headache, and dizziness. Splenomegaly is present in about one-half of patients.

Etiology While the precise cause of this disorder is not known, some patients have been shown to have inherited it as an autosomal dominant genetic trait.

Epidemiology Men and women are affected in equal numbers, usually in their 50s or 60s, although symptoms can occur at any age.

Related Disorders See *Thrombocytopenia, Essential.*

Treatment—Standard Hydroxyurea is the treatment of choice, since other effective agents (e.g., radioactive phosphorus) have been associated with risk of neoplasms.

Other therapy depends on symptoms. In cases of genetic transmission, patients and their families should receive genetic counseling.

Treatment—Investigational An orphan drug, Anagrelide, is being tested for use against essential thrombocythemia. The manufacturer is Bristol-Myers, 5 Research Parkway, P.O. Box 5100, Wallingford, Connecticut 06492.

Plateletpheresis is also being used experimentally to treat this disorder, but its safety and effectiveness over the long term have not yet been determined.

Please contact the agencies listed under Resources, below, for the most current information.

Resources

For more information on essential thrombocythemia: National Organization for Rare Disorders (NORD); Myeloproliferative Disease Foundation; NIH/National Heart, Lung and Blood Institute (NHLBI).

For genetic information and genetic counseling referrals: March of Dimes Birth Defects Foundation; NIH/National Center for Education in Maternal and Child Health (NCEMCH).

References

Mendelian Inheritance in Man, 9th ed.: V.A. McKusick; The Johns Hopkins University Press, 1990, pp. 910–911.

Internal Medicine, 3rd ed.: J.H. Stein, ed.-in-chief; Little, Brown and Company, 1990, p. 1128.

Essential Thrombocythemias. Clinical Evolutionary and Biological Data: S. Bellucci, et al.; Cancer, December 1986, issue 58(11), pp. 2440–2447.

Essential Thrombocythemia and Leukemic Transformation: S. M. Sedlacek, et al.; Medicine (Baltimore), November 1986, issue 65(6), pp. 353–364.

Clinical Presentation and Natural History of Patients with Essential Thrombocythemia and the Philadelphia Chromosome: D.B. Stoll, et al.; Am. J. Hematol., February 1988, issue 27(2), pp. 77–83.

THROMBOCYTOPENIA, ESSENTIAL

Description Essential thrombocytopenia is a rare blood platelet disorder characterized by an abnormally small number of circulating platelets (less than 150 x 10^9 per liter) that survive for a shorter than normal time (10 days). Excessive hemorrhaging in the mucous membranes or skin, especially at the time of menstruation, also is characteristic.

Signs and Symptoms Excessive hemorrhaging is the chief symptom, especially purpura under the skin, in the eyes, and in the mucous membranes of the mouth, and, in extreme cases, hemorrhaging in the skull. Patients bruise easily and have sudden nosebleeds. Tiny petechiae form in mild cases around the ankles and feet, but become more widespread and enlarged in more severe cases. Uncontrolled hemorrhaging causes anemia, fatigue, weakness, and symptoms of congestive heart failure. However, massive extravasation such as happens in hemophilia does not occur in thrombocytopenia.

Etiology The major causes of thrombocytopenia are decreased platelet production, increased platelet destruction, and platelet sequestration by the spleen.

Platelet production can be impaired as a result of B12 or folate deficiency, generalized disease in the bone marrow, viral infections, a toxic reaction or hypersensitivity to drugs, systemic infections, malignant disease, or aplastic anemia.

Increased platelet destruction can be immune-mediated, induced by drugs such as hydrocortisone, aspirin, thiazide diuretics, quinine, cyclophosphamide, prednisone, azathioprine, tricyclic antidepressants, indomethacin, phenylbutazone, antihistamines, vincristine, or phenothiazines; or there may be alloantibody or autoantibody precipitants. Nonimmune-related platelet destruction may result from disorders such as thrombotic thrombocytopenic purpura or disseminated intravascular coagulation, or be related to extracorporeal circulation or prosthetic intravascular devices.

Sequestration of platelets by the spleen causes thrombocytopenia and results in splenomegaly.

Epidemiology Both males and females are equally affected by this disorder.

Related Disorders See *Chédiak-Higashi Syndrome; Anemia, Fanconi;*

Hemophilia; May-Hegglin Anomaly; von Willebrand Disease; Thrombocy-topenia-Absent Radius (TAR) Syndrome.

Kasabach-Merritt syndrome is characterized by hemorrhages in the eyes and skin, hemangiomas, and some cutaneous features of thrombocytopenic purpura.

Treatment—Standard Transfusions of normal platelets are given to control hemorrhage, and intravenous injections of immune globulin are given to stimulate platelet production. In rare instances, splenectomy is performed. When the underlying cause of thrombocytopenia is another disease, platelet production improves with successful treatment of that disease. Patients should avoid drugs that inhibit platelet function, such as antiinflammatory agents and certain salicylates.

Treatment—Investigational Plasmapheresis has been used experimentally for extreme cases, but its safety and efficacy are still being investigated. The orphan drug Anagrelide is also being tried experimentally for thrombocytopenia. The manufacturer is Bristol-Myers, 5 Research Parkway, P.O. Box 5100, Wallingford, Connecticut 06492.

Please contact the agencies listed under Resources, below, for the most current information.

Resources

For more information on essential thrombocytopenia: National Organization for Rare Disorders (NORD); NIH/National Heart, Lung and Blood Institute (NHLBI).

For more information on TAR syndrome only, not other forms of thrombocytopenia: Thrombocytopenia-Absent Radius Syndrome Association (TARSA).

For genetic information and genetic counseling referrals: March of Dimes Birth Defects Foundation; NIH/National Center for Education in Maternal and Child Health (NCEMCH).

References

Internal Medicine, 3rd ed.: J.H. Stein, ed.-in-chief; Little, Brown and Company, 1990, pp. 1044–1048.

Successful Intravenous Immune Globulin Therapy for Human Immunodeficiency Virus-Associated Thrombocytopenia: A.N Pollak, et al.; Arch. Intern. Med., March 1988, issue 148(3), pp. 695–697.

Splenectomy for Thrombocytopenia due to Secondary Hypersplenism: W.W. Coon; Arch. Surg., March 1988, issue 148(3), pp. 369–371.

Successful Conservative Management of Thrombocytopenia in Adult Hemophiliacs: J.C. Goldsmith, et al.; Transfusion, January–February 1988, issue 28(1), pp. 68–69.

TONGUE CARCINOMA

Description Tongue carcinoma is a malignant oral neoplasm characterized by an ulcerating squamous cell tumor that is usually located on the side of the tongue and which can metastasize to the same side of the neck.

Synonyms
Cancer of the Tongue

Signs and Symptoms The lesion that appears bleeds easily, fails to heal, and may become painful. The pain may eventually spread throughout the side of the face. The patient's tongue may become restricted in movement. About one-half of patients experience ipsilateral lymph-node enlargement if the tumor metastasizes to the neck.

Etiology Increased risk for tongue carcinoma is associated with excessive alcohol consumption, excessive use of tobacco, syphilis, herpes simplex virus, and human papillomavirus. Leukoplakia and erythroplasia are precancerous lesions that may progress to carcinoma.

Epidemiology Tongue carcinoma is rare. Males are affected more often than females, although the number of females affected has risen in recent years. Age at onset is generally between 40 and 60, and the incidence tends to increase with age.

Related Disorders Carcinoma of the floor of the mouth, another rare malignant neoplasm, is characterized by a hard tumor often felt with the tip of the patient's tongue. Symptoms include increased salivation, ear pain, difficulty in speaking, and, ultimately, bleeding. Lymph nodes in the neck are frequently affected. Poor oral hygiene and tobacco use are suspected causes.

Carcinoma of the cheek (mouth or buccal mucosa) is a malignant neoplasm marked by a buccal lesion, trismus, pain, mucosal bleeding, and difficulty in chewing. The neoplasm can metastasize to lymph glands beneath the jaw.

Treatment—Standard Treatment may be by surgical excision of the lingual muscle and cervical lymph nodes, possibly combined with pre- or postoperative radiation therapy. Interstitial irradiation and chemotherapy may also be beneficial. Twenty-eight percent of patients survive 5 years. Early diagnosis and treatment are keys to survival, particularly if the patient is under 20 years of age.

Treatment—Investigational Please contact the agencies listed under Resources, below, for the most current information.

Resources
For more information on tongue carcinoma: National Organization for Rare Disorders (NORD); American Cancer Society; NIH/National Cancer Institute PDQ (Physician Data Query) phoneline.

References
Harrison's Principles of Internal Medicine, 12th ed.: J.D. Wilson, et al., eds.; McGraw-Hill, 1991, pp. 245–248.

Surgical Treatment of Early-Stage Carcinoma of the Oral Tongue–Would Wound Adjuvant Treatment be Beneficial? Head and Neck Surgery, July–August 1986, issue 8(6), pp. 401–408.

Changing Trends in the Management of Squamous Carcinoma of the Tongue: C.D. Callery, et al.; Amer. J. of Surgery, October 1984, issue 148(4), pp. 449–454.

What You Need to Know about Cancer of the Mouth: U.S. Department of Health and Human Services, Public Health Service, National Institutes of Health, National Cancer Institute; March 1985.

VON WILLEBRAND DISEASE

Description An inherited coagulation disease that usually arises in infancy or early childhood, von Willebrand disease is characterized by prolonged bleeding and abnormally slow blood clotting time due a deficiency of factor VIII and von Willebrand factor protein combined with a morphologic defect of platelets.

Synonyms
> Angiohemophilia
> Constitutional Thrombopathy
> Minot-von Willebrand Disease
> Pseudohemophilia
> Vascular Hemophilia
> Willebrand-Juergens Disease

Signs and Symptoms Prolonged bleeding usually occurs in the nose or gastrointestinal tract. Patients bruise easily and bleed excessively after injury, menstruation, childbirth, surgery, and some dental procedures. Hemarthrosis also occurs, but rarely.

Etiology Inheritance is both autosomal dominant and recessive, and an X-linked form has also been reported. Abnormal coagulation and excessive bleeding result from deficiency in the production of factor VIII and von Willebrand factor plus a platelet abnormality. A similar disorder, acquired in adulthood, results from overproduction of von Willebrand factor antibodies. Associated disorders include certain renal diseases, congenital cardiac disease that involves a defective heart valve, and one type of leukemia.

Epidemiology Onset is usually in infancy or early childhood, although some nonhereditary forms can be acquired in adulthood. The disease tends to affect more females than males.

Related Disorders See *Hemophilia.*

Treatment—Standard Intravenous injections of frozen or stored plasma or whole blood are administered to increase the levels of factor VIII and von Willebrand factor in the patient's blood to aid coagulation. Transfusions of blood or plasma before childbirth or surgery or after an accident or unexplained bleeding are given to reduce the risk of hemorrhage. Patients with mild cases have been given daily doses of the synthetic blood agent desmopressin acetate (**DDAVP**) before surgery to shorten clotting time by stimulating the release of factor VIII molecules from cells that line the blood vessels. Injectable DDAVP, which is an antidiuretic peptide, is available from Rorer Pharmaceutical Corp., Fort Washington, Pennsylvania.

Cryoprecipitates may be given to control excess bleeding in some cases, but careful monitoring of dosage is required. For severe cases, cryoprecipitates are the most effective means of replacing factor VIII. Aminocaproic acid can also be given to reduce bleeding.

Patients are advised to wear a medical identification bracelet that includes information about the medications used to treat the disease. Patients should also avoid drugs that prolong bleeding, aspirin, and any activities that are likely to result in injury. Most patients can lead a normal life if they receive proper treatment and take the necessary precautions. Generally, the bleeding tendencies will decrease with age. Patients and their families should receive genetic counseling.

Treatment—Investigational Under investigation as a treatment for von Willebrand disease is intranasal administration of a form of DDAVP. In addition, the use of coagglutinin is being studied by Marjorie Read, Ph.D., at the University of North Carolina in Chapel Hill, under a grant from the Food and Drug Administration.

Please contact the agencies listed under Resources, below, for the most current information.

Resources
For more information on von Willebrand disease: National Organization for Rare Disorders (NORD); NIH/National Heart, Lung and Blood Institute (NHLBI).

Although von Willebrand disease is not a form of hemophilia, national health agencies providing information, referrals, and support groups for von Willebrand disease are organizations that are primarily concerned with hemophilia: National Hemophilia Foundation; Canadian Hemophilia Society; World Federation of Hemophilia; The Haemophilia Society.

For genetic information and genetic counseling referrals: March of Dimes Birth Defects Foundation; National Center for Education in Maternal and Child Health (NCEMCH).

References
Mendelian Inheritance in Man, 9th ed.: V.A. McKusick; The Johns Hopkins University Press, 1990, pp. 972–976, 1530–1531, 1732.

A Human Myeloma-Produced Monoclonal Protein Directed Against the Active Subpopulation of von Willebrand Factor: E.G. Bovill, et al.; Am. J. Clin. Pathol., January 1986, issue 85(1), pp. 115–123.

Von Willebrand's Disease and Pregnancy: Management During Delivery and Outcome of Offspring: J.R. Chediak, et al.; Am. J. Obstet. Gynecol., September 1986, issue 155(3), pp. 618–624.

Von Willebrand Syndrome: I. Scharrer; Behring Inst. Mitt., February 1986, issue 79, pp. 12–23.

WEGENER GRANULOMATOSIS

Description Wegener granulomatosis is a multisystem disease characterized primarily by necrotizing vasculitis of the lung and upper respiratory tract, and glomerulonephritis. There is a range of symptom severity, and the disease can be limited to one or more systems.

Synonyms
Lethal Midline Granuloma
Necrotizing Respiratory Granulomatosis
Pathergic Granulomatosis

Signs and Symptoms Upper respiratory tract involvement is usually the initial presentation, with sinusitis and bloody and purulent discharge that do not respond to antibiotics. Accompanying early symptoms and signs include fever, malaise, and weight loss. Nasal mucosal ulceration may be present, with septal deterioration that results in saddle nose deformity.

The eyes may be involved, with findings that include conjunctivitis, episcleritis, optic neuritis, ciliary vessel vasculitis, and occlusion of the retinal artery. Aseptic meningitis and cranial nerve lesions have been reported. Cardiac involvement includes pericarditis and myocardial infarctions due to coronary arteritis. Skin lesions occur in a variety of forms that include papules, a purpuric rash, and ulcers. Arthralgias occur in about half of the cases. Pulmonary cavitations are seen on x-ray.

Renal disease, present in 85 percent of patients, is the most grave development. Hematuria, proteinuria, and red cell casts may be seen initially, but without treatment the initial mild glomerulonephritis progresses to rapid renal failure.

Some patients with the limited form of the disorder have only nasal and pulmonary lesions with little or no systemic involvement.

Etiology The cause is not determined. Delayed hypersensitivity and immune complex mediation seem to be associated. No viral, bacterial, or other causative agent has been identified.

Epidemiology Wegener granulomatosis can occur at any age. Males are affected twice as often as females.

Related Disorders These include glomerulonephritis, the other vasculitides, Goodpasture syndrome, and some granulomatous diseases.

Treatment—Standard Early diagnosis and treatment are important because of the possible rapid progression to renal failure. Cyclophosphamide is the drug of choice, but azathioprine and chlorambucil are useful also. Today, 90 percent of those treated with cyclophosphamide and prednisone experience complete remission.

Duration of therapy depends on the patient's response. Leukocytes are monitored closely, and therapeutic dosages are reduced gradually to prevent leukopenia. When the patient has been free of symptoms for one year, attempts should be made to discontinue therapy. When medications are being reduced or discontinued, careful monitoring for relapse of the kidney disease should be conducted. Complete, longterm remissions are often achieved with drug therapy, even in cases of advanced disease. Kidney transplantation has been successful in cases with kidney failure.

For nonrenal symptoms, corticosteroids can be used intermittently in conjunction with the cytotoxic drugs. Pulmonary symptoms may improve or worsen spontaneously.

Treatment—Investigational The National Institute of Allergy and Infectious Diseases is studying treatment for Wegener granulomatosis. NIH will pay for treatment and travel for patients who are at least 14 years old and who have recently developed symptoms. For more information, contact Gary S. Hoffman, M.D., or Randi Y. Levitt, M.D., at NIH/National Institute of Allergy and Infectious Diseases, Building 10, Room 11813, 9000 Rockville Pike, Bethesda, Maryland 20892; (301) 496-1124.

Please contact the agencies listed under Resources, below, for the most current information.

Resources

For more information on Wegener granulomatosis: National Organization for Rare Disorders (NORD); Wegener Granulomatosis Support Group; Wegener Foundation; National Heart, Lung and Blood Institute (NHLBI); The National Kidney Foundation; American Lung Association.

References
Harrison's Principles of Internal Medicine, 12th ed.: J.D. Wilson, et al., eds.; McGraw-Hill, 1991, pp. 1460–1461.

WILMS TUMOR

Description Wilms tumor, the most common malignant renal neoplasm in children, is characterized by abdominal pain and swelling. Current therapy results in a longterm survival rate of close to 80 percent, depending on the child's general health and his or her age at the time of detection.

Synonyms
> Embryoma Kidney
> Embryonal Adenomyosarcoma Kidney
> Embryonal Carcinosarcoma Kidney
> Embryonal Mixed Tumor Kidney
> Nephroblastoma

Signs and Symptoms Initially, patients are usually asymptomatic, but in later stages of the disease, pallor, appetite loss, weight loss, low-grade fever, lethargy, hematuria, and abdominal swelling occur, along with pain that may be sudden or sharp, or intermittent and slight. The child may also have developmental anomalies, including hemihypertrophy (in approximately 3 percent of patients), genitourinary defects (in about 5 percent), and aniridia (in about 10 percent).

Etiology While the cause of Wilms tumor is unknown, evidence suggests that both hereditary and nonhereditary forms exist. It is believed that the hereditary type affects both kidneys or several areas of one kidney, with onset at an early age due to a genetic abnormality that results in a fetal kidney defect. Studies suggest a link between the growth of Wilms tumor and a deleted section of chromosome 11 (p13); the location of the gene that controls this growth is still being sought.

Epidemiology Wilms tumor comprises 6 to 8 percent of all malignant neoplasms in children; it strikes about 1:10,000 children in the United States. The disease affects equal numbers of boys and girls, who are mainly under age 7 and most frequently between ages 1 and 4.

Treatment—Standard Surgery (including nephrectomy) combined with radiation therapy and chemotherapy has proved to be successful in treating most patients. The antineoplastic drugs vincristine and actinomycin D are used to reduce the tumors. Two-year survival without recurrence of disease is considered a cure; 70 to 80 percent of treated patients survive for 2 years or more. The outlook is less promising, however, for a small number of children who have aggressive or widespread forms of the disease; but intensive therapy can lead to longterm survival.

Treatment—Investigational The National Cancer Institute has funded The National Wilms Tumor Study among a group of hospitals and clinics nationwide. Findings of this study are the basis for treatment standards for this disease. Present research is investigating ways to improve care for patients with metastatic disease or who are at high risk because they have certain cell types.

Please contact the agencies listed under Resources, below, for the most current information.

Resources

For more information on Wilms tumor: National Organization for Rare Disorders (NORD); The National Kidney Foundation; American Cancer Society; NIH/National Cancer Institute PDQ (Physician Data Query) phoneline.

References

Adult Kidney Cancer and Wilms' Tumor. Research Report: U.S. Department of Health and Human Services, Public Health Service, National Cancer Institute, National Institutes of Health.

X-LINKED LYMPHOPROLIFERATIVE (XLP) SYNDROME

Description A rare genetic disease, XLP syndrome is a life-threatening condition of the immune system in males that exposes them to death from mononucleosis caused by Epstein-Barr virus.

Synonyms

Duncan Disease
Epstein-Barr Infection, Familial Fatal
Immunodeficiency 5

Signs and Symptoms Patients are usually asymptomatic until they are infected with the Epstein-Barr virus. Symptoms include fever, pharyngitis, lymphadenopathy, and hepatosplenomegaly. The mononucleosis can be life-threatening and the patients are vulnerable to other potentially fatal disorders, such as hypogammaglobulinemia and lymphoma. Death can result in 60 to 75 percent of XLP patients after they contract one of these diseases.

Etiology A rare inherited recessive defect on the X chromosome is believed to be the cause; however, scientists have not yet found the precise location of the defect. Only males who carry the defect and are infected by Epstein-Barr virus are affected.

Related Disorders See *Agammaglobulinemias, Primary.*

Infectious mononucleosis is caused by the Epstein-Barr virus. It is characterized by extreme fatigue, fever, swollen lymph glands, and an unusual proliferation of leukocytes in the blood. Tests are sometimes necessary to distinguish these leukocytes from certain leukemia cells. Mild forms are difficult to diagnose. Patients usually recover after 6 to 8 weeks or longer without treatment.

Malignant lymphoma is a malignant neoplasm that arises from the normal sites containing lymphoreticular cells, such as the spleen and lymph nodes. The disease may infiltrate the blood and mimic leukemia or it can be found in virtually any part of the body. The different varieties of lymphoma are distinguished by their nodular pattern, degrees of differentiation, and cell type.

Treatment—Standard Treatment depends on symptoms. Gammaglobulin is given to boost the patient's immune system when hypogammaglobulinemia occurs. Patients and their families should receive genetic counseling.

Treatment—Investigational Interferon-gamma is under investigation as a treatment, but further study is necessary. DNA probes are being used to try to determine the location of the defective gene.

Please contact the agencies listed under Resources, below, for the most current information.

Resources

For more information on X-linked lymphoproliferative syndrome: National Organization for Rare Disorders (NORD); NIH/National Institute of Allergy and Infectious Diseases.

For information on participation in genetic studies: James Skare, M.D., Boston University School of Medicine, Center for Human Genetics, Boston, Massachusetts 02118.

For genetic information and genetic counseling referrals: March of Dimes Birth Defects Foundation; NIH/National Center for Education in Maternal and Child Health (NCEMCH).

References

Mendelian Inheritance in Man, 9th ed.: V.A. McKusick; The Johns Hopkins University Press, 1990, pp. 1654–1655.

Markers Mapped for Life-Threatening Disorder: James Skare, Research Resources Reporter, National Institutes of Health, June 1989, issue XIII(6), pp. 6–7.

Malignant Lymphoma in the X-Linked Lymphoproliferative Syndrome: D.S. Harrington, et al.; Cancer, April 15, 1987, issue 59(8), pp. 1419–1429.

Epstein-Barr Virus Infections in Males with the X-Linked Lymphoproliferative Syndrome: H. Grierson, et al.; Ann. Intern. Med., April 1987, issue 106(4), pp. 538–545.

X-Linked Lymphoproliferative Disease: A Karyotype Analysis: A. Harris, et al.; Cytogenet. Cell Genet., 1988, issue 47(1-2), pp. 92–94.

Interferon-Gamma in a Family with X-Linked Lymphoproliferative Syndrome with Acute Epstein-Barr Virus Infection: M. Okano, et al.; J. Clin. Immunol., January 1989, issue 9(1), pp. 48–54.

6 | IMMUNOLOGIC DISORDERS AND INFECTIOUS DISEASES
By Robert Fekety, M.D.

The approach to diagnosis of rare infectious and immunologic diseases is no different from that of other diseases. Taking a complete history from the patient plus doing a thorough physical examination will often point to the salient feature of the illness. The differential diagnosis can then be built around that feature. Attention to the family history and social history may add important clues. Where has the patient traveled? What birds or animals have been contacted? What is the patient at risk of acquiring because of his or her occupation and hobbies? Also, the importance of an expert, detailed, and sensitive sexual history cannot be overemphasized. Patients should be asked whether they ever have sexual relations with members of the same sex, not whether they are gay or homosexual.

The travel history may help to suggest diseases indigenous to certain countries. A good up-to-date textbook of tropical and geographic medicine is useful for browsing once a few likely diseases have come to mind. What other diseases are listed in the differential of that disease? Do they occur in the countries visited by the patient? What other diseases are known to occur in that country?

Armed with these clues, one can peruse the standard texts on those conditions. The clinician can then begin to order pertinent common laboratory tests and radiologic studies, or even begin some empiric therapy, depending upon the patient's condition.

A special plea should be made at this point for obtaining a consult from clinical microbiology or clinical immunology laboratory personnel. They can often suggest an additional diagnosis or two. Even more important is the fact that if they know what diseases are under consideration, they can obtain cultures in the most appropriate media and incubate them for an appropriate time and at the proper temperature and atmospheric conditions. In a mixed culture, the suspect organism is less likely to be overlooked if it is suspected beforehand.

The serology laboratory may also be able to suggest the best serologic or skin tests for diagnosing the diseases in question.

Patients with eosinophilia often have immunologic or parasitic diseases. Proper ways to obtain and transport stool specimens are critical in making many of these diagnoses. The Parasitology Branch of the Centers for Disease Control in Atlanta can provide a battery of special serologic tests designed to aid in diagnosis of diseases causing eosinophilia. Their help may be invaluable.

In many cases, it may be necessary to obtain one or more biopsies for diagnosis. The pathologist should become a close collaborator in the elucidation of the problem.

Empiric therapy is, for the most part, a poor way to reach a diagnosis. "Gut reactions" or "shotgun approaches" are to be discouraged.

It has been said that "You don't have to be smart to be a good doctor. What you have to do if you're not brilliant is to apply to the diagnostic problem the simple system all of us learned in medical school." This is what is outlined above. If you do this, "The System" will make the brilliant diagnosis for you. Try it.

IMMUNOLOGIC DISORDERS AND INFECTIOUS DISEASES
Listings in This Section

ACANTHOCHEILONEMIASIS

Description Acanthocheilonemiasis is a mild parasitic infection caused by the tissue nematode *Acanthocheilonema perstans*, and found most commonly in Africa.

Synonyms
Dipetalonemiasis

Signs and Symptoms Infection with *A. perstans* is usually asymptomatic. Symptoms appear to be more frequent in visitors to endemic regions, rather than in native populations. One common presentation is asymptomatic eosinophilia in a tourist on return from an endemic region.

When symptoms occur they may include pruritis, abdominal pain, chest pain, myalgias, and subcutaneous swellings. Physical examination may reveal hepatosplenomegaly, and eosinophilia is the rule. The adult worm lodges in the subserous tissues of the abdomen and thorax, where local inflammatory and immune reactions give rise to pleuritis, pericarditis, and the symptoms described above.

Microfilariae of *A. perstans* can be isolated from the blood. The usual means of diagnosis is examination of a thick blood smear for these organisms.

Etiology The causative organism is a filarial worm, *Acanthocheilonema perstans*, also referred to as *Dipetalonema perstans*. It is transmitted by a small black midge, *A. Cailicoides.*

Epidemiology *A. perstans* is common in central Africa, and in some areas of South America.

Treatment—Standard Diethylcarbamazine is the treatment of choice. Surgical removal of large adult worms is occasionally necessary. Mild cases do not require treatment.

Treatment—Investigational Please contact the agencies listed under Resources, below, for the most current information.

Resources
   For more information on acanthocheilonemiasis: National Organization for Rare Disorders (NORD); NIH/National Institute of Allergy and Infectious Diseases; Centers for Disease Control (CDC).

References
Diethylcarbamazine and New Compounds for the Treatment of Filariasis: Adv. Pharmacol. Chemother., 1979, vol. 16(129), p. 94.

ACQUIRED IMMUNE DEFICIENCY SYNDROME (AIDS)

Description AIDS is an immunosuppressive disorder caused by infection with the human immunodeficiency virus (**HIV**). The immune deficiency results from viral infection and destruction of specific T cells. HIV infection is characterized initially by a long asymptomatic period. This may be followed by the development of generalized lymphadenopathy. Eventually most patients experience a syndrome of constitutional symptoms (fatigue, weight loss, rashes), which has been referred to as the AIDS-related complex or **ARC**. The endstage of HIV infection is marked by progressive depression of T cell immunity; superinfections, particularly *Pneumocystis carinii* pneumonia; neoplasms; and a wide variety of neurologic abnormalities, most notably the AIDS dementia complex, which appears to be a direct result of HIV nervous system infection.

Signs and Symptoms HIV infection is acquired years before signs of immunodeficiency appear. There are usually no symptoms at the time the infection is acquired, but in some patients an acute, mononucleosislike illness can be clearly identified a few weeks after exposure.

Most infected individuals experience a long asymptomatic period of variable length. At 7 years from exposure, 75 percent of patients have developed some type of symptoms, although only a third manifest the fullblown immunosuppressive syndrome. Some develop persistent generalized lymphadenopathy without evidence of superinfection. Later, a constitutional syndrome of wasting, fatigue, fever, oral thrush, and rashes develops which is considered by some investigators to represent a manifestation of fullblown AIDS, and by others to be an AIDS-related complex (ARC).

The best-known stage of HIV infection is characterized by superinfection with opportunistic organisms. However, patients with HIV infection appear to be unusually susceptible to certain infections before they reach this stage, most notably candida and tuberculosis.

Thrombocytopenia is common, and infection may initially be manifested by symptoms of idiopathic thrombocytopenic purpura.

The final stages of HIV infection are marked by superinfection, malignant neoplasms, and neurologic disease. Superinfection, the hallmark of the disease, results from progressive destruction of the T4 helper cell population. Most commonly, the infected individual succumbs to one or more opportunistic infections, particularly *Pneumocystis carinii*. These infections are frequently difficult to treat and impossible to eradicate, and consequently recurrences are the rule. They may be due to viral, bacterial, fungal, or protozoan agents:

Viral: cytomegalovirus (**CMV**); herpes simplex virus, types I and II; Epstein-Barr virus; varicella zoster; papovavirus.

Bacterial: *Mycobacterium tuberculosis; Mycobacterium avium-intracellulare; Legionella pneumophila; Klebsiella pneumoniae; Salmonella* species.

Fungal: *Candida albicans; Cryptococcus neoformans; Aspergillus* species; *Histoplasma capsulatum.*

Protozoan: *Pneumocystis carinii; Toxoplasma gondii; Entamoeba histolytica; Giardia lamblia; Cryptosporidium; Isospora belli.*

Many infections due to the agents listed above present differently in patients with HIV infection than in immunocompetent individuals.

The most common opportunistic infection in patients with AIDS is an interstitial pneumonia caused by *Pneumocystis carinii*. The symptoms, fever and dyspnea, usually develop gradually over several weeks. Also very common is CMV infection, especially CMV retinitis and enteritis. Tuberculosis, particularly with extrapulmonary manifestations, is common in AIDS. Common central nervous system infections include cryptococcal meningitis, and toxoplasmosis, which usually presents as a mass lesion with focal signs or seizures.

Malignant neoplasms are also characteristic of AIDS. Kaposi's sarcoma is especially common in homosexuals with AIDS, occurring in as many as 37 percent of these patients. It is much less frequent in heterosexuals for reasons that are unclear. It is also seen in homosexual males lacking HIV infection. In this type of cancer the skin, and often the viscera, develop small purple plaques and nodules representing vascular tumors. Patients who have only Kaposi's sarcoma have a somewhat better prognosis than those with opportunistic infections, apparently because their immune systems have retained slightly better function up to that point. Other cancers associated with AIDS include certain malignant lymphomas (e.g., Hodgkin's lymphoma) and primary B cell lymphoma of the brain.

There are a variety of neurologic manifestations of AIDS which may become apparent before the immunodeficiency is recognized. The most devastating neurologic complication is HIV encephalopathy, or AIDS-related dementia complex. Recent research suggests that as many as 60 percent of AIDS patients develop dementia that cannot be attributed to superinfection. Ataxia, spastic paraplegia, and peripheral neuropathies have also been recognized as neurologic complications of AIDS.

Peripheral neuropathy may affect 10 percent or more of patients with AIDS, but the clinical and pathological features are not completely characterized. The spectrum of symptom complexes includes sensory and motor neuropathies and multiple mononeuropathy.

Developmental abnormalities in children with AIDS, characterized by loss of cognitive ability and progressive long-tract signs, are now encountered with increasing frequency. An AIDS-associated dysmorphic syndrome in children, the result of intrauterine infection, has also been described (see **Acquired Immunodeficiency Dysmorphic Syndrome).**

Etiology AIDS is caused by a human T cell lymphotrophic virus (originally called HTLV-III) known as **HIV** (human immunodeficiency virus). It is a retrovirus. There are now known to be two human immunodeficiency viruses, HIV-1 and HIV-2. HIV-1 causes the vast majority of AIDS cases worldwide. HIV-2 occurs in West Africa and may be less virulent than HIV-1.

Epidemiology Several populations are at risk for HIV infection, the 2 major ones being homosexuals and intravenous drug abusers. Other groups at risk include recipients of blood transfusion and blood products (including hemophiliacs), although the risk of new infection should be dramatically reduced since the advent of blood screening. Finally, sexual partners and children of individuals in high-risk groups are also at risk for acquiring HIV infection.

There are 3 major routes of transmission: sexual contact, bloodborne transmission, and perinatal transmission. Worldwide, sexual contact is the most common mode of transmission; in the United States, this accounts for the spread of disease among homosexuals. In central Africa, sexual transmission occurs primarily in heterosexuals.

The next most common means of spread worldwide is the bloodborne route, which includes transfusions of blood and blood products, needlestick and other occupational accidents among health care workers, and intravenous drug abuse that involves sharing contaminated needles. The high incidence of the disease among hemophiliacs is due to their need for factor VIII concentrate, which is derived from pooled plasma. Blood screening for HIV antibody, which began in 1985, will drastically reduce the risk of acquiring AIDS through transfusions and blood products.

HIV-infected mothers may transmit the virus in utero and perinatally, through breast milk and possibly delivery. The majority of pediatric AIDS cases result from perinatal transmission, the mothers either being intravenous drug abusers or sexual partners of drug abusers. The risk of the child acquiring infection by this route is estimated to be about 30 to 40 percent. To date (1990), approximately 2000 cases of AIDS have been reported in children under the age of 13 in the United States.

In young children, the incubation period of HIV infection is much shorter than in adults. Most develop symptoms within 2 years.

About 55 percent of the homosexual population in certain communities have been found to have antibodies to HIV, suggesting that, although exposure to it has been widespread, some other cofactors may be necessary for HIV infection to develop. Coinfection with other microbial agents has been postulated as a cofactor.

Kaposi's sarcoma, immunologic evidence of exposure or infection with HIV, and AIDS-like syndromes are exceptionally common among both sexes in central Africa, where the disease is thought to have originated. Here the major route of transmission is sexual contact between heterosexuals.

In the United States, transmission through heterosexual intercourse is thought to account for about 2 percent of all cases. Intravenous drug addicts and their sex partners are the primary sources of AIDS infection among heterosexuals. Four out of 5 cases reported among this group are women. Among immigrant cases in this country, the proportion attributed to heterosexual contact is 4 percent. Three percent of cases seem to be idiopathic but there are questions as to accurate admission by these patients of past drug use and/or sexual practices.

Data from blood donors screened from April through December 1985 in New York City revealed that 0.08 percent had antibodies to the AIDS virus. Further investigation revealed 90 percent of those with the virus belonged to one of the high-risk groups mentioned above. In only 11 cases could the source of infection not be identified.

In tests of military applicants in New York City from October 1985 through July 1986, 1.06 percent of men and 0.83 percent of women had evidence of AIDS infection. Most of these infections could be traced to homosexual contact or drug use, and the proportion attributed to heterosexual relations was "minor."

The exact risk of virus transmission between males and females during intercourse is unclear. Two new studies on risks of unprotected intercourse with a virus carrier have described a higher rate of transmission (50 to 80 percent over months to years) than was previously thought possible for ordinary vaginal intercourse. In addition, one of these studies describes 2 cases of transmission from an infected male in spite of the use of condoms. This may be attributed to oral sex with semen discharge.

Some studies find inconsistent rates of transmission through intercourse depending on how the first partner became infected. One study found that drug abusers were much more effective transmitters than persons infected through contaminated blood products. In addition, rates of infection may vary among individuals or in the same person over time.

Available evidence indicates that the likelihood of viral transmission in a single heterosexual encounter is less than 1 percent. The virus probably spreads more easily in anal intercourse, which more often involves tearing of tissue, with resultant entry of the virus into the bloodstream. Promiscuity also increases risk.

Recent evidence suggests the AIDS virus can survive in insect hosts such as mosquitoes and other blood-sucking insects. However, there is no evidence that these insects can propagate the virus and transfer it to humans. To date, no case of AIDS has been linked to an insect bite in the United States.

There is currently a worldwide epidemic of AIDS and HIV infection. Areas with a high incidence include North America, central Africa, western Europe, and South America, particularly Brazil. Although there is a high incidence in Haiti, Haitians in the United States are not a high-risk group.

In the United States, over 1 million persons are thought to be infected, with the major cities having the highest reporting rates. Given this prevalence rate, AIDS can no longer be regarded as a disease restricted to certain populations.

Diagnosis The diagnosis of HIV infection usually begins with the screening test, the enzyme-linked immunosorbent assay (**ELISA),** for antibody to HIV. Because this test has a fairly high rate of false-positive results, any positive test should be repeated and confirmed by the western blot test for specific viral antibodies.

These tests will miss those cases of HIV infection where antibody is absent or undetectable, which may be the case in the first few months of infection. Cases have been reported in which antibody takes years to develop in infected individuals. Detection of these cases requires a test for the virus itself; such tests are currently under investigation.

The diagnosis of AIDS, rather than HIV infection, is made on the basis of documented HIV infection and the presence of one of the clinical syndromes discussed above, opportunistic infection, neoplasm, and neurologic disease being the major categories.

Treatment—Standard The treatment of choice for AIDS is the orphan drug zidovudine, brand name Retrovir (formerly known as azidothymidine or **AZT).** It is currently used for patients, symptomatic or not, with CD4+ lymphocytes at levels of less than 500 cells per microliter. The drug appears to slow the progression of AIDS (and in some cases allows the immune system to rebuild itself) by inhibiting production of an essential enzyme necessary for the AIDS virus to replicate. (A $30 million emergency fund to help low-income AIDS patients buy AZT has been established by the Health Resources and Services Administration. Eligibility will be determined by states. For more information, call [800] 843-9388.) In 1990, AZT was approved by the FDA for treatment of pediatric AIDS patients as young as 6 months old. The drug was approved in 1987 for patients 13 years of age and older.

A variety of nucleoside analogues have been under investigation for the treatment of HIV infection, including dideoxyinosine **(ddI),** and dideoxycytydine **(ddC).** Initial reports indicate that while ddC may reduce viral antigen levels, AZT remains the only drug that improves longterm survival. It has been reported that ddI can cause pancreatitis in patients with AIDS. Therefore, patients taking ddI should avoid alcoholic beverages and seek medical help immediately if they have abdominal pain, nausea, or vomiting. As of March 13, 1990, of the 8,300 AIDS patients taking ddI, 78 developed pancreatitis and 7 of them died.

Treatment with suramin, interleukin-2 to promote T lymphocyte growth, and various types of interferon (an antiviral protein), have not been effective, nor has treatment with acyclovir, vidarabine, various other drugs, white cell transfusions, thymic factors, and thymus and bone marrow transplants.

Many of the infections associated with AIDS respond to antibiotics, antifungals, etc., although recurrences are very common. Nystatin, clotrimazole, and ketoconazole are used to control episodes of esophageal and oral candidiasis. Severe candidiasis, as well as the other major fungal infection of AIDS, cryptococcal meningitis, will respond to amphotericin B or fluconazole. 5-Fluorocytosine may be used in combination with amphotericin in cryptococcal disease. Herpes simplex has responded to a course of treatment with acyclovir. Toxoplasmosis may be controlled with sulfadiazine and pyrimethamine, although these drugs have side effects that can limit their usefulness. Cryptosporidiosis may be treated symptomatically with tincture of opium, diphenoxylate, or cholestyramine. Spiramycin, an antibiotic used in Canada and Europe but not yet approved in the United States, appears to resolve or diminish diarrhea associated with cryptosporidiosis. (See Orphan and Experimental Drugs, below, for further mention of spiramycin.) A combination of quinine and clindamycin has also been reported to be effective.

Pneumocystis carinii pneumonia is more difficult to treat. At present, trimethoprim-sulfamethoxazole and pentamidine are the 2 drugs known to be effective. Intravenous pentamidine has been associated with serious side effects including hypoglycemia, hyperglycemia, hypocalcemia, hypotension, and renal and hepatic dysfunction. These functions must be monitored very closely in any patient on pentamidine. Currently, aerosolized pentamidine is recommended for prophylaxis against *P. carinii* infection. Patients with very low CD4+ counts (under 200 cells per microliter), as well as patients who have had one episode of *P. carinii* pneumonia, are recommended to receive aerosolized pentamidine on a monthly basis. Pentamidine is commercially available in the United States from Lyphomed, Inc., in inhalant (NebuPent) and injectable (Pentam 300) forms. (See under Treatment—Investigational, below, for information on other studies of pentamidine.)

No reliably effective treatment has been found for some kinds of AIDS-related infections. These include *Mycobacterium avium-intracellulare,* CMV, and Epstein-Barr virus. The drug ganciclovir (dihydroxypropoxymethyl guanine—**DHPG**) is effective against CMV retinitis in AIDS patients. The patient's eyesight often can be protected by this treatment, which is, however, complicated by toxic reactions, usually hematologic.

Kaposi's sarcoma responds to chemotherapy. Drugs have included vinblastine, etoposide, doxorubicin, bleomycin, and combinations of these. Interferon-alpha in high doses is moderately effective in treating Kaposi's sarcoma. Also reportedly effective in this cancer is vincristine, which has antitumor activity without causing further immunosuppression due to bone marrow suppression. Radiation therapy may also be used to palliate the lesions of Kaposi's sarcoma. Generally, however, treatment is not recommended for Kaposi's sarcoma unless the lesions are cosmetically unacceptable to the patient or are producing significant symptoms.

Prevention is the key to slowing the AIDS epidemic. Among the precautions against HIV transmission recommended by the Public Health Service are the following:

1) Sexual contact with persons known or suspected to be HIV carriers should be avoided. Multiple sex partners increase the probability of acquiring infection. 2) No members of high-risk groups should donate blood or blood products. 3) Blood transfusions should only be performed when absolutely necessary. 4) Screening procedures for plasma or blood likely to transmit AIDS have been developed, and safer blood products are available for hemophilia patients. 5) Health care personnel, laboratory workers, and others in frequent contact with AIDS patients should take great care with needles and similar sharp objects, and with blood-soiled materials.

Treatment—Investigational (See above under Treatment—Standard for a comparison of some investigational therapies with AZT.)

Tests to identify individuals infected with the AIDS virus before they develop the disease have shown an increase in virus-infected white blood cells in the year before AIDS symptoms become apparent. Present methods to detect these cells (peripheral blood mononuclear cells or monocytes) are very time-consuming and expensive, and simpler tests are currently under development. Treatment of asymptomatic infection, when identified early enough, may be more effective than treating the disease after symptoms appear.

The Food and Drug Administration gave a 1987 orphan drug research grant to John E. Conte, Jr., M.D., for studies on pentamidine pharmacokinetics related to AIDS patients on hemodialysis. Another grant was given for studies on the drug diethyldithiocarbamate for treatment of AIDS to Evan M. Hersh, M.D., of the University of Arizona.

Various vaccines are currently under investigation for the prevention of HIV infection.

Orphan and Experimental Drugs (see also the Orphan Drug Directory elsewhere in the Guide): Patients and doctors wishing to apply for admission into clinical trials of any AIDS drug should call the FDA at 1-800-TRIALS-A (see under Resources, below, for further information on this service).

Clinical trials are being conducted on the following orphan drugs for treatment of AIDS: diethyldithiocarbamate (Imuthiol), by Merieux Institute, Inc.; and 2'3'-

dideoxycytidine, by the National Cancer Institute.

Experimental orphan drugs for the treatment of AIDS include HPA-23, and others. For additional information about HPA-23, contact Rhone-Poulenc Pharmaceuticals. (See below for a further listing of experimental drugs and their indications and manufacturers.)

Two orphan drugs are undergoing clinical trials for treatment of AIDS-related Kaposi's sarcoma: interferon alfa-nf (Wellferon), Burroughs Wellcome Company; and interferon alfa-2B (Intron A), Schering Corporation. Other drugs being investigated for treating Kaposi's sarcoma include lymphoblastoid interferon and piritrexim isethionate, Burroughs Wellcome Company; doxorubicin, National Institute of Allergy and Infectious Diseases; tumor necrosis factor, Genentech, Inc.; and menogaril, National Cancer Institute.

Reports about the possibility of cyclosporine being an effective treatment for AIDS were released prematurely from researchers in France in 1985. This drug is commonly used for immunosuppression in patients who have received a transplanted organ. The French reports were issued after the drug had been used for only 6 days on a very limited number of patients, all of whom died after transient initial improvement.

More than 80 ongoing human studies have been approved by the FDA to test potential drug treatments for opportunistic infections and cancers often found in AIDS patients, based on investigational new drug **(IND)** applications. They are listed below by what they are designed to treat, their names, and the manufacturers, respectively.

Anti-infective agents

For *Pneumocystis carinii* pneumonia:

> aerosol pentamidine, Fisons Corporation and the National Institute of Allergy and Infectious Diseases;
>
> dapsone, Jacobus Pharmaceutical Co., Inc.;
>
> diethyldithiocarbamate (Imuthiol), Merieux Institute, Inc.;
>
> eflornithine (DMFO), Merrell Dow Pharmaceuticals Inc.;
>
> pentamidine isethionate, Rhone Poulenc Pharmaceuticals;
>
> piritrexim, Burroughs Wellcome Company;
>
> trimetrexate, Warner-Lambert Company and the National Institute of Allergy and Infectious Diseases;

For CMV retinitis:

> foscarnet sodium IV (Foscavir), Astra Pharmaceutical Products, Inc. and the National Institute of Allergy and Infectious Diseases.

For *Mycobacterium avium-intracellulare*:

> ansamycin, also called rifabutin (no brand name as yet established), in combination with other drugs, Adria Laboratories;
>
> clofazimine (Lamprene—Geigy Pharmaceuticals), San Francisco General Hospital.

For cryptosporidiosis:

> spiramycin, Rhone-Poulenc Pharmaceuticals;

For opportunistic infections:

immune globulin IG-IV, Sandoz Pharmaceuticals Corporation; Alpha Therapeutic Corporation; and Miles, Inc. Also involved are the National Institutes of Health and the National Institute of Child Health and Human Development.

Experimental antineoplastic agents
For primary lymphoma:
M-BACOD (**m**ethotrexate; **b**leomycin; **A**driamycin [doxorubicin]; **c**yclophosphamide; **O**ncovin [vincristine]; **d**examethasone), National Institute of Allergy and Infectious Diseases (NIAID).

Other experimental agents
For oral candidiasis prevention:
nystatin, E.R. Squibb and Sons, Inc;
For AIDS-related diarrhea:
octreotide acetate (Sandostatin), Sandoz Pharmaceuticals Corporation;
For cryptosporidial diarrhea:
diclazuril, Janssen Pharmaceutica Inc.;
For toxoplasmic encephalitis:
clindamycin, Mark Jacobson, M.D., San Francisco, CA;
For toxoplasmosis prevention:
pyrimethamine (Daraprim), Burroughs Wellcome Company;
For histoplasmosis:
itraconazole (Sporanox), Janssen Pharmaceutica Inc.

Please contact the agencies listed under Resources, below, for the most current information.

Resources

For more information on AIDS: National Organization for Rare Disorders (NORD); American Foundation for AIDS Research; National Gay Task Force (NGTF—provides a handbook listing support groups, fund-raising organizations, etc.); National Gay Task Force Crisis Line; National Hemophilia Foundation; NIH/National Institute of Allergy and Infectious Diseases (NIAID); Centers for Disease Control (CDC); National Sexually Transmitted Diseases Hotline; AIDS Information Clearinghouse; National Cancer Institute Physician Data Query (PDQ) phoneline; AIDSLINE—National Library of Medicine.

Information on privately funded clinical trials of drugs and biologics used to treat AIDS and AIDS-related illnesses is now available through a toll-free telephone service **(1-800-TRIALS-A).** This service is staffed by specially trained information specialists, including some who speak Spanish. Service for the hearing-impaired is also available, at **(800) 243-7012.** Callers can find out where studies are located and the eligibility criteria for participants, the name of the product being studied and the purpose of the study, and a contact person and phone number for the company sponsoring the clinical trials. All inquiries are kept confidential. Information from the phone service is also accessible through DIRLINE, the National Library of Medicine's online computer database.

References

Reports on AIDS have been published in the Morbidity and Mortality Weekly Report from June 1981 through the present by the Centers for Disease Control.

Justification of Appropriation Estimates for Committee on Appropriations. Public Health Service Supplementary Budget Data (Moyer Material) A through L: Fiscal Year 1986, vol. VII. This publication contains information on all AIDS research being funded by NIH.

National Institutes of Health Conference. Acquired Immunodeficiency Syndrome: Epidemiologic, Clinical, Immunologic, and Therapeutic Considerations: A.S. Fauci, et al.; Ann. Intern. Med., January 1983, vol. 100(1), pp. 92–106.

Acquired Immunodeficiency Syndrome: A.M. Macher; Am. Fam. Phys., December 1984, vol. 30(6), pp. 131–144.

Acquired Immune Deficiency Syndrome: An Update and Interpretation: C.B. Daul, et al.; Ann. Allergy, September 1983, vol. 51(3), pp. 351–361.

The Acquired Immune Deficiency Syndrome: A.J. Pinching; Clin. Exp. Immunol., April 1984, vol. 56(1), pp. 1–13.

Treatment of Kaposi's Sarcoma and Thrombocytopenia with Vincristine in Patients with the Acquired Immunodeficiency Syndrome: D.M. Mintzer, et al.; Ann. Intern. Med., February 1985, vol. 102(2), pp. 200–202.

Treatment of Intestinal Cryptosporidiosis with Spiramycin: D. Portnoy, et al.; Ann. Intern. Med., August 1984, vol. 101(2), pp. 202–204.

ACQUIRED IMMUNODEFICIENCY DYSMORPHIC SYNDROME

Description AIDS dysmorphic syndrome is a constellation of craniofacial anomalies accompanied by developmental delay. The syndrome has been reported in some infants with intrauterine human immunodeficiency virus (**HIV**) infection. HIV is thought to be transmitted transplacentally by an infected woman who may or may not have symptoms of AIDS. Children with AIDS dysmorphic syndrome are infected with HIV and hence are prone to develop all the other manifestations of AIDS.

Synonyms

AIDS Dysmorphic Syndrome
Dysmorphic Acquired Immune Deficiency Syndrome
Embryopathy

Signs and Symptoms Signs of AIDS dysmorphic syndrome become apparent before one year of age. It is characterized by growth failure, microcephaly, and dysmorphic craniofacial features including wide-set eyes, prominent box-like forehead, flat nasal bridge, mild upward or downward slant of the eyes, long eyelid fissures, a blue tinge to the whites of the eyes, a shortened nose, a triangular groove in the upper lip, and patulous lips. These features vary in severity and may not be noticeable until the child is a few months old.

The degree of physical and mental developmental delay in affected children varies.

The typical infections of pediatric AIDS usually develop later in infancy. Affected infants are highly susceptible to infections such as *Pneumocystis carinii* pneumonia, meningitis, urinary infections, or soft tissue infections.

Etiology The syndrome is thought to be caused by intrauterine transmission of the HIV virus from an AIDS-infected mother.

Epidemiology Dysmorphic AIDS usually becomes apparent among affected children between 3 weeks and 23 months of age. The disorder affects males and females in equal numbers.

Treatment—Standard Fetal HIV infection can be diagnosed prenatally by testing for the presence of the HIV virus in the fetus after the 14th week of pregnancy. Blood from the umbilical cord may also be tested for the virus. After birth, HIV antibody is present, but it is likely to have been passively transferred from the mother.

In children with dysmorphic AIDS, treatment with intravenous immunoglobulin **(IG-IV)** helps restore the immune system, thus decreasing the chance of infections. Treatment with zidovudine (formerly known as AZT) may help prevent developmental delay. The longterm outcome of these treatments is unknown at this time.

Treatment—Investigational Please contact the agencies listed under Resources, below, for the most current information.

Resources

For more information on AIDS dysmorphic syndrome: National Organization for Rare Disorders (NORD); American Foundation for AIDS Research; Computerized AIDS Information Network (CAIN); NIH/National Institute of Allergy and Infectious Diseases (NIAID); Centers for Disease Control.

References
AIDS in Children: Barbara J. Proujan; Research Resources Reporter, January 1988, vol. 12(1), pp. 1–5.

Fetal AIDS Syndrome Score: R.W. Marion, et al.; Am. J. Dis. Child., 1987, vol. 141, pp. 429–431.

Pediatric AIDS: A. Rubinstein; Curr. Probl. Pediatr., 1986, vol. 16, pp. 364–409.

Human T-Cell Lymphotropic Virus Type III (HTLV-III) Embryopathy: R.W. Marion, et al.; Am. J. Dis. Child., July 1986, vol. 140(7), pp. 638–640.

Intravenous Gamma-Globulin in Infant Acquired Immunodeficiency Syndrome: T.A. Calvelli, et al.; Pediatr. Infect. Dis., 1986, vol. 5, pp. S207–S210.

ANAPHYLAXIS

Description Anaphylaxis is a type I IgE-mediated hypersensitivity reaction. It is an immediate systemic response triggered by IgE-antigen interaction, and mediated by mast cells, basophils, and their products. Major symptoms may include pruritis, urticaria, flushing, angioedema, vomiting, diarrhea, dyspnea, and shock.

Synonyms

Anaphylactic Reaction

Anaphylactic Shock
Generalized Anaphylaxis

Signs and Symptoms Anaphylaxis is mediated by prostaglandins and histamine, substances that can evoke angioedema, urticaria, bronchiolar constriction, laryngeal edema, and vascular collapse. The respiratory symptoms may include wheezing, chest tightness, stridor, and dyspnea. Urticarial eruptions may be local or generalized, and are very pruritic. Angioedema represents edema and reaction at deeper layers of the skin, and includes the subcutaneous tissue. It is generally not pruritic but may be accompanied by a burning sensation.

Anaphylactic reactions occur within seconds or minutes and can be rapidly fatal. When death occurs, it may be due to upper airway obstruction, or shock, or both.

The diagnosis is made on the basis of the history and clinical appearance of the patient.

Etiology Anaphylaxis is a hypersensitivity reaction to an antigen. The most common triggers include penicillin, insect venom, pollen extracts, fish, shellfish, and nuts. Various other foods, drugs, radiographic dyes, food additives (particularly sulfites), and chemicals are known to cause anaphylactic reactions in hypersensitive individuals.

Epidemiology The sexes and all age groups are affected equally. There are approximately 50 to 100 deaths from anaphylaxis caused by insect stings each year in the United States.

Related Disorders Other hypersensitivity reactions that are IgE-mediated include atopy and urticaria. Repeated contact with a particular antigen may result in more serious reactions at a later time. See **Dermatitis, Atopic; Dermatitis, Contact; Arachnoiditis.**

Treatment—Standard The major drug used in the treatment of anaphylaxis is epinephrine. It should be given as early as possible and may be required in repeated doses. Bronchospasm may benefit from aminophylline in addition to epinephrine, and supplemental oxygen will be required in most cases where there is respiratory compromise. Diphenhydramine may be used to treat urticarial and angioedematous reactions. Desensitization may reduce hypersensitivity to some substances.

Treatment—Investigational Please contact the agencies listed under Resources, below, for the most current information.

Resources

For more information on anaphylaxis: National Organization for Rare Disorders (NORD); NIH/National Institute of Allergy & Infectious Diseases (NIAID); Asthma & Allergy Foundation of America.

References
Internal Medicine, 2nd ed.: J.H. Stein, ed.-in-chief; Little, Brown and Company, 1987, pp. 1249–1250.

Anaphylactic Shock. Guidelines for Immediate Diagnosis and Treatment: A.J. Costa; Postgrad. Med., March 1988, vol. 83(4), pp. 368–369, 372–373.

Fatal Food-Induced Anaphylaxis: J.W. Yunginger, et al.; JAMA, September 9, 1988, vol. 260(10), pp. 1450–1452.

Anaphylaxis, an Allergic Reaction that Can Kill: M. Segal; FDA Consumer, May 1989, pp. 21–23.

ASPERGILLOSIS

Description Aspergillosis is an infection with a species of the fungus *Aspergillus,* the most common pathogen being *A. fumigatus.* Infections may be focal or systemic, and most commonly occur in the lung; the brain and sinuses are also common sites. There are several distinct types of *Aspergillus* infection that occur in different circumstances: these are allergic bronchopulmonary aspergillosis, aspergilloma, and invasive aspergillosis. Immunosuppressed patients, particularly acute leukemics, are prone to fulminant invasive forms of aspergillosis. Other types of aspergillus infection include endocarditis, skin ulcers, and bone involvement.

Signs and Symptoms Allergic bronchopulmonary aspergillosis **(ABPA)** is one of the syndromes associated with pulmonary infiltrates and **eosinophilia** (**PIE** syndrome). It occurs in patients with asthma, and is characterized by infiltrates on chest x-ray, eosinophilia, elevated serum IgE, and serum precipitins to *A. fumigatus.* This form of aspergillosis is not invasive, but may lead to central bronchiectasis. Patients complain of worsening asthma, cough, and expectorating mucus plugs.

Pulmonary mycetoma, also known as aspergilloma or "fungus ball," is a form of noninvasive aspergillosis that often occurs as a result of fungal colonization of a pulmonary cavity. This may complicate tuberculosis, sarcoidosis, histoplasmosis, and many chronic pulmonary diseases. The patient's symptoms are usually referrable to the underlying lung disease, rather than to the fungus, but complications can occur. These include hemoptysis, bronchopleural fistula, and bacterial superinfection. Fungus balls are usually diagnosed on chest x-ray.

Invasive aspergillosis commonly originates in the lung or the sinuses, and tends to occur in immunosuppressed patients, particularly those with severe neutropenia. *Aspergillus* pneumonia is a rapidly progressive infection with fever, pulmonary symptoms, and rapidly enlarging infiltrates on chest x-ray. Hematogenous spread throughout the body is common and the patient usually succumbs. A fulminant, invasive sinusitis can also occur in immunosuppressed patients, particularly acute leukemics.

The diagnosis of invasive aspergillosis is rarely made on blood culture. Since *Aspergillus* is ubiquitous, positive sputum and nasal cultures may represent contamination, colonization, or invasion; the interpretation rests on the clinical appearance of the patient.

Aspergillus is also a cause of infective endocarditis, and madura foot.

Etiology There are several pathogenic species of *Aspergillus,* the most frequent being *A. fumigatus,* followed by *A. flavus,* and others.

Epidemiology *Aspergillus* infection or colonization is acquired by inhalation. The spores of this fungus are ubiquitous, and may be found in decaying vegetable matter, grains, grass, leaves, soil, wet paint, air conditioning systems, and construction and fireproofing materials, and on refrigerator walls. Nosocomial infections may be associated with potted plants in the patient's room, and hospital construction.

Related Disorders Related diseases include other fungal infections of the lung, including histoplasmosis, cryptococcosis, blastomycosis, and coccidioidomycosis. *Aspergillus* infections of the sinus and nasal cavity may resemble rhinocerebral mucormycosis.

ABPA is one of the PIE syndromes; the others are eosinophilic pneumonia, Churg-Strauss allergic granulomatosis, Loeffler syndrome, and the hypereosinophilic syndrome. ABPA may be distinguished by its association with asthma, elevated serum IgE, and serum precipitins and skin reactions to *A. fumigatus.*

Treatment—Standard The treatment of ABPA is with systemic steroids. Amphotericin B is used for invasive disease. Surgery is often indicated in cases of aspergillus endocarditis, as well as invasive disease of the sinuses and brain. Aspergillomas do not ordinarily require treatment, except if life-threatening hemoptysis complicates the picture. Surgical excision is the treatment of choice in these cases.

Treatment—Investigational Studies are currently being conducted on the effectiveness of the therapeutic agents itraconazole, imidazoles, ketoconazole, and fluconazole in aspergillosis.

Please contact the agencies listed under Resources, below, for the most current information.

Resources

For more information on aspergillosis: National Organization for Rare Disorders (NORD); NIH/National Institute of Allergy and Infectious Diseases (NIAID); Centers for Disease Control (CDC).

References
Internal Medicine, 2nd ed.: J.H. Stein, ed.-in-chief; Little, Brown and Company, 1987, p. 1765.

Pulmonary Diseases and Disorders, vol. 2, 2nd ed.: A.P. Fishman, ed.-in-chief; McGraw-Hill, 1980, p. 1639.

Rapid Diagnosis of Candidiasis and Aspergillosis: J. Bennett; Rev. Infect. Dis., March–April 1987, vol. 9(2), pp. 398–402.

Allergic Bronchopulmonary Aspergillosis: P. Bock; Am. Fam. Phys., January 1988, vol. 37(1), pp. 177–182.

Invasive Aspergillosis in Children: E. Golladay, et al.; J. Pediatr. Surg., June 1987, vol. 22(6), pp. 504–505.

Aspergilloma in Sarcoid and Tuberculosis: J. Tomlinson, et al.; September 1987, vol. 92(3), pp. 505–508.

Aspergillosis: S. Levitz; Infect. Dis. Clin. North Am., March 1989, vol. 3(1), pp. 1–18.

BABESIOSIS

Description Babesiosis is primarily a disease of animals, caused by protozoan organisms of the genus *Babesia*. The disease is similar to malaria in its pathophysiology and symptoms. It is most severe in splenectomized individuals who develop fulminant, frequently fatal infection.

Signs and Symptoms Most human *Babesia* infections are probably asymptomatic. Patients who experience symptoms tend to be older (over 50), or asplenic.

Babesiosis has a 1- to 3-week incubation period. Patients then complain of fever, malaise, fatigue, and myalgias. Nausea, vomiting, and abdominal pain are also common. Laboratory examination reveals evidence of hemolytic anemia; thrombocytopenia and leukopenia may also be seen. In severe cases jaundice and renal failure may occur.

The diagnosis of babesiosis is made by examination of thick and thin blood smears for parasitic forms inside the erythrocytes. The diagnosis may also be serologically confirmed by indirect immunofluorescent antibody testing.

Etiology *Babesia* are protozoa. There are many species, but only 3 are pathogenic in man: *B. microti*, *B. bovis*, and *B. divergens*. Of these, the first is the major cause of babesiosis in the United States, whereas the other 2 have been found in European infection. *Babesia* are erythrocytic parasites, like the *Plasmodium* species that causes malaria. Both have a reproductive cycle inside the red blood cell, with cell rupture and subsequent hemolysis. Unlike most species of *Plasmodium*, *Babesia* do not rupture in a synchronous fashion, and so periodic paroxysms do not occur.

Epidemiology Babesiosis is transmitted by the *Ixodes dammini* tick, which also transmits Lyme disease. In the United States, most cases are confined to the Northeastern coast. The disease is rare; only about 200 cases were reported in the United States in the 1980s.

Related Disorders Babesiosis is closely related to malaria, although the 2 are easily distinguished by the geographic history of the patient.

Treatment—Standard Most cases of babesiosis will resolve spontaneously. Severe disease is treated with a regimen of clindamycin and quinine.

Treatment—Investigational Please contact the agencies listed under Resources, below, for the most current information.

Resources

For more information on babesiosis: National Organization for Rare Disorders; NIH/ National Institute of Allergy and Infectious Diseases; Centers for Disease Control (CDC).

References
Report of the Committee on Infectious Diseases, 21st ed.: G. Peter, et al., eds.; American Academy of Pediatrics, 1988, p. 131.

Babesia: J.A. Gelfand; *in* Principles and Practice of Infectious Diseases: G.L. Mandell et al., eds.; Churchill Livingstone, 1990, pp. 2119–2121.

BALANTIDIASIS

Description Balantidiasis is an intestinal infection with *Balantidium coli*, a ciliated protozoan parasite that frequently infects pigs. On the rare occasions it is transmitted to man, it produces a disease that resembles amebic dysentery.

Synonyms
> Balantidial Dysentery
> Ciliary Dysentery

Signs and Symptoms *B. coli* infection may be asymptomatic or mild, or the patient may be acutely ill with fever, nausea, vomiting, abdominal pain, and bloody diarrhea. The symptoms are caused by mucosal invasion of the intestinal wall, creating ulcers. In fulminating infections, perforation through the ulcer occurs, resulting in peritonitis.

In dysentery, the trophozoite form of the organism is usually recoverable from the stool. Another diagnostic method involves scraping the ulcer base and examining the scrapings for trophozoites.

Etiology Balantidiasis is caused by the ciliated protozoan parasite *B. coli*.

Epidemiology This disease occurs in tropical regions such as Brazil, New Guinea, and southern Iran. It is primarily a disease of people in close contact with pigs. Transmission is fecal-oral, through direct contact with pig feces, or indirectly from contaminated drinking water.

Related Disorders Balantidiasis must be distinguished from amebic dysentery, *Shigella* dysentery, and ulcerative colitis.

Treatment—Standard The treatment of choice is tetracycline. Alternatives include iodoquinol or metronidazole. Prevention is accomplished by good hygiene.

Treatment—Investigational Please contact the agencies listed under Resources, below, for the most current information.

Resources
For more information on balantidiasis: National Organization for Rare Disorders (NORD); NIH/National Institute of Allergy and Infectious Diseases (NIAID); Centers for Disease Control (CDC).

References
Cecil Textbook of Medicine, 18th ed.: J.B. Wyngaarden and L.H. Smith, Jr., eds.; W.B. Saunders Company, 1988, p. 1889.

BARTONELLOSIS

Description Bartonellosis is a disease caused by *Bartonella bacilliformis* and transmitted by sandflies. It is characterized by fever, hemolytic anemia, and a chronic skin rash.

Synonyms
> Carrion's Disease
> Oroya Fever
> Verruga Peruana

Signs and Symptoms There are 2 phases of *B. bacilliformis* infection. In the first, called Oroya fever, there is fever, anemia, headache, and severe bone and joint pain. Physical examination reveals hepatosplenomegaly and generalized lymphadenopathy. The anemia is hemolytic and results from parasitization of erythrocytes by the bacteria, with subsequent rupture. Neurologic involvement may also occur, with meningoencephalitis. The mortality of untreated disease is high, and often due to superinfection with *Salmonella* and other microorganisms.

The 2nd phase of infection, referred to as verruga peruana, usually but not necessarily follows the Oroya fever phase. It is characterized by fever, pains, and an eruption on the skin. The rash consists of multiple small nodular lesions, usually on the face and extremities. Lesions may also appear in the gastrointestinal and genitourinary tracts, where they occasionally make their presence known by bleeding.

The diagnosis of bartonellosis during the first phase is made on microscopic examination of a peripheral blood smear; the bacteria may be seen inside the red blood cells. During the 2nd phase of illness, organisms may be seen on a smear of material from a skin lesion.

Etiology The cause of bartonellosis is the gram-negative bacterium, *Bartonella bacilliformis*. This organism parasitizes erythrocytes, cells of the reticuloendothelial system, and the endothelial cells of blood vessels. Invasion of the skin and subcutaneous tissues characterizes the verruga peruana phase.

Epidemiology The geography of bartonellosis is limited by the range of its mosquito vector, which lives at certain altitudes in the Andes. The populations of Peru, Ecuador, Colombia, Chile, and Guatemala may be affected, particularly in the spring.

Treatment—Standard The treatment of choice is chloramphenicol. Preventative measures include the use of mosquito netting, adequate clothing, and insect repellents.

Treatment—Investigational Please contact the agencies listed under Resources, below, for the most current information.

Resources
> **For more information on bartonellosis:** National Organization for Rare Dis-

orders (NORD); NIH/National Institute of Allergy and Infectious Diseases (NIAID); Centers for Disease Control (CDC).

References
  Manson's Tropical Diseases, 19th ed.: P.E.C. Manson-Bahr and D.R. Bell; Ballière Tindall, 1987, pp. 246-251.

BEJEL

Description Bejel is a treponemal disease that is very similar to syphilis but is not transmitted sexually. Also referred to as **endemic syphilis,** bejel is a disease of stages, the late stage being the most clinically significant. The disease consists of skin and bone lesions.

Synonyms
    Dichuchwa
    Endemic Syphilis
    Frenga
    Njovera
    Nonvenereal Syphilis
    Siti

Signs and Symptoms The primary lesion is an ulcer on a mucous membrane, frequently inside the mouth. It usually occurs in childhood and is rarely noticed. Secondary disease involves adenopathy, ulcers, and a rash, generally on the trunk, arms, and legs. Lesions may also be concentrated in the axilla, groin, and rectum. The late lesion is the gumma, which appears in the skin and bones. The diagnosis is based on the geographic history of the patient, with darkfield examination of material from the lesions, or serology (Venereal Disease Research Laboratory [VDRL] test; the fluorescent treponemal antibody-absorption [FTA-ABS] test).

Etiology Bejel is caused by a spirochete, *Treponema pallidum II*. It is morphologically indistinguishable from the agent that causes syphilis.

Epidemiology Transmission is by direct, nonsexual contact, or indirectly, through shared eating utensils. It is rare in the United States, but occurs in the Middle East; Africa; parts of Europe, particularly Yugoslavia; Southeast Asia; and Australia.

Related Disorders Bejel is a treponematosis, and as such is related to syphilis, pinta, and yaws. These organisms are morphologically similar, but their epidemiologies and clinical characteristics differ.

Treatment—Standard Bejel is treated with benzathine penicillin G.

Treatment—Investigational Please contact the agencies listed under Resources, below, for the most current information.

Resources

For more information on bejel: National Organization for Rare Disorders (NORD); NIH/National Institute of Allergy and Infectious Diseases (NIAID); Centers for Disease Control (CDC).

References

Cecil Textbook of Medicine, 18th ed.; J.B. Wyngaarden and L.H. Smith, Jr., eds.; W.B. Saunders Company, 1988, p. 1723.

BLASTOMYCOSIS

Description Blastomycosis is a systemic fungal infection caused by *Blastomyces dermatitidis*. The lungs, skin, bones, and genitourinary tract are most frequently involved.

Synonyms

Gilchrist's Disease
North American Blastomycosis

Signs and Symptoms The initial infection is pulmonary. Fever, chills, cough, and dyspnea may occur; alternatively, the acute pulmonary infection may be asymptomatic. The chronic phase of blastomycosis may involve the lung, skin, bones, joints, genitourinary tract, or central nervous system.

Involvement of the skin is most common; papulopustular and verrucous lesions are common. The color may be violaceous and microabscesses may form around the periphery of the lesion. Subcutaneous nodules may appear, usually accompanied by active pulmonary disease.

Chronic pulmonary disease usually takes the form of chronic pneumonia. Consolidation or cavitation may be evident on chest x-ray.

Bone lesions commonly involve the long bones, ribs, and vertebrae, the most frequent lesion being a painless lytic lesion that may present with an overlying abscess or sinus.

Genitourinary tract involvement is common in men; prostate and epididymal disease is seen in up to a third of cases.

Involvement of the central nervous system, liver, spleen, gastrointestinal tract, thyroid, adrenals, and other organs has been reported.

The diagnosis of blastomycosis is initially made by direct microscopic examination of infected material (pus, sputum, urine, or biopsy material). Preparation with potassium hydroxide usually renders the yeast cells easily visible. Culture will confirm the diagnosis. Skin testing and serologic tests are not helpful.

Etiology Blastomycosis is caused by the dimorphic fungus *Blastomyces dermatitidis*. It grows in the yeast form at body temperature, and the mycelial form at room temperature.

Epidemiology Blastomycosis is endemic in the south central and southeastern United States. It is also found around the perimeter of the Great Lakes, and along the St. Lawrence River in Canada. Elsewhere, blastomycosis has been reported in South and Central America and parts of Africa.

The natural habitat of this fungus is unclear but may be in the soil. Farmers, construction workers, and others who work with soil appear to be at increased risk.

Related Disorders Pulmonary blastomycosis may be mistaken for malignancy, and bronchoscopy may be required to confirm the diagnosis. Cutaneous blastomycosis may also resemble malignancy.

Treatment—Standard Oral ketoconazole is now the treatment of choice for all but severe cases of blastomycosis. When the central nervous system is involved, amphotericin B is required.

Treatment—Investigational Please contact the agencies listed under Resources, below, for the most current information.

Resources
  For more information on blastomycosis: National Organization for Rare Disorders (NORD); Centers for Disease Control (CDC); NIH/National Institute of Allergy and Infectious Diseases (NIAID).

References
  Cecil Textbook of Medicine, 18th ed.: J.B. Wyngaarden and L.H. Smith, Jr., eds.; W.B. Saunders Company, 1988, pp. 1838–1843, 2334.
  Blastomyces Dermatitidis: S.W. Chapman; *in* Principles and Practice of Infectious Diseases: G.L. Mandell, et al., eds.; Churchill Livingstone, 1990, pp. 1999–2007.

BOTULISM

Description Botulism is a paralytic syndrome caused by an enterotoxin elaborated by *Clostridium botulinum.* There are 3 different forms: foodborne, in which food containing the toxin is ingested; wound botulism, where the wound becomes contaminated with *C. botulinum,* which then produces the toxin; and infant botulism, in which food contaminated with the bacteria is ingested, and the toxin is elaborated after ingestion. The toxin produces symptoms by blocking transmission at the neuromuscular junction.

Signs and Symptoms In **foodborne botulism,** the most common form, food containing preformed toxin is ingested. Symptoms start approximately 12 to 36 hours later, although the incubation period varies from 4 hours to 8 days. The initial manifestations are nonspecific, including weakness, headache, and dizziness. There may be gastrointestinal symptoms such as nausea, vomiting, diarrhea, and abdominal pain.

  When neurotransmission in the autonomic system is blocked, extreme dryness of the mouth and pharynx occurs. The same pathophysiologic process may give rise to urinary retention, ileus, and constipation.

  The neurologic manifestations of botulism may accompany the anticholinergic symptoms, or may be delayed as long as 3 days. When neurologic symptoms begin they do so in a descending fashion, starting with the cranial nerves. Patients may experience blurred vision and photophobia, then dysarthria and dysphagia, followed by variable degrees of muscle weakness, descending down the body. When death occurs, it is usually a result of respiratory muscle paralysis.

Physical examination usually reveals a fully conscious patient. Fever is generally absent. Postural hypotension is a relatively frequent finding. The pupils are dilated and fixed, and a variety of cranial nerve abnormalities may be present. The pharynx may be so erythematous and dry that bacterial pharyngitis is suspected. Neurologic examination reveals muscle weakness with variable deep tendon reflexes and normal sensation.

Recovery is generally slow, and some symptoms, such as constipation, dry mouth, and intermittent diplopia have been known to persist for months.

The diagnosis of botulism is made on the clinical features described above, although a characteristic electromyographic picture supports the diagnosis. Diagnosis may be confirmed by demonstrating the toxin in the blood, stool, or gastric contents.

Wound botulism generally appears 4 to 14 days after the injury. It is characterized by the same neurologic symptoms as foodborne botulism; however, gastrointestinal symptoms are absent, and wound infection may be associated with fever.

Infant botulism is seen most often between the ages of 2 and 3 months. Constipation occurs initially in approximately two-thirds of cases. This may be followed by varying degrees of neuromuscular paralysis—the so-called floppy infant syndrome. The diagnosis is made by demonstrating the organism in the stool.

Milk is not usually the source of infant botulism. Cases have been related to the ingestion of honey, vacuum cleaner dust, and soil.

Etiology Botulism is the result of ingestion and absorption of toxin produced by the anaerobic bacillus, *Clostridium botulinum.* The toxin blocks neurotransmission at the neuromuscular junction by inhibiting the release of the neurotransmitter, acetylcholine.

There are 8 distinct types of the toxin, but human poisoning is usually caused by only 3, types A, B, and E. Wound and infant botulism tend to be associated only with types A and B.

Clostridium botulinum spores are highly resistant to heat and may survive for several hours at 100° C (212° F), but not at 120° C (248° F). On the other hand, the toxins are readily destroyed by heat; cooking at 80° C (176° F) for 30 minutes protects against botulism.

Epidemiology Home-canned food is the most common source of botulism; however, commercially prepared foods have been implicated in about 10 percent of cases. A wide variety of foods may cause botulism, including vegetables, fish, fruits, beef, milk products, pork, and poultry.

The different types of toxins have different geographic distributions: type A is the most common in the United States, and is the most frequent type west of the Mississippi River. Type B is more frequent in the Eastern states, and type E is more prevalent in Alaska and the Great Lakes region. Worldwide, type E is frequent in northern latitudes and Japan.

Treatment—Standard Botulism requires careful attention to respiratory status. Monitoring with frequent determinations of vital capacity is recommended, and early institution of mechanical ventilation may be lifesaving.

A trivalent antitoxin (A, B, E) is available through the Centers for Disease Control in Atlanta, Georgia. Antitoxin is also available for outbreaks due to types C, D, or F. Treatment should be initiated as soon as possible; it may still be beneficial even weeks after toxin ingestion. However, the risks of treatment must be weighed against potential benefits. The antitoxins are made from horse serum, and may cause serious allergic reactions. Patients should be tested for hypersensitivity and desensitized if necessary prior to administration of the antitoxin.

The antitoxin does not reverse preexisting neurologic impairment although it may slow or halt further progression of disease.

Guanidine has been advocated by some in the treatment of botulism; it is thought to enhance release of acetylcholine at the synapse. However, results have been inconsistent and the effectiveness of the drug remains unproved.

Treatment—Investigational Please contact the agencies listed under Resources, below, for the most current information.

Resources

For more information on botulism: National Organization for Rare Disorders (NORD); NIH/National Institute of Allergy and Infectious Diseases (NIAID); Centers for Disease Control; Food and Drug Administration.

References

Cecil Textbook of Medicine, 18th ed.: J.B. Wyngaarden and L.H. Smith, Jr., eds.; W.B. Saunders Company, 1988, pp. 1633–1634, 1663, 1666.

Clostridium Botulinum (Botulism): W. Schaffner; in Principles and Practice of Infectious Diseases: G.L. Mandell, et al., eds.; Churchill Livingstone, 1990, pp. 1847–1849.

BRUCELLOSIS

Description Brucellosis is a ubiquitous infection of livestock that may be transmitted to man. It is caused by different species of the genus *Brucella*. Initial infection may result in an acute flulike illness, or may evolve insidiously over months. Untreated cases may take months to resolve, and some cases become chronic.

Synonyms

Bang Disease
Cyprus Fever
Febris Melitensis
Febris Sudoralis
Febris Undulans
Gibraltar Fever
Goat Fever
Maltese Fever
Mediterranean Fever

Melitensis Septicemia
Melitococcosis
Neapolitan Fever
Rock Fever
Undulant Fever

Signs and Symptoms Brucellosis has a very wide range of manifestations. Asymptomatic infection occurs, particularly in children. Acute brucellosis is a flulike illness without localizing symptoms. Typically there is gradual onset of fever, weakness, headache, myalgias, nightsweats, and fatigue. Examination generally reveals few abnormalities; occasionally there may be lymphadenopathy, splenomegaly, or hepatomegaly. In untreated cases, the symptoms may persist intermittently for several weeks. Occasionally, chronic disease develops, with repeated waves of fever (the so-called undulant fever) recurring for more than a year.

Localized forms of brucellosis may occur anywhere in the body. The most frequent focal infections are osteomyelitis (usually of the lumbar vertebrae), splenic abscess, orchitis, endocarditis, and lung infection.

Endocarditis is an uncommon complication but is the most frequent cause of death. A wide variety of central nervous system complications may also occur.

Laboratory tests are not distinctive and generally do not help to distinguish brucellosis from other conditions with similar symptoms.

The diagnosis of brucellosis is occasionally made by isolating the organism from the blood, bone marrow, or other sites (lymph nodes, spleen, liver). However, *Brucella* is hazardous to culture in the laboratory, and only certain laboratories will undertake the task. Most infections are confirmed serologically using agglutination tests. A 4-fold rise in antibody titer of specimens drawn a few weeks apart is diagnostic of acute infection. The presence of IgG antibodies against *Brucella* may be used to indicate ongoing infection, since with effective treatment they should disappear.

Etiology *Brucella* are small gram-negative coccobacilli. There are several species, but human brucellosis is caused by only 4 of these: *B. abortus* (carried by cattle), *B. suis* (carried by hogs), *B. melitensis* (transmitted by sheep and goats), and *B. canis,* carried by dogs. Of these, *B. melitensis* is the most frequent pathogen, and causes the most severe disease.

Epidemiology Domestic livestock are the major source of human infection. As an infection of livestock, brucellosis occurs worldwide. There are 2 major routes of transmission. Direct contact with infected secretions may transmit the disease, as may occur with veterinarians, abbatoir employees, meat packers, and farmers. More commonly, infection occurs by ingestion of unpasteurized milk or milk products.

Brucellosis is rare in the United States, since pasteurization is routine and cattle are vaccinated against the disease. It is much more common in the U.S.S.R., Africa, South America, and the Middle East. Less than 200 cases are reported annually in the U.S., most cases being either imported from endemic regions or related to consumption of unpasteurized goats' milk.

Treatment—Standard The treatment of choice for brucellosis is a combination of tetracycline and streptomycin. Trimethoprim/sulfamethoxazole is an adequate alternative, but it is not as effective. In serious infections, such as meningitis or endocarditis, rifampin may be added to the regimen. Endocarditis generally warrants valve replacement in addition to antibiotic therapy.

Human infection can be prevented by a variety of measures. A vaccine is available for cattle, sheep, and goats. Workers handling meat or milk products that are likely to be infected should use protective clothing and gloves. Finally, pasteurization kills the bacteria.

Treatment—Investigational Please contact the agencies listed under Resources, below, for the most current information.

Resources
For more information on brucellosis: National Organization for Rare Disorders (NORD); Centers for Disease Control (CDC); Food and Drug Administration.

References
Brucella Species: A.J. Mikolich; *in* Principles and Practice of Infectious Diseases: G.L. Mandell, et al., eds.; Churchill Livingstone, 1990, pp. 1735–1742.

Cecil Textbook of Medicine, 18th ed.: J.B. Wyngaarden and L.H. Smith, Jr., eds.; W.B. Saunders Company, 1988, pp. 1676–1679.

CHAGAS DISEASE

Description Chagas disease is a systemic parasitic infection caused by *Trypanosoma cruzi* and transmitted by the bite of an insect, or by blood transfusion. Acute infection is usually contracted in childhood and is a mild illness. However, this is generally followed by chronic, low grade parasitemia, and in 10 to 30 percent of patients, chronic Chagas disease develops. The heart and gastrointestinal systems are most frequently involved; heart failure, megaesophagus, and megacolon are the most common features of endstage disease.

Synonyms
American Trypansomiasis
Brazilian Trypansomiasis

Signs and Symptoms Acute Chagas disease initially becomes manifest with a local reaction at the inoculation site, referred to as a chagoma. Occasionally the parasite enters through the conjunctiva of the eye, which produces a periorbital swelling referred to as Romana's sign. This is followed by fever and malaise and facial and leg edema. Physical examination may reveal generalized lymphadenopathy and hepatosplenomegaly. Severe cases may be complicated by meningoencephalitis or myocarditis, either of which may be fatal, but in the vast majority of cases symptoms resolve spontaneously without treatment.

T. cruzi infection then enters an indeterminate, or asymptomatic phase. During this phase parasitemia persists and the organisms may be transmitted by blood transfusion.

Many years after initial infection the symptoms of chronic Chagas disease develop. The heart is the most common organ involved; it becomes dilated as a result of atrophy of the myocardial cells and diffuse fibrosis. The symptoms are those of a dilated cardiomyopathy: arrhythmia, thromboembolism, and congestive heart failure.

Esophageal involvement, or megaesophagus, presents with dysphagia, chest pain, regurgitation, and aspiration. Megacolon generally produces constipation and abdominal pain and may be complicated by obstruction or volvulus.

In the acute stage, Chagas disease is diagnosed by microscopic examination of fresh anticoagulated blood, or thick and thin blood smears. Chronic infection may be confirmed serologically by either enzyme-linked immunosorbent assay (**ELISA**), or complement fixation tests.

Etiology Chagas disease is caused by the protozoan *Trypanosoma cruzi.*

Epidemiology *T. cruzi* is transmitted in nature by reduviid bugs. The bug bites the host; and then its feces, which contain the trypanosomes, contaminate the bite wound. Reduviid bugs tend to live in thatched and mud houses in rural environments of Latin America. The acute disease is mostly seen in children living in such environments, but the organism is also transmitted by blood transfusion, and this is its major route of spread in urban areas.

T. cruzi infection is very common in Central and South America; it has been estimated that 10 to 12 million people are parasitemic in these regions. Infection does not occur in the United States through reduviid bug transmission, but transfusion-associated cases have been reported. With increasing numbers of immigrants from endemic areas, transfusion-associated Chagas disease may become a more significant problem in the United States.

Related Disorders There are 2 species of trypanosomes that are pathogenic in man. *T. brucei* causes African trypanosomiasis. There are several subspecies, each of which causes different disease syndromes in different regions of Africa. The best known is African sleeping sickness, which is transmitted by the tsetse fly.

Treatment—Standard Acute Chagas disease may be treated with nifurtimox (a derivative of nitrofurazone), which reduces the morbidity and mortality of the acute illness. In most cases, however, the parasite survives and chronic parasitemia ensues. There are no satisfactory antimicrobial drugs for the treatment of the indeterminate and chronic stages of Chagas disease.

Chagas disease can be prevented by eliminating the insect that transmits the disease. Various insecticides can be used to spray houses. Improvements in housing are also helpful in preventing transmission.

Treatment—Investigational Allopurinol riboside is currently undergoing clinical trials. For more information, physicians can contact Burroughs Wellcome Co., 3030 Cornwallis Rd., Research Triangle Park, NC 27709.

A French pharmaceutical manufacturer, Fournier, is developing the drug

LF1695, for the treatment of Chagas and other diseases. Fournier may be contacted at Fournier Labs; BP90, Daix; 21121 Fontaine; Les Dijon, France.

Please contact the agencies listed under Resources, below, for the most current information.

Resources
For more information on Chagas disease: National Organization for Rare Disorders (NORD); Centers for Disease Control (CDC); NIH/National Institute of Allergy and Infectious Diseases (NIAID).

References
Cecil Textbook of Medicine, 18th ed.: J.B. Wyngaarden and L.H. Smith, Jr., eds.; W.B. Saunders Company, 1988, pp. 352–353, 1865–1869, 1920.
Is *Trypanosoma cruzi* a New Threat to our Blood Supply? L.V. Kirschoff; Ann. Int. Med., November 1989, vol. 110(10), pp. 773–774.

CHIKUNGUNYA

Description Chikungunya is one of several arthropod-borne viral diseases characterized by a rash, fever, and severe arthralgias. (Others include o'nyong-nyong fever and Mayaro virus disease.)

Signs and Symptoms Clinical disease begins with fever, headache, and arthralgias that may be so severe as to immobilize the patient. The joints involved include the knees, elbows, wrists, ankles, and fingers. Backache and a rash are also common. The fever usually abates before the 10th day, but the joint symptoms may take several weeks to resolve. Permanent joint damage does not occur.

Etiology Chikungunya is caused by a virus belonging to the group A arboviruses.

Epidemiology Chikungunya affects mostly children and young adults in Africa, Southeast Asia, and India. It is transmitted by various species of mosquitoes. Monkeys may also be infected.

Treatment—Standard Chikungunya resolves spontaneously. There is no specific treatment, but bed rest and antiinflammatory agents may be useful.

Treatment—Investigational Please contact the agencies listed under Resources, below, for the most current information.

Resources
For more information on chikungunya: National Organization for Rare Disorders (NORD); Centers for Disease Control (CDC); NIH/National Institute of Allergy and Infectious Diseases (NIAID).

References
Cecil Textbook of Medicine, 18th ed.: J.B. Wyngaarden and L.H. Smith, Jr., eds.; W.B. Saunders Company, 1988, p. 1819.

CHOLERA

Description Cholera is an acute illness caused by *Vibrio cholerae*, which colonizes but does not invade the small intestine. The major symptom, massive watery diarrhea, results from a bacterial enterotoxin that stimulates the intestinal cells to secrete fluid. There are several strains of *V. cholerae*, which differ somewhat in their virulence.

Cholera is not difficult to treat; most patients recover well with appropriate oral hydration alone. Without treatment, it can be a rapidly fatal disease.

Synonyms
    Asiatic Cholera
    Epidemic Cholera

Signs and Symptoms The symptoms of cholera vary in severity. Infection may be symptomatic, or the patient may only experience a few days of mild diarrhea. Alternatively, the initial fluid loss may be so great that the patient develops shock and dies within hours of onset.

The initial symptoms consist of a sudden painless diarrhea associated with vomiting. The diarrhea becomes progressively watery and large volumes of fluid, sodium, chloride, potassium, and bicarbonate are lost. Subsequent symptoms are all a result of dehydration and electrolyte imbalance. Intense thirst, decreased urine output, muscle cramps, and weakness can develop. Hypotension and hypokalemia are common; acidosis and shock may intervene if treatment is not provided. Renal failure may develop, but this generally responds to fluid replacement.

Etiology Cholera is caused by *Vibrio cholerae*, a gram-negative rod with several variably virulent biotypes. The symptoms represent the effects of a bacterial toxin.

Epidemiology Cholera is endemic in India and parts of the Middle East, Asia, and Africa. In these areas children are affected most often, with outbreaks occurring during the warmest part of the year. In addition it occasionally spreads to Europe, Japan, Australia, and South America, where epidemics can occur at any time of the year and affect persons of all ages equally.

Cholera is primarily a waterborne disease. During epidemics, spread may be particularly rapid as increasing numbers of individuals excrete large volumes of infected stool. If sanitation standards are less than optimal, drinking, washing, and cooking water becomes rapidly contaminated.

Related Disorders Cholera is one of several enterotoxigenic diarrheal diseases. *Escherichia coli* and some salmonella and shigella infections also produce similar clinical features. Other bacteria of the *Vibrio* genus that cause gastroenteritis include *V. parahaemolyticus*.

Pancreatic cholera is not a bacterial disease, but a result of pancreatic dysfunction leading to severe diarrhea.

Treatment—Standard In mild cases, cholera resolves spontaneously within 3 to 6 days of onset, and the bacteria disappear within 2 weeks. Most cases will require fluid replacement, and if started early, the majority of patients can do this orally. Intravenous fluids are necessary in very severe cases (with stool output that exceeds 7 liters a day), for patients in shock, and in cases where vomiting prohibits oral intake. Various solutions containing salts, bicarbonate, and glucose are available in packet form and can be administered easily without medical personnel.

Antibiotics will shorten the course of the disease. Tetracycline is the drug of choice, and ampicillin is an acceptable substitute for pregnant women and children. Furazolidone is effective against resistant strains.

The most important methods of prevention and control are a clean water supply and adequate sewage disposal. Boiling all water and food prior to consumption is also effective but is expensive and impractical in many areas of the world where the disease is endemic.

Vaccines are available but are not 100 percent effective, and require booster injections every 6 months. Tetracycline may be used prophylactically to protect against cholera if a patient is exposed to contaminated food or water.

Persons living in endemic areas usually develop immunity. Travelers to endemic regions should be vaccinated against this disorder.

Treatment—Investigational Please contact the agencies listed under Resources, below, for the most current information.

Resources

For more information on cholera: National Organization for Rare Disorders (NORD); Centers for Disease Control (CDC); National Institute of Allergy and Infectious Diseases (NIAID).

References
The Merck Manual, 15th ed.: R. Berkow, ed.-in-chief; Merck Sharp & Dohme Research Laboratories, 1987, pp. 91, 773, 1064.

Cecil Textbook of Medicine, 18th ed.: J.B. Wyngaarden and L.H. Smith, Jr., eds.; W.B. Saunders Company, 1988, pp. 1388–1389, 1651–1653.

COWPOX

Description Cowpox, a viral disease normally affecting the udders and teats of cows, is occasionally transmitted to man, in whom it produces a characteristic rash and enlarged lymph nodes. Cowpox also produces an immunity to smallpox, a fact that was massively exploited in the 19th century through widespread use of the virus, or virus-infected material, in vaccination programs. As a result, smallpox has been eradicated. The cause of cowpox, now called vaccinia virus, has been noted to produce systemic reactions in certain individuals following vaccination. This is referred to as generalized vaccinia.

Synonyms
Bovine Smallpox
Vaccinia

Signs and Symptoms The rash characteristic of human cowpox infection consists of numerous vesicles which may become inflamed or may bleed or ulcerate. The rash occurs on exposed skin (i.e., the face and extremities), and may be accompanied by lymphadenopathy.

When an immunosuppressed individual (particularly with agammaglobulinemia or chronic lymphocytic leukemia) is inadvertently vaccinated, a more severe form of infection may occur. Called vaccinia necrosum, or progressive vaccinia, this syndrome is characterized by progressive necrosis of the vaccination site, and a generalized eruption of metastatic lesions. It can be fatal.

Patients with severe eczema may also experience a generalized vaccinia eruption on vaccination or on contact with someone recently vaccinated.

A mild form of generalized vaccinia occurs in normal individuals following vaccination. Typically, a vesicular rash develops 7 to 12 days after vaccination; there are no other symptoms and the rash resolves spontaneously.

Other complications of smallpox vaccination include bacterial superinfection of vesicular lesions, postinfectious encephalitis, myocarditis, pericarditis, and arthritis.

Etiology Cowpox is caused by vaccinia virus.

Epidemiology Cowpox can be transmitted to humans directly by handling infected cows' udders, and can result from vaccination against smallpox, or, in some cases, from contact with a person with a vaccination lesion.

Currently, disease resulting from vaccination has become rare because the eradication of smallpox has rendered vaccination unnecessary, and it is no longer routine. However, vaccinia is being considered as a vector for immunization against other types of infectious agents; more widespread use of this virus will increase the prevalence of its adverse reactions.

Related Disorders Smallpox, caused by the variola virus, is a far more severe and disfiguring disease. Smallpox no longer occurs, although the virus is still retained in a few laboratories.

Treatment—Standard As in the case of most viral infections, there is no specific treatment for most cases. Vaccinia hyperimmune globulin is used to treat some complications of vaccinia. Other complications are treated symptomatically.

Treatment—Investigational Please contact the agencies listed under Resources, below, for the most current information.

Resources

For more information on vaccinia: National Organization for Rare Disorders (NORD); Centers for Disease Control (CDC); NIH/National Institute of Allergy and Infectious Diseases (NIAID).

References
Cecil Textbook of Medicine, 18th ed.: J.B. Wyngaarden and L.H. Smith, Jr., eds.; W.B. Saunders Company, 1988, pp. 1792–1793.

CRYPTOCOCCOSIS

Description Cryptococcosis is a systemic fungal infection caused by *Cryptococcus neoformans*. It is a common infection in patients with AIDS, and occasionally occurs in immunocompetent individuals. The most frequent systems involved are the central nervous system and the lungs.

Synonyms
> Busse-Buschke Disease
> European Blastomycosis
> Torulosis

Signs and Symptoms The most common presentation is meningoencephalitis. The onset is usually gradual and symptoms often are mild. The usual complaints include headache, confusion, nausea, dizziness, irritability, gait abnormalities, and behavioral changes.

There may be few specific findings on physical examination. Fever is frequently absent, as is meningismus. Papilledema is present in about one-third of cases, and even fewer patients have cranial nerve deficits. Other neurologic findings are rare.

The diagnosis is made on lumbar puncture. The cerebrospinal fluid usually shows elevated protein levels, low glucose levels, and a leukocytosis. An india ink stain of the fluid will reveal the organism in about 50 percent of cases. However, approximately 90 percent of samples will contain the cryptococcal capsular antigen.

Pulmonary infection is frequently inapparent. Chest pain and cough occur occasionally. The chest x-ray picture frequently resembles a malignancy. Diagnosis of pulmonary cryptococcosis often requires a biopsy, since sputum cultures are frequently negative, and are difficult to interpret when positive (many patients with other types of lung disease may be colonized).

C. neoformans may also cause skin lesions and osteolytic bone lesions. Cryptococcal pyelonephritis, chorioretinitis, endocarditis, adrenalitis, and hepatitis have also been reported, but these are rare.

Etiology Cryptococcosis is caused by the fungus *Cryptococcus neoformans*.

Epidemiology Cryptococcosis occurs worldwide. It is found in the soil and in pigeon feces, although patients generally have no history of exposure to pigeons. Transmission is thought to be by inhalation. Most patients with cryptococcosis have an underlying immunodeficiency such as AIDS or lymphoma. The disease tends to occur more often in males than females.

Treatment—Standard The antibiotic regimen used to treat cryptococcal meningoencephalitis includes amphotericin B, either alone or in combination with flucytosine. Fluconazole is a useful alternative to amphotericin. Hematologic side effects and rashes are very common in AIDS patients on flucytosine. The time course of therapy is determined by repeated lumbar puncture and cultures. Patients with AIDS are notoriously difficult to cure and may require some form of treatment for life, such as weekly intravenous injections of amphotericin B, or regular doses of flucytosine orally.

Other forms of cryptococcal disease are also treated with amphotericin B, with or without flucytosine. Some forms in immunocompetemt individuals may not require treatment, or may respond to surgical excision alone.

Treatment—Investigational Please contact the agencies listed under Resources, below, for the most current information.

Resources

For more information on cryptococcosis: National Organization for Rare Disorders (NORD); NIH/National Institute of Allergy and Infectious Diseases (NIAID); Centers for Disease Control (CDC); NIH/National Institute of Neurological Disorders & Stroke (NINDS).

References

Cryptococcal Meningitis: T.L. Tjia, et al.; J. Neurol. Neurosurg. Psychiatry, 1985, vol. 48(9), pp. 853–858.

Cryptococcal Meningitis: R. Biniek, et al.; Nervenarzt, 1986, vol. 57(1), pp. 47–55.

Clinical Spectrum of Infections in Patients with HTLV-III–Associated Diseases: J.W. Gold; Cancer Res., 1985, vol. 45(9 Suppl.), pp. 4652s–4654s.

CYSTICERCOSIS

Description Cysticercosis is one type of infection with the pork tapeworm, *Taenia solium*. Humans may be infected with 2 different stages of *T. solium,* and each produces a different syndrome.

In the life cycle of this parasite, pork containing encysted *T. solium* larvae are ingested by man, and the larvae develop into mature worms in the intestinal tract. This results in a tapeworm infection, which is usually mild or asymptomatic. The adult passes eggs in the stool, and these are ingested by the pig, develop into larvae, and the cycle continues. If man ingests the eggs (not the larvae), these will penetrate into the bloodstream and disseminate throughout various tissues of the body, where they encyst, resulting in cysticercosis.

Once in the tissues, they develop into cysticerci, which evoke a granulomatous reaction until they start to die. Dying cysts stimulate an acute inflammatory response that can produce tissue damage. While the cysticerci may appear anywhere in the body, preferred sites are the skeletal muscles, the eye, and brain. Other less common sites include the liver, heart, and lungs. Eventually, larvae will calcify.

Signs and Symptoms Cysts outside the brain and eye are generally asymptomatic. Cerebral cysticercosis causes seizures, which may be focal or generalized. Less common manifestations include headache, transient neurologic deficits, and psychosis. Ocular symptoms include visual disturbances, uveitis, and retinitis. Rarely, muscular infection may produce the symptoms of a myopathy.

Once the larvae calcify, they may be easily seen on skull x-rays, as well as CT scan. The radiologic appearance is diagnostic in some cases, and in others the disease may be confirmed serologically, although a large number of patients have false negative tests. Surgery is often necessary to provide a definitive diagnosis.

Etiology Cysticercosis develops when the eggs of the pork tapeworm *T. solium* are ingested. Egg ingestion occurs through consumption of food or water contaminated with human feces, and may occur by autoingestion. This results when the patient harbors the adult worm in the intestine; the eggs are passed in the feces, and through poor hygiene are transferred to the mouth of the same individual.

Epidemiology Cysticercosis is common in Mexico, Africa, and South America.

Related Disorders Tapeworms can be acquired from various uncooked meats, including beef *(Taenia saginata)* and fish *(Diphyllobothrium latum)*, but *T. solium* appears to be the only tapeworm that produces larvae capable of invading human muscle and forming cysts. The roundworm *Trichinella spiralis* also has a larval stage that invades the tissues and encysts; the resulting disease, trichinosis, is predominantly characterized by a diffuse myositis.

Treatment—Standard Praziquantel is the treatment of choice for both adult and larval stages of *T. solium.* Niclosamide may be used as an alternative. Steroids may be necessary to control edema surrounding cerebral lesions. Surgery may be required in some cases.

Treatment—Investigational Please contact the agencies listed under Resources, below, for the most current information.

Resources

For more information on cysticercosis: National Organization for Rare Disorders (NORD); Centers for Disease Control (CDC); NIH/National Institute of Allergy and Infectious Diseases (NIAID).

References

Cecil Textbook of Medicine, 18th ed.: J.B. Wyngaarden and L.H. Smith, Jr., eds.; W.B. Saunders Company, 1988, p. 1892.

Manson's Tropical Diseases, 19th ed.: P.E.C. Manson-Bahr and D.R. Bell; Ballière Tindall, 1987, pp. 536–540.

DENGUE FEVER

Description Dengue fever is an acute viral illness primarily consisting of fever, severe myalgias, and a rash. It is caused by a flavivirus and transmitted by mosquitoes. A severe form of dengue, known as dengue hemorrhagic fever, is characterized by thrombocytopenia, bleeding, and shock.

Synonyms

Breakbone Fever
Dandy Fever
Duengero
Seven-Day Fever

Signs and Symptoms Dengue fever begins abruptly after an incubation period of 5 to 8 days. Symptoms include fever, weakness, prostration, severe headache, retroorbital pain, and severe myalgias. The temperature rises rapidly, sometimes to as high as 40°C (104°F), and may be accompanied by a relative bradycardia. There may be lymphadenopathy and a maculopapular rash on physical examination. The rash typically begins on the trunk and spreads peripherally. The symptoms usually persist for 7 days.

Dengue hemorrhagic fever appears to occur in individuals already immunized against one dengue virus serotype, who are infected with another. It usually begins with fever, nausea, vomiting, and abdominal pain. Then thrombocytopenia develops, accompanied by petechiae, purpura, epistaxis, gastrointestinal hemorrhage, and in severe cases, shock **(dengue shock syndrome)**. Fibrinogen, and clotting factors V, VII, IX, and X are also reduced.

The diagnosis of dengue may be confirmed by virus isolation from the blood, or by serologic testing.

Etiology The dengue fever virus is a flavivirus. There are several distinct serotypes.

Epidemiology Dengue fever occurs mainly in the subtropical or tropical regions of southern Asia, South America (particularly Brazil), and the Caribbean, including Puerto Rico and the U.S. Virgin Islands. Dengue fever virus has also been imported into the United States by tourists from endemic areas.

Severe forms of dengue, including dengue hemorrhagic fever and dengue shock syndrome, usually occur in young children who have previously been infected with a different serotype. Infants may also develop the severe forms; they acquire immunity to one serotype passively either transplacentally or through breast milk. Infection with a new serotype produces the severe disease. Massive outbreaks have occurred when a new serotype is introduced to a susceptible population.

Dengue is transmitted by the *Aedes aegypti* mosquito.

Related Disorders There are a number of viral hemorrhagic fevers. The best known is yellow fever. Others include Lassa fever, Machupo fever (Bolivian hemorrhagic fever), Junin fever (Argentinian hemorrhagic fever), lymphocytic choriomeningitis, Marburg virus (hemorrhagic fever), and Ebola virus (hemorrhagic fever). Most of these can be distinguished on epidemiologic grounds.

Treatment—Standard There is no specific treatment for dengue, or dengue hemorrhagic fever. Supportive care, particularly intravenous fluid administration, may be lifesaving in severe cases. Transfusions of packed red blood cells or platelets may control bleeding.

Treatment—Investigational Interferon has been under investigation for the treatment of dengue hemorrhagic fever. In addition there have been attempts to develop a vaccine.

Please contact the agencies listed under Resources, below, for the most current information.

Resources

For more information on dengue fever: National Organization for Rare Disorders (NORD); Centers for Disease Control (CDC); NIH/National Institute of Allergy and Infectious Diseases (NIAID).

References

Dengue Fever in the United States. A Report of a Cluster of Imported Cases and Review of the Clinical, Epidemiologic, and Public Health Aspects of the Disease: M.D. Malison, et al.; JAMA, 1983, vol. 249(4), pp. 496–500.

Dengue Virus Type 2 Vaccine: Reactogenicity and Immunogenicity in Soldiers: W.H. Bancroft, et al.; J. Infect. Dis., 1984, vol. 149(6), pp. 1005–1010.

Dengue and Hepatic Failure: M.E. Alvarez, et al.; Amer. J. Med., 1985, vol. 79(5), pp. 670–674.

Effect of Interferons on Dengue Virus Multiplication in Cultured Monocytes/Macrophages: H. Hotta, et al.; Biken Journal, 1984, vol. 27(4), pp. 189–193.

DRACUNCULIASIS

Description Dracunculiasis is an infection caused by the tissue nematode *Dracunculus medinensis*, the guinea worm. Infection begins by drinking water containing infected crustaceans. Once in the stomach, the larvae are released and pass into the intestine. From there they migrate into the retroperitoneum where they mature. The adult females migrate out into the subcutaneous tissues and produce ulcers in the overlying skin. On contact with water, larvae are discharged from the ulcer.

Synonyms

Dracontiasis
Dracunculosis
Fiery Serpent Infection
Guinea Worm Infection

Signs and Symptoms Dracunculiasis is characterized by chronic skin ulcers in which the worms may be visible. Skin involvement begins with a painful, stinging papule on the skin, usually on the legs. This may be accompanied by nausea, vomiting, and diarrhea. Later the papule ulcerates and the female worm discharges her larvae. Gradually the worm is extruded over several weeks and then the ulcers heal.

Diagnosis of dracunculiasis is made on finding the larvae during microscopic examination of ulcer fluid.

Etiology Dracunculiasis is caused by swallowing water containing small, barely visible water fleas which carry the larva of the parasitic guinea worm, *Dracunculus medinensis*.

Epidemiology Dracunculiasis affects people in regions of Africa, the Middle East, and India, where drinking water is contaminated with *D. medinensis*.

Treatment—Standard This disorder is treated with niridazole, or the antihelmintic drugs thiabendazole or metronidazole. Treatment with these drugs promptly relieves symptoms and reduces the inflammation, but does not affect the worms. However, once the inflammation has subsided, the worms can be easily removed.

Chlorination, boiling, and straining of contaminated drinking water in areas of the world with poor sanitation can prevent transmission of dracunculiasis.

Treatment—Investigational Please contact the agencies listed under Resources, below, for the most current information.

Resources

For more information on dracunculiasis: National Organization for Rare Disorders (NORD); NIH/National Institute of Allergy and Infectious Diseases (NIAID); Centers for Disease Control (CDC).

References

The Comparative Study of Patterns of Guinea Worm Prevalence as a Guide to Control Strategies: S.J. Watts, et al.; Soc. Sci. Med., 1986, vol. 23(10), pp. 975–982.

Dracunculus Orchitis: A Case Report: A.K. Pendse, et al.; J. Trop. Med. Hyg., 1987, vol. 90(3), pp. 153–154.

Controlled Comparative Trial of Thiabendazole and Metronidazole in the Treatment of Dracontiasis: O.O. Kale, et al.; Ann. Trop. Med. Parasitol., 1983, vol. 77(2), pp. 151–157.

ELEPHANTIASIS

Description Elephantiasis is characterized by massive hypertrophy of a limb. It is caused by lymphatic obstruction. In tropical regions, it is most commonly associated with filariasis. In temperate regions, it has been reported rarely in individuals with recurrent streptococcal infections.

Synonyms

Elephantiasis Nostras

Signs and Symptoms The patient provides a history of recurrent streptococcal lymphangitis and cellulitis. There may have been initially an episode of thrombophlebitis. With successive infections, the impairment to lymphatic drainage worsens, and the edema progresses. The skin and subcutaneous tissue become thickened and fibrotic. The skin color becomes brawny and ulcerations may develop. Ultimately, the skin becomes pebbly and verrucous in appearance. The reason for the skin responding in this way to chronic lymphedema is unclear.

In filariasis the external genitalia may also be involved.

Etiology Elephantiasis nostras is the end result of a cycle of repeated streptococcal infections, each followed by progressive edema, occurring over many years. Impairment of lymphatic drainage is known to be a risk factor for streptococcal infection, and while the initial insult to the lymphatics may have been noninfectious, each bout of infection worsens the lymphatic obstruction, and therefore continues the cycle.

Tinea pedis has been associated with streptococcal infection of the leg. First reported in men following saphenous vein resection for coronary bypass surgery, the lesions of tinea pedis are thought to be the portal of entry for the streptococcus. The combination of superficial foot wound and lymphatic obstruction sets the stage for infection. However, in spite of the prevalence of minor degrees of lymphatic obstruction in the population, progression to elephantiasis nostras is very rare.

Epidemiology Elephantiasis is most common in Africa, where filariasis is the usual cause. Elephantiasis nostras occurs very rarely in temperate climates.

Related Disorders

Hereditary lymphedema is a genetic disorder of the lymphatic system in which the lymphatic channels are obstructed or underdeveloped.

Filariasis is the most common cause of elephantiasis worldwide.

Treatment—Standard The infections are treated with penicillin. Erythromycin is the major alternative in penicillin-allergic patients. Once elephantiasis develops, surgery may be necessary to remove excess tissue.

Treatment—Investigational Please contact the agencies listed under Resources, below, for the most current information.

Resources

For more information on elephantiasis: National Organization for Rare Disorders; NIH/National Institute of Allergy and Infectious Diseases; Centers for Disease Control (CDC).

References

Elephantiasis Nostras: An Eight-Year Observation of Progressive Nonfilarial Elephantiasis of the Lower Extremity: L.J. Sanders, et al.; Cutis, November 1988, vol. 42(5), pp. 406–411.

Elephantiasis Nostras—A Case Report: S.A. Baughman et al.; Angiology, February 1988, vol. 39(2), pp. 164–168.

ENCEPHALITIS, HERPETIC

Description Herpetic encephalitis is caused by herpes simplex virus **(HSV),** and is the most common form of acute, sporadic encephalitis in the United States. It is characterized clinically by fever, headache, and focal neurologic symptoms, usually due to a focus of infection in the temporal lobe.

Synonyms

Herpes Encephalitis

Herpes Simplex Encephalitis

Herpetic Meningoencephalitis

Signs and Symptoms The onset of herpes encephalitis is usually abrupt, with fever, headache, behavior disturbances, personality changes, and focal seizures. In some cases there is a prodrome of malaise, fever, anorexia, and other nonspecific symptoms. Focal neurologic deficits may occur, including hemiparesis, dysphasia, and cranial nerve deficits, and later in the course of illness stupor and coma may develop.

The cerebrospinal fluid characteristically shows elevated protein levels, lymphocytosis, and the presence of red blood cells. The most common electroencephalographic abnormality is a diffuse slowing over the involved temporal lobe. CT scanning may reveal swelling in the temporal lobe. None of these is diagnostic, and brain biopsy has been the method of choice for confirming the diagnosis of herpes encephalitis. Assays for HSV antigens in the cerebrospinal fluid are under investigation, and should they become available, the diagnosis may require only a lumbar puncture.

Etiology The vast majority of cases of herpes encephalitis are caused by HSV-1. Encephalitis may result from primary HSV infection, or more commonly there is evidence of past mucocutaneous infection.

Epidemiology Herpes encephalitis usually occurs during childhood or early adulthood. There is no seasonal variation.

Related Disorders The differential diagnosis of herpes encephalitis includes other viral encephalitides, meningitis, and focal intracerebral processes such as abscess, tumor, and vascular accidents.

Treatment—Standard The treatment of choice for herpetic encephalitis is intravenous acyclovir. This improves survival but does not always correct all neurologic deficits; significant residual neurologic impairment is common. Vidarabine (arabinosyl adenine, Ara-A) is also useful, but less effective than acyclovir.

Treatment—Investigational Several new antiviral agents are currently under investigation.

Please contact the agencies listed under Resources, below, for the most current information.

Resources

For more information on herpes encephalitis: National Organization for Rare Disorders (NORD); NIH/National Institute of Allergy and Infectious Diseases (NIAID); Centers for Disease Control (CDC); NIH/National Institute of Neurological Disorders & Stroke (NINDS).

References

Herpetic Encephalitis: Prognostic Elements in Adults and Children (49 Cases): A. Foucher, et al.; Rev. Electroencephalogr. Neurophysiol. Clin., 1985, vol. 15(2), pp. 185–193.

Ocular Infection With Herpes Simplex Virus Type 1: Prevention of Acute Herpetic Encephalitis by Systemic Administration of Virus-Specific Antibody: W.B. Taylor, et al.; J. Infect. Dis., 1979, vol. 140(4), pp. 534–540.

ENCEPHALITIS, JAPANESE

Description Japanese encephalitis is caused by a flavivirus, the Japanese B encephalitis virus (**JBEV**), and transmitted by mosquitoes in certain areas of the world, particularly Asia. This disorder most commonly affects children and tends to be more actively spread during the summer.

Synonyms
> Japanese B Encephalitis
> Russian Autumnal Encephalitis
> Summer Encephalitis

Signs and Symptoms Most JBEV infections are mild or asymptomatic, but in a small percentage of cases, severe encephalitis occurs. After an incubation period of 4 to 14 days the patient is suddenly stricken with fever, headache, nausea, vomiting, behavioral changes, and neurologic deficits. The patient may be stuporous or comatose by the 4th day. The mortality rate is high, particularly in the elderly, and residual neurologic deficits are common among those who survive.

The cerebrospinal fluid may be normal, or may show a pleocytosis and elevated protein. The diagnosis may be confirmed serologically, using complement fixation or hemagglutination inhibition tests.

Etiology Japanese encephalitis is caused by a flavivirus (group B arbovirus). Symptoms are due to viral invasion and destruction of neurons. Necrosis is most marked in the thalamus and substantia nigra.

Epidemiology Japanese encephalitis afflicts approximately 20,000 people annually. Epidemics occur during the summer months in India, Bangladesh, the eastern part of Russia, China, Korea, Nepal, Burma, Vietnam, and northern Thailand. In tropical areas of southeast Asia, southern India, southern Thailand, and Sri Lanka, the disease is present year-round. Sporadic outbreaks occur throughout the year until the tropical rainy season, when the illness can be transmitted in epidemic proportions.

The virus is transmitted by mosquitoes that breed in rice fields. Pigs and birds are the major reservoirs.

Related Disorders The symptoms of Japanese encephalitis are similar to those of other viral encephalitides. JBEV is antigenically related to the viruses of Murray Valley encephalitis and St. Louis encephalitis, and to West Nile virus.

Murray Valley encephalitis, also known as **Australian X disease,** is a severe encephalitis which is found in Australia and New Guinea. Like Japanese encephalitis, the Murray Valley type is also transmitted by mosquitoes. Cases among children tend to be most severe, and permanent brain damage may result.

Saint Louis encephalitis is less severe. Caused by a group B arbovirus and transmitted by mosquitoes, this type of encephalitis occurs in sporadic outbreaks in urban areas of Missouri, Arizona, Colorado, Nevada, Texas, Indiana, Illinois, Kentucky, Florida, New Jersey, Pennsylvania, and the Ohio Valley. It tends to be more prevalent during midsummer to early fall. The symptoms are typical of encephalitis.

West Nile encephalitis, also known as **West Nile fever,** is characterized by severe headaches, high fever, enlargement of the lymph nodes, and meningismus. Symptoms of this disorder may last only a few weeks, but it may cause permanent neurologic damage.

Treatment—Standard In Asian nations, an effective vaccination is available for Japanese encephalitis. In the United States, the vaccination is not available to civilian personnel. For information on availability of vaccines against Japanese encephalitis, please contact the Division of Vector-Borne Viral Diseases, Department of Health and Human Services, Public Health Service, Centers for Disease Control. Short-term travelers to Asian urban centers are at low risk to contract this disorder. The mosquitoes which transmit the virus are most concentrated in rural areas where there is standing water. They feed at sunset. Precautions include adequate clothing, sleeping in screened quarters under mosquito netting, and the use of insect repellents on exposed skin. Repellents containing over 30 percent active ingredient N,N-diethyl-meta-toluamide (DEET) are recommended.

Treatment—Investigational The antiviral agent carboxymethylacridanone (**CMA**) is currently under investigation for the treatment of Japanese encephalitis. It has shown benefit in JBEV-infected laboratory animals. More research is needed before it can be recommended for use in humans.

Please contact the agencies listed under Resources, below, for the most current information.

Resources

For more information on Japanese encephalitis: National Organization for Rare Disorders (NORD); Centers for Disease Control (CDC); World Health Organization.

References

The Pathogenesis of Acute Viral Encephalitis and Postinfectious Encephalomyelitis: R.T. Johnson; J. Infect. Dis., 1987, vol. 155(3), pp. 359–364.

Clinical Aspects of Japanese B Encephalitis in North Vietnam: D.H. Le; Clin. Neurol. Neurosurg., 1986, vol. 88(3), pp. 189–192.

Trial of Inactivated Japanese Encephalitis Vaccine in Children with Underlying Diseases: A. Yamada, et al.; Vaccine 1986, vol. 4(1), pp. 32–34.

ENCEPHALITIS, RASMUSSEN

Description Rasmussen encephalitis is a rare central nervous system disorder characterized by seizures, progressive hemiparesis, and mental deterioration.

Synonyms

Chronic Encephalitis and Epilepsy
Chronic Localized Encephalitis
Epilepsy, Hemiplegia, and Mental Retardation

Signs and Symptoms Rasmussen encephalitis usually begins in childhood. Some cases are thought to follow viral infections such as influenza and measles. Typically, the child develops seizures that are usually focal but may become generalized. Hemiparesis and mental retardation generally have their onset early in childhood and progress slowly.

The diagnosis of encephalitis may not be made until surgery is performed or postmortem brain tissue is examined.

Etiology The etiology of Rasmussen encephalitis is unknown. It may be a postviral phenomenon or a slow virus infection.

Epidemiology Fewer than 30 cases of Rasmussen encephalitis have been described in the medical literature since this disorder was first identified in 1958. The number of unidentified cases may be much higher.

Related Disorders See *Subacute Sclerosing Panencephalitis;* its course and symptoms may be similar to those of Rasmussen encephalitis.

Treatment—Standard Treatment consists of anticonvulsants and other symptomatic measures.

Treatment—Investigational Surgery is currently under investigation for the treatment of Rasmussen encephalitis. The procedure involves resection of the areas of the brain affected by encephalitis, in an attempt to control the seizures and progressive neurologic degeneration. For more information, please contact Ben Carson, M.D., Chief of Pediatric Neurosurgery, Children's Center, Johns Hopkins Hospital, Baltimore, MD 21205.

Please contact the agencies listed under Resources, below, for the most current information.

Resources

For more information on Rasmussen encephalitis: National Organization for Rare Disorders (NORD); NIH/National Institute of Neurological Disorders & Stroke (NINDS); Centers for Disease Control (CDC); Theodore Rasmussen, M.D., Montreal Neurological Hospital; Ben Carson, M.D., Johns Hopkins Hospital.

References
Focal Seizures Due to Chronic Localized Encephalitis: T. Rasmussen, et al.; Neurology, 1958, vol. 8(6), pp. 435–445.

Further Observations on the Syndrome of Chronic Encephalitis and Epilepsy: T. Rasmussen; Applied Neurophysiology, 1978, vol. 41, pp. 1–12.

Smoldering Encephalitis in Children: P.C. Gupta, et al.; Neuropediatrics, 1984, vol. 15(4), pp. 191–197.

ENCEPHALOMYELITIS, MYALGIC (ME)

Description Myalgic encephalomyelitis is a disorder that affects the central, peripheral, and autonomic nervous systems and the muscles. It is thought to be infectious in nature, possibly viral, but the exact etiology is unknown. The major symptoms may include fatigue, headache, myalgias, weakness, and emotional lability.

Synonyms
Akureyri Disease
Benign Myalgic Encephalomyelitis
Epidemic Myalgic Encephalomyelitis
Epidemic Neuromyasthenia
Iceland Disease
Raphe Nucleus Encephalopathy
Royal Free Disease
Tapanui Flu

Signs and Symptoms There may be a prodromal phase consisting of one or more of the following: headache, fatigue, sore throat, coughing, diarrhea or vomiting, malaise, and depression. These symptoms may persist up to 3 weeks. Then myalgias and arthralgias may develop, with or without a low-grade fever. Mental symptoms such as emotional lability, memory loss, depression, and difficulty in concentrating may be present. Other symptoms may include visual disturbances and paresthesias, urinary retention, and respiratory symptoms. Symptoms may be aggravated by strenuous exercise or emotional stress.

The aches and pains may subside after several days, but can persist intermittently for months or years.

Physical examination may reveal hepatomegaly, hyperactive tendon reflexes, muscle twitching, sensory loss, and cranial nerve paralysis. Certain laboratory abnormalities have been reported, such as an elevated lactic dehydrogenase (LDH), abnormal lymphocytes, and an elevated cerebrospinal fluid protein level.

Etiology The etiology of myalgic encephalomyelitis is unknown. It is thought to be a viral illness, possibly related to Epstein-Barr virus (**EBV**), although this relationship is unproven.

Epidemiology Myalgic encephalomyelitis occurs most often in the summer. It affects young adults, and is more common in females than in males. Epidemics have been reported worldwide, but sporadic cases are the rule.

Related Disorders Symptoms of the following disorders can be similar to myalgic encephalomyelitis. Comparisons may be useful for a differential diagnosis.

Chronic EBV infection, the protracted form of infectious mononucleosis that occurs in some patients, resembles myalgic encephalomyelitis in many respects.

See ***Multiple Sclerosis (MS),*** which may manifest in a similar fashion to ME, with intermittent neurologic deficits. MS has a characteristic picture on nuclear magnetic resonance scanning that will easily distinguish it from ME.

See ***Polymyalgia Rheumatica,*** which is also characterized by muscle pain and may be accompanied by fever, fatigue, and depression; it, however, usually occurs in older individuals.

Treatment—Standard The treatment of myalgic encephalomyelitis is supportive.

Antidepressant drugs may be helpful. Drugs such as pizotifen and carbamazepine may alleviate headache and myalgias.

Treatment—Investigational Research is underway to determine if a coxsackie B virus and tryptophan deficiency may be etiologic factors in myalgic encephalomyelitis.

Please contact the agencies listed under Resources, below, for the most current information.

Resources

For more information on myalgic encephalomyelitis: National Organization for Rare Disorders (NORD); American Encephalomyelitis Society; Myalgic Encephalomyelitis Association; NIH/National Institute of Allergy and Infectious Diseases (NIAID); Centers for Disease Control (CDC); Chronic Fatigue Syndrome Society; National Chronic Fatigue Syndrome Association.

References

Epidemiolgical Approaches to 'Epidemic Neuromyasthenia': Syndromes of Unknown Etiology (Epidemic Myalgic Encephalopathies): M. Thomas; Postgrad. Med. J., 1978, vol. 54(637), pp. 768–770.

Raphe Nucleus Encephalopathy (Myalgic Encephalomyelitis, Epidemic Neuromyasthenia): C.P. Maurizi; Med. Hypotheses, 1985, vol. 16(4), pp. 351–354.

FASCIOLIASIS

Description Fascioliasis is caused by the liver fluke, *Fasciola hepatica.* The clinical syndrome is caused by parasitization of the bile ducts. A subtype of fascioliasis **(Halzoun syndrome)** affects the pharynx.

Signs and Symptoms Initial symptoms may include fever, epigastric pain, arthralgias, diarrhea, pruritis, and jaundice. There may be hepatosplenomegaly and facial edema, and eosinophilia is evident on laboratory examination. In untreated cases cirrhosis may occur, but only after very prolonged infection. Subclinical infections are probably common in some parts of the world.

The diagnosis rests on finding the parasite ova in the feces.

Etiology The cause of fascioliasis is infection with *F. hepatica.*

Epidemiology *F. hepatica* infection is a zoonosis; sheep are the usual host. Consequently, fascioliasis is most common in sheep-raising areas, particularly in South America, Australia, China, and Africa. Infection has been reported in the southern and western United States. The intermediate host is the snail, and encysted forms of the parasite may be found attached to aquatic plants. Man usually acquires infection by ingestion of contaminated plants. Adequate cooking is generally sufficient to prevent infection.

Related Disorders Other liver flukes capable of producing infection in man are *Clonorchis sinensis,* and *Opisthorchis* species.

Halzoun syndrome, a variant of fascioliasis, affects the throat. It is caused by *F. hepatica, F. gigantica,* or other parasites known as linguatulid larvae.

Treatment—Standard Praziquantel has been used to treat fascioliasis, although recent studies show that bithionol (see below) may be more effective. Preventative measures include boiling vegetables and water purification.

Treatment—Investigational Studies of bithionol are being conducted by the Centers for Disease Control **(CDC).** Although this drug is available for experimental use through the CDC, its longterm effectiveness and toxicity have yet to be determined.

The drug Niclofolan, a biphenyl anthelmintic compound, is being investigated in West Germany as a treatment for fascioliasis. Further testing is needed to determine effectiveness and possible side effects of this drug.

Please contact the agencies listed under Resources, below, for the most current information.

Resources

For more information on fascioliasis: National Organization for Rare Disorders (NORD); American Liver Foundation; The United Liver Foundation; Children's Liver Foundation; NIH/National Institute of Allergy and Infectious Diseases; Centers for Disease Control (CDC).

References

Treatment of Human Fascioliasis with Niclofolan: T. Eckhardt, et al.; Gastroenterology, October 1981, issue 81(4), pp. 795–798.

FILARIASIS

Description The term filariasis usually refers to disease caused by either the *Wuchereria bancrofti* or *Brugia malayi* worms. It is characterized by lymphadenopathy and chronic lymphatic obstruction, which over prolonged periods may result in elephantiasis (see ***Elephantiasis),*** especially of the legs and genitalia.

The larval forms of the pathogen are inoculated by the mosquito. These make their way to the lymphatics, where they mature and reproduce microfilariae. Disease is primarily a response to adult worms, which elicit a granulomatous inflammatory reaction. The chronic inflammation progresses to fibrosis and obstruction of the lymph flow.

Synonyms

Filarial Elephantiasis
Wuchereriasis

Signs and Symptoms Filariasis may be asymptomatic. Alternatively, there may be bouts of lymphangitis with fever, aches, and pain in the involved lymph nodes. Edema of the involved limb may occur but it resolves after the attack. Acute funiculitis, epididymitis, and orchitis may accompany these attacks. Characteristically, eosinophilia may be found during acute episodes, but when the inflammation subsides, the eosinophil count returns to normal.

Another common presentation of filariasis is chronic lymphadenopathy without other findings.

Longstanding lymphatic obstruction has several consequences. These include hydrocele, chyluria (due to rupture of lymph into the urinary tract), lymph varices, and progressive edema of the scrotum, vulva, breast, or limbs, i.e., elephantiasis. Chronic edema is ultimately accompanied by a thickened, warty appearance of the skin.

The diagnosis of filariasis requires examination of a blood smear for microfilariae. Since parasitemia tends to occur at night, the specimen is best obtained at night. When parasitemia cannot be demonstrated, the adult worms may occasionally be found in a lymph node biopsy. In the late stages of disease, the diagnosis is often made by exclusion.

Etiology Filariasis is caused by the tissue nematodes *W. bancrofti* and *B. malayi*. Symptoms result primarily from inflammatory reactions to the adult worms, as described above. Hypersensitivity reactions to the microfilariae may also develop.

Epidemiology Filariasis is common in tropical regions of the world. *W. bancrofti* is widely distributed throughout Africa, Asia, China, and South America. *B. malayi* is found in southern and southeast Asia. The disease does not occur in North America, although cases are occasionally imported from tropical regions. The infection is transmitted by several tropical mosquito species which transfer the larval stage (microfilariae) from one host to another.

Related Disorders The term "filariasis" has been used here in its narrower sense. In its broad sense, filariasis refers to infections with various species of nematodes, whose adult forms have a hairlike appearance. In addition to the lymphatic filariasis described in this chapter, there are subcutaneous types (onchocerciasis and loiasis) and those associated with serous cavity infection, chiefly acanthocheilonemiasis (see *Acanthocheilonemiasis*). Others include dirofilariasis. All of these except dirofilariasis are common tropical diseases.

Treatment—Standard Diethylcarbamazine is the most effective agent for filariasis. It removes microfilariae from the circulation and kills or impairs the reproductive capacity of the adult worms. A somewhat less effective drug, levamisole, has also been investigated. The elimination of adult worms must be undertaken with care because the dead worms can provoke dangerous allergic reactions and abscesses. Antihistamines and corticosteroids are used to control such hypersensitivity reactions. Surgery may be used to treat hydrocele, or to remove the remains of adult worms and calcifications developing around them.

Treatment—Investigational Please contact the agencies listed under Resources, below, for the most current information.

Resources
    For more information on filariasis: National Organization for Rare Disor-

ders (NORD); Centers for Disease Control (CDC); NIH/National Institute of Allergy and Infectious Diseases.

References

Tropical Diseases of Importance to the Traveler: K.R. Brown, S.M. Phillips; Adv. Intern. Med., 1984, vol. 29, pp. 59–84.

Efficacy of the Vermectins Against Filarial Parasites: A Short Review: W.C. Campbell; Vet. Res. Commun., May 1982, vol. 5(3), pp. 251–262.

Recent Advances in Research on Filariasis. Chemotherapy: L.G. Goodwin; Trans. R. Soc. Trop. Med. Hyg., 1984, 78 suppl., pp. 1–8.

Diethylcarbamazine and New Compounds for the Treatment of Filariasis: F.Hawking; Adv. Pharmacol. Chemother., 1979, vol. 16, pp. 129–194.

Use of Levamisole in Parasitic Infections: M.J.Miller; Drugs, August 1980, vol. 20(2), pp. 122–130.

Tropical Eosinophilia: C.J.Spry, V. Kumaraswami; Semin. Hematol., April 1982, vol. 19(2), pp. 107–115.

GIARDIASIS

Description Giardiasis is an infection of the duodenum and jejunum caused by the protozoan *Giardia lamblia*. The primary manifestation of symptomatic infection is malabsorption, but many infections are asymptomatic.

Synonyms

Beaver Fever
Lambliasis

Signs and Symptoms Within 3 weeks of exposure, crampy abdominal discomfort, watery diarrhea, flatulence, and foul-smelling stools may appear. Acute attacks usually last approximately 3 or 4 days, although symptoms may persist for several weeks.

In longterm infestation, patients may experience chronic diarrhea, malabsorption of nutrients, weight loss, epigastric cramping, anorexia, nausea, and vomiting. Children with chronic giardiasis may experience growth retardation.

The diagnosis of giardiasis is usually made by demonstrating the parasites in the stool. Occasionally a duodenal aspirate or jejunal biopsy is required.

Etiology Giardiasis is caused by the protozoan parasite known as *Giardia lamblia*. Humans are infected by the parasites in the cyst stage.

Epidemiology This disorder occurs worldwide. Epidemics in the United States have been linked to the excretion of cysts into public water reservoirs by infected beavers. Outbreaks have also occurred in daycare centers and custodial institutions such as prisons and longterm care facilities, where transmission occurs directly from person to person.

Other populations at risk include homosexuals practicing anilingus, immunocompromised individuals, travelers from endemic areas, and campers who drink untreated water.

Related Disorders Related disorders include other parasitic infections of the intestine: amebiasis, hookworm infection, and strongyloidiasis. Disorders with similar symptoms include those that produce malabsorption.

Amebiasis is a disease of the intestinal tract caused by the protozoan parasite *Entamoeba histolytica.* It is transmitted person-to-person and by food- and water-borne routes. The organism invades the colon and rectum producing ulcers and inflammation. Symptoms begin gradually with an increasing number of stools reaching as many as 15 per day. Stools may be semi-solid to liquid and may be bloody. Abdominal pain is common, but fever is unusual. In the United States, amebiasis primarily affects visitors returning from countries with poor sanitation. Treatment with the drug metronidazole is often effective in eliminating the disorder.

Hookworm is a parasitic organism that penetrates the skin and migrates to the intestines where it attaches and sucks blood. Abdominal pain may occur, but the most prominent symptoms are those related to chronic blood loss: iron deficiency anemia and hypoalbuminemia. Approximately 25 percent of the world population may be infected with hookworms. Infection is acquired by walking barefoot in soil contaminated with parasites that penetrate the skin.

Strongyloidiasis is a parasitic intestinal disorder which, when severe, produces epigastric pain and tenderness, vomiting, and diarrhea. The causative agent is the intestinal nematode *Strongyloides stercoralis.* This disorder is usually found in the tropics in areas of poor sanitation. It can exist in crowded, unsanitary institutions anywhere, can persist for decades, and may recrudesce in fulminant form should the host become immunocompromised. Treatment with thiabendazole is often effective for patients with strongyloidiasis.

Treatment—Standard The treatment of choice for giardiasis patients is quinacrine or metronidazole (however, the latter is not yet approved for giardiasis in the United States). Furazolidone is especially useful in the treatment of children. The most important factor for preventing this disorder is proper treatment of infected water. Chlorination may not kill cysts; sedimentation, flocculation, and filtration should also be performed. Water can be boiled for 1 minute or mixed with halazone or iodine to eliminate contamination. Travelers to areas with contaminated water should drink only boiled or treated water and should not consume uncooked fruit or vegetables.

Treatment—Investigational Treatment with tinidazole or ornidazole for giardiasis may be effective. However, these medications have not yet been approved for use in the United States for this condition.

Please contact the agencies listed under Resources, below, for the most current information.

Resources

For more information on giardiasis: National Organization for Rare Disorders (NORD); NIH/National Institute of Allergy and Infectious Diseases (NIAID); Centers for Disease Control (CDC).

References

Internal Medicine, 2nd ed.: J.H. Stein, ed.-in-chief; Little, Brown and Company, 1987, pp. 1785–1786.

Management of Giardiasis: E.D. Gorski; Am. Fam. Phys., 1985, vol. 32(5), pp. 157–164.

Selective Primary Health Care: Strategies for Control of Disease in the Developing World. XIX. Giardiasis: D.P. Stevens; Rev. Infect. Dis., 1985, vol. 7(4), pp. 530–535.

Treatment of Intestinal E. Histolytica and G. Lamblia with Metronidazole, Tinidazole and Ornidazole: A Comparative Study: S. Bassily, et al.; J. Trop. Med. Hyg., 1987, vol. 90(1), pp. 9–12.

HAND-FOOT-MOUTH SYNDROME

Description Hand-foot-mouth syndrome is a relatively common mild viral disease that occurs in young children. It is characterized by a vesicular rash that appears on the hands and feet and in the mouth. It is usually caused by coxsackieviruses.

Synonyms

Hand, Foot, and Mouth Disease

Vesicular Stomatitis with Exanthem

Signs and Symptoms The most prominent feature of the syndrome is a rash, which begins as a macular or papular eruption. The lesions become vesicular and ulcerate. The intraoral lesions are ulcerative and painful and occur on the tongue and buccal mucosa. The lesions on the hands and feet, usually vesicular, occur most often dorsally. Occasionally lesions appear on the buttocks as well. The rash generally resolves in a week, but chronic and recurrent forms occur. The rash may be accompanied by fever, malaise, and headache. Hand-foot-mouth syndrome may be epidemic in certain geographic areas.

More severe forms of hand-foot-mouth syndrome have been associated with enterovirus 71; these may be complicated by central nervous system involvement (aseptic meningitis or encephalitis).

Hand-foot-mouth disease is generally diagnosed clinically, and usually can be distinguished from other exanthems by its distribution.

Etiology Hand-foot-mouth syndrome is caused by a virus, the coxsackievirus A16 or enterovirus 71.

Epidemiology The syndrome affects males and females in equal numbers and is common in young children.

Related Disorders The differential diagnosis of hand-foot-mouth disease includes chickenpox, herpangina, and exanthems caused by coxsackie- and echoviruses.

Herpangina is an acute viral infection that usually affects infants and young children. Fever is often the initial complaint. Sore throat, anorexia, and diffuse myalgias may occur, as well as vomiting and convulsions. In the first 24 hours a small number (average, 5) of small lesions appear in the oropharangeal area. These lesions eventually become shallow ulcers and will heal within 5 days. In contrast to hand-foot-mouth disease, the extremities are generally not involved.

The skin lesions of **chickenpox** may resemble hand-foot-mouth disease, but the distributions are quite different. The rash of chickenpox is more extensive and more centrally located.

Echoviruses and coxsackieviruses are also associated with vesicular eruptions, although the distributions are more central.

Encephalitis may be associated with hand-foot-mouth syndrome. It can also be caused by viruses such as the St. Louis, western equine, California, mumps, ECHO, and several coxsackieviruses.

Treatment—Standard Treatment is supportive. Calamine lotion and acetaminophen (not aspirin in children) may be helpful.

Treatment—Investigational At the present time, a study is being conducted on the effectiveness of murine interferon as a treatment for coxsackievirus type A 16 (CA-16) or enterovirus type 71 (EV 71). More research must be conducted to determine longterm safety and effectiveness of this drug.

Please contact the agencies listed under Resources, below, for the most current information.

Resources

For more information on hand-foot-mouth syndrome: National Organization for Rare Disorders (NORD); Centers for Disease Control (CDC); NIH/National Institute of Allergy and Infectious Diseases (NIAID).

References

Internal Medicine, 2nd ed.: J.H. Stein, ed.-in-chief; Little, Brown and Company, 1987, p. 1569.

Outbreak of Enterovirus 71 Infection in Victoria, Australia, with a High Incidence of Neurological Involvement: G. Gilbert, et al.; Pediatr. Infect. Dis. J., 1988, vol. 7(7), pp. 484–488.

Hand, Foot, and Mouth Disease: A. Buchner, 1976, vol. 41(3), pp. 333–337.

Protective Effect of Interferon on Infections with Hand, Foot and Mouth Disease Virus in Newborn Mice; D. Sasaki, et al.; J. Infect. Dis., 1986, vol. 153(3), pp. 498–502.

HEPATITIS B

Description Hepatitis B is a form of infectious hepatitis caused by the hepatitis B virus **(HBV)**. There are 5 known viruses capable of producing infectious hepatitis; these have been named hepatitis A, B, C, D (or delta agent) and E. All 5 can produce an acute hepatitis syndrome. HBV infection may be asymptomatic or can produce an acute hepatitis ranging from mild to fulminant. HBV infection can also persist in an asymptomatic carrier state which has been implicated in the development of hepatocellular carcinoma, or as chronic active hepatitis, which can progress to cirrhosis.

Synonyms

Hepatitis
Viral Hepatitis

Signs and Symptoms The incubation period of HBV is 2 to 6 weeks. There may be a prodrome prior to the onset of jaundice with variable symptoms including cough, pharyngitis, nausea, vomiting, arthralgias, myalgias, and low-grade fever. Once jaundice appears, hepatomegaly and occasionally splenomegaly can be detected on examination. The liver is usually tender. In severe cases, ascites, edema, bleeding, and signs of hepatic encephalopathy may occur.

Hepatitis B usually runs its course in 4 to 8 weeks, except in some variations of the disease. (For information on these, please see the Related Disorders section of this discussion.)

The diagnosis of hepatitis B is based on serologic studies.

Immunologically, the virus has several detectable components. Those of major diagnostic importance are the surface antigen (**HBsAg**) and the core antigen (**HBcAg**). A 3rd distinct antigen, the e antigen, is associated with a high degree of infectivity.

The first antigen to appear in the blood in measurable quantities is the s antigen, and this appears before clinical illness. This antigen may persist beyond the acute phase of disease and can be used to diagnose the carrier state. More typically, HBsAg disappears and antibody (**anti-HBs**) subsequently develops. Anti-HBs antibody is the protective antibody.

The c antigen is not usually detectable, but antibody to the c antigen (**anti-HBc**) appears early in infection and remains elevated long after the fall in HBsAg levels. This antibody is an important diagnostic aid, and is used to diagnose those cases where the HBsAg levels are no longer detectable and anti-HBs antibody is not yet detectable.

Etiology HBV is a DNA virus composed of a surface coat and a core. These components are immunologically distinct, as described above.

Epidemiology HBV has been found in virtually all body fluids and may be transmitted in several different ways. Worldwide, its most important mode of transmission is perinatal. Perinatal infection is associated with the chronic carrier state and development of hepatocellular carcinoma in later years.

HBV may be transmitted through transfusion of blood and blood products; this well-established fact led to the original but now outmoded term "serum hepatitis." Since the advent of bloodbank screening, the risk of acquiring hepatitis B from a transfusion has diminished markedly.

Hepatitis B is common among intravenous drug abusers and may occur with other types of percutaneous exposure such as in patients on hemodialysis and needle-stick accidents in health care workers. Currently it is recommended that all workers at risk be vaccinated against HBV.

A 3rd important route of infection is by sexual transmission, which accounts for the high rate of infection among male homosexuals. Perinatal infection is also important as was mentioned above; it occurs usually with HBV carrier mothers either in utero or during delivery.

HBV is present in saliva as well as other body fluids, and infection is probably spread through oral contact in some cases, although this is not thought to be a very effective route of transmission.

Once HBV infection has occurred, the individual is susceptible to **delta agent**

(HDV) superinfection. HDV is a defective virus which cannot replicate or produce disease in the absence of HBV infection. HDV hepatitis is not clinically distinguishable from HBV hepatitis; however, delta superinfection on chronic hepatitis B is more likely to be fulminant.

Related Disorders There are 5 major types of viral hepatitis: A, B, C, D, and E. As was described above, they are frequently indistinguishable clinically.

Hepatitis A (HAV) virus infection is the most common form of hepatitis. Symptoms are much the same as with hepatitis B infection. HAV infection is spread through fecal-oral contact, and outbreaks have been associated with contaminated milk and shellfish. Water- and foodborne epidemics of hepatitis A are common, especially in developing countries. Hepatitis A virus can quickly spread through institutions and daycare facilities if personal hygiene is less than adequate. HAV infection has generally been thought of as a mild hepatitis, but this is because most infections take place in childhood where asymptomatic and mild illness is the rule. As hygiene improves, the childhood infection rate declines. Consequently more infections are now appearing in susceptible adults, in whom illness is more severe and may even be fulminant.

Hepatitis C infection constitutes the majority of what used to be referred to as **non-A, non-B** infections. It is clinically and epidemiologically similar to HBV, and is now the most common form of transfusion-associated hepatitis in the U.S. It is diagnosed serologically, but antibodies may not be detected for long periods after the onset of hepatitis. (See *Hepatitis, Non-A, Non-B.*)

Hepatitis D (also known as delta hepatitis), and **hepatitis E** infections may be clinically indistinguishable from hepatitis C in the acute phase. They are both viral illnesses although D is an incomplete virus that requires B for full expression and replication. Hepatitis E resembles hepatitis A epidemiologically. (See *Hepatitis, Non-A, Non-B.*)

Fulminant hepatitis is a rare syndrome more common with hepatitis D and B coinfection. Rapid physical deterioration and the onset of liver degeneration may be initial symptoms. There is massive liver cell necrosis. Bleeding is common; encephalopathy and coma frequently ensue. The hepatorenal syndrome may develop. Massive doses of corticosteroids and exchange transfusions have not proved effective. Rarely, patients may recover completely with no permanent liver damage, but the majority are very seriously ill with little hope of full recovery. Transplantation has been successful in a few cases.

Chronic active hepatitis, characterized histologically by bridging necrosis, can progress to cirrhosis of the liver. It can follow hepatitis B or C infection. Hepatitis A may be followed by a relapsing syndrome, relapsing hepatitis, or cholestatic hepatitis, a syndrome of prolonged cholestasis. While chronic, both of these are histologically distinct from chronic active hepatitis and do not progress to cirrhosis. The clinical picture of chronic active hepatitis may also be seen in noninfectious diseases such as systemic lupus erythematosus.

Hepatitis induced by longterm alcoholism is marked by anorexia, nausea with or without vomiting, weight loss, and a general feeling of discomfort. Other symptoms of hepatitis include jaundice and weakness. Hepatomegaly and ascites nay be present. Abstinence from alcohol will usually bring about great improvement in liver function, which may possibly even return to normal. With continued drinking, the hepatitis may evolve into cirrhosis.

Toxic, drug, or chemically induced hepatitis may be caused by inhalation, ingestion, or skin penetration of chemical agents or industrial toxins such as carbon tetrachloride, yellow phosphorus, toxic cyclic peptides of the mushroom *Amanita phalloides,* or pharmacologic agents used in medical therapy. Typical initial symptoms of this form of hepatitis may include anorexia, nausea, vomiting, and diarrhea. Timely withdrawal of the toxic substance is important in treating this disorder. If left untreated, this form of hepatitis can cause serious liver damage and in some cases, death.

Treatment—Standard The best treatment of hepatitis B infection is prevention. The first genetically engineered hepatitis vaccine—hepatitis B vaccine (recombinant)—was approved by the Food and Drug Administration during the mid-1980s. The FDA urges that the new vaccine be used by individuals who are at high risk of becoming infected with hepatitis B, including dental and medical workers, homosexuals, drug users, and personnel who work with mentally disabled individuals in institutional or daycare settings.

Vaccination of newborn infants of IIBsAg carrier mothers will prevent some 90 percent of newborn infections. (It is presumed that the other 10 percent of infections were acquired in utero—as opposed to during delivery—and were already well established at the time of birth.)

An appropriate formulation of the new vaccine for kidney patients on dialysis is not yet available.

The treatment of acute viral hepatitis is symptomatic and supportive. Blood precautions should be maintained carefully to guard against transmission. Fulminant hepatitis requires intensive supportive therapy. Specific treatments such as glucocorticoids, plasmapheresis, and exchange transfusion have not been proven to be effective. Liver transplantation has been successful.

Treatment—Investigational Experimental treatment of viral hepatitis B infection with recombinant human alpha-interferon therapy is being investigated and may be of benefit in chronic active hepatitis.

Please contact the agencies listed under Resources, below, for the most current information.

Resources

For more information on hepatitis B: National Organization for Rare Disorders (NORD); American Liver Foundation; The United Liver Foundation; Children's Liver Foundation; Centers for Disease Control (CDC); NIH/National Institute of Allergy and Infectious Diseases (NIAID).

References

Pilot Study of Recombinant Human Alpha-Interferon for Chronic Type B Hepatitis: J.S. Dooley, et al., eds.; Gastroenterology, 1986, vol. 90(1), pp. 150–157.

Weighing the Risks of the Raw Bar: Carol Ballantine; FDA Consumer, September 1986.

HEPATITIS, NEONATAL

Description Neonatal hepatitis is one of several cholestatic disorders which present in the first month of life. It is the most common cause of neonatal intrahepatic cholestasis. The histologic picture is characterized by diffuse hepatocellular disease with giant cell transformation of the hepatocytes.

Synonyms
  Congenital Liver Cirrhosis
  Giant Cell Cirrhosis of Newborn
  Giant Cell Disease
  Giant Cell Hepatitis
  Idiopathic Neonatal Hepatitis

Signs and Symptoms The symptoms of neonatal hepatitis usually become apparent 2 to 4 weeks after birth. The clinical picture is that of bile duct obstruction, with jaundice, pale stools, dark urine, and hepatomegaly. By the age of 2 to 3 months, slow growth, irritability from pruritus, and signs of portal hypertension may be present. These signs and symptoms do not differentiate neonatal hepatitis from other causes of neonatal cholestasis.

The first step in establishing a diagnosis depends on the finding of conjugated hyperbilirubinemia, indicating the presence of cholestasis. Following this, infectious causes of cholestasis (such as sepsis) should be ruled out, as well as specific inherited metabolic diseases (alpha-1-antitrypsin deficiency, tyrosinemia, Gaucher disease, galactosemia, and others). Ultrasonography and hepatobiliary scintigraphy help to distinguish neonatal hepatitis from biliary atresia and other forms of extrahepatic biliary obstruction. Liver biopsy is frequently diagnostic. Occasionally laparotomy with intraoperative cholangiography is necessary.

Etiology The cause of neonatal hepatitis is unknown in the majority of cases.

Epidemiology Infants of both sexes may be affected by neonatal hepatitis.

Related Disorders The clinical syndrome of neonatal cholestasis may be produced by a wide variety of diseases including infections (most commonly sepsis or a viral infection), and inherited metabolic disorders, but the most common cause is either biliary atresia or idiopathic neonatal hepatitis.

Related disorders include intrahepatic bile duct hypoplasia or paucity, Alagille syndrome, and Zellweger syndrome. The latter 2 syndromes usually have associated congenital anomalies. See *Alagille Syndrome; Zellweger Syndrome.*

Treatment—Standard Cholestyramine, which binds bile salts in the intestine, can be administered if pruritis is suspected. Malabsorption of long-chain triglycerides can be corrected by special formulas containing medium-chain triglycerides, and fat-soluble vitamins should be replaced.

With progression of disease, portal hypertension, ascites, and cirrhosis develop. Transplantation is the treatment of choice for signs of impending liver failure.

Treatment—Investigational Please contact the agencies listed under Resources,

below, for the most current information.

Resources
For more information on neonatal hepatitis: National Organization for Rare Disorders (NORD); American Liver Foundation; National Institute of Diabetes, Digestive & Kidney Diseases Information Clearinghouse; The United Liver Foundation; Children's Liver Foundation.

References
The Merck Manual, 15th ed.: R. Berkow, ed.-in-chief; Merck Sharp & Dohme Research Laboratories, 1987, pp. 1913, 1943.

HEPATITIS, NON-A, NON-B (HEPATITIS C)

Description Non-A, non-B hepatitis is currently thought to consist of 2 distinct viral illnesses which will hereafter be referred to as hepatitis C and hepatitis E. Hepatitis C is caused by the hepatitis C virus (**HCV**) and is a bloodborne infection. **HEV** is transmitted enterically like hepatitis A.

Hepatitis C resembles hepatitis B clinically, but the risk of progression to chronic hepatitis is much higher. As with HBV infection, a carrier state, chronic active hepatitis and cirrhosis may occur.

Synonyms
Hepatitis
Hepatitis C

Signs and Symptoms Symptoms of hepatitis C and B are indistinguishable, although C tends to be less severe in the acute phase. Influenzalike symptoms (fever, aches, eye-ear-nose-throat involvement, weakness, nausea, vomiting, etc.) and jaundice usually occur. The incubation period of this form of hepatitis is usually from 4 to 25 weeks. A carrier form of HCV infection (asymptomatic) occurs more frequently than in HBV infection, and the rate of progression to chronic hepatitis is almost 50 percent.

A specific antibody test is available for diagnosis of hepatitis C. However, this test may not become positive until up to 3 months after infection. An alternative method, diagnosis by exclusion, can be used by testing for HBsAg, IgM antiHBc, and IgM antiHAV. If all of these are negative, then HCV infection is more likely.

Etiology Hepatitis C is caused by a DNA virus transmitted predominantly by blood transfusion, inoculation, medical procedures which involve penetration of the skin, and other percutaneous routes (intravenous drug abuse).

Epidemiology To date there are approximately 150,000 cases of hepatitis C in the United States each year, according to the Centers for Disease Control. Approximately 8 to 11 percent of these cases are due to transfusions of infected blood. (During 1990 the FDA approved an antibody test for hepatitis C, which is now used to screen blood for transfusion.) The vast majority of persons are infected through other types of contact, including intravenous drug use or sexual contact.

Hemodialysis patients are also at risk. This disease can occur worldwide, and may equally affect males and females of all age groups.

Related Disorders The chapter *Hepatitis B* further mentions hepatitis A, D, and E, and briefly discusses fulminant hepatitis, chronic active hepatitis, hepatitis induced by longterm alcoholism, and toxic, drug, or chemically induced hepatitis. See also *Hepatitis, Neonatal.*

Treatment—Standard Treatment for acute hepatitis C is symptomatic and supportive. Personal hygiene should be carefully maintained and blood precautions are appropriate.

Treatment—Investigational Effective immunization against hepatitis C does not exist at this time. Interferon-alfa-2b (Intron A) is being investigated as a treatment for the chronic active form of hepatitis C. The drug appears to return liver function to near normal, but there is controversy as to whether high or low doses are needed. Patients may relapse after the alpha-interferon is discontinued. More research is needed to determine the longterm safety and effectiveness of this drug.

Please contact the agencies listed under Resources, below, for the most current information.

Resources

For more information on non-A, non-B hepatitis (hepatitis C): National Organization for Rare Disorders (NORD); National Sexually Transmitted Diseases Hotline; Centers for Disease Control (CDC); American Liver Foundation; Children's Liver Foundation; The United Liver Foundation; NIH/National Institute of Allergy and Infectious Diseases (NIAID).

References

Non-A, Non-B Hepatitis: Evolving Epidemiologic and Clinical Perspective: J.L. Dienstag, et al.; Semin. Liver Dis., 1986, vol. 6(1), pp. 67–81.

Non-A, Non-B Hepatitis: An Update: J.A. Hellings; Vox Sang., 1986, Supplement 51(1), pp. 63–66.

Hepatitis in Clinical Practice: D.K. Sarver; Postgrad. Med., 1986, vol. 79(4), pp. 229–230.

Weighing the Risks of the Raw Bar: C. Ballantine; FDA Consumer, 1986, vol. 90(1), pp. 150–157.

Treatment of Chronic Hepatitis C with Recombinant Interferon Alfa: A Multicenter Randomized, Controlled Trial: G.L. Davis, et al.; New Engl. J. Med., 1989, vol. 321(221), pp. 1501–1506.

Recombinant Interferon Alfa Therapy for Chronic Hepatitis C. A Randomized, Double-Blind, Placebo Controlled Trial: Di Bisceglie, M. Adrian, et al.; New Engl. J. Med., 1989, vol. 321(2), pp. 1406–1410.

LEPROSY

Description Leprosy is a progressive, chronic infection caused by *Mycobacterium leprae.* It affects the peripheral nerves, skin, mucous membranes, and eyes. In severe cases, sensory loss, disfigurement, and blindness may result. Leprosy occurs in several forms: tuberculoid (minor and major; benign Hansen's disease); lepromatous (malignant Hansen's disease); dimorphous (borderline leprosy); and indeterminate leprosy.

Synonyms

Elephantiasis Graecorum
Hansen's Disease
Lepra

Signs and Symptoms Leprosy is a slowly progressive disease that involves the nerves and skin of the face, hands, lower legs, and feet. Symptoms of nerve involvement include paresthesias, anesthesia, weakness, paralysis, and muscular atrophy. Nerve lesions tend to occur in the skin and along the nerve trunks. Skin lesions include macules, plaques (which may be erythematous or hypopigmented), papules, and nodules.

Leprosy is classified into the subtypes **lepromatous** and **tuberculoid,** and **intermediate subtypes** between these two. The most limited subtype is the tuberculoid, which is manifested by large plaques that are anesthetic, dry, and hairless. The intermediate or borderline subtype is characterized by more numerous skin lesions but less sensory loss. Patients with intermediate or borderline disease tend to progress toward either the tuberculoid or the lepromatous form over time.

Lepromatous disease also has less severe sensory loss; but both skin and nerve involvement are more extensive, and invasive. Nodular skin lesions are characteristic of this subtype. Complications, with eye involvement and deformities of the face, hands, and feet may occur. Facial deformities are a direct result of mycobacterial destruction of the nasal septum, cartilage, and other facial tissues. In addition to this, the eyebrows and eyelashes are usually lost, and the earlobes enlarge. In the hands and feet, deformities result from repeated trauma sustained in the face of sensory loss.

Ocular complications include conjunctivitis, keratitis, and iridocyclitis that may lead to cataract formation. Corneal anesthesia, due to trigeminal nerve involvement, may lead to inadvertent corneal injury and blindness.

Another serious complication of lepromatous leprosy is erythema nodosum leprosum **(ENL).** This is a syndrome of high fever, necrosis of skin nodules, and a painful neuritis. This may be associated with polyarthralgias and glomerulonephritis.

Some patients with intermediate or tuberculoid leprosy experience a worsening of disease while on therapy (reversal reaction). Pathologically this appears to be a local immune reaction. Clinically, the lesions become indurated and may ulcerate, and associated neurologic symptoms may deteriorate.

Amyloidosis is a complication of leprosy, although its prevalence varies from one geographic region to another.

The pathologic lesion of leprosy is the granuloma. These may be seen in the dermis, lymph nodes, liver, and spleen. The diagnosis is made on skin biopsy, and it is important to examine a fairly large specimen in order to be certain of the diagnosis. An excisional biopsy is preferred over a punch biopsy.

Etiology Leprosy is caused by the bacterium *Mycobacterium leprae*. This is an acid-fast bacillus that grows only in vivo.

Epidemiology The mode of transmission is not clear. Spread may be by direct skin contact, or by inhalation, but prolonged exposure is usually necessary. Breast feeding and vector transmission by insects have also been implicated.

Worldwide, 12 million to 15 million people are affected. Children are more susceptible. Leprosy is a major problem in tropical regions of Asia, Africa, and South America, and is also prevalent in some islands of the South Pacific. In the United States, native leprosy occurs in the south (i.e., around the Gulf of Mexico), but the majority of cases are imported. North American Indians appear to be immune.

The incidence of leprosy is currently rising in the United States, a result of large waves of immigrants from endemic regions, particularly Southeast Asia. The exact incidence is unknown, since many patients may not seek or have access to health care.

Related Disorders Symptoms of the following disorders can be similar to those of leprosy. Comparisons may be useful for a differential diagnosis.

Lupus miliaris disseminatus faciei is a chronic skin infection caused by *Mycobacterium tuberculosis*. It is characterized by soft, brownish-red papules that may appear singularly or in clusters. The face, neck, mouth, and nose may be involved. Healing is slow and scarring is common.

Lupus vulgaris, another cutaneous form of tuberculosis, is a progressive infection that may cause scarring and deformities of the face. The lesions are small, soft, yellowish-brown tubercles and crusted ulcers. Lupus vulgaris is more common in children and young adults.

Treatment—Standard The treatment of leprosy may include the use of dapsone, rifampin, ethionamide, and the orphan drug clofazimine (Lamprene). Combination therapy is currently recommended. A typical regimen would include dapsone, rifampin, and clofazimine. Therapy must be continued for 2 years in all cases, and longer in some. Reversal reactions and ENL are treated with steroids.

Corneal dryness is treated with eye drops and ophthalmic mucin substitutes. Ocular complications of ENL must be treated promptly to prevent permanent damage to the eyes. Local atropine and hydrocortisone may be used to keep the pupils dilated and reduce the inflammation until the reaction subsides. Supportive care is important. Anesthetic areas (eyes and limbs) must be protected from injury and infection.

Treatment—Investigational Solasulphone and acedapsone are currently under investigation. Vaccines are also being studied. Progress is hampered by the inability to culture the organism in vitro. Please contact the agencies listed under Resources, below, for the most current information.

Resources

For more information on leprosy: National Organization for Rare Disorders (NORD); National Hansen's Disease Center; NIH/National Institute of Allergy and Infectious Diseases; Centers for Disease Control (CDC).

References

Internal Medicine, 3rd ed.: J.H. Stein, ed.-in-chief; Little, Brown and Company, 1990, pp. 1552–1556.

LEPTOSPIROSIS

Description Leptospirosis is an acute systemic disease of domestic and wild animals which is caused by spirochetes of the genus *Leptospira*. Human leptospirosis is rare. The disease usually occurs in 2 stages: the first, a leptospiremic phase with flulike symptoms; and the second, a widespread vasculitis thought to be of immune etiology. The most severe form of leptospirosis is referred to as **Weil syndrome.**

Synonyms
>   Canefield Fever
>   Canicola Fever
>   Field Fever
>   Mud Fever
>   Seven-Day Fever
>   Spirochetosis
>   Swineherd Disease

Signs and Symptoms Leptospirosis is characteristically a biphasic illness. The first phase begins after an incubation period of 2 to 20 days, with fever, severe headache, myalgias, chills, coughing, chest pain, and gastrointestinal symptoms including nausea, vomiting, and abdominal pain. The symptoms last a week or less and then abate. After an afebrile period of 1 to 2 days, the 2nd phase begins, with severe headache, myalgias, nausea, vomiting, and abdominal pain. In severe cases there is jaundice, hepatic and renal dysfunction, and vascular collapse; this is called Weil syndrome (see **Weil Syndrome**).

Physical examination frequently reveals signs of meningitis, hepatosplenomegaly, muscle tenderness, and conjunctival hemorrhage. Except in severe cases, fever is minimal. Rashes and uveitis may also be seen. The cerebrospinal fluid generally shows a pleocytosis, normal glucose, and elevated protein levels. The bacteria cannot be isolated from either blood or cerebrospinal fluid; at this stage, however, antibodies appear in the serum. The diagnosis of leptospirosis is usually made by serology. Agglutination tests, and an enzyme-linked immunosorbent assay (**ELISA**) are available for diagnosis. The spirochetes may be found in the blood and cerebrospinal fluid, but only in the early phase of illness. They may also be found in the urine for up to a month.

Etiology Leptospirosis is caused by spirochetes of the genus *Leptospira*. There is one species, *L. interrogans,* which has several serotypes.

Epidemiology Leptospirosis is distributed worldwide. It is primarily a disease of animals; and in the United States, dogs, cats, livestock, and rodents are the usual sources of human infection. Infected animals may pass leptospira in the urine for many months, which can contaminate soil and water.

Approximately 75 percent of cases occur in young men, and may be related to occupational or recreational transmission (e.g., swimming in contaminated water). At particular risk are farmers, veterinarians, and abbatoir and sewer workers.

Leptospirosis may occur in people of all ages. Breaks in the skin and exposed mucous membranes (such as the conjunctiva, nose, or mouth) are the usual portals of entry.

Related Disorders Aseptic meningitis may be caused by a variety of viruses.

See **Weil Syndrome,** a severe, icteric form of leptospirosis which appears to be due to extensive vasculitis.

Treatment—Standard The treatment of leptospirosis is doxycycline, intravenous penicillin, or ampicillin, but this must be started by the 4th day of illness if it is to have any effect. Mild cases may be treated with tetracycline, which has the added advantage of eradicating the bacteria in the urine, which the penicillins do not. Intensive supportive care, including ventilatory assistance, dialysis, and other measures may be required in severe cases.

A vaccine is available for domestic animals but it is not very effective.

Treatment—Investigational Please contact the organizations listed under Resources, below, for the most current information.

Resources

For more information on leptospirosis: National Organization for Rare Disorders (NORD); Centers for Disease Control (CDC); NIH/National Institute of Allergy and Infectious Diseases (NIAID).

References

Leptospiral Exposure in Detroit Rodent Control Workers: Demers; Am. J. Pub. Health, 1985, vol. 75(9), pp. 1090–1091.

LISTERIOSIS

Description Listeriosis is an infection caused by *Listeria monocytogenes*. This organism produces several different clinical syndromes, depending on various host factors. In pregnant women, and probably in other immunocompetent hosts, asymptomatic infection, or mild nonspecific illness occurs. Transplacental transmission is associated with a severe disseminated disease known as granulomatosis infantiseptica. Two additional syndromes, primary *Listeria* sepsis, and meningoencephalitis occur in immunosuppressed adults and in neonates. Focal infections with *L. monocytogenes* have also been reported but these are very rare.

Signs and Symptoms The majority of listeria infections are mild. The major disease syndromes of listeriosis will be described individually here.

Listeriosis of pregnancy may be asymptomatic or may be marked only by a fever and back pain. It is most common in the last trimester when it may be mistaken for pyelonephritis. The diagnosis can be confirmed by blood culture. If untreated, the fetus is at risk for developing granulomatous infantiseptica.

Granulomatous infantiseptica is a fetal listeria infection that results from transplacental transmission. This form of listeriosis is characterized by widespread abscesses and granulomas, usually involving the liver, spleen, kidneys, lungs, skin, eyes, and brain. Such infants should be extensively cultured, including lumbar puncture, and treated immediately, but even with treatment the prognosis is poor.

Listeria sepsis may occur in infants infected during vaginal delivery or postnatally, and in immunosuppressed adults. Such patients show all the signs of bacterial sepsis, and shock may intervene. There are no focal signs and few clues as to the exact nature of the illness. Blood cultures confirm the diagnosis.

Listeria meningoencephalitis can occur in immunosuppressed patients or newborns. Predisposing factors include cirrhosis, malignancy, and organ transplantation, and cases also occur in immunocompetent individuals. Unlike most cases of bacterial meningoencephalitis, listeria often presents in a subtle or subacute fashion with anorexia, lethargy, behavioral changes, and/or low-grade fever. Focal neurologic signs such as cranial nerve palsies may be present, as well as other signs of meningitis and encephalitis. The cerebrospinal fluid shows variable abnormalities. The organism may not be seen on a Gram stain, which may be misleading, but cultures are diagnostic.

Localized listeria infection may follow direct contact with *L. monocytogenes* on the skin or conjunctiva. Other cases may result from the bacteremia. In these cases, arthritis, osteomyelitis, endocarditis, or peritonitis may occur.

Etiology Listeriosis is caused by *Listeria monocytogenes*, a gram-positive, aerobic bacillus.

Epidemiology *L. moncytogenes* appears to be ubiquitous. It is found worldwide in soil, water, and dust, and in the meat of many wild and domestic animals. It has also been isolated from feces of normal humans, and it has been cultured from the vagina and the urethra.

Several epidemics have been traced to ingestion of contaminated food products such as improperly pasteurized milk, cheese, unwashed vegetables, and raw meat. An epidemic in California in 1985 affected nearly 200 persons and was attributed to contaminated cheese manufactured in Mexico. Other cases have been transmitted through contact with other infected persons or animals, but most patients have no history of such contact.

Listeriosis occurs most often in the summer months. According to the Centers for Disease Control, approximately 1,600 cases are reported annually in the United States.

Related Disorders Listeria sepsis resembles gram-negative sepsis. Similarly, listeria meningoencephalitis is usually clinically indistinguishable from other types of meningitis or encephalitis. (See also Signs and Symptoms, above.)

Treatment—Standard The treatment of choice for listeriosis usually includes high-dose intravenous penicillin G, or ampicillin with or without an aminoglycoside. Alternative drugs include trimethoprim/sulfamethoxazole, tetracycline, erythromycin, or chloramphenicol. Supportive therapy is important in severe cases.

Treatment—Investigational DNA probes that can detect the presence of *L. monocytogenes* in food samples are currently under investigation. This technique is much faster than conventional culture techniques, and may be useful in controlling foodborne outbreaks of listeriosis. New pasteurization procedures to eliminate the presence of *L. monocytogenes* in milk and milk products are also under study.

Please contact the agencies listed under Resources, below, for the most current information.

Resources

For more information on listeriosis: National Organization for Rare Disorders (NORD); NIH/National Institute of Allergy & Infectious Diseases (NIAID); Centers for Disease Control (CDC); Food and Drug Administration (FDA).

References

Perinatal Listeriosis (Early-Onset): Correlation of Antenatal Manifestations and Neonatal Outcome: M. Boucher, et al.; Obstet. Gynecol., 1986, vol. 68(5), pp. 593–597.

Clinical Manifestations of Epidemic Neonatal Listeriosis: A.J. Teberg, et al.; Pediatr. Infect. Dis. J., September 1987, vol. 6(9), pp. 817–820.

Listeria: Battling Back Against One 'Tough Bug': K.J. Skinner; FDA Consumer, July–August 1988, pp. 12–15.

MESENTERITIS, RETRACTILE

Description Retractile mesenteritis (mesenteric panniculitis) is a poorly understood inflammatory disorder of the mesentery. It appears to begin with lipodystrophy in the mesenteric fat, and then progresses to inflammation and marked fibrosis. The major symptoms include abdominal pain, nausea, vomiting, and fever, and the major complication is intestinal obstruction.

Synonyms

Mesenteric Panniculitis
Nodular Mesenteritis
Nonspecific Sclerosing Mesenteritis
Sclerosing Panniculitis

Signs and Symptoms The onset of retractile mesenteritis is characterized by malaise, fever, vague abdominal pain, nausea, vomiting, and weight loss. As the inflammation progresses, the mesentery becomes thickened and may distort and retract the intestines, which eventually may lead to obstruction of the lymphatics, veins, or the intestines themselves. Ultimately, malabsorption, steatorrhea, ascites, and symptoms of partial or complete intestinal obstruction complicate the picture.

The diagnosis of retractile mesenteritis is usually made at laparotomy, and biopsy is confirmatory.

Etiology The exact cause of retractile mesenteritis is not known.

The mesentery initially develops lipodystrophy, then becomes infiltrated with inflammatory cells. Fibrosis, scarring, and calcifications follow. The initial insult may be infectious, vascular, or related to another underlying process.

IMMUNOLOGIC DISORDERS AND INFECTIOUS DISEASES | 679

Epidemiology Retractile mesenteritis is more common in the elderly, and in men.

Related Disorders See *Weber-Christian Disease,* which is characterized by fever and the development of subcutaneous nodules. The pathology of these nodules is similar to that found in the mesentery in retractile mesenteritis, and for this reason, retractile mesenteritis is also called mesenteric Weber-Christian disease. However, Weber-Christian disease has a different epidemiology; it usually affects young adult women.

Treatment—Standard The treatment of retractile mesenteritis most often consists of prednisone and immunosuppressants such as azathioprine. Surgery is usually necessary for complete intestinal obstruction. Other treatment is symptomatic and supportive.

Treatment—Investigational Please contact the agencies listed under Resources, below, for the most current information.

Resources
   For more information on retractile mesenteritis: National Organization for Rare Disorders (NORD); National Digestive Diseases Information Clearinghouse.

References
   Successful Treatment of a Patient with Retractile Mesenteritis with Prednisone and Azathioprine: G.N. Tytgat, et al.; Gastroenterology, 1980, vol. 79(2), pp. 352–356.
   Sclerosing Mesenteritis. Response to Cyclophosphamide: R.W. Bush, et al.; Arch. Intern. Med., 1986, vol. 146(3), pp. 503–505.
   Retractile Mesenteritis Involving the Colon: Barium Enema, Sonographic, and CT Findings: F.J. Perez-Fontan, et al.; AJR, 1986, vol. 147(5), pp. 937–940.

NOCARDIOSIS

Description Nocardiosis is an infectious disease caused by *Nocardia asteroides,* now classified as bacteria. This organism typically produces chronic, smoldering infections, most frequently in the lung, though the brain, soft tissues, and many other organs may be involved.

Signs and Symptoms Pulmonary infection is the most common form of nocardiosis. Pneumonia, cavitation, and abscess are common presentations. Frequent complications include empyema, and extension into the chest wall. In most patients, infection is chronic and dominated by nonspecific symptoms: weight loss, anorexia, weakness, cough, chest pain, and occasionally hemoptysis. In the immunocompromised host, the course tends to be more acute.

   Hematogenous spread is common, resulting in brain abscesses in about one-third of cases, or, less frequently, abscesses in the kidney, intestines, or other organs. Symptoms associated with brain abscesses may include severe headache and focal neurologic deficits.

   Skin abscesses occur in approximately one-third of all cases of nocardiosis. Iliopsoas, ischiorectal, and perirectal abscesses are also relatively common forms of nocardial infection.

Nocardiosis may last from several months to years, but it is not difficult to diagnose. A Gram stain and modified acid-fast stains of pus or sputum are often diagnostic.

Etiology Nocardiosis is caused by *Nocardia asteroides*. While it is classified as a bacterium, it is able to grow in filaments like fungi.

Epidemiology Nocardiosis occurs worldwide. It is most common in the southern United States, and South America. It is more common in males than in females, and it is increasingly seen in patients with underlying diseases such as malignancy, chronic obstructive pulmonary disease, cirrhosis, ulcerative colitis, and other chronic diseases. Transplant recipients, and patients on steroids and other forms of immunosuppressive therapy are also at risk.

Related Disorders The clinical features of nocardiosis may resemble tuberculosis, actinomycosis, and malignancy. (See *Tuberculosis.*)

The hallmark of **actinomycosis** is the draining sinus. The organism produces small abscesses that spread without regard for anatomic boundaries. Pulmonary and abdominal disease may occur, and chronic smoldering infections are frequent.

Treatment—Standard Nocardia organisms are usually resistant to penicillin. Sulfonamides are the drugs of choice for nocardiosis: sulfisoxazole or trimethoprim-sulfamethoxazole are the most commonly used. Minocycline and cycloserine have also been used to treat this infection. Usually treatment must be continued for 6 to 12 months. In addition, surgery is often required to drain abscesses or empyema.

Treatment—Investigational Please contact the agencies listed under Resources, below, for the most current information.

Resources

For more information on nocardiosis: National Organization for Rare Disorders (NORD); American Lung Association; NIH/National Institute of Allergy and Infectious Diseases (NIAID); Centers for Disease Control (CDC).

References
Pleuropulmonary Manifestations of Actinomycosis and Nocardiosis: J.E. Heffner; Semin. Respir. Infect., 1988, vol. 3(4), pp. 352–361.

Nocardiosis: A Neglected Chronic Lung Disease in Africa: G.G. Baily, et al.; Thorax, 1988, vol. 43(11), pp. 905–910.

Presumed Intraocular Nocardiosis in a Cardiac-Transplant Patient: N. Mamalis, et al.; Ann. Ophthalmol., 1988, vol. 20(7), pp. 271–273, 276.

PARACOCCIDIOIDOMYCOSIS (PCM)

Description PCM is a chronic, systemic infection caused by the fungus *Paracoccidioides brasiliensis*. The initial infection is in the lungs, but dissemination to the skin, mucous membranes, and reticuloendothelial system is common.

Synonyms
Lutz-Splendore-Almeida Disease
Paracoccidioidal Granuloma
South American Blastomycosis

Signs and Symptoms After a prolonged incubation period of at least 5 years, patients present with one or more types of disease. Mucocutaneous PCM involves the mouth and nose most frequently, with ulcerative granulomatous lesions.

In pulmonary PCM, the patient commonly notes cough, dyspnea, and chest pain. The chest x-ray may show areas of patchy infiltration. In older patients, fibrosis and emphysema are evident, with progression to cor pulmonale in some cases.

In the lymphatic form of PCM there is generalized lymphadenopathy, most prominent in the neck. Suppuration may occur, with sinus tract formation.

Other visceral lesions may occur in the liver, spleen, intestines, and adrenals.

The diagnosis is made by examination of infected material. Sputum or pus may be examined with potassium hydroxide and found to reveal the fungus. Biopsy specimens may also be diagnostic. Cultures are confirmatory.

Serologic tests are useful but cannot distinguish between active and past infection. Skin tests are available but are unreliable.

Etiology The cause of PCM is the dimorphic fungus, *Paracoccidioides brasiliensis.*

Epidemiology This disease is largely limited to the state of Sao Paolo in Brazil. Sporadic cases have occurred in other regions of South and Central America. Men are affected about 10 times as frequently as women.

Related Disorders PCM may resemble and even coexist with **Tuberculosis.**

Treatment—Standard The most effective therapy for PCM is amphotericin B. Sulfonamides have also been used; these halt the progress of the disease but do not eliminate the fungus.

Treatment—Investigational Ketoconazole and itraconazole are currently under investigation for the treatment of PCM and other systemic mycoses. They seem to be as effective as amphotericin B in most reported series.

Please contact the agencies listed under Resources, below, for the most current information.

Resources
For more information on paracoccidioidomycosis: National Organization for Rare Disorders (NORD); Centers for Disease Control (CDC); NIH/National Institute of Allergy and Infectious Diseases (NIAID).

References
Manson's Tropical Diseases, 19th ed.: P.E.C. Manson-Bahr and D.R. Bell; Baillière Tindall, 1987, pp. 708–712.

Pertussis

Description Pertussis is an acute respiratory disease caused by *Bordetella pertussis*. The illness has 3 stages: catarrhal, paroxysmal, and convalescent. The paroxysmal phase is characterized by a cough with an inspiratory whoop, which gives the disease its common name, whooping cough. With widespread use of the DPT (Diphtheria, Pertussis, Tetanus) vaccine, the incidence of pertussis has diminished substantially.

Synonyms
>Whooping Cough

Signs and Symptoms The incubation period is 7 to 10 days. Following this, the catarrhal stage begins with the nonspecific symptoms of the common cold: malaise, rhinorrhea, sneezing, and lacrimation. Low-grade fever may or may not be present. Toward the end of this phase a cough appears, becoming increasingly persistent.

The paroxysmal stage is characterized by recurrent bouts of coughing. A paroxysm consists of a series of coughs in rapid succession, with inadequate attempts at inspiration between them. Typically, the patient expectorates copious amounts of thick mucus, which may induce vomiting. This phase is associated with very high white blood cell counts, predominantly a lymphocytosis.

The convalescent stage of pertussis begins approximately 4 weeks after onset. By then paroxysms are less frequent and severe, but occasionally they will recur sporadically for months. Complications include epistaxis and scleral hemorrhage, due to sudden increases in venous pressure associated with a paroxysm. Other complications associated with paroxysms include seizures, atelectasis, bronchiectasis, subcutaneous emphysema, and inguinal hernia. Bacterial superinfection and, rarely, encephalitis may occur.

The diagnosis of pertussis is confirmed by isolating the organism from the sputum. Samples are best obtained using a swab placed through the nose into the posterior pharynx.

Etiology Pertussis is caused by the gram-negative coccobacillus, *Bordetella pertussis*.

Epidemiology Pertussis is most frequent in young children; in adolescents and adults the symptoms are much less severe and the disease may not be recognized as pertussis.

The disease has a worldwide distribution, and the World Health Organization has estimated that 60 million cases occur worldwide each year, with 500,000 to 1,000,000 deaths.

Related Disorders Bronchitis and influenza often resemble pertussis in the catarrhal stage.

Treatment—Standard Antibiotic therapy for pertussis rapidly clears the bacteria but does not change the symptoms. Erythromycin is the drug of choice, and is routinely given because it halts transmission of the disease to others. Trimetho-prim-sulfamethoxazole is an alternative. Exposed contacts are also given ery-thromycin if nasopharyngeal cultures grow the organism.

Human hyperimmune pertussis globulin is recommended by some, but its effi-cacy is the subject of controversy.

Intensive supportive care may be lifesaving in severe cases, particularly in infants. Meticulous pulmonary toilet and prompt ventilatory assistance are critical, as is adequate nutrition.

The pertussis vaccine has been in widespread use since the late 1940s. Since then, the incidence of pertussis has fallen from 250,000 to less than 3000 cases annually. The vaccine is not 100 percent effective in preventing disease; in out-breaks, susceptibility to infection rises with time elapsed since immunization.

Adverse reactions have been associated with vaccination, and the risk rises with age. Vaccination is contraindicated over the age of 7 years in most circumstances. Adverse reactions may be local or systemic. Local reactions include pain, erythe-ma, and swelling. Fever is a common systemic reaction. Rarely, fever over 40.5° C (104.9° F), seizures, encephalopathy, shock, and severe hypersensitivity reactions occur. The Centers for Disease Control estimate the risk of serious complications to be 1:100,000 to 1:300,000 for the vaccine, and 1:9500 for the disease. Unfortu-nately, local outbreaks of pertussis have occurred because parents have refused vaccination.

Treatment—Investigational Acellular pertussis vaccines are currently under investigation in Sweden and Japan. Their success rates are not as high as was ini-tially hoped.

Please contact the agencies listed under Resources, below, for the most current information.

Resources

For more information on pertussis: National Organization for Rare Disor-ders (NORD); NIH/National Institute of Allergy and Infectious Diseases; Centers for Disease Control (CDC); Dissatisfied Parents Together (DPT).

References
Cecil Textbook of Medicine, 18th ed.: J.B. Wyngaarden and L.H. Smith, Jr., eds.: W.B. Saunders Company, 1988, pp. 1624–1626.

PINTA

Description Pinta, a skin disease caused by the spirochete *Treponema carateum,* is characterized by rashes and skin discoloration.

Synonyms
Azul
Carate
Empeines

Iota
Mal del Pinto
Tina

Signs and Symptoms The earliest lesions are small papules which occur at the site of inoculation. Within several months secondary lesions appear; these are small, reddish or purplish, and psoriatic (pintids). They occur most often on the face, hands, and feet. Gradually the color of these lesions changes to slate blue. These colored patches eventually undergo depigmentation and become vitiligoid. The skin on the soles and palms may become somewhat thickened.

The lesions are susceptible to secondary infection by other organisms, but the skin is the only organ affected.

The diagnosis of pinta may be made on darkfield examination of fluid from the skin lesions, which usually reveals spirochetes. Serologic tests (VDRL; fluorescent treponemal antibody absorption—FTA-ABS) usually become positive after the secondary lesions appear.

Etiology Pinta is caused by the spirochete *Treponema carateum.*

Epidemiology Predominantly a disease of remote rural areas, pinta is common in the tropical lowlands of South and Central America, such as Mexico and Colombia. It is rare in the United States. Transmission is by direct, nonsexual contact with pinta lesions.

Related Disorders See *Yaws; Bejel.* The treponematoses—bejel (endemic syphilis), venereal syphilis, pinta, and yaws—are caused by identical-looking treponemes and are capable of producing chronic disease syndromes. However, their clinical and epidemiologic characteristics are quite distinct.

Treatment—Standard The lesions of pinta respond to antibiotics such as benzathine penicillin G, given in a single dose of 1.2 million units. Alternatives include tetracyclines and chloramphenicol.

Treatment—Investigational Please contact the agencies listed under Resources, below, for the most current information.

Resources

For more information on pinta: National Organization for Rare Disorders (NORD); Centers for Disease Control (CDC); NIH/National Institute of Allergy and Infectious Diseases (NIAID).

References
Cecil Textbook of Medicine, 18th ed.: J.B. Wyngaarden and L.H. Smith, Jr., eds.; W.B. Saunders Company, 1988, p. 1723.

Q FEVER

Description Q fever is a rickettsial disease that primarily occurs in animals, and is caused by *Coxiella burnetti*. It is most commonly an acute febrile illness with headache, chills, and myalgias. Pneumonia, hepatitis, and endocarditis may also occur.

Synonyms
> Q Fever Pneumonia

Signs and Symptoms Q fever usually begins with sudden severe headache and high fever. Chills and mylagias are also common. Occasionally, gastrointestinal symptoms are prominent, with nausea, vomiting, and diarrhea. Examination frequently shows hepatosplenomegaly.

Q fever has a wide variety of clinical manifestations. In addition to the above, patients may present with pneumonitis, hepatitis, or endocarditis. Q fever endocarditis is a chronic infection with symptoms characteristic of infective endocarditis: fatigue, fever, and cardiac murmurs, typically of the aortic valve.

The diagnosis of Q fever is based on the clinical picture and the history of possible exposure. Unlike other rickcttsia, *C. burnetti* does not produce a positive Weil-Felix reaction. Diagnosis may be confirmed retrospectively by demonstrating a rise in antibody titer.

Etiology The cause of Q fever is the rickettsia *Coxiella burnetti*.

Epidemiology Q fever is primarily a disease of cattle, sheep, and goats, although infection has been reported in cats, rats, rabbits, and ticks. The organism is distributed worldwide, but human infection usually occurs only in those with occupational exposure to animals. Infection is usually transmitted by inhalation of aerosolized organisms, from contaminated urine, feces, milk, or dust. These are most concentrated in the placenta and milk of an infected animal. Those at risk include veterinarians, abattoir workers, farmers, wool sorters, dairy workers, and researchers working in close proximity to the organism. Infection can also occur through a tick bite.

Related Disorders Related disorders include other rickettsioses and diseases with similar presentations. Mild forms of Q fever without significant focal symptoms (such as those of pneumonitis or hepatitis) resemble viral illness. Q fever pneumonia is an atypical pneumonia, and must be distinguished from *Mycoplasma* pneumonia, legionellosis, psittacosis, and viral pneumonias. Q fever endocarditis should be suspected in cases of culture-negative subacute endocarditis.

Other rickettsioses include Rocky Mountain spotted fever; endemic, epidemic, and scrub typhus; and rickettsialpox. These differ from Q fever in that they are associated with rashes, arthropod transmission, and a positive Weil-Felix reaction.

Treatment—Standard Q fever is treated with tetracyclines or chloramphenicol. Endocarditis may require treatment for years, as it is rarely cured without surgery. A vaccine is available for individuals with occupational risk of contracting Q fever.

Treatment—Investigational Please contact the agencies listed under Resources, below, for the most current information.

Resources

For more information on Q fever: National Organization for Rare Disorders (NORD); NIH/National Institute of Allergy and Infectious Diseases (NIAID); Centers for Disease Control (CDC).

References

Poker Player's pneumonia: An Urban Outbreak of Q Fever Following Exposure to a Parturient Cat: Joanne M. Langley, et al.; N. Engl. J. Med., August 11, 1988, issue 319(6), pp. 354–56.

Q Fever: Current Concepts: L.A. Sawyer, et al.; Rev. Infect. Dis., September-October 1987, issue 9(5), pp. 935–946.

REYE SYNDROME

Description Reye syndrome is a childhood disease characterized by acute hepatic failure, encephalopathy, and hypoglycemia. It usually follows a viral infection, typically influenza or varicella, and is associated with the use of salicylates. In addition to these factors, deficiencies of urea cycle enzymes have been implicated as contributing factors in the development of Reye syndrome.

Synonyms

Fatty Liver with Encephalopathy

Signs and Symptoms Reye syndrome usually follows an upper respiratory tract infection and begins with vomiting. In very young children (under 2 years of age), diarrhea and/or hyperventilation may be the first signs of illness. The initial stage is rapidly followed by signs of central nervous system involvement: listlessness, somnolence, irritability, and other behavioral changes. The neurologic disturbance progresses quickly to involve seizures, stupor, and then coma, usually within 3 to 5 days of onset. These symptoms are due to cerebral edema, which is a prominent feature of the disease. Hepatomegaly is usually seen on physical examination, but jaundice is minimal.

Laboratory data usually reveal elevated serum aminotransferases, prolonged prothrombin time, hypoglycemia, hyperammonemia, and metabolic acidosis.

The mortality rate of Reye syndrome is very high, but complete recovery is possible. Residual brain damage may occur.

Etiology Reye syndrome may be caused by a mitochondrial insult, precipitated by certain toxins, specifically salicylates, in individuals with a deficiency of urea cycle enzymes. The use of aspirin is relatively contraindicated in children with viral illnesses. The FDA has also warned that antiemetics such as the phenothiazines may increase the severity of Reye syndrome or mask its early symptoms.

Reye syndrome may occur in the absence of salicylate ingestion; however, one recent study indicated that 90 percent of affected children had taken salicylate-containing drugs during the preceding viral illness.

Epidemiology Reye syndrome occurs almost exclusively in children under the age of 16 years with a recent viral upper respiratory tract illness (most frequently chickenpox or influenza). It has also been reported in newborns and the middle-aged. The incidence of Reye syndrome in teenagers has been rising in recent years, possibly because of self-medication with aspirin.

The incidence of Reye syndrome varies with the pattern of influenza virus activity from year to year, according to the National Reye Syndrome Surveillance System. However, in 1984, the incidence of influenza rose while reported cases of Reye syndrome in children under 10 years of age decreased. There were decreases in both influenza- and varicella-associated cases.

Related Disorders See *Medium-Chain Acyl-CoA Dehydrogenase Deficiency,* a very rare metabolic disorder with similar clinical features to Reye syndrome. The enzyme medium-chain acyl-CoA dehydrogenase is important in triglyceride metabolism. Hypoglycemia and central nervous system involvement (lethargy and possibly coma) occur, associated with fatty changes in the liver. During hypoglycemic periods, tests usually show massive urinary levels of dicarboxylic acid.

Treatment—Standard There is no specific treatment for Reye syndrome; however, intensive supportive measures addressing both the hepatic failure and the cerebral edema have improved survival. Permanent neurologic sequelae, such as mental impairment, have been reported.

Treatment—Investigational Please contact the agencies listed under Resources, below, for the most current information.

Resources
   For more information on Reye syndrome: National Organization for Rare Disorders (NORD); National Reye Syndrome Society; American Reye Syndrome Association; Reye Syndrome Society; NIH/National Institute of Neurological Disorders & Stroke (NINDS); Centers for Disease Control (CDC); Food and Drug Administration.

References
   Reye Syndrome: D.C. DeVivio; Neurol. Clin., 1985, vol. 3, pp. 95–115.

RHEUMATIC FEVER

Description Rheumatic fever is an inflammatory syndrome that appears to represent an inappropriate immune response to streptococcal infection. It is characterized by symptoms known as the Jones criteria; the major criteria include carditis, polyarthritis, chorea, a skin rash referred to as erythema marginatum, and subcutaneous nodules. Of these, the cardiac manifestations are ultimately the most serious, since damage inflicted on the cardiac valves during a bout of rheumatic fever continues chronically, long after the acute episode. Affected individuals are susceptible to recurrent attacks with each subsequent streptococcal infection; they are also at risk for infective endocarditis with any episode of bacteremia, such as might occur during a dental procedure. These patients require prophylactic antibiotics for recurrent streptococcal infections, as well as infective endocarditis.

Synonyms
Acute Rheumatic Fever
Inflammatory Rheumatism
Rheumatic Arthritis

Signs and Symptoms Acute rheumatic fever (**ARF**) follows an episode of streptococcal pharyngitis, which is usually, but not always, symptomatic. (In as many as one-third of cases, the preceding streptococcal infection may be either asymptomatic or so mild that the patient does not seek medical attention.) Approximately 1 to 5 weeks later the attack of ARF begins, usually with polyarthritis and fever. Arthralgias or arthritis may develop, classically with a migratory pattern.

Other common manifestations include carditis, which may only be evident by the appearance of a new murmur, or may be symptomatic. Endocarditis, myocarditis, or pericarditis may occur, alone or in combination. In severe cases congestive heart failure may occur, which can be fatal.

Serious disease of the cardiac valves may evolve over the years following the acute episode. Inflammation of the valves, most frequently the mitral valve, is followed by scarring, turbulent flow, and further damage. The end result may not be evident for 20 or 30 years, when the patient presents with symptoms of progressive valvular dysfunction. Because the initial insult may have been silent, this end result may be the first sign of a problem.

Chorea is much less common. It consists of involuntary, abrupt, purposeless movements, and inappropriate crying or laughter. It typically persists for 2 to 4 months.

Rashes and subcutaneous nodules are also less common. The characteristic rash, erythema marginatum, occurs mainly on the trunk and may only last for hours. Subcutaneous nodules are small and painless. They appear on bony prominences.

The diagnosis of ARF is made on clinical grounds by a set of criteria. The Jones criteria include major and minor manifestations of ARF. The diagnosis is considered highly probable if the patient meets either 2 major, or 1 major and 2 minor criteria, and has evidence of a recent streptococcal infection (positive throat culture; elevated titers of anti-streptococcal antibodies such as antistreptolysin-O).

The major criteria are carditis, polyarthritis, chorea, erythema marginatum, and subcutaneous nodules. The minor criteria include fever, arthralgia, elevated C-reactive protein (CRP) or erythrocyte sedimentation rate (ESR), a prolonged PR interval on electrocardiogram, and a history of rheumatic fever in the past.

Etiology Although rheumatic fever is clearly linked to Group A streptococcal infections, the exact mechanism causing the disorder is not well understood. It is thought to be an autoimmune phenomenon, triggered by cross-reactivity between streptococcal antigens and host tissue, but this is not proven.

Certain strains of *Streptococcus pyogenes* are known to be more rheumatogenic than others and have been associated with outbreaks. However, only a small percentage of patients with pharyngitis will develop ARF. Why this occurs in some individuals and not in others remains a mystery.

Following a primary episode of ARF, recurrences develop with each subsequent streptococcal infection. These are progressively more severe and are preventable with antibiotic prophylaxis.

Epidemiology Rheumatic fever is epidemic in India, the Middle East, and regions of South America and Africa, where it accounts for a major percentage of heart disease. In the United States, the incidence of ARF has declined steadily over the 20th century, but outbreaks were reported in the mid 1980s, apparently related to a resurgence of the rheumatogenic serotypes of S. *pyogenes*.

Rheumatic fever usually affects children between 5 and 15 years of age, but may occur among young adults as well. In the United States the delayed sequelae of ARF generally do not appear before the 4th or 5th decade; in the developing world where recurrences are common, these sequelae may become evident much earlier.

Related Disorders There are a number of diseases that may be manifested by fever and polyarthritis, and several may resemble ARF. Juvenile rheumatoid arthritis (Still's disease), is associated with fever, arthritis, and skin rash, as may be rheumatoid arthritis and other autoimmune disorders. These may often be distinguished from ARF by the appearance of rheumatoid factor and antinuclear antigens which do not occur in ARF, as well as by their symptom evolution.

Treatment—Standard There is no specific therapy for ARF. It can be prevented by timely treatment of streptococcal pharyngitis, although as stated above, this will only prevent those cases that are preceded by a symptomatic pharyngitis.

When rheumatic fever first develops, a course of penicillin is recommended to ensure eradication of any remaining streptococci. Following this, patients require longterm antibiotic prophylaxis, such as a monthly injection of 1.2 million units of benzathine penicillin G. Exactly how long such a regimen should be continued is controversial; some argue that it should be lifelong. Antibiotic prophylaxis against infective endocarditis is also necessary for any instrumental procedure with a risk of bacteremia.

Arthritic symptoms may be treated with antiinflammatory and analgesic drugs. When carditis is present, steroids may be prescribed although their benefit has yet to be demonstrated by controlled clinical trials. Chorea does not respond to steroids or antiinflammatory drugs. Sedatives may be useful.

Treatment—Investigational Researchers at Rockefeller University have identified 2 monoclonal antibodies that have the potential to be used as a screen to detect those at risk for rheumatic fever. It is hoped that when fully developed, this screen might be used to select candidates for immunization against streptococcal pharyngitis.

Please contact the agencies listed under Resources, below, for the most current information.

Resources

For more information on rheumatic fever: National Organization for Rare Disorders (NORD); NIH/National Institute of Allergy and Infectious Diseases (NIAID); Centers for Disease Control (CDC).

References

Resurgence of Acute Rheumatic Fever in the Intermountain Area of the United States: L.G. Veasy, et al.; N. Engl. J. Med., 1987, vol. 316(8), pp. 421–427.

Rheumatic Fever in the Eighties: M. Markowitz; Pediatr. Clin. North Am., 1986, vol. 33(5), pp. 1141–1150.

Rheumatic Fever: Down but Not Out: Evelyn Zamula; FDA Consumer, July–August 1987, pp. 26–28.

ROCKY MOUNTAIN SPOTTED FEVER (RMSF)

Description Rocky Mountain spotted fever is an acute disease caused by a rickettsia and transmitted by ticks. The illness is initially manifested by fever and rash, but progresses to multisystem involvement. Pathologically, it is a diffuse vasculitis. Early diagnosis and treatment are vital to avoid serious complications, but the disease lacks distinctive features in the early stages, frequently thwarting early diagnosis.

Synonyms

Black Fever
Black Measles
Blue Disease
Blue Fever
Mexican Spotted Fever
Sao Paulo Fever
Tobia Fever

Signs and Symptoms The incubation period of RMSF is 2 to 12 days, with an average of 7 days. The usual clinical picture then begins suddenly, with fever, severe headache, and myalgias. Nausea, vomiting, and abdominal pain may accompany these early symptoms. On about the 4th day, a rash develops, classically beginning on the wrists and ankles and spreading centrally. The rash is the most helpful diagnostic sign, but it may not occur in as many as 10 percent of cases, and in fulminant cases, death may intervene before the rash develops. The lesions are macular at the outset, but the rash generally becomes petechial within a few days. As the disease progresses, the skin lesions may become purpuric, ulcerative, necrotic, and finally gangrenous in severe cases.

Extensive vasculitis may occur throughout the body, with subsequent capillary leak syndrome. As fluid leaks out into the tissue, edema becomes prominent in the face, hands, and feet. Pulmonary edema may also develop. Other manifestations seen in severe cases include myocarditis and renal and liver dysfunction. Capillary leakage also results in hypotension, which compounds the ischemic effect of vasculitis and may progress to shock.

The central nervous system manifestations of RMSF include delirium, agitation, and meningismus, which frequently leads to a diagnosis of meningitis. Seizures and coma can occur in severe cases.

Laboratory data usually reveal a normal white blood cell count and thrombocytopenia. Signs of disseminated intravascular coagulation (**DIC**) may be present.

Etiology The cause of RMSF is the rickettsial organism *Rickettsia rickettsii*. It is transmitted by ticks, specifically *Dermacentor variabilis* in the eastern United States, and *Dermacentor andersoni* in the west.

Epidemiology RMSF was initially reported in the Rocky Mountains, the region that gave rise to its name, but it has been reported in almost all 50 states. Currently, the areas of greatest prevalence are in the eastern states. RMSF is a disease that concentrates in certain specific localities, such as Cabarrus and Rowan counties in North Carolina, Cape Cod in Massachusetts, and Long Island, New York. While it is normally thought of as a rural disease, an epidemic was reported in New York City in 1988, related to tick infestation of a park in the Bronx.

The tick that transmits RMSF has a marked preference for crevices in the skin, such as the axilla and gluteal regions. It attaches, feeds for several hours, and only then does it release the rickettsia into the bite wound.

Approximately 1000 cases are reported in the United States each year, with the greatest number occurring in the spring and summer. By law, all cases of RMSF must be reported to the Centers for Disease Control.

Related Disorders Related disorders include other rickettsial diseases and other infections that may resemble RMSF. The differential diagnosis commonly includes measles, meningococcemia, meningitis, typhoid fever, and other riskettsial diseases, particularly epidemic typhus. A wide variety of other illnesses may occasionally resemble RMSF: thrombotic thrombocytopenic purpura (TTP), septic shock, rubella, leptospirosis, and typhoid fever, to mention a few.

Meningococcemia may resemble RMSF, but the purpuric rash of this disease occurs very early in its course, whereas in RMSF the rash does not become petechial or purpuric until several days after onset of the illness.

Measles and epidemic typhus frequently are the most similar. In children, measles is a common misdiagnosis, which can be disastrous since no specific treatment is given for measles. The rash of measles characteristically starts on the neck and face, and there is also often a history of measles exposure; these features may distinguish it from RMSF.

Epidemic, or louse-borne typhus, caused by *Rickettsia prowazecki,* begins similarly to RMSF. A rash appears on the trunk on about the 5th day. Multisystem involvement occurs, as in RMSF, although it is usually not as severe.

Typhus and RMSF may be distinguished epidemiologically. Typhus is rare in the United States, and recent cases have been either recrudescent cases, initially acquired outside the United States, or in association with flying squirrels.

Typhus and RMSF may also be distinguished by the Weil-Felix reaction, a test for rickettsial antigens.

The diagnosis of RMSF is based on the clinical picture. The Weil-Felix reaction provides supportive evidence of RMSF, but the test is considered insufficiently sensitive to be confirmatory. A direct immunofluorescence test for skin biopsy specimens is available in some laboratories, and this may reveal rickettsia in the specimen by the 3rd or 4th day of illness.

The diagnosis of RMSF is generally confirmed by serologic testing, comparing acute and convalescent antibody titers. Obviously this is not useful in the acute illness.

Treatment—Standard Rocky Mountain spotted fever is treated with tetracycline, doxycycline, or chloramphenicol. Tetracyclines are preferred except in pregnant women and young children.

Preventative measures include the use of protective clothing, insect repellents, and regular hourly checks for ticks.

Treatment—Investigational A vaccine is currently under investigation.

Please contact the agencies listed under Resources, below, for the most current information.

Resources

For more information on Rocky Mountain spotted fever: National Organization for Rare Disorders (NORD); NIH/National Institute of Allergy & Infectious Diseases (NIAID); Centers for Disease Control (CDC).

References

Rocky Mountain Spotted Fever Presenting as Thrombotic Thrombocytopenic Purpura: R.C. Turner, et al.; Am. J. Med., 1986, vol. 81(1), pp. 153–157.

Rocky Mountain Spotted Fever: C.A. Kamper, et al.; Clin. Pharm., 1988, vol. 7(2), pp. 109–116.

Staphylococcus Aureus Septicemia Mimicking Fulminant Rocky Mountain Spotted Fever: M.R. Milunski, et al.; Am. J. Med., 1987, vol. 83(4), pp. 801–803.

The Sensitivity of Various Serologic Tests in the Diagnosis of Rocky Mountain Spotted Fever: J.E. Kaplan, et al.; Am. J. Trop. Med. Hyg., 1986, vol. 35(4), pp. 840–844.

Cloned Gene of Rickettsia Rickettsii Surface Antigen: Candidate Vaccine for Rocky Mountain Spotted Fever: G.A. McDonald, et al.; Science, 1987, vol. 235(4784), pp. 83–85.

ROSEOLA INFANTUM

Description Roseola infantum is an acute infectious disease of infants and very young children. Its major characteristics are high fever, and a rash that appears as the fever dissipates.

Synonyms

Exanthem Subitum
Pseudorubella
Sixth Disease

Signs and Symptoms Following an incubation period of approximately 5 to 15 days, roseola begins with high fever. The fever usually lasts for 3 to 5 days, and may be accompanied by febrile seizures, but apart from this the child does not look particularly ill. There may be cervical and posterior auricular adenopathy.

Defervescence of the fever is followed within 48 hours by appearance of a maculopapular rash, usually on the trunk and neck. The sequence and timing of these symptoms is diagnostic of roseola.

Etiology Roseola infantum is caused by herpesvirus type 6.

Epidemiology Roseola infantum usually affects children between 6 months and 3 years of age. It occurs most often in the spring and fall. Epidemics have been reported.

Related Disorders The differential diagnosis of roseola includes rubella, rubeola, and allergic rashes. The child with rubeola usually looks more toxic, and the pattern of fever and rash are different. Coryza, Koplik spots, and conjunctivitis, which occur in measles, further help to distinguish it from roseola. Atypical measles, particularly occurring in individuals vaccinated prior to 1980 who may have received an inadequate vaccine, may be milder than typical measles and resemble roseola more closely in this regard.

Rubella is distinguished from roseola chiefly by the presence of high fever prior to development of the rash in roseola.

Treatment—Standard There is no specific therapy for roseola infantum, and in most cases, specific treatment is not necessary. Antipyretics are recommended, although salicylates should be avoided because of the risk of Reye syndrome. Children who are at risk for febrile seizures may be sedated or prescribed prophylactic medication.

Treatment—Investigational Please contact the agencies listed under Resources, below, for the most current information.

Resources

For more information on roseola infantum: National Organization for Rare Disorders (NORD); NIH/National Institute of Allergy and Infectious Diseases (NIAID); Centers for Disease Control (CDC).

References

Identification of Human Herpesvirus-6 as a Causal Agent for Exanthem Subitum: K. Yamanishi, et al.; Lancet, May 14, 1988, issue 1(8594), pp. 1065–1067.

Acute Exanthems in Children. Clues to Differential Diagnosis of Viral Disease: C.A. Bligard, et al.; Postgrad. Med., April 1986, issue 79(5), pp. 150–154, 159–167.

Viral Exanthems: J.D. Cherry; Curr. Probl. Pediatr., April 1983, issue 13(6), pp. 1–44.

RUBELLA

Description Rubella is a viral infection that produces a different clinical syndrome depending on whether it is contracted pre- or postnatally. The congenital form (see *Rubella, Congenital*) has devastating manifestations, but postnatally, the disease rarely entails more than a rash with adenopathy.

Synonyms
> German Measles
> Three-Day Measles

Signs and Symptoms This discussion will be limited to postnatal rubella. The majority of rubella infections are asymptomatic. When symptoms occur, they follow a 12- to 23-day incubation period. In adults there may be a prodrome of malaise and fever which precedes the major characteristic manifestations of the disease, but this is not seen in children.

Rubella is predominantly an exanthem with adenopathy. Characteristically, posterior auricular, posterior cervical, and occipital nodes are involved. The rash begins on the face and then spreads to the trunk and extremities, lasting 3 to 5 days. Fever is unusual at this stage. In adults, this phase may be accompanied by headache, malaise, and anorexia.

The most common complication of postnatal rubella is joint involvement, which consists of arthralgias as well as frank arthritis. This occurs in women, but is rare in children and men. Thrombocytopenia with subsequent hemorrhage has occurred in children as a complication of rubella. Encephalitis has been reported in epidemics but is very rare.

The diagnosis of rubella is usually confirmed by serologic testing, most often using the hemagglutination-inhibition technique.

Etiology Rubella is caused by an RNA virus of the *Togaviridae* family.

Epidemiology Rubella is a disease of childhood; however, as more and more children are vaccinated against the disease it may become increasingly frequent in older age groups.

Transmission is by droplet spread from respiratory secretions. An infected individual can spread the disease in this manner from 10 days before the rash appears, until 15 days after it fades. (Patients with congenital rubella can spread the disease for months).

Related Disorders Measles (rubeola), scarlet fever (scarlatina), secondary syphilis, drug eruptions, erythema infectiosum (5th disease), infectious mononucleosis, and echo-, coxsackie-, and adenovirus infections may be considered in the differential diagnosis, with varying emphasis, depending on the age of the patient.

Rubella may be distinguished from measles by the following characteristics: the patient with measles looks considerably more toxic, has coryza, fever, and respiratory symptoms, and may be observed to have Koplik spots.

Like measles, scarlet fever has more constitutional symptoms; and, in addition to the rash, there is a marked pharyngitis.

The diagnoses of syphilis and infectious mononucleosis are best confirmed by laboratory tests (the VDRL, white blood cell count and differential, heterophil antibody), which will easily distinguish them from rubella.

The diagnosis of rubella may be confirmed by serologic testing, which may be extremely important if the patient is pregnant.

Treatment—Standard There is no treatment for rubella. An effective vaccine is available (the measles-mumps-rubella vaccine), and is routinely given at the age of

15 months. Women of childbearing age with insufficient antibody titer against rubella should be immunized. It is a live virus vaccine, which theoretically could produce congenital rubella in a fetus if given during pregnancy. Therefore vaccination is contraindicated during pregnancy, and it is recommended that conception be prevented for a minimum of 3 months following vaccination.

Treatment—Investigational Please contact the agencies listed under Resources, below, for the most current information.

Resources

For more information on rubella: National Organization for Rare Disorders (NORD); NIH/National Institute of Allergy and Infectious Diseases (NIAID); Centers for Disease Control (CDC).

References

Rubella: Public Health Education Information Sheet: March of Dimes Birth Defects Foundation, 1984.

Rubella Virus: A.A. Gershon; in Principles and Practice of Infectious Diseases, 3rd ed.: G.L. Mandell, et al., eds.; Churchill Livingston, 1990, pp. 1242–1247.

RUBELLA, CONGENITAL

Description When rubella is contracted during pregnancy the virus may be transmitted transplacentally. Congenital rubella is associated with a wide variety of birth defects as well as fetal demise.

Synonyms

Congenital German Measles
Expanded Rubella Syndrome

Signs and Symptoms The symptoms of congenital rubella may be transient or permanent. Among the transient symptoms are low birth weight, thrombocytopenia, hepatosplenomegaly, and meningoencephalitis. The permanent symptoms include deafness, cataracts, microphthalmia, retinopathy, cardiac malformations, mental retardation, and microcephaly. Infants who appear to be asymptomatic at birth may manifest symptoms, such as hearing loss and psychomotor retardation, later in childhood.

The diagnosis of congenital rubella is confirmed by serologic testing. The presence of IgM antibody to rubella in the fetus indicates transplacental infection occurred. Also, rising rubella titers in the infant suggest that active rubella infection, rather than passive antibody transfer, has occurred.

Etiology Congenital rubella results from the transplacental transmission of the rubella virus, an RNA virus of the *Togaviridae* family.

Epidemiology Not all maternal infections are transmitted transplacentally. The risk of fetal infection is highest early in pregnancy, as is the risk of severe manifestations. There is a 40 to 60 percent risk of infection with multiple sequelae in the first 8 weeks of gestation; however, by the 16th week the risk has declined to 10 percent. The risks of fetal defects with infection at 8, 12, 13 to 20, and over 20 weeks of gestation are 85, 50, 15, and 0 percent, respectively.

Widespread vaccination against rubella has dramatically reduced the incidence of the congenital disease. There have been no epidemics since vaccination has become routine.

Treatment—Standard There is no treatment for either maternal or congenital rubella. Vaccination is currently required at the age of 15 months. Because the vaccine is a live virus vaccine, there is a theoretical risk of developing congenital rubella following vaccination in pregnancy. Currently vaccination is contraindicated during pregnancy, and conception should be avoided for at least 3 months following vaccination.

Treatment—Investigational Please contact the agencies listed under Resources, below, for the most current information.

Resources

For more information on congenital rubella: National Organization for Rare Disorders (NORD); NIH/National Institute of Child Health and Human Development.

For genetic information and genetic counseling referrals: March of Dimes Birth Defects Foundation; National Center for Education in Maternal and Child Health.

References
Rubella; Public Health Education Information Sheet: March of Dimes Birth Defects Foundation, 1984.

Rubella Virus: A.A. Gershon; *in* Principles and Practice of Infectious Diseases, 3rd ed.: G.L. Mandell, et al., eds.; Churchill Livingston, 1990, pp. 1242–1247.

SEVERE COMBINED IMMUNODEFICIENCY (SCID)

Description SCID comprises a group of congenital syndromes in which there appears to be little or no specific cellular or humoral immune response. Thus, the patient is susceptible to recurrent infections with bacteria, viruses, fungi, and other infectious agents. Untreated, SCID results in frequent, severe infections, growth retardation, and a short life span. Several causes and types of SCID have been identified: autosomal recessive, X-linked recessive, adenosine deaminase deficiency (ADA), bare lymphocyte syndrome, SCID with leukopenia (reticular dysgenesis), and Swiss-type agammaglobulinemia.

Signs and Symptoms Maternal antibodies usually continue to protect young infants with SCID in the first few months of life. Afterwards, however, infections occur and recur frequently, e.g., pneumonia, sepsis, otitis media, diarrhea, and skin infections. Weight loss, weakness, and drastic growth retardation ensue.

Opportunistic organisms that may cause fatal infections include *Candida albicans,* vaccinia, varicella, measles, cytomegalovirus, and the live bacteria in the BCG (bacille Calmette-Guérin) vaccine against tuberculosis. The pneumonia caused by *Pneumocystis carinii* is common and is very difficult to treat.

The fact that SCID patients do not reject foreign tissue has several effects. Immunocompetent cells introduced into the patient's body (e.g., by a blood transfusion) may cause graft-versus-host (**GvH**) disease, reacting primarily against the recipient's skin, liver, gut, and bone marrow. However, since transplants are not rejected, bone marrow transplantation, one of the only effective treatments in this disorder, is facilitated. After immunization, antibodies are not formed; if immunization is with a live vaccine, fatal infections may result. Patients do not have cutaneous reactions to antigens and do not develop allergic reactions.

In SCID patients, T and B lymphocytes and serum immunoglobulins are usually severely reduced in number or are absent; even if present, function is severely impaired. The thymus is small and underdeveloped; lymph nodes are lacking in lymphocytes; and tonsils, adenoids, and other lymphoid organs are poorly developed or absent.

In SCID with leukopenia (reticular dysgenesis), granulocytes are also absent or greatly reduced in number. These patients also have virtually no means of removing invading organisms from the body.

Etiology Hereditary SCID occurs in autosomal recessive and X-linked recessive forms. Approximately 50 percent of autosomal recessive cases of SCID have adenosine deaminase (**ADA**) deficiency. This results in high levels of adenosine in the plasma. Lymphocytes trap unusually high levels of this adenosine. Intracellularly, adenosine and its metabolites interfere with a variety of cell functions.

In the bare lymphocyte syndrome, clinical SCID is associated with a lack of histocompatibility antigens and B2 microglobulin on the lymphocytes. In the absence of these proteins, T cells cannot be activated.

Epidemiology SCID is estimated to occur with a frequency of about 1:100,000 to 1:500,000 live births.

Related Disorders Various other forms of immunodeficiency exist. They include the acquired immune deficiency syndrome, isolated defects of T cell function, and various antibody disorders. (See *Acquired Immune Deficiency Syndrome [AIDS]).*

Treatment—Standard Bone marrow transplantation, which can cure this disorder if an identical donor match can be found, has been facilitated greatly by the use of haplo-identical bone marrow cells, treated to remove those cells likely to cause GvH disease but leave stem cells intact.

Fetal liver grafts, which contain lymphoid and white blood stem cells, have sometimes been effective in restoring T cell function, but not antibody production. Fetal thymus grafts have usually been unsuccessful.

In isolated cases, agents such as transfer factor, thymosin, and levamisole may augment existing cellular immunity.

In 1990 the FDA approved PEG-ADA, an orphan drug that replaces the ADA enzyme deficiency in SCID. Children taking PEG-ADA through a weekly injection have had a normal immune system restored, and they are recovering from infections that might previously have been deadly. For more information on PEG-ADA, please contact Enzon Inc.

Infections in persons with SCID must be treated vigorously with antifungal, antibiotic, and supportive measures. *P. carinii* pneumonia can be particularly difficult to treat; the 2 drugs used are usually trimethoprim-sulfamethoxazole and the orphan drug pentamidine idethionate. (For further information on treatment of *P. carinii* pneumonia, see *Acquired Immune Deficiency Syndrome [AIDS]*). Cytomegalovirus and generalized herpes simplex infections are preferentially treated with idoxuridine, floxuridine, or cytarabadine. Severe candidiasis and other fungal infections usually respond to amphotericin B therapy.

Treatment—Investigational Scientists at Johns Hopkins University in Maryland are studying the use of thalidomide as a treatment for GVH disease. Preliminary studies indicate it may have beneficial side effects on skin and hair symptoms. The major side effects of thalidomide are sedation and teratogenesis. More research is necessary to determine longterm safety and effectiveness of this treatment for GvH disease.

Scientists at the National Institutes of Health are using an experimental gene therapy procedure in combination with the orphan drug PEG-ADA, to enhance the immune system of children with ADA-deficient SCID. The procedure involves implanting the ADA gene into an activated virus. When the virus merges into the patient's cells, it manufactures the human enzyme. The corrected cells will be infused into the patient every few months. Patients interested in participating in this experimental protocol should ask their physicians to contact Dr. Nelson Wivel, Office of Recombinant DNA Activities, National Institutes of Health, Building 31, Room 4B11, Bethesda, MD 20892.

The FDA Orphan Products Division awarded a grant in 1988 to Carol Michele Paradise, M.D., of Cetus Corporation, Emeryville, CA, for her treatment of SCID with interleukin-2.

Please contact the agencies listed under Resources, below, for the most current information.

Resources

For more information on SCID: National Organization for Rare Disorders (NORD); Immune Deficiency Foundation; M. Hershfield, M.D., Duke University Hospital; NIH/National Institute of Allergy and Infectious Diseases (NIAID).

References

Immunodeficiency: Buckley, R.H.; J. Allergy Clin. Immunol., 1983, vol. 72(6), pp. 627–641.

Metabolic Defects in Immunodeficiency Diseases: A.D.B. Webster; Clin. Exp. Immunol., 1982, vol. 49(1), pp. 1–10.

Combined Immunodeficiency and Thymic Abnormalities; A.D.B. Webster; J. Clin. Pathol., Suppl., 1979, vol. 13, pp. 10–14.

SIMIAN B VIRUS INFECTION

Description Simian B virus is a type of herpesvirus which causes infection in monkeys. Human infections have occurred through monkey bites and laboratory accidents. In humans, the virus produces a severe encephalitis.

Synonyms

Herpesvirus Simiae, B Virus
Herpesvirus Simiae Encephalomyelitis
Monkey B Virus

Signs and Symptoms Infection with simian B virus produces the clinical picture of severe encephalitis, with fever, headache, malaise, vomiting, and meningismus. Associated neurologic abnormalities may include neuromuscular dysfunction, visual disturbances, cranial nerve dysfunction, psychiatric symptoms, seizures, paralysis, and coma. Respiratory function may be affected.

Encephalomyelitis and meningitis may occur. The mortality rate is high.

Etiology This disease is caused by the simian B virus, a herpesvirus.

Epidemiology Simian B virus infection occurs in laboratory workers who are bitten or scratched by infected monkeys, or accidentally exposed to virus-infected simian tissue cultures. It is rare; it has been estimated that 24 cases of the disorder occurred in the United States between 1932 and 1972.

Related Disorders The symptoms of simian B virus infection are common to the viral encephalitides. The epidemiologic setting of simian B virus infection is the major diagnostic clue to the nature of the disease. The syndrome of acute disseminated encephalomyelitis may also be caused by viruses other than simian B virus.

Treatment—Standard Protective clothing is recommended for those working with infected monkeys or tissues. Once a laboratory worker is bitten or scratched, there is some evidence that transmission may be prevented by intravenous acyclovir. Intravenous acyclovir may also be helpful once the disease has developed. Otherwise treatment is supportive.

Treatment—Investigational A vaccine is under investigation, but it is not yet available for general use.

Please contact the agencies listed under Resources, below, for the most current information.

Resources

For more information on simian B virus infection: National Organization for Rare Disorders (NORD); NIH/National Institute of Allergy and Infectious Diseases (NIAID); Centers for Disease Control (CDC).

References

B Virus, Herpesvirus Simiae: Historical Perspective: A.E. Palmer; J. Med. Primatol., 1987, issue 16(2), pp. 99–130.

The Spectrum of Antiviral Activities of Acyclovir in Vitro and in Vivo: P. Collins; J. Antimicrob. Chemother., September 1983, issue 12(suppl. B), pp. 19–27.

Successful Treatment of Experimental B Virus (Herpesvirus Simiae) Infection with Acyclovir: E.A. Boulter, et al.; Br. Med. J., March 8, 1980, issue 280(6215), pp. 681–683.

STEVENS-JOHNSON SYNDROME

Description Stevens-Johnson syndrome is the most severe form of erythema multiforme and is characterized by bullous lesions on the skin and mucous membranes.

Synonyms

> Dermatostomatitis
> Ectodermosis Erosiva Pluriorificialis
> Erythema Multiforme Major
> Febrile Mucocutaneous Syndrome
> Herpes Iris

Signs and Symptoms Typical Stevens-Johnson syndrome affects the mucous membranes of the oral cavity, pharynx, nares, eyes, and anogenital region. It may or may not be associated with erythema multiforme elsewhere on the body. The bullous lesions are generally painful; oropharyngeal lesions may be so intolerable as to prevent eating. A painful conjunctivitis occurs, frequently with a purulent discharge, and can lead to corneal scarring and loss of vision. In addition to the mucous membrane lesions, fever and prostration are usual.

Approximately one-third of patients have pulmonary involvement with cough and patchy infiltrates on chest x-ray. In fatal cases, renal failure and pneumonia may occur.

The diagnosis of Stevens-Johnson syndrome is usually based on the clinical appearance and distribution of the lesions.

Etiology The Stevens-Johnson syndrome has been associated with a variety of infectious and pharmacologic agents. Coxsackie-, echo-, and, most commonly, herpes simplex viruses as well as mycoplasma have precipitated the syndrome. Vaccines, such as those for tuberculosis, smallpox, and polio have also been implicated. Penicillin, sulfonamides, anticonvulsants, and barbiturates are the most frequently associated drugs. In approximately 50 percent of cases no cause can be identified.

Epidemiology Stevens-Johnson syndrome is more frequent in children and young adults but occurs in all ages. Males are affected more frequently than females.

Related Disorders See *Behçet Syndrome.* Other diseases that may resemble Stevens-Johnson syndrome include the following.

Allergic stomatitis is characterized by an intense, painful erythema which may be related to food or cosmetic hypersensitivity. **Herpetic stomatitis** is characterized by pruritis followed by the appearance of small, tense blisters on a red base.

Mikulicz syndrome (aphthous stomatitis) is also limited to the oral cavity; it consists of recurrent ulcerative lesions. The 3 diseases mentioned above tend not to have systemic manifestations.

Treatment—Standard Every attempt should be made to identify a precipitating agent, and to remove it if possible. Antibiotics are appropriate if superinfection is suspected, or if bacterial disease, such as mycoplasma, is suspected to be the cause. Intensive supportive care is important in severe cases. Fluid replacement is often required, and meticulous oral hygiene is necessary to prevent superinfection. Examination by an ophthalmologist is recommended for patients with eye lesions so that precautions can be taken to avoid permanent eye damage.

Treatment—Investigational Please contact the agencies listed under Resources, below, for the most current information.

Resources

For more information on Stevens-Johnson syndrome: National Organization for Rare Disorders (NORD); NIH/National Institute of Allergy and Infectious Diseases (NIAID); The National Arthritis and Musculoskeletal and Skin Diseases Information Clearinghouse; NIH/National Eye Institute.

References
Erythema Multiforme: W. Stewart, et al., eds.; *in* Dermatology, Diagnosis and Treatment of Cutaneous Disorders, 3rd ed.: Mosby, 1984.

SUBACUTE SCLEROSING PANENCEPHALITIS (SSPE)

Description SSPE is a progressive neurologic disorder caused by an inappropriate immune response to the measles virus. Onset of SSPE often occurs 2 to 10 years after the original attack.

Synonyms
Decerebrate Dementia

Signs and Symptoms SSPE is a disease of childhood or young adulthood. The first signs are behavioral changes: failing schoolwork, memory loss, and irritability. Myoclonic jerks, involuntary movements, and generalized seizures follow. The course is one of progressive dementia and neurologic deterioration. Spasticity, cortical blindness, and optic atrophy may occur. In advanced cases, signs of hypothalamic involvement are present, with hyperthermia and other disturbances of homeostasis.

The disease is usually fatal within 1 to 3 years, the terminal event often being pneumonia. Sometimes prolonged remissions occur.

Laboratory abnormalities include a characteristic EEG picture, and high serum levels of measles antibody. The cerebrospinal fluid shows elevated levels of gammaglobulin and measles antibody. The diagnosis of SSPE is based on these abnormalities.

Etiology SSPE is thought to be a form of measles encephalitis, associated with an inappropriate immune response to rubeola (measles virus). Usually there is a history of measles 2 to 10 years prior to the onset. There have been cases where patients have had contact with pets such as monkeys, dogs, or kittens that later died from the illness.

Epidemiology SSPE occurs in children and adolescents; almost all cases appear before the age of 20 years. Males are affected more often than females.

Related Disorders Progressive multifocal leukoencephalopathy is a polyoma virus infection of the brain seen in immunosuppressed patients. Symptoms include ataxia, paralysis, blindness, and, ultimately, coma.

Inclusion-body encephalitis is an infection with gradual onset, mostly in children under 12 years of age. Symptoms include behavioral changes, myoclonus of the trunk and extremities, and aphasia.

Treatment—Standard There is no specific treatment for SSPE as yet. A number of antiviral agents have been investigated with little success. Isolated reports about the effectiveness of isoprinosine have not been confirmed by controlled clinical trials. Supportive measures and anticonvulsants are useful.

Treatment—Investigational Please contact the agencies listed under Resources, below, for the most current information.

Resources

For more information on SSPE: National Organization for Rare Disorders (NORD); National SSPE Registry (University of Alabama School of Medicine); NIH/National Institute of Allergy and Infectious Diseases (NIAID).

References
The Merck Manual, 15th ed.: Robert Berkow, ed.-in-chief; Merck Sharp & Dohme Research Laboratories, 1987, pp. 1401, 2023, 2041.

Cecil Textbook of Medicine, 18th ed.: J.B. Wyngaarden and L.H. Smith, Jr., eds.; W.B. Saunders Company, 1988, pp. 2203, 2206–2207.

SUTTON DISEASE II

Description Sutton disease II, also known as recurrent aphthous stomatitis, is a disease of uncertain etiology characterized by recurrent painful episodes of aphthous stomatitis.

Synonyms
>Aphthous Ulcer
>Periadenitis Mucosa Necrotica
>Recurrent Aphthous Stomatitis
>Ulcerative Stomatitis
>von Mikulicz Aphthae
>von Zahorsky Disease

Signs and Symptoms This disease is marked by oral ulcers of varying size, often 7 to 15mm. They may be numerous; as many as 15 may be present at any one time. At the start they are shallow erosions covered with inflammatory exudate. As healing progresses, scarring may occur. Lesions heal in one to two weeks, but recurrence is the rule.

The diagnosis is based on the clinical appearance of the ulcers, as well as the history of recurrence.

Etiology The precise etiology of Sutton disease II is unknown, but local disturbances in immunity may contribute. Iron, vitamin B12, and folic acid deficiencies increase susceptibility to the disease. Attacks are usually triggered by stress.

Epidemiology Before puberty, males and females are equally affected; after puberty, women are more often affected. The disease occurs most frequently in malnourished children and debilitated adults.

Related Disorders Pemphigus may resemble Sutton disease II. Herpetic oral ulcers are similar but they occur mainly on the hard palate and immovable mucosa, while the aphthae of Sutton disease II rarely appear in these locations. Recurrent mouth ulcers also occur in the cyclic neutropenia syndrome and in B12, folate, and iron deficiency syndromes.

Treatment—Standard An anesthetic oral rinse and topical steroids give symptomatic relief, and a tetracycline oral suspension may reduce the lesions. However, use of antibiotics and steroids may promote the development of oral candidiasis. When therapy is begun promptly, relief is rapid. Subsequent attacks require renewed efforts at treatment.

Treatment—Investigational Please contact the agencies listed under Resources, below, for the most current information.

Resources

For more information on Sutton disease II: National Organization for Rare Disorders (NORD); NIH/National Institute of Dental Research.

References

Cecil Textbook of Medicine, 18th ed.: J.B. Wyngaarden and L.H. Smith, Jr., eds.; W.B. Saunders Company, 1988, pp. 675–676, 1664, 2347.

TORCH SYNDROME

Description The term TORCH is a mnemonic referring to 4 infectious agents that are capable of causing serious intrauterine infection, leading to both disease and/or malformations. The agents are: *TO*xoplasma gondii, *R*ubella virus, *C*ytomegalovirus, and *H*erpes virus. The mnemonic is useful in the diagnostic workup of any neonate with hepatosplenomegaly, chorioretinitis, or fetal malformations; these 4 agents will rank high on the list of diagnostic possibilities.

Synonyms

Toxoplasmosis-Rubella-Cytomegalovirus-Herpes Syndrome

Signs and Symptoms Congenital toxoplasmosis may be asymptomatic or may be present at birth with a wide variety of symptoms such as hepatosplenomegaly, chorioretinitis, jaundice, thrombocytopenia, and numerous central nervous system abnormalities. Those cases that are asymptomatic at birth may manifest evidence of infection at a later date.

The symptoms of congenital rubella are hepatosplenomegaly, thrombocytopenia, meningoencephalitis, microcephaly, cardiac malformations, cataracts, hearing loss, and mental retardation, to mention a few. (See *Rubella, Congenital.*)

Cytomegalovirus infection (**CMV**) is associated with hepatosplenomegaly, jaundice, petechiae, chorioretinitis, and a variety of central nervous system abnormalities. The clinical syndrome ranges in severity from asymptomatic to fulminant and fatal.

Neonatal herpes can be characterized by hepatosplenomegaly, jaundice, a bleeding diathesis, and central nervous system abnormalities. There is considerable variation in the severity of symptoms. Unlike the above disorders, herpes appears to be transmitted during delivery, by passage through an infected genital tract.

Etiology The etiologic agents are *Toxoplasma gondii*, rubella virus, cytomegalovirus, and herpes virus, usually herpes simplex virus, type II.

Epidemiology These infections occur worldwide. Transmission to the fetus is transplacental in rubella, toxoplasmosis, and cytomegalovirus, and appears to be at the time of delivery in the case of herpes.

Treatment—Standard Congenital toxoplasmosis may be treated with pyrimethamine and sulfadiazine, or spiramycin. There is some evidence that treatment reduces the chance of developing further symptoms during postnatal life.

There is no effective treatment for congenital rubella or congenital CMV, but ganciclovir may be of some benefit in the latter.

The first step in the approach to neonatal herpes is prevention; if the mother develops symptoms of herpes infection, or vaginal or cervical cultures done late in pregnancy show herpes virus, the fetus is best delivered by cesarean section. When this is not possible and infection results, acyclovir has been used with success in neonatal herpes.

Treatment—Investigational Please contact the agencies listed under Resources, below, for the most current information.

Resources

For more information on the TORCH diseases: National Organization for Rare Disorders (NORD); NIH/National Institute of Allergy and Infectious Diseases (NIAID); NIH/National Institute of Neurological Disorders & Stroke (NINDS); Centers for Disease Control (CDC).

For genetic information and genetic counseling referrals: March of

Dimes Birth Defects Foundation; National Center for Education in Maternal and Child Health.

References

The TORCH Syndrome, A Clinical Review: J.D. Fine and K.A. Arndt; J. Amer. Acad. Dermatol., 1985, vol. 12(4), pp. 2477–2478.

TORCH, A Literature Review and Implications for Practice: L. Haggerty; J. Obstet. Gynecol. Nurs., 1985, vol. 14(2), pp. 124–129.

TOXIC SHOCK SYNDROME (TSS)

Description TSS, produced by a toxin elaborated by *Staphylococcus aureus*, is a multisystem disease with widespread manifestations. Characteristic features include high fever, vomiting, diarrhea, hypotension, and a skin rash that typically resembles a sunburn. Most, but not all, cases occur in menstruating females in association with the use of tampons. TSS also may develop as a consequence of relatively minor postoperative wound infections, sometimes in association with nasal packing.

Signs and Symptoms Onset of TSS is usually sudden. Initially, there is a high fever, accompanied by headache, sore throat, and conjunctivitis. The classic "sunburn" rash appears early and desquamates on the palms and soles over several days. Gastrointestinal involvement, with vomiting and diarrhea, is common. Central nervous system dysfunction may be noted, with disorientation. Hypotension is common and frank shock occurs in severe cases. There may be acute renal failure, hepatic insufficiency, myositis, and disseminated intravascular coagulation, as well as development of adult respiratory distress syndrome.

Diagnosis of toxic shock syndrome is based on clinical criteria that include fever, rash with desquamation, hypotension, and involvement of at least 3 organ systems (typically gastrointestinal, hepatic, renal, hematologic, muscular, or central nervous system). *S. aureus* may be isolated from the vagina or from focal lesions, but blood cultures are usually negative.

The mortality rate is approximately 3 percent, though this figure may be excessive, reflecting heavy reporting of severe cases. Recurrences have occurred, chiefly during subsequent menses of women using tampons.

Etiology Toxic shock syndrome is caused by one or more toxins (TSST-1) elaborated by certain strains of *S. aureus*. Approximately 70 to 75 percent of cases are associated with vaginal infections of *S. aureus* and the use of hyperabsorbent tampons. Other associated types of staphylococcal infection include postoperative and postpartum wound infections, abscesses, pneumonia, osteomyelitis, and skin infections.

Epidemiology The major risk group for toxic shock syndrome is menstruating women. The combination of vaginal *S. aureus* infection and continuous tampon use sets the stage for TSS. However, TSS has been reported in association with a wide variety of other infections occurring in nonmenstruating women, children, and men. The incidence is estimated to be 3 cases per 100,000 menstruating women. Cases have been reported from all 50 states.

TSS has also been reported in association with the use of the vaginal contraceptive sponge. According to Food and Drug Administration reports, 12 cases have been confirmed out of an estimated 600,000 regular users, although none were fatal. To minimize the risk it is recommended that the sponge not be worn for more than 30 hours continuously, and that it not be used during menstruation or during the first 3 months postpartum.

Treatment—Standard Aggressive fluid and electrolyte replacement is essential. In severe cases, intensive supportive care will be necessary to address pulmonary and renal insufficiency, hypotension, and other complications. In nonmenstrual TSS the wound, abscess, or other focus needs to be treated appropriately. The drug of choice is a beta-lactamase–resistant antistaphylococcal penicillin.

Prevention involves judicious use of tampons; intermittent use and avoidance of highly absorbent brands is advised.

Treatment—Investigational Please contact the agencies listed under Resources, below, for the most current information.

Resources
For more information on toxic shock syndrome: National Organization for Rare Disorders (NORD); NIH/National Institute of Allergy and Infectious Diseases; Centers for Disease Control (CDC).

References
Cecil Textbook of Medicine, 18th ed.: J.B. Wyngaarden and L.H. Smith, Jr., eds.: W.B. Saunders Company, 1988, pp. 1598, 2323.

TOXOCARIASIS

Description Toxocariasis is a systemic helminthic infection caused by the dog ascarid *Toxocara canis*.

Synonyms
Visceral Larva Migrans

Signs and Symptoms The majority of infections are probably asymptomatic, but severe and even fatal infection is possible. When symptoms occur, they vary with the migratory patterns of the parasite. Common complaints include fever, cough, wheezing, and abdominal pain. Involvement of the central nervous system, particularly the eye, occurs. Hepatomegaly is common, and lung examination frequently reveals rales and wheezes. The chest x-ray may be abnormal. Marked eosinophilia is the rule.

The diagnosis of toxocariasis is usually made on the clinical picture. An enzyme-linked immunosorbent assay (**ELISA**) may be used to confirm the diagnosis.

Etiology Toxocariasis is caused by the helminth *Toxocara canis*. Infection is acquired by eating the eggs of the organism. The larvae invade the tissues of the body where they elicit granuloma formation.

Epidemiology The adult worms inhabit the intestines of dogs, and the eggs are passed in the stool. Young children are at risk, particularly in areas where geophagia is common. Toxocariasis has been reported mostly in the United States (south central and southeastern regions) and in Europe.

Related Disorders Disorders that can produce similar symptoms with eosinophilia include other nematode infections such as *Ascaris lumbricoides* and *Strongyloides stercoralis*, as well as schistosomes and hookworm. Ocular infection is unique to toxocariasis, but may require differentiation from other diseases of the eye, such as malignancy.

Treatment—Standard Toxocariasis may be treated with diethylcarbamazine or thiabendazole, but neither of these is uniformly effective. Most cases are self-limited and do not warrant specific therapy. Preventative measures consist of deworming dogs, preventing geophagia, and good hygiene. Retinal infection may be treated with laser photocoagulation.

Treatment—Investigational Please contact the agencies listed under Resources, below, for the most current information.

Resources

 For more information on toxocariasis: National Organization for Rare Disorders (NORD); National Institute of Allergy & Infectious Diseases (NIAID); Centers for Disease Control (CDC).

References

Serologic and Intradermal Test for Parasitic Infections: D.A. Bruckner; Pediatr. Clin. North Am., August 1985, issue 32(4), pp. 1063–1075.

Human Toxocariasis. Review with Report of a Probable Case: P.D. Morris, et al.; Postgrad. Med., January 1987, issue 81(1), pp. 263–267.

Internal Medicine, 2nd ed.: J.H. Stein, ed.-in-chief; Little, Brown and Company, 1987, pp. 1801–1802.

TOXOPLASMOSIS

Description Toxoplasmosis is an infectious disease caused by the protozoan parasite, *Toxoplasma gondii*. The infection produces several different syndromes depending on host factors, and whether it occurs pre- or postnatally. Congenital toxoplasmosis produces a range of fetal abnormalities, including spontaneous abortion, central nervous system damage, hepatitis, and chorioretinitis. In immunocompetent adults, toxoplasmosis is usually a benign mononucleosislike illness. Immunocompromised patients are more likely to develop a severe, disseminated form of infection that may be fatal.

Synonyms

 Disseminated Toxoplasmosis

Lymphadenopathic Toxoplasmosis

Signs and Symptoms The 3 different syndromes of toxoplasmosis will be described separately.

The majority of **toxoplasma infections in immunocompetent individuals** are asymptomatic. In symptomatic cases the most frequent abnormality is lymphadenopathy, usually cervical; however, regional adenopathy in other locations, and generalized adenopathy, occur. Fever, malaise, hepatosplenomegaly, and laboratory features of a mononucleosislike syndrome may also be present. The course is generally benign but may be protracted. Since toxoplasmosis often cannot be distinguished clinically from infectious mononucleosis, lymphoma, and other diseases, diagnosis should be confirmed by serologic testing.

Toxoplasmosis in the immunosuppressed patient: Patients with AIDS, hematologic malignancies, and organ transplants are at risk for a disseminated, more serious form of toxoplasmosis. Involvement of the central nervous system is the most common manifestation; mass lesions, encephalitis, and meningoencephalitis may occur. A common presentation is a generalized seizure, produced by a ring-enhancing lesion seen on CT scan. Brain biopsy may be necessary to distinguish cerebral toxoplasmosis from other lesions in the immunosuppressed host (lymphoma, tuberculoma, and others). Myocarditis and pneumonitis may also develop.

Congenital toxoplasmosis results from maternal infection, which is usually asymptomatic. When infection is acquired early in pregnancy, the risk of transmission to the fetus is lower, but the chance of severe fetal disease resulting from infection is higher. The manifestations of fetal toxoplasmosis may be evident before birth, with spontaneous abortion; at birth, in which case the disease is usually severe; or may be mild and not become evident until some time after birth. The clinical picture may include any of the following: microcephaly, hydrocephalus, chorioretinitis, blindness, mental retardation, seizures, anemia, jaundice, and a rash.

In cases where fetal infection is mild or asymptomatic at birth, early treatment can markedly reduce the risk of developing symptoms at a later date.

Etiology Toxoplasmosis is caused by an intracellular protozoan parasite, *T. gondii*. This organism is ubiquitous in nature. Its life cycle involves a sexual stage that occurs in cats. Humans become infected by cysts, either oocysts, which are excreted in the cat feces, or tissue cysts, present in a variety of foodstuffs.

Infection may be asymptomatic but persist in a latent form, only to be reactivated in the event of immunosuppression.

Epidemiology Toxoplasmosis affects men and women in equal numbers worldwide. The incidence varies widely from country to country, and within different regions of the United States. The incidence of congenital infection is 0.25 to 5.0 per 100,000 live births.

Toxoplasmosis is acquired transplacentally or by oral ingestion. Cysts may be present in lamb, pork, and eggs, and probably contaminate vegetables and other food products. As was mentioned above, cysts are also present in cat feces, and may be transmitted during routine care of cat litter. Pregnant women are advised to avoid cat litter in order to minimize the risk of transmission.

Related Disorders The **mononucleosis** syndrome is most frequently caused by Epstein-Barr virus, or occasionally cytomegalovirus. Hepatitis B may produce a similar clinical picture (see *Hepatitis B.)*

Chorioretinitis may also be caused by cytomegalovirus. Related congenital infections include those of the TORCH complex: Toxoplasmosis-Rubella-Cytomegalovirus-Herpes (see *TORCH Syndrome.)*

Treatment—Standard Specific treatment of toxoplasmosis in immunocompetent individuals is rarely necessary. In pregnancy, spiramycin is the preferred drug, since pyrimethamine may be teratogenic. Immunocompromised patients are generally treated with pyrimethamine and sulfadiazine (clindamycin may be substituted for sulfadiazine); infected neonates may be treated with these or spiramycin. Since these drugs are associated with significant hematologic toxicity, periodic monitoring is recommended.

Treatment—Investigational The Food and Drug Administration has awarded a research grant to Rima McLeod, M.D., Michael Reese Hospital & Medical Center, Chicago, Illinois, for comparison studies on treatments for congenital toxoplasmosis. Included in the studies are pyrimethamine and sulfadiazine, spiramycin, and pyrimethamine and sulfadoxine.

Please contact the agencies listed under Resources, below, for the most current information.

Resources

For more information on toxoplasmosis: National Organization for Rare Disorders (NORD); Centers for Disease Control (CDC); NIH/National Institute of Allergy and Infectious Diseases (NIAID).

References

Toxoplasma Gondii: R.E. McCabe and J.S. Remington; *in*Principles and Practice of Infectious Diseases: G.L. Mandell, et al., eds.; Churchill Livingstone, 1990, pp. 2090–2102.

TUBERCULOSIS (TB)

Description Tuberculosis is a bacterial disease caused by *Mycobacterium tuberculosis* or *Mycobacterium bovis*. Pathologically, the hallmark of TB is the granuloma. Clinically, typical TB is characterized by an initial asymptomatic infection followed by a latent period of years, with the possibility of reactivation in later adulthood.

TB is usually a chronic infection with protean manifestations. The lungs are most often affected, where the most common manifestation is cavitary pneumonia. The tubercle bacillus is remarkably adept at setting up infection in virtually any organ of the body.

Signs and Symptoms The signs and symptoms of TB depend on the site of infection. Tuberculosis is usually thought of as a disease that occurs in stages. The initial, or primary, infection is in the lungs. It frequently occurs in childhood and is most often asymptomatic. When symptomatic, the syndrome is one of lower lobe pneumonia. However, if primary infection does not occur until adulthood, the disease may progress so quickly that the clinical syndrome is indistinguishable from reactivation disease.

Reactivated or secondary TB is most commonly a chronic, slowly progressive disease which begins insidiously with nonspecific constitutional symptoms. Weight loss, night sweats, fever, and fatigue are prominent. In the lungs, a cavity usually develops, which may be seen on chest x-ray. The major symptom at this stage is coughing, and the secretions are infectious. Hemoptysis may also occur late in the disease.

Extrapulmonary TB is increasingly common because of a resurgence of tuberculosis in patients with AIDS. The organs most commonly affected are the pleura, genitourinary tract, kidney, meninges, bones, and pericardium. The symptoms vary with the organ involved.

Miliary TB may be a fulminant disease with severe lung disease and pleural, peritoneal, and meningeal involvement.

The diagnosis of TB requires demonstrating the organism in tissues or body fluids. The presence of a cavity on chest x-ray, with the appropriate clinical picture, points strongly to the diagnosis, and sputum smears for acid-fast bacilli are confirmatory. In the past gastric aspirates have been used to obtain smears for microbiological staining, but these are regarded as unreliable.

Asymptomatic infection is diagnosed using the Mantoux, or tuberculin, test. This involves an intradermal injection of purified protein derivative (PPD) and observing for a reaction 48 to 72 hours later. A positive test is considered to be 10 mm or more induration (not erythema).

The diagnosis of extrapulmonary TB may require acid-fast staining of the cerebrospinal fluid and pleural, peritoneal, or bone marrow biopsy, depending on the site of suspected disease. Often cultures are necessary, particularly for determining antibiotic resistances. These are time-consuming, as growth of the organism in vitro requires 4 to 6 weeks.

Etiology In the United States today, *M. tuberculosis* is the most common cause of tuberculosis. This organism may also be referred to as the tubercle bacillus, or as acid-fast bacilli (**AFB**). In the past the disease was often caused by *M. bovis*, which is transmitted through dairy products; in countries where milk pasteurization is not routine, *M. bovis* is still a principal source of infection.

Epidemiology Tuberculosis is spread by droplets in the secretions from individuals with active cavitary disease. Patients with TB but without pulmonary cavities are generally regarded as noninfectious. TB is generally not highly contagious, and prolonged periods of close contact are usually required for spread of the disease.

Tuberculosis is associated with advanced age, poverty, alcoholism, and AIDS. In the United States, it remains a serious health problem, particularly in urban areas with high concentrations of AIDS patients and immigrants from the third world. Recently, the southeast area of the United States and states bordering Mexico reported the highest number of TB cases. In addition, recent immigrants from

Southeast Asia now constitute 3 to 5 percent of new cases.

Since 1984 the incidence of TB in the United States has been rising. Over 22,000 cases have been reported each year, with approximately 2000 deaths.

Worldwide, TB is a major health problem with as many as 4 million new cases and 3 million deaths each year. The Centers for Disease Control currently estimate that ten million people are infected worldwide, and while they are not all symptomatic, for each there is a lifelong risk of developing active TB.

Related Disorders See also *Nocardiosis* and *Paracoccidioidomycosis*, which may resemble TB.

Following is a list of the various subtypes of tuberculosis:

Childhood tuberculosis (primary TB) is the initial infection, and typically produces a lower lobe pneumonia in symptomatic cases.

Disseminated hematogenous TB (miliary TB) is a more fulminant form of TB occurring mostly during early childhood. Multisystem involvement is the rule.

Tuberculous lymphadenitis is only rarely associated with significant symptoms. Most patients have no sign of TB elsewhere in the body, and most have involvement of a single node. Lymph node biopsy is required for diagnosis.

Cutaneous TB. There are a variety of different skin lesions associated with tuberculous infection. Skin infection occurs through direct inoculation from an exogenous source, or through hematogenous or local spread from elsewhere in the body. Tuberculous warts and chancres are associated with inoculation; gummas, scrofuloderma, and many other lesions may result from endogenous infection.

Bone involvement is most frequent in the spine (Pott's disease, tuberculous spondylitis). It produces a characteristic deformity (gibbus). If it spreads to the surrounding area it may impinge on the spinal cord and cause paralysis. Other forms of bony involvement include osteomyelitis and arthritis, usually monoarticular.

Central nervous system TB may be manifested by meningitis, or by a tuberculoma in the brain, which behaves as a space-occupying lesion. Tuberculous meningitis is generally a problem of young children aged 1 to 5 years although it may occur at any age. Approximately 25 percent of children will develop sequelae, including convulsive disorders, communicating hydrocephalus, mental retardation, and other neurologic abnormalities.

Pleural TB can occur in at least 2 forms, one in conjunction with active pulmonary TB, and the other shortly after primary infection. Stains of pleural fluid for AFB are not useful, although the yield on culture is higher. The diagnostic procedure of choice is a pleural biopsy. Surgical drainage may be required in addition to antituberculous drugs.

Genitourinary TB may involve the kidneys, bladder, seminal vesicles, prostate, fallopian tubes, or ovaries. In renal tuberculosis urinary symptoms usually, but not invariably, occur. The urinary sediment is abnormal in 90 percent of cases.

Tuberculous peritonitis may spread from the lymph nodes, gastrointestinal tract, or uterine tube and ovary to surrounding areas. Local tenderness, fever, and weight loss are symptomatic of this type of TB. In most cases the onset is insidious, but a more fulminant course resembling typical bacterial peritonitis may also occur. A peritoneal biopsy may be required for diagnosis.

Tuberculous pericarditis is usually due to spread from infected mediastinal nodes. Pericardiectomy is necessary in cases where the pericarditis becomes constrictive, or if the effusion threatens to progress to tamponade.

Silicotuberculosis is the result of TB infection in a patient with silicosis. Patients with silicosis run a much higher risk of contracting tuberculosis than the general population.

Chronic hematogenous TB is a bloodborne reactivated infection, usually spread from an extrapulmonary source. It occurs years after primary infection and tends to be superimposed on other chronic illness. The symptoms are vague and the diagnosis very difficult.

Treatment—Standard The tubercle bacillus is remarkably hardy, and is capable of long periods of metabolic inactivity. Successful eradication requires multiple drugs administered over many months. Fortunately, infectivity is dramatically reduced after 10 to 14 days of effective therapy; and significant symptomatic improvement occurs in the first 2 to 3 weeks. Unfortunately, lengthy treatment regimens depend heavily on patient compliance for their success, and relapses are a problem in incompletely treated cases.

There are several currently recommended regimens. The precise regimen used initially depends on the likelihood of drug resistance, the likelihood of compliance, and other patient factors such as the presence of renal insufficiency or pregnancy.

The most effective regimen is isoniazid and rifampin for 9 to 12 months. Ethambutol is frequently added initially until the drug sensitivities of the organism are known. Less toxic, and recommended for pregnant women, is a regimen of isoniazid and ethambutol for 12 to 18 months.

In cases where the patient can be closely monitored and compliance is likely to be high, a short-course regimen may be suitable. There are several regimens, all starting with 2 months of isoniazid, rifampin, pyrazinamide, and a 4th drug (either streptomycin or ethambutol), followed by 4 to 6 months of double or triple drug therapy.

In all these regimens the drugs must be taken daily. When daily therapy over a long period is not a reasonable option, there is an effective regimen of twice weekly therapy which may begin after the first month: isoniazid, at triple the usual dosage, and rifampin twice weekly for 8 months.

Patients with concurrent HIV infection are treated with the same regimens as other individuals, but because of their underlying immunodeficiency the potential for relapse is probably lifelong in spite of therapy. Patients with renal failure require significant dose reductions and close monitoring for toxicity.

Drug toxicity is an important factor in the choice and modification of treatment regimens. Hepatotoxicity is common to isoniazid, rifampin, and pyrazinamide, and when symptomatic hepatitis develops, the offending drugs should be discontinued. Monitoring liver enzymes has been recommended in the past but is no longer thought to be necessary.

Prophylaxis: Tuberculin-positive patients without evidence of active disease are recommended to take isoniazid daily for one year. Since the risk of hepatotoxicity rises with age, this recommendation is frequently limited to patients under the age of 35 years. Household contacts, particularly children, should be treated for 3 months. After 3 months, if their skin test is positive, treatment should continue for a full 12 months.

The vaccine for tuberculosis, the bacille Calmette-Guérin **(BCG),** has been widely used in some countries, but its efficacy is the subject of controversy. It is not currently recommended in the United States since not only is its protective value in doubt, but it interferes with the interpretation of the tuberculin skin test, the major test for detection of asymptomatic infections.

Treatment—Investigational Please contact the agencies listed under Resources, below, for the most current information.

Resources

For more information on TB: National Organization for Rare Disorders (NORD); American Lung Association; NIH/National Institute of Allergy and Infectious Diseases (NIAID); Centers for Disease Control (CDC).

References

Curable, Preventable, but Still a Killer: Tuberculosis: Annabel Hecht; FDA Consumer, December 1986–January 1987, pp. 7–10.

Mycobacterium Tuberculosis: R.M. Des Prez and C.R. Heim; in Principles and Practice of Infectious Diseases: G.L. Mandell, et al., eds.; Churchill Livingstone, 1990, pp. 1877–1905.

TYPHOID

Description Typhoid fever is an acute systemic infection caused by *Salmonella typhi*. Major symptoms reflect involvement of the gastrointestinal, hematologic, neurologic, and respiratory systems. Complications are common and may be life-threatening.

Synonyms

Enteric Fever

Typhoid Fever

Signs and Symptoms The symptoms of typhoid fever begin after an incubation period of 1 to 3 weeks. Onset is usually insidious and the initial symptoms are characteristically vague, with fever, headache, myalgias, and malaise. Respiratory symptoms are common at this stage. By the end of the first week of illness, the fever is high and may be associated with a relative bradycardia. Diarrhea is common, but constipation may also occur. Neurologic symptoms may be present, such as seizures, psychosis, or delirium, the symptom for which the disease was originally named *(typhos,* Greek for cloud, referring to a clouded consciousness).

Physical examination may reveal the rash classically associated with typhoid fever: rose spots. These are erythematous lesions, usually 2 to 4 mm in size, that appear transiently on the upper abdomen. There may be rales on chest examination. The abdomen is tender and may be distended, and hepatosplenomegaly is common.

There are a number of laboratory abnormalities in typhoid fever. Anemia is common, as is neutropenia. There may be evidence of subclinical disseminated intravascular coagulation (DIC), and elevated hepatic enzymes.

Complications of typhoid fever include gastrointestinal hemorrhage and perforation, myocarditis, transient bone marrow suppression, and rarely, hepatic failure. Relapses may occur in untreated cases.

S. typhi infection can persist in a chronic carrier state. In these cases there is asymptomatic shedding of bacteria in the stool or urine.

The diagnosis of typhoid fever is made by isolation of the bacteria from blood cultures. The majority of patients will have detectable bacteremia in the first week of illness but the rate of blood culture positivity falls to 20 to 30 percent of untreated patients by the 3rd week. Stool cultures may be diagnostic in regions where the prevalence of asymptomatic carriers is extremely low. Bone marrow cultures may also be used to diagnose typhoid fever. Serologic tests, such as the Widal test for agglutinins against typhoid O antigen, are not sufficiently reliable for diagnosis.

Etiology Typhoid fever is caused by the gram-negative rod, *Salmonella typhi*.

Epidemiology Man is the only reservoir for *S. typhi;* therefore infection is usually spread by contact with symptomatic individuals (carriers) or with food contaminated by a chronic carrier, or by sewage contamination of the water supply.

There are approximately 500 cases reported annually in the United States; the majority of these are imported from elsewhere, particularly Mexico and India. Outbreaks have occurred in the United States, and these are usually traced to a carrier involved in food preparation. Typhoid fever remains a serious health problem, with a mortality rate of 10 percent per year in many parts of the world (Central and South America, Asia, Africa, and the Middle East).

Related Disorders The differential diagnosis of typhoid fever varies with the stage and presenting symptoms of the illness. Depending on which symptoms are prominent, typhoid fever can resemble a respiratory illness such as influenza, or pneumonia; a neurologic infection such as meningitis; an acute abdomen, such as appendicitis or intestinal infarction; or dysentery and other forms of infectious diarrhea. In longstanding untreated cases the differential may include brucellosis, bacterial endocarditis, inflammatory bowel disease, and malaria.

Related diseases include those caused by other species of *Salmonella,* including paratyphoid, which resembles typhoid fever but is usually milder, and acute enterocolitis. *Salmonella* species may also produce a primary bacteremia; patients with sickle cell anemia, hemolytic diseases, and AIDS are susceptible to this type of infection.

Treatment—Standard The treatment of typhoid fever involves administration of chloramphenicol, ampicillin, ceftriaxone, pefloxacin, or co-trimoxazole (trimethoprim-sulfamethoxazole). Vaccines are available but of debatable efficacy; and precautions regarding food and water are necessary when traveling in developing countries where typhoid is prevalent.

Treatment—Investigational Please contact the agencies listed under Resources, below, for the most current information.

Resources
  For more information on typhoid: National Organization for Rare Disorders (NORD); Centers for Disease Control (CDC); NIH/National Institute of Allergy and Infectious Diseases (NIAID).

References
Internal Medicine, 2nd ed.: J.H. Stein, ed.-in-chief; Little, Brown and Company, 1987, pp. 1664–1691, 1696.

Salmonella Typhi Infections in the United States, 1975–1984: Increasing Role of Foreign Travel: C.A. Ryan, et al.; Rev. Infect. Dis., January–February 1989, vol. 11(1), pp. 1–8.

Cefoperazone Compared with Chloramphenicol in the Treatment of Typhoid Fever: F. Paradisi; Chemotherapy, 1988, vol. 34(1), pp. 71–76.

Clinical Experience with Pefloxacin in the Therapy of Typhoid Fever: P. Christiano, et al.; Infection, March–April 1989, vol. 17(2), pp. 86–67.

Assessment on Antimicrobial Treatment of Acute Typhoid and Paratyphoid Fevers in Britain and the Netherlands 1971–1980: R.J. Fallon, et al.; J. Infect., March 1988, vol. 16(2), pp. 129–134.

Mary Mallon's Trail of Typhoid: C. Cary; FDA Consumer, April 1989, pp. 18–21.

URTICARIA, CHOLINERGIC

Description Cholinergic urticaria is an immediate-type hypersensitivity disorder induced by heat, emotional stress, or exercise in susceptible individuals. It is characterized by the wheal-and-flare reaction and pruritus, and may be associated with systemic symptoms.

Synonyms
  Physical Urticaria

Signs and Symptoms The disorder is characterized by pruritic, erythematous macules and hives (the wheal-and-flare reaction) that are usually 2 to 5 cm in diameter. These lesions may coalesce. The eyelids, lips, hands, and feet may become swollen, and this may be accompanied by abdominal cramps, diarrhea, faintness, weakness, and sweating.

  The diagnosis may be established by provocative testing, such as an intradermal injection of methacholine. Heat, as in immersing an arm in warm water, or exercise may also be used provocatively to diagnose cholinergic urticaria.

Etiology Cholinergic urticaria is an IgE-mediated hypersensitivity reaction which may be produced by anything that raises the skin temperature, such as hot baths, warm rooms, physical exercise, and exposure to the sun. Irritants in products such as cosmetics or drugs may contribute to the reaction. Eating hot foods, excitement, sweating, and possibly hypersensitivity to acetylcholine, may also induce an urticarial reaction in this syndrome.

Related Disorders See *Dermatitis, Contact.*

Treatment—Standard Hydroxyzine is the drug of choice for cholinergic urticaria. Antihistamines may ameliorate the pruritis. Protective clothing, sunscreens, and avoiding direct sunlight may be helpful.

Treatment—Investigational Please contact the agencies listed under Resources, below, for the most current information.

Resources

For more information on cholinergic urticaria: National Organization for Rare Disorders (NORD); Allergy and Asthma Foundation of America; NIH/National Institute of Allergy and Infectious Diseases (NIAID).

References

Cecil Textbook of Medicine, 18th ed.: J.B. Wyngaarden and L.H. Smith, Jr., eds.; W.B. Saunders Company, 1988, pp. 1948–1951, 2334–2335.

URTICARIA, COLD

Description Cold urticaria is a chronic disorder in which exposure to cold precipitates urticaria and, in some cases, angioedema. It is a type of physical urticaria.

Signs and Symptoms In cold urticaria the skin develops pruritis, hives, and in some cases, angioedema, when exposed to cold. Systemic manifestations including fever, headache, anxiety, fatigue, and, sometimes, syncope, may occur. Palpitations and wheezing are other occasional complaints.

Familial cold urticaria is usually precipitated by generalized cold, rather than a local stimulus. It usually develops about 30 minutes after exposure, and may persist for up to 48 hours. It may be accompanied by systemic symptoms, including fever, headache, fatigue, and arthralgias, and leukocytosis may be evident on laboratory testing.

Acquired cold urticaria is classified into primary, secondary, delayed, localized, and reflex types.

Primary acquired cold urticaria occurs within minutes of exposure to cold. The reaction often develops during rewarming rather than during the cold phase itself. Usually the initial symptoms are pruritis and erythema, followed by a burning sensation and urticaria, which lasts 30 minutes. The systemic symptoms mentioned above may also occur.

In delayed cold urticaria, the reaction may be delayed for several hours after exposure.

Localized cold urticaria is similar to the primary type described above, except the reaction is limited to previous sites of immunologic challenge, such as ragweed injection sites or insect bites.

In reflex cold urticaria, generalized urticaria occurs when a local cold stimulus is applied (such as an ice pack). The local stimulus precipitates a fall in body temperature which prompts the generalized response.

Secondary cold urticaria can occur in the presence of cryoglobulins and other cryoproteins, which may appear in association with lymphoproliferative disorders.

Etiology Cold urticaria can be idiopathic or it may rarely be transmitted as an autosomal dominant trait. It may also be associated with autoimmune disorders. Exposure to cold weather or water triggers mast cell degranulation in the dermis and subcutaneous tissue.

Epidemiology Cold urticaria affects males and females in equal numbers. The familial autosomal dominant form is rare.

Related Disorders The symptoms of Raynaud's disease, like those of cold urticaria, are precipitated by exposure to cold. However, the pathophysiology and symptoms themselves are different. Raynaud's disease, discussed elsewhere in the Guide in **Raynaud's Disease and Phenomenon,** is a vasospastic disorder characterized by pain and pallor; urticaria is not a feature. Other diseases in which symptoms are precipitated by cold include **cold agglutinin disease,** which may be associated with infectious mononucleosis, mycoplasma pneumonia, or lymphoproliferative disorders. The cold agglutinins are usually hemolytic; rarely they produce red cell agglutination with local cyanosis. They are not associated with urticaria. **Paroxysmal cold hemoglobinuria** is a rare disorder that can be associated with infectious diseases (syphilis, measles); it is a hemolytic disorder precipitated by exposure to cold. Urticaria may occur.

Urticaria should be distinguished from other skin lesions, such as contact dermatitis. The diagnosis is generally confirmed by attempting to elicit the symptoms with cold exposure (e.g., immersing the arm in cold water).

Treatment—Standard The treatment of cold urticaria includes the use of antihistamines and sympathomimetics: diphenhydramine, cyproheptadine, cetirizine, and epinephrine. Prevention involves the use of warm clothing during cold weather and avoiding cold environments, particularly swimming in cold water, since syncope, followed by drowning, may occur.

Treatment—Investigational Please contact the agencies listed under Resources, below, for the most current information.

Resources

For more information on cold urticaria: National Organization for Rare Disorders (NORD); NIH/National Institute of Allergy & Infectious Diseases (NIAID); Asthma & Allergy Foundation of America.

For information about Raynaud's disease: Raynaud Association Trust.

For genetic information and genetic counseling referrals: March of Dimes Birth Defects Foundation; NIH/National Center for Education in Maternal and Child Health (NCEMCH).

References
Internal Medicine, 2nd ed.: J.H. Stein, ed.-in-chief; Little, Brown and Company, 1987, pp. 945, 1058.

Clinical Characteristics of Cold-Induced Systemic Reactions in this Complication and a Proposal for a Diagnostic Classification of Cold Urticaria: A.A. Wanderer, et al.; J. Allergy Clin. Immunol., September 1986, vol. 78(3, Pt. 1), pp. 417–423.

Cold Urticaria: Release into the Circulation of Histamine and Eosinophil Chemotactic Factor of Anaphylaxis During Cold Challenge: N.A. Soter, et al.; N. Engl. J. Med., March 1975, vol. 294(13), pp. 687–690.

Inhibiting Effect of Cetirizine on Histamine-Induced and 48/80-Induced Wheals and Flares, Experimental Dermographism, and Cold-Induced Urticaria: L. Juhlin, et al.; J. Allergy Clin. Immunol., October 1987, vol. 80(4), pp. 599–602.

WALDENSTROM MACROGLOBULINEMIA

Description Waldenstrom macroglobulinemia is a malignant lymphocytic disorder in which the malignant lymphocytes secrete IgM. The major clinical manifestations are those of the hyperviscosity syndrome which results from macroglobulinemia.

Synonyms

> Hyperglobulinemic Purpura
> Macroglobulinemia
> Waldenstrom Purpura
> Waldenstrom Syndrome

Signs and Symptoms The clinical manifestations of Waldenstrom macroglobulinemia are weakness, fatigue, epistaxis, and a variety of neurologic symptoms including visual disturbances, peripheral neuropathy, dizziness, and headache. Bleeding occurs because the high level of IgM interferes with platelet function. On examination there is usually hepatosplenomegaly and lymphadenopathy, and retinal examination may reveal segmentation of the veins due to hyperviscosity of the blood.

The initial complaint may be related to a peripheral neuropathy. Other neurologic manifestations include hearing loss, muscular atrophy, and leukoencephalopathy.

Anemia is common, and there is significant paraproteinemia (the serum M component). Cryoglobulins are often present, and these may be associated with Raynaud's phenomenon.

The diagnosis of Waldenstrom macroglobulinemia is based on 2 findings: an elevated monoclonal IgM level (over 3 gm/dl), and histologic examination of the bone marrow aspirate.

Etiology Waldenstrom macroglobulinemia is a malignancy of plasma cells that produce IgM. The precise etiology is unknown.

Epidemiology The disorder is slightly more common in males than in females. Its frequency is highest in the 7th decade.

Related Disorders Waldenstrom macroglobulinemia is very similar to chronic lymphocytic leukemia, lymphocytic lymphoma, and multiple myeloma. The disease IgM myeloma differs only in that lytic bone lesions appear in myeloma.

Other entities associated with hypergammaglobulinemia include benign monoclonal gammopathy, and chronic cold agglutinin disease. It may not be possible to distinguish these from asymptomatic Waldenstrom macroglobulinemia; the diagnosis in this case can only be clarified later when symptoms appear.

Treatment—Standard This disease is commonly diagnosed while asymptomatic. These cases do not require treatment until symptoms appear. When symptomatic, those symptoms related directly to elevated IgM levels are treated by plasmapheresis alone.

The standard chemotherapy of Waldenstrom macroglobulinemia consists of repeated courses of an alkylating agent, such as cyclophosphamide or chlorambucil, and prednisone. Treatment is administered every 4 to 6 weeks for 1 to 2 years, and doses are titrated against bone marrow toxicity.

Treatment—Investigational Please contact the agencies listed under Resources, below, for the most current information.

Resources

For more information on Waldenstrom macroglobulinemia: National Organization for Rare Disorders (NORD); American Cancer Society; NIH/National Cancer Institute Physician Data Query (PDQ) phoneline; NIH/National Heart, Lung and Blood Institute (NHLBI).

References

Polyneuropathy in Waldenstrom Macroglobulinemia: Reduction of Endoneural IgM Deposits after Treatment with Chlorambucil and Plasmapheresis: C. Meier, et al.; Acta Neuropathol. (Berlin), 1984, vol. 64(4), pp. 297–307.

Alleviation of Ocular Complications of the Hyperviscosity Syndrome in Waldenstrom Macroglobulinemia Using Plasma Exchange: F. Malecaze, et al.; Journal Fr. Ophtalmol., 1986, vol. 9(5), pp. 367–371.

Plasma Exchange and Moderate Dose of Cytostatics in Advanced Macro(cryo)-globulinemia: P. Pihlstedt; Acta Med. Scand., 1982, vol. 212(3), pp. 187–190.

WEIL SYNDROME

Description Weil syndrome, the severe icteric form of leptospirosis, is characterized by hepatic and renal dysfunction, with alterations in consciousness, hemorrhage, and shock. Leptospirosis, a systemic, spirochetal infection of animals, occasionally transmitted to man, is discussed in a separate chapter.

Synonyms

Fiedler Disease
Icterohemorrhagic Leptospirosis
Lancereaux-Mathieu-Weil Spirochetosis
Leptospiral Jaundice
Spirochetal Jaundice
Weil Disease

Signs and Symptoms Leptospirosis is typically a disease with 2 phases. The first phase consists of fever, headache, severe myalgias, nausea, vomiting, and abdominal pain. During this phase of the illness, spirochetes may be isolated from the blood.

The 2nd phase of leptospirosis, known as the immune phase, follows the first phase after an asymptomatic period of 1 to 3 days. Weil syndrome is a severe form of the 2nd phase; patients with this syndrome experience the first phase routinely. Weil syndrome is characterized by fever, jaundice, tender hepatomegaly, renal insufficiency with proteinuria and hematuria, thrombocytopenia, hemorrhage, and alterations of consciousness. Hepatic enzymes are moderately elevated, but the creatine phosphokinase is markedly elevated, which is characteristic and of diagnostic importance. Cardiac involvement may occur with hemorrhagic myocarditis. Shock and adult respiratory distress syndrome may also occur. Hepatic and renal functions eventually return to normal if the patient survives.

The definitive diagnosis of leptospirosis requires isolation of the organism or a rise in antibody titer. Since isolation demands special techniques and media not found in many laboratories, specimens must be sent to the appropriate authorities.

The diagnosis of Weil syndrome is based on the clinical features described above, in the setting of leptospirosis.

Etiology Leptospirosis is caused by spirochetes of the genus *Leptospira.* Until recently there were thought to be several species of *Leptospira,* but these variants are currently considered to be serotypes of a single species, *L. interrogans.* Weil syndrome can be seen with any of the *Leptospira* serotypes.

Leptospirosis is a biphasic illness, as described above, in which the first phase is the septic phase, namely a direct result of bacterial action, and the 2nd phase is thought to be an immune reaction. Weil syndrome is a severe form of the 2nd phase and is probably due to diffuse vasculitis.

Epidemiology Leptospirosis is primarily a disease of animals. In the United States, human infection is usually contracted from livestock, dogs, rodents, and cats. Those at increased risk are veterinarians, abattoir workers, and farmers. Swimming in infected water has also been known to cause this infection.

Related Disorders Rickettsial diseases such as typhus, and viral diseases such as the hemorrhagic fever with renal syndrome (HFRS), as well as a host of bacterial diseases, particularly those progressing to septic shock, may resemble Weil syndrome.

Treatment—Standard The treatment of Weil syndrome itself is largely supportive. Dialysis, exchange transfusion, and other intensive measures may be appropriate.

Early treatment of leptospirosis may prevent its progression to Weil syndrome. The treatment of choice is doxycycline, intravenous penicillin, or ampicillin. Streptomycin, tetracyclines, chloramphenicol, and erythromycin have also been used effectively. A vaccine is available for animal use, but it is not 100 percent effective.

Treatment—Investigational Please contact the agencies listed under Resources, below, for the most current information.

Resources

For more information on Weil syndrome: National Organization for Rare

Disorders (NORD); Centers for Disease Control (CDC); NIH/National Institute of Allergy and Infectious Diseases (NIAID).

References

Adult Respiratory Distress Syndrome in Leptospira Icterohaemorrhagiae Infection: H.D. Chee, et al.; Intensive Care Medicine, 1985, issue 11(5), pp. 254–256.

Leptospira Species (Leptospirosis): W.E. Farrar; in Principles and Practice of Infectious Diseases: G.L. Mandell, et al., eds.; Churchill Livingstone, 1990, pp. 1813–1815.

WISKOTT-ALDRICH SYNDROME

Description Wiskott-Aldrich syndrome is an X-linked hereditary disorder characterized by immune deficiency primarily affecting B cells, eczema, and thrombocytopenia. The course is variable but those affected usually succumb to the complications of thrombocytopenia and immunodeficiency before adulthood.

Synonyms

Aldrich Syndrome
Immunodeficiency with Thrombocytopenia and Eczema

Signs and Symptoms Wiskott-Aldrich syndrome generally presents in infancy. Hemorrhage from circumcision or minor trauma is a common form of presentation. Gastrointestinal bleeding, which may be severe, also begins in infancy. Thrombocytopenic purpura and petechiae may be evident on examination. In addition, the skin shows a chronic eczematous eruption.

Affected boys have defects in both cell-mediated and humoral immunity, although the T cell abnormalities are thought to be secondary. The most prominent defect is in the synthesis of antibody to polysaccharide antigens. Patients are highly susceptible to infections with encapsulated organisms such as the pneumococcus and *Hemophilus influenzae*. Otitis media, pneumonia, meningitis, and sepsis are common problems.

Cell-mediated immunity becomes progressively dysfunctional with age; fungal and viral infections become significant later in the course of the disorder. *Pneumocystis carinii* and herpes virus infections are also common.

Additional features of the Wiskott-Aldrich syndrome include splenomegaly and anemia. There is a 10 percent incidence of malignancy, predominantly leukemia and lymphoma.

Serum antibody concentrations are normal, although the proportions between the different antibody classes are not, and as was mentioned above, antibody function is distinctly abnormal. Platelet precursors appear normal, but circulating platelets have both structural and functional abnormalities.

Etiology Wiskott-Aldrich syndrome is hereditary. It is transmitted by an X-linked recessive mechanism.

Related Disorders Similar immune deficiency syndromes include ataxia telangiectasia, immunodeficiency with short-limbed short stature, and immunodeficiency with thymoma. See *Ataxia Telangiectasia.*

Treatment—Standard A lymphocyte-derived transfer factor has been used to restore hematologic and immunologic function. This factor, which also improves the eczema, is only effective in about 50 percent of cases. Bone marrow transplantation from a histocompatible sibling has also been used with some success.

Alternative forms of therapy for the platelet disorder include splenectomy and platelet transfusions. While effective in reducing the risk of bleeding, splenectomy does further increase the risk of serious infection with encapsulated organisms, and most of such patients will require prophylactic antibiotics. Platelet transfusions are not without problems, since repeated transfusions are likely to stimulate the formation of platelet antibodies. Corticosteroids and immunosuppressant drugs have no role in the therapy of thrombocytopenia in Wiskott-Aldrich syndrome.

Intravenous gammaglobulin and antibiotics may be useful in preventing and combating infection.

Vincristine may be a useful drug in the treatment of malignancy in this disorder, because it tends to improve platelet function and is not an immunosuppressant.

Infections require vigorous therapy with antifungal, antibiotic, and supportive measures. As in the case of AIDS, *P. carinii* pneumonia can be particularly difficult to treat; the 2 drugs usually used are trimethoprim-sulfamethoxazole and pentamidine isethionate. (For more information on treatment of *P. carinii* pneumonia, see *Acquired Immune Deficiency Syndrome [AIDS].)* Cytomegalovirus and generalized herpes simplex infections may be treated with acyclovir, ganciclovir (DHPG), idoxuridine, floxuridine, or cytarabine. Amphotericin B therapy remains the treatment of choice for severe fungal infections.

Prevention is important and every attempt should be made to protect affected patients from infection. Immunization with live virus vaccines should probably be avoided.

Treatment—Investigational Please contact the agencies listed under Resources, below, for the most current information.

Resources
For more information on Wiskott-Aldrich syndrome: National Organization for Rare Disorders (NORD); NIH/National Institute of Allergy and Infectious Diseases (NIAID); Immune Deficiency Foundation; American Cancer Society; NIH/National Cancer Institute Physician Data Query (PDQ) phoneline.

For genetic information and genetic counseling referrals: March of Dimes Birth Defects Foundation; National Center for Education in Maternal and Child Health.

References
Immunodeficiency: R.H. Buckley; J. Allergy Clin. Immunol., December 1983, vol. 72(6), pp. 627–641.

YAWS

Description Yaws is an infectious disease caused by the spirochete *Treponema pertenue*. It is characterized by 3 stages of symptoms. The first consists of skin lesions; the later 2 stages, of bone, joint, and skin involvement. The late forms of the disease are known as gangosa (also referred to as ogo, or rhinopharyngitis mutilans) and goundou (henpue; henpuye; gundo; anakhre).

Synonyms
> Bouba
> Breda Disease
> Charlouis Disease
> Frambesia
> Parangi
> Pian
>> note: Pian differs from pian bois (also called forest yaws, a form of leishmaniasis) and hemorrhagic pian (verruga peruana, one of the manifestations of bartonellosis).

Signs and Symptoms The first stage of yaws occurs in early childhood. A papillomatous lesion appears at the site of inoculation, usually on the leg or foot. The lesion grows, becomes crusted, and then heals slowly over several months, leaving a scar.

Stage 2 follows several weeks or months after the first. Similar skin lesions appear on the face, legs, and arms, and around the anus and genitals. Healing is slow, and relapses occur. On the soles of the feet, the lesions may become keratotic with painful cracks and ulcerations, resulting in a crablike gait called crab yaws.

The tertiary stage of yaws does not always occur. Several years after the initial stages, destructive lesions of the skin and bone may develop. Cutaneous plaques, nodules, and ulcers occur, and can cause facial disfigurement. Painful, gummatous lesions of the bones develop, especially of the tibia. Painful and destructive nodules may appear around the joints.

Tertiary yaws may produce 2 distinct syndromes. **Goundou** is a painless but marked symmetrical paranasal swelling due to hypertrophic osteitis. It is accompanied by headache and nasal discharge. **Gangosa, or rhinopharyngitis mutilans,** consists of destruction of the nose, the pharynx, and the hard palate.

The diagnosis of stage 1 and 2 yaws is made by darkfield examination of material from the skin lesions. Tertiary yaws may be diagnosed by serologic tests (VDRL, treponemal antibodies), in the presence of the appropriate clinical picture.

Etiology Yaws is caused by the spirochete *Treponema pertenue*.

Epidemiology Yaws is common among children in tropical Africa, South and Central America, the West Indies, and the Far East, but is rare in the United States. It is usually transmitted by direct contact with infected skin lesions, but insect transmission occurs in some regions, and sexual transmission has been reported.

Related Disorders See *Bejel; Pinta.* The treponematoses—yaws, bejel (endemic syphilis), pinta, and venereal syphilis—are all caused by identical-looking spirochetes. While the organisms are related, the diseases they produce differ in distribution, mode of transmission, and clinical characteristics. The treponematoses do have 2 things in common: protracted chronic phases of illness, and response to penicillin.

Treatment—Standard Antimicrobial drugs such as benzathine penicillin G, given as a single dose of 1.2 million units, are very effective. Such drugs can also be used preventatively for close contacts of affected individuals. There is no treatment for the destructive bony lesions, or for scars.

Treatment—Investigational Please contact the agencies listed under Resources, below, for the most current information.

Resources

For more information: National Organization for Rare Disorders (NORD); Centers for Disease Control (CDC); NIH/National Institute of Allergy and Infectious Diseases (NIAID).

References
Cecil Textbook of Medicine, 18th ed.: J.B. Wyngaarden and L.H. Smith, Jr., eds.; W.B. Saunders Company, 1988, p. 1723.

The Merck Manual, 15th ed.: R. Berkow, ed.-in-chief; Merck Sharp & Dohme Research Laboratories, 1987, p. 132.

7 | DERMATOLOGIC DISORDERS
By D. Martin Carter, M.D., Ph.D.

This section has been prepared to assist in arriving at an accurate diagnosis of the rare dermatological disorders. Based upon the presumptive diagnosis, the practitioner will be making selections of which descriptive passages to read, making decisions concerning referral to other physicians, and subjecting patients to diagnostic and therapeutic procedures.

The history may be particularly informative for rare disorders in this field. When was the dermatosis first observed? Was it present at birth? Was it first noticed in the neonatal period? At puberty? Are other family members similarly affected? Does the eruption persist or is it only present periodically? Is it associated with exposure to environmental agents? Do such physical elements as sunlight, heat, or cold cause the eruption to exacerbate or remit? Is it associated with the ingestion of drugs or foods? Does the patient have any other significant medical illnesses or complaints?

The entire skin including the epidermal appendages should next be inspected. In a thorough examination, it is necessary to assess the scalp, nail, mucous membranes, and body folds. It is not sufficient to look only at those portions of the uncovered skin which can be revealed by partially removing a skirt, blouse, or trouser. The patient must be completely undressed in order to determine the extent of the eruption and to assess the character of the individual lesions. What is the color and texture of the skin in general? Is jaundice, pallor, or cyanosis evident? Is the skin warm, moist, or cold to the touch?

Distribution of the lesions is important. Is the eruption bilateral and symmetrical? Does it localize to exposed or unexposed skin? Does it involve body folds? Intertriginous areas? Hairy skin? Mucous membranes? Do lesions occur in groups or clusters? In lines? In sites of previous trauma? In a dermatome? The following glossary of terms should be used to describe the pattern of lesions:

distribution—Where are the lesions located?

arrangement—Are the lesions grouped, single, linear, or follicular, or associated with body folds or a vascular or nerve distribution?

size—What are the dimensions of the lesions?

margins—Are the margins sharp or indistinct, and do they correspond to exposure to some environmental agent?

shape—Are the lesions round, gyrate, targetoid, polygonal, or polycyclic?

Careful assessment of a primary lesion is needed. There may be few such primary lesions, and therefore a complete examination may again be required. In addition, one must characterize secondary lesions which may have developed with the passage of time and represent a change from the primary lesion. Have lesions formed crusts, ulcers, or plaques? Do they coalesce? Do they hyper- or hypo-pigment or develop scars? It is appropriate to use precise adjectives, so that an accurate word picture of the skin eruption is presented.

The following glossary of terms should be used to describe individual lesions.

atrophy—Loss of cutaneous elements producing flaccid or sclerotic scars.

bulla—A large vesicle, tense or flaccid.

crust—Dried secretions on the surface of a lesion.

erosion—Loss of epidermal cells from the surface of the skin.

excoriation—Loss of skin secondary to scratching.

fissure—Linear separation or split in the skin.

keratosis—Firmly adherent, horny growth.

macule—A flat lesion with a different color from surrounding skin; may be brown, black, red, white; may have sharply defined or indistinct margins.

nodule—Large papule; a circumscribed lesion that represents a collection of inflammatory or neoplastic cells in the dermis.

papule—Elevated lesion caused by cellular proliferation or infiltration; 0.1 to 1.0 cm in diameter.

pustule—A vesicle containing purulent fluid.

scale—Desquamated epidermal cells.

scar—Permanent fibrous lesion of the skin secondary to resolution of a previous skin lesion.

tumor—A particularly large nodule which may be benign or malignant.

ulcer—Larger, deeper lesion than an erosion, caused by loss of epidermal and dermal skin cells.

vesicle—A small, fluid-filled blister.

wheal—Transient, raised lesion (these are also called hives), which represents extravasation of fluid from vessels into the perivascular skin; may be pink, red, or white.

The accuracy of dermatological diagnosis is greatly enhanced by obtaining a specimen of skin from an appropriate lesion and subjecting the biopsy specimen to histopathological examination. Dermatopathology is a highly specialized field, and diagnosis may require the use of immunohistochemical as well as electronmicroscopic techniques.

Other laboratory tests commonly used in dermatological diagnosis include examination by Wood's light to enhance the evaluation of pigmentation; potassium hydroxide (KOH) examination of scale to identify yeast and fungal elements; darkfield microscopy to identify spirochetal organisms; Gram stain to identify bacteria; and Giemsa stain to identify epidermal cells infected with virus (such as the herpes virus) or cells which have become separated from their neighbors (because of antibodies—characteristic of pemphigus).

DERMATOLOGIC DISORDERS
Listings in This Section

ACANTHOSIS NIGRICANS

Description Acanthosis nigricans is a disorder in which the skin in sites of predilection becomes hyperkeratotic and thickened with brown-gray pigmentation. Several forms are recognized, including a benign, inherited form (Miescher syndrome); a benign, possibly hereditary, generalized form prevalent in young adult females (Gougerot-Carteaud syndrome); a benign juvenile form associated with obesity or endocrine disorders (pseudoacanthosis nigricans); and an adult form often associated with an internal carcinoma.

Synonyms
Keratosis Nigricans

Signs and Symptoms The eruption is bilateral and symmetrical. Characteristic lesions are hyperpigmented, velvety, papillomatous, warty plaques with indistinct margins. Lesions appear in the skin of the face, neck, axillae, backs of hands, forearms, the area between the breasts, the inner thighs, and the groin. Other susceptible sites are the genitals, buttocks, and the perianal area. The oral and anal mucous membranes and other mucous membranes may be involved. In **Miescher syndrome,** an increase in the number of lesions during adolescence is followed by regression after puberty. Regression is characteristic except in the **adult types,** in which the lesions tend to increase and the skin may become hairless and the fingernails may be affected. In the **adult form related to malignancy,** progression correlates with that of the neoplasm.

Histology: The epidermis is thickened and papillomatous, and may resemble that of a seborrheic keratosis.

Etiology The cause is unknown but may be related to increased response to trophic growth factors in connection with associated disorders. Miescher syndrome is thought to be autosomal dominant. Gougerot-Carteaud syndrome may also be hereditary. Pseudoacanthosis nigricans is associated with pituitary adenoma, Addison's disease, diabetes mellitus, and ovarian disorders such as Stein-Leventhal syndrome, and with obesity.

Epidemiology Miescher syndrome may be present at birth. Gougerot-Carteaud syndrome is prevalent in young adult females. Pseudoacanthosis nigricans affects obese individuals and those with endocrine disorders. The adult form is most common in patients with visceral carcinoma, but it may occur with breast or lung cancers, as well.

Treatment—Standard Pseudoacanthosis nigricans responds to treatment of the underlying problem. Lesions usually regress as an obese patient loses weight, or a thyroid dysfunction or other endocrine disorder is brought under control. The adult form related to malignancy regresses upon remission or cure of the neoplastic disease.

Treatment—Investigational Please contact the agencies listed under Resources, below, for the most current information.

Resources

For more information on acanthosis nigricans: National Organization for Rare Disorders (NORD); The National Arthritis and Musculoskeletal and Skin Diseases Information Clearinghouse.

For genetic information and genetic counseling referrals: March of Dimes Birth Defects Foundation; National Center for Education in Maternal and Child Health (NCEMCH).

References

Dermatology, 3rd ed.: O. Braun-Falco, et al.; Springer-Verlag, 1991.

Skin Signs of Systemic Disease: I.M. Braverman; W.B. Saunders Company, 1981.

Dermatology in General Medicine: Textbook and Atlas, 3rd ed.: T.B. Fitzpatrick, et al., eds.; McGraw-Hill, 1987.

Dermatology, 2nd ed. (3rd ed., 1992): S.L. Moschella and H.J. Hurley, eds.; W.B. Saunders Company, 1985.

Textbook of Dermatology, 4th ed.: A. Rook, et al., eds.; Blackwell Scientific Publications, 1986.

Cecil Textbook of Medicine, 18th ed.: J.B. Wyngaarden and L.H. Smith, Jr., eds.; W.B. Saunders Company, 1988, p. 1112.

Mendelian Inheritance in Man, 9th ed.: V.A. McKusick; The Johns Hopkins University Press, 1990, p. 5.

ACNE ROSACEA

Description Acne rosacea is a skin disorder in which flushing, acneiform pustules, erythema, and telangiectasia are seen on the central face.

Synonyms

> Acne Erythematosa
> Hypertrophic Rosacea
> Rhinophyma
> Rosacea

Signs and Symptoms In acne rosacea, the primary lesion is erythema distributed diffusely on the face. At the onset there is periodic flushing; but with time the skin of the forehead, nose, and cheeks becomes oily and progressively erythematous, and telangiectasia develops. Small papules and perifollicular pustules develop in the affected areas. In very severe cases, rhinophyma, conjunctivitis, and keratitis may be found.

Etiology The cause is not known, although a genetic predisposition is believed to exist. Vasodilatory symptoms can be intensified by hot liquids, spicy foods, vitamin deficiencies, and alcohol consumption; heat and vigorous exercise; certain endocrine disturbances; and emotional stress. Reactions to the follicular mite, *Demodex folliculorum,* have been implicated.

Epidemiology Onset usually is between 30 and 50 years of age. Females are affected more often than males, but males may be more severely affected.

Related Disorders Acne vulgaris is primarily a disease of the follicular structure and is not related. In the common form of adolescent acne, the skin eruptions primarily appear on the face, upper back, and chest.

Acne conglobata is a severe, chronic variant of acne vulgaris in which many skin eruptions become abscessed and cysts form, often containing purulent liquid. Scarring is common. The eruptions occur most often on the neck and upper trunk; they also occur on the upper arms, lower back, buttocks, and thighs. Acne conglobata is seen most often in males, with onset usually at puberty but continuing in later years. This form of acne resists treatment with systemic antibiotics. In some cases symptoms may be controlled by the use of isotretinoin.

Acne fulminans is a rare variant of acne seen mostly in adolescent males. The skin lesions initially are similar to mild acne vulgaris but progress to severely inflamed and painful ulcerations on the upper trunk and occasionally the face. Systemic symptoms and signs may be associated, e.g., fever, weight loss, polyarthritis, leukocytosis, anemia, and elevated erythrocyte sedimentation rate. Treatment usually involves isotretinoin, with or without systemic corticosteroid drugs and antibiotics.

Excoriated acne results from excessive manipulation of acne lesions, with resulting increased scarring. Although it is often found among young women, it can be seen in any age group and both sexes.

Chloracne is a skin eruption that resembles acne and may occur as a result of exposure to chlorinated hydrocarbons. Treatment must include removal of the irritating substance from the environment.

Atypical acneiform eruptions may result from certain drugs (corticosteroids, androgens, progesterone, diphenylhydantoin, and lithium); ingestion of iodine or bromine salts; or skin contact with certain machine oils. These eruptions can occur in any age group and are not always limited to sebaceous glands.

Treatment—Standard There is no cure for acne rosacea. Topical and systemic antibiotics can reduce microbial flora. Mild topical steroids can reduce inflammation. The orphan drug metronidazole (Metrogel—Curatek Pharmaceuticals of Elk Village, Illinois) was approved in 1988 by the FDA for treatment of acne rosacea.

In rhinophyma, carbon dioxide laser and conventional surgery are used to remove excess skin growth. Argon lasers have been effective in reducing erythema in the nose area in mild cases that have not progressed to rhinophyma. Other treatment is symptomatic and supportive.

Treatment—Investigational Please contact the agencies listed under Resources, below, for the most current information.

Resources
For more information on acne rosacea: National Organization for Rare Disorders (NORD); Acne Research Institute; The National Arthritis and Musculoskeletal and Skin Diseases Information Clearing House.

References
Dermatology, 3rd ed.: O. Braun-Falco, et al.; Springer-Verlag, 1991.
Skin Signs of Systemic Disease: I.M. Braverman; W.B. Saunders Company, 1981.

Dermatology in General Medicine: Textbook and Atlas, 3rd ed.: T.B. Fitzpatrick, et al., eds.; McGraw-Hill, 1987.

Dermatology, 2nd ed. (3rd ed., 1992): S.L. Moschella and H.J. Hurley, eds.; W.B. Saunders Company, 1985.

Textbook of Dermatology, 4th ed.: A. Rook, et al., eds.; Blackwell Scientific Publications, 1986.

Internal Medicine, 3rd ed.: J.H. Stein, ed.-in-chief; Little, Brown and Company, 1990, p. 1840.

Topical Metronidazole Therapy for Rosacea: P.A. Bleicher, et al.; Arch. Dermatol., May 1987, issue 123(5), pp. 609–614.

Treatment of the Red Nose with the Argon Laser: C.H. Dicken; Mayo Clin. Proc., November 1986, issue 61(11), pp. 893–895.

Surgical Treatment of Rhinophyma with the Shaw Scalpel: R.F. Eisen, et al.; Arch. Dermatol., March 1986, issue 122(3), pp. 307–309.

Treatment of Rosacea with Isotretinoin: E. Hoting, et al.; Int. J. Dermatol., December 1986, issue 25(10), pp. 660–663.

Combined Carbon Dioxide Laser Excision and Vaporization in the Treatment of Rhinophyma: R.G. Wheeland, et al.; J. Dermatol. Surg. Oncol., February 1987, issue 13(2), pp. 172–177.

ACRODERMATITIS ENTEROPATHICA (AE)

Description AE is characterized by dermatitis, diarrhea, and alopecia. The disorder is inherited and congenital; in extremely rare cases, it may be acquired.

Synonyms
> Brandt Syndrome
> Danbolt-Closs Syndrome
> Zinc Deficiency, Congenital

Signs and Symptoms Minor or significant chronic diarrhea and steatorrhea in infancy are hallmarks of inherited AE. Onset is gradual, usually occurring during weaning. Pustular dermatitis appears around the mouth, anus, eyes, and nails; also affected is the skin on the elbows, knees, hands, and feet. Initially the skin is blistered, but eventually drying produces lesions resembling those of psoriasis. Inflammatory lesions around the nail may result in chronic paronychia and nail dystrophy. Alopecia involving the scalp, eyelids, and eyebrows may occur. Conjunctivitis is usually present.

When the disorder is acute, atrophy of the cerebral cortex may lead to irritability and mental disturbances.

Long remissions of congenital AE are common, usually beginning at puberty. Rarely, the disorder may recur during pregnancy. With treatment, patients may enjoy a normal life.

Etiology Inherited AE is an autosomal recessive disorder in which the serum alkaline phosphatase is deficient and the serum zinc is also low, perhaps because of a congenital lack of a pancreatic zinc-binding factor. It is thought that these combined factors cause jejunal malabsorption of zinc.

Acquired AE is the result of a nutritional lack of zinc.

Epidemiology The congenital form is rare. Males and females are affected in equal numbers. Women with inherited AE who breast-feed their infants have milk that is deficient in this factor. Consequently, healthy infants may become zinc-deficient and symptomatic.

Acquired AE is extremely rare.

Related Disorders See *Celiac Sprue.*

Treatment—Standard Zinc sulfate supplements are indicated upon diagnosis of inherited AE and must be continued throughout life. Iodoquinol obtains a response within a week. Genetic counseling is suggested.

For acquired AE, the addition of zinc supplements to the nutritional regimen is both prophylactic and therapeutic.

Treatment—Investigational Please contact the agencies listed in Resources, below, for the most current information.

Resources

For more information on acrodermatitis enteropathica: National Organization for Rare Disorders (NORD); National Digestive Diseases Information Clearinghouse; Research Trust for Metabolic Diseases in Children.

For genetic information and genetic counseling referrals: March of Dimes Birth Defects Foundation; National Center for Education in Maternal and Child Health (NCEMCH).

References
Dermatology, 3rd ed.: O. Braun-Falco, et al.; Springer-Verlag, 1991.

Skin Signs of Systemic Disease: I.M. Braverman; W.B. Saunders Company, 1981.

Dermatology in General Medicine: Textbook and Atlas, 3rd ed.: T.B. Fitzpatrick, et al., eds.; McGraw-Hill, 1987.

Dermatology, 2nd ed. (3rd ed., 1992): S.L. Moschella and H.J. Hurley, eds.; W.B. Saunders Company, 1985.

Textbook of Dermatology, 4th ed.: A. Rook, et al., eds.; Blackwell Scientific Publications, 1986.

Abnormal Immune Responses During Hypozincaemia in Acrodermatitis Enteropathica: P.H. Anttila, et al., Acta Paediatr. Scand., November 1986, issue 75(6), pp. 988–992.

Mendelian Inheritance in Man, 9th ed.: V.A. McKusick; The Johns Hopkins University Press, 1990, pp. 999–1000.

Ocular Histopathology of Acrodermatitis Enteropathica: J.D. Cameron, et al.; Br. J. Ophthalmol., September 1986, issue 70(9), pp. 662–667.

ALBINISM

Description Albinism comprises a cluster of syndromes with the common denominator of the congenital absence of pigmentation in the skin, hair, and eyes. Associated with the disorders are several ocular defects. The syndromes are primarily categorized as tyrosinase-negative oculocutaneous albinism, tyrosinase-positive oculocutaneous albinism (albinoidism), and ocular albinism.

Signs and Symptoms In oculocutaneous albinism, the integument and the eyes are affected. The tyrosinase-negative and -positive forms are similar at birth, with pinkish-white skin, white hair, and pink, light gray, blue, or hazel eyes. However, those children who are tyrosinase-positive will develop pigmentation in the skin, hair, and eyes as they grow. Children with both forms of oculocutaneous albinism may have nystagmus, astigmatism, strabismus, and myopia, and photophobia will be a problem. Squamous cell carcinomas may develop in these patients.

A form of oculocutaneous albinism (albinoidism, partial albinism) has been described that is characterized by hypomelanism of the skin and hair and certain pigmentation abnormalities of the eyes, but without other visual defects such as nystagmus.

In ocular albinism, the skin and hair are relatively normal, but are fair. Photophobia and the ocular abnormalities of oculocutaneous albinism are present, and there may be retinal mosaicism.

The various syndromes of oculocutaneous albinism have distinctive characteristics. In Hermansky-Pudlak syndrome, for example, lipid- and platelet-storage abnormalities are associated with retarded mental and physical development and microphthalmos. Chédiak-Higashi syndrome is marked by leukocytic disease, proneness to infections, and a high rate of lymphoreticular malignancies.

Types of ocular albinism include Nettleship-Falls syndrome (X-linked), and Forsius-Eriksson syndrome (X-linked).

Etiology A lack of tyrosinase, which catalyzes the incorporation of tyrosine to melanin, explains the pigmentary aspect of albinism. There is even distribution of the melanocytes per se, but the melanosomes, which normally become filled with melanin prior to transfer to keratinocytes, are empty. Most of the oculocutaneous forms are autosomal recessive; an autosomal dominant form (the partial albinism, or albinoidism mentioned above) has been described. Ocular types may be autosomal dominant, recessive, or X-linked.

Epidemiology The incidence of all forms of albinism is approximately 1:10,000. The disorder is more common in some isolated communities, such as the Amish or Mennonite groups in the United States.

Related Disorders See *Vitiligo* for discussion of an unrelated, depigmenting disorder.

Treatment—Standard The basic metabolic abnormality in albinism is incurable. Protection from sunlight, especially for those patients with oculocutaneous syndromes, is essential. Sunglasses, protective clothing, and sun-protective lotions are beneficial. Visual aids may be helpful. Surgery for strabismus provides cosmetic improvement but none in vision; the optic decussation is abnormal. Treatment of other disorders of the syndromes is symptomatic. In Chédiak-Higashi syndrome, it is reported that high doses of ascorbic acid may lessen some of the consequences of the lipid storage abnormalities.

Treatment—Investigational Please contact the agencies listed under Resources, below, for the most current information.

Resources
For more information on albinism: National Organization for Rare Disor-

ders (NORD); National Organization for Albinism and Hypopigmentation (NOAH); NIH/National Institute of Child Health and Human Development (NICHHD).

For genetic information and genetic counseling referrals: March of Dimes Birth Defects Foundation; National Center for Education in Maternal and Child Health (NCEMCH).

References
Dermatology, 3rd ed.: O. Braun-Falco, et al.; Springer-Verlag, 1991.

Skin Signs of Systemic Disease: I.M. Braverman; W.B. Saunders Company, 1981.

Dermatology in General Medicine: Textbook and Atlas, 3rd ed.: T.B. Fitzpatrick, et al., eds.; McGraw-Hill, 1987.

Dermatology, 2nd ed. (3rd ed., 1992): S.L. Moschella and H.J. Hurley, eds.; W.B. Saunders Company, 1985.

Textbook of Dermatology, 4th ed.: A. Rook, et al., eds.; Blackwell Scientific Publications, 1986.

Cecil Textbook of Medicine, 18th ed.: J.B. Wyngaarden and L.H Smith, Jr., eds.: W.B Saunders Company, 1988, pp. 152–153, 2344–2345.

Mendelian Inheritance in Man, 9th ed.: V.A. McKusick; The Johns Hopkins University Press, 1990, pp. 266, 1017–1021, 1554–1556.

ALOPECIA AREATA

Description Alopecia areata is marked by the development of non-tender patches of hair loss. As a rule, the bald patches are limited to the scalp and facial hair, but they may be generalized (alopecia universalis) or complete (alopecia totalis).

Synonyms
Alopecia Celsi
Alopecia Circumscripta
Cazenave Vitiligo
Celsus Vitiligo
Jonston Alopecia
Porrigo Decalvans
Vitiligo Capitis

Signs and Symptoms Onset is frequently sudden; oval or round hairless areas develop, usually on the head. These are painless, are not inflamed, and do not itch. The bald spots appear pale and smooth and slowly enlarge. New patches may abut existing bald spots, and this joining of the bald spots may occur during regrowth in established bald spots. Loss of hair may be permanent in patients, however. While hair follicles may degenerate, the sebaceous glands usually remain stable. This condition is non-scarring. A few patients may become totally bald. When alopecia areata develops in children, it is likely to be more severe and more refractory to treatment than that which starts in adulthood.

Etiology Alopecia areata is idiopathic, but there are microscopic signs of inflammation. An autoimmune disorder is suggested. In addition, some cases are associated with an endocrine disorder.

Epidemiology Males and females are affected in equal numbers in either childhood or adulthood. A 1983 study at the Mayo Clinic in Rochester, Minnesota, estimated there were 2 million cases in the United States at that time.

Related Disorders The following conditions may be confused with alopecia areata but are not related.

In **hypotrichiasis (hypotrichosis, alopecia congenitalis, alopecia adnata, congenital alopecia, congenital baldness)** the newborn is hairless. Hypotrichiasis is hereditary and either dominant or recessive. Frequently, there are other ectodermal abnormalities.

Alopecia medicamentosa, characterized by significant hair loss, usually of the scalp, occurs in individuals who are hypersensitive or allergic to a drug. Chemotherapy is another cause.

Alopecia mucinosa (follicular mucinosis) appears in children and young adults as roseate, discrete plaques under the bald spots. Histologically, there are deposits of mucinous material in the hair follicles. Small scales may form on the face, scalp, trunk, arms, or legs. Plaque growth may be accompanied by numbness in the area. The disorder is idiopathic; it may be due to a cutaneous inflammation. Prognosis is guarded. Resolution is frequently spontaneous within a few months. In some patients, however, this is an early sign of a lymphoma.

Scarring alopecias: In contrast to alopecia areata, the bald skin is scarred or atrophic. Scarring alopecias develop after many types of inflammatory conditions of the scalp, including infections from bacteria or fungi. Among the noninfectious causes of scarring alopecias are lichen planopilaris (related to lichen planus); systemic lupus erythematosus; pseudopelade (of Brocq); and sarcoidosis.

Androgenetic alopecia: Both males and females, with age, develop gradual hair loss, the extent of which is genetically determined. Because it sometimes starts at a young age, it may be confused with some of the pathologic conditions mentioned in these lists. In males, the pattern is usually patchy, involving the temporal, frontal, or occipital scalp. In females, the pattern of alopecia is usually diffuse. Treatment with topical minoxidil may be useful.

In **trichotillomania,** patches of hair loss caused by hair pulling are a manifestation of psychological disturbance. Prognosis is good in children for whom counseling is sought.

Telogen effluvium: Temporary hair loss, often very extensive, is associated with an acute febrile illness, administration of certain medicines, severe psychological stress, and the postpartum period.

Treatment—Standard Many cases of alopecia areata are self-limited. The goal of treatment is regrowth of hair. Systemic corticosteroids may achieve this, but a longterm course may have unacceptable side effects. Triamcinolone acetonide suspension administered sublesionally is usually effective for discrete patches. Application of potent topical steroids is sometimes useful. Wigs and hairpieces may be indicated.

Treatment—Investigational A combination of 8-methoxypsoralen ointment and ultraviolet light exposure is being tried experimentally; it may not be effective in every patient. Some investigators consider that ultraviolet light may produce immunomodulation, which might control hair loss.

Synthetic immunomodulator drugs such as isoprinosine and diphencyprone are also being studied. A clinical trial of low-dose spironolactone, which is given to control hirsutism in females with hormonal imbalance, is ongoing. Minoxidil was ineffective in a trial with patients with alopecia areata. Other tests compared dinitrochlorobenzene ointment with squaric acid dibutylester, but the former is not recommended because some study participants developed undesirable side effects.

Cyclosporine may have potential in treating alopecia areata, but the possibly dangerous side effects must be considered. Relapse may occur upon stopping the drug.

Please contact the agencies listed under Resources, below, for the most current information.

Resources

For more information on alopecia areata: The National Organization for Rare Disorders (NORD); National Alopecia Areata Foundation; Help Alopecia International Research, Inc. (HAIR); The National Arthritis and Musculoskeletal and Skin Diseases Information Clearinghouse.

References

Dermatology, 3rd ed.: O. Braun-Falco, et al.; Springer-Verlag, 1991.

Skin Signs of Systemic Disease: I.M. Braverman; W.B. Saunders Company, 1981.

Dermatology in General Medicine: Textbook and Atlas, 3rd ed.: T.B. Fitzpatrick, et al., eds.; McGraw-Hill, 1987.

Dermatology, 2nd ed. (3rd ed., 1992): S.L. Moschella and H.J. Hurley, eds.; W.B. Saunders Company, 1985.

Textbook of Dermatology, 4th ed.: A. Rook, et al., eds.; Blackwell Scientific Publications, 1986.

Clinical and Immunologic Response to Isoprinosine in Alopecia Areata and Alopecia Universalis: Association with Autoantibodies: M. Lowy, et al.; J. Am. Acad. Dermatol., January 1985, issue 12(1 pt. 1), pp. 78–84.

Low-Dose Spironolactone in the Treatment of Female Hirsutism: Int. J. Fertil., January–February 1987, issue 32(1), pp. 41–45.

Topical Photochemotherapy for Alopecia Areata: A.J. Mitchell, et al.,; J. Am. Acad. Dermatol., April 1985, issue 12(4), pp. 644–649.

Bowen Disease

Description Bowen disease, often referred to as squamous cell carcinoma in situ, is a psoriasiform squamous cell carcinoma of the skin with the potential for invasion. Its advance is slow, and it may appear anywhere on the skin or in the mucous membranes.

Synonyms

Intraepidermal Squamous Cell Carcinoma

Signs and Symptoms The initial sign of Bowen disease is an epidermal or intraepidermal scaly patch. Irregularly formed pink or brown crusty papules develop. An exudative red surface lies under the crust. Misdiagnosis of the disorder as psoriasis, actinic keratosis, or other dermatitis is possible.

Etiology Bowen disease is idiopathic. Frequent exposure to the sun may be a contributing factor. Arsenic exposure has also been implicated, especially when the lesion occurs in body areas protected from light or in the mucous membranes. Human papillomavirus 16 DNA has been isolated from the lesions and may be significant in etiology.

Epidemiology Bowen disease affects both males and females at any age, but it is very seldom seen in children. In women, the incidence of the disorder in the genital area is 3 times that of men.

Related Disorders See *Malignant Melanoma; Squamous Cell Carcinoma, Cutaneous.*

Paget disease of the breast is marked by unilateral malignancy of the nipples in either men or women. The nipple is inflamed and has an exudative crusty surface. This finding usually signals adenocarcinoma of the breast. A form of the disorder also affects the genital area, more often in women. This form is easily treatable when it is on the skin's surface, but when associated with carcinoma of the rectum, treatment becomes more challenging and prognosis is guarded.

Treatment—Standard Treatment commonly requires surgical removal of the cutaneous carcinoma. Carbon dioxide lasers are being utilized as are other destructive modes of treatment for skin lesions. For other types of tumors, various surgical procedures are indicated. Otherwise, therapy is symptomatic and supportive.

Treatment—Investigational Please contact the agencies listed under Resources, below, for the most current information.

Resources

For more information on Bowen disease: National Organization for Rare Disorders (NORD); The Skin Cancer Foundation; American Cancer Society; NIH/National Cancer Institute PDQ (Physician Data Query); NIH/National Institute of Arthritis, Musculoskeletal and Skin Diseases (NIAMS) Information Clearinghouse.

References
Dermatology, 3rd ed.: O. Braun-Falco, et al.; Springer-Verlag, 1991.

Skin Signs of Systemic Disease: I.M. Braverman; W.B. Saunders Company, 1981.

Dermatology in General Medicine: Textbook and Atlas, 3rd ed.: T.B. Fitzpatrick, et al., eds.; McGraw-Hill, 1987.

Dermatology, 2nd ed. (3rd ed., 1992): S.L. Moschella and H.J. Hurley, eds.; W.B. Saunders Company, 1985.

Textbook of Dermatology, 4th ed.: A. Rook, et al., eds.; Blackwell Scientific Publications, 1986.

Bowenoid Papulosis in a Three-Year-Old Girl: C. Halsz, et al.; J. Am. Acad. Dermatol., February 1986, issue 14(2 pt. 2), pp. 326–330.

Bowen's Disease of the Feet. Presence of Human Papillomavirus 16 DNA in Tumor Tissue: M.S. Stone, et al.; Arch. Dermatol., November 1987, issue 123(11), pp. 1517–1520.

Bowen's Disease and Internal Malignant Diseases. A Study of 581 Patients: F. Reymann, et al.; Arch. Dermatol., May 1988, issue 124(5), pp. 677–679.

CAVERNOUS HEMANGIOMA

Description Cavernous hemangioma, a vascular tumor composed of large blood-filled spaces, can occur at any site in the body and is present at birth or shortly thereafter. It grows rapidly and, after several years, spontaneously regresses or disappears.

Synonyms
- Cavernomas
- Cavernous Angioma
- Congenital Vascular Cavernous Malformations
- Hemangioma, Familial
- Nevus Cavernosus
- Vascular Erectile Tumor

Signs and Symptoms In the skin, lesions vary in size from one to 50 cm or more. They are red, purple-red, or gray, depending upon their depth and state of regression. The most common extracutaneous site for cavernous hemangioma is the liver, but these lesions have been found in the rectum, kidney, eyes, nerves, spinal cord, and brain as well.

Etiology Most cases are spontaneous and nonheritable and arise for unknown reasons, although cavernous hemangioma can be inherited as an autosomal dominant trait. Some may be acquired as a result of injury to a particular area of the body. Growth factors may be responsible for the proliferation of vascular tissue.

Epidemiology Males and females of all ages are affected equally.

Related Disorders Arteriovenous malformations of the brain may cause headaches, seizures, strokes, or bleeding into the brain. They may affect arteries, veins, and midsized blood vessels. See *Moyamoya Disease; Blue Rubber Bleb Nevus; von Hippel-Lindau Disease.*

Treatment—Standard Because these lesions usually disappear spontaneously, treatment is often not necessary. If, however, they impinge upon body orifices or cause bleeding, treatment may be required.

Various imaging diagnostic methods such as magnetic resonance imaging **(MRI),** computed tomography **(CT)** scans, and x-rays are useful in determining the extent of the lesions. There is some question as to the effectiveness of surgical treatment of hemangioma. Cryotherapy, systemic corticosteroids, and radiotherapy have their places in treatment of hemangiomas. Lasers are often useful for small lesions.

Treatment—Investigational Please contact the agencies listed under Resources, below, for the most current information.

Resources

For more information on cavernous hemangioma: National Organization for Rare Disorders (NORD); NIH/National Heart, Lung and Blood Institute (NHLBI).

For genetic information and genetic counseling referrals: March of Dimes Birth Defects Foundation; NIH/National Center for Education in Maternal and Child Health (NCEMCH).

References

Dermatology, 3rd ed.: O. Braun-Falco, et al.; Springer-Verlag, 1991.

Skin Signs of Systemic Disease: I.M. Braverman; W.B. Saunders Company, 1981.

Dermatology in General Medicine: Textbook and Atlas, 3rd ed.: T.B. Fitzpatrick, et al., eds.; McGraw-Hill, 1987.

Dermatology, 2nd ed. (3rd ed., 1992): S.L. Moschella and H.J. Hurley, eds.; W.B. Saunders Company, 1985.

Textbook of Dermatology, 4th ed.: A. Rook, et al., eds.; Blackwell Scientific Publications, 1986.

Mendelian Inheritance in Man, 9th ed.: V.A. McKusick; The Johns Hopkins University Press, 1990, p. 391.

Colorectal Hemangioma; Radiologic Findings: A.H. Dachman, et al.; Radiology, April 1988, issue 167(1), pp. 31–34.

Cavernous Hemangioma of the Optic Nerve: N. Maruoka, et al.; J. Neurosurg., August 1988, issue 69(2), pp. 292–294.

Cavernous Hemangioma of the Liver; Role of Percutaneous Biopsy: J.J. Cronan, et al.; Radiology, January 1988, issue 166(1 pt. 1), pp. 135–138.

Cavernous Angiomas of the Spinal Cord: G.R. Cosgrove, et al.; J. Neurosurg., January 1988, issue 68(1), pp. 31–36.

CUTIS LAXA

Description Cutis laxa is a congenital or acquired connective tissue disorder marked by limp or slack skin. The affected areas of skin may be thickened and dark.

Synonyms

Chalasodermia
Dermatochalasia
Dermatolysis
Dermatomegaly

Signs and Symptoms Congenital cutis laxa is diagnosed at birth or during an infant's early months. Transient edema is often an initial sign. The skin is inelastic, and folds appear in the areas of loose skin. These are most apparent on the face, giving the infant a sad expression. The disease advances during infancy and is less noticeable postpuberty. The voice may deepen because of vocal cord laxity. As a rule, patients develop normally, but in some males the genitalia may remain immature into adulthood and the patient may be impotent. Cardiorespiratory complications can be severe. Other complications include inguinal hernia, and diverticula of the gastrointestinal tract and the urinary bladder.

The onset of acquired cutis laxa is slow. It may not manifest until puberty or later. Transient angioedema and inflammation are frequent precursors. Skin changes emerge slowly and may be generalized or localized to the face, body, or neck. Blood vessels are subject to rupture, and purpura results. Potential dangers are aortic rupture, pulmonary complications, respiratory insufficiency due to emphysema, or gastroenteric problems.

Etiology The autosomal recessive form of cutis laxa is the most common, but autosomal dominant and X-linked forms exist. Acquired cutis laxa may develop following a severe illness involving fever, polyserositis, and erythema multiforme. The patient is frequently a child or an adolescent. Acquired cutis laxa also may have an autoimmune association.

Treatment—Standard No specific treatment exists. Plastic surgery may be indicated as a cosmetic measure in patients with the congenital form. The surgery may be less effective in patients with the acquired form. Otherwise, treatment is confined to that for any cardiorespiratory or other complications that may develop.

Treatment—Investigational Please contact the agencies listed under Resources, below, for the most current information.

Resources
For more information on cutis laxa: National Organization for Rare Disorders (NORD); The National Arthritis and Musculoskeletal and Skin Diseases Information Clearinghouse.

For information on genetics and genetic counseling referrals: March of Dimes Birth Defects Foundation; National Center for Education in Maternal and Child Health (NCEMCH).

References
Dermatology, 3rd ed.: O. Braun-Falco, et al.; Springer-Verlag, 1991.
Skin Signs of Systemic Disease: I.M. Braverman; W.B. Saunders Company, 1981.
Dermatology in General Medicine: Textbook and Atlas, 3rd ed.: T.B. Fitzpatrick, et al., eds.; McGraw-Hill, 1987.
Dermatology, 2nd ed. (3rd ed., 1992): S.L. Moschella and H.J. Hurley, eds.; W.B. Saunders Company, 1985.
Textbook of Dermatology, 4th ed.: A. Rook, et al., eds.; Blackwell Scientific Publications, 1986.
Syndromes of the Head and Neck, 3rd ed.: R.J. Gorlin, et al.; Oxford University Press, 1990, pp. 422–425.
Mendelian Inheritance in Man, 9th ed.: V.A. McKusick; The Johns Hopkins University Press, 1990, pp. 242–243, 1117–1118, 1582–1583.

DARIER DISEASE

Description Darier disease is a gradually progressive, hereditary skin disorder characterized by widespread keratotic papules on the skin and mucous membranes, and by nail dystrophy.

Synonyms
Dyskeratosis Follicularis
White-Darier Disease

Signs and Symptoms The onset of Darier disease is gradual, beginning with burning and itching of the skin in the seborrheic areas, and extending elsewhere. Papules appear, becoming larger and darker and covered with gray-brown scales or crusts. The enlarging papules eventually coalesce to form larger patches. Sites of predilection include the scalp, forehead, trunk, and extremities. The hyperkeratotic plaques are often foul-smelling as a result of bacterial colonization. Nails show longitudinal ridging, splits, and subungual keratoses. Hyperkeratotic white plaques in the oral cavity are characteristic. Patients complain of severe pruritus. Symptoms tend to be more severe during periods of emotional stress and with exposure to sunlight, and may decrease during the winter. Some but not all patients are mentally retarded.

Etiology Darier disease is inherited as a dominant trait. The cause is unknown. Histologically there is suprabasal acantholysis with evidence of premature cornification of individual keratinocytes.

Epidemiology Onset usually is during childhood, but the disease may appear as late as the 7th decade of life. Males are more commonly affected. In Denmark the incidence has been estimated at 1:10,000 persons.

Related Disorders Acrokeratosis verruciformis of Hopf is a dominant, hereditary skin disorder typified by flat or convex, smooth, firm papules distributed symmetrically on the backs of the hands, feet, wrists, and ankles. The number, size, and coloration of the papules vary. Other symptoms include hyperkeratosis of the palms and soles, and nail abnormalities such as opacity and brittleness.

Hyperkeratosis follicularis in cutem penetrans (Kyrle disease) is a rare dermatologic disorder occurring mostly in female adults. It is characterized by painful, scattered eruptions with horn-like cone-shaped plugs, on the extremities, buttocks, and cheeks.

Keratosis pilaris (follicular ichthyosis) is a common skin disorder of adolescence that is characterized by mild erythema and the development of irregularly distributed keratotic papules. The thighs and arms also may have the appearance of gooseflesh.

Treatment—Standard The cutaneous manifestations of Darier disease sometimes respond to etretinate *(NOTE: This drug should not be taken by pregnant women.)* Surgical debridement may be helpful in certain cases. Keratolytics and antibiotics are useful.

Treatment—Investigational Please contact the agencies listed under Resources, below, for the most current information.

Resources
For more information on Darier disease: National Organization for Rare Disorders (NORD); Foundation for Ichthyosis and Related Skin Types (F.I.R.S.T.); The National Arthritis and Musculoskeletal and Skin Diseases Infor-

mation Clearinghouse.

For genetic information and genetic counseling referrals: March of Dimes Birth Defects Foundation; National Center for Education in Maternal and Child Health (NCEMCH).

References

Dermatology, 3rd ed.: O. Braun-Falco, et al.; Springer-Verlag, 1991.

Skin Signs of Systemic Disease: I.M. Braverman; W.B. Saunders Company, 1981.

Dermatology in General Medicine: Textbook and Atlas, 3rd ed.: T.B. Fitzpatrick, et al., eds.; McGraw-Hill, 1987.

Dermatology, 2nd ed. (3rd ed., 1992): S.L. Moschella and H.J. Hurley, eds.; W.B. Saunders Company, 1985.

Textbook of Dermatology, 4th ed.: A. Rook, et al., eds.; Blackwell Scientific Publications, 1986.

Genetically Transmitted, Generalized Disorders of Cornification: The Ichthyoses: M.L. Williams, et al.; in Dermatologic Clinics, January 1987, issue 5(1), pp. 173–175.

Etretinate: Effect of Milk Intake on Absorption: J.J. DiGiovanna, et al.; J. Invest. Dermatol., June 1984, issue 82(6), pp. 636–640.

The Surgical Treatment of Hypertrophic Darier's Disease: R.G. Wheeland, et al.; J. Dermatol. Surg. Oncol., April 1985, issue 11(4), pp. 420–423.

DERMATITIS, ATOPIC

Description Atopic dermatitis, a common, chronic form of eczematous dermatitis, is usually seen in persons with a history of allergy.

Synonyms

Atopic Eczema

Besnier Prurigo

Constitutional Eczema

Signs and Symptoms The disorder is characterized by itching with cutaneous erythema, and crusted, scaling, and oozing lesions. Lichenification is often present. The irritants that trigger atopic dermatitis are many, and include harsh soaps, detergents, medications; extremes of heat and cold; wool and silk clothing; and emotional stress. Distribution of skin lesions to the flexor surfaces of the arms and legs, neck, and face is common.

Patients with active skin lesions are susceptible to skin infection with bacteria, especially *Staphylococcus aureus,* and with viruses, especially herpes, vaccinia, and molluscum contagiosum.

Measurement of serum immunoglobulin E may help in diagnosis, although findings do not always clearly correlate with the clinical picture.

Etiology The cause is not known but is immunologically mediated. Susceptibility to eczema is believed to be an inherited trait.

Epidemiology Atopic dermatitis primarily affects infants and children, with improvement or resolution by age 10 years. In severe cases, however, the disorder may persist into adulthood as a chronic problem. Occasionally the onset is in adult life. Males and females are affected in equal numbers.

Related Disorders See *Dermatitis, Contact.*

Pompholyx, a disorder of unknown cause, is characterized initially by deep-seated itchy blisters or elevated spots usually on the sides of the fingers and the palms. Later, the skin of the hands may become dry, scaly, hardened, and fissured. The feet may also be affected.

Treatment—Standard Treatment includes emollient creams to keep the skin lubricated. When the lesions are oozing or weeping, wet compresses may help. Corticosteroid creams and antihistamines may relieve the pruritus. Oral antibiotics may be required for secondary bacterial infections.

Other recommendations include tar preparations or ultraviolet light therapy, mild lanolin-based soaps and bath oils for bathing, and the use of mild laundry detergents.

Treatment—Investigational Please contact the agencies listed under Resources, below, for the most current information.

Resources

For more information on atopic dermatitis: National Organization for Rare Disorders (NORD); NIH/National Institute of Arthritis, Musculoskeletal & Skin Disorders (NIAMS) Information Clearinghouse.

References

Dermatology, 3rd ed.: O. Braun-Falco, et al.; Springer-Verlag, 1991.

Skin Signs of Systemic Disease: I.M. Braverman; W.B. Saunders Company, 1981.

Dermatology in General Medicine: Textbook and Atlas, 3rd ed.: T.B. Fitzpatrick, et al., eds.; McGraw-Hill, 1987.

Dermatology, 2nd ed. (3rd ed., 1992): S.L. Moschella and H.J. Hurley, eds.; W.B. Saunders Company, 1985.

Textbook of Dermatology, 4th ed.: A. Rook, et al., eds.; Blackwell Scientific Publications, 1986.

Internal Medicine, 3rd ed.: J.H. Stein, ed.-in-chief; Little, Brown and Company, 1990, pp. 1837–1838.

DERMATITIS, CONTACT

Description Contact dermatitis is an inflammatory reaction in the skin in response to irritants and allergens. It may be acute or chronic. Primary irritant contact dermatitis affects all persons who contact the irritating substance. Allergic contact dermatitis affects only those individuals who contact an irritating substance to which they have been previously sensitized and to which they have developed a delayed hypersensitivity reaction.

Synonyms

Delayed Hypersensitivity

Dermatitis Medicamentosa

Dermatitis Venenata

Drug Hypersensitivity

Signs and Symptoms Contact dermatitis is marked by inflamed skin and, possibly, blisters at the site of contact with an offending agent. If acute, the area may be edematous, crusty, scaly, and exudative. The patient complains of burning pain and, as a rule, pruritus. Irritating the site by scratching or rubbing may cause lichenification.

Allergic contact dermatitis is a delayed reaction to an allergen such as poison ivy or a medication. The lapse between exposure and manifestation may be a few hours, days, or weeks. Patients may suddenly become allergic to a skin medication or cosmetic that they have been applying for years.

Irritant contact dermatitis caused by contact with a potent chemical substance usually develops immediately. When the irritant is weaker, the onset of dermatitis may be delayed.

Photoallergic and phototoxic contact dermatitis develops following exposure to light after use of certain chemicals. The effect of sunlight on the patient seems exaggerated. Common culpable chemicals in photoallergic contact dermatitis include aftershave lotions, perfumes, and topical sulfonamides. Certain ingredients in perfumes or drugs—psoralens, coal tar, and cutting oils—may also cause dermatitis. Hypersensitivity to sunlight due to certain drugs, usually antibiotics, is *not* a form of photoallergic contact dermatitis; the abnormal reactions to sun are a side effect of the drugs.

Etiology The irritants, allergens, and substances that can cause contact dermatitis are innumerable. They include medications; cosmetics; natural irritants such as Rhus oleoresin (found in poison ivy and poison oak); chemicals such as solvents; biological substances such as the saliva of house pets, and parasites such as mites and fleas; and physical agents (sunlight, temperature extremes).

Epidemiology Contact dermatitis affects males and females of all ages in equal numbers. As a rule, each succeeding contact increases hypersensitivity. Forms of contact dermatitis constitute 90 percent of the occupational skin disorders in the United States.

Related Disorders See *Dermatitis, Atopic*.

Treatment—Standard Serum immunoglobulin testing and patch tests for specific agents help in diagnosis. Prophylaxis is usually successful if the patient employs a combination of environmental, personal, and medical measures.

Avoidance of the causative agent is the key in treatment. Prednisone is indicated in acute severe cases. Antihistamines may lessen itching, and antibiotics are required in secondary bacterial infections. Topical corticosteroids are indicated for chronic forms of contact dermatitis. Topical treatment for acute exudative dermatitis includes wet compresses (water or aluminum subacetate) and cortisone lotions.

Treatment—Investigational Please contact the agencies listed under Resources, below, for the most current information.

Resources

For more information about contact dermatitis: National Organization for Rare Disorders (NORD); Allergy Foundation of America; Asthma & Allergy

Foundation of America; NIH/National Arthritis, Musculoskeletal & Skin (NIAMS) Information Clearinghouse; Eczema Association for Science and Education; Allergy Information Association.

References
Dermatology, 3rd ed.: O. Braun-Falco, et al.; Springer-Verlag, 1991.
Skin Signs of Systemic Disease: I.M. Braverman; W.B. Saunders Company, 1981.
Dermatology in General Medicine: Textbook and Atlas, 3rd ed.: T.B. Fitzpatrick, et al., eds.; McGraw-Hill, 1987.
Dermatology, 2nd ed. (3rd ed., 1992): S.L. Moschella and H.J. Hurley, eds.; W.B. Saunders Company, 1985.
Textbook of Dermatology, 4th ed.: A. Rook, et al., eds.; Blackwell Scientific Publications, 1986.
Allergic Contact Dermatitis in Children: W.L. Weston, et al.; Am. J. Dis. Child., October 1984, issue 138(10), pp. 932–936.
Internal Medicine, 3rd ed.: J.H. Stein, ed.-in-chief; Little, Brown and Company, 1990, p. 1837.
Household Treatment for "Chili Burns" of the Hands: L.A. Jones, et al.; J. Toxicol. Clin. Toxicol., 1987, issue 25(61), pp. 483–491.
Local and Systemic Desensitization Induced by Repeated Epicutaneous Hapten Application: G.H. Boerrigter, et al.; J. Invest. Dermatol., January 1987, issue 88(1), pp. 3–7.

DERMATITIS HERPETIFORMIS (DH)

Description A chronic disorder, DH is marked by groups of severely itching blisters and papules and is often associated with gluten-sensitive enteropathy.

Synonyms
Brocq-Duhring Disease
Dermatitis Multiformis
Duhring Disease
Gluten-Sensitive Enteropathy

Signs and Symptoms A slow onset is typical in adult life, but children can be affected also. Small blisters, discrete papules, and itchy, smooth lesions resembling hives appear symmetrically on the head, elbows, knees, lower back, and buttocks. Quite often blisters and papules occur on the face and neck. Itching and burning may be almost intolerable, and the need to scratch irresistible. Over three-quarters of patients have a gluten-sensitive, gastrointestinal atrophy similar to that in celiac disease. Malabsorption generally does not occur.

The direct immunofluorescence test for IgA in normal skin is positive.

Etiology Dermatitis herpetiformis is idiopathic, but several immunologic abnormalities have been detected. The presence in lesions of IgA and complement components supports an immunoregulatory disturbance. Iodide and other halides can cause a flare.

Epidemiology Onset may be at any age, but it usually occurs in middle adult life; it is rare in the pediatric group. Males are affected more often than females (3:2).

Treatment—Standard Dapsone frequently treats the rash successfully and brings symptomatic relief within 1 or 2 days. The urgent need to scratch usually abates in 1 to 3 days. Dapsone can be associated with severe hematologic disturbances and must be closely monitored.

Treatment—Investigational Please contact the agencies listed under Resources, below, for the most current information.

Resources

For more information on dermatitis herpetiformis: National Organization for Rare Disorders (NORD); Gluten Intolerance; The National Arthritis and Musculoskeletal and Skin Diseases Information Clearinghouse.

References

Dermatology, 3rd ed.: O. Braun-Falco, et al.; Springer-Verlag, 1991.

Skin Signs of Systemic Disease: I.M. Braverman; W.B. Saunders Company, 1981.

Dermatology in General Medicine: Textbook and Atlas, 3rd ed.: T.B. Fitzpatrick, et al., eds.; McGraw-Hill, 1987.

Dermatology, 2nd ed. (3rd ed., 1992): S.L. Moschella and H.J. Hurley, eds.; W.B. Saunders Company, 1985.

Textbook of Dermatology, 4th ed.: A. Rook, et al., eds.; Blackwell Scientific Publications, 1986.

Internal Medicine, 3rd ed.: J.H. Stein, ed.-in-chief; Little, Brown and Company, 1990, p. 1831.

DYSPLASTIC NEVUS SYNDROME

Description Dysplastic nevus syndrome is characterized by the appearance in adolescence or young adulthood of typical nevi or moles having variation in size, shape, and color. They are considered by many people to be precursors of melanoma. Sporadic, multiple heritable, and multiple nonheritable forms exist.

Synonyms

B-K Mole Syndrome
Familial Atypical Mole-Malignant Melanoma Syndrome

Signs and Symptoms Dysplastic nevi have irregular edges and are pink to reddish-brown in color. They appear in variable numbers, especially on the trunk. Histologically, these nevi have marked atypical melanocytic hyperplasia. When frankly malignant histologic features are present, dysplastic nevi are then said to be melanomas.

Etiology The cause is unknown. Heritable forms are transmitted as autosomal dominant genes.

Epidemiology Symptoms usually first appear in young adulthood. Males and females are affected in equal numbers.

Treatment—Standard Periodic examination of lesions for change suggesting malignancy is indicated. Questionable lesions should be excised. Patients should use sunscreen and avoid sunburn.

Treatment—Investigational Please contact the agencies listed under Resources, below, for the most current information.

Resources
 For more information on dysplastic nevus syndrome: National Organization for Rare Disorders (NORD); Skin Cancer Foundation; American Cancer Society; NIH/National Cancer Institute PDQ (Physician Data Query) phoneline.
 For genetic information and genetic counseling referrals: March of Dimes Birth Defects Foundation; National Center for Education in Maternal and Child Health (NCEMCH).

References
Dermatology, 3rd ed.: O. Braun-Falco, et al.; Springer-Verlag, 1991.
Skin Signs of Systemic Disease: I.M. Braverman; W.B. Saunders Company, 1981.
Dermatology in General Medicine: Textbook and Atlas, 3rd ed.: T.B. Fitzpatrick, et al., eds.; McGraw-Hill, 1987.
Dermatology, 2nd ed. (3rd ed., 1992): S.L. Moschella and H.J. Hurley, eds.; W.B. Saunders Company, 1985.
Textbook of Dermatology, 4th ed.: A. Rook, et al., eds.; Blackwell Scientific Publications, 1986.
The Efficacy of Histopathological Criteria Required for Diagnosing Dysplastic Naevi: P.M. Steijlen, et al.; Histopathology, March 1988, issue 12(3), pp. 289–300.
Dysplastic Nevus Syndrome: Ultraviolet Hypermutability Confirmed in Vitro by Elevated Sister Chromatid Exchanges: E.G. Jung, et al.; Dermatologica, 1986, issue 173(6), pp. 297–300.
Role of Topical Tretinoin in Melanoma and Dysplastic Nevi: F.L. Meyskens Jr., et al.; J. Am. Acad. Dermatol., October 1986, issue 15(4 pt. 2), pp. 822–825.
Mendelian Inheritance in Man, 8th ed.: V.A. McKusick; The Johns Hopkins University Press, 1988, pp. 485–486.

EPIDERMOLYSIS BULLOSA (EB)

Description EB refers to a group of rare, hereditary skin diseases characterized by fragile skin in which blisters and vesicles develop following minor trauma. In some forms of EB the mucous membranes are involved. Healing is impaired in some forms, causing mutilating scars or contractures.

Synonyms
 Dowling-Meara Syndrome
 Hallopeau-Siemens Disease
 Herlitz Syndrome
 Koebner Disease
 Localized Epidermolysis
 Weber-Cockayne Disease

Signs and Symptoms Classification of the major types of EB depends upon the depth of the blisters.
 In **EB simplex (nonscarring),** the blisters occur within the epidermis. The Weber-Cockayne form of EB simplex is characterized by the development of blis-

ters following minor trauma to the hands and feet and other friction points. It is autosomal dominant. In EB herpetiformis (Dowling-Meara), which is another form of EB simplex, there is extensive blistering and much of the body may be affected. This is probably autosomal dominant. The mucous membranes are seldom involved. Blisters usually heal without scars; secondary infection is the primary complication. Warm weather may aggravate the condition. Patients with the simplex form usually have normal mental and physical development.

In **junctional EB,** the blisters occur within the lamina lucida of the basement membrane zone. The Herlitz type (EB lethalis) has extensive blisters of skin and mucous membranes and is usually fatal in the newborn period. In other junctional forms of EB, such as the generalized junctional form, there may be extensive facial erosions and loss of nails. All junctional forms are probably autosomal recessive diseases.

EB dystrophic (scarring) is characterized by blisters that develop beneath the basement membrane zone of the skin. All forms cause scarring. There are both autosomal dominant and recessive types. The recessive dystrophic form (Hallopeau-Siemens) is the most severe. Blisters appear on extremities and are widespread, affecting mucous membranes and skin. Blisters leave scars and miliary cysts after healing. The tongue, eyes, and esophagus are often affected; teeth may be malformed. Nails may be lost. Scars leave mitten deformities of the digits. In some cases, hair follicles may be destroyed and alopecia develops. Malnutrition, anemia, and growth retardation can result from chronic blood loss and poor food intake.

Etiology Various forms of epidermolysis bullosa are inherited as either autosomal dominant or recessive traits (see Signs and Symptoms, above). The mechanism involved may be related to structural abnormalities of keratin and collagen and/or to defects with the reparative dermal enzyme, collagenase.

Epidemiology About 25,000 to 50,000 persons in the United States are thought to be affected by all forms of epidermolysis bullosa.

Treatment—Standard Therapy is symptomatic and supportive. Antibiotics are useful, and a high-protein diet is helpful in cases where malnutrition develops. A cool environment is usually more comfortable for patients suffering from this disease.

Treatment—Investigational Research is ongoing in the areas of orphan drugs, wound-healing antibiotics, and the inhibition of blister formation. Phenytoin blocks collagenase in vitro, but has not proved to be clinically useful in reducing blistering.

Epidermal cells cultured to form sheets of skin have been successfully transplanted onto the damaged skin of patients with epidermolysis bullosa. Approximately 50 percent of the grafted tissue attached successfully, with no sign of infection, rejection, or recurrent blistering during a 4-year follow-up period.

Please contact the agencies listed under Resources, below, for the most current information.

Resources
For more information on epidermolysis bullosa: National Organization for Rare Disorders (NORD); Dystrophic Epidermolysis Bullosa Research Association of America, Inc. (DEBRA); D.E.B.R.A. (England); Eugene Bauer, M.D., Stanford University School of Medicine, Department of Dermatology; The National Arthritis and Musculoskeletal and Skin Diseases Information Clearinghouse.

For genetic information and genetic counseling referrals: March of Dimes Birth Defects Foundation; National Center for Education in Maternal and Child Health (NCEMCH).

References
Dermatology, 3rd ed.: O. Braun-Falco, et al.; Springer-Verlag, 1991.

Skin Signs of Systemic Disease: I.M. Braverman; W.B. Saunders Company, 1981.

Dermatology in General Medicine: Textbook and Atlas, 3rd ed.: T.B. Fitzpatrick, et al., eds.; McGraw-Hill, 1987.

Dermatology, 2nd ed. (3rd ed., 1992): S.L. Moschella and H.J. Hurley, eds.; W.B. Saunders Company, 1985.

Textbook of Dermatology, 4th ed.: A. Rook, et al., eds.; Blackwell Scientific Publications, 1986.

Mendelian Inheritance in Man, 9th ed.: V.A. McKusick; The Johns Hopkins University Press, 1990, pp. 303–305.

Dermatologic Clinics: The Genodermatoses: J. Alper, ed.; W.B. Saunders Company, 1987, vol. 5(1), pp. 27–30.

EPIDERMOLYTIC HYPERKERATOSIS

Description Epidermolytic hyperkeratosis is a hereditary skin disorder characterized by hyperkeratosis and erythroderma.

Synonyms
Bullous Congenital Ichthyosiform Erythroderma

Signs and Symptoms Symptoms are present at birth and may range from mild to severe. The skin appears warty, blistery, and thick over most of the body surface, and particularly in the skin creases over joints. The disorder can be detected by amniocentesis.

Etiology Epidermolytic hyperkeratosis is inherited as an autosomal dominant trait. The cause is unknown. There is degeneration of the granular layer; increased epidermal proliferation and reduced epidermal transit time.

Epidemiology Males and females are affected in equal numbers.

Related Disorders See *Ichthyosis Congenita; Ichthyosis Hystrix, Curth-Macklin Type; Darier Disease; Sjögren-Larsson Syndrome; Netherton Syndrome.*

Treatment—Standard Symptoms can be alleviated by the application of keratolytics and emollients, including plain petroleum jelly. This can be especially effective after bathing while the skin is still moist. Salicylic acid gel, applied under occlusion, is useful in some instances for removal of scales. Lactate lotion also can be an effective keratolytic. Topical and systemic retinoids can be beneficial in some cases but must be used with caution because of adverse side effects including those to fetal development in pregnant women.

Treatment—Investigational Please contact the agencies listed under Resources, below, for the most current information.

Resources

For more information on epidermolytic hyperkeratosis: National Organization for Rare Disorders (NORD); Foundation for Ichthyosis and Related Skin Types (F.I.R.S.T.); The National Arthritis and Musculoskeletal and Skin Diseases Information Clearinghouse.

For genetic information and genetic counseling referrals: March of Dimes Birth Defects Foundation; National Center for Education in Maternal and Child Health (NCEMCH).

References

Dermatology, 3rd ed.: O. Braun-Falco, et al.; Springer-Verlag, 1991.

Skin Signs of Systemic Disease: I.M. Braverman; W.B. Saunders Company, 1981.

Dermatology in General Medicine: Textbook and Atlas, 3rd ed.: T.B. Fitzpatrick, et al., eds.; McGraw-Hill, 1987.

Dermatology, 2nd ed. (3rd ed., 1992): S.L. Moschella and H.J. Hurley, eds.; W.B. Saunders Company, 1985.

Textbook of Dermatology, 4th ed.: A. Rook, et al., eds.; Blackwell Scientific Publications, 1986.

Genetically Transmitted, Generalized Disorders of Cornification. The Icthyoses: M.L. Williams, et al.; Dermatol. Clin., January 1987, issue 5(1), pp. 155–178.

Therapeutic Activity of Lactate 12% Lotion in the Treatment of Ichthyosis. Active Versus Vehicle and Active Versus a Petroleum Cream: M. Buxman, et al.; J. Am. Acad. Dermatol., December 1986, issue 15(6), pp. 1253–1258.

ERYTHEMA MULTIFORME

Description Erythema multiforme is an allergic inflammatory skin disorder, caused by various agents, producing characteristic lesions that develop on the skin and mucous membranes.

Synonyms

Stevens-Johnson Syndrome

Signs and Symptoms Usually the initial lesions are erythematous macules or papules, possibly with vesicular centers and progressing to bullae. Target or iris lesions are characteristic. Mild pruritus may be present. Distribution of the lesions is usually on the hands, forearms, and feet, and the mucous membranes of the mouth, nose, and genitals. The skin lesions are bilateral and symmetrical and tend to resolve in 2 to 6 weeks, but may recur.

Systemic symptoms include fever, arthralgia, malaise, cough, and sore throat.

See **Stevens-Johnson Syndrome,** which is a severe, bullous form of erythema multiforme.

Etiology Several infectious agents have been identified as the cause of erythema multiforme. These include viruses (e.g., herpes simplex, coxsackie, and echo); and other agents such as *Mycoplasma pneumoniae; Histoplasma capsulatum;* or *Coccidioides immitis.*

The disorder can also be induced by drugs (e.g., sulfonamides, penicillins, phenytoin, barbiturates); by occult malignancies; and by radiation therapy in persons being treated for malignancies.

Epidemiology Individuals of both sexes and any ages can be affected.

Related Disorders See *Pemphigoid, Bullous; Dermatitis Herpetiformis; Pemphigus*—which are among the many disorders producing blisters that are to be distinguished from erythema multiforme.

Treatment—Standard The underlying cause should be identified and treated. Other therapy for mild erythema multiforme is symptomatic. Systemic corticosteroids may be required for severe cases, although care should be used where there is a danger of respiratory infections. Systemic antibiotics may be needed in some cases.

Treatment—Investigational Please contact the agencies listed under Resources, below, for the most current information.

Resources

For more information on erythema multiforme: National Organization for Rare Disorders (NORD); The National Arthritis and Musculoskeletal and Skin Diseases Information Clearinghouse.

References

Dermatology, 3rd ed.: O. Braun-Falco, et al.; Springer-Verlag, 1991.

Skin Signs of Systemic Disease: I.M. Braverman; W.B. Saunders Company, 1981.

Dermatology in General Medicine: Textbook and Atlas, 3rd ed.: T.B. Fitzpatrick, et al., eds.; McGraw-Hill, 1987.

Dermatology, 2nd ed. (3rd ed., 1992): S.L. Moschella and H.J. Hurley, eds.; W.B. Saunders Company, 1985.

Textbook of Dermatology, 4th ed.: A. Rook, et al., eds.; Blackwell Scientific Publications, 1986.

Harrison's Principles of Internal Medicine, 12th ed.: J.D. Wilson, et al., eds.; McGraw-Hill, 1991, p. 331.

ERYTHROKERATODERMIA SYMMETRICA PROGRESSIVA

Description Erythrokeratodermia symmetrica progressiva is a rare hereditary skin disorder characterized by sharply marginated, red, hyperkeratotic plaques with hyperpigmented margins.

Signs and Symptoms The hyperkeratotic plaques are distributed symmetrically and may appear on the head, arms, legs, and buttocks. The lesions may be pruritic. Usually, this disorder stabilizes after 1 to 2 years, and partially regresses during puberty. Palms and soles are spared.

Etiology This rare disorder is probably transmitted through an autosomal dominant gene.

Epidemiology Males and females are affected in equal numbers.

Related Disorders See *Ichthyosis; Ichthyosis Congenita; Ichthyosis Hystrix, Curth-Macklin Type; Ichthyosis, Lamellar Recessive; Ichthyosis, X-Linked; Darier Disease; Epidermolytic Hyperkeratosis; Netherton Syndrome; Sjö-gren-Larsson Syndrome.*

Treatment—Standard Symptoms can be alleviated by the application of keratolytic and emollient ointments, including plain petroleum jelly. These can be especially effective after bathing while the skin is still moist. Salicylic acid gel applied under occlusive dressings is useful in some instances for removal of scales. Lactate lotion can also be an effective keratolytic agent. Topical and systemic retinoids can be beneficial in some cases but must be used with caution because of adverse side effects including those to fetal development in pregnant women.

Treatment—Investigational Please contact the agencies listed under Resources, below, for the most current information.

Resources

For more information on erythrokeratodermia symmetrica progressiva: National Organization for Rare Disorders (NORD); Foundation for Ichthyosis and Related Skin Types, Inc. (F.I.R.S.T.); NIH/National Arthritis, Musculoskeletal & Skin (NIAMS) Information Clearinghouse.

For genetic information and genetic counseling referrals: March of Dimes Birth Defects Foundation; National Center for Education in Maternal and Child Health (NCEMCH).

References

Dermatology, 3rd ed.: O. Braun-Falco, et al.; Springer-Verlag, 1991.

Skin Signs of Systemic Disease: I.M. Braverman; W.B. Saunders Company, 1981.

Dermatology in General Medicine: Textbook and Atlas, 3rd ed.: T.B. Fitzpatrick, et al., eds.; McGraw-Hill, 1987.

Dermatology, 2nd ed. (3rd ed., 1992): S.L. Moschella and H.J. Hurley, eds.; W.B. Saunders Company, 1985.

Textbook of Dermatology, 4th ed.: A. Rook, et al., eds.; Blackwell Scientific Publications, 1986.

Genetically Transmitted, Generalized Disorders of Cornification. The Ichthyoses: M.L. Williams, et al.; Dermatol. Clin., January 1987, issue 5(1), pp. 155–178.

Therapeutic Activity of Lactate 12% Lotion in the Treatment of Ichthyosis. Active Versus Vehicle and Active Versus a Petroleum Cream: M. Buxman, et al.; Journ. Am. Acad. Dermatol., December 1986, issue 15(6), pp. 1253–1258.

Progressive Symmetric Erythrokeratodermia. Histological and Ultrastructural Study of Patient Before and After Treatment with Etretinate: V. Nazzaro, et al.; Arch. Dermatol., April 1986, issue 122(4), pp. 434–440.

ERYTHROKERATODERMIA VARIABILIS

Description Erythrokeratodermia variabilis is a form of ichthyosis characterized by sharply marginated erythematous scaling plaques with a shifting configuration, and by fixed hyperkeratotic plaques.

Synonyms
> Keratosis Rubra Figurata
> Mendes Da Costa Syndrome

Signs and Symptoms The eruption begins early in childhood and persists throughout life. The erythematous areas may develop after exposure to heat, cold, wind, or emotional upset, and they may rapidly change shape or position. The keratotic plaques usually are limited to small areas but in some cases appear over the entire body surfaces, including the palms and soles. The disorder may improve in the summer.

Etiology The disorder appears to be transmitted by autosomal dominant genes. The cause is unknown.

Epidemiology Erythrokeratodermia variabilis is a rare form of ichthyosis, present at birth or in childhood, that affects males and females in equal numbers.

Related Disorders See *Ichthyosis; Ichthyosis Congenita; Ichthyosis, Harlequin Type; Ichthyosis Hystrix, Curth-Macklin Type; Ichthyosis, Lamellar Recessive; Ichthyosis Vulgaris; Darier Disease; Epidermolytic Hyperkeratosis; Erythrokeratodermia Symmetrica Progressiva; Erythrokeratolysis Hiemalis; Multiple Sulfatase Deficiency; Netherton Syndrome; Refsum Syndrome; Sjögren-Larsson Syndrome.*

Treatment—Standard Symptoms can be alleviated by the application of emollient and keratolytic ointments, including plain petroleum jelly. This can be especially effective after bathing while the skin is still moist. Salicylic acid gel and lactate lotions are useful in some instances for removal of scales, especially when used under occlusion. The retinoids, topically or systemically, and topical steroids may be indicated but must be used with caution to avoid side effects.

Treatment—Investigational Please contact the agencies listed under Resources, below, for the most current information.

Resources

For more information on **erythrokeratodermia variabilis:** National Organization for Rare Disorders (NORD); Foundation for Ichthyosis and Related Skin Types, Inc. (F.I.R.S.T.); National Arthritis, Musculoskeletal & Skin (NIAMS) Information Clearinghouse.

For **genetic information and genetic counseling referrals:** March of Dimes Birth Defects Foundation; National Center for Education in Maternal and Child Health (NCEMCH).

References

Dermatology, 3rd ed.: O. Braun-Falco, et al.; Springer-Verlag, 1991.

Skin Signs of Systemic Disease: I.M. Braverman; W.B. Saunders Company, 1981.

Dermatology in General Medicine: Textbook and Atlas, 3rd ed.: T.B. Fitzpatrick, et al., eds.; McGraw-Hill, 1987.

Dermatology, 2nd ed. (3rd ed., 1992): S.L. Moschella and H.J. Hurley, eds.; W.B. Saunders Company, 1985.

Textbook of Dermatology, 4th ed.: A. Rook, et al., eds.; Blackwell Scientific Publications, 1986.

Mendelian Inheritance in Man, 9th ed.: V.A. McKusick; The Johns Hopkins University Press, 1990, pp. 311–312.

Erythrokeratodermia Variabilis Treated with Isotretinoin. A Clinical, Histologic, and Ultrastructural Study: I.P. Rappaport, et al.; Arch. Dermatol., April 1986, issue 122(4), pp. 441–445.

Progressive Symmetric Erythrokeratodermia. Histological and Ultrastructural Study of Patient Before and After Treatment with Etretinate: V. Nazzaro, et al.; Arch. Dermatol., April 1986, issue 122(4), pp. 434–440.

Erythrokeratodermia Variabilis: Immunohistochemical and Ultrastructural Studies of the Epidermis: N. McFadden, et al.; Acta Derm. Venereol., Stockholm, 1987, issue 67(4), pp. 284–288.

Genetically Transmitted, Generalized Disorders of Cornification. The Icthyoses: M.L. Williams, et al.; Dermatol. Clin., January 1987, issue 5(1), pp. 155–178.

ERYTHROKERATOLYSIS HIEMALIS

Description Erythrokeratolysis hiemalis is a heritable eruption of the palms and soles with recurrent episodes in cold weather of scaling erythematous plaques which peel from the center outwards.

Synonyms
Keratolytic Winter Erythema
Oudtshoorn Skin

Signs and Symptoms Lesions are symmetrical red scaling, peeling plaques. In most cases only the palms and soles are affected, but in severe cases the plaques may involve the skin of the back or elsewhere. Appearance of new plaques may be precipitated by fever or surgery. Onset of symptoms ranges from infancy to adolescence.

Etiology The disorder is inherited as an autosomal dominant trait.

Epidemiology The syndrome primarily affects descendants of farmers from the Oudtshoorn district in South Africa. Males and females are affected in equal numbers.

Related Disorders See *Ichthyosis; Ichthyosis Congenita; Icythyosis, X-Linked; Ichthyosis Hystrix, Curth-Macklin Type; Epidermolytic Hyperkeratosis; Darier Disease; Netherton Syndrome; Sjögren-Larsson Syndrome.*

Treatment—Standard None is curative. Symptoms can be alleviated by the application of keratolytic and emollient ointments, including plain petroleum jelly. This can be especially effective after bathing while the skin is still moist. Salicylic acid gel and lactate lotion, applied under occlusion, are useful in some instances for removal of scales. Topical and systemic retinoids can be beneficial in some cases but must be used with caution because of adverse side effects including those to fetal development in pregnant women.

Treatment—Investigational Please contact the agencies listed under Resources, below, for the most current information.

Resources
   For more information on erythrokeratolysis hiemalis: National Organization for Rare Disorders (NORD); Foundation for Ichthyosis and Related Skin Types, Inc. (F.I.R.S.T.); NIH/National Arthritis, Musculoskeletal & Skin (NIAMS) Information Clearinghouse.
   For genetic information and genetic counseling referrals: March of Dimes Birth Defects Foundation; National Center for Education in Maternal and Child Health (NCEMCH).

References
Dermatology, 3rd ed.: O. Braun-Falco, et al.; Springer-Verlag, 1991.
Skin Signs of Systemic Disease: I.M. Braverman; W.B. Saunders Company, 1981.
Dermatology in General Medicine: Textbook and Atlas, 3rd ed.: T.B. Fitzpatrick, et al., eds.; McGraw-Hill, 1987.
Dermatology, 2nd ed. (3rd ed., 1992): S.L. Moschella and H.J. Hurley, eds.; W.B. Saunders Company, 1985.
Textbook of Dermatology, 4th ed.: A. Rook, et al., eds.; Blackwell Scientific Publications, 1986.
Genetically Transmitted, Generalized Disorders of Cornification. The Ichthyoses: M.L. Williams, et al.; Dermatol. Clin., January 1987, issue 5(1), pp. 155–178.
Therapeutic Activity of Lactate 12% Lotion in the Treatment of Ichthyosis. Active Versus Vehicle and Active Versus a Petroleum Cream: M. Buxman, et al.; J. Am. Acad. Dermatol., December 1986, issue 15(6), pp. 1253–1258.

ERYTHROMELALGIA

Description Erythromelalgia is characterized by episodes of severe burning pain and increased temperature in the extremities. It occurs both as a primary disorder and secondarily to organic disease.

Synonyms
   Gerhardt Disease
   Mitchell Disease
   Weir-Mitchell Disease

Signs and Symptoms The patient complains of burning pain and redness of the feet, which worsen during hot weather; less frequently, the hands may be involved. Severity of symptoms may increase over the years, with eventual disability for the patient.

Etiology Primary erythromelalgia may be inherited as an autosomal dominant trait.

The underlying disorder in secondary erythromelalgia may be proliferative bone marrow disease, polycythemia vera, diabetes mellitus, venous insufficiency, or hypertension. The condition has been attributed to intravascular platelet aggregation and to disturbances in prostaglandin metabolism, but the cause is unknown.

Epidemiology Males are affected more often than females.

Related Disorders Causalgia syndrome (traumatic erythromelalgia) is associated with persistent diffuse burning pain, particularly in the palms and the soles. Friction and heat and other minor stimuli intensify the discomfort.

Treatment—Standard Cold packs or immersion in ice water, rest, and elevation of the extremity can relieve symptoms. In primary erythromelalgia aspirin may be beneficial, as may ephedrine, propranolol, or methysergide. In the secondary form, the primary disorder is treated.

Treatment—Investigational IV sodium nitroprusside (sodium nitroferricyanide) has been used, but its potential side effects are severe.

Please contact the agencies listed under Resources, below, for the most current information.

Resources

For more information on erythromelalgia: National Organization for Rare Disorders (NORD); Erythromelalgia Association of America.

For genetic information and genetic counseling referrals: March of Dimes Birth Defects Foundation; National Center for Education in Maternal and Child Health (NCEMCH).

References
Dermatology, 3rd ed.: O. Braun-Falco, et al.; Springer-Verlag, 1991.
Skin Signs of Systemic Disease: I.M. Braverman; W.B. Saunders Company, 1981.
Dermatology in General Medicine: Textbook and Atlas, 3rd ed.: T.B. Fitzpatrick, et al., eds.; McGraw-Hill, 1987.
Dermatology, 2nd ed. (3rd ed., 1992): S.L. Moschella and H.J. Hurley, eds.; W.B. Saunders Company, 1985.
Textbook of Dermatology, 4th ed.: A. Rook, et al., eds.; Blackwell Scientific Publications, 1986.
Mendelian Inheritance in Man, 9th ed.: V.A. McKusick; The Johns Hopkins University Press, 1990, p. 309.
Sodium Nitroprusside Treatment in Erythromelalgia: S. Ozsoylu, et al.; Euro. J. Pediatr., 1984, issue 141, pp. 185–187.

GIANOTTI-CROSTI SYNDROME

Description Gianotti-Crosti syndrome is an inflammatory condition affecting children in which there are a lichenoid papular skin eruption, enlarged lymph nodes, and an intercurrent viral infection, often with hepatitis B.

Synonyms
Acrodermatitis, Infantile Lichenoid

Acrodermatitis Papular Infantile
Crosti-Gianotti Syndrome

Signs and Symptoms Onset of Gianotti-Crosti syndrome, often preceded by a viral infection, is usually between ages 9 months and 9 years. Infections with Epstein-Barr and hepatitis B viruses and coxsackie- and cytomegalovirus, and vaccination with a live virus, may be precursors. Large flat papules appear, most commonly on the face, buttocks, arms, or legs. The papules may not be pruritic, and their usual duration is 20 to 25 days; recurrence is uncommon. Upon palpation, enlarged lymph nodes are often found in the truncal area. Patients may have a slight fever.

Etiology The cause is unknown. The trigger is considered to be a reaction to a prior viral infection, but the mechanism is not known. In many countries the precursor is most frequently infection with the hepatitis B virus. In North America other viruses are more commonly involved.

Epidemiology Boys and girls are affected in equal numbers.

Related Disorders Coxsackievirus infections are summer-associated illnesses. Young children, especially boys, are most prone to the disease. Characteristic are fever, sore throat, vomiting, headache, respiratory signs and symptoms, diarrhea, abdominal pain, rash, and earache.

Infectious mononucleosis, caused by the Epstein-Barr virus, has an incubation period of 30 to 50 days in young adults, and a briefer one in children. Symptoms include flulike malaise for a few days, headache, fever, and sore throat, with marked fatigue. Signs include generalized lymphadenopathy, eyelid and orbital edema, and perhaps rash. Tonsillitis, anorexia, photosensitivity, and hepato- and splenomegaly may be present. Other organs in the body may become involved.

Treatment—Standard Spontaneous resolution, usually within 20 to 25 days, is the rule. Meanwhile, treatment is symptomatic and supportive.

Treatment—Investigational Please contact the agencies listed under Resources, below, for the most current information.

Resources
   For more information on Gianotti-Crosti syndrome: National Organization for Rare Disorders (NORD); The National Arthritis and Musculoskeletal and Skin Diseases Information Clearinghouse; NIH/National Institute of Allergy and Infectious Disease; Centers for Disease Control (CDC).

References
Dermatology, 3rd ed.: O. Braun-Falco, et al.; Springer-Verlag, 1991.
Skin Signs of Systemic Disease: I.M. Braverman; W.B. Saunders Company, 1981.
Dermatology in General Medicine: Textbook and Atlas, 3rd ed.: T.B. Fitzpatrick, et al., eds.; McGraw-Hill, 1987.
Dermatology, 2nd ed. (3rd ed., 1992): S.L. Moschella and H.J. Hurley, eds.; W.B. Saunders Company, 1985.
Textbook of Dermatology, 4th ed.: A. Rook, et al., eds.; Blackwell Scientific Publications, 1986.

Gianotti-Crosti Syndrome: D. Rubenstein, et al.; Pediatrics, March 1978, issue 61(3), pp. 433–437.
Gianotti-Crosti Syndrome: A Review of Ten Cases Not Associated With Hepatitis-B: K.L. Spear, et al.; Arch. Dermatol., July 1984, issue 120(7), pp. 891–896.
Gianotti-Crosti Syndrome: A Study of 26 Cases: A. Taieb, et al.; Br. J. Dermatol., July 1986, issue 115(1), pp. 49–59.

GRANULOMA ANNULARE

Description Granuloma annulare is a benign dermatologic disease characterized by ringlike papules or nodules that may be confined to certain areas or disseminated over a large part of the body. It may be self-limited or chronic and recurrent.

Signs and Symptoms The circular lesions are indurated and reddish brown, yellow, or flesh-colored, with centers of normal or slightly depressed skin. Usually the lesions appear on the dorsa of the hands and feet, and on the ankles, knees, or elbows. The disorder's chronicity may have a pattern of remissions and recurrence.

The diagnosis is established histopathologically where there are granulomas with necrobiotic destruction of collagen resembling rheumatoid nodules. A disseminated form may be associated with sun exposure.

Etiology Granuloma annulare is idiopathic, and the cause is unknown. The disseminated form may occur in diabetes mellitus or as a complication of pseudorheumatoid nodules or herpes zoster. Some types of the disorder are familial, but the trait is undetermined.

Epidemiology Both children and adults may develop the disorder. Females are affected more often than males.

Related Disorders The condition must be distinguished from sarcoidosis and syphilis. Also to be differentiated is **eruptive xanthoma,** marked by groups of tiny yellow or yellow-brown elevated spots, perhaps ringed in red, in generalized distribution.

Treatment—Standard Spontaneous remission is common. Isotretinoin and dapsone are indicated in chronic types of the disorder. *(NOTE: Care should be taken in prescribing these drugs for pregnant and nursing women.)*

Treatment—Investigational Please contact the agencies listed under Resources, below, for the most current information.

Resources
  For more information on granuloma annulare: National Organization for Rare Disorders (NORD); The National Arthritis and Musculoskeletal and Skin Diseases Information Clearinghouse.

References
Dermatology, 3rd ed.: O. Braun-Falco, et al.; Springer-Verlag, 1991.
Skin Signs of Systemic Disease: I.M. Braverman; W.B. Saunders Company, 1981.

Dermatology in General Medicine: Textbook and Atlas, 3rd ed.: T.B. Fitzpatrick, et al., eds.; McGraw-Hill, 1987.

Dermatology, 2nd ed. (3rd ed., 1992): S.L. Moschella and H.J. Hurley, eds.; W.B. Saunders Company, 1985.

Textbook of Dermatology, 4th ed.: A. Rook, et al., eds.; Blackwell Scientific Publications, 1986.

Localized Granuloma Annulare Associated with Insulin-Dependent Diabetes Mellitus: M.F. Muhlemann, et al., Brit. J. Dermatol., September 1984, issue 111(3), pp. 325–329.

Resolution of Disseminated Granuloma Annulare Following Isotretinoin Therapy: S.M. Schleicher, et al.; Cutis, August 1985, issue 36(2), pp. 147–148.

Sulfone Treatment of Granuloma Annulare: A. Steiner, et al.; J. Am. Acad. Dermatol., December 1985, issue 13(6), pp. 1004–1008.

HAIRY TONGUE

Description Hairy tongue is a disorder characterized by discoloration of the tongue and excessive growth of the filiform papillae.

Synonyms
Black Hairy Tongue
Lingua Nigra

Signs and Symptoms The tongue appears yellow, brown, black, or blue, and the papillae form a V shape at its rear. These signs may disappear spontaneously and, in some cases, recur. There is often a bad taste in the mouth.

Etiology The disorder may result from changes in the oral flora caused by antibiotics or be due to the excessive use of certain mouthwashes. Some cases seem to be the result of reduced saliva, or of fever. Tobacco can stain the papillae.

Epidemiology Onset and duration of hairy tongue are variable. The disorder can affect both males and females, and is seen in children and adults.

Related Disorders Differential diagnosis includes the following disorders.

Glossitis (inflammation of the tongue) may occur in association with candidiasis, anemia, diabetes mellitus, latent nutritional deficiencies, and malignancies.

Geographic tongue is characterized by migratory lesions of smooth, sore, and sometimes itchy patches on the tongue. Episodes typically may remit and then recur. The cause is unknown; the disorder may be familial.

In **Moeller's glossitis** the tongue is slick, glossy, or glazed. The lesions are often a concomitant sign of pernicious anemia. They can cause great discomfort and are persistent.

Severe acute glossitis can occasionally be the result of local infection, burns, or injury to the tongue, with ensuing pain and tenderness, and swelling that in severe cases blocks air passages.

In **burning tongue (burning mouth) syndrome** patients experience a burning sensation. There is no obvious clinical evidence of inflammation. The disorder may be one of the first signs of vitamin B12 deficiency. A *Candida albicans* infection or denture irritation may also be responsible. Other suggested etiologies include allergic reactions to pollen, cereals, and metals, and materials used in the manufacture of dentures. The disorder may be a hysterical symptom and an early sign of depression in middle-aged or older women.

Treatment—Standard Treatment includes avoidance of irritants and substances that can sensitize the tongue. Discontinuation of antibiotics or mouthwashes usually results in disappearance of symptoms as normal oral flora regenerate. In some cases the symptoms disappear spontaneously.

Treatment—Investigational Please contact the organizations listed under Resources, below, for the most current information.

Resources

For more information on hairy tongue: National Organization for Rare Disorders (NORD); NIH/National Institute of Dental Research; Clinical Smell and Taste Research Center, University of Pennsylvania Hospital; Connecticut Chemosensory Clinical Research Center, University of Connecticut Health Center.

References
Dermatology, 3rd ed.: O. Braun Falco, et al.; Springer-Verlag, 1991.

Skin Signs of Systemic Disease: I.M. Braverman; W.B. Saunders Company, 1981.

Dermatology in General Medicine: Textbook and Atlas, 3rd ed.: T.B. Fitzpatrick, et al., eds.; McGraw-Hill, 1987.

Dermatology, 2nd ed. (3rd ed., 1992): S.L. Moschella and H.J. Hurley, eds.; W.B. Saunders Company, 1985.

Textbook of Dermatology, 4th ed.: A. Rook, et al., eds.; Blackwell Scientific Publications, 1986.

HIDRADENITIS SUPPURATIVA

Description Hidradenitis suppurativa is a chronic inflammatory process with scarring associated with bacterial infection of the apocrine glands. Subcutaneous nodules in the involved area are similar to furuncles.

Synonyms
Apocrinitis
Hidrosadenitis Axillaris

Signs and Symptoms Patients commonly complain of pain in the involved sites, which are usually axillary or inguinal but are sometimes anogenital. Examination shows subcutaneous inflamed nodules that resemble boils. Tenderness and a purulent exudate are present. Patients may be febrile and lose weight. Eventually, scarring of tissue in inflamed sites may produce a tender, bound-down mass. The lesions may recur.

Etiology Hidradenitis is idiopathic, and the cause for destruction of the apocrine glands is unknown. Hidradenitis suppurativa has been associated with endocrine disorders and the use of depilatories or deodorants.

Epidemiology Onset is commonly during puberty. Men and women are affected in equal numbers.

Related Disorders Differential diagnosis includes the following disorders.

Furunculosis, the common boil, usually stems from a staphylococcal infection of hair follicles or the sebaceous glands. The erythematous, painful nodules may burst and emit pus, and they may recur. Among the settings in which they occur are inadequate hygiene, obesity, diabetes mellitus, blood disorders, poor health, and malnutrition.

Aural furunculosis can develop from a scratch in the ear or discharge of pus from the middle ear. Frequently the patient has boils elsewhere, has diabetes mellitus, or is in poor health. Symptoms include mild hearing impairment, a feeling of pressure on the ear from a swollen mass, and fever. The mass eventually ruptures and drains. When treated, lasting injury to the ear is unlikely.

American cutaneous leishmaniasis is due to the bite of a sandfly *(Phlebotomus)*, which is indigenous to Central and South America. The lesions itch intensely, and are accompanied by joint pain, weight loss, and poor health.

Pyoderma gangrenosum, cutaneous inflammatory bowel disease (Crohn's disease), and **actinomycosis** may also resemble hidradenitis suppurativa.

Treatment—Standard The patient should avoid antiperspirants or other skin irritants such as depilatories. Rest and local moist heat are helpful. Oral antibiotic therapy is required. Excision and/or plastic surgery may be necessary in the most persistent cases.

Recurrence at the same location after surgical removal is likely. Recurrences are fewer when excision is followed by split skin grafting or local skin flap cover.

Treatment—Investigational An antiandrogen (cyproterone acetate) in combination with estrogen therapy is being tried in women with longstanding severe cases of hidradenitis suppurativa. At times, cyproterone acetate alone has achieved control.

Please contact the agencies listed under Resources, below, for the most current information.

Resources

For more information on hidradenitis suppurativa: National Organization for Rare Disorders (NORD); NIH/National Institute of Allergy and Infectious Diseases; The National Arthritis and Musculoskeletal and Skin Diseases Information Clearinghouse.

References
Dermatology, 3rd ed.: O. Braun-Falco, et al.; Springer-Verlag, 1991.
Skin Signs of Systemic Disease: I.M. Braverman; W.B. Saunders Company, 1981.
Dermatology in General Medicine: Textbook and Atlas, 3rd ed.: T.B. Fitzpatrick, et al., eds.; McGraw-Hill, 1987.
Dermatology, 2nd ed. (3rd ed., 1992): S.L. Moschella and H.J. Hurley, eds.; W.B. Saunders Company, 1985.
Textbook of Dermatology, 4th ed.: A. Rook, et al., eds.; Blackwell Scientific Publications, 1986.

Control of Hidradenitis Suppurativa in Women Using Combined Antiandrogen (Cyproterone Acetate) and Oestrogen Therapy: R.S. Sawers, et al.: Br. J. Dermatol., September 1986, issue 115(3), pp. 269–274.

Hidradenitis Suppurativa–A Clinical Review: J.D. Watson; Br. J. Plast. Surg., October 1985, issue 38(4), pp. 567–569.

HYPERHIDROSIS

Description This condition is characterized by constitutional hyperactivity of the eccrine sweat glands. The disorder may be generalized and consist of excessive body sweating, or localized, with sweating confined to the palms, soles, armpits, groin, and under the breasts.

Synonyms
Excessive Perspiration
Excessive Sweating
Genuine Hyperhidrosis

Signs and Symptoms As a rule, onset is in childhood or during puberty. Patients experience a heightened reaction to sweating stimuli such as anxiety, pain, exercise, tension, caffeine, and nicotine. The sweat-prone areas may be localized or generalized. When the palms and soles are involved, the skin may appear pink or blue-white, and may even macerate, crack, or scale, particularly on the feet. Patients often experience spontaneous relief in adult life.

Etiology The etiology is unknown. However, one must distinguish idiopathic hyperhidrosis from excess sweating due to malfunction of the thyroid or pituitary gland, infection, diabetes mellitus, tumors, gout, menopause, and drunkenness.

Related Disorders See *Frey Syndrome.*

Epidemiology The disorder affects males and females in equal numbers.

Treatment—Standard Before treating generalized hyperhidrosis, a primary disorder must be ruled out.

For patients with palmar-plantar-type hyperhidrosis, cotton socks and shoes that promote the circulation of air prevent overheating of the feet. Alternating footwear is helpful. Applications of medicated powder formulated to hamper bacterial growth and absorb moisture may be beneficial, but cornstarch is not recommended.

For refractory cases, topical agents, such as aluminum chloride in ethyl alcohol, may be indicated. Short-term courses of anticholinergic drugs are also useful in severely afflicted patients, but the side effects of dry mouth, drowsiness, and constipation frequently occur.

Sympathectomy will not completely overcome the excessive sweating, and recurrence is not unlikely. Furthermore, the sequela may be Horner syndrome, in which nerve paralysis results in drooping eyelids.

Biofeedback has met with varying degrees of success.

Treatment—Investigational Iontophoresis, in which ions are electrically driven into the skin, is being used to treat the condition.

Please contact the agencies listed under Resources, below, for the most current information.

Resources

For more information on hyperhidrosis: National Organization for Rare Disorders (NORD); National Institute of Diabetes, Digestive & Kidney Diseases Information Clearinghouse.

References

Dermatology, 3rd ed.: O. Braun-Falco, et al.; Springer-Verlag, 1991.

Skin Signs of Systemic Disease: I.M. Braverman; W.B. Saunders Company, 1981.

Dermatology in General Medicine: Textbook and Atlas, 3rd ed.: T.B. Fitzpatrick, et al., eds.; McGraw-Hill, 1987.

Dermatology, 2nd ed. (3rd ed., 1992): S.L. Moschella and H.J. Hurley, eds.; W.B. Saunders Company, 1985.

Textbook of Dermatology, 4th ed.: A. Rook, et al., eds.; Blackwell Scientific Publications, 1986.

Sweating it out: The Problem of Profuse Perspiration: D. Farley, FDA Consumer, December 1985–January 1986, pp. 21–25.

ICHTHYOSIS

Description The ichthyoses are a group of cutaneous disorders of keratinization.

Signs and Symptoms Ichthyosis is characterized by dry, scaly, itchy, erythematous skin, often over large areas of the body. Symptoms range from mild to severe, and remissions can occur.

Etiology Most known forms of ichthyosis are inherited, some as dominant traits, some as recessive.

Epidemiology Most ichthyoses are present at birth and affect males and females in equal numbers. X-linked ichthyosis affects only males.

Related Disorders See *Ichthyosis Congenita; Ichthyosis, Harlequin Type; Ichthyosis Hystrix, Curth-Macklin Type; Ichthyosis, Lamellar Recessive; Ichthyosis Vulgaris; Ichthyosis, X-Linked.*

See also *Conradi-Hünermann Syndrome; Darier Disease; Epidermolytic Hyperkeratosis; Erythrokeratodermia Symmetrica Progressiva; Erythrokeratodermia Variabilis; Erythrokeratolysis Hiemalis; Keratosis Follicularis Spinulosa Decalvans; Sjögren-Larsson Syndrome; Tay Syndrome.*

Treatment—Standard Symptoms can be alleviated by application of keratolytics and emollients, including plain petroleum jelly. This can be especially effective after bathing while the skin is still moist. Salicylic acid gel, applied under occlusion, is useful in some instances for removal of scales. Lactate lotion can also be an effective keratolytic. Topical and systemic retinoids can be beneficial in some cases but must be used with caution because of adverse side effects, including those to fetal development in pregnant women.

Treatment—Investigational Please contact the agencies listed under Resources, below, for the most current information.

Resources

For more information on ichthyosis: National Organization for Rare Disorders (NORD); Foundation for Ichthyosis and Related Skin Types, Inc. (F.I.R.S.T.); National Arthritis, Musculoskeletal & Skin (NIAMS) Information Clearinghouse.

For genetic information and genetic counseling referrals: March of Dimes Birth Defects Foundation; National Center for Education in Maternal and Child Health (NCEMCH).

References

Dermatology, 3rd ed.: O. Braun-Falco, et al.; Springer-Verlag, 1991.

Skin Signs of Systemic Disease: I.M. Braverman; W.B. Saunders Company, 1981.

Dermatology in General Medicine: Textbook and Atlas, 3rd ed.: T.B. Fitzpatrick, et al., eds.; McGraw-Hill, 1987.

Dermatology, 2nd ed. (3rd ed., 1992): S.L. Moschella and H.J. Hurley, eds.; W.B. Saunders Company, 1985.

Textbook of Dermatology, 4th ed.: A. Rook, et al., eds.; Blackwell Scientific Publications, 1986.

Genetically Transmitted, Generalized Disorders of Cornification. The Ichthyoses: M.L. Williams, et al., Dermatol. Clin., January 1987, issue 5(1), pp. 155–178.

Therapeutic Activity of Lactate 12% Lotion in the Treatment of Ichthyosis. Active Versus Vehicle and Active Versus a Petroleum Cream: M. Buxman, et al., J. Am. Acad. Dermatol., December 1986, issue 15(6), pp. 1253–1258.

ICHTHYOSIS CONGENITA

Description Ichthyosis congenita comprises a group of inherited skin disorders characterized by dry, rough, and erythematous skin of various degrees of severity.

Synonyms

      Collodion Baby
      Congenital Ichthyosiform Erythroderma
      Desquamation of Newborn
      Harlequin Fetus

Signs and Symptoms The skin over most of the body typically is red, dry, and rough, and also may be scaly and itchy. The skin on the palms of the hands and soles of the feet may be abnormally thick.

Etiology The ichthyosis congenita syndromes are all probably transmitted as autosomal recessive inherited disorders, with some forms being sex-linked.

Epidemiology The ichthyosis congenita syndromes are rare. Symptoms onset is pre- or postnatal.

Related Disorders See *Ichthyosis Vulgaris; Ichthyosis, X-Linked; Epider-*

molytic Hyperkeratosis.

Treatment—Standard The symptoms may be alleviated by application of kera-tolytics and emollients, including plain petroleum jelly. This can be especially effective after bathing while the skin is still moist. Salicylic acid gel is useful in some instances for removal of scales. Lactate lotion also can be an effective kera-tolytic. Topical and systemic retinoids can be beneficial in some cases but must be used with caution because of potentially adverse side effects.

Treatment—Investigational Investigational approaches include the local applica-tion of cholesterol and of therapeutic agents that can hydrolyze the cholesterol sul-fate bond.

Please contact the agencies listed under Resources, below, for the most current information.

Resources

For more information on ichthyosis congenita: National Organization for Rare Disorders (NORD); Foundation for Ichthyosis and Related Skin Types, Inc. (F.I.R.S.T.); The National Arthritis and Musculoskeletal and Skin Diseases Infor-mation Clearinghouse.

For genetic information and genetic counseling referrals: March of Dimes Birth Defects Foundation; National Center for Education in Maternal and Child Health (NCEMCH).

References

Dermatology, 3rd ed.: O. Braun-Falco, et al.; Springer-Verlag, 1991.

Skin Signs of Systemic Disease: I.M. Braverman; W.B. Saunders Company, 1981.

Dermatology in General Medicine: Textbook and Atlas, 3rd ed.: T.B. Fitzpatrick, et al., eds.; McGraw-Hill, 1987.

Dermatology, 2nd ed. (3rd ed., 1992): S.L. Moschella and H.J. Hurley, eds.; W.B. Saunders Company, 1985.

Textbook of Dermatology, 4th ed.: A. Rook, et al., eds.; Blackwell Scientific Publications, 1986.

Mendelian Inheritance in Man, 9th ed.: V.A. McKusick; The Johns Hopkins University Press, 1990, p. 1272.

Cecil Textbook of Medicine, 18th ed.: J.B. Wyngaarden and L.H. Smith, Jr., eds.; W.B. Saunders Company, 1988, pp. 2326–2329.

ICHTHYOSIS, HARLEQUIN TYPE

Description This rare, autosomal recessive skin disorder is characterized by the appearance at birth of very large, thick skin plates causing facial distortion and var-ious other constricting deformities.

Synonyms

> Harlequin Fetus
> Ichthyosis Congenita, Harlequin Fetus Type

Signs and Symptoms Newborns with the disease have massive, thick scales on the skin. The top layer of skin reveals an abnormally large number of squames, thought to be caused by a defect in the metabolism of the corneocytes. Constriction of the chest and abdomen causes respiration and feeding difficulties. Harlequin-type ichthyosis can be detected by fetoscopy.

Etiology The disorder is transmitted through autosomal recessive genes that cause formation of abnormal keratins.

Epidemiology The disorder is evident in utero. Males and females are affected in equal numbers.

Related Disorders See *Ichthyosis; Ichthyosis Congenita; Ichthyosis Hystrix, Curth-Macklin Type; Ichthyosis, Lamellar Recessive.*

See also *Epidermolytic Hyperkeratosis; Netherton Syndrome; Sjögren-Larsson Syndrome.*

Treatment—Standard Treatment is only palliative. Symptoms can be alleviated by application of keratolytics and emollients, including plain petroleum jelly. This can be especially effective after bathing while the skin is still moist. Salicylic acid gel is useful in some instances for removal of scales.

Treatment—Investigational Please contact the agencies listed under Resources, below, for the most current information.

Resources

For more information on harlequin-type ichthyosis: National Organization for Rare Disorders (NORD); Foundation for Ichthyosis and Related Skin Types, Inc. (F.I.R.S.T.); The National Arthritis and Musculoskeletal and Skin Diseases Information Clearinghouse.

For genetic information and genetic counseling referrals: March of Dimes Birth Defects Foundation; National Center for Education in Maternal and Child Health (NCEMCH).

References
Dermatology, 3rd ed.: O. Braun-Falco, et al.; Springer-Verlag, 1991.

Skin Signs of Systemic Disease: I.M. Braverman; W.B. Saunders Company, 1981.

Dermatology in General Medicine: Textbook and Atlas, 3rd ed.: T.B. Fitzpatrick, et al., eds.; McGraw-Hill, 1987.

Dermatology, 2nd ed. (3rd ed., 1992): S.L. Moschella and H.J. Hurley, eds.; W.B. Saunders Company, 1985.

Textbook of Dermatology, 4th ed.: A. Rook, et al., eds.; Blackwell Scientific Publications, 1986.

Genetically Transmitted, Generalized Disorders of Cornification. The Ichthyoses: M.L. Williams, et al.; Dermatol. Clin., January 1987, issue 5(1), pp. 155–178.

Therapeutic Activity of Lactate 12% Lotion in the Treatment of Ichthyosis. Active Versus Vehicle and Active Versus a Petroleum Cream: M. Buxman, et al.; J. Am. Acad. Dermatol., December 1986, issue 15(6), pp. 1253–1258.

ICHTHYOSIS HYSTRIX, CURTH-MACKLIN TYPE

Description Ichthyosis hystrix, Curth-Macklin type, is a rare inherited skin disorder characterized by ichthyosis that can range from mild to severe. Keratoderma may be limited to the palms and soles or may extend to other parts of the body surface.

Signs and Symptoms In ichthyosis hystrix, Curth-Macklin type, the skin on the soles of the feet and the palms of the hands is abnormally thick and hard. In some cases, widespread hyperkeratosis is also seen. Microscopic examination reveals many corneocytes with 2 nuclei and prominent nuclear shells.

Etiology The disorder is transmitted by autosomal dominant genes.

Epidemiology Onset is at birth. Males and females are affected in equal numbers.

Related Disorders See *Ichthyosis Congenita; Ichthyosis Vulgaris; Epidermolytic Hyperkeratosis.*

Treatment—Standard The cutaneous symptoms of ichthyosis hystrix, Curth-Macklin type, can be alleviated by the application of keratolytics and emollient ointments, including plain petroleum jelly. This can be especially effective after bathing while the skin is still moist. Salicylic acid gel and lactate lotion can be useful. Topical and systemic retinoids are beneficial in some cases but must be used with caution because of potentially adverse side effects.

Treatment—Investigational Please contact the agencies listed under Resources, below, for the most current information.

Resources

For more information on ichthyosis hystrix, Curth-Macklin type: National Organization for Rare Disorders (NORD); Foundation for Ichthyosis and Related Skin Types, Inc. (F.I.R.S.T.); The National Arthritis and Musculoskeletal and Skin Diseases Information Clearinghouse.

For genetic information and genetic counseling referrals: March of Dimes Birth Defects Foundation; National Center for Education in Maternal and Child Health (NCEMCH).

References
Dermatology, 3rd ed.: O. Braun-Falco, et al.; Springer-Verlag, 1991.
Skin Signs of Systemic Disease: I.M. Braverman; W.B. Saunders Company, 1981.
Dermatology in General Medicine: Textbook and Atlas, 3rd ed.: T.B. Fitzpatrick, et al., eds.; McGraw-Hill, 1987.
Dermatology, 2nd ed. (3rd ed., 1992): S.L. Moschella and H.J. Hurley, eds.; W.B. Saunders Company, 1985.
Textbook of Dermatology, 4th ed.: A. Rook, et al., eds.; Blackwell Scientific Publications, 1986.
Genetically Transmitted, Generalized Disorders of Cornification. The Ichthyoses: M.L. Williams, et al.; Dermatol. Clin., January 1987, issue 5(1), pp. 155–178.
Ichthyosis Hystrix (Curth-Macklin). Light and Electron Microscopic Studies Performed Before and After Etretinate Treatment: L. Kanerva, et al.; Arch. Dermatol., September 1984, issue 120(9), pp. 1218–1223.
Therapeutic Activity of Lactate 12% Lotion in the Treatment of Ichthyosis. Active Versus Vehicle and Active Versus a Petroleum Cream: Buxman, et al.; J. Am. Acad. Dermatol., December 1986, issue 15(6), pp. 1253–1258.

Mendelian Inheritance in Man, 9th ed.: V.A. McKusick; The Johns Hopkins University Press, 1990, p. 507.

ICHTHYOSIS, LAMELLAR RECESSIVE

Description Lamellar recessive ichthyosis is characterized by extreme hyperkeratosis over the entire body surface.

Signs and Symptoms Large, dark, platelike scales appear over the entire body surface. Ectropion of the eyelids and lips may be present. Erythroderma may underlie the scales, and keratoderma may occur on the palms of the hands and soles of the feet. Lamellar recessive ichthyosis in a newborn resembles the collodion baby type of ichthyosis congenita. Sweating is impaired and patients have secondary bacterial infections in their skin. Lipid analysis of the stratum corneum shows increased free sterols and ceramides but normal hydrocarbon content.

Etiology The disorder is transmitted through autosomal recessive genes.

Epidemiology Lamellar recessive ichthyosis is very rare, affecting fewer than 1:100,000 births. Males and females are affected in equal numbers.

Related Disorders See *Ichthyosis Congenita; Ichthyosis Hystrix; Epidermolytic Hyperkeratosis; Sjögren-Larsson Syndrome.*

Treatment—Standard The discomfort of the dry, scaly skin can be alleviated by application of keratolytics and emollients, including plain petroleum jelly. This can be especially effective after bathing while the skin is still moist. Salicylic acid gel is useful in some instances for removal of scales. Topical and systemic retinoids can be beneficial in some cases but must be used with caution because of potentially adverse side effects. Surgical correction of the ectropion is of some benefit in severe cases. Topical and systemic antibiotics may be useful.

Treatment—Investigational Please contact the agencies listed under Resources, below, for the most current information.

Resources

For more information on lamellar recessive ichthyosis: National Organization for Rare Disorders (NORD); Foundation for Ichthyosis and Related Skin Types, Inc. (F.I.R.S.T.); The National Arthritis and Musculoskeletal and Skin Diseases Information Clearinghouse.

For genetic information and genetic counseling referrals: March of Dimes Birth Defects Foundation; National Center for Education in Maternal and Child Health (NCEMCH).

References
Dermatology, 3rd ed.: O. Braun-Falco, et al.; Springer-Verlag, 1991.
Skin Signs of Systemic Disease: I.M. Braverman; W.B. Saunders Company, 1981.
Dermatology in General Medicine: Textbook and Atlas, 3rd ed.: T.B. Fitzpatrick, et al., eds.; McGraw-Hill, 1987.

Dermatology, 2nd ed. (3rd ed., 1992): S.L. Moschella and H.J. Hurley, eds.; W.B. Saunders Company, 1985.

Textbook of Dermatology, 4th ed.: A. Rook, et al., eds.; Blackwell Scientific Publications, 1986.

Genetically Transmitted, Generalized Disorders of Cornification. The Ichthyoses: M.L. Williams, et al.; Dermatol. Clin., January 1987, issue 5(1), pp. 155–178.

Ichthyosis Hystrix (Curth-Macklin). Light and Electron Microscopic Studies Performed Before and After Etretinate Treatment: L. Kanerva, et al.; Arch. Dermatol., September 1984, issue 120(9), pp. 1218–1223.

Therapeutic Activity of Lactate 12% Lotion in the Treatment of Ichthyosis. Active Versus Vehicle and Active Versus a Petroleum Cream: Buxman, et al.; Journ. Am. Acad. Dermatol., December 1986, issue 15(6), pp. 1253–1258.

Mendelian Inheritance in Man, 9th ed.: V.A. McKusick; The Johns Hopkins University Press, 1990, p. 507.

ICHTHYOSIS VULGARIS

Description Ichthyosis vulgaris is an inherited disorder characterized by firmly adherent scales on the skin.

Synonyms
Ichthyosis Simplex

Signs and Symptoms Symptoms usually begin during the first year of life, and may vary from mild to severe. Features of this disorder include hyperkeratosis and the development of fish-scale–like skin on the back and over extensor surfaces. Pronounced palm and sole markings are commonly seen. In approximately 50 percent of patients, atopic dermatitis also is observed. Hay fever, asthma, or eczema may be present. Symptoms tend to improve with age and change of season, and in moist, warm climates.

Etiology The disorder is transmitted through autosomal dominant inheritance. The cause is unknown, but epidermal proliferation rate and transit time are normal. Thus, the symptoms are thought to be due to abnormal retention and decreased shedding of scales.

Epidemiology Ichthyosis affects approximately 1:250 persons in the United States. The disorder occurs in males and females in equal numbers.

Related Disorders See *Ichthyosis Congenita; Ichthyosis Hystrix, Curth-Macklin Type; Epidermolytic Hyperkeratosis; Netherton Syndrome; Sjögren-Larsson Syndrome.*

Treatment—Standard Cutaneous symptoms can be alleviated by application of keratolytics and emollient ointments, including plain petroleum jelly. This can be especially effective after bathing while the skin is still moist. Salicylic acid gel and lactate lotion are also effective. Topical and systemic retinoids can be beneficial in some cases but must be used with caution because of potentially adverse side effects.

Treatment—Investigational Please contact the agencies listed under Resources,

below, for the most current information.

Resources

For more information on ichthyosis vulgaris: National Organization for Rare Disorders (NORD); Foundation for Ichthyosis and Related Skin Types, Inc. (F.I.R.S.T.); The National Arthritis and Musculoskeletal and Skin Diseases Information Clearinghouse.

For genetic information and genetic counseling referrals: March of Dimes Birth Defects Foundation; National Center for Education in Maternal and Child Health (NCEMCH).

References

Dermatology, 3rd ed.: O. Braun-Falco, et al.; Springer-Verlag, 1991.

Skin Signs of Systemic Disease: I.M. Braverman; W.B. Saunders Company, 1981.

Dermatology in General Medicine: Textbook and Atlas, 3rd ed.: T.B. Fitzpatrick, et al., eds.; McGraw-Hill, 1987.

Dermatology, 2nd ed. (3rd ed., 1992): S.L. Moschella and H.J. Hurley, eds.; W.B. Saunders Company, 1985.

Textbook of Dermatology, 4th ed.: A. Rook, et al., eds.; Blackwell Scientific Publications, 1986.

Genetically Transmitted, Generalized Disorders of Cornification. The Ichthyoses: M.L. Williams, et al.; Dermatol. Clin., January 1987, issue 5(1), pp. 155–178.

Therapeutic Activity of Lactate 12% Lotion in the Treatment of Ichthyosis. Active Versus Vehicle and Active Versus a Petroleum Cream: M. Buxman, et al.; J. Am. Acad. Dermatol., December 1986, issue 15(6), pp. 1253–1258.

ICHTHYOSIS, X-LINKED

Description X-linked ichthyosis is a genetic skin disorder of males linked to an inborn error of metabolism.

Synonyms

Steroid Sulfatase Deficiency

Signs and Symptoms Symptoms usually begin between 1 and 3 weeks of age with development of large, tightly adherent brownish scales. These are most prominent on the skin covering extensor surfaces, but the flexor surfaces may also be involved. The back of the neck is almost always scaly, and the skin in the hollows of the elbows and knees is less commonly affected. The trunk may be involved, but the face, scalp, palms, and soles are usually spared.

Symptoms often greatly improve in the summer.

Clouding of the cornea occurs in approximately 50 percent of adult men with X-linked ichthyosis. Affected males develop cryptorchidism in about 12 to 25 percent of cases, and may also be at increased risk of testicular malignancies. Normal functioning of sex hormones does not appear to be affected.

Diminished estrogen production may occur if a female carrier is pregnant with an affected male, and there may be a delay in labor and difficulties with cervical dilation. The disorder can be detected by amniocentesis.

Etiology X-Linked genes transmit the disorder. This is a retention hyperkeratosis with normal epidermal proliferation rate and transit times. The condition is associated with a deficiency of steroid sulfatase, resulting in several biochemical alterations in keratocyte biology and in steroid sex hormone metabolism. Maternal estrogen production is diminished in late pregnancy in carrier females. Cholesterol sulfate may accumulate in the blood and skin.

Epidemiology X-linked ichthyosis is rare, affecting slightly more than 1:6000 males. Female carriers are usually asymptomatic but may have mild scaling and clouding of corneas.

Related Disorders See *Ichthyosis Congenita; Ichthyosis Hystrix, Curth-Macklin Type; Ichthyosis, Lamellar Recessive; Darier Disease; Epidermolytic Hyperkeratosis; Netherton Syndrome; Sjögren-Larsson Syndrome.*

Treatment—Standard Cutaneous manifestations of X-linked ichthyosis can be alleviated by the application of keratolytics and emollients, including plain petroleum jelly. This can be especially effective after bathing while the skin is still moist. Salicylic acid gel is useful in some instances for removal of scales. Topical and systemic retinoids can be beneficial in some cases but must be used with caution because of potentially adverse side effects.

Treatment—Investigational Please contact the agencies listed under Resources, below, for the most current information.

Resources

For more information on X-linked recessive ichthyosis: National Organization for Rare Disorders (NORD); Foundation for Ichthyosis and Related Skin Types, Inc. (F.I.R.S.T.); The National Arthritis and Musculoskeletal and Skin Diseases Information Clearinghouse.

For genetic information and genetic counseling referrals: March of Dimes Birth Defects Foundation; National Center for Education in Maternal and Child Health (NCEMCH).

References
Dermatology, 3rd ed.: O. Braun-Falco, et al.; Springer-Verlag, 1991.

Skin Signs of Systemic Disease: I.M. Braverman; W.B. Saunders Company, 1981.

Dermatology in General Medicine: Textbook and Atlas, 3rd ed.: T.B. Fitzpatrick, et al., eds.; McGraw-Hill, 1987.

Dermatology, 2nd ed. (3rd ed., 1992): S.L. Moschella and H.J. Hurley, eds.; W.B. Saunders Company, 1985.

Textbook of Dermatology, 4th ed.: A. Rook, et al., eds.; Blackwell Scientific Publications, 1986.

Genetically Transmitted, Generalized Disorders of Cornification. The Ichthyoses: M.L. Williams, et al.; Dermatol. Clin., January 1987, issue 5(1), pp. 155–178.

Therapeutic Activity of Lactate 12% Lotion in the Treatment of Ichthyosis. Active Versus Vehicle and Active Versus a Petroleum Cream: M. Buxman, et al.; Journ. Am. Acad. Dermatol., December 1986, issue 15(6), pp. 1253–1258.

Topical Cholesterol Treatment of Recessive X-Linked Ichthyosis: G. Lykkesfeldt, et al.; Lancet, December 1983, issue 2(8363), pp. 1337–1338.

INCONTINENTIA PIGMENTI

Description The disorder is characterized by unusual patterns of discolored skin caused by excessive deposits of melanin. Developmental abnormalities are sometimes seen; and oral, visual, and neurologic symptoms may occur.

Synonyms
> Bloch-Siemens-Sulzberger Syndrome
> Bloch-Sulzberger Syndrome

Signs and Symptoms There are 4 stages of progression in incontinentia pigmenti. Onset of the first stage is typically between birth and 6 months. The skin is inflamed and red, with spiral or linear patterns of small, fluid-filled blisters. The white cell count is usually elevated.

The skin in the 2nd stage is characterized by rough, warty growths following the same patterns as the blisters in the first stage. The lesions more commonly are found on the arms and legs, less often on the head or trunk. These lesions generally resolve during early childhood, although the condition has been reported as persisting in some patients to age 16.

The 3rd stage generally begins between 3 months and 2 years, often as the lesions of the first 2 stages are resolving. Abnormal deposits of melanin cause spots of discoloration that may be brown or gray. These spots appear in linear or spiral patterns in areas previously unaffected. This stage generally resolves by adolescence, although the condition persists into adulthood in occasional cases.

A 4th stage sometimes occurs, consisting of loss of pigmentation and atrophy in areas of discoloration. Hair loss and scarring are seen rarely.

Approximately 50 percent of affected persons also have nondermatologic symptoms and signs. These include dental abnormalities such as tooth decay or loss, diminished vision, and neurologic findings such as seizures or mild paralysis.

Developmental abnormalities may accompany incontinentia pigmenti but are not typical: short stature, clubfoot, spina bifida, skull and ear deformities, cleft lip or palate, hemiatrophy, chondrodystrophy, syndactyly, and congenital dislocation of the hip. There also have been very rare reported cases of woolly hair nevus and immune system dysfunction.

Etiology The cause is unknown. The disorder is thought to be inherited as an X-linked dominant trait that may be lethal to males.

Epidemiology Approximately 600 cases have been reported in this century. The condition affects females almost exclusively.

Related Disorders Incontinentia pigmenti achromians is unrelated to incontinentia pigmenti. It is inherited as an autosomal dominant trait and is characterized by a swirling pattern of skin hypopigmentation that resembles, in pattern only, the discolorations of incontinentia pigmenti. A variety of other developmental abnormalities may occur in conjunction with the disorder. Skin color tends to normalize as the individual ages.

Naegeli-Franceschetti-Jadassohn syndrome, inherited as an autosomal dominant trait, is characterized by reticulated skin pigmentation in childhood in previously normal children, that resembles incontinentia pigmenti. However, there are no inflammatory skin changes. Skin may thicken on the hands and feet, the ability to sweat may become impaired, and yellow mottling of the teeth may occur.

Treatment—Standard The cutaneous abnormalities generally resolve without treatment by adolescence or adulthood. The other aspects of the condition can usually be treated effectively by the appropriate specialist intervention. Treatment is otherwise symptomatic and supportive, and genetic counseling may be of benefit.

Treatment—Investigational Please contact the agencies listed under Resources, below, for the most current information.

Resources

For more information on incontinentia pigmenti: National Organization for Rare Disorders (NORD); The National Arthritis and Musculoskeletal and Skin Diseases Information Clearinghouse.

For genetic information and genetic counseling referrals: March of Dimes Birth Defects Foundation; National Center for Education in Maternal and Child Health (NCEMCH).

References

Dermatology, 3rd ed.: O. Braun-Falco, et al.; Springer-Verlag, 1991.

Skin Signs of Systemic Disease: I.M. Braverman; W.B. Saunders Company, 1981.

Dermatology in General Medicine: Textbook and Atlas, 3rd ed.: T.B. Fitzpatrick, et al., eds.; McGraw-Hill, 1987.

Dermatology, 2nd ed. (3rd ed., 1992): S.L. Moschella and H.J. Hurley, eds.; W.B. Saunders Company, 1985.

Textbook of Dermatology, 4th ed.: A. Rook, et al., eds.; Blackwell Scientific Publications, 1986.

Incontinentia Pigmenti. Study of 3 Families: B. Garcia-Bravo, et al.; Ann. Dermatol. Venereol., 1986, issue 113(4), pp. 301–308.

Dominant Disorders with Multiple Organ Involvement: M.F. Kegel; Dermatologic Clinics, January 1987, issue 5(1), pp. 210–214.

KERATOSIS FOLLICULARIS SPINULOSA DECALVANS

Description The disorder is a form of ichthyosis characterized by keratosis of the hair follicles, which leads to progressive scarring and alopecia.

Synonyms
Siemens Syndrome

Signs and Symptoms Keratosis around the hair follicles results in scarring and baldness. Atopy, photophobia, and keratitis may occur.

Etiology The disorder is inherited as an X-linked trait.

Epidemiology Female carriers usually have a milder form of the disease than affected males.

Related Disorders See *Ichthyosis Congenita; Ichthyosis, X-Linked.*

Treatment—Standard Symptoms can be alleviated by applications of keratolytics and emollients, including plain petroleum jelly. This can be especially effective after bathing while the skin is still moist. Salicylic acid gel is useful in some instances for removal of scales. Lactate lotion can also be an effective keratolytic. Topical and systemic retinoids are beneficial in some cases but must be used with caution because of potentially adverse side effects.

Treatment—Investigational Please contact the agencies listed under Resources, below, for the most current information.

Resources

For more information on **keratosis follicularis spinulosa decalvans:** National Organization for Rare Disorders (NORD); Foundation for Ichthyosis and Related Skin Types, Inc. (F.I.R.S.T.); The National Arthritis and Musculoskeletal and Skin Diseases Information Clearinghouse.

For **genetic information and genetic counseling referrals:** March of Dimes Birth Defects Foundation; National Center for Education in Maternal and Child Health (NCEMCH).

References

Dermatology, 3rd ed.: O. Braun-Falco, et al.; Springer-Verlag, 1991.

Skin Signs of Systemic Disease: I.M. Braverman; W.B. Saunders Company, 1981.

Dermatology in General Medicine: Textbook and Atlas, 3rd ed.: T.B. Fitzpatrick, et al., eds.; McGraw-Hill, 1987.

Dermatology, 2nd ed. (3rd ed., 1992): S.L. Moschella and H.J. Hurley, eds.; W.B. Saunders Company, 1985.

Textbook of Dermatology, 4th ed.: A. Rook, et al., eds.; Blackwell Scientific Publications, 1986.

Trichostasis Spinulosa: M.C. Young, et al.; Int. J. Dermatol., November 1985, issue 24(9), pp. 575–580.

Keratosis Spinulosa Decalvans. Report of Two Cases and Literature Review: Arch. Dermatol., January 1983, issue 119(1), pp. 22–26.

Genetically Transmitted, Generalized Disorders of Cornification. The Ichthyoses: M.L. Williams, et al.; Dermatol. Clin., January 1987, issue 5(1), pp. 155–178.

Therapeutic Activity of Lactate 12% Lotion in the Treatment of Ichthyosis. Active Versus Vehicle and Active Versus a Petroleum Cream: M. Buxman, et al.; J. Am. Acad. Dermatol., December 1986, issue 15(6), pp. 1253–1258.

LEINER DISEASE

Description Leiner disease is a skin disorder that typically appears during early infancy as seborrheic dermatitis and extends to erythroderma. A reddish patch of thickened skin appears on the buttocks, then spreads and is accompanied by scaling and peeling, itching, anemia, and diarrhea. Symptoms usually decrease after a few weeks with treatment.

Synonyms

Erythrodermia Desquamativa Leiner
Leiner-Moussous Desquamative Erythroderma
Severe Infantile Dermatitis

Signs and Symptoms The initial manifestation is the appearance of thick, reddish skin on the buttocks. The erythema soon involves the entire body, and after a few days may be followed by the appearance of crusty, dry, moist, or greasy scaling on the scalp. Scaling may also appear behind the ears, on the nose or eyebrows, or around the mouth. In some cases, thin sheets of skin may peel from these areas. Itching, anemia, and diarrhea are other typical findings. Loss of protein or electrolytes can result if skin infections are left untreated.

Etiology The etiology is unknown. It has been suggested that the disorder may be caused by toxic substances passed to infants through breast milk or originating in their intestinal tracts. A deficiency in C5 inhibitor may be a causative factor.

Epidemiology The disorder usually begins during the first 2 months of life. Breast-fed infants have a higher incidence. Males and females are affected in equal numbers.

Related Disorders Ritter disease (dermatitis exfoliativa neonatorum) is a skin disorder of infants, usually caused by a bacterial infection, and characterized by erythematous skin that may peel, leaving raw areas that heal in dry, crusty, yellow patches. This disorder may follow upper respiratory tract infections, impetigo, or other improperly treated infections.

Treatment—Standard Treatment usually involves hospitalization, to provide a controlled environment and to avoid nutritional deficiencies and skin infections. After a few weeks of careful treatment, redness and scaliness decrease and do not usually recur. However, 10 percent of cases may be fatal as a result of uncontrolled infection or severe electrolyte loss.

Treatment—Investigational Please contact the agencies listed under Resources, below, for the most current information.

Resources

For more information on Leiner disease: National Organization for Rare Disorders (NORD); The National Arthritis and Musculoskeletal and Skin Diseases Information Clearinghouse.

For genetic information and genetic counseling referrals: March of Dimes Birth Defects Foundation; National Center for Education in Maternal and Child Health (NCEMCH).

References

Dermatology, 3rd ed.: O. Braun-Falco, et al.; Springer-Verlag, 1991.

Skin Signs of Systemic Disease: I.M. Braverman; W.B. Saunders Company, 1981.

Dermatology in General Medicine: Textbook and Atlas, 3rd ed.: T.B. Fitzpatrick, et al., eds.; McGraw-Hill, 1987.

Dermatology, 2nd ed. (3rd ed., 1992): S.L. Moschella and H.J. Hurley, eds.; W.B. Saunders Company, 1985.

ATLAS OF VISUAL DIAGNOSIS

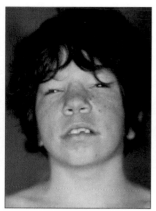

18p- syndrome (see p. 11)

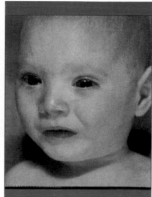

Cri du chat syndrome
(see p. 46)

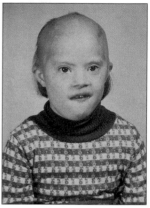

Down syndrome with alopecia
(see p. 55)

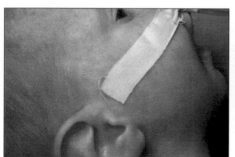

Trisomy 18 syndrome (see p. 143)

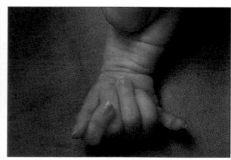

Trisomy 18 syndrome—typical hand (see p. 143)

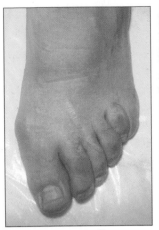

Laurence-Moon-Biedl
syndrome (see p. 85)

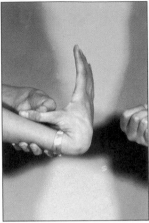

Marfan syndrome (see p. 92)

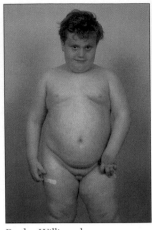

Prader-Willi syndrome
(see p. 113)

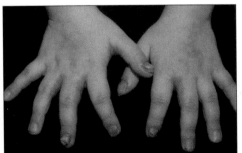

Moniliasis secondary to hypoparathyroidism
(see DiGeorge syndrome, p. 54)

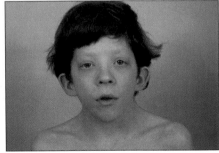

Noonan syndrome (see p. 102)

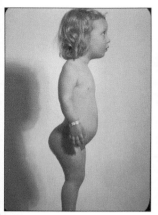

Spondyloepiphyseal dysplasia
(see pp. 128, 129)

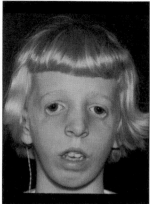

Treacher Collins syndrome
(see p. 135)

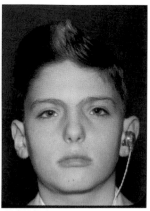

Waardenburg syndrome
(see p. 149)

Williams syndrome
(see p. 152)

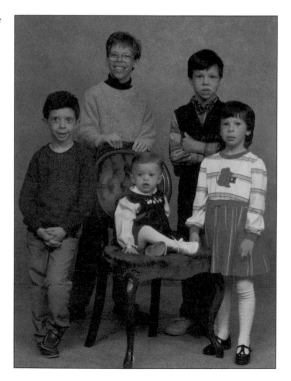

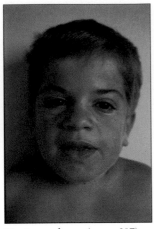
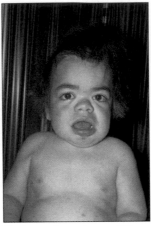
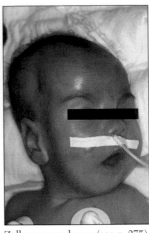

Hunter syndrome (see p. 207)   Hurler syndrome (see p. 209)   Zellweger syndrome (see p. 275)

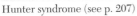

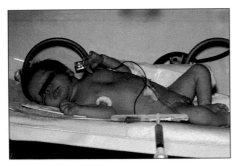

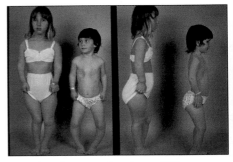

Catastrophically ill newborn with citrullinemia (see p. 186). This degree of hypotonia is typical of hyperammonemia.

Hypophosphatemic rickets (see p. 891)

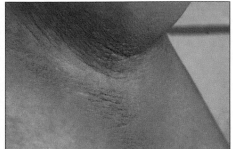

Acanthosis nigricans (see p. 731)

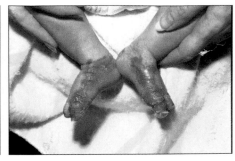

Acrodermatitis enteropathica (see p. 734)

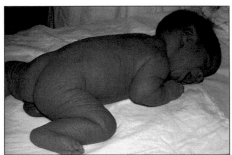

Cutis laxa (see p. 742)

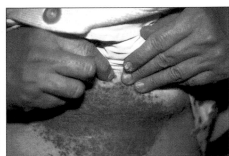

Darier disease (see p. 743)

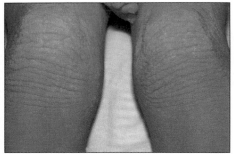

Epidermolytic hyperkeratosis (see p. 752)

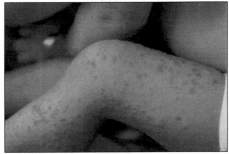

Gianotti-Crosti syndrome (see p. 759)

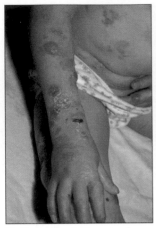

Epidermolysis bullosa simplex
(see p. 750)

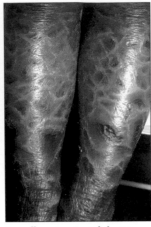

Lamellar recessive ichthyosis
(see p. 771)

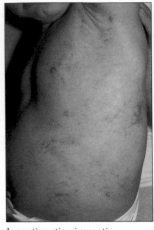

Incontinentia pigmenti
(see p. 775)

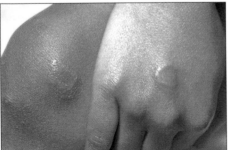

Granuloma annulare (see p. 761)

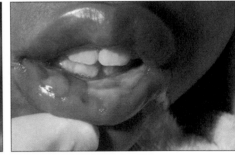

Benign mucosal pemphigoid (see p. 782)

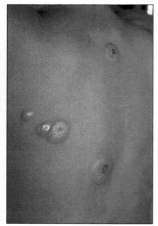

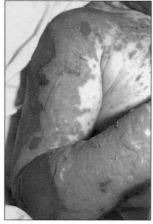

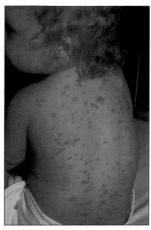

Sweet syndrome (see p. 793)

Toxic epidermal necrolysis (see p. 796)

Urticaria pigmentosa (see p. 798)

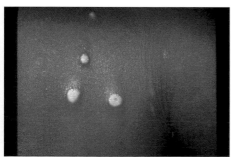

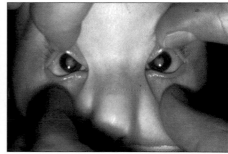

Yaws—multiple papillomata of two weeks' duration (see p. 723)

Congenital rubella—typical pearly, nuclear bilateral rubella cataracts (see p. 695)

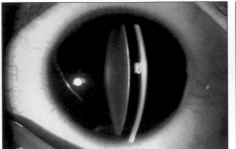

Aniridia (see p. 969)

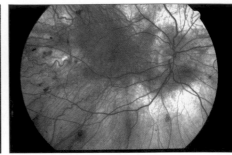

Choroideremia (see p. 971)

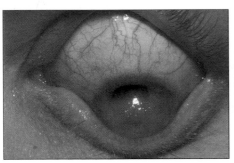

Keratoconus with acute hydrops (see p. 974)

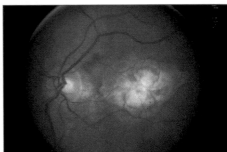

Disciform macular degeneration (see p. 976)

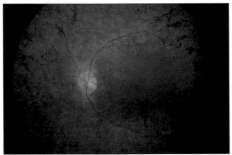

Retinitis pigmentosa (see p. 969)

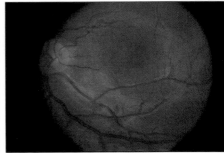

Juvenile X-linked retinoschisis (see p. 984)

Textbook of Dermatology, 4th ed.: A. Rook, et al., eds.; Blackwell Scientific Publications, 1986.

Inherited Disorders of Complement: L. Guenther; J. Am. Acad. Dermatol., December 1983, issue 9(6), pp. 815–839.

Yeast Opsonization Defect and Immunoglobulin Deficiency in Severe Infantile Dermatitis (Leiner's Disease): D.I. Evans, et al.; Arch. Dis. Child., September 1977, issue 52(9), pp. 691–695.

LEOPARD SYNDROME

Description LEOPARD syndrome is a rare heritable disorder caused by an autosomal gene of variable expressivity whose characteristics include the presence of **L**entigenes, **E**lectrocardiogram abnormalities, **O**cular hypertelorism, **P**ulmonary stenosis, **A**nomalies of the genital organs, **R**etarded growth, and **D**eafness.

Synonyms
Cardiomyopathic Lentiginosis
Multiple Lentigines Syndrome

Signs and Symptoms LEOPARD syndrome is most visibly characterized by small, dark cutaneous spots (lentigines) that resemble freckles but are unrelated to exposure to the sun. The lentigines range between 1 and 5mm in size and are usually spread across the neck and torso but can occur anywhere on the skin. They tend to increase with age.

Other abnormalities associated with LEOPARD syndrome include cardiomyopathy, hypertelorism, prominent ears, winged scapulae, mild growth retardation, cryptorchidism, and late onset of adolescence. An impaired sense of smell, deafness, and ovarian and renal hypoplasia or agenesis are among other characteristics that may also be present.

Etiology The syndrome is inherited as an autosomal dominant trait.

Epidemiology Males and females are affected in equal numbers.

Treatment—Standard No specific therapy is available. Undescended testes may require surgery. Cardiac abnormalities must be monitored and treated as required. Other treatment is symptomatic and supportive. Genetic counseling may be beneficial.

Treatment—Investigational Please contact the agencies listed under Resources, below, for the most current information.

Resources
For more information on LEOPARD Syndrome: National Organization for Rare Disorders (NORD); NIH/National Institute of Child Health and Human Development.

For genetic information and genetic counseling referrals: March of Dimes Birth Defects Foundation; NIH/National Center for Education in Maternal and Child Health (NCEMCH).

References

Dermatology, 3rd ed.: O. Braun-Falco, et al.; Springer-Verlag, 1991.

Skin Signs of Systemic Disease: I.M. Braverman; W.B. Saunders Company, 1981.

Dermatology in General Medicine: Textbook and Atlas, 3rd ed.: T.B. Fitzpatrick, et al., eds.; McGraw-Hill, 1987.

Dermatology, 2nd ed. (3rd ed., 1992): S.L. Moschella and H.J. Hurley, eds.; W.B. Saunders Company, 1985.

Textbook of Dermatology, 4th ed.: A. Rook, et al., eds.; Blackwell Scientific Publications, 1986.

Mendelian Inheritance in Man, 9th ed.: V.A. McKusick, The Johns Hopkins University Press, 1990, pp. 565–566.

Smith's Recognizable Patterns of Human Malformation, 4th ed.: K.L. Jones; W.B. Saunders Company, 1988, pp. 470–471.

LICHEN SCLEROSUS ET ATROPHICUS (LSA)

Description LSA is a chronic dermatologic disease characterized by the progressive development of white, atrophic skin lesions of the neck, arms, trunk, vulva, and other areas. LSA is not a premalignant disease.

Synonyms

Lichen Sclerosus

White Spot Disease

Signs and Symptoms LSA is characterized by the appearance in the skin of pale patches that become thin, shiny, and parchment-like. On close inspection, the patches contain clusters of minute white lesions that coalesce. There may be a violaceous color to the borders. Fissures, cracks, and ecchymoses may appear. Distribution is on the neck, under the breast, in body folds, and in the perianal and vulvar areas. Patients may complain of pruritus. Atrophy and shrinkage of the skin of the vagina and vulva may cause painful sexual intercourse.

Females are affected most often. In the rare cases of LSA in males, it is generally the foreskin that is affected, making retraction of the foreskin impossible. The condition is progressive and the atrophy does not regress. If leukoplakia is present, then squamous cell carcinoma must be suspected also. Some cases are associated with diabetes mellitus.

Etiology The cause is not known. LSA may be due to an autoimmune process or an injury. A genetic predisposition may exist.

Epidemiology The disorder most often affects females between the ages of 40 and 60, although cases involving younger females and males have been reported.

Related Disorders See *Scleroderma.* Symptoms of lichen planus may be similar to those of LSA.

Treatment—Standard Treatment consists of topical applications of antipruritics, corticosteroids, and testosterone to the affected areas. Surgical removal of affected skin layers may be of benefit in severe cases.

Treatment—Investigational Etretinate is being evaluated as a treatment; the drug must not be used by pregnant women.

Please contact the agencies listed under Resources, below, for the most current information.

Resources

For more information on LSA: National Organization for Rare Disorders (NORD); The National Arthritis and Musculoskeletal and Skin Diseases Information Clearinghouse.

References

Dermatology, 3rd ed.: O. Braun-Falco, et al.; Springer-Verlag, 1991.

Skin Signs of Systemic Disease: I.M. Braverman; W.B. Saunders Company, 1981.

Dermatology in General Medicine: Textbook and Atlas, 3rd ed.: T.B. Fitzpatrick, et al., eds.; McGraw-Hill, 1987.

Dermatology, 2nd ed. (3rd ed., 1992): S.L. Moschella and H.J. Hurley, eds.; W.B. Saunders Company, 1985.

Textbook of Dermatology, 4th ed.: A. Rook, et al., eds.; Blackwell Scientific Publications, 1986.

Cecil Textbook of Medicine, 18th ed.: J.B. Wyngaarden and L.H. Smith, Jr., eds.; W.B. Saunders Company, 1988, pp. 1419, 2341.

NETHERTON SYNDROME

Description Netherton syndrome is a rare skin condition in which cornification leads to the distinctive circular scaling pattern of ichthyosis linearis circumflexa. Atopy and abnormalities of the hair are also associated with the syndrome.

Synonyms

Ichthyosis Linearis Circumflexa

Netherton Disease

Signs and Symptoms At birth, characteristic findings include generalized redness and the presence of a parchment-like membrane that can be peeled off. Later, hyperkeratosis and shedding may lead to ichthyosis linearis circumflexa, or in some cases, a rash similar to lamellar ichthyosis. Itching may be mild to severe.

Various allergic disorders often accompany the cutaneous findings, and lichenification on one side of the arms and legs may be an allergic reaction.

Abnormalities of the hair that are characteristic of Netherton syndrome include trichorrhexis invaginata ("bamboo" hair), pili torti (twisted hair), and trichorrhexis nodosa.

Etiology The syndrome is transmitted through autosomal recessive genes.

Epidemiology Males and females are affected equally in this rare condition.

Related Disorders See *Ichthyosis Congenita; Ichthyosis, Lamellar Recessive; Tay Syndrome.*

Treatment—Standard Cutaneous symptoms can be alleviated by application of keratolytics and emollients, including plain petroleum jelly. This can be especially effective after bathing while the skin is still moist. Salicylic acid gel is useful in some instances for removal of scales.

Foods that are known to cause an allergic skin reaction should be avoided.

Treatment—Investigational Please contact the agencies listed under Resources, below, for the most current information.

Resources
For more information on Netherton syndrome: National Organization for Rare Disorders (NORD); Foundation for Ichthyosis and Related Skin Types, Inc. (F.I.R.S.T.); The National Arthritis and Musculoskeletal and Skin Diseases Information Clearinghouse.

For genetic information and genetic counseling referrals: March of Dimes Birth Defects Foundation; National Center for Education in Maternal and Child Health (NCEMCH).

References
Dermatology, 3rd ed.: O. Braun-Falco, et al.; Springer-Verlag, 1991.

Skin Signs of Systemic Disease: I.M. Braverman; W.B. Saunders Company, 1981.

Dermatology in General Medicine: Textbook and Atlas, 3rd ed.: T.B. Fitzpatrick, et al., eds.; McGraw-Hill, 1987.

Dermatology, 2nd ed. (3rd ed., 1992): S.L. Moschella and H.J. Hurley, eds.; W.B. Saunders Company, 1985.

Textbook of Dermatology, 4th ed.: A. Rook, et al., eds.; Blackwell Scientific Publications, 1986.

Netherton Syndrome. Report of a Case and Review of the Literature: S.L. Greene, et al.; J. Am. Acad. Dermatol., August 1985, issue 13(2 pt. 2), pp. 329–337.

Genetically Transmitted, Generalized Disorders of Cornification. The Ichthyoses: M.L. Williams, et al.; Dermatol. Clin., January 1987, issue 5(1), pp. 155–178.

Therapeutic Activity of Lactate 12% Lotion in the Treatment of Ichthyosis. Active Versus Vehicle and Active Versus a Petroleum Cream: M. Buxman, et al.; J. Am. Acad. Dermatol., December 1986, issue 15(6), pp. 1253–1258.

PEMPHIGOID, BENIGN MUCOSAL

Description Benign mucosal pemphigoid is a rare chronic disease characterized by blisters and scarring on the mucous membranes. The oral cavity and the conjunctiva are the most commonly affected areas.

Synonyms
Cicatricial Pemphigoid
Mucous Membrane Pemphigoid

Signs and Symptoms Presenting symptoms may include erythema and blistering of the oral mucosa, or redness and inflammation of the eyes and conjunctiva. Conjunctival scarring may occur, and the formation of scar tissue between the eyelid and eyeball. Blisters also may develop in the mucous membranes of the pharynx and esophagus, nose, urethra, and vulva, but are uncommon on the external skin.

Subepidermal blisters are seen histologically with deposits of immunoglobulins IgG and IgA and of C3 in the cutaneous basement membrane zone. The pattern resembles that of bullous pemphigoid.

Benign mucosal pemphigoid is a persistent condition that remits and recurs.

Etiology The cause is not known.

Epidemiology Middle-aged and elderly persons, males and females equally, are most often affected. However, cases involving children and adolescents have been reported.

Related Disorders See *Pemphigoid, Bullous; Pemphigus.*

Localized cicatricial pemphigoid (Brunsting-Perry syndrome) is a chronic scarring disease characterized by blisters on the head and neck that are caused by trauma or other factors.

Vegetating mucous membrane pemphigoid combines features of benign mucosal pemphigoid and **pemphigus vegetans** (a variation of **pemphigus vulgaris**). Blisters that are large and fast-growing are usually seen in the axillary and inguinal areas.

Intermittent mucosal pemphigoid is characterized by oral blisters that are sparse, occur only intermittently, and heal without forming scars.

Epidermolysis bullosa acquisita is an acquired autoimmune skin disorder in which blisters that leave scars occur on the skin of extensor areas, and sometimes the skull. Eyes may also be affected. There usually is IgG activity around the blisters. Middle-aged and elderly persons are most often affected.

Treatment—Standard Treatment is not satisfactory. Topical corticosteroids such as fluocinonide can relieve inflammation and itching, and systemic corticosteroids such as prednisone relieve inflammation and can suppress the immune system. Immunosuppressive drugs such as cyclophosphamide or azathioprine may also be used. Dapsone may be given to relieve inflammation. *All of these drugs require careful monitoring.* Other treatment is symptomatic and supportive.

Treatment—Investigational Aldesulfonsodium is being investigated to treat childhood benign mucosal pemphigoid.

Please contact the agencies listed under Resources, below, for the most current information.

Resources

For more information on benign mucosal pemphigoid: National Organization for Rare Disorders (NORD); NIH/National Institute of Arthritis, Musculoskeletal and Skin Diseases (NIAMS) Clearinghouse.

References

Dermatology, 3rd ed.: O. Braun-Falco, et al.; Springer-Verlag, 1991.

Skin Signs of Systemic Disease: I.M. Braverman; W.B. Saunders Company, 1981.

Dermatology in General Medicine: Textbook and Atlas, 3rd ed.: T.B. Fitzpatrick, et al., eds.; McGraw-Hill, 1987.

Dermatology, 2nd ed. (3rd ed., 1992): S.L. Moschella and H.J. Hurley, eds.; W.B. Saunders Company, 1985.

Textbook of Dermatology, 4th ed.: A. Rook, et al., eds.; Blackwell Scientific Publications, 1986.

Mucosal Involvement in Bullous and Cicatricial Pemphigoid. A Clinical and Immunopathological Study: V.A. Venning, et al.; Br. J. Dermatol., January 1988, issue 118(1), pp. 7–15.
Ocular Cicatricial Pemphigoid with Granular IgG and Complement Deposition: A.D. Proia, et al.; Arch. Ophthalmol., November 1985, issue 103(11), pp. 1669–1672.
Immunosuppressive Therapy in Ocular Cicatricial Pemphigoid: B.J. Mondino, et al.; Am. J. Opthalmol., October 1983, issue 96(4), pp. 453–459.

PEMPHIGOID, BULLOUS

Description A chronic, cutaneous, relatively benign blistering disease more common in elderly persons, bullous pemphigoid is marked by generalized subepidermal blisters. It usually subsides spontaneously in several months or years, but it may recur. Infrequently, complications such as pneumonia develop which are potentially fatal.

Synonyms
    Benign Pemphigus
    Old Age Pemphigus
    Parapemphigus
    Pemphigoid
    Senile Dermatitis Herpetiformis

Signs and Symptoms The initial finding is erythema surrounding a lesion, scar, or the umbilicus. Within weeks bullae appear on the flexor surfaces, axillae, abdomen, and groin. The disorder usually spares mucous areas, such as the mouth; when these are affected, healing is rapid. The bullae are sizable and rigid, contain clear or blood-tinged fluid, and do not rupture easily. If rupture occurs pain may result, but healing is rapid.

The white cell count rises, but the patient is not likely to have fever. Immunofluorescent microscopic examination of the skin reveals subepidermal blisters and binding of IgG to the basement membrane zone. The serum will reveal antibodies directed against the basement membrane in approximately 70 percent of the patients. The significance of the antibody titre in relation to the degree of the symptoms is unknown, because titres do not correlate well with disease activity.

Etiology The disease is idiopathic; an autoimmune association has been suggested. Certain drug reactions can produce the picture of bullous pemphigoid.

Related Disorders See *Pemphigus; Erythema Multiforme; Pemphigoid, Benign Mucosal; Dermatitis Herpetiformis.*

Treatment—Standard Corticosteroids reduce the number of lesions, and doses required are lower than those needed in pemphigus. The drug (usually prednisone) can be discontinued in approximately 50 percent of cases because the patients go into remission. The balance of the patients need maintenance therapy. Some patients have a self-limited course and, because many are elderly, decisions about whether to treat with systemic steroids must be individualized.

Treatment—Investigational Immunosuppressive agents, e.g., azathioprine and methotrexate, have been used experimentally as adjuncts to the corticosteroid. Cyclosporine may be useful in bullous pemphigoid.

Please contact the agencies listed under Resources, below, for the most current information.

Resources

For more information on bullous pemphigoid: National Organization for Rare Disorders (NORD); The National Arthritis and Musculoskeletal and Skin Diseases Information Clearinghouse.

References

Dermatology, 3rd ed.: O. Braun-Falco, et al.; Springer-Verlag, 1991.
Skin Signs of Systemic Disease: I.M. Braverman; W.B. Saunders Company, 1981.
Dermatology in General Medicine: Textbook and Atlas, 3rd ed.: T.B. Fitzpatrick, et al., eds.; McGraw-Hill, 1987.
Dermatology, 2nd ed. (3rd ed., 1992): S.L. Moschella and H.J. Hurley, eds.; W.B. Saunders Company, 1985.
Textbook of Dermatology, 4th ed.: A. Rook, et al., eds.; Blackwell Scientific Publications, 1986.
Internal Disorders Associated with Bullous Disease of the Skin. A Critical Review: J.P. Callen; J. Am. Acad. Dermatol., August 1980, issue 3(2), pp. 107–119.
Mechanism of Lesion Production in Pemphigus and Pemphigoid: W.M. Sams, Jr.; J. Am. Acad. Dermatol., April 1982, issue 6(4 pt. 1), pp. 431–452.
Pemphigus and Pemphigoid. A Review of the Advances Made Since 1964: W.F. Lever; J. Am. Acad. Dermatol., July 1979, issue 1(1), pp. 2–31.

PEMPHIGUS

Description Pemphigus encompasses a group of autoimmune skin disorders characterized by the development of blisters in the epidermis and mucous membranes. The location and type of blisters vary according to the type of pemphigus. Untreated, pemphigus is often fatal.

Signs and Symptoms Blisters resulting from acantholysis (separation of epidermal cells from one another) are common to all types of pemphigus, explaining the development of intraepidermal blisters. The blisters generally occur on the neck, scalp, mucous membranes, and inguinal and axillary areas, and are usually flaccid. Most patients have deposits of IgG around keratinocytes in skin in the areas of the blisters. Antiepidermal antibodies are present in the serum. Diagnosis requires histologic identification of acantholytic blisters as well as detection of the IgG antibodies.

Pemphigus vulgaris may begin with isolated blisters on the scalp, and then in the mouth. These may persist for several months and then be followed by blistering of the esophagus, nose, conjunctiva, and rectum. The blisters are soft, break easily, and heal poorly. Pressure on their borders causes them to spread. Pressure on normal-looking skin causes it to blister **(Nikolsky sign). Pemphigus vegetans**

is a variation of pemphigus vulgaris. The blisters are large and fast-growing and have hypertrophic lesions which are usually located in the axillary and inguinal areas.

Pemphigus foliaceus is less severe and less common. Soft blisters occur closer to the surface of the skin, and when they break they ooze and become crusty, scaly, and susceptible to infection. They may occur on the scalp, face, upper chest, and back, but the mucous membranes are usually spared. Small, horny plugs attached to the undersurface of the affected skin also may be seen. Another type of pemphigus foliaceus occurs in South America, particularly Brazil and Colombia, and is called **fogo selvagem.**

When patients have features of both pemphigus foliaceus and systemic lupus erythematosus, they are said to have **pemphigus erythematosus.** Pemphigus may occur as an adverse reaction to drugs such as D-penicillamine and rifampin, with symptoms resembling those of pemphigus foliaceus rather than pemphigus vulgaris. Some research indicates that **pemphigus herpetiformis** is a discrete form of pemphigus with its own characteristic blisters, but blisters that form during a relapse may resemble those of pemphigus foliaceus.

In **benign familial pemphigus (Hailey-Hailey disease),** recurrent blisters are seen primarily on the neck, groin, and axillae. Precipitating factors include heat, sweating, skin infection, and ultraviolet radiation.

Etiology Most forms of pemphigus are generally considered to be autoimmune-related. Benign familial pemphigus (Hailey-Hailey disease) is inherited as an autosomal dominant trait.

Fogo selvagem (Brazilian pemphigus foliaceus) is an autoimmune disorder with blistering that is thought to be triggered by a substance transmitted by the bite of blackflies.

Pemphigus may also occur following x-ray exposure or as an adverse reaction to drugs such as D-penicillamine or rifampin.

Epidemiology Pemphigus is most common in the middle-aged and elderly, but cases involving children have been observed. It has been found in all ethnic groups and races, but is more common in persons of Jewish or Mediterranean origin. Pemphigus occurs once in every 100,000 live births, with males and females being affected equally.

Fogo selvagem occurs in Brazil in the rural, central areas heavily infested with a species of blackfly.

Related Disorders See *Bullous Pemphigoid; Darier Disease; Epidermolysis Bullosa; Epidermolytic Hyperkeratosis; Erythema Multiforme; Dermatitis Herpetiformis.*

Epidermolysis bullosa acquisita is an autoimmune disorder affecting the middle-aged and elderly. Injuries may cause blisters on the skin of extensor areas such as elbows, knees, pelvis, and buttocks, and on the scalp. Increased levels of IgG are usually found around the blisters, and scars remain after healing.

Treatment—Standard Corticosteroids are widely used for treating pemphigus. Topical corticosteroids can relieve inflammation and itching, and systemic corticosteroids such as prednisone relieve inflammation and suppress the immune system.

Immunosuppressive drugs such as cyclosporine, cyclophosphamide, azathioprine, or methotrexate may be prescribed. Cytotoxic drugs are used to suppress the immune system. Gold compounds such as auranofin may be given to relieve inflammation and, possibly, to suppress the immune system. Dapsone is also given. *These drugs should be used with extreme caution.* To reduce immediate or longterm side effects, drug therapy may have to be stopped temporarily or changed.

Antibiotic drugs or creams may be given to manage infection and relieve inflammation. Silver sulfadiazine cream also may be used. Dusting the patient and the bedsheets with talcum powder may relieve the discomfort of raw skin. Other treatment is symptomatic and supportive. Genetic counseling may be beneficial for patients with hereditary pemphigus, and their families.

Treatment—Investigational Two methods of plasmapheresis are under investigation, as is the use of extracorporeal photopheresis. Surgery is being investigated for use in nonresponsive cases, with removal of blistered skin and application of skin grafts.

Please contact the agencies listed under Resources, below, for the most current information.

Resources

For more information on pemphigus: National Organization for Rare Disorders (NORD); The National Arthritis and Musculoskeletal and Skin Diseases Information Clearinghouse.

For genetic information and genetic counseling referrals: March of Dimes Birth Defects Foundation; NIH/National Center for Education in Maternal and Child Health (NCEMCH).

References
Dermatology, 3rd ed.: O. Braun-Falco, et al.; Springer-Verlag, 1991.
Skin Signs of Systemic Disease: I.M. Braverman; W.B. Saunders Company, 1981.
Dermatology in General Medicine: Textbook and Atlas, 3rd ed.: T.B. Fitzpatrick, et al., eds.; McGraw-Hill, 1987.
Dermatology, 2nd ed. (3rd ed., 1992): S.L. Moschella and H.J. Hurley, eds.; W.B. Saunders Company, 1985.
Textbook of Dermatology, 4th ed.: A. Rook, et al., eds.; Blackwell Scientific Publications, 1986.
Mendelian Inheritance in Man, 9th ed.: V.A. McKusick; The Johns Hopkins University Press, 1990, pp. 717–718.
Dermatologic Clinics: The Genodermatoses, vol. 5, no. 1: J.C. Alper, ed.; W.B. Saunders Company, 1987, pp. 160–161, 171–173.
Pemphigus: N. Korman; J. Am. Acad. Dermatol., June 1988, issue 18(6), pp. 1219–1238.
The Pathogenic Effect of IgG 4 Autoantibodies in Endemic Pemphigus Foliaceus (Fogo Selvagem): J. Terblanche, et al.; New Eng. J. of Med., June 1989, issue 320(22), pp. 1463–1469.

PITYRIASIS RUBRA PILARIS (PRP)

Description PRP is a chronic skin disorder characterized by pruritus and numerous coalescent, perifollicular papules that increase in size and eventually connect, producing large red scaling plaques.

Signs and Symptoms The follicular papules are itchy, sharply pointed, horn-like, and brownish-red to rosy yellow or salmon in color. They usually occur on the scalp, axillae, forearms, elbows, wrists, hands, fingers, and knees. Over time the papules increase in size and connect, resulting in large dry, scaly, rough, and red plaques. Islands of normal skin may be present in so-called "skip" areas. Palms and soles may be severely affected with scaling. The nails may be gray and brittle and the scalp seborrheic. Ectropion of the eyelids may be present. The course can be limited to a few weeks or months or prolonged for many years. PRP can usually be distinguished from psoriasis.

Etiology The cause is unknown. An autosomal dominant inheritance is suspected in some families. An acquired form of the disease may be associated with a deficiency of vitamin A. Some cases are exacerbated by exposure to light.

Epidemiology Males and females of all ages are affected equally.

Related Disorders Symptoms of lichen planus, psoriasis, and pityriasis rosea may be similar to those of PRP.

Treatment—Standard Some cases resolve with only topical lubricants and topical corticosteroids. PRP may respond to treatment with vitamin A, either orally or in alcohol as an ointment. Phototherapy must be considered cautiously because light exacerbates some cases.

Treatment—Investigational The disease has been treated with retinoid drugs such as isotretinoin, and the antineoplastic drug methotrexate, but these agents must be used cautiously because of their toxic side effects.

Research on PRP is being conducted at New York University Medical Center. For information please contact Irwin M. Freedberg, M.D., NYU Medical Center, Department of Dermatology, 550 First Avenue, New York, NY 10016, (212) 340-5245.

Please contact the agencies listed under Resources, below, for the most current information.

Resources

For more information on pityriasis rubra pilaris: National Organization for Rare Disorders (NORD); Foundation for Ichthyosis and Related Skin Types (F.I.R.S.T.); NIH/National Institute of Arthritis, Musculoskeletal and Skin (NIAMS) Diseases Information Clearinghouse.

For genetic information and genetic counseling referrals: March of Dimes Birth Defects Foundation; National Center for Education in Maternal and Child Health (NCEMCH).

References

Dermatology, 3rd ed.: O. Braun-Falco, et al.; Springer-Verlag, 1991.
Skin Signs of Systemic Disease: I.M. Braverman; W.B. Saunders Company, 1981.
Dermatology in General Medicine: Textbook and Atlas, 3rd ed.: T.B. Fitzpatrick, et al., eds.; McGraw-Hill, 1987.
Dermatology, 2nd ed. (3rd ed., 1992): S.L. Moschella and H.J. Hurley, eds.; W.B. Saunders Company, 1985.
Textbook of Dermatology, 4th ed.: A. Rook, et al., eds.; Blackwell Scientific Publications, 1986.
Childhood-Onset Pityriasis Rubra Pilaris with Immunologic Abnormalities: D. Shvili, et al.; Pediatr. Dermatol., May 1987, issue 4(1), pp. 21–23.
Pityriasis Rubra Pilaris, Vitamin A and Retinol-Binding Protein: A Case Study: P.C. van Voorst Vader, et al.; Acta Derm. Venereol. (Stockholm), 1984, issue 64(5), pp. 430–432.
Isotretinoin Treatment of Pityriasis Rubra Pilaris: C.H. Dicken; J. Am. Acad. Dermatol., February 1987, issue 16(2 part 1), pp. 297–301.

PSEUDOXANTHOMA ELASTICUM (PXE)

Description Pseudoxanthoma elasticum describes a group of inherited connective tissue disorders involving the skin, eyes, and cardiovascular system.

Synonyms
Elastosis Dystrophica Syndrome
Groenblad-Strandberg Syndrome
Systemic Elastorrhexis of Touraine

Signs and Symptoms Plaques and papules appear most often on the face and neck and in the axillary, antecubital, and inguinal areas. These areas are reddish-purple at first and later become yellow or white. They thicken and become inelastic because of the connective tissue abnormalities. Skin folds may droop and the surface resemble the plucked skin of a chicken. Retinal angioid streaks may be evident, and retinal hemorrhage and vision loss may develop. Vascular changes include peripheral, coronary, and cerebral arterial occlusion, which may be apparent on x-rays early in the course, even though other symptoms may appear years later. The condition is progressive, but in many cases progression is slow.

Etiology The cause is unknown. There is a generalized abnormality in elastic tissue with fragmentation in skin, eye, and vessels. Autosomal recessive inheritance is the most common pattern observed, although a dominant pattern has also been described.

Epidemiology The disease affects approximately 1:100,000 persons worldwide. It is estimated that there are 2,500 cases in the United States.

Treatment—Standard Only symptomatic treatment is available.
General therapeutic strategies include regular exercise, weight control, and avoidance of smoking, aspirin, and excessive calcium. Activities likely to cause head trauma (e.g., rough sports) should be avoided because of the danger of retinal bleeding.
Cosmetic surgery may be useful for improving the appearance of the skin. Laser

coagulation may be required for retinal hemorrhage. Genetic counseling is recommended for patients and families.

Treatment—Investigational Please contact the agencies listed under Resources, below, for the most current information.

Resources

For more information on pseudoxanthoma elasticum: National Organization for Rare Disorders (NORD); National Association for Pseudoxanthoma Elasticum; The National Arthritis and Musculoskeletal and Skin Diseases Information Clearinghouse; NIH/National Eye Institute.

For information on clinics: Mark Lebwohl, M.D., Mount Sinai School of Medicine; Kenneth H. Nelder, M.D., Texas Tech University Health Sciences Center.

For genetic information and genetic counseling referrals: March of Dimes Birth Defects Foundation; National Center for Education in Maternal and Child Health (NCEMCH).

References

Dermatology, 3rd ed.: O. Braun-Falco, et al.; Springer-Verlag, 1991.

Skin Signs of Systemic Disease: I.M. Braverman; W.B. Saunders Company, 1981.

Dermatology in General Medicine: Textbook and Atlas, 3rd ed.: T.B. Fitzpatrick, et al., eds.; McGraw-Hill, 1987.

Dermatology, 2nd ed. (3rd ed., 1992): S.L. Moschella and H.J. Hurley, eds.; W.B. Saunders Company, 1985.

Textbook of Dermatology, 4th ed.: A. Rook, et al., eds.; Blackwell Scientific Publications, 1986.

Cecil Textbook of Medicine, 18th ed.: J.B. Wyngaarden and L.H. Smith, Jr., eds.; W.B. Saunders Company, 1988, pp. 1181–1182.

PYODERMA GANGRENOSUM

Description Pyoderma gangrenosum is an ulcerative skin disease of unknown etiology. It is not caused by cutaneous bacterial or other infection. It may occur sporadically alone or as a severe complication of one of a variety of underlying diseases.

Signs and Symptoms Pyoderma gangrenosum is characterized by an extremely painful, ulcerative, purplish skin lesion which may rapidly expand to 20 cm in size. The ulcers most frequently develop on the legs but may appear anywhere on the body. They can appear at sites of trauma (**pathergy**). Biopsy of these lesions reveals nonspecific inflammation; therefore the diagnosis of pyoderma gangrenosum is largely one of exclusion.

Etiology The cause is not known; an autoimmune etiology is suspected. Approximately 50 percent of all cases are idiopathic. The remainder are associated with an underlying disease; ulcerative colitis and Crohn's disease are the most common. In these cases, the course of the skin lesion usually parallels the course of the bowel disease, but appearance during remission does occur. Other disorders associated with pyoderma gangrenosum include rheumatoid arthritis, chronic active hepatitis, and various hematologic malignancies such as acute and chronic myelogenous leukemia, polycythemia vera, and myeloma.

Epidemiology Males and females are affected equally. The disease is least common in children and most common in middle-aged women.

Related Disorders The ulcers of pyoderma gangrenosum may resemble those seen in necrotizing vasculitis, spider bites (such as those of the brown recluse spider), and certain deep fungal diseases.

Treatment—Standard Treatment is not satisfactory. Debridement, wet dressings, and topical application of disodium cromoglycate or zinc sulfate may be helpful. The skin must be protected from trauma which could result in development of other ulcers. In severe cases, systemic steroids, antibiotics, and antimetabolites may be indicated.

Treatment—Investigational Thalidomide and clofazamine are being tested for treatment of pyoderma gangrenosum. Thalidomide, especially, is contraindicated in pregnancy because it causes severe birth defects. For information on the use of thalidomide, contact Pediatric Pharmaceutical, 379 Thornall St., Edison, New Jersey 08837.

Please contact the agencies listed under Resources, below, for the most current information.

Resources

For more information on pyoderma gangrenosum: National Organization for Rare Disorders (NORD); The National Arthritis and Musculoskeletal and Skin Diseases Information Clearinghouse.

For information about colitis or Crohn's disease: National Foundation for Ileitis and Colitis.

References

Dermatology, 3rd ed.: O. Braun-Falco, et al.; Springer-Verlag, 1991.

Skin Signs of Systemic Disease: I.M. Braverman; W.B. Saunders Company, 1981.

Dermatology in General Medicine: Textbook and Atlas, 3rd ed.: T.B. Fitzpatrick, et al., eds.; McGraw-Hill, 1987.

Dermatology, 2nd ed. (3rd ed., 1992): S.L. Moschella and H.J. Hurley, eds.; W.B. Saunders Company, 1985.

Textbook of Dermatology, 4th ed.: A. Rook, et al., eds.; Blackwell Scientific Publications, 1986.

Pyoderma Gangrenosum Associated with Ulcerative Colitis; Treatment with Disodium Cromoglycate: D.R. Cave, et al.; Am. J. Gastroenterol., August 1987, issue 82(8), pp. 802–804.

Pyoderma Gangrenosum Complicating Ulcerative Colitis; Successful Treatment with Methylprednisolone Pulse Therapy and Dapsone: E. Galun, et al.; Am. J. Gastroenterol., October 1986, issue 81(10), pp. 988–989.

Pustular Pyoderma Gangrenosum Associated with Ulcerative Colitis in Childhood. Report of Two Cases and Review of the Literature: L. Barnes, et al.; J. Am. Acad. Dermatol., October 1986, issue 15(4 pt. 1), pp. 608–614.

SJÖGREN-LARSSON SYNDROME

Description Sjögren-Larsson syndrome is a rare autosomal recessive inherited disorder characterized by ichthyosis and hyperkeratosis, ocular and speech abnormalities, seizures, spasticity, and mental retardation.

Signs and Symptoms Onset of symptoms usually is in infancy. There is variably severe erythroderma accompanied by fine scales on the neck and lower abdomen; larger, thicker, platelike scales may appear later in infancy, developing into dark, nonerythematous lesions, especially in the flexures of the arms and legs. Speech abnormalities, mental retardation, and seizures usually begin in the first 2 or 3 years of life. Glistening spots in the fundus may be an early sign of the disorder. About half of patients have retinal pigmentary degeneration. Patients may be short of stature.

The syndrome can be detected in utero.

Etiology Sjögren-Larsson syndrome is transmitted through autosomal recessive genes.

Epidemiology The syndrome occurs in approximately 8.3:100,000 persons in northern Sweden. It is less prevalent in the United States. Males and females are affected in equal numbers, and all races are affected.

Related Disorders See *Ichthyosis Congenita; Ichthyosis Hystrix, Curth-Macklin Type; Ichthyosis, Lamellar Recessive; Ichthyosis, X-Linked; Darier Disease; Epidermolytic Hyperkeratosis.*

Treatment—Standard Cutaneous symptoms can be alleviated by application of keratolytics and emollients, including plain petroleum jelly. This can be especially effective after bathing while the skin is still moist. Salicylic acid gel is useful in some instances for removal of scales. Lactate lotion can also be an effective keratolytic. Topical and systemic retinoids can be beneficial in some cases but must be used with caution because of adverse side effects.

Anticonvulsant medications may be needed to control seizures. Speech therapy and special education services may be helpful. Other treatment is symptomatic and supportive.

Treatment—Investigational Clinical improvement has been reported following limitation of dietary fat to medium-chain triglycerides.

Please contact the agencies listed under Resources, below, for the most current information.

Resources

For more information on **Sjögren-Larsson syndrome:** National Organization for Rare Disorders (NORD); Foundation for Ichthyosis and Related Skin Types, Inc. (F.I.R.S.T.); The National Arthritis and Musculoskeletal and Skin Diseases Information Clearinghouse.

For **genetic information and genetic counseling referrals:** March of Dimes Birth Defects Foundation; National Center for Education in Maternal and

Child Health (NCEMCH).

References

Dermatology, 3rd ed.: O. Braun-Falco, et al.; Springer-Verlag, 1991.
Skin Signs of Systemic Disease: I.M. Braverman; W.B. Saunders Company, 1981.
Dermatology in General Medicine: Textbook and Atlas, 3rd ed.: T.B. Fitzpatrick, et al., eds.; McGraw-Hill, 1987.
Dermatology, 2nd ed. (3rd ed., 1992): S.L. Moschella and H.J. Hurley, eds.; W.B. Saunders Company, 1985.
Textbook of Dermatology, 4th ed.: A. Rook, et al., eds.; Blackwell Scientific Publications, 1986.
Genetically Transmitted, Generalized Disorders of Cornification. The Ichthyoses: M.L. Williams, et al.; Dermatol. Clin., January 1987, issue 5(1), pp. 155–178.
Therapeutic Activity of Lactate 12% Lotion in the Treatment of Ichthyosis. Active Versus Vehicle and Active Versus a Petroleum Cream: M. Buxman, et al.; J. Am. Acad. Dermatol., December 1986, issue 15(6), pp. 1253–1258.
Treatment of the Ichthyosis of the Sjögren-Larsson Syndrome with Etretinate (Tigason): S. Jagell, et al.; Acta Derm. Venereol., Stockholm, 1983, issue 63(1), pp. 89–91.
Mendelian Inheritance in Man, 9th ed.: V.A. McKusick; The Johns Hopkins University Press, 1990, p. 1478.

SWEET SYNDROME

Description Sweet syndrome is a rare skin disorder characterized by the explosive appearance of multiform, painful erythematous lesions on the skin of the arms, face, neck, and legs, accompanied by fever and malaise.

Synonyms

Febrile Neutrophilic Dermatosis, Acute

Signs and Symptoms Malaise and other constitutional complaints including high fever accompany the widespread painful skin lesions. These may be up to 1 inch in diameter and are usually bluish-red, sharply demarcated, indurated, and circular, and may be flat or raised. Tiny blisters or bacteria-free pustules may cover the plaques. Central clearing associated with a trailing collarette of scale is sometimes noted. Scarring may appear, especially in infants.

Sweet syndrome is usually preceded by a systemic febrile, infectious, or other inflammatory illness. Histologically, there is a massive neutrophilic infiltration in the dermis. A high ESR and leukocytosis with a predominance of neutrophils are present. Remission may occur after a few weeks, but recurrences are possible.

Etiology The cause is not known; an allergic reaction to an unknown infectious agent is often suspected. Leukemia may be associated, as may a skin injury such as vaccination or a scrape. An upper respiratory or skin infection may precede by 1 to 3 weeks the precipitation of the syndrome.

Epidemiology Sweet syndrome is seen most often in middle-aged females, but men, children, and infants have been affected in rare cases.

Related Disorders See *Erythema Multiforme; Leiner Disease.*

Erythema elevatum diutinum (possibly a variant of erythema multiforme) is a rare, chronic skin disorder usually seen in adults between ages 30 and 60. It may be associated with recurrent polyarthritis and is characterized by symmetric nodules and plaques near the joints and on the backs of the hands and feet. The size of the lesions may vary over the course of a day.

Treatment—Standard Systemic corticosteroid drugs may produce dramatic improvement, but the syndrome may go into spontaneous remission after a few weeks without treatment.

Treatment—Investigational Dapsone has been used experimentally to treat the syndrome, but more research is needed to determine safety and effectiveness.

Please contact the agencies listed under Resources, below, for the most current information.

Resources

For more information on Sweet syndrome: National Organization for Rare Disorders (NORD); The National Arthritis and Musculoskeletal and Skin Diseases Information Clearinghouse.

References

Dermatology, 3rd ed.: O. Braun-Falco, et al.; Springer-Verlag, 1991.
Skin Signs of Systemic Disease: I.M. Braverman; W.B. Saunders Company, 1981.
Dermatology in General Medicine: Textbook and Atlas, 3rd ed.: T.B. Fitzpatrick, et al., eds.; McGraw-Hill, 1987.
Dermatology, 2nd ed. (3rd ed., 1992): S.L. Moschella and H.J. Hurley, eds.; W.B. Saunders Company, 1985.
Textbook of Dermatology, 4th ed.: A. Rook, et al., eds.; Blackwell Scientific Publications, 1986.
Acute Febrile Neutrophilic Dermatosis. Sweet's Syndrome: M.A. Bechtel, et al.; Arch. Dermatol., October 1981, issue 117(10), pp. 664–666.
Sweet's Syndrome: Histological and Immunohistochemical Study of 15 Cases: J.J. Going, et al.; J. Clin. Pathol., February 1987, issue 40(2), pp. 175–179.
Acute Febrile Neutrophilic Dermatosis. Sweet's Syndrome: H. Chmel, et al.; South. Med. J., November 1978, issue 71(11), pp. 1350–1352.

TAY SYNDROME

Description Tay syndrome is a hereditary disorder characterized by erythroderma and ichthyosis, sparse and brittle hair, delayed physical development, mental retardation, and the look of progeria.

Synonyms

Congenital Ichthyosis with Trichothiodystrophy
Ichthyosiform Erythroderma with Hair Abnormality and Growth and Mental Retardation
Trichothiodystrophy with Congenital Ichthyosis

Signs and Symptoms Erythroderma may be present at birth.

Ichthyosis characterized by fine, dark scales covers most of the body. The hair **(trichothiodystrophy)** and nails are sulfur-deficient; the hair is sparse and brittle and the finger- and toenails dysplastic. Facial features include a beaked nose, receding chin, and protruding ears. Loss of subcutaneous fat results in a prematurely aged-looking face.

Low birth weight, short stature, and mental retardation are typical, and there may be an increased susceptibility to infection. Central nervous system abnormalities include neurosensory deafness, seizures, tremors, and ataxia. Cryptorchidism may be seen in males, and female genitalia may be underdeveloped. In women, normal nipple development may occur with absence of other breast tissue. Small cataracts and bone and teeth abnormalities may be found.

Etiology The syndrome is transmitted through autosomal recessive genes.

Epidemiology Abnormalities are usually present at birth. Males and females are affected in equal numbers.

Related Disorders See *Ichthyosis Congenita; Ichthyosis, Lamellar Recessive; Netherton Syndrome.*

Amish brittle hair syndrome (hair-brain syndrome) usually is found in persons of Amish descent. It is characterized by brittle hair, intellectual impairment, decreased fertility, and short stature. The condition lacks the skin and facial abnormalities of Tay syndrome.

Pollitt syndrome (trichorrhexis nodosa syndrome) is characterized by microcephaly, mental and physical retardation, and fragile hair (trichorrhexis nodosa). The skin is usually scaly and the nails are underdeveloped and spoon-shaped.

Treatment—Standard The discomfort of the dry, scaly skin can be alleviated by application of keratolytics and emollients, including plain petroleum jelly. This can be especially effective after bathing while the skin is still moist. Salicylic acid gel is useful in some instances for removal of scales. Lactate lotion can also be an effective keratolytic. Topical and systemic retinoids can be beneficial in some cases, but must be used with caution.

Other treatment is symptomatic and supportive. Genetic counseling may be beneficial.

Treatment—Investigational Please contact the agencies listed under Resources, below, for the most current information.

Resources

For more information on Tay syndrome: National Organization for Rare Disorders (NORD); Foundation for Ichthyosis and Related Skin Types, Inc. (F.I.R.S.T.); National Arthritis, Musculoskeletal & Skin (NIAMS) Information Clearinghouse.

For genetic information and genetic counseling referrals: March of Dimes Birth Defects Foundation; National Center for Education in Maternal and Child Health (NCEMCH).

References

Dermatology, 3rd ed.: O. Braun-Falco, et al.; Springer-Verlag, 1991.

Skin Signs of Systemic Disease: I.M. Braverman; W.B. Saunders Company, 1981.

Dermatology in General Medicine: Textbook and Atlas, 3rd ed.: T.B. Fitzpatrick, et al., eds.; McGraw-Hill, 1987.

Dermatology, 2nd ed. (3rd ed., 1992): S.L. Moschella and H.J. Hurley, eds.; W.B. Saunders Company, 1985.

Textbook of Dermatology, 4th ed.: A. Rook, et al., eds.; Blackwell Scientific Publications, 1986.

Mendelian Inheritance in Man, 9th ed.: V.A. McKusick; The Johns Hopkins University Press, 1990, p. 1272.

Genetically Transmitted, Generalized Disorders of Cornification. The Ichthyoses: M.L. Williams, et al.; Dermatol. Clin., January 1987, issue 5(1), pp. 155–178.

The Tay Syndrome (Congenital Ichthyosis with Trichothiodystrophy): R. Happle, et al.; Eur. J. Pediatr., January 1984, issue 141(3), pp. 147–152.

TOXIC EPIDERMAL NECROLYSIS (TEN)

Description TEN is characterized by severe epidermal erythema, blisters, and peeling. Onset can occur at any age. The infantile form (**Lyell's syndrome**) usually follows a staphylococcal infection, but in adults the cause is often a drug reaction.

Synonyms

    Acute Toxic Epidermolysis
    Dermatitis Exfoliativa
    Lyell's Syndrome
    Ritter Disease
    Ritter-Lyell Syndrome
    Scalded Skin Syndrome
    Staphylococcal Scalded Skin Syndrome

Signs and Symptoms Infantile or childhood-onset TEN may have a preliminary stage marked by fever, sore throat, conjunctivitis, nasal discharge, vomiting, diarrhea, and back pain. Crusted lesions appear around the nose or ears, and are followed within 24 hours by intense erythema in the same area. The redness may spread, and tenderness, itching, and separation of skin layers may be seen within 36 to 48 hours. Skin may peel away in large sheets when touched, and blisters may form. Severe discomfort and anorexia may occur. With healing, peeled areas may become dried, and yellowish crusts may appear.

The first apparent symptom of adult-onset TEN may be large, easily broken blisters. Slight injury or even touching can cause large sheets of skin to peel. The mucous membranes may also be involved. The condition usually progresses rapidly and within a few days may be severe. Up to 40 percent of cases are fatal. Loss of skin barrier may lead to sepsis; fluid loss may result in dehydration. Scars resembling those of burns may develop when the skin begins to heal.

Etiology Childhood TEN is often associated with a staphylococcal infection, usually phage type 71, and may be preceded by impetigo. The staph produce an exotoxin which causes epidermal cleavage just below the stratum corneum. Rarely, childhood TEN may be due to an allergic drug reaction.

The adult form is often the result of a delayed-type drug reaction. Many drugs have been associated, including phenytoin, sulfonamides, and barbiturates.

Epidemiology Males and females are affected in equal numbers. The childhood syndrome may occur sporadically or in epidemic proportions in nurseries.

Related Disorders See *Epidermolysis Bullosa; Stevens-Johnson Syndrome.*

Treatment—Standard Symptoms of childhood TEN may progress rapidly, and early treatment is important. Hospitalization and, if necessary, isolation are needed to ensure a sterile environment. Treatment includes antibiotics and correction of fluid and electrolyte imbalance. Patients should be closely observed to prevent touching of the blistered skin. With appropriate treatment, healing may be rapid.

Treatment of adult-onset TEN is similar to therapy for severe burns. Contact with peeled skin surface should be minimal. Hospitalization with isolation may be necessary, and ongoing fluid and electrolyte replacement may be needed to correct severe fluid loss. If the disease is caused by a drug reaction, systemic corticosteroids may control the reaction but do not seem to alleviate the skin symptoms. Septicemia and pulmonary infections should be anticipated. Other therapy is symptomatic and supportive.

Treatment—Investigational Plasmapheresis may be of benefit in cases caused by a severe reaction to drugs, but the procedure is still investigational. Research is under way in the areas of new wound-healing drugs, antibiotics, and inhibition of blister formation.

Please contact the agencies listed under Resources, below, for the most current information.

Resources

For more information on TEN: National Organization for Rare Disorders (NORD); The National Arthritis and Musculoskeletal and Skin Diseases Information Clearinghouse; Dystrophic Epidermolysis Bullosa Research Association of America (DEBRA); D.E.B.R.A. (England).

For information on clinical facilities: University of Washington School of Medicine, St. Louis, Missouri; Rockefeller University, New York, New York; Children's Hospital, Philadelphia, Pennsylvania; University of Pennsylvania, Philadelphia, Pennsylvania.

References
Dermatology, 3rd ed.: O. Braun-Falco, et al.; Springer-Verlag, 1991.
Skin Signs of Systemic Disease: I.M. Braverman; W.B. Saunders Company, 1981.
Dermatology in General Medicine: Textbook and Atlas, 3rd ed.: T.B. Fitzpatrick, et al., eds.; McGraw-Hill, 1987.
Dermatology, 2nd ed. (3rd ed., 1992): S.L. Moschella and H.J. Hurley, eds.; W.B. Saunders Company, 1985.
Textbook of Dermatology, 4th ed.: A. Rook, et al., eds.; Blackwell Scientific Publications, 1986.
Improved Burn Center Survival of Patients with Toxic Epidermal Necrolysis Managed without Corticosteroids: P.H. Halebian, et al.; Ann. Surg., November 1986, issue 204(5), pp. 503–512.
Plasmapheresis in Severe Drug-Induced Toxic Epidermal Necrolysis: D. Kamanabroo, et al.; Arch. Dermatol., December 1985, issue 121(12). pp. 1548–1549.

URTICARIA PIGMENTOSA

Description Urticaria pigmentosa is the name of a cutaneous form of mastocytosis, a disorder of excessive mast cell proliferation. Urticaria pigmentosa is generally benign and self-limiting.

Synonyms
Infantile Mastocytosis

Signs and Symptoms Reddish-brown, pruritic macules and papules appear on the epidermis overlying dermal collections of mast cells. Lesions may rarely be present in bone or other organs. The skin lesions become urticarial when they are touched or exposed to heat. Sometimes lesions are bullous. Other symptoms of mastocytosis include headache, malaise, flushing, abdominal pain, and diarrhea, but these are uncommon in urticaria pigmentosa.

Etiology The etiology is not known. The symptoms are those of release of histamine and other vasodilatory substances from the mast cell infiltrates.

Epidemiology Onset is generally during the first year of life. Lesions usually disappear by adolescence.

Related Disorders See *Mastocytosis*, in which there is multisystem mast cell infiltration.

Treatment—Standard Treatment is symptomatic and supportive. Topical steroids may be useful, as may antihistamines given systemically.

Treatment—Investigational Urticaria pigmentosa has been treated experimentally with oral disodium cromoglycate, cimetidine (sometimes combined with chlorpheniramine or propantheline), and with ketotifen.

Please contact the agencies listed under Resources, below, for the most current information.

Resources
For more information on urticaria pigmentosa: National Organization for Rare Disorders (NORD); The National Arthritis and Musculoskeletal and Skin Diseases Information Clearinghouse.

References
Dermatology, 3rd ed.: O. Braun-Falco, et al.; Springer-Verlag, 1991.
Skin Signs of Systemic Disease: I.M. Braverman; W.B. Saunders Company, 1981.
Dermatology in General Medicine: Textbook and Atlas, 3rd ed.: T.B. Fitzpatrick, et al., eds.; McGraw-Hill, 1987.
Dermatology, 2nd ed. (3rd ed., 1992): S.L. Moschella and H.J. Hurley, eds.; W.B. Saunders Company, 1985.
Textbook of Dermatology, 4th ed.: A. Rook, et al., eds.; Blackwell Scientific Publications, 1986.
Cecil Textbook of Medicine, 18th ed.: J.B. Wyngaarden and L.H. Smith, Jr., eds.; W.B. Saunders Company, 1988, pp. 1948–1951, 2334–2335.

VITILIGO

Description Vitiligo is an acquired disorder characterized by an absence of melanocytes, which results in decreased or absent pigmentation in patches of skin. Vitiliginous patches may be localized or widespread.

Synonyms
White Spot Disease

Signs and Symptoms The areas of decreased pigmentation appear white under a Wood's light. They are usually sharply demarcated and symmetric in shape, and typically appear on the face, neck, hands, abdomen, and thighs, although they can occur anywhere on the skin. They are common around body orifices and on palms and soles. The hair in affected areas is usually white. The depigmented lesions burn easily in the sun, and should be protected by application of sunscreens.

Etiology The cause is unknown. Vitiligo is sometimes familial, and although the exact mode of inheritance is not determined, vitiligo often is transmitted as an autosomal dominant gene. The disorder is 10 to 15 times more common in patients with autoimmune diseases, and has been associated with pernicious anemia, Addison disease, hypothyroidism, and alopecia areata. Organ-specific antibodies have recently been detected in patients with vitiligo, indicating that destruction of melanocytes may have an immune basis. The disorder also is associated with head trauma. Vitiligo sometimes is associated with melanoma, and patients should be screened for these malignant tumors.

Epidemiology Onset is usually before age 20.

Treatment—Standard Small lesions may be camouflaged with cosmetic creams. Para-aminobenzoic acid solution or gel protects against sunburn. In larger areas, patients may use psoralen photochemotherapy (PUVA), with systemic psoralens administered orally followed by exposure to UV-A from sunlight or an artificial source.

Treatment—Investigational Please contact the agencies listed under Resources, below, for the most current information.

Resources
   For more information on vitiligo: National Organization for Rare Disorders (NORD); Frontier's International Vitiligo Foundation; National Foundation for Vitiligo & Pigment Disorders; The National Arthritis and Musculoskeletal and Skin Diseases Information Clearinghouse.

References
   Dermatology, 3rd ed.: O. Braun-Falco, et al.; Springer-Verlag, 1991.
   Skin Signs of Systemic Disease: I.M. Braverman; W.B. Saunders Company, 1981.
   Dermatology in General Medicine: Textbook and Atlas, 3rd ed.: T.B. Fitzpatrick, et al., eds.; McGraw-Hill, 1987.
   Dermatology, 2nd ed. (3rd ed., 1992): S.L. Moschella and H.J. Hurley, eds.; W.B. Saunders Company, 1985.

Textbook of Dermatology, 4th ed.: A. Rook, et al., eds.; Blackwell Scientific Publications, 1986.

Harrison's Principles of Internal Medicine, 12th ed.: J.D. Wilson, et al., eds.: McGraw-Hill, 1991, pp. 326–328.

Mendelian Inheritance in Man, 9th ed.: V.A. McKusick; The Johns Hopkins University Press, 1990, p. 969.

Cecil Textbook of Medicine, 18th ed.: J.B. Wyngaarden and L.H. Smith, Jr., eds.; W.B. Saunders Company, 1988, pp. 2344–2345.

WEBER-CHRISTIAN DISEASE

Description Weber-Christian disease is characterized by recurrent febrile episodes with formation of nonsuppurating subcutaneous fat nodules.

Synonyms
>Nodular Nonsuppurative Panniculitis
>Pfeiffer-Weber-Christian Syndrome

Signs and Symptoms Onset of Weber-Christian disease usually is gradual, with nodules appearing in the subcutaneous tissue of the arms, legs, thighs, buttocks, and abdomen. The overlying skin usually is erythematous. Accompanying symptoms may include fever, enlargement of the spleen and lymph nodes, malaise, sore throat, chills, nausea, and anemia, and pain in the joints, muscles, or abdomen. Symptoms may subside spontaneously after days or weeks, but may recur weeks, months, or years later.

Etiology The cause is unknown; allergic factors may be involved, or a predisposition of fatty tissue to a granulomatous reaction. Weber-Christian disease must be differentiated from similar nodular lesions associated with diabetes mellitus, systemic lupus erythematosus, subacute bacterial endocarditis, tuberculosis, iodide and bromide therapy, withdrawal from large doses of corticosteroids, and pancreatitis.

Epidemiology Weber-Christian disease most often affects adult women, usually between the ages of 20 and 40 years.

Related Disorders See *Mesenteritis, Retractile.*

Treatment—Standard Treatment is symptomatic and supportive. If the disorder is associated with an underlying condition, treatment of that disorder can alleviate the symptoms of Weber-Christian disease.

Treatment—Investigational Treatment with oral cyclophosphamide has shown some promise in preliminary clinical trials. Thalidomide is being tested as a treatment, although this drug must not be taken by pregnant women.

Please contact the agencies listed under Resources, below, for the most current information.

Resources
>**For more information on Weber-Christian disease:** National Organization

for Rare Disorders (NORD); The National Arthritis and Musculoskeletal and Skin Diseases Information Clearinghouse; NIH/National Institute of Allergy and Infectious Diseases.

References

Dermatology, 3rd ed.: O. Braun-Falco, et al.; Springer-Verlag, 1991.

Skin Signs of Systemic Disease: I.M. Braverman; W.B. Saunders Company, 1981.

Dermatology in General Medicine: Textbook and Atlas, 3rd ed.: T.B. Fitzpatrick, et al., eds.; McGraw-Hill, 1987.

Dermatology, 2nd ed. (3rd ed., 1992): S.L. Moschella and H.J. Hurley, eds.; W.B. Saunders Company, 1985.

Textbook of Dermatology, 4th ed.: A. Rook, et al., eds.; Blackwell Scientific Publications, 1986.

Cyclophosphamide-Induced Remission in Weber-Christian Panniculitis: W. Kirch, et al.; Rheumatol. Int., 1985, 5(5), pp. 239–240.

XERODERMA PIGMENTOSUM

Description Xeroderma pigmentosum is a rare skin disorder that begins during early childhood. It is characterized by photosensitivity to sunlight, and the early development of hyper- and hypopigmentation in exposed skin. Cutaneous malignancies are common, and patients have numerous basal cell and squamous cell carcinomas as well as melanomas.

Signs and Symptoms The first sign of xeroderma pigmentosum is severe infantile photosensitivity followed by extensive freckling in exposed skin. Telangiectasia as well as diffuse hyper- and hypopigmentation appears in the exposed skin.

Malignancies of the skin may occur before age 5, and the face and skin may appear old. Growth retardation, short stature, neurologic dysfunction, and mental retardation may occur in some persons.

Ocular findings include photophobia, excessive lacrimation, keratitis, corneal opacities, and tumors of the eyelid or cornea.

Etiology The disorder is transmitted as an autosomal recessive trait. Several forms exist, but each is caused by impaired excisional repair of photo-damage to DNA. Thymine dimer excision is defective in most forms of xeroderma pigmentosum, as is repair of chemically induced DNA damage.

Epidemiology Xeroderma pigmentosum affects approximately 1:100,000 persons, and there are an estimated 250,000 cases in the United States. Children of both sexes may be affected as early as the first year of life.

Related Disorders See *Malignant Melanoma.*

Treatment—Standard Total protection of the skin from sunlight is necessary for patients with xeroderma pigmentosum, to prevent the development of additional skin lesions. In some cases surgery has been performed with limited success. Other treatment is symptomatic and supportive.

Treatment—Investigational Application of a catalase cream appears to prevent tumors in some children. Ointments containing vitamin A derivatives are also being investigated. Isotretinoin has been shown to reduce the recurrence of tumors, but the drug is very toxic and many patients find the side effects intolerable. T4 endonuclease V.B. liposome encapsulated (T4N5) is an orphan drug being used to prevent the skin cancers and other skin abnormalities of xeroderma pigmentosum. The drug is available from Applied Genetics, Inc., 205 Buffalo Avenue, Freeport, New York 11520.

Please contact the agencies listed under Resources, below, for the most current information.

Resources

For more information on xeroderma pigmentosum: National Organization for Rare Disorders (NORD); Xeroderma Pigmentosum Registry; The Skin Cancer Foundation; NIH/National Cancer Institute PDQ (Physician Data Query) phoneline; The National Arthritis and Musculoskeletal and Skin Diseases Information Clearinghouse.

References

Dermatology, 3rd ed.: O. Braun-Falco, et al.; Springer-Verlag, 1991.

Skin Signs of Systemic Disease: I.M. Braverman; W.B. Saunders Company, 1981.

Dermatology in General Medicine: Textbook and Atlas, 3rd ed.: T.B. Fitzpatrick, et al., eds.; McGraw-Hill, 1987.

Dermatology, 2nd ed. (3rd ed., 1992): S.L. Moschella and H.J. Hurley, eds.; W.B. Saunders Company, 1985.

Textbook of Dermatology, 4th ed.: A. Rook, et al., eds.; Blackwell Scientific Publications, 1986.

Xeroderma Pigmentosum, Defective DNA Repair–and Schistosomiasis?: J. German; Annales de Genetique, Paris 1980, issue 23(2), pp. 69–72.

Microinjection of Human Cell Extracts Corrects Xeroderma Pigmentosum Defect: A.J. de Jonge, et al.; EMBO Journal, 1983, issue 2(5), pp. 637–641.

8 GASTROINTESTINAL DISORDERS
By William F. Balistreri, M.D.

There are a number of rare disorders which can affect various portions of the gastrointestinal tract, including disorders of the upper and lower intestine, the liver, and the pancreas. The clinical consequences primarily relate to altered digestion and metabolism. These disorders may present with malabsorption and, therefore, failure to thrive or weight loss. Watery diarrhea may be a manifestation of disorders of carbohydrate transport; the degree of severity can range from troublesome to life-threatening. Chronic blood loss from the gastrointestinal tract may be seen in polyposis syndromes.

Disorders that affect the liver may present with mild degrees of unconjugated hyperbilirubinemia that have little consequence (e.g., Gilbert syndrome). However, a severe form of unconjugated hyperbilirubinemia (Crigler-Najjar syndrome) is life-threatening, with relentless accumulation of bilirubin and the development of kernicterus and death without liver transplantation. The presence of conjugated hyperbilirubinemia (cholestasis) is never benign—this always indicates hepatobiliary dysfunction. Cholestasis is the presenting sign of biliary atresia.

Recognition of these rare disorders of the gastrointestinal tract is important, since certain ones are responsive to specific or supportive therapy. Patients with achalasia will be cured with dilatation or surgical myotomy. Persons with the Budd-Chiari syndrome can be recognized by the development of hepatomegaly, often with ascites; surgical therapy is required. The recognition of gluten-sensitive enteropathy (celiac sprue) will allow the institution of a gluten-free diet, which will (1) reverse the gut injury; (2) allow for more effective absorption of dietary nutrients; and (3) decrease the potential for malignant degeneration. The malignant potential of the familial polyposis syndromes and Gardner syndrome must also be recognized so that early, aggressive surgery can be performed.

Early detection of biliary atresia is also critical, since the successful establishment of bile flow is dependent upon the age at which surgical drainage is performed. Prompt diagnosis of Hirschsprung disease is also imperative because delayed discovery can result in abdominal distention and poor weight gain, with the potential complication of toxic megacolon with perforation and death. Patients with Caroli disease, plagued by persistent cholangitis with infection of the dilated biliary ductal system, may benefit from early, aggressive antibiotic therapy.

Eosinophilic gastroenteritis is a poorly understood disorder; it may, however, respond to dietary or steroid therapy. Patients with inborn errors of carbohydrate transport, such as glucose-galactose malabsorption and sucrase-isomaltase deficiency, will require restriction of the offending carbohydrate from the diet, thereby diminishing the diarrhea.

Patients with intestinal pseudoobstruction can present with a lifelong history of constipation, and while no effective therapy has yet been defined, palliative procedures are available.

GASTROINTESTINAL DISORDERS
Listings in This Section

ACHALASIA

Description A motor disorder of the esophagus, achalasia is distinguished by dilation of the esophagus, impaired peristalsis, and failure to relax the lower esophageal sphincter.

Synonyms
> Cardiospasm
> Dyssynergia Esophagus
> Esophageal Aperistalsis
> Megaesophagus

Signs and Symptoms Onset is gradual. Patients are likely to complain of dysphagia and of chest pain, which may range from transient discomfort to overwhelming agony. Gastric contents may be regurgitated or may enter the tracheobronchial tree. Nighttime regurgitation is reported in approximately one-third of cases. Significant weight loss may occur in untreated cases. A nocturnal cough may also be present.

Pneumonia, pulmonary infections, and strangulation can occur from aspiration of the esophageal contents. Esophageal carcinoma occurs in approximately 5 percent of cases.

Radiology is often useful in diagnosis, as dilation of the esophagus and retention of food, secretions, and barium can be seen. Manometric examination may also be useful. Pharmacologic stimulation and endoscopy are not advised.

Etiology The cause of achalasia is not known. The condition may be caused by degeneration of Auerbach's plexus.

Epidemiology While achalasia affects mainly adults between the ages of 20 and 40 years, the disorder may occur at any age.

Treatment—Standard Treatment is directed at removing the obstruction caused by failure of the lower esophageal sphincter to relax. This may be done pharmacologically, manipulatively, or surgically.

Isosorbide, a long-acting nitrate, or nifedipine, a calcium channel blocker, may provide some relief.

Balloon dilation aimed at the lower esophageal sphincter, effective in about 85 percent of cases, can be complicated by bleeding and perforation. The success rate of Heller myotomy, in which the muscular fibers in the lower esophageal sphincter are cut, is also about 85 percent.

Treatment—Investigational Please contact the agencies listed under Resources, below, for the most current information.

Resources
For more information on achalasia: National Organization for Rare Disorders (NORD); National Digestive Diseases Information Clearinghouse.

References

Harrison's Principles of Internal Medicine, 12th ed.: J.D. Wilson, et al., eds.; McGraw-Hill, 1991, pp. 1224–1225.
Cecil Textbook of Medicine, 18th ed.: J.B. Wyngaarden and L.H. Smith, Jr., eds.; W.B. Saunders Company, 1988, pp. 359–360, 1198–1203.

ALAGILLE SYNDROME

Description Alagille syndrome, a genetic liver disorder, is characterized by insufficient bile flow due to a congenital paucity of intrahepatic bile ducts.

Synonyms
> Arteriohepatic Dysplasia
> Cholestasis with Peripheral Pulmonary Stenosis
> Intrahepatic Bile Duct Paucity
> Syndromatic Hepatic Ductular Hypoplasia

Signs and Symptoms Jaundice is usually present at birth. The hepatic malformation is accompanied by other anomalies, including structural abnormalities of the eye, cardiac valve and arterial malformations, and abnormally shaped (butterfly) vertebrae. Facial characteristics include a broad forehead, a straight nose with a bulbous tip, deep-set eyes spaced widely apart, and a pointed jaw. Fingers may be short. Symptoms can range from mild to severe.

Etiology The syndrome is thought to be inherited as an autosomal dominant trait.

Epidemiology Alagille syndrome is a rare disorder that frequently occurs in more than one person in a family and in many generations of an affected family.

Related Disorders See *Alpha-1-Antitrypsin Deficiency; Zellweger Syndrome.*

Cholestasis-lymphedema syndrome is a genetic disorder characterized by impaired bile flow and jaundice at birth, which tends to recur throughout life. Hypoplasia of lymph vessels results in edema of the legs, usually at 5 or 6 years of age.

Byler disease (progressive familial intrahepatic cholestasis) is an inherited liver disorder with an early onset. It is characterized by loose, foul-smelling stools, jaundice, hepatomegaly, splenomegaly, and short stature.

Treatment—Standard Treatment of Alagille syndrome is symptomatic and supportive. Genetic counseling is recommended for patients and their families.

Treatment—Investigational Please contact the agencies listed under Resources, below, for the most current information.

Resources

For more information on Alagille syndrome: National Organization for Rare Disorders (NORD); American Liver Foundation; The United Liver Foundation; Children's Liver Foundation; National Institute of Diabetes, Digestive & Kidney Diseases Information Clearinghouse.

For genetic information and genetic counseling referrals: March of Dimes Birth Defects Foundation; National Center for Education in Maternal and Child Health (NCEMCH).

References
Journal of Pediatrics, vol. 110, 1987, p. 195.

Mendelian Inheritance in Man, 9th ed.: V.A. McKusick; Johns Hopkins University Press, 1990, p. 187.

Arteriohepatic Dysplasia (Alagille Syndrome): Extreme Variability Among Affected Family Members: S.A. Shulman, et al.; Am. J. Med. Genet.; October 1984, vol. 19(2), pp. 325–332.

BILIARY ATRESIA

Description The most common form of extrahepatic biliary atresia is the closure of bile ducts near the porta hepatis; distal biliary atresia is much less common.

Signs and Symptoms Signs of biliary atresia (jaundice, pale stools, dark urine, and hepatomegaly) usually are not evident until the infant is 2 weeks old. Within 6 to 10 weeks, however, certain features may have developed: irritability (from itchiness), growth delay, and portal hypertension.

Other abnormalities that may be present in children with biliary atresia include renal and cardiac malformations.

Liver biopsy, laparotomy, and cholangiography are used in diagnosis.

Etiology The etiology is unknown.

Epidemiology The incidence is 1:10,000 to 1:15,000 live births. Males and females are both affected.

Related Disorders See *Hepatitis, Neonatal,* in which the intrahepatic bile ducts are underdeveloped, unlike the extrahepatic abnormality seen in biliary atresia.

Treatment—Standard The type of surgical repair performed, including Kasai hepatoportoenterostomy, depends on the type and area of abnormality found. Even with successful surgical intervention, some hepatic dysfunction may remain. The Kasai procedure may be used as an early intermediate procedure to support the child's growth until liver transplantation is feasible.

Treatment—Investigational Please contact the agencies listed under Resources, below, for the most current information.

Resources
For more information on biliary atresia: National Organization for Rare Disorders (NORD); American Liver Foundation; The United Liver Foundation; Children's Liver Foundation; National Institute of Diabetes, Digestive & Kidney Diseases Information Clearinghouse.

References
Mendelian Inheritance in Man, 9th ed.: V.A. McKusick; The Johns Hopkins University Press, 1990, pp. 1064–1065.

Nelson Textbook of Pediatrics, 13th ed.: R.E. Behrman and V.C. Vaughan, III, eds.; W.B. Saunders Company, 1987, pp. 831–834.

Cecil Textbook of Medicine, 18th ed.: J.B. Wyngaarden and L.H. Smith, Jr., eds.; W.B. Saunders Company, 1988, p. 846.

BUDD-CHIARI SYNDROME

Description Budd-Chiari syndrome is a rare hepatic vascular disorder characterized by abnormal enlargement of the liver due to occlusion of the major hepatic veins. The obstruction usually results from thrombosis or congenital webs that form at the junction of the hepatic veins and the inferior vena cava.

Synonyms
> Hepatic Veno-Occlusive Disease
> Rokitansky Disease

Signs and Symptoms Abdominal pain is common and usually accompanied by ascites, edema of the legs, and mild jaundice. Hepatomegaly is present. Hemoglobinuria also may be observed. When the obstruction is severe, onset of the disorder can be sudden and acute. The chronic form of Budd-Chiari syndrome is characterized by an insidious onset and less severe pain; liver enlargement occurs gradually. The associated portal hypertension that develops causes impaired liver function and serious liver damage.

Routine biochemical testing is of little diagnostic value. Liver biopsy tests can reveal central cell deterioration, development of fibrous growths, and occlusion of the terminal hepatic veins.

Etiology In about 70 percent of cases, the cause of the blockage is due to an underlying disorder. The syndrome can be associated with hypercoagulable states (polycythemia vera or another myeloproliferative disorder; oral contraceptives or pregnancy), or with a tumor in the inferior vena cava. Other potential causes include exposure to radiation and arsenic; trauma; sepsis; certain chemotherapy drugs; and in some parts of the world, drinking a beverage made from pyrrolidizine plant alkaloids (bush tea).

Epidemiology Males and females are equally affected. Patients between the ages of 20 and 40 years tend to be most susceptible.

Related Disorders Lesions of the hepatic artery or of the hepatic venous system may produce symptoms similar to Budd-Chiari syndrome.

Treatment—Standard Treatment depends on the underlying disorder and the location and extent of the occlusion. Diagnostic procedures such as x-ray, CT scanning, MRI, and ultrasound are useful for this purpose. Liver biopsy reveals changes in cell structure. Therapeutic choices include medical treatment of ascites, angioplasty, shunting, and in some cases, liver transplantation.

Treatment—Investigational Please contact the agencies listed under Resources,

below, for the most current information.

Resources
For more information on Budd-Chiari syndrome: National Organization for Rare Disorders (NORD); American Liver Foundation; The United Liver Foundation; Children's Liver Foundation; National Institute of Diabetes, Digestive and Kidney Diseases Information Clearinghouse (NDIC).

References
Internal Medicine, 3rd ed.: J.H. Stein, ed.-in-chief; Little, Brown and Company, 1990, pp. 516–517.

Treatment of the Budd-Chiari Syndrome with Percutaneous Transluminal Angioplasty. Case Report and Review of the Literature: J. Sparano, et al.; Am. J. Med., April 1987, issue 82(4), pp. 821–828.

Results of Portal Systemic Shunts in Budd-Chiari Syndrome: C. Vons, et al.; Ann. Surg., April 1986, issue 203(4), pp. 366–370.

Comparison of Ultrasonography, Computed Tomography and 99mTc Liver Scan in Diagnosis of Budd-Chiari Syndrome: S. Gupta, et al.; Gut, March 1987, issue 38(3), pp. 242–247.

CAROLI DISEASE

Description In Caroli disease the intrahepatic bile ducts are characterized by segmental cystic dilatation. Complications often occur, and include stone formation, recurrent cholangitis, and hepatic abscesses.

Synonyms
Acute Cholangitis
Congenital Dilatation of Intrahepatic Bile Ducts

Signs and Symptoms Abdominal pain, sepsis, fever, and jaundice occur in individuals with Caroli disease. Symptoms may manifest in childhood, or as late as the 6th decade of life.

Etiology This rare disorder is believed to result from abnormal prenatal development of the intrahepatic bile ducts. Caroli disease may be associated with cystic disease of the kidney or other organs.

Epidemiology Males are affected by Caroli disease more often than females.

Related Disorders Benign tumors of the extrahepatic bile ducts, including papillomas, adenomas, fibroadenomas, adenomyomas, leiomyomas, granular cell myoblastomas, neurinomas, and hamartomas may occur. Surgical removal of the neoplasm is the appropriate treatment.

Carcinoma of the extrahepatic bile ducts, although rare, may occur.

Helminthiasis of the bile ducts caused by the parasite *Ascaris lumbricoides* has been reported.

Treatment—Standard Surgical resection of cysts and removal of stones may be appropriate. Antibiotics and drainage are supportive but seldom successful treatments. Death may result from gram-negative septicemia.

Treatment—Investigational Please contact the agencies listed under Resources, below, for the most current information.

Resources
 For more information on Caroli disease: National Organization for Rare Disorders (NORD); National Digestive Diseases Information Clearinghouse; American Liver Foundation; The United Liver Foundation; Children's Liver Foundation.
 For genetic information and genetic counseling referrals: March of Dimes Birth Defects Foundation; National Center for Education in Maternal and Child Health (NCEMCH).

References
Caroli's Disease; New Diagnostic and Therapeutic Approaches: S. L. Newman, et al.; South. Med. J., December 1986, issue 79(12), pp. 1587–1590.
Successful Treatment of Caroli's Disease by Hepatic Resection. Report of Six Patients: N. Nagasue; Ann. Surg., December 1984, issue 200(6), pp. 718–723.
Scintigraphic and Radiographic Findings in Caroli's Disease: A.J. Moreno, et al.; Am. J. Gastroenterol., April 1984, issue 79(4), pp. 299–303.

CELIAC SPRUE

Description Celiac sprue is an inherited intestinal malabsorption disorder associated with intolerance to gluten.

Synonyms
   Celiac Disease
   Gee-Herter Disease
   Gee-Thaysen Disease
   Gluten Enteropathy
   Huebner-Herter Disease
   Nontropical Sprue

Signs and Symptoms Symptoms range from severe to mild; celiac sprue can be asymptomatic. Age at onset also varies, with the disease becoming evident in infancy or adulthood.
 Affected children from 6 months to 3 years of age may have diarrhea, projectile vomiting, and a bloated abdomen. Growth is retarded. Frequent symptoms in adults include weight loss, chronic fatty diarrhea, abdominal cramping and distention, and myopathy. Food craving, weakness, and fatigue are also common.
 In patients with celiac sprue, the intestinal villi are partially or totally absent, and the absorptive surface is flattened or reduced. Symptoms depend on the degree of mucosal damage and the duration of nutrient malabsorption. Vitamin and mineral deficiencies may result in anemia, mucous membrane deterioration, follicular hyperkeratosis, osteomalacia, osteoporosis, decreased blood coagulation, or muscle cramps. Malabsorption of protein, salt, and water can produce dehydration, electrolyte depletion, growth retardation, and edema. Lactose intolerance,

peripheral neuropathy, and central nervous system lesions can also occur. Less commonly, dermatitis herpetiformis may be seen. Behavioral changes such as irritability and crankiness may be noted, especially in children. Difficulty in concentration, decreased mental alertness, and impaired memory may also occur.

Etiology The genetic inheritance is probably dominant with incomplete penetrance. HLA-B8 antigen has been identified in 80 percent of persons with the disease. Typical mucosal abnormalities can appear in healthy siblings of affected persons.

Epidemiology Celiac sprue occurs equally in males and females. Although the disorder begins in infancy, it may not be diagnosed until adulthood.

Related Disorders Celiac sprue can be differentiated from **Whipple's disease** and **tropical sprue** by a jejunal biopsy that shows flat or absent villi and by clinical improvement after withdrawal of dietary gluten.

Treatment—Standard Over 75 percent of patients respond to a gluten-free diet, with symptoms usually improving within weeks. Intestinal histological improvement may not be evident for months. Appropriate dietary supplementation may be indicated, with fat-soluble vitamins, minerals, and hematinics. Patients who do not respond initially to gluten withdrawal may benefit from limited treatment with oral steroids.

Treatment—Investigational Please contact the agencies listed under Resources, below, for the most current information.

Resources

For more information on celiac sprue: National Organization for Rare Disorders (NORD); American Celiac Society; Celiac Sprue Association/USA; Gluten Intolerance Group; National Digestive Diseases Information Clearinghouse.

For genetic information and genetic counseling referrals: March of Dimes Birth Defects Foundation; National Center for Education in Maternal and Child Health (NCEMCH).

References

Nelson Textbook of Pediatrics, 13th ed.: R.E. Behrman and V.C. Vaughan, III, eds.; W.B. Saunders Company, 1987, pp. 804–805.

Harrison's Principles of Internal Medicine, 12th ed.: J.D. Wilson, et al., eds.; McGraw-Hill, 1991, pp. 1264–1265.

CHOLESTASIS

Description Cholestasis, the stoppage or suppression of the flow of bile, results from intra- or extrahepatic causes. The condition may occur as a symptom or complication of other disorders. Subdivisions of the disorder include familial progressive cholestasis (Byler disease—see Related Disorders, below); syndromatic paucity of intrahepatic bile ducts (see *Alagille Syndrome);* benign recurrent intrahepatic cholestasis (BRIC or Summerskill syndrome); estrogen-related cholestasis (cholestasis of pregnancy and of oral contraceptive users); and postoperative cholestasis.

Signs and Symptoms Symptoms of cholestasis include jaundice, dark urine, light or acholic stools, pruritus, steatorrhea, hypoprothrombinemia, and hyperlipidemia. If cholestasis is longstanding, muddy skin pigmentation and excoriations from pruritus may occur, as well as bone pain, osteoporosis or osteomalacia, a bleeding diathesis, and xanthelasma or xanthomas. When cholestasis occurs in infants, symptoms are generally evident about 2 weeks after birth; and by age 2 to 3 months, signs of portal hypertension, irritability (from pruritus), and growth retardation may be observed.

Benign recurrent intrahepatic cholestasis (BRIC or Summerskill syndrome) is characterized by the classic symptoms of cholestasis, as well as fatigue, anorexia, and, occasionally, hepatomegaly. Prolonged recurrent attacks lasting weeks to months occur, sometimes with regularity. Symptoms generally manifest in childhood or adolescence.

Estrogen-related cholestasis may result from pregnancy or from the use of oral contraceptives. In pregnancy, symptoms of cholestasis may occur late in the 3rd trimester, and subside after childbirth. Cholestasis resulting from the use of oral contraceptives may begin soon after use; the condition usually subsides upon termination of the medication. Both variants of estrogen-related cholestasis carry an increased risk of cholelithiasis.

Postoperative cholestasis may occur after surgery with multiple blood transfusions. In the most severe cases, shock, hemorrhage, and acute renal failure may occur.

Etiology The most common intrahepatic causes of cholestasis are genetic, viral (e.g., hepatitis), drug-related, and metabolic (e.g., tyrosinemia).

Extrahepatic causes of the condition are bile duct injury or obstruction.

Epidemiology Cholestasis is believed to be a rare condition that may affect both males and females at any age.

Related Disorders See *Alagille Syndrome; Dubin-Johnson Syndrome.*

Byler disease is a lethal form of intrahepatic cholestasis. Symptoms and signs include steatorrhea, growth retardation, hepatosplenomegaly, and cirrhosis that can lead to death in the first 10 years of life.

Treatment—Standard In cases of intrahepatic cholestasis, treatment should be directed at the underlying cause of the condition. Extrahepatic biliary obstruction requires surgery. In affected infants, surgery on atretic ducts may be successful, but medical problems may persist. Permanent damage may result from cholestasis caused by neonatal hepatitis.

Treatment—Investigational S-Adenosylmethionine is under investigation for treatment of estrogen-related cholestasis.

The orphan drug ursodeoxycholic acid (UDCA) is being studied for treating neonatal cholestasis. William Balistreri, M.D., Children's Hospital Medical Center, Cincinnati, Ohio, may be contacted.

Replacement of vitamin E in children with cholestasis through a drug termed TPGS is being studied by Ronald Sokol, M.D., at the University of Colorado.

Please contact the agencies listed under Resources, below, for the most current information.

Resources

For more information on cholestasis: National Organization for Rare Disorders (NORD); American Liver Foundation; The United Liver Foundation; Children's Liver Foundation; National Digestive Diseases Information Clearinghouse; William Balistreri, M.D., Children's Hospital Medical Center, Cincinnati, Ohio.

For genetic information and genetic counseling referrals: March of Dimes Birth Defects Foundation; NIH/National Center for Education in Maternal and Child Health (NCEMCH).

References

Mendelian Inheritance in Man, 9th ed.: V.A. McKusick; The Johns Hopkins University Press, 1990, pp. 187–188, 530, 1065, 1072, 1094, 1278–1279.

Nelson Textbook of Pediatrics, 13th ed.: R.E. Behrman and V.C. Vaughan, III, eds.; W.B. Saunders Company, 1987, pp. 829–835.

Vitamin E Deficiency Linked to Liver Disease in Children: C. Pierce; Research Resources Reporter, October 1986, National Institutes of Health, pp. 7–9.

CRONKHITE-CANADA DISEASE

Description Cronkhite-Canada disease, allergic granulomatous angiitis, is characterized by generalized gastrointestinal polyposis, alopecia, hyperpigmentation, and nail atrophy.

Synonyms
Gastrointestinal Polyposis with Ectodermal Changes
Canada-Cronkhite Disease

Signs and Symptoms Polyps composed of dilated cystic glands appear on the walls of the large and small intestines. Alactasia, diarrhea, malabsorption, hypoproteinemia, and intestinal loss of electrolytes occur. Lung involvement, cutaneous lesions, and large ecchymotic plaques may be seen in affected individuals.

Etiology There is some evidence that this rare disease is hereditary.

Epidemiology Middle-aged and elderly women are more frequently affected than men.

Related Disorders See *Familial Polyposis; Gardner Syndrome; Peutz-Jeghers Syndrome.*

Treatment—Standard Medical treatment is not helpful in the management of

Cronkhite-Canada disease; surgical removal of polyps or gastric resection may be necessary.

Treatment—Investigational Please contact the agencies listed under Resources, below, for the most current information.

Resources

For more information on Cronkhite-Canada disease: National Organization for Rare Disorders (NORD); National Digestive Diseases Information Clearinghouse.

References

Cecil Textbook of Medicine, 18th ed.: J.B. Wyngaarden and L.H. Smith, Jr., eds.; W.B. Saunders Company, 1988, p. 768.

Scientific American MEDICINE: E. Rubinstein and D. Federman, eds.; Scientific American, Inc., 1978–1991, pp. 4:XIII:1,5,90.

DUBIN-JOHNSON SYNDROME

Description Dubin-Johnson syndrome is a familial chronic form of nonhemolytic jaundice. The presence of a brown, coarsely granular pigment in the centrilobular hepatocytes is pathognomonic of the condition.

Synonyms

Conjugated Hyperbilirubinemia

Hyperbilirubinemia II

Chronic Idiopathic Jaundice

Signs and Symptoms In individuals affected by Dubin-Johnson syndrome, the liver is deeply pigmented owing to the intracellular presence of a melanin-like substance; otherwise, the organ is histologically normal. Conjugated hyperbilirubinemia occurs, and bile appears in the urine.

Etiology The syndrome, probably inherited as an autosomal recessive genetic trait, is thought to result from a defect in the excretion of conjugated bilirubin and certain other organic anions (e.g., sulfobromophthalein) by the liver. Bile salt excretion is not impaired. The cause of pigment deposition in the liver is unknown.

Epidemiology Dubin-Johnson syndrome affects males and females in equal numbers. Age at onset of symptoms may be 10 weeks to 56 years. Individuals of Middle Eastern Jewish descent are affected disproportionately to other populations or ethnic groups.

Related Disorders See *Primary Biliary Cirrhosis.*

Treatment—Standard No treatment may be necessary, although symptomatic and supportive modalities may be appropriate.

Treatment—Investigational Please contact the agencies listed under Resources, below, for the most current information.

Resources

For more information on Dubin-Johnson syndrome: National Organization for Rare Disorders (NORD); American Liver Foundation; The United Liver Foundation; Children's Liver Foundation; National Institute of Diabetes, Digestive & Kidney Diseases Information Clearinghouse; Jewish National Foundation for Genetic Diseases.

For genetic information and genetic counseling referrals: March of Dimes Birth Defects Foundation; NIH/National Center for Education in Maternal and Child Health (NCEMCH).

References

Mendelian Inheritance in Man, 9th ed.: V.A. McKusick; The Johns Hopkins University Press, 1990, pp. 1253–1254.

The Metabolic Basis of Inherited Disease, 6th ed.: C.R. Scriver, et al., eds.; McGraw-Hill, 1989, pp. 1391–1408.

Bile Salt Transport in the Dubin-Johnson Syndrome: J.G. Douglas, et al.; Gut, October 1980, issue 21(10), pp. 890–893.

FAMILIAL POLYPOSIS

Description Familial polyposis is characterized by initially benign polyps in the mucous lining of the gastrointestinal tract.

Synonyms

Adenomatous Polyposis of the Colon

Signs and Symptoms Bleeding and diarrhea are the most common symptoms. Cramping abdominal pain and weight loss may also occur. Chronic rectal bleeding may result in secondary anemia. Untreated patients develop bowel cancer, usually by their late 30s. Some patients are asymptomatic until a malignancy is diagnosed.

Etiology Familial polyposis is inherited through an autosomal dominant gene believed to be on chromosome 5. The gene may control the manufacture of a cell growth substance.

Epidemiology Familial polyposis occurs in one of 5,000 to 10,000 individuals and accounts for about one percent of colorectal cancers. The greatest incidence of the disorder occurs between ages 20 and 45 years, although diagnosis has been made in teenage patients and in persons older than 45.

Related Disorders See *Peutz-Jeghers Syndrome; Gardner Syndrome; Cronkhite-Canada Syndrome.*

Treatment—Standard Early diagnosis is important to prevent malignancy. All children and siblings of a patient should undergo lifelong periodic rectal examination from puberty onward. Surgical removal of the colon may prevent cancer. Surgical methods include joining the ileum and rectum and monitoring for rectal polyps, removing the rectum and an ileostomy, removing the lining of the rectum and developing a reservoir from the ileum, and removing the rectum and constructing an internal abdominal pouch with a nipple valve.

Treatment—Investigational Please contact the agencies listed under Resources, below, for the most current information.

Resources
   For more information on familial polyposis: National Organization for Rare Disorders (NORD); Familial Polyposis Registry (for information on national and international familial polyposis and colon cancer registries, please check with NORD); National Digestive Diseases Information Clearinghouse; National Foundation of Ileitis and Colitis, Inc.; United Ostomy Association.
   For genetic information and genetic counseling referrals: March of Dimes Birth Defects Foundation; National Center for Education in Maternal and Child Health (NCEMCH).

References
   Mendelian Inheritance in Man, 9th ed.: V.A. McKusick; The Johns Hopkins University Press, 1990, pp. 769–773.
   Cecil Textbook of Medicine, 18th ed.: J.B. Wyngaarden and L.H. Smith, Jr., eds.; W.B. Saunders Company, 1988, pp. 767–768.

GARDNER SYNDROME

Description Gardner syndrome is a rare variant of familial polyposis of the large bowel, associated with supernumerary teeth, fibrous dysplasia of the skull, osteomas of the skull and mandible, fibromas, and epithelial cysts.

Synonyms
      Bone Tumor-Epidermoid Cyst-Polyposis
      Intestinal Polyposis III
      Polyposis-Osteomatosis-Epidermoid Cyst Syndrome

Signs and Symptoms Symptoms generally appear during late childhood or after puberty. Multiple colonic adenomas are accompanied by rectal bleeding, diarrhea or constipation, abdominal pain, and weight loss. Osteomas, soft tissue tumors, and abnormal dentition are evident. Affected individuals have a propensity to develop a variety of extra-colonic malignant tumors, and the risk of colon cancer is close to 100 percent.

Etiology The syndrome is inherited as an autosomal dominant trait.

Related Disorders See *Familial Polyposis; Peutz-Jeghers Syndrome; Cronkhite-Canada Disease.*

Treatment—Standard Cancer prevention is the major goal in Gardner syndrome. Resection of the colon and rectum or ileoproctostomy may be necessary. New polyps must be excised or fulgurated.

Treatment—Investigational Please contact the agencies listed under Resources,

below, for the most current information.

Resources
For more information on Gardner syndrome: National Organization for Rare Disorders (NORD); National Digestive Diseases Information Clearinghouse; American Cancer Society; NIH/National Cancer Institute; The National Cancer Institute Physician Data Query (PDQ) phoneline.

For genetic information and genetic counseling referrals: March of Dimes Birth Defects Foundation; National Center for Education in Maternal and Child Health (NCEMCH).

References
Mendelian Inheritance in Man, 9th ed.: V.A. McKusick; The Johns Hopkins University Press, 1990, pp. 769–773.

Cecil Textbook of Medicine, 18th ed.: J.B. Wyngaarden and L.H. Smith, Jr., eds.; W.B. Saunders Company, 1988, pp. 767–771, 2337.

GASTRITIS, GIANT HYPERTROPHIC

Description Giant hypertrophic gastritis is a chronic disorder distinguished by the presence of large, coiled ridges or folds, which may resemble polyps, in the stomach's inner wall. Inflammation may or may not occur.

Synonyms
Ménétrier's Disease
Protein-Losing Gastroenteropathy

Signs and Symptoms The most obvious clinical manifestation is pain or discomfort, accompanied by tenderness, in the upper middle region of the abdomen. Associated symptoms are anorexia, nausea, vomiting, diarrhea, and, in 40 percent of cases, hematemesis. Less frequently, ulcer-like pains are reported following eating.

If protein seeps into the abdominal cavity, hypoproteinuria and edema result. Because the risk of gastric carcinoma may be increased in patients with this condition, periodic examination is necessary.

Biopsy or x-rays, and sometimes endoscopy, are generally necessary for differential diagnosis.

Etiology The cause is unknown.

Epidemiology The disorder usually affects adults between the ages of 30 and 60 years, though a childhood variety has been described. Men are affected more often than women.

Treatment—Standard A high-protein diet, anticholinergic drugs, and acid blockers may correct hypoproteinemia. Gastric resection is rarely necessary.

Treatment—Investigational Please contact the agencies listed under Resources, below, for the most current information.

Resources

For more information on giant hypertrophic gastritis: National Organization for Rare Disorders (NORD); National Digestive Diseases Information Clearinghouse.

References

Cecil Textbook of Medicine, 18th ed.: J.B. Wyngaarden and L.H. Smith, Jr., eds.; W.B. Saunders Company, 1988, pp. 691–692.

GASTROENTERITIS, EOSINOPHILIC (EG)

Description This form of gastritis is distinguished by heavy infiltration of eosinophils in the lining of the stomach, small intestine, and/or large intestine. The infiltration generally causes cramping abdominal pain, diarrhea, and vomiting. The disorder is classified into patterns I, II, and III.

Signs and Symptoms Pattern I is distinguished by extensive infiltration of eosinophils in the area below the submucosa and muscle wall. It commonly involves the stomach but may affect the small intestine or colon as well. Nausea, vomiting, and abdominal pain, and sometimes obstruction are among the symptoms.

In pattern II, eosinophilic infiltration occurs mainly in the mucous and submucosal membranes. In children the gastric mucosa is usually involved, while in adults pattern II tends to affect the small intestine. Symptoms include diarrhea, abdominal and back pain, edema, and mild-to-moderate malabsorption. Laboratory analysis may reveal iron-deficiency anemia, hypoproteinemia, steatorrhea, and other abnormalities.

Pattern III, the rarest form of EG, usually involves the subserosal and serosal membranes of the stomach and is characterized by an accumulation of eosinophil-containing fluid in the abdomen. This fluid can infiltrate the serous membrane of the lungs. Chest pain, fever, shortness of breath, and limited motion of the chest wall are among the symptoms.

Etiology The precise cause is unknown, but some cases may be the result of hypersensitivity to certain foods or other unknown allergens.

Epidemiology Individuals with a history of allergies, eczema, and seasonal asthma are more likely to develop EG, which affects males and females in equal numbers. The disease usually occurs between the ages of 30 and 60 years.

Related Disorders See *Celiac Sprue.*

Treatment—Standard Prednisone is usually effective. Eliminating foods that cause an allergic reaction may help some patients. In severe cases, surgery may be required to remove intestinal obstructions. Additional treatment is symptomatic and supportive.

Treatment—Investigational Sodium chromoglycate is being investigated.

Please contact the agencies listed under Resources, below, for the most current information.

Resources

For more information on eosinophilic gastroenteritis: National Organization for Rare Disorders (NORD); National Digestive Diseases Clearinghouse.

References
Cecil Textbook of Medicine, 18th ed.: J.B. Wyngaarden et al., eds.; W.B. Saunders Company, 1988, p. 807.

Near Fatal Eosinophilic Gastroenteritis Responding to Oral Sodium Chromoglycate: R. Moots, et al.; Gut, September 1988, issue 29(9), pp. 1282–1285.

Eosinophilic Gastroenteritis: Ultrastructural Evidence for a Selective Release of Eosinophil Major Basic Protein: G. Torpier, et al.; Clin. Exp. Immunol., December 1988, issue 74(3), pp. 404–408.

Eosinophilic Gastroenteritis Presenting with Biliary and Duodenal Obstruction: M. Rumans, et al.; Am. Gastroenterol., August 1987, issue 82(8), pp. 775–778.

GLUCOSE-GALACTOSE MALABSORPTION

Description Glucose-galactose malabsorption is a familial disorder of transport produced by deficient intestinal monosaccharidase. The condition is clinically identical to disaccharide intolerance.

Synonyms
Carbohydrate Intolerance
Complex Carbohydrate Intolerance

Signs and Symptoms In children, the inability to digest carbohydrates causes diarrhea and failure to gain weight. In adults the disorder manifests as abdominal distention, nausea, diarrhea, cramps, borborygmus, and flatus.

Etiology Glucose-galactose intolerance is inherited as an autosomal recessive trait.

Epidemiology No statistics on the epidemiology of this extremely rare disorder are available.

Related Disorders See *Galactosemia, Classic; Lactose Intolerance.*

Treatment—Standard Treatment consists of a lactose-free diet with oral calcium supplementation. Fructose (and sometimes sucrose) may be substituted as a source of carbohydrate calories.

Treatment—Investigational Please contact the agencies listed under Resources, below, for the most current information.

Resources

For more information on glucose-galactose intolerance: National Organization for Rare Disorders (NORD); National Digestive Diseases Information Clearinghouse.

For genetic information and genetic counseling referrals: March of

Dimes Birth Defects Foundation; NIH/National Center for Education in Maternal and Child Health (NCEMCH).

References
Mendelian Inheritance in Man, 9th ed.: V.A. McKusick; The Johns Hopkins University Press, 1990, pp. 1208–1209.
The Metabolic Basis of Inherited Disease, 6th ed.: C.R. Scriver, et al., eds.; McGraw-Hill, 1989, pp. 2463–2471.
Glucose-Galactose Malabsorption: Demonstration of Specific Jejunal Brush Membrane Defect: I.W. Booth, et al.; Gut, December 1988, issue 29(12), pp. 1661–1665.
Complex Carbohydrate Intolerance: Diagnostic Pitfalls and Approach to Management: J.D. Loyd-Still, et al., J. Pediatr., May 1988, issue 112(5), pp. 709–713.

HIRSCHSPRUNG DISEASE

Description Congenital Hirschsprung disease is characterized by the absence at birth of myenteric ganglion cells in a distal segment of the large bowel. Peristaltic activity in the involved segment is absent or abnormal, causing continuous spasm, obstruction, and massive hypertrophic dilatation of the normal proximal colon. The aganglionic segment usually remains narrowed, but may dilate passively.

Synonyms
Congenital Megacolon
Megacolon, Aganglionic

Signs and Symptoms Symptoms of Hirschsprung disease appear soon after birth, with constipation, abdominal distention, and vomiting evident in affected neonates. Older infants may become anorexic, lose the physiologic urge to defecate, and have a palpable colon, visible peristalsis, and failure to thrive. The longer the disorder persists untreated, the greater the risk of toxic enterocolitis, which may be fatal.

Etiology It has been suggested that Hirschsprung disease results from a defect in early fetal development caused by maternal hyperthermia. The condition may also be inherited as an autosomal recessive trait, or as an X-linked disorder.

Epidemiology Males are affected more often than females.

Related Disorders Patients with Down syndrome and Waardenburg syndrome may have aganglionic megacolon.

Treatment—Standard The initial treatment of Hirschsprung disease in infants is colostomy at a site proximal to the aganglionic segment. Resection of the colon and definitive repair may be deferred until the infant is larger. Prognosis after surgery is generally good, with most infants achieving satisfactory bowel control.

Treatment—Investigational Please contact the agencies listed under Resources, below, for the most current information.

Resources

For more information on Hirschsprung Disease: National Organization for Rare Disorders (NORD); NIH/National Digestive Diseases Information Clearinghouse; American Hirschsprung Disease Association; Pull-Through Network; Support Group for Parents of Ostomy Children (SPOC).

For genetic information and genetic counseling referrals: March of Dimes Birth Defects Foundation; NIH/National Center for Education in Maternal and Child Health (NCEMCH).

References

Mendelian Inheritance in Man, 9th ed.: V.A. McKusick; The Johns Hopkins University Press, 1990, pp. 1313–1314.

Management of Hirschsprung's Disease in Adolescents: R.R. Ricketts, et al.; Am. Surg., April 1989, issue 55(4), pp. 219–225.

Hirschsprung's Disease. Identification of Risk Factors for Enterocolitis: D.H. Teitelbaum, et al.; Ann. Surg., March 1988, issue 207(3), pp. 240–244.

Adult Hirschsprung's Disease. An experience with the Duhamel-Martin Procedure with Special Reference to Obstructed Patients: N.B. Natsikas, et al.; Dis. Colon Rectum, March 1987, issue 30(3), pp. 204–206.

Segmental Intestinal Muscular Thinning. A Possible Cause of Intestinal Obstruction in the Newborn: J.F. Johnson, et al.; Radiology, December 1987, issue 165(3), pp. 659–660.

INTESTINAL PSEUDOOBSTRUCTION

Description Intestinal pseudoobstruction is characterized by hypomotility of the intestinal walls. The condition resembles a true obstruction, but no evidence of organic obstruction is present at laparotomy.

Synonyms
>Congenital Short Bowel Syndrome
>Hypomotility Disorder
>Pseudointestinal Obstruction Syndrome

Signs and Symptoms Constipation, colicky pain, vomiting, and weight loss or failure to thrive are characteristic of this condition, which may be present at birth. Central nervous system deterioration, speech disturbances, and neuromuscular symptoms may also occur.

Etiology Intestinal pseudoobstruction may occur as a complication of other disorders, including scleroderma, myxedema, amyloidosis, muscular dystrophy, hypokalemia, chronic renal failure, and diabetes mellitus. The cause of the condition is unknown. An autosomal dominant inheritance has been suggested.

Epidemiology Males and females are affected in equal numbers in this rare disorder.

Related Disorders Megacystis microcolon intestinal hypoperistalsis syndrome is characterized by bowel and bladder dysfunction. Catheterization and anticholinergic drugs may be helpful in management, producing temporary asymptomatic periods. Surgery followed by enteral or parenteral nutrition may, however, be necessary.

Paralytic ileus results from paralysis of the bowel wall caused by peritonitis or shock. Symptoms are similar to those of intestinal pseudoobstruction.

Acute colonic pseudoobstruction (Ogilvie syndrome) is characterized by hypomotility of the colon. Decompression of the enlarged colon is appropriate treatment.

A **tumor, abscess, or other mechanical blockage** may cause intestinal obstruction.

The following disorders may precede the development of intestinal pseudoobstruction (see also *Amyloidosis; Scleroderma*): **Myxedema** is characterized by hypothyroidism accompanied by coarse, dry hair and skin, evidence of intellectual impairment, and numerous other anomalies. Affected individuals have a dull facial expression. The condition may be treated with a variety of thyroid hormone preparations. **Anticholinergic toxicity** and **opiate toxicity** are adverse drug reactions that may produce intestinal pseudoobstruction.

Treatment—Standard If intestinal pseudoobstruction has occurred as a secondary effect of another disorder, treatment of the underlying condition is the goal of therapy. The administration of antibiotics, enteral or parenteral nutrition, and, sometimes, surgical removal of the dilated sections of intestine may help to control malabsorption and diarrhea, improve nutrition, and relieve pain.

Treatment—Investigational The orphan drug cisapride, which induces peristalsis in intestinal pseudoobstruction, is being tested. For more information, contact Paul Hyman, M.D., at Harbor UCLA Medical Center's Pediatric Gastrointestinal Motility Center, or Janssen Pharmaceutica, Inc.

Please contact the agencies listed under Resources, below, for the most current information.

Resources

For more information on intestinal pseudoobstruction: National Organization for Rare Disorders (NORD); North American Pediatric Pseudoobstruction Society; National Diabetes, Digestive and Kidney Diseases Information Clearinghouse; Frances Harley, M.D., University of Alberta, Canada.

For information on parenteral or enteral nutrition: PEN Parent Education Network.

For genetic information and genetic counseling referrals: March of Dimes Birth Defects Foundation; National Center for Education in Maternal and Child Health (NCEMCH).

References
Problems of Trace Elements and Vitamins During Long-Term Parenteral Nutrition: A Case Report of Idiopathic Intestinal Pseudo-Obstruction: H. Kadowski, et al.; JPEN, 11(3), pp. 322–325.

Chronic Idiopathic Intestinal Pseudo-Obstruction Caused by Visceral Neuropathy Localised in the Left Colon: Report of Two Cases: H. Suzuki, et al.; Jpn. J. Surg., 17(4), pp. 302–306.

Familial Intestinal Pseudoobstruction Dominated by a Progressive Neurologic Disease at a Young Age: J. Faber, et al.; Gastroenterology, 92(3), pp. 786–790.

Familial Visceral Neuropathy with Autosomal Dominant Transmission: E.A. Mayer, et al.; Gastroenterology, 91(6), 1528–1535.

Chronic Idiopathic Intestinal Pseudo-Obstruction: Clinical and Intestinal Manometric Findings: V. Stanghellini, et al.; Gut, 28(1), pp. 5–12.

MALLORY-WEISS SYNDROME

Description Mallory-Weiss syndrome is characterized by slitlike lacerations of the gastric mucosa, longitudinally placed at or slightly below the esophagogastric junction.

Synonyms
Gastroesophageal Laceration-Hemorrhage Syndrome

Signs and Symptoms Hematemesis or melena generally follows hours or days of vomiting, retching, or hiccups.

Etiology The esophagogastric lacerations of Mallory-Weiss syndrome are usually caused by vomiting, but they may also result from trauma to the chest or abdomen, intense snoring, hiccups, gastritis, or cancer chemotherapy.

Epidemiology The disorder was originally described in alcoholics, but it may occur in other situations as described above.

Related Disorders Boerhaave syndrome is characterized by esophageal rupture, an emergency situation with a high mortality rate. Mediastinitis and pleural effusion should be treated immediately by surgical repair and drainage.

Peptic ulcer is a common disorder that is recurrent and chronic. The goal of treatment is to neutralize or decrease gastric activity.

Esophageal varices occur in the azygos and portal veins in individuals with portal hypertension.

Treatment—Standard Most episodes of bleeding from Mallory-Weiss syndrome stop spontaneously. However, ligation of the lacerations or an angiographically guided infusion of vasopressin into the left gastric artery may be required.

Treatment—Investigational The effectiveness of embolization is being evaluated as a treatment for massive uncontrolled bleeding of the esophagus.

The orphan drug sodium tetradecyl sulfate (Sotradecol) is being used as an experimental treatment for bleeding esophageal varices. For more information contact Elkins-Sinn, Inc., 2 Esterbrook Lane, Cherry Hill, New Jersey 08003-4099.

Please contact the agencies listed under Resources, below, for the most current information.

Resources
For more information on Mallory-Weiss syndrome: National Organization for Rare Disorders (NORD); NIH/National Digestive Diseases Information Clearinghouse.

References

Internal Medicine, 3rd ed.: J.H. Stein, ed.-in-chief; Little, Brown and Company, 1990, pp. 310–311.

Upper Gastrointestinal Bleeding: J. Lancaster; Prim. Care, March 1988, issue 15(1), pp. 31–41.

Multipolar Electrocoagulation in the Treatment of Active Upper Gastrointestinal Tract Hemorrhage. A Prospective Controlled Trial: L. Laine; New Eng. J. Med., June 1987, issue 316(26), pp. 1613–1617.

Mallory-Weiss Tear. A Complication of Cancer Chemotherapy: M. Fishman, et al.; Cancer, December 1983, issue 52(11), pp. 2031–2032.

Snore-Induced Mallory-Weiss Syndrome: J. Merrill; J. Clin. Gastroenterol., February 1987, issue 9(1), pp. 88–89.

Mallory-Weiss Syndrome. A Study of 224 Patients: C. Sugawa, et al.; Am. J. Surg., January 1983, issue 145(1), pp. 30–33.

Percutaneous Transhepatic Embolization of Gastroesophageal Varices: Results in 400 Patients: C.L. Hermine, et al.; April 1989, issue 152(4), pp. 775–760.

MICROVILLUS INCLUSION DISEASE

Description Microvillus inclusion disease is a progressive intestinal disease characterized by chronic, severe, watery diarrhea occurring in infants at or soon after birth.

Synonyms
Familial Enteropathy

Signs and Symptoms Diarrhea persists after oral feeding. Dehydration, acidosis, growth retardation, and developmental delay may be observed in affected infants.

Etiology Microvillus inclusion disease is a congenital defect in the intestinal wall that is inherited as an autosomal recessive trait.

Epidemiology Males and females are affected in equal numbers.

Related Disorders See *Lactose Intolerance.*

Familial chloride diarrhea is characterized by profuse watery stools with excessive chloride content. Infants born with this autosomal recessive disorder are often premature.

Infantile diarrhea with abnormal hair is a progressive malabsorption syndrome that develops around the 3rd week of life. Affected infants have dark, kinky hair that falls out easily, large low-set ears, a flat nasal bridge, and a large mouth. The disorder is inherited as an autosomal recessive trait.

Congenital sodium diarrhea results from defective sodium exchange in the bowels. This recessive disorder is present at birth.

Treatment—Standard Microvillus inclusion disease is treated with intravenous feeding. Genetic counseling is recommended.

Treatment—Investigational An analogue of somatostatin being tested for treatment of prolonged diarrhea shows some promise.

Please contact the agencies listed under Resources, below, for the most current

information.

Resources

For more information on microvillus inclusion disease: National Organization for Rare Disorders (NORD); National Institute of Diabetes, Digestive & Kidney Diseases Information Clearinghouse.

For genetic information and genetic counseling referrals: March of Dimes Birth Defects Foundation; NIH/National Center for Education in Maternal and Child Health (NCEMCH).

References

Microvillus Inclusion Disease: An Inherited Defect of Brush-Border Assembly and Differentiation: E. Cutz, et al.; New Eng. J. of Med., March 9, 1989, issue 320(10), pp. 646–651.

Biochemical Abnormality in Brush Border Membrane Protein of a Patient with Congenital Microvillus Atrophy: L. Carruthers, et al.; J. Pediatr. Gastroenterol. Nutr., December 1985, issue 4(6), pp. 902–907.

Microvillus Inclusion Disease: Specific Diagnostic Features Shown by Alkaline Phosphatase Histochemistry: B.D. Lake; J. Clin. Pathol., August 1988, issue 41(8), pp. 880–882.

PEUTZ-JEGHERS SYNDROME

Description Peutz-Jeghers syndrome is a hereditary disorder characterized by polyps on the mucous lining of the intestinal wall and dark discolorations on the skin and mucous membrane surfaces.

Synonyms

Hutchinson-Weber-Peutz Syndrome
Intestinal Polyposis II
Intestinal Polyposis-Cutaneous Pigmentation Syndrome
Jeghers Syndrome
Melanoplakia-Intestinal Polyposis
Peutz-Touraine Syndrome

Signs and Symptoms Intussusception and bleeding are the most common symptoms. Discrete brown-to-black macules occur around the lips; inside the mouth on the mucosal lining of the cheeks; on the fingers, palms of the hands, forearms, and toes; and around the naval. Polyps occur most often in the jejunum and ileum but may be present anywhere in the gastrointestinal tract. Severe bleeding can cause anemia and recurrent pain that disappears with massage, physical manipulation, or contorting the body. Intussusception can cause complications such as intestinal obstruction and gangrene. The polyps are benign hamartomas, but about 50 percent of patients develop intestinal and nonintestinal malignancies, particularly in the pancreas, ovaries, and breast, as adults.

Etiology Peutz-Jeghers syndrome is an inherited autosomal dominant trait.

Related Disorders See *Familial Polyposis; Gardner Syndrome; Cronkhite-*

Canada Disease.

Treatment—Standard Periodic x-rays of the gastrointestinal tract from childhood through adolescence monitor changes in size and number of polyps. Large individual polyps or particularly heavily affected sections of the intestine can be removed surgically. If intestinal gangrene develops, the involved section must be resected.

Treatment—Investigational Please contact the agencies listed under Resources, below, for the most current information.

Resources

For more information on Peutz-Jeghers syndrome: National Organization for Rare Disorders (NORD); National Digestive Diseases Information Clearinghouse.

For genetic information and genetic counseling referrals: March of Dimes Birth Defects Foundation; National Center for Education in Maternal and Child Health (NCEMCH).

References

Smith's Recognizable Patterns of Human Malformation, 4th ed.: K.L. Jones; W.B. Saunders Company, 1988, p. 462.

Cecil Textbook of Medicine, 18th ed.: J.B. Wyngaarden and L.H. Smith, Jr., eds.; W.B. Saunders Company, 1988, pp. 767, 771.

PRIMARY BILIARY CIRRHOSIS

Description Primary biliary cirrhosis is a chronic, progressive disease occurring in 4 stages and thought to be related to abnormalities in the immune system. In later stages of the disease, cholestasis of the intrahepatic bile ducts results in jaundice. Excessive amounts of copper accumulate in the liver (but the relationship of these elevated levels to the disease is not understood), and fibrous or granular induration of the soft liver tissue develops.

Synonyms

Hanot Cirrhosis

Signs and Symptoms Commonly, the patient with primary biliary cirrhosis is a woman of about 50 who complains of persistent, generalized itching, dark urine, pale stools, and jaundice. The disease has 4 symptomatic stages stemming from unrelieved obstruction of the extrahepatic bile ducts.

In stage I, hepatomegaly, centrilobular bile stasis, cell degeneration, and focal areas of necrosis occur. Unexplained itching is common and is often worse at night. Increased amounts of melanin pigmentation appear in the skin, and excoriation occurs. Fatigue and unexplained weight loss are common.

In stage II, proliferation and dilatation of the portal ducts and ductules are more widespread but less specific. Biopsy shows loss of normal bile ducts and increased numbers of those with irregularly shaped lumens. Fibrous cells infiltrate and spread within the liver. Bile stoppage is limited to portal areas.

In stage III, cholestasis of bile acids, bilirubin, copper, and other substances normally excreted into bile cause progressive damage. The medium-sized bile ducts become inflamed and distorted. Over a period of time the itching, jaundice, and hyperpigmentation increase. Xanthomas may be noticeable on the skin and may occur in internal organs. Excessive amounts of lipids and cholesterol are found circulating in the blood. The bile acid concentration in the intestines is inadequate for complete digestion and absorption of triglycerides in the diet. Additionally, normal absorption of vitamins A, D, E, and K as well as calcium may be diminished, and iron-deficiency anemia may develop. Muscle wasting, spider angiomas, palmar erythema, ascites and edema, and in about 25 percent of patients, the bony tenderness of osteoporosis and osteomalacia occur.

Stage IV represents the endstage of lesion formation, with widespread cirrhosis and regenerative nodules. Jaundice becomes pronounced.

Patients may die within 5 to 10 years of the first appearance of the disease, primarily because of the development of portal hypertension.

Etiology The cause is not known. An immunologic relationship is suspected because IgG is present in the sera of 95 percent of patients with primary biliary cirrhosis; however, these circulating antibodies, which react with mitochondrial antibodies, are seldom present in other forms of liver disease. Since 90 percent of those affected with the disease are women over age 50, an endocrine contribution is also suggested.

Epidemiology The disease, a rare form of biliary cirrhosis, affects females over 50 years of age in approximately 90 percent of cases.

Related Disorders **Extrahepatic bile duct obstruction** originates outside the liver but may produce symptoms similar to those of primary biliary cirrhosis. **Obstructive biliary cirrhosis** is characterized by fibroid or granular hardening of the soft liver tissue due to bile duct obstruction rather than the deterioration inside the liver that is typical of primary biliary cirrhosis.

Alcoholic cirrhosis is characterized by gradual hardening of the soft tissue of the liver, a condition that frequently develops in alcoholics. The early stage is marked by liver enlargement due to fatty infiltration with mild fibrosis. In late stages, normal liver lobes are replaced with small nodules, separated by a framework of fine fibrous tissue strands (hobnail liver).

Treatment—Standard Since this is a prolonged, chronic, and incurable disease, treatment is often directed at relieving itching, malabsorption, fluid retention, portal hypertension, and late-stage hepatic insufficiency. Topical menthol lotions, sedation, and cholestyramine relieve itching in almost all patients. Large-volume plasmapheresis may relieve itching in patients who do not respond to drug treatment. A balanced high-calorie diet is adequate, but fat intake may be reduced to below 30 to 40 gm per day if the patient complains of diarrhea. Malabsorption of fat-soluble vitamins may be treated with vitamins K1, A, and D, and with calcium. Iron-deficiency anemia responds to oral iron supplements. Folic acid is recommended for patients taking cholestyramine because the drug may produce a folic acid deficiency. Folic acid and cholestyramine should be taken several hours apart. In severe cases, liver transplantation may be considered.

Treatment—Investigational Several drugs including colchicine, prednisolone, D-penicillamine, azathioprine, ursodeoxycholic acid, cyclosporine A, and chlorambucil are being evaluated for therapy.

Please contact the agencies listed under Resources, below, for the most current information.

Resources

For more information on primary biliary cirrhosis: National Organization for Rare Disorders (NORD); Primary Biliary Cirrhosis Patient Support Network; American Liver Foundation; The United Liver Foundation; Children's Liver Foundation; NIH/National Institute of Diabetes, Digestive & Kidney Diseases Clearinghouse.

References

Clinical and Statistical Analyses of New and Evolving Therapies for Primary Biliary Cirrhosis: R.H. Wiesner, et al.; Hepatology, May–June 1988, issue 8(3), pp. 668–676.

Treatment of Pruritis in Primary Biliary Cirrhosis with Rifampin. Results of a Double-Blind, Crossover, Randomized Trial: C.N. Ghent, et al.; Gastroenterology, February 1988, issue 94(2), pp. 488–493.

Transplantation of Liver, Heart, and Lungs for Primary Biliary Cirrhosis and Primary Pulmonary Hypertension: J. Wallwork, et al.; Lancet, July 1987, issue 2(8552), pp. 182–185.

SUCROSE-ISOMALTOSE MALABSORPTION, CONGENITAL

Description Congenital sucrose-isomaltose malabsorption results from an inborn deficiency of the enzyme sucrase-isomaltase. Characteristic symptoms result from the ingestion of table sugar or certain other carbohydrates.

Synonyms

> Disaccharide Intolerance I
> Sucrase-Alpha-Dextrinase Deficiency, Congenital

Signs and Symptoms Diarrhea is the major symptom. Affected children may be unable to gain weight on a normal diet, since the diarrhea can be severe enough to purge other nutrients before they can be absorbed. Adults may experience abdominal cramps, bloating, and flatus.

Etiology The disorder is transmitted through autosomal recessive genes.

Epidemiology Congenital sucrose-isomaltose malabsorption is rare, affecting children from birth, and males and females in equal numbers. Some patients may be only mildly affected; others may have moderate to severe forms of the disorder.

Related Disorders See *Lactose Intolerance.*

Treatment—Standard Symptoms are prevented by avoiding sucrose and sucrose-containing foods.

Treatment—Investigational Please contact the agencies listed under Resources, below, for the most current information.

Resources

For more information on congenital sucrose-isomaltose malabsorption: National Organization for Rare Disorders (NORD); National Digestive Diseases Information Clearinghouse; Research Trust for Metabolic Diseases in Children (RTMDC).

For genetic information and genetic counseling referrals: March of Dimes Birth Defects Foundation; National Center for Education in Maternal and Child Health (NCEMCH).

WALDMANN DISEASE

Description Waldmann disease is characterized by dilatation of the lymphatics of the intestinal lamina propria. The disorder may be congenital or acquired.

Synonyms

> Familial Dysproteinemia
> Familial Hypoproteinemia with Lymphangiectatic Enteropathy
> Hypercatabolic Protein-Losing Enteropathy
> Hypoproteinemia, Idiopathic
> Intestinal Lymphangiectasia
> Lymphangiectatic Protein-Losing Enteropathy
> Neonatal Lymphedema due to Exudative Enteropathy

Signs and Symptoms Gross, often asymmetric edema, intermittent diarrhea, nausea, vomiting, and abdominal pain occur in children or young adults. Protein-losing enteropathy, steatorrhea, chylous effusions, lymphopenia, and ascites may also be present. Serum albumin, IgA, and IgG are markedly reduced.

Etiology Waldmann disease may be inherited as an autosomal dominant trait characterized by congenital malformation of the lymphatics. The condition may also be acquired as a secondary effect of tuberculous enteritis, granulomatous enteritis, lymphoma, retroperitoneal fibrosis, pancreatitis, or constrictive pericarditis.

Epidemiology Both males and females are affected.

Related Disorders See *Hemolytic-Uremic Syndrome.*

Treatment—Standard Treatment of Waldmann disease is accomplished with a low-fat diet supplemented by medium-chain triglycerides. Sodium restriction and diuretic therapy may be helpful in some patients. Occasionally surgical resection of the involved intestinal segment may be necessary.

Treatment—Investigational Please contact the agencies listed under Resources,

below, for the most current information.

Resources

For more information on Waldmann disease: National Organization for Rare Disorders (NORD); National Lymphatic and Venous Diseases Foundation, Inc.; National Digestive Diseases Information Clearinghouse.

References

Dietary Management of Intestinal Lymphangiectasia Complicated by Short Gut Syndrome: J.M. Thompson, et al.; Human Nutrition and Applied Nutrition, April 1986, issue 40(2), pp. 136–140.

9 | INHERITED RENAL AND GENITOURINARY DISORDERS
By Russell W. Chesney, M.D.

The kidney and genitourinary tract can be afflicted by more than 235 inherited disorders and 75 chromosomal abnormalities resulting in renal defects. Some inherited renal disorders are reasonably common, including diabetic nephropathy or familial nephrolithiasis, which can affect a substantial portion of the population (0.5 to 1 percent). But many are quite rare, with an incidence of 1:10,000 to 1:100,000.

Clinical manifestations of these disorders comprise a broad spectrum; e.g., hematuria, proteinuria, hydronephrosis, nephrolithiasis, renal dysplasia, mono- or polycystic kidneys, tubulointerstitial nephritis, and renal medullary disease. Other abnormalities include renal vascular stenosis, aminoaciduria, glycosuria, and various other tubular abnormalities which result in the hyperexcretion of organic solutes or ions. A common final development is renal insufficiency, which leads to the symptom complex called uremia, further known as "endstage renal disease."

Although it is difficult to generalize about the diversity of genetic renal disorders, the following universal principles concerning inherited renal disease can be identified.

1. More than one child in a family may be affected; a family history should be obtained.

2. The child with hereditary renal disease frequently presents with growth failure.

3. The inherited pattern is usually autosomal recessive, but it may

also be autosomal dominant, X-linked recessive, or X-linked dominant.

Inherited renal disease is diagnosed by conventional nephrological diagnostic procedures including a physical history, a family history, urinalysis, renal ultrasonography, pyelography, and percutaneous renal biopsy. The techniques used to diagnose inborn errors of metabolism are also necessary to discern those conditions which include a renal component as part of their systemic involvement. For example, several lysosomal storage diseases include renal abnormalities; thus, lysosomal enzyme activity must be measured and a renal biopsy must be performed to detect changes in the renal tubule or glomerulus. Many renal disorders also influence the serum concentration of electrolytes, blood urea nitrogen, and creatinine. Various acid-base disturbances occur, including metabolic acidosis with a normal anion gap, hyperchloremia (found in proximal or distal renal tubular acidosis), metabolic acidosis with an increased anion gap (found in diabetic nephropathy), and hypokalemic metabolic alkalosis (common in Bartter syndrome). These disorders may also impair several normal functions of the kidney: plasma filtration so as to reduce glomerular filtration rate; reabsorption by the proximal or distal tubule or collecting duct resulting in excessive excretion of ions or organic solutes; secretion, which results in retention of excreted substances such as uric acid; production of kidney-derived hormones including erythropoietin and 1,25-dihydroxyvitamin D_3; concentration and dilution of the final urine, which is observed in nephrogenic diabetes insipidus or sickle cell nephropathy; and the regulation of blood pressure.

The child who presents with either acute or chronic oliguric renal failure poses the greatest dilemma. A diagnosis must be made in the face of life-threatening hyperkalemia, volume overload, congestive heart failure, and hypertension. The accompanying diagram offers an approach to such a child. This chart lists only the more common disorders and is not exhaustive. Oliguria has four major causes: obstruction, prerenal azotemia as observed in dehydration, and acute or chronic renal failure. The child with acute renal failure will usually exhibit physical findings which point to the cause of renal failure, such as pyoderma or pharyngitis associated with poststreptococcal glomerulonephritis, or a facial rash and arthralgia associated with systemic lupus erythematosus. The child with chronic renal failure will present with short stature, anemia,

Figure 9.1. Clinical presentation of oliguric renal failure.

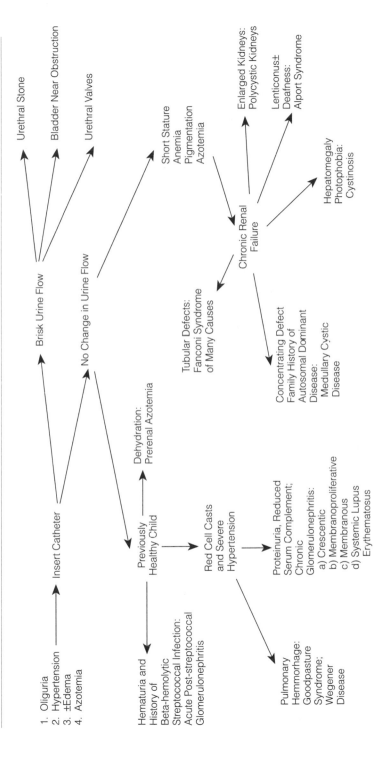

anorexia, and hyperpigmentation because of the deposition in skin of nitrogenous waste products not excreted by failing kidneys. Other physical features pointing to chronic renal failure are enlarged kidneys in polycystic kidney disease, lenticonus and deafness in Alport hereditary nephritis, photophobia and hepatomegaly in cystinosis, and polyuria and anemia in medullary cystic disease. Inherited diseases are far more likely to result in chronic rather than acute renal failure.

Therapy is now available for a variety of inherited renal diseases. Cystinuria can be treated with D-penicillamine or alpha-methylpropinylglycine, which reduces the excretion of relatively insoluble cystine by the formation of more solubly mixed disulfides. The progression toward endstage renal disease can be slowed by cysteamine in patients with cystinosis. Indomethacin can improve the profound hypokalemia of Bartter syndrome. Tight metabolic control of hyperglycemia will probably forestall nephropathy in diabetes, although this needs to be proven.

Patients with nephrogenic diabetes insipidus will have a marked reduction in urine volume if placed on a sodium chloride-restricted diet in conjunction with a thiazide diuretic. For children who develop uremia because of an inherited renal disorder, the techniques of hemo- and peritoneal dialysis and renal transplantation are successful in reversing uremia.

References

Renal Diseases in Children: Clinical Evaluation and Diagnosis: A.Y. Barakat; Springer-Verlag, 1990.

Inherited Renal Tubular Disorders: R.W. Chesney and A.L. Friedman; in Diseases of the Kidney, 5th ed.: R.L. Schrier and C.M. Gottschalk; Little, Brown and Company, 1988, pp. 663–688.

INHERITED RENAL AND GENITOURINARY DISORDERS
Listings in This Section

ALPORT SYNDROME

Description The syndrome encompasses a group of hereditary renal disorders marked by progressive deterioration of the glomerular basement membrane, which in a high proportion of cases leads to chronic renal failure, uremia, and the development of endstage renal disease **(ESRD).** Uremia and renal failure may cause cardiac disturbances and renal osteodystrophy. In some forms of Alport syndrome vision and hearing are also impaired.

Alport syndrome is classified according to its mode of inheritance, the age of onset of uremia, and features other than renal abnormalities. Six types of the disorder, designated I-VI, have been described. Juvenile forms are characterized by the development of ESRD before age 31. In adult forms, ESRD occurs after age 31.

Synonyms
> Epstein Syndrome (Type V)
> Hereditary Nephritis
> Nephritis and Nerve Deafness, Hereditary
> Nephropathy and Deafness, Hereditary

Signs and Symptoms The characteristic renal glomerular basement membrane abnormality probably causes hematuria and proteinuria. When chronic renal failure, uremia, or ESRD develops, other signs and symptoms appear. Symptoms of uremia and chronic renal failure (see below) begin insidiously.

Renal failure may lead to abnormalities of bone formation, calcium and phosphorus metabolism, and conversion of vitamin D to its active metabolite, as well as excessive parathyroid hormone secretion. Hypocalcemia and hyperphosphatemia are characteristic findings.

Ocular abnormalities may occur in the juvenile forms of Alport syndrome. Lenticonus or spherophakia may be noted. Cataracts, retinal macular flecks, or fundus albipunctatus may also be present. Children with Alport syndrome may be myopic.

Acoustic nerve or cochlear deafness also occurs in some forms of the syndrome, with high-tone hearing loss being a prominent feature.

Signs and symptoms of uremia include anorexia, nausea and vomiting, peptic ulcer disease, weakness, fatigue, hypersomnia, lassitude, dry skin, and pruritus. A urine-like breath odor is frequently noted in association with pallor, dyspnea, hypertension, fluid retention, and edema. Nerve conduction defects and attention deficits are common.

Etiology Alport syndrome may be inherited as an autosomal dominant or an X-linked dominant trait, or it may occur through gene mutation. An autosomal recessive inheritance has also been reported. The 6 types of syndrome and their modes of inheritance are as follows:

Type I, a juvenile form characterized by renal disease with nerve deafness and ocular abnormalities, is an autosomal dominant disorder.

Type II, a juvenile form that includes renal disease with nerve deafness and ocular abnormalities, is X-linked dominant.

Type III, an adult form that includes renal disease with nerve deafness, is X-linked dominant.

Type IV, an adult form that affects only the kidney, is X-linked dominant. No vision or hearing impairment is present.

Type V (Epstein syndrome), which includes nerve deafness and thrombocytopathia, is an autosomal dominant disorder. This rare type has not yet been classified as a juvenile or an adult form.

Type VI, a juvenile form that includes kidney disease with nerve deafness and ocular abnormalities, is autosomal dominant.

Epidemiology Approximately 1:50,000 Americans carries the gene for Alport syndrome, although not all of them develop the syndrome. About 15 to 18 percent of affected newborns have no family history of renal disease. These cases may represent spontaneous gene mutation. The syndrome is more frequent and more severe in men. No racial preponderance or geographic clusters have been noted.

Related Disorders See *Fabry Disease; Medullary Cystic Disease.*

See also *Hematuria, Benign Familial*. The abnormalities of the glomerular basement membrane that characterize Alport syndrome are not found in benign familial hematuria, and proteinuria is not a feature.

Glomerulonephritis is characterized by inflammatory changes in the glomeruli. Manifestations include hematuria and proteinuria, facial edema, oliguria, and hypertension. Nephrotic syndrome and chronic renal failure may also occur.

Treatment—Standard Chronic renal failure caused by Alport syndrome must be treated vigorously. Renal function and certain components in the blood are regularly monitored. Fluid intake and diet, particularly salt and protein content, may be restricted and drugs prescribed. Control of hypertension and prompt and aggressive treatment of urinary tract and ear infections are important to maintain function of either organ.

Dialysis or renal transplantation may be used to treat chronic renal failure and ESRD. Because of the slight or inapparent disease in some female family members, care must be taken in selecting living related kidney donors.

In some cases, successful kidney transplantation has halted the progression of hearing loss. Transplantation of the cornea or removal of the lens may be helpful in patients with visual problems.

Other treatment is symptomatic and supportive. Genetic counseling is indicated for patients and their families.

Treatment—Investigational Calcium acetate is a new orphan drug being used in the treatment of hyperphosphatemia in ESRD. It is manufactured by Pharmedic Co.

Please contact the agencies listed under Resources, below, for the most current information.

Resources

For more information on Alport syndrome: National Organization for Rare Disorders (NORD); Hereditary Nephritis Foundation; Alport Syndrome Study; National Kidney and Urologic Diseases Information Clearinghouse; National Kidney Foundation; American Kidney Fund.

For genetic information and genetic counseling referrals: March of Dimes Birth Defects Foundation; NIH/National Center for Education in Maternal and Child Health.

References

Hereditary Nephropathies: M.C. Gregory, et al.; *in* Textbook of Internal Medicine; Lippincott, 1988, Ch. 118.

Alport Syndrome: C.L. Atkins, et al.; *in* Diseases of the Kidney, 4th ed.; Little, Brown & Company, 1988, pp. 617–641.

Mendelian Inheritance in Man, 9th ed.: V.A. McKusick; The Johns Hopkins University Press, 1990, pp. 47–49, 1025, 1561.

Internal Medicine, 3rd ed.: J.H. Stein, ed.-in-chief; Little, Brown & Company, 1990, pp. 913–914.

EXSTROPHY OF THE BLADDER

Description Exstrophy of the bladder is a congenital anomaly characterized by the absence of a portion of the lower abdominal wall and the anterior vesical wall, and eversion of the posterior vesical wall through the opening. Urine is excreted through this opening.

Synonyms

Ectopia Vesicae

Signs and Symptoms The anomaly results in incontinence. The pubic arch is open, and the ischia are widely separated and connected by a fibrous band. The connection between the ureter and the bladder is constricted, and the ureters are dilated. If the defect is not corrected, ureteral reflux will occur, and pyelonephritis and renal failure are likely to develop.

Etiology Exstrophy of the bladder may result from rupture of the fetal bladder or from transposition of the earliest embryologic form of the organ due to a change in position of the vitelline duct.

Epidemiology The incidence of the abnormality is 7 times higher in males than in females.

Treatment—Standard Treatment consists of primary closure of the exstrophic bladder, often using a segment of colon to form the anterior and superior portion of the bladder wall. An alternative but rarely used procedure to correct the defect is by ureterosigmoidostomy, with or without a colostomy. A third corrective procedure is ileal or colon loop urinary diversion.

Reconstruction of the genitalia, when necessary, is usually begun before the age of 2 years. The outlook for maintaining normal renal function is relatively good.

Treatment—Investigational Please check with the agencies listed under Resources, below, for the most current information.

Resources
   For more information on exstrophy of the bladder: National Organization for Rare Disorders (NORD); National Support Group for Exstrophy of the Bladder; National Kidney and Urologic Diseases Information Clearinghouse; Simon Foundation; Help for Incontinent People (H.I.P.).

References
   Cecil Textbook of Medicine, 18th ed.: J.B. Wyngaarden and L.H. Smith, Jr., eds.; W.B. Saunders Company, 1988, pp. 2107, 650.
   Nelson Textbook of Pediatrics, 13th ed.: R.E. Behrman and V.C. Vaughan, III, eds.; W.B. Saunders Company, 1987, p. 1159.

HEMATURIA, BENIGN FAMILIAL

Description Benign familial hematuria is a hereditary nonprogressive renal disorder that begins in childhood. It is characterized by episodes of hematuria and scattered thinning of the glomerular basement membrane.

Synonyms
      Hematuria, Benign Recurrent
      Hematuria, Essential

Signs and Symptoms The hematuria may be macro- or microscopic and is often preceded by a respiratory infection. Little or no proteinuria occurs, and renal function is unaffected. In children, the urine may clear after each episode; in adults, the hematuria may be more persistent.

Etiology The cause is unknown. A genetic predisposition transmitted through autosomal dominant genes is suspected. The disorder's frequent appearance after respiratory infections may be significant.

Epidemiology Benign familial hematuria occurs more frequently in males than females, and more often in children and young adults.

Related Disorders See *IGA Nephropathy; Alport Syndrome.*
   Chronic renal failure can be a complication of many kidney diseases or a symptom of a variety of diseases and conditions. It occurs gradually when the kidneys can no longer filter waste products from the blood. Polyuria, hematuria, proteinuria, hypertension, and anemia may occur.

Treatment—Standard Treatment may not be necessary, or is symptomatic and supportive. Genetic counseling may be helpful.

Treatment—Investigational Please check with the agencies listed under Resources, below, for the most current information.

Resources

For more information on benign familial hematuria: National Organization for Rare Disorders (NORD); National Kidney Foundation; American Kidney Fund; National Kidney and Urological Diseases Information Clearinghouse.

For genetic information and genetic counseling referrals: March of Dimes Birth Defects Foundation; NIH/National Center for Education in Maternal and Child Health (NCEMCH).

References

Mendelian Inheritance in Man, 9th ed.: V.A. McKusick; The Johns Hopkins University Press, 1990, p. 392.

Internal Medicine, 3rd ed.: J.H. Stein, ed.-in-chief; Little, Brown and Company, 1990, p. 914.

Establishing the Diagnosis of Benign Familial Hematuria. The Importance of Examining the Urine Sediment of Family Members: S. Blumenthal, et al.; JAMA, April 15, 1988, issue 259(15), pp. 2263–2266.

Benign Familial Hematuria: N. Yoshikawa, et al.; Arch. Pathol. Lab. Med., August 1988, issue 112(8), pp. 794–797.

HEMOLYTIC-UREMIC SYNDROME (HUS)

Description HUS is a syndrome of diverse etiologies defined as a microangiopathic hemolytic anemia, thrombocytopenia, and acute kidney failure with hematuria and proteinuria.

Synonyms

Gasser Syndrome

Signs and Symptoms Onset usually is abrupt; in most cases the first sign is diarrhea, with or without blood in the stool (hematochezia). Other characteristics include vomiting, dehydration, labored breathing, hematemesis, melena, petechiae, hypertension, and seizures. Thrombocytopenia and anemia usually occur. The kidneys are primarily affected, and anuria may be present. The onset of anemia (pallor) and oliguria may occur abruptly during the course of the diarrhea.

Approximately 60 percent of children with HUS develop acute kidney failure, which usually reverses after dialysis. Chronic kidney failure occurs in approximately 10 percent of children, who require lifelong dialysis or transplantation. Kidney involvement is generally more severe in adults, and cortical necrosis may occur.

Etiology The cause is unknown. An association with *Escherichia coli* infection is found in 70 percent of cases in North America and 35 percent of cases in the United Kingdom. The *E. coli* strains associated with HUS (1057:H7;0157:H— and others) produce verocytotoxins similar to the toxins produced by *Shigella dysenteriae*. HUS usually appears abruptly in children 3 to 10 days after an episode of gastroenteritis or viral upper respiratory tract infections. In adults, it most commonly affects women and is often associated with pregnancy or the use of birth control pills.

Epidemiology The syndrome occurs rarely, and most frequently in children under the age of 4 years, and in pregnant or postpartum women. It is occasionally seen in older children and nonpregnant adults. Some areas of the world (e.g., Argentina) have a much higher incidence than North America, but the west coast of the United States appears to be an endemic region.

Related Disorders See *Purpura, Thrombotic Thrombocytopenic.*

Treatment—Standard Infants and children recover more easily than adults. Dialysis may be necessary for children and postpartum women. Fresh frozen plasma transfusions may be used. The orphan drug erythropoetin (EPO), used in the treatment of anemia related to kidney dialysis, should not be prescribed.

Treatment—Investigational Plasmapheresis may be beneficial in severe cases, but is still under investigation to analyze side effects and effectiveness.

Please check with the agencies listed under Resources, below, for the most current information.

Resources
   For more information on hemolytic-uremic syndrome: National Organization for Rare Disorders (NORD); NIH/National Kidney and Urologic Diseases Information Clearinghouse; National Kidney Foundation; American Kidney Fund.

References
   Illnesses Associated with Escherichia Coli 0157:H7 Infections. A Broad Clinical Spectrum: P.M. Griffin, et al.; Ann. Intern. Med., November 1, 1988, issue 109(9), pp. 705–712.
   Cytoxin-Producing Escherichia Coli and the Hemolytic-Uremic Syndrome: T.G. Cleary; Pediatr. Clin. North Am., June 1988, issue 35(5), pp. 485–501.
   Hemolytic-Uremic Syndrome Associated with an Infection by Verotoxin-Producing Escherichia Coli 0111 in a Woman on Oral Contraceptives: K.O. Stenger, et al.; Clin. Nephrol., March 1989; issue 29(3), pp. 153–158.

HEPATORENAL SYNDROME

Description Hepatorenal syndrome develops as a result of severe liver disease; the kidneys appear normal. The disorder is seen in 2 forms, one milder than the other.

Signs and Symptoms Unique circulatory abnormalities occur in hepatorenal syndrome. Cardiac output is increased. The arteries of the symtemic circulation widen. The renal arteries narrow, causing a decrease in renal blood flow.

The more severe form of the syndrome is characterized by ascites, jaundice, and rapidly progressive renal failure, with oliguria and azotemia and, in some cases, proteinuria and hematuria. The jaundice may be accompanied by dark urine and an enlarged and tender liver. Anorexia, fever, fatigue, and weakness may be present. Hepatic or portosystemic encephalopathy may develop, possibly causing changes in mental acuity, personality changes, inappropriate behavior, depression, and sleep disturbances.

In the 2nd form of the syndrome, jaundice is milder, renal failure advances less rapidly, and hepatic encephalopathy does not occur.

Etiology Reported causes of the syndrome include hepatitis, advanced cirrhosis, obstructive jaundice, liver cancer, and tumors of the bile ducts.

In many cases a precipitating factor can be identified, such as an infection or gastrointestinal bleeding.

Epidemiology The syndrome occurs equally in males and females with severe liver disease.

Related Disorders Most cases of acute renal failure are distinguished from hepatorenal syndrome by underlying renal abnormalities, such as renovascular disease; glomerular disturbances associated with infections, Goodpasture syndrome, polycystic kidney disease, or Wegener granulomatosis; acute interstitial nephritis, commonly related to drugs or infections; intratubular obstruction; or acute tubular necrosis. (See *Goodpasture Syndrome; Polycystic Kidney Diseases; Wegener Granulomatosis.*)

Treatment—Standard Treatment is primarily directed toward correcting the characteristic circulatory disturbances. Three methods have been used: head-out water immersion (immersion of the body in water, leaving the head out, which redistributes the blood from the arms and legs to the trunk); paracentesis; and peritoneovenous shunting.

Other treatment is symptomatic and supportive.

Treatment—Investigational Liver transplantation has been used for patients who do not respond to other therapies.

The effectiveness of transfusion with fresh frozen plasma and the use of lumbar sympathectomy in treating the acute renal failure are being evaluated. The therapeutic roles of drugs such as atrial natriuretic peptide, calcium channel blockers, prostaglandins, and the liver hormone glomerulopressin are under investigation.

Please check with the agencies listed under Resources, below, for the most current information.

Resources

For more information on hepatorenal syndrome: National Organization for Rare Disorders (NORD); American Liver Foundation; Children's Liver Foundation; National Kidney and Urologic Diseases Information Clearinghouse.

References

The Hepatorenal Syndrome: P.S. Kellerman & S.L. Linas; AKF Nephrology Letter, November 1988, issue 5(4), pp. 47–54.

Pathophysiology of the Hepatorenal Syndrome and Potential for Therapy: M. Levy; Am. J. Cardiol., December 14, 1987, issue 60(17), pp. 66I–72I.

HYPOPHOSPHATEMIC RICKETS

Description Hypophosphatemic rickets is a rare genetic form of rickets characterized by a renal tubular defect in transport of phosphate and altered renal metabolism of vitamin D. Additionally, intestinal absorption of calcium and phosphate is decreased, which compounds hypophosphatemia and leads to osteomalacia. Major manifestations include skeletal changes and retarded growth.

Synonyms

Familial Hypophosphatemic (Vitamin D-Resistant) Rickets
Hereditary Type II Hypophosphatemia
Phosphate Diabetes
X-Linked Hypophosphatemia
X-Linked Vitamin D-Resistant Rickets

Signs and Symptoms Signs and symptoms are usually first noticed after 12 to 18 months of age. Dental problems may develop, such as delayed eruption of teeth, or caries and abscesses, especially of the dental pulp. Skeletal abnormalities include softening or thinning of bones, fractures, and abnormal bony extensions at the site of muscular attachments. Other characteristics include weakness, intermittent muscle cramps, a waddling walk due to abnormalities in the hip joint, pain in the knees, knock-knees or bowlegs, diminished growth (especially of the legs), and abnormal skull or rib development.

The symptoms and signs range from mild to severe. Some patients may have no noticeable symptoms, while others have pain and stiffness of the back, hips, and shoulders, possibly limiting mobility. Very rarely, some hair loss may occur. One rare acquired form of this disorder may be associated with a benign tumor that secretes a phosphaturic substance.

Etiology The most common form of hypophosphatemic rickets is inherited as an X-linked dominant trait. Symptoms are caused by altered metabolism of phosphorus, calcium, and vitamin D, although the exact mechanism for this is unclear. One important factor in the pathogenesis of this disease is impaired reabsorption of phosphorus by the renal proximal tubules, with resultant hypophosphatemia. Because of the hypophosphatemia, mineralization of bone is impaired.

Epidemiology The disorder occurs in males and females in equal numbers, but is usually more severe in males. Asymptomatic hypophosphatemic adult carriers are always females.

Related Disorders Rickets occurs in several forms, either acquired or inherited, all of which are characterized by weakening of bones due to abnormal calcium metabolism as well as possible decreases in magnesium or phosphorus levels.

Rickets is due to vitamin D deficiency resulting in deficient calcification of osteoid. This condition can develop at any age and can be successfully treated with high doses of vitamin D.

Pseudovitamin D deficiency rickets (vitamin D-dependent rickets, type I) is characterized by more severe skeletal changes and weakness than those of hypophosphatemic rickets, and onset is earlier. This disorder is caused by abnormal vitamin D metabolism and is inherited as an autosomal recessive trait. Serum calcium levels are decreased, although phosphate levels may be normal or only slightly decreased. Aminoaciduria occurs because of a proximal tubule abnormality. Intermittent muscle cramps are due to hypocalcemia. Convulsions and abnormalities of the spine and pelvis may also develop.

Osteomalacia is characterized by gradual softening and bending of the bones. Pain may occur in varying degrees of severity. Softening is due to defective calcification of bone, resulting from vitamin D deficiency or renal dysfunction. Osteomalacia is more common in women than in men, and often develops during pregnancy. It can exist alone or in association with other disorders, such as hypophosphatemic rickets.

Fanconi syndrome is characterized by renal proximal tubular dysfunction and bone abnormalities similar to those of hypophosphatemic rickets. Excess amounts of phosphate, amino acids, bicarbonate, glucose, and uric acid are excreted in the urine. This rare disorder is thought to be inherited in an autosomal recessive pattern. Bone abnormalities include rickets in children and osteomalacia in adults. Fanconi syndrome may be associated with a variety of inherited metabolic disorders. See *Cystinosis; Lowe Syndrome; Fructose Intolerance, Hereditary; Wilson Disease; Galactosemia, Classic.* Other associated disorders include a form of tyrosinemia and a glycogen storage disorder.

Treatment—Standard Hypophosphatemic rickets is treated with both oral phosphate and vitamin D, usually in the form of calcitriol. The dosage of calcitriol is gradually increased until bone healing occurs. This treatment must be carefully monitored to prevent hypercalciuria and nephrocalcinosis. Vitamin D alone reduces renal loss of phosphate but does not affect the patient's growth rate, the intestinal absorption of phosphate, or renal function. Phosphate alone may improve intestinal absorption of calcium and phosphate as well as enhance bone healing, but these effects may not be sustained without concomitant administration of vitamin D.

Covering teeth with chrome crowns may be effective in preventing spontaneous dental abscesses. Genetic counseling may benefit patients and their families. Those rare cases of hypophosphatemic rickets that are caused by bone tumors can be treated through surgical removal of the tumor, whenever feasible.

Treatment—Investigational Bone growth abnormalities associated with hypophosphatemic rickets can be surgically corrected in an attempt to prevent further shortening or deformities of affected arms or legs. However, this should not be attempted before hypophosphatemia has been corrected with phosphate and calcitriol therapy.

Please check with the agencies listed under Resources, below, for the most current information.

Resources

For more information on hypophosphatemic rickets: National Organization for Rare Disorders (NORD); National Institute of Diabetes, Digestive & Kidney Diseases Information Clearinghouse.

For genetic information and genetic counseling referrals: March of Dimes Birth Defects Foundation; National Center for Education in Maternal and Child Health.

References

Prophylactic Dental Treatment for a Patient with Vitamin D-Resistant Rickets. Report of Case: G.H. Breen; J. Dent. Child., January–February 1986, vol. 53(1), pp. 38–43.

Early Diagnosis and Early Treatment of Hypophosphatemic Vitamin D-Resistant Rickets: E. Schaumberger, et al.; Klin. Pediatr., January–February 1986, vol. 198(1), pp. 44–48.

Tibial Bowing Exacerbated by Partial Premature Epiphyseal Closure in Sex-linked Hypophosphatemic Rickets: W.H. McAlister, et al.; Radiology, February 1987, vol. 162(2), pp. 461–463.

IGA NEPHROPATHY

Description IgA nephropathy occurs during childhood and young adulthood. Hematuria related to IgA nephropathy usually occurs after a viral infection of the upper respiratory or gastrointestinal tract.

Synonyms

> Berger Disease
> Idiopathic Renal Hematuria
> Mesangial IgA Nephropathy

Signs and Symptoms The first recognizable sign of IgA nephropathy is hematuria due to acute nephritis or glomerulonephritis. There is often mild proteinuria with slowly progressive renal changes. Loin pain may occur, but hypertension or edema is unusual during the initial phase of the disease.

IgA nephropathy may progress slowly for several decades and can result in progressive renal failure in 35 percent of cases.

Etiology A postinfectious process is suspected as the cause of IgA nephropathy. An immune association is postulated because of an increase in the immunoglobulin IgA factor, but the mechanisms leading to glomerular immune deposit formation are unclear.

Epidemiology IgA nephropathy affects males 2 or 3 times more often than females and usually occurs between the ages of 15 and 35. It is one of the leading causes of acute nephritis in young people in the United States, Europe, and Japan. The incidence is significantly higher in American Indians than in any other ethnic group studied, and it is more prevalent in whites than in blacks. A study showed an occurrence rate of approximately 94 cases per 100,000 young men tested upon induction into the military.

Related Disorders See *Purpura, Schoenlein-Henoch; Systemic Lupus Erythematosus.*

Treatment—Standard No specific treatment for IgA nephropathy has been shown to be effective for all patients. Some have responded to oral steroid therapy, especially in the early stages of the disease. Longterm remission of symptoms has been achieved with the use of cyclophosamide, even after therapy was withdrawn. Kidney transplantation has been successful for many persons.

Treatment—Investigational Please contact the organizations listed under Resources, below, for the most current information.

Resources

    For more information on IgA nephropathy: National Organization for Rare Disorders (NORD); American Kidney Fund; National Kidney Foundation; National Kidney and Urologic Diseases Information Clearinghouse.

References

Steroid Therapy in IgA Nephropathy: A Retrospective Study in Heavy Proteinuric Cases: Y. Kobayaski, et al.; Nephron, 1988, vol. 48(1), pp. 12–17.

Tonsillar Distribution of IgA and IgG Immunocytes and Production of IgA Subclasses and J Chain in Tonsillitis Vary with the Presence or Absence of IgA Nephropathy: J. Nagy, et al.; Scand. J. Immunol., April 1988, vol. 27(4), pp. 393–399.

Proteinuria in IgA Nephropathy: K. Neelakantappa, et al.; Kidney Int., March 1988, vol. 33(3), pp. 716–721.

IgA Nephropathy, the Most Common Glomerulonephritis Worldwide. A Neglected Disease in the United States?: Am. J. Med., January 1988, vol. 84(1), pp. 129–32.

Cyclosporin in the Treatment of Steroid-Responsive and Steroid-Resistant Nephrotic Syndrome in Adults: E. Maher, et al.; Nephrol. Dial. Transplant., 1988, vol. 3(6).

MEDULLARY CYSTIC DISEASE

Description Medullary cystic disease is a genetic or congenital nephropathy that usually appears in children or young adults **(juvenile nephronopthisis)** and progresses gradually to the onset of uremia, either in childhood or adulthood.

Synonyms

    Familial Juvenile Nephronophthisis
    Renal-Retinal Dysplasia

Signs and Symptoms The initial manifestation is often a severe polyuria and sodium wasting. Metabolic acidosis with or without hyperchloremia may be present. Affected children frequently have growth retardation and signs of bone disease. Many patients compensate so well during the development of the disorder that medullary cystic disease goes unrecognized until uremia develops. Anemia may be an early clue to medullary cystic disease.

    Laboratory findings are similar to those in chronic renal failure, although proteinuria is not evident. Intravenous urography reveals small kidneys; medullary cysts may be seen with ultrasonography or arteriography.

    A subset of patients have retinal changes and are difficult to fit for corrective glasses. These patients fit into the category of **renal-retinal dysplasia.**

Etiology The disease may be inherited as a recessive or a dominant trait.

Epidemiology Fifty percent of cases are diagnosed in childhood; however, the disease may not develop until adulthood and has appeared as late as the 7th decade.

Related Disorders See *Medullary Sponge Kidney; Polycystic Kidney*

Diseases.

Treatment—Standard The polyuria is resistant to vasopressin. Treatment consists of management of uremia when it occurs. Diet is monitored. An increase in caloric intake should be accompanied by a reduction in total dietary protein. Sufficient carbohydrates and fats should be consumed to provide energy and prevent the body from metabolizing its own proteins.

Treatment—Investigational Please check with the agencies listed under Resources, below, for the most current information.

Resources
   For more information on medullary cystic disease: National Organization for Rare Disorders (NORD); National Kidney and Urologic Diseases Information Clearinghouse; The National Kidney Foundation.
   For genetic information and genetic counseling referrals: March of Dimes Birth Defects Foundation; National Center for Education in Maternal and Child Health.

References
   Cecil Textbook of Medicine, 18th ed.: J.B. Wyngaarden and L.H. Smith, Jr., eds.; W.B. Saunders Company, 1988, pp. 645–648.

MEDULLARY SPONGE KIDNEY

Description Medullary sponge kidney is a hereditary congenital defect occurring in one or both kidneys and characterized by marked dilatation of the collecting tubules. Nephrolithiasis and hematuria may be associated.

Synonyms
   Sponge Kidney
   Tubular Ectasia

Signs and Symptoms Urinary tract infections often are the first sign of the underlying abnormality.
   Nephrolithiasis with renal colic, loin pain, and the excretion of small stones is a prominent feature of medullary sponge kidney. The stones, which form in the dilated portions of the collecting tubules, consist of calcium oxalate, calcium phosphate, and other calcium salts. About 13 percent of all patients who develop renal calculi have medullary sponge kidney. The disorder seldom progresses to end-stage renal failure, although reduced glomerular filtration rates have been observed.
   The most common functional abnormalities include the loss of urinary concentrating capacity and metabolic acidosis secondary to renal tubular acidosis.

Etiology The disorder is inherited in an autosomal dominant pattern. A possible relationship between hyperparathyroidism and medullary sponge kidney has been proposed. Medullary sponge kidney is also found in individuals with the Beckwith-

Wiedemann syndrome.

Epidemiology The incidence is higher in males than in females.

Treatment—Standard Patients should take in sufficient fluids in order to excrete about 2 liters of urine daily. Those with hypercalciuria may benefit from longterm therapy with thiazide diuretics as well as a high fluid intake. For patients with calcium urolithiasis and normal calcium excretion, oral phosphate therapy may be useful. A low calcium diet may prevent stone formation. Yearly urinalysis and urine culture are advisable.

Many patients with medullary sponge kidney have recurrent urinary tract infections and should probably receive prophylactic antibiotics.

Treatment—Investigational Please check with the agencies listed under Resources, below, for the most current information.

Resources

For more information on medullary sponge kidney: National Organization for Rare Disorders (NORD); National Kidney and Urologic Diseases Information Clearinghouse; The National Kidney Foundation.

For genetic information and genetic counseling referrals: March of Dimes Birth Defects Foundation; National Center for Education in Maternal and Child Health.

References
Cecil Textbook of Medicine, 18th ed.: J.B. Wyngaarden and L.H. Smith, Jr., eds.; W.B. Saunders Company, 1988, pp. 645–648.

POLYCYSTIC KIDNEY DISEASES (PKD)

Description The presence of bilateral renal cysts characterizes these inherited diseases. Renal cystic enlargement over time results in encroachment on normal renal tissue, with lost of renal function. The enlargement of renal tissue also stretches renal vasculature and results in hypertension.

Infantile and adult forms of PKD exist.

Signs and Symptoms Onset of the infantile form is soon after birth. The abdomen is enlarged and the kidneys are palpable. Dehydration and emaciation are frequently noted. Fibrosis of the liver associated with hypertension and splenomegaly often occurs in infants and children with PKD.

In the adult form, symptoms usually develop in the 30s and result from cystic pressure; they include lumbar pain, hematuria, and colic. Hypertension may be present. Splenomegaly is often found, and hepatic cysts occur in about one-third of cases. Most patients with severe cystic kidneys develop endstage renal failure and require dialysis.

Etiology The infantile form is an autosomal recessive disorder. The adult form, which is autosomal dominant, has been found to be caused by more than one defective gene. The defective genes are located on chromosome 16 and are so closely linked on the short arm of the chromosome that they are usually inherited together, although this is not the case in about 5 percent of affected persons. These variations may account for clinical differences in patients with PKD.

Epidemiology Approximately 500,000 persons in the United States are affected. The disorder accounts for 8 to 10 percent of cases of endstage renal disease.

Related Disorders See *Medullary Cystic Disease; Medullary Sponge Kidney.*

Glomerular cystic disease is similar to PKD, but the liver and spleen are unaffected.

Treatment—Standard Treatment consists of management of urinary infections and secondary hypertension. When uremia occurs, it is managed by an increase in caloric intake combined with a reduction in total dietary protein. Sufficient carbohydrates and fat must be provided to meet energy requirements.

With dialysis, a normal hematocrit can be achieved. Renal transplantation is sometimes indicated, but the use of parental and sibling donors may be impractical because of the familial nature of the disease. Genetic counseling is recommended for affected families.

Treatment—Investigational Please check with the agencies listed under Resources, below, for the most current information.

Resources
For more information on polycystic kidney diseases: National Organization for Rare Disorders (NORD); Polycystic Kidney Disease Research Foundation; National Kidney and Urologic Diseases Information Clearinghouse; The National Kidney Foundation; National Association of Patients on Hemodialysis and Transplantation.

For genetic information and genetic counseling referrals: March of Dimes Birth Defects Foundation; National Center for Education in Maternal and Child Health.

References
Cecil Textbook of Medicine, 18th ed.: J.B. Wyngaarden and L.H. Smith, Jr., eds.: W.B. Saunders Company, 1988, pp. 148, 506, 644–647.

RENAL AGENESIS, BILATERAL

Description The failure of both kidneys to develop in utero results in oligohydramnios. The lack of amniotic fluid may cause compression of the fetus and further fetal malformations. Bilateral renal agenesis is more common in infants with a parent who has a renal anomaly, particularly unilateral renal agenesis. Studies have shown that unilateral and bilateral renal agenesis may be genetically related.

Signs and Symptoms Premature labor, breech delivery, and a disproportionately low birth weight are often associated with bilateral renal agenesis.

A typical facies includes ocular hypertelorism, a "parrot beak" nose, a receding chin, and large, low-set ears deficient in cartilage (the so-called **Potter facies**). Other characteristics may include excess and dehydrated skin, prominent epicanthal folds, the facial expression of an older infant, and deformities of the hands and feet. The uterus and upper vagina may be absent in females; males may lack the seminal vesicles and spermatic duct. Gastrointestinal anomalies include the absence of a rectum, esophagus, and duodenum. Other abnormalities that may occur are the presence of only one umbilical artery and major deformities of the lower trunk and lower limbs. Pulmonary hypoplasia and pneumothorax are common associated findings.

Etiology The disorder has an autosomal dominant mode of inheritance.

Epidemiology Bilateral renal agenesis occurs more frequently in males than in females. It is a very rare disorder.

Related Disorders See *Sirenomelia Sequence; Fraser Syndrome.*

Oligohydramnios sequence (Potter syndrome) is characterized by an insufficient level of amniotic fluid, which may be due to the absence of urinary output to the fetus or to chronic leakage of fluid from the amniotic sac.

Cat-eye syndrome (coloboma of iris-anal atresia syndrome) is a genetic disorder that is marked by a fissure in the iris and the absence of an anal opening. Associated abnormalities may include renal agenesis.

Melnick-Fraser syndrome (branchio-oto-renal syndrome) is a genetic disorder characterized by hearing loss and kidney malformations, including renal agenesis.

MURCS association (müllerian duct, renal, and cervical vertebral defects) is a rare disorder characterized by malformation of the vertebrae and absence of a vagina and kidneys.

Rokitansky sequence is a disorder in which the vagina and uterus are incompletely formed.

Treatment—Standard Treatment is symptomatic and supportive for patients with this disorder. Most children will die of renal insufficiency.

Treatment—Investigational Please check with the agencies listed under Resources, below, for the most current information.

Resources

For more information on bilateral renal agenesis: National Organization for Rare Disorders (NORD); American Kidney Fund; National Kidney Foundation; National Institute of Diabetes and Digestive and Kidney Diseases Information Clearinghouse.

For genetic information and genetic counseling referrals: March of Dimes Birth Defects Foundation; NIH/National Center for Education in Maternal and Child Health (NCEMCH).

References

Mendelian Inheritance in Man, 9th ed.: V.A. McKusick; The Johns Hopkins University Press, 1990, pp. 958–960.

RENAL GLYCOSURIA

Description Renal glycosuria is a rare metabolic disorder in which abnormal amounts of glucose are excreted into the urine when the blood glucose levels are normal or low. There are 2 types: primary and congenital.

Synonyms
> Diabetes, True Renal
> Glucosuria

Signs and Symptoms Primary renal glycosuria occurs without any apparent functional or structural abnormalities of the kidney. It tends to occur in pregnant women and almost always disappears after childbirth.

Congenital renal glycosuria is a rare inherited disorder characterized by (1) the intestines' inability to absorb glucose and (2) an excessive amount of glucose in the urine. Since glycosuria is the primary symptom of this disorder, a fasting blood glucose test and a glucose oxidase test must be performed to differentiate renal glycosuria from diabetes mellitus.

Etiology The cause is probably a defect in the renal glucose transport protein. Renal glycosuria is recognized as a metabolic disorder and is believed to be inherited as an autosomal recessive trait. Because some patients eventually develop diabetes mellitus, some believe the disorder may precede the onset of diabetes, but this has not been proved.

Epidemiology Males and females are equally affected. The incidence in women is higher during pregnancy, with the glycosuria subsiding after delivery. Some patients with severe renal failure also have renal glycosuria.

Related Disorders See *Cystinosis; Hypophosphatemic Rickets.*

Treatment—Standard Treatment may not be necessary. Since an excessive loss of glucose can occur with this disorder, fasting should be avoided; theoretically it could lead to hypoglycemia. Severe diarrhea in infants with renal glycosuria must be treated to avoid dehydration. Genetic counseling may be beneficial. Other treatment is symptomatic and supportive.

Treatment—Investigational Please check with the agencies listed under Resources, below, for the most current information.

Resources
> **For more information on renal glycosuria:** National Organization for Rare Disorders (NORD); American Kidney Fund; National Kidney Foundation; National Digestive Diseases Information Clearinghouse.
>
> **For genetic information and genetic counseling referrals:** March of Dimes Birth Defects Foundation; NIH/National Center for Education in Maternal and Child Health (NCEMCH).

References

Mendelian Inheritance in Man, 8th ed.: V.A. McKusick; The Johns Hopkins University Press, 1986, pp. 971.

The Metabolic Basis of Inherited Disease, 5th ed.: J.B. Stanbury, et al., eds.; McGraw-Hill, 1983, p. 1806.

Internal Medicine, 2nd ed.: J.H. Stein, ed.-in-chief; Little, Brown & Company, 1987, pp. 880–881.

Complete Absence of Tubular Glycose Reabsorption; A New Type of Renal Glucosuria: B.S. Oemar et al.; Clin. Nephrol., March 1987; vol. 27(3), pp. 156–160.

10 | ENDOCRINE DISORDERS
By Inese Z. Beitins, M.D.

During the past few decades there have been dramatic advances in the science of endocrinology, leading to better understanding of the impact of genetic and environmental factors upon inherited endocrine disorders as well as pathophysiologic processes which disrupt endocrine function. The contributions of these discoveries to diagnostic and therapeutic potentials are extraordinary and have made endocrinology a discipline in which diagnoses can be made with precision, and appropriate, safe treatment prescribed.

The classic definition of endocrinology as the integration and communication between endocrine tissues which release chemical signals into the circulation that act on distant target tissues is too limited. The definition now needs to incorporate the modification of action (amplification or inhibition) and independent function of tissue growth factors and regulatory peptides as well as classic hormones as local mediators via autocrine and paracrine mechanisms. Increasing amalgamation of other systems with the endocrine system has led to new fields of study such as psychoneuroendocrinology, immunopathoendocrinology, and reproductive endocrinology.

Molecular biology coupled with new immunological and biochemical approaches has provided a profound influence and new insights into the study and classification of endocrine disorders. It is now possible to identify patients with rare disorders who were previously assigned the term "an experiment in nature," to identify the inherent problem at the level of the responsible gene, and to study the problem in terms of deletion or mutation for the transcription of the hormones themselves, hormonal receptors, or post-receptor functions. To further delineate results of hormonal excesses or transcription of genes with single point mutations, transgenic animals can be produced, bred, and studied. Through these types of studies, mechanisms of both inherited and acquired endocrine disease can be studied in exquisite detail at the cellular and molecular levels.

Endocrine problems themselves are common in the practices of internal medicine and pediatrics. Some, such as non-insulin-dependent diabetes and hypothyroidism, are readily treated by medical practitioners. Others have vague symptomatology leading to a delay in appropriate diagnosis or, especially in young children, rapid onset of catastrophic proportions requiring immediate appropriate diagnosis and treatment. Medical practitioners therefore must continually consider the possibility of an underlying endocrine cause for commonly observed symptoms such as loss of energy, nausea, diarrhea, skin turgor, and changes in skin pigmentation and texture, as well as those related to reproduction-ambiguity, loss of libido, and amenorrhea. Because of the relative variety of many of the conditions described in this section, prompt consultation with an appropriate specialist in adult or pediatric endocrinology or in reproductive endocrinology needs to be obtained.

If an endocrine cause is found and promptly treated, preservation of good health can be expected. Especially in the pediatric age group, unrecognized endocrine disorders related to adverse changes in serum electrolyte and fluid balance, calcium and phosphorus relationships, and hypoglycemia can lead to irreparable health hazards and retardation.

Therefore, in this age of rapid expansion of our knowledge base—diagnostic potentials as well as therapeutic possibilities through hormonal and synthetic analogue therapies—the practitioner needs to be aware of the symptoms of uncommon disease as well as the consultants (specialists, disease-focused self-help groups, or governmental agencies) through whom important, pertinent information can be acquired. In addition, these rare conditions deserve not only study as medical curiosities but also full support from insurance companies and the pharmaceutical industry to furnish the hormones and medications required to provide the potential of total replacement therapies and restoration of optimal health for a lifetime.

ENDOCRINE DISORDERS
Listings in This Section

ACROMEGALY

Description Acromegaly is an insidious disorder of growth hormone excess, which manifests itself in abnormal enlargement of bones of the extremities and head, especially the frontal bone and jaws, and thickening of soft tissues, including those of the heart.

Synonyms

Marie Disease

Signs and Symptoms Symptoms are slowly progressive after puberty, becoming prominent in middle age. Facial features coarsen with the growth of soft tissues and cartilage. Facial bones are prominent, the jaw protrudes, and overbite leads to wide separation of the teeth. The voice usually deepens and sounds husky. Osseous overgrowth and cartilage hypertrophy lead to osteoarthritis; kyphoscoliosis may occur. Enlargement of the hands and feet is gradual. Compression of the spinal nerve root may lead to functional abnormalities and pain. Darkening of the skin and hirsutism may be apparent. Cardiomegaly (which may lead to congestive heart failure), hepatomegaly, splenomegaly, and renal enlargement may occur. At times there is enlargement of the thyroid and adrenal glands.

Approximately 25 percent of patients are hypertensive. Pituitary enlargement can produce headache, visual abnormalities, and hormonal imbalances. Since excessive growth hormone (**GH**) influences insulin, 50 percent of patients have elevated glucose levels. The metabolic rate may quicken, and the activity of the sweat and sebaceous glands may increase.

At a late stage, myopathy and peripheral neuropathy may develop. Visual impairment may progress, even to blindness. Left untreated, 25 percent of patients have glycosuria, polydipsia, and polyphagia.

Etiology Hypersecretion of GH is most often due to a pituitary adenoma involving the somatotrophic cells of the anterior lobe; less often, ineffective control of these cells by the hypothalamus is responsible. GH-secreting tumors may sometimes be due to overstimulation by the hypothalamus.

Epidemiology Acromegaly affects males and females in equal numbers.

Related Disorders Gigantism, also caused by hypersecretion of GH, occurs prepubertally. It is associated with enlarged soft tissues and late epiphyseal closure, which produces excessive growth during childhood; height may reach 7 or 8 feet. Onset of hypopituitarism later in the course may result in myopathy and hypogonadism. Sexual development may be normal, or it may be affected by associated hypogonadism. In some cases peripheral neuropathy may develop.

The hereditary **Wermer syndrome (type I multiple endocrine neoplasia; polyendocrine adenomatosis)** has the hallmarks of excessive growth and multiple tumors or endocrine hypersecretion. The patient may have diarrhea and abdominal pain. A child may have hypoglycemia, and an adult, peptic ulcers. At times epileptic seizures occur.

See *Marfan Syndrome; McCune-Albright Syndrome; Sotos Syndrome.*

Treatment—Standard The usual treatment of acromegaly is partial or total surgical removal of the pituitary gland, perhaps supplemented by irradiation. If the entire gland is removed, lifelong hormonal replacement therapy is essential. GH suppressors, including estrogen, medroxyprogesterone, chlorpromazine, and somatostatin (the latter must be given intravenously), have had only limited success. In mild cases or in elderly patients, dopamine agonists such as bromocryptine have been used adjunctively.

Treatment—Investigational Treatment of acromegaly is now possible with somatostatin analog (SMS 201-995). This medication significantly lowers the mean plasma GH concentrations and when given preoperatively causes a significant shrinkage of invasive pituitary macroadenomas with improved surgical remission rates. Treatment with somatostatin analog is available in many research-oriented medical centers within the United States.

Please contact the agencies listed under Resources, below, for the most current information.

Resources

For more information on acromegaly: National Organization for Rare Disorders (NORD); National Arthritis and Musculoskeletal and Skin Diseases Information Clearinghouse; Human Growth Foundation (HGF).

References

Preoperative Treatment of Acromegaly with Long-Acting Somatostatin Analog SMS 201-995: Shrinkage of Invasive Pituitary Macroadenomas and Improved Surgical Remission Rate: A.L. Barkan, et al.; J. Clin. Endo. and Metab., vol. 67(5), pp. 1040–1047.

Treatment of Acromegaly with the Long-Acting Somatostatin Analog SMS 201-995: A.L. Barkan, et al.; J. Clin. Endo. and Metab., vol. 66(1), pp. 16–23.

Plasma Insulin-Like Growth Factor-I/Somatomedin-C in Acromegaly: Correlation with the Degree of Growth Hormone Hypersecretion: A.L. Barkan, et al.; J. Clin. Endo. and Metab., vol. 67(1) pp. 69–73.

Acromegalic Heart Disease: Influence of Treatment of the Acromegaly on the Heart: R.P. Hayward, et al.; Q.J. Med., January 1987, issue 62(237), pp. 41–58.

Acromegaly: J.D. Nabarro; Clin. Endocrinol. (Oxford), April 1987, issue 26(4), pp. 481–512.

Somatomedin-C Levels in Treated and Untreated Patients with Acromegaly: F. Roelfsema, et al.; Clin. Endocrinol. (Oxford), February 1987, issue 26(2), pp. 137–144.

Somatostatin Proves Effective in Treating Resistant Acromegaly: A.J. Clark; Res. Resource Rep., April 1988, pp. 5–7.

The Pathogenesis of Acromegaly: Clinical and Immunocytochemical Analysis in 75 Patients: E.R. Laws, Jr., et al.; J. Neurosurg., July 1985, issue 63(1), pp. 35–38.

ACTH DEFICIENCY

Description Decreased or absent adrenocorticotropic hormone (**ACTH**) and abnormally low levels of cortisol and steroid hormones mark this disorder.

Synonyms

Adrenocorticotropic Hormone Deficiency, Isolated

Signs and Symptoms ACTH deficiency usually manifests during adulthood; a few cases in children have been identified. The patient may experience weight loss, anorexia, muscle weakness, nausea, vomiting, and hypotension. As a rule, hypoglycemia, hyponatremia, and hyperkalemia are present. Blood tests may show no detectable level of ACTH, and cortisol levels may be subnormal. Urinary 17-hydroxy- and 17-ketosteroid concentrations are low, as are androgen levels. Although the male distribution of body hair is usually normal, females have sparse pubic and axillary hair. Decreased skin pigmentation is the norm, but in some it may be normal or even increased. Emotionally, patients may range from being depressed to exhibiting frank psychosis.

Etiology ACTH deficiency is idiopathic; hypothalamic or pituitary abnormalities have been suggested. The symptoms are a reflection of understimulation of the adrenal cortex by ACTH, which results in insufficient hormone secretion.

Epidemiology Males and females are affected in equal numbers. Symptoms usually become apparent in adulthood, but laboratory tests can reveal ACTH deficiency in asymptomatic infants.

Related Disorders Secondary adrenal insufficiency stems from insufficient production or release of ACTH. Causes range from prolonged corticosteroid therapy and adenomas and granulomas of the pituitary gland to postpartum pituitary necrosis.

Treatment—Standard Replacement with cortisone constitutes therapy. Replacement enables patients to lead a normal life with the exception that they require increased doses of cortisone replacement therapy in the presence of moderate and severe stress..

Treatment—Investigational Please contact the agencies listed under Resources, below, for the most current information.

Resources

For more information on ACTH deficiency: National Organization for Rare Disorders (NORD); National Institute of Diabetes, Digestive & Kidney Diseases Information Clearinghouse; The Endocrine Society.

References
Internal Medicine, 2nd ed.: J.H. Stein, et al., eds.; Little, Brown and Company, 1987, p. 1899.

ADDISON DISEASE

Description Addison disease is the result of chronic, usually progressive, hypofunction of the adrenal cortex. Deficiencies of cortisol and aldosterone lead to electrolyte imbalance (low sodium and chloride, and high potassium levels). The imbalance causes increased water excretion, and hypotension and dehydration follow. Major characteristics are fatigability, gastrointestinal discomfort, and changes in skin pigmentation.

Synonyms
> Adrenocortical Insufficiency
> Primary Adrenal Insufficiency
> Schmidt Syndrome

Signs and Symptoms Weakness, fatigue, anorexia, increased water excretion, hypotension, and darkened pigmentation of scars, skin folds, and mucous membranes are early symptoms and signs. In addition, there may be black freckles over the head and shoulder areas.

Later developments are nausea, dehydration from vomiting and diarrhea, dizziness, cold intolerance, syncopal attacks, apathy, mental confusion, fever, abdominal pain, and hypoglycemia. Adrenal crisis may occur, signaled by a marked sudden loss of strength; severe abdominal, lower back, or leg pain; and/or renal failure.

Etiology Idiopathic atrophy, perhaps autoimmune-related, accounts for about three-quarters of cases; the rest are due to partial destruction of the gland by such factors as tuberculosis, tumor, or amyloidosis. Acute infection, trauma, surgery, or sodium loss through heavy sweating can trigger adrenal crisis.

Epidemiology Males and females are affected in equal numbers. Onset may occur at any age.

Treatment—Standard In chronic adrenal insufficiency, replacement therapy consists of cortisone and fludrocortisone, taken with meals. To avert adrenal crisis during infection, trauma, surgery, and other stress, the dosage is increased. Adrenal crisis demands *immediate* intravenous administration of high-dose hydrocortisone succinate or phosphate and fluid and electrolyte replacement; a short-term course of a vasopressor may be indicated to maintain blood pressure. Patients should carry a card or wear a tag stating that they have Addison disease.

Treatment—Investigational The National Institute of Diabetes, Digestive & Kidney Diseases (NIDDK) is conducting a study on Addison disease. For more information, contact Joan Chamberlain, Deputy Director, NIH/National Institute of Diabetes, Digestive & Kidney Diseases, Building 31, Room 9A-04, 9000 Rockville Pike, Bethesda, Maryland 20892.

Please contact the agencies listed under Resources, below, for the most current information.

Resources
For more information on Addison disease: National Organization for Rare Disorders (NORD); National Addison Disease Foundation; NIH/National Institute of Diabetes, Digestive & Kidney Disease Information Clearinghouse; The Endocrine Society.

References
Harrison's Principles of Internal Medicine, 12th ed.: J.D. Wilson, et al., eds.; McGraw-Hill, 1991, pp. 1729–1731.

ADRENAL HYPERPLASIA, CONGENITAL (CAH)

Description CAH comprises a group of disorders resulting from defective synthesis of adrenal corticosteroids. Lack of glucocorticoids, especially cortisol, causes various kinds of metabolic problems. The response to low levels of cortisol is increased production of corticotropin **(ACTH)**. Lack of mineralocorticoids, primarily aldosterone, causes sodium and water imbalance which, in some cases, can be fatal. The various forms of CAH represent defects in the different stages of corticosteroid synthesis, usually hydroxylation reactions at certain positions on the original cholesterol molecule.

CAH can result from congenital lipoid hyperplasia (adrenal cortex with male pseudohermaphroditism; 20-22–desmolase deficiency); 3-beta–hydroxy-steroid **(HSD)** dehydrogenase deficiency; 17–hydroxylase deficiency; 21–hydroxylase deficiency; 17-20–desmolase deficiency; 11-beta–hydroxylase deficiency; 17-alpha–hydroxylase deficiency.

Synonyms
Adrenal Virilism
Hydroxylase Deficiency

Signs and Symptoms In several forms of CAH in which adrenomegaly produces abnormally large amounts of androgen, abnormalities of sexual development may be the most conspicuous consequence, particularly masculinization of the external genitalia in females. Deficiencies of glucocorticoids occur in some cases despite the adrenal hypertrophy, causing symptoms of Addison disease. These include weakness, nausea, vomiting, anorexia, irritability, depression, darkening or pigmentation of the skin, hypotension, lack of resistance to cold, and inability to respond physiologically to stress; even patients who produce adequate corticosteroids under normal conditions usually cannot meet the increased requirement. Life-threatening Addisonian crisis can then occur. A deficiency of aldosterone can lead to sodium depletion, dehydration, and circulatory collapse.

In **congenital lipoid hyperplasia (adrenal cortex with male pseudohermaphroditism; 20-22–desmolase deficiency),** the most prominent feature is male pseudohermaphroditism. The disorder is characterized by failure of the external male genitalia to masculinize, and by hypospadias. There is accompanying impaired androgen action. Infant survival is very poor in this form of CAH.

3-Beta–HSD deficiency occurs early in the chain of reactions required to produce adrenal corticosteroid hormones. Androgens, glucocorticoids, and mineralocorticoids are not synthesized. In males, there is pseudohermaphroditism and hypospadias. Virilization of females is not as noticeable or does not occur at all. Salt loss is a frequent cause of adrenal crisis. Infants usually survive no more than a few hours unless diagnosed and treated rapidly. A few patients with incomplete forms of this defect have been described. These fail to be symptomatic until later in childhood (first menstruation at age 4 to 6, clitorimegaly, acne, and advanced maturation of the skeleton) or until adulthood. The late-onset form is characterized by menstrual irregularity and hirsutism.

17–Hydroxylase deficiency deprives genetic males of androgens during fetal development. As a consequence, they are born with female external genitalia; the testes are buried within the abdominal cavity. Cryptorchidism may become malignant later in life. Other characteristics are failure to develop secondary sexual traits, amenorrhea, hypertension, and hypokalemia.

17-20–Desmolase deficiency results in genetic males having female or ambiguous external genitalia. The adrenal glands are normal in size, and production of gluco- and mineralocorticoids is adequate.

21–Hydroxylase deficiency: Female pseudohermaphroditism is the most common form of CAH. Although both males and females are affected, this disorder is not usually apparent in males until later in life. Females are born with abnormalities of the external genitalia that range from mild clitorimegaly to fusion of the labia so that the infant appears to have a phallus with undescended testes. Internally, the female reproductive organs are present; however, labial fold fusion may seal off the vagina from the exterior. These children are often raised as boys until the small size of the phallus becomes apparent at about age 4. Very rarely, genetic females have lived their lives as males. Untreated females do not menstruate and are infertile. Physical growth may initially be rapid, but retardation occurs fairly soon, and adult stature is short. Untreated affected females may have psychological problems.

Male infants appear normal. At age 3 to 4 certain characteristics become apparent: unusually rapid growth, acne, voice deepening, penile enlargement, and pubic and axillary hair growth. High levels of androgens suppress hormones required for normal puberty, testicular development, and spermatogenesis. Since the disorder is not initially apparent in boys, there is risk of an unanticipated, potentially fatal gluco- or mineralocorticoid deficiency crisis.

About one-third of patients with 21–hydroxylase deficiency also have a deficiency of aldosterone, which results in natriuresis and possible dehydration, hypovolemia, and hypotension. Symptoms develop 5 to 10 days after birth, and include lethargy, vomiting, diarrhea, and circulatory collapse. Untreated, the disorder is rapidly fatal.

11-Beta–hydroxylase deficiency causes female virilization. Both males and females have hypertension and short stature. Precocious puberty occurs in males.

17-Alpha–hydroxylase deficiency usually goes undetected until adolescence when there is a lack of secondary sexual development in males and females. Genetic males have female external genitalia. Females fail to menstruate or develop breasts. There is no production of androgens by the testes, and the ovaries fail to produce estrogen. Low levels of blood potassium and hypertension are other important characteristics of the disorder.

Symptoms of **nonclassical adrenal hyperplasia (NAH)** include infertility, premature sexual development, severe acne, excessive facial hair in women, and short stature in men. Symptoms of NAH are all caused by excess androgen before or at birth.

Etiology Most of the adrenal hyperplasias are inherited as autosomal recessive disorders, and in some, the gene location is known. However, in 17-beta–HSD, the disorder may also be inherited as an X-linked recessive trait.

Epidemiology The most common form of CAH, 21–hydroxylase deficiency, is estimated to affect between 1:5,000 and 1:15,000 persons in the United States and Europe. In the Yupik Eskimo, however, the incidence of the salt-wasting form of CAH may be as high as 1:282. Other forms of CAH are much rarer.

Related Disorders Virilization of female fetuses and children, or accelerated sexual maturity in males, may also result from androgen-producing tumors or maternal ingestion of androgenic substances. The congenital absence of gonads and cryptorchidism can also result in abnormal sexual development.

Hermaphroditism is characterized by the presence of both ovaries and testes in the same individual. The reproductive organs can contain eggs or sperm. Most affected persons have a mixture of female and male external genitalia.

Klinefelter's syndrome results from an excess of X chromosomes. It is characterized in males by small testes, lack of sperm, enlarged mammary glands, and an abnormally small penis. Other symptoms include retarded development of sex organs, an absence of beard and body hair, a high-pitched voice, and lack of muscular development.

See *Turner Syndrome; Addison Disease.*

Treatment—Standard Early diagnosis and genetic sex determination are extremely important to prevent unexpected circulatory crises and to permit any necessary surgical modification of the external genitalia. Oral corticosteroid therapy corrects the endocrine deficiency and must continue throughout life. If the mineralocorticoid deficiency is not corrected, intravenous therapy, or desoxycorticosterone acetate or fludrocortisol, is necessary to maintain proper sodium and water balance. Treated girls menstruate and may have normal pregnancies. In boys, androgen suppression permits normal puberty, testicular development, and the production of viable sperm.

A decrease in the quantity of androgens may cause some regression of enlarged genital structures, but in many cases (especially when therapy begins late), surgical reconstruction of the external genitalia of girls is necessary.

Once identified, individuals with the defective genes for **nonclassical adrenal hyperplasia** can be treated with cortisol orally to reverse most of the symptoms, including infertility.

Treatment—Investigational Treatment of female fetuses affected with **21–hydroxylase deficiency** has been started during early pregnancy with dexamethasone and continued until birth. This experimental treatment suppresses the adrenal glands, and the external sex organs are normal at birth. Further study is needed to determine the longterm safety and effectiveness of this treatment.

Please contact the agencies listed under Resources, below, for the most current information.

Resources

For more information on CAH: National Organization for Rare Diseases (NORD); Congenital Adrenal Hyperplasia Support Group; NIH/National Institute of Child Health and Human Development (NICHHD); Research Trust for Metabolic Diseases in Children.

For information on genetics and genetic counseling referrals: March of Dimes Birth Defects Foundation; National Center for Education in Maternal and Child Health (NCEMCH).

References

Congenital Adrenal Hyperplasia: M.I. New and L.S. Levine; *in* Monographs on Endocrinology, vol. 26, Springer Verlag, vol. 198, p. 4.

Diurnal Variation in Blood 17–Hydroxyprogesterone Concentrations in Untreated Congenital Adrenal Hyperplasia: J. Slonim; Arch. Dis. Child., vol. 59(8), pp. 743–747.

Prenatal Treatment of Congenital Adrenal Hyperplasia Resulting from 21–Hydroxylase Deficiency: R. David, et al.; J. Pediatr., vol. 105(5), pp. 799–803.

Recent Advances in 21–Hydroxylase Deficiency: M.I. New, et al.; Ann. Rev. Med., vol. 35, pp. 649–663.

AHUMADA-DEL CASTILLO SYNDROME

Description Ahumada-del Castillo syndrome represents a dysfunction of the pituitary-hypothalamic axis. It is one of a group of disorders affecting women and is not correlated with pregnancy.

Synonyms
> Amenorrhea-Galactorrhea Syndrome
> Galactorrhea-Amenorrhea Without Pregnancy
> Nonpuerperal Galactorrhea-Amenorrhea

Signs and Symptoms Symptoms consist of galactorrhea and amenorrhea. The breasts and nipples are of normal size and appearance, as are the secondary sexual characteristics.

Laboratory tests reveal elevated levels of prolactin and low gonadotropin secretion.

Etiology The underlying abnormality is unknown. Evidence suggests that small tumors in the pituitary-hypothalamic region are sometimes responsible. The tumors are frequently microscopic and difficult to detect.

Rarer causes of galactorrhea-amenorrhea syndromes are hypothyroidism, chronic use of dopamine-antagonistic drugs such as chlorpromazine, and discontinuance of oral contraceptive agents.

Related Disorders Galactorrhea-amenorrhea syndromes include **Chiari-Frommel Syndrome,** which is correlated with pregnancy, and **Forbes-Albright Syndrome,** which is associated with demonstrable tumors in the sella turcica.

Treatment—Standard Drugs such as bromocriptine and lergotrile mesilate lower prolactin levels, thereby stopping abnormal milk secretion and often restoring menstrual function. Small tumors may in some cases be excised; others may respond to irradiation. When another underlying disorder is the cause, the galactorrhea-amenorrhea syndrome resolves upon successful treatment of the disorder.

Treatment—Investigational Please contact the agencies listed under Resources, below, for the most current information.

Resources

For more information on Ahumada-del Castillo syndrome: National Organization for Rare Disorders (NORD); NIH/National Institute of Child Health and Human Development (NICHHD).

AMENORRHEA, PRIMARY

Description Absence of menses by age 18 or older constitutes primary amenorrhea. Menarche is usually within 2 years after the onset of puberty.

Signs and Symptoms The sole symptom is absence of menarche. Signs include lack of secondary sexual characteristics and incomplete or underdeveloped external genitalia and breasts. Laboratory tests may reflect ovarian deficiency or hypopituitarism. The hymen may be imperforate.

Etiology Simple physiologic delay may explain why a patient as old as age 18 has not experienced menarche. If so, secondary sexual characteristics are usually present and the genitalia normal.

The cause of primary amenorrhea is usually an excess or a deficiency of hypothalamic gonadotropic-releasing hormone **(GnRH).** Anorexia nervosa, crash dieting, emotional stress (especially depression), obesity, and disorders such as tuberculosis or lymphoma can alter hypothalamic function.

Chromosomal abnormalities (e.g., Turner syndrome) may cause primary ovarian failure. Ovarian destruction may be due to infection or, possibly, autoimmunity or premenarchal menopause.

An anatomic abnormality may be responsible for primary amenorrhea. Possibilities include the congenital absence of the vagina, uterus, or ovaries; an atrophic endometrium; and hermaphroditism. Furthermore, an imperforate hymen or a transverse vaginal septum may obstruct the menstrual flow.

A number of drugs can cause amenorrhea. The list includes barbiturates, opiates, corticosteroids, chlordiazepoxide, phenothiazines, and progesterone.

Epidemiology Menstrual disorders are among the most common form of endocrinopathy in women.

Related Disorders See *Acromegaly* and *Adrenal Hyperplasia, Congenital,* which are among the disorders that may be related to primary amenorrhea. Others include **hypogonadotropic hypogonadism, polycystic ovary disease, pituitary tumors, Cushing disease, hyperthyroidism, and hypothyroidism.**

Treatment—Standard The patient should be examined by an endocrinologist or gynecologist. If the amenorrhea is a result of physiologic delay, as a rule no therapy is indicated before age 18. If secondary sexual development is lacking by age

14, however, a thorough investigation is warranted.

Progesterone, estrogen, and corticosteroids are effective in some types of amenorrhea. The patient may benefit from emotional support and counseling. Imperforate hymen, other obstructions, and neoplasm may require surgery.

Treatment—Investigational Please contact the agencies listed under Resources, below, for the most current information.

Resources

For more information on primary amenorrhea: National Organization for Rare Disorders (NORD); National Women's Health Network; NIH/National Institute of Child Health and Human Development (NICHHD).

References
Cecil Textbook of Medicine, 18th ed.: J.B. Wyngaarden and L.H. Smith, Jr., eds.; W.B. Saunders Company, 1988, pp. 1435–1440.

BARTTER SYNDROME

Description Bartter syndrome is a disorder of renal metabolism.

Synonyms
>Aldosteronism with Normal Blood Pressure
>Hyperaldosteronism with Hypokalemic Alkalosis
>Hyperaldosteronism without Hypertension
>Juxtaglomerular Hyperplasia

Signs and Symptoms The majority of symptoms reflect a large urinary loss of potassium due to hypersecretion of renin. The patient may experience polydipsia, polyuria, mental retardation, weakness, short stature, and cramps in the muscles of the extremities.

Etiology The syndrome is thought to be inherited as an autosomal recessive trait. Investigations suggest the involvement of 2 renal dysfunctions: increased prostaglandin synthesis or a defect in chloride reabsorption.

Epidemiology Bartter syndrome affects males and females in equal numbers. While more frequent in children than in adults, it can occur at any age.

Related Disorders Renal tubular acidosis is a disorder in which renal secretion of hydrogen and reabsorption of bicarbonate are deficient. Sequelae may be chronic metabolic acidosis and potassium depletion, osteomalacia, or rickets.

See *Anemia, Fanconi.*

Treatment—Standard Counteraction of potassium loss is usually achieved with albumin and aldosterone antagonists. Other drug therapy may employ aspirin, indomethacin plus spironolactone, or triamterene. Otherwise, treatment is symptomatic and supportive. Patients and their families may benefit from genetic counseling.

Treatment—Investigational Enalapril has raised serum potassium levels in trials dealing with patients with this disorder.

Please contact the agencies listed under Resources, below, for the most current information.

Resources

For more information on Bartter syndrome: National Organization for Rare Disorders (NORD); National Kidney Foundation; American Kidney Fund; National Institute of Diabetes, Digestive & Kidney Diseases Information Clearinghouse.

For genetic information and genetic counseling referrals: March of Dimes Birth Defects Foundation; NIH/National Center for Education in Maternal and Child Health (NCEMCH).

References

Mendelian Inheritance in Man, 9th ed.: V.A. McKusick; The Johns Hopkins University Press, 1990, pp. 1267–1268, 1061.

Renal Tubular Reabsorption of Chloride in Bartter's Syndrome and Other Conditions with Hypokalemia: J.A. Rodriguez-Portales, et al.; Clin. Nephrol., December 1986, issue 26(6), pp. 269–272.

The Juxtaglomerular Apparatus in Bartter's syndrome and Related Tubulopathies. An Immunocytochemical and Electron Microscopic Study: R. Raugner, et al.; Virchows Arch. [A], 1988, issue 412(5), pp. 459–470.

Total Body Potassium in Bartter's Syndrome Before and During Treatment with Enalapril: A. van de Stolpe, et al.; Nephron 1987, issue 45(2), pp. 122–125.

CARCINOID SYNDROME

Description Carcinoid syndrome is a rare malignant disease affecting the small bowel, stomach, and/or pancreas. Slow-growing tumors can metastasize to the liver, lungs, and ovary.

Synonyms

Carcinoid Tumor
Endocrine Tumors
Malignant Carcinoid Syndrome
Metastatic Carcinoid Tumor

Signs and Symptoms Initially asymptomatic, the carcinoid syndrome usually becomes manifest after years of growth. It is most often characterized by flushing, wheezing, and diarrhea, which can be debilitating. The diarrhea may be severe enough to cause life-threatening dehydration and electrolyte imbalance. Abdominal pain, blockage of hepatic arteries, and excessive urinary peptide excretion may be present. Congestive heart failure may occur, associated with right-sided valvular cardiac disease. A **carcinoid crisis** may develop rarely, with life-threatening hypotension.

Etiology Carcinoid syndrome is idiopathic. It has been suggested that the tumors develop from endocrine cells in the gastrointestinal tract, usually the ileum, the gonads, the bronchi, or the pancreas.

Epidemiology The incidence of carcinoid tumors is approximately 8:100,000. Males and females of all ages are equally affected. It may be that prevalence is greater than suspected because of lack of diagnosis; not all patients have the initial triad of flushing, wheezing, and diarrhea.

Related Disorders See *Zollinger-Ellison Syndrome.*

Pancreatic cholera (vipoma) is characterized by watery diarrhea, hypokalemia, and acidosis. In most cases the disorder is due to a non-B islet cell pancreatic tumor that secretes vasoactive intestinal polypeptide **(VIP)** and peptide histidine isoleucine. The episodes of diarrhea in association with profound loss of potassium, hypochlorhydria, and metabolic acidosis can be life-threatening.

Treatment—Standard Therapy may involve the use of doxorubicin, 5-fluorouracil, dacarbazine, dactinomycin, or cisplatin. It may also employ a combination of drugs for malignant carcinoid tumors including streptozocin and 5-fluorouracil or streptozocin and cyclophosphamide. Other drug therapy may include parachlorophenylalanine, cyproheptadine, tamoxifen, and interferon. Surgical removal of the tumors has proven successful in some patients, as has hepatic artery ligation or occlusion.

A somatostatin analogue has proven effective in blocking flushing and relieving diarrhea and wheezing; symptoms usually improve within a few days. This drug has also been successful in the prophylaxis of carcinoid crisis and as an adjunct for patients undergoing surgery or starting chemotherapy.

Treatment—Investigational Please contact the agencies listed under Resources, below, for the most current information.

Resources

For more information on carcinoid syndrome: National Organization for Rare Disorders (NORD); American Cancer Society; NIH/National Cancer Institute PDQ (Physician Data Query) phoneline.

References

Advances in Diagnostic and Treatment Methods in Carcinoids: B. Hyde; Res. Resources Rept., 1989, vol. 13(1), pp. 1–4.

Carcinoid Crisis during Anesthesia: Successful Treatment with a Somatostain Analogue: H.M. Marsh, et al.; Anesthesiology, 1987, vol. 66(1), pp. 89–91.

Effect of Somatostatin Analog on Water and Electrolyte Transport and Transit Time in Human Small Bowel: M. Duano, et al.; Digest. Disease and Sciences, 1987, vol. 32(10), pp. 1092–1096.

Effect of a Long-Acting Somatostatin Analogue in a Patient with Pancreatic Cholera: P.N. Maton, et al.; New Engl. J. Med., January 3, 1985, vol. 312, pp. 17–21.

The Carcinoid Syndrome: A Treatable Malignant Disease: L. Kvols; Oncology, 1988, vol. 2(2), pp. 33–39.

Treatment of the Malignant Carcinoid Syndrome: L. Kvols, et al.; New Engl. J. Med., September 11, 1986, vol. 315(11), pp. 663–666.

Vipoma Syndrome: H.S. Mekhuian, et al.; Sem. in Onc., September 1987, vol. 14(3), pp. 282–289.

Vipoma Syndrome: Effect of a Synthetic Somatostatin Analogue: W.C. Santangelo, et al.; Scand. J. Gastroentero., 1986, vol. 21(119), pp. 187–190.

CHIARI-FROMMEL SYNDROME

Description Chiari-Frommel syndrome is a postpartum endocrine disorder in which lactation, anovulation, and amenorrhea persist long after childbirth. The absence of normal hormonal cycles may eventually lead to uterine atrophy. Some cases resolve spontaneously, with return of normal hormone levels and reproductive function.

Synonyms
>   Chiari I Syndrome
>   Frommel-Chiari Syndrome
>   Lactation-Uterus Atrophy

Signs and Symptoms The pregnancy preceding the onset of Chiari-Frommel syndrome is typically normal, and childbirth and initial lactation are uneventful. However, normal menses and ovulation do not resume, and persistent discharge from the nipples occurs, sometimes lasting for years. Other clinical findings include emotional lability, headache, backache, abdominal pain, visual deficits, occasionally obesity, and, in longstanding cases, uterine atrophy. Laboratory findings include high levels of prolactin and low urinary levels of estrogen and gonadotropins.

Etiology The cause of the abnormality of the hypothalamic-pituitary axis underlying Chiari-Frommel syndrome is not known. Most cases are attributable to pituitary tumors. Tiny hypothalamic lesions may also be involved. An association with oral contraceptive use has been suggested.

Epidemiology

Related Disorders See *Ahumada-del Castillo Syndrome; Forbes-Albright Syndrome.*

Treatment—Standard Medical and surgical therapy may be used to treat Chiari-Frommel syndrome. Large pituitary tumors causing the disorder may be removed surgically, but excision of small tumors may not be feasible. Bromocriptine is prescribed to reduce prolactin levels and restore ovulatory cycles.

Treatment—Investigational Please contact the agencies listed under Resources, below, for the most current information.

Resources
   For more information on Chiari-Frommel syndrome: National Organization for Rare Disorders (NORD); NIH/National Institute of Child Health and Human Development (NICHHD).

CONN SYNDROME

Description Conn syndrome is a rare metabolic endocrine disorder characterized by oversecretion of aldosterone, causing hypervolemia, hypernatremia, and hypokalemic alkalosis. Aldosterone causes transfer of sodium in exchange for potassium and hydrogen in the kidneys, salivary and sweat glands, and in the cells of the mucous membranes of the intestines. The renin-angiotensin mechanism and, to a lesser extent, the adrenocorticotropin hormone (ACTH) regulate aldosterone secretion. The sodium and water retention resulting from increased aldosterone secretion not only causes hypervolemia but also reduces renin secretion.

Synonyms
> Aldosteronism, Primary
> Hyperaldosteronism, Primary

Signs and Symptoms Hypernatremia, hypervolemia, and hypokalemic alkalosis can cause periods of weakness, unusual sensations such as tingling and warmness, a transient paralysis, and muscle spasms. Hypertension, polyuria, and polydipsia can also occur.

Etiology The most frequent cause is a unilateral adenoma of the adrenal cortex glomerulosa cells. The origin of the tumor is unknown. Less commonly an adrenal carcinoma or hyperplasia underlies Conn syndrome.

Related Disorders Secondary aldosteronism is characterized by increased adrenal cortex production of aldosterone resulting from stimuli exogenous to the adrenal glands, probably the result of excessive secretion of renin secondary to constriction of the renal vessels. The disorder is similar to Conn syndrome and related to hypertension and disorders with fluid retention and/or edema, such as congestive heart failure and cirrhosis with ascites. This syndrome also occurs as a symptom of other renal disorders, but unlike Conn syndrome, it is marked by decreased sodium levels and increased plasma-renin activity.

See also ***Bartter syndrome.***

Treatment—Standard A search for adenoma in both adrenal glands is essential, although there is most often a unilateral lesion. Therapy consists of removal of the tumor. Among the choices for follow-up drug therapy are mitotane, spironolactone, or hydrochlorothiazide.

Treatment—Investigational Please contact the agencies listed under Resources, below, for the most current information.

Resources
> **For more information on Conn syndrome:** National Organization for Rare Disorders (NORD); NIH/National Institute of Diabetes, Digestive & Kidney Diseases; NIH/National Heart, Lung, and Blood Institute (NHLBI).

References
Aging and Aldosterone: R. Hegstad, et al.; Amer. J. Med., 1983, vol. 74(3), pp. 442–448.

Clinical Implications of Primary Aldosteronism with Resistant Hypertension: E.L. Bravo, et al.; Hypertension, 1988, vol. 11(2 Pt.2), pp. 1207–1211.

Isolated Clinical Syndrome of Primary Aldosteronism in Four Patients with Adrenocortical Carcinoma: D. Farge, et al.; Amer. J. Med., 1987, vol. 83(4), pp. 635–640.

Pure Primary Hyperaldosteronism due to Adrenal Cortical Carcinoma: D.J. Greathouse, et al.; Amer. J. Med., 1984, vol. 76(6), pp. 1132–1136.

CUSHING SYNDROME

Description Cushing syndrome consists of a myriad of clinical abnormalities. The many problems are the result of hypersecretion of corticosteroids by the adrenal cortex.

Synonyms
    Adrenal Hyperfunction
    Adrenal Neoplasm
    Ectopic ACTH Syndrome

Signs and Symptoms Excessive weight gain produces fat deposits in the face, causing a rounded shape, and in the supraclavicular and dorsal cervical areas. The trunk is obese, but the arms and legs remain slender. The face is reddened, and the skin is thin, fragile, and slow to heal if wounded. Weakened connective tissue causes reddish-blue stretch marks to appear on the arms, breasts, axillae, abdomen, buttocks, and thighs.

In women hirsutism affects the face, neck, chest, abdomen, and thighs, and menstrual disorders are common. In men, fertility is often decreased and the sex drive diminished or absent.

Hypertension occurs in 85 percent of patients. Bones become brittle and easily broken, a result of osteoporosis. Hyperglycemia, severe weakness and fatigue, and psychiatric disturbances also may be present.

Etiology Cushing syndrome is caused by excessive secretion of cortisol, often due to hormone-secreting benign adrenal or pituitary tumors. Adrenocorticotropin (ACTH) stimulates the adrenals to overproduce cortisol. **Ectopic ACTH syndrome** is caused by hormone-secreting malignant tumors, especially oat cell or small cell lung carcinomas.

An exogenous cause of elevated cortisol levels is corticosteroid therapy.

Epidemiology Cushing syndrome affects 5 times more women than men. Onset is most commonly at age 30 to 40 years; women who have just given birth are at higher risk. Cushing disease accounts for about 70 percent of all reported cases; ectopic ACTH syndrome is responsible for about 17 percent; adrenal tumors underlie 13 percent of the cases.

Treatment—Standard Pituitary tumors may be removed by transphenoidal adenomectomy, with a success rate of over 80 percent. After surgery, the expected drop in the production of ACTH can be temporarily compensated with hydrocortisone. Therapy usually lasts for less than one year. If the patient is not a candidate for surgery or surgery proves unsuccessful, irradiation of the pituitary gland for 6 weeks is indicated. The rate of improvement is 40 to 50 percent for adults and 80 percent for children.

Mitotane alone or in combination with irradiation is used to inhibit cortisol and speed recovery. Aminoglutethimide, metyrapone, or ketoconazole also controls the production of cortisol.

The orphan drug trilostane (Modrastane) has been approved for treatment of Cushing syndrome.

The destruction of ACTH-secreting tumor cells is essential to reverse the effects of ectopic ACTH syndrome. Adrenal tumors are usually removed by surgery, and a course of mitotane is given.

If cortisol levels are elevated because of corticosteroid therapy, the dosage should be reduced until the symptoms are under control.

Treatment—Investigational A glucocorticoid antagonist, RU 486, is undergoing clinical trials in the treatment of Cushing syndrome.

George P. Chrousos, M.D., at the Developmental Endocrinology Branch, National Institutes of Health, is studying patients with Cushing syndrome. The address is Building 10, Room 10N262, Bethesda, Maryland 20892; (301) 4964686.

Please contact the agencies listed under Resources, below, for the most current information.

Resources

For more information on Cushing syndrome: National Organization for Rare Disorders (NORD); National Cushing Syndrome Association; National Institute of Diabetes, Digestive & Kidney Diseases; Brain and Pituitary Foundation of America.

References

The Merck Manual, 15th ed.: R. Berkow, ed.-in-chief; Merck Sharp & Dohme Research Laboratories, 1987, pp. 1056–1058.

Internal Medicine, 2nd ed.: J.H. Stein, ed.-in-chief; Little, Brown and Company, 1987, pp. 1947–1951.

DERCUM DISEASE

Description Dercum disease is characterized by subcutaneous lipomas that exert pressure on nerves, causing extreme pain and weakness.

Synonyms

Adiposa Dolorosa

Juxta-Articular Adiposis Dolorosa

Signs and Symptoms Painful, irregularly shaped soft fatty tissue deposits occur most frequently in the trunk, forearms, knees, and thighs. These deposits may spontaneously resolve, leaving hardened tissue or pendulous folds of skin. In some cases, severe asthenia is present. Some patients may experience depression, but it is not known whether depression is a symptom of the disorder or a response to the pain of chronic illness.

Etiology Dercum disease is idiopathic. It has been suggested that it may be genetic or associated with an unidentified endocrine abnormality.

Epidemiology Dercum disease usually affects obese females age 45 to 60. It has been recorded in more than one member of the same family, and has been known to affect persons of normal weight. Rare cases of men affected by Dercum disease have been reported in the literature.

Related Disorders Symptoms of Dercum disease are similar to those of arthritis.

Treatment—Standard Treatment is directed primarily at easing painful episodes. Surgical excision of fatty tissue deposits around joints may temporarily relieve symptoms; recurrence is common. Intravenous infusions of lidocaine bring temporary relief, but periodic infusions may be necessary to sustain the effect. Mexiletine, taken orally, may also eliminate pain for variable periods. Psychotherapy may help patients cope with longterm intense pain. Other treatment is symptomatic and supportive.

Treatment—Investigational Please contact the agencies listed under Resources, below, for the most current information.

Resources

For more information on Dercum disease: National Organization for Rare Disorders (NORD); National Institute of Diabetes, Digestive & Kidney Diseases Information Clearinghouse; American Chronic Pain Association, Inc; National Chronic Pain Outreach Association.

References

Mendelian Inheritance in Man, 9th ed.: V.A. McKusick; The Johns Hopkins University Press, 1990, p. 31.

A Case of Adiposis Dolorosa: Lipid Metabolism and Hormone Secretion: A. Taniguchi, et al.; Int. J. Obes., 1986, vol. 10(4), pp. 277–281.

Dercum Disease (Adiposa Dolorosa), A Case Report and Review of the Literature: T.J. Bonatus, et al.; Clin. Orthrop., 1986, vol. 205, pp. 251–253.

Dercum Disease (Adiposa Dolorosa). Treatment of Severe Pain with Intravenous Lidocaine: P. Petersen, et al.; Pain, 1987, vol. 28(1), pp. 77–80.

DIABETES INSIPIDUS (DI)

Description Diabetes insipidus, a disorder of the neurohypophyseal system, is characterized by the excretion of large amounts of urine of low specific gravity and by dehydration and excessive thirst. The more common form, which can be inherited, acquired, or idiopathic, is due to a deficiency of antidiuretic hormone (**ADH; vasopressin**). The rarer congenital nephrogenic diabetes insipidus (**NDI**) is caused by failure of the renal tubules to respond to ADH, preventing reabsorption of water.

Synonyms
>Vasopressin-Sensitive Diabetes Insipidus (Central or Neurogenic Diabetes Insipidus)
>Vasopressin-Resistant Diabetes Insipidus (Nephrogenic Diabetes Insipidus)

Signs and Symptoms In central or neurogenic diabetes insipidus, increased thirst, polydipsia, and polyuria vary in severity among patients. Symptoms may also include weakness, fatigue, and dryness of the mouth and skin. Other physical symptoms and signs are usually those of the underlying disorder.

In nephrogenic diabetes insipidus, infants develop polydipsia and polyuria. Since infants cannot communicate thirst, severe dehydration with hypernatremia, fever, vomiting, or convulsions should signal the possibility of NDI. Mental retardation may result.

Etiology Central or neurogenic DI can be inherited (X-linked forms as well as autosomal dominant forms), acquired (the result of malignancy, granuloma, infection, trauma, vascular abnormalities), or idiopathic.

Nephrogenic DI usually occurs as an X-linked recessive trait. It may occasionally be acquired.

Epidemiology The inherited forms of diabetes insipidus usually affect males. Females can be carriers.

Treatment—Standard Effective control of DI may be obtained with several commercially available preparations of synthetic ADH. These include lypressin, a nasal spray, the simplest form for self-administration, and the longer-acting desmopressin acetate (DDAVP), which appears to enhance antidiuretic activity with minimal adverse effects on the vascular system or smooth muscles. Both lypressin and DDAVP may be inhaled or blown high into the nasal passages with an insufflator. In many patients, nasal irritation may be a drawback to this form of treatment.

An intramuscular (*never intravenous*) injection of vasopressin tannate in oil usually controls polyuria and polydipsia for 1 to 3 days. An aqueous posterior pituitary hormone injection is of little use in chronic treatment of DI, but an intramuscular injection may give an antidiuretic response lasting usually 6 hours or less.

Chlorpropamide, used to treat hyperglycemia in diabetes mellitus, is effective in reducing polyuria in neurogenic DI patients. Clofibrate and carbamazepine also have been used successfully.

Thiazide diuretics are effective for treating the polyuria in patients with both neurogenic and nephrogenic DI.

Treatment—Investigational Research in treating DI is ongoing. Prostaglandin synthesis inhibitors under investigation have not shown uniform effectiveness. Use of hydrochlorothiazide-amiloride in the treatment of congenital NDI has indicated that treatment with both of these compounds may possibly be more effective than hydrochlorothiazide alone and can be a satisfactory alternative to the hydrochlorothiazide-prostaglandin synthetase inhibitor combination in the treatment of NDI.

Please contact the agencies listed under Resources, below, for the most current information.

Resources

For more information on diabetes insipidus: National Organization for Rare Diseases (NORD); American Diabetes Association; National Diabetes Information Clearinghouse.

For genetic information and genetic counseling referrals: March of Dimes Birth Defects Foundation; National Center for Education in Maternal and Child Health (NCEMCH).

References

Hydrochlorothiazide-Amiloride in the Treatment of Congenital Nephrogenic Diabetes Insipidus: V. Alon and J.C. Chan; Am. J. Nephrol., 1985, vol. 5(1), pp. 9–13.

Treatment of Nephrogenic Diabetes Insipidus with Prostaglandin Synthesis-Inhibitors: S. Libber, et al., eds; J. Pediatr., February 1986, vol. 108(2), pp. 305–311.

FORBES-ALBRIGHT SYNDROME

Description Forbes-Albright syndrome is one of a group of disorders associated with hypersecretion of prolactin by the pituitary.

Synonyms

Galactorrhea-Amenorrhea Syndrome
Nonpuerperal Amenorrhea-Galactorrhea
Nonpuerperal Galactorrhea

Signs and Symptoms Onset of galactorrhea and amenorrhea in women and galactorrhea and other changes in men is usually during the patient's 20s or 30s. Women with galactorrhea and amenorrhea have breasts and nipples of normal size and appearance, but the pattern of body hair may change and the libido decrease. Obesity and exceptionally oily skin are characteristics in some patients.

Men not only have enlarged breasts but they may begin to secrete milk. Even in the absence of galactorrhea, men may experience a lessening of libido and impotence, and a decrease in sperm.

High levels of prolactin and low concentrations of gonadotropins, e.g., follicle-stimulating hormone **(FSH),** are typical findings.

Etiology The primary cause of the syndrome is a hormone-secreting pituitary tumor or, at times, a tumor in the hypothalamus. Also to blame may be hypothyroidism, chronic use of dopamine antagonists (e.g., chlorpromazine), and discontinuation of oral contraceptives.

Epidemiology Forbes-Albright syndrome occurs in individuals whose pituitary hypersecretes prolactin.

Related Disorders See *Chiari-Frommel Syndrome; Ahumada-del Castillo*

Syndrome.

Treatment—Standard Surgical removal of neoplasm is usually curative. For smaller or inoperable tumors, irradiation or treatment with bromocriptine or lergotrile mesilate is indicated. These drugs lower prolactin levels, thereby preventing abnormal lactation, and often produce normal menses.

Treatment—Investigational Please contact the agencies listed under Resources, below, for the most current information.

Resources
  For more information on **Forbes-Albright syndrome:** National Organization for Rare Disorders (NORD); NIH/National Institute of Child Health and Human Development (NICHHD).

FRÖLICH SYNDROME

Description Frölich syndrome is characterized by delayed puberty, small testes, and obesity; it primarily affects males. In recent years, Frölich syndrome has referred exclusively to such features in boys who have lesions in the hypothalamus. Teenagers with this disorder must be differentiated from those who simply have a familiar trait of slower-than-normal growth or **Prader-Willi syndrome.**

Synonyms
  Adiposogenital Dystrophy
  Babinski-Frölich Syndrome
  Dystrophia Adiposogenitalis
  Hypothalamic Infantilism-Obesity
  Launois-Cleret Syndrome
  Sexual Infantilism

Signs and Symptoms Obesity accompanies delayed puberty. Body growth may also be slow, and patients often remain short in stature. Fingernails are often malformed or undersized. Headaches are common. Some patients may have mental retardation, visual disturbances, and, rarely, diabetes mellitus.

Etiology In some cases the anterior pituitary fails to secrete the hormones necessary for puberty because of a lesion, usually caused by a tumor or inflammation resulting from an infection such as tuberculosis or encephalitis. Frölich syndrome is due to lesions in the hypothalamus, which produces substances that stimulate the pituitary and is also believed to regulate the appetite.

Related Disorders Hypogonadotropic hypogonadism is a disorder of the development of the region of the hypothalamus that regulates the production of gonadotropins.
  See also *Laurence-Moon-Biedl Syndrome; Prader-Willi Syndrome.*

Treatment—Standard Hormonal replacement therapy is indicated, but hypothalamic tumors should be removed if possible. The patient's appetite makes it difficult to achieve weight control.

Treatment—Investigational Please contact the agencies listed under Resources, below, for the most current information.

Resources
   For more information on Frölich syndrome: National Organization for Rare Disorders (NORD); NIH/National Institute of Neurological Disorders & Stroke (NINDS); Human Growth Foundation.

References
   Regulation of the Endocrine Hypothalamus: S. Reichlin; S. Med. Clin. North Am., 1978, vol. 62(2), pp. 235–250.

GRAVES DISEASE

Description Hyperthyroidism, goiter, exophthalmos, and dermopathy are the major characteristics of Graves disease.

Synonyms
    Basedow Disease
    Exophthalmic Goiter
    Parry Disease
    Thyrotoxicosis

Signs and Symptoms The major features of Graves disease do not necessarily occur together and often run courses independent of each other. There may be periods of remission. The diffusely enlarged goiter may be asymmetric, with an enlarged pyramidal lobe. Besides exophthalmos, the other often characteristic ocular findings include inflammation and conjunctival edema; ophthalmoplegia may occur in the more severe cases. Diplopia and photophobia may also be present. The dermopathy most often presents as erythematous, pruritic swelling over the pretibial area.

   Other findings include hyperactivity and tachycardia and, less often, clubbing of the fingers and toes, and gynecomastia.

Etiology The cause of Graves disease is unknown. Both recessive and autosomal dominant inheritances have been reported. The disease is strongly suspected to have an autoimmune association, with thyroid-stimulating antibodies a factor.

Epidemiology Graves disease can occur at any age but is most common in the 20s and 30s. Females are affected more often than males. A 1987 survey of 924 hyperthyroid patients from 17 thyroid centers in 6 European countries indicated that 60 percent of hyperthyroid patients have Graves disease.

Related Disorders See *Hashimoto Syndrome.*

Treatment—Standard Antithyroid drugs are preferred initially by many physicians, since ablative procedures more often produce hypothyroidism. Antithyroid drugs are also preferred for children, teenagers, and pregnant women. These drugs, however, seem to result in fewer lasting remissions.

Radioactive iodine is preferred by many centers because of its effectiveness in treating thyrotoxicosis without the possible complications of surgical procedures. The hypothyroidism that ensues must be anticipated and treated.

Surgery is usually reserved for patients refractory to other therapies. Lifelong followup is indicated postthyroidectomy.

Genetic counseling may benefit patients and their families. Other treatment is symptomatic and supportive.

Treatment—Investigational Please contact the agencies listed under Resources, below, for the most current information.

Resources

For more information on Graves disease: National Organization for Rare Disorders (NORD); Graves Disease Foundation; The Thyroid Foundation of America, Inc.; The Thyroid Foundation of Canada; NIH/National Institute of Diabetes, Digestive & Kidney Diseases Information Clearinghouse.

For genetic information and genetic counseling referrals: March of Dimes Birth Defects Foundation; NIH/National Center for Education in Maternal and Child Health (NCEMCH).

References

Graves Disease Associated with Histologic Hashimoto's Thyroiditis: S.A. Falk, et al.; Otolaryngol. Head Neck Surg., 1985, vol. 93(1), pp. 86–91.

Graves Disease. Manifestations and Therapeutic Options: K.F. McFarland, et al.; Postgrad. Med., 1988, vol. 83(4), pp. 275–282.

High Serum Progesterone in Hyperthyroid Men with Graves Disease: K. Nomura, et al.; J. Clin. Endocrinol. Metab., 1988, vol. 66(1), pp. 230–232.

Internal Medicine, 3rd ed.: J.H. Stein, ed.-in-chief; Little, Brown and Company, 1990, pp. 2174–2178.

Mendelian Inheritance in Man, 9th ed.: V.A. McKusick; The Johns Hopkins University Press, 1990, pp. 1509–1510.

GROWTH DELAY, CONSTITUTIONAL

Description Constitutional growth delay is a term describing a temporary slowdown in the skeletal growth and height of a child who has no other physical abnormalities that might cause the delay. Growth eventually resumes at a normal rate. The delay may be familial or sporadic.

Synonyms

Constitutional Delay in Growth and Puberty
Constitutional Short Stature
Idiopathic Growth Delay
Idiopathic Short Stature

Physiologic Delayed Puberty
Sporadic Short Stature

Symptoms and Signs

The child who eventually has a delay in growth is born at a normal height and weight and may grow at a normal rate for as much as 2 years. During the period of slowdown the child's height on a growth chart is usually below the 5th percentile. When testing is done, no physical impairment is found to cause the delay.

Normally puberty begins when the bone age reaches 10.5 years in females and 11.5 years in males. The chronologic age of puberty in children with constitutional growth delay is usually later. The normal age for epiphyseal fusion to occur is age 15 in females and age 18 in males. Female adolescents with constitutional growth delay typically continue growing until they are 17 or 18, while males may continue to grow into their early 20s. Puberty is normal in adolescents with constitutional growth delay except for the later age. Adult height is within the normal range.

In some patients skeletal age is not delayed as much as height age.

Etiology The cause is not known. There is often a history of this delay in growth occurring in other members of the family. On the other hand, some children may experience a period of delayed growth for no known reason. A deficiency of growth hormone can be ruled out through laboratory tests in cases where other physical and genetic factors are not apparent.

Epidemiology Approximately 35 percent of all children with short stature have constitutional growth delay. Both males and females are affected, although many more boys than girls seek help.

Related Disorders See *Growth Hormone Deficiency; Rickets, Vitamin D-Deficiency; Turner Syndrome.*

Conditions often associated with short stature include juvenile diabetes, cystic fibrosis, kidney diseases, and asthmatics who have inhaled steroids.

Hypochondroplasia is a rare inherited skeletal disorder. The major feature is short stature that is not evident until mid childhood. Other characteristics include a head of normal size, and small but normally shaped hands and feet. Affected children appear normal at birth, but their limbs fail to develop properly.

Treatment—Standard Treatment is not recommended, since affected children will eventually grow to a height within the normal range. A child generally will get through this lull in growth with no problems. Occasionally there may be psychological difficulties associated with short stature, and counseling as well as family and peer support may be necessary.When severe psychological symptoms are apparent, drugs may be prescribed in conjunction with counseling. These may include male hormones, including anabolic steroids. This treatment should be done with caution under careful medical supervision, and frequent x-rays should be taken to make sure that the skeletal age is not being advanced too much. When bone development is increased faster than height, the growing period can be reduced, with ultimate reduction of the patient's adult height. Since steroids have potentially severe physical and behavioral side effects, this form of therapy is rarely recommended.

Treatment—Investigational Treatment with recombinant human growth hormone **(hGH)** is recommended only for children with documented growth hormone deficiency as confirmed through laboratory tests. The use of hGH on healthy short children is controversial, since longterm consequences are unknown.

The orphan drug testosterone (sublingual) is currently being tested for treatment of constitutional delay of growth and puberty in boys. The orphan drug oxandrolone is currently being tested for use in the treatment of constitutional delay of growth and puberty. Both drugs are sponsored by Gynex, Inc., 1175 Corporate Woods Parkway, Deerfield, Illinois 60015.

Please contact the agencies listed under Resources, below, for the most current information.

Resources

For more information on constitutional growth delay: National Organization for Rare Disorders (NORD); Human Growth Foundation; Short Stature Foundation; National Institute of Child Health and Human Development (NICHHD).

References
Internal Medicine, 2nd ed.: J.H. Stein, ed.-in-chief; Little, Brown and Company, 1987, pp. 1986–1988.

Cecil Textbook of Medicine, 19th ed.: J.B. Wyngaarden and L.H. Smith, Jr., eds.; W.B. Saunders Company, 1990, p. 1418.

Clinical Pediatric Endocrinology: S.A. Kaplan; W.B. Saunders Company, 1990, pp. 10, 49–53.

Growth Hormone Therapy: L. Shulman, et al.; Am. Family Physician, May 1990, issue 41(5), pp. 1541–1546.

Testosterone Treatment in Adolescent Boys with Constitutional Delay in Growth and Development: R.A. Richman, et al.; N. Engl. J. Med., December 15, 1988, issue 319(24), pp. 1563–1567.

Double Blind Placebo Controlled Trial of Low Dose Oxandrolone in the Treatment of Boys with Constitutional Delay of Growth and Puberty: R. Stanhope, et al.; Arch. Dis. Child, May 1988, issue 63(5), pp. 501–505.

Treatment of Short Stature and Delayed Adolescence: D.M. Wilson, et al.; Pediatr. Clin. North Am., August 1987, issue 34(4), pp. 865–879.

GROWTH HORMONE DEFICIENCY (GHD)

Description A sufficient quantity of growth hormone **(GH),** manufactured in the pituitary, is required during infancy or childhood to maintain growth and normalize sexual maturity. Growth hormone deficiency causes an absence or delay of lengthening and widening of the skeletal bones inappropriate to the chronological age of the child.

There are several types of GHD: IA, IB, IIB, and III.

Signs and Symptoms Growth increments are the most important criteria in the diagnosis of GHD. Normal levels of growth usually follow a pattern, and if growth during a recorded 6- to 12-month period is within those levels, it is unlikely that a growth disorder exists.

Growth in the first 6 months of life is usually 16 to 17 cm, and in the second 6 months, about 8 cm. During the second year, 10 or more cm are normal. Growth in the third year should equal 8 cm or more, and in the fourth year, 7 cm. In the years between ages 4 and 10, an average of 5 or 6 cm is normal. Ten percent deviation in these norms is the standard in assessing a growth abnormality. If a child falls below the 10 percent deviation in growth, he or she should then be tested for abnormally low levels of growth hormone.

The infant with GHD is usually of normal weight and length at birth. During the newborn period the infant may become hypoglycemic. Micropenis may be present in males. Signs and symptoms common to children with GHD are abnormal rates of development of facial bones, slow tooth eruption, delayed skeletal development, fine hair, and poor nail growth. They may also experience truncal obesity, a high-pitched voice, and delayed closure of the fontanelles.

GHD IA is characterized by prenatal growth retardation. The infant usually has a normal response to administration of GH at first, then develops antibodies to the hormone. The child is small in relation to his or her siblings, and becomes a very short adult.

GHD IB is similar to IA, but some growth hormone is present at birth. The child may respond to treatment with GH.

GHD IIB is similar to IB, but with a different inheritance.

GHD III is similar to the above, but also with a different inheritance.

Laboratory testing is necessary before a diagnosis of GHD is made, because growth and maturity delays can be caused by a wide variety of factors, including normal genetic influences.

Etiology The growth hormone gene is located on the long arm of chromosome 17. In some children, GHD occurs for no apparent reason; in others, it may be inherited or familial. GHD IA and IB are inherited as autosomal recessive traits. GHD IIB inheritance is autosomal dominant. GHD III is inherited through X-linked transmission, affecting only males.

Epidemiology For all forms except GHD III, males and females are affected equally. Growth hormone deficiency is closely associated with other disorders such as Down syndrome, CHARGE association, cystic fibrosis, chronic renal failure, and Turner syndrome. There may be approximately 10,000 to 15,000 children in the United States with pituitary dwarfism caused by GHD.

Related Disorders See *Turner Syndrome; Down Syndrome; CHARGE Association.*

Cystic fibrosis, an inherited disorder that involves the exocrine glands, affects children and young adults. Mucus is secreted that is thick and sticky, and clogs and obstructs air passages in the lungs and pancreatic bile ducts. Dysfunction of salivary and sweat glands is also present. There may be digital clubbing, decreased tolerance for exercise, decreased appetite, weight loss, and failure to gain weight or grow normally.

Laron short stature is characterized by proportionate severe short stature which is evident at birth or soon after. Along with growth retardation, there are delays in tooth eruption. There is also disproportion between the growth of the head and jaw, a saddle nose, and deep-set eyes. Sexual development is slow but does occur. The usual age of sexual maturation in boys with this disorder is about 22 years of age. In females, sexual maturation usually takes place between 16 to 19 years of age. Hands and feet are smaller than normal. Obesity and a high-pitched voice may also be present. This is a disorder of growth hormone receptors, in which the body is unable to use the growth hormone that it produces. A high percentage of patients have extremely low blood sugar levels.

Treatment—Standard Determination as to whether the child with growth retardation does indeed have GHD is most important. Tests used include insulin-arginine-estrogen, GH-plasma-exercise, clonidine, or L-dopa and propranolol.When a diagnosis of GHD can be made, treatment can then be instituted. The question of whether short children whose levels of growth hormone have not been tested should be treated with human growth hormone (**hGH**) is controversial, since commercially available biotechnology-engineered hGH is very expensive and many health insurance companies will not reimburse for the product unless laboratory tests confirm GHD. Moreover, adverse effects of hGH on healthy short children without GHD have not been adequately assessed.

Recombinant hGH is available on the United States market as Protropin (Genentech) and Humatrope (Eli Lilly), as an injection. Children with GHD are usually started on small doses of recombinant hGH as soon as the condition is recognized. The dosage is gradually increased to its highest during puberty, and discontinued by approximately age 17.

Treatment—Investigational Please contact the agencies listed under Resources, below, for the most current information.

Resources

For more information on growth hormone deficiency: National Organization for Rare Disorders (NORD); Human Growth Foundation; Short Stature Foundation; Little People of America; NIH/National Institute of Child Health and Human Development (NICHHD).

For genetic information and genetic counseling referrals: March of Dimes Birth Defects Foundation; NIH/National Center for Education in Maternal and Child Health (NCEMCH).

References
Mendelian Inheritance in Man, 9th ed.: V.A. McKusick; The Johns Hopkins University Press, 1990, pp. 377–380, 887–888, 1426–1427.

Diagnostic Recognition of Genetic Disease: W.L. Nyhan, et al.; Lea & Febiger, 1987, pp. 706–709, 712, 718.

Smith's Recognizable Patterns of Human Malformation, 4th ed.: K.L. Jones; W.B. Saunders Company, 1988, pp. 614–618, 762–763.

Cecil Textbook of Medicine, 18th ed.: J.B. Wyngaarden and L.H. Smith, Jr., eds.; W.B. Saunders Company, 1988, pp. 1290–1297, 2205.

Clinical Pediatric Endocrinology: S.A. Kaplan; W.B. Saunders Company, 1990, pp. 1–56.

Growth Hormone Therapy: L. Shulman, et al.; Am. Fam. Physician, May 1990, issue 41(5), pp. 1541–1546.

Biosynthetic Human Growth Hormone in the Treatment of Growth Hormone Deficiency: J.H. Holcombe, et al.; Acta Paediatr. Scand. Suppl., 1990, issue 367, pp. 44–48.

Urinary Growth Hormone Excretion as a Screening Test for Growth Hormone Deficiency: J.M. Walker, et al.; Arch. Dis. Child, January 1990, issue 65(1), pp. 89–92.

Growth Hormone for Short Stature not due to Classic Growth Hormone Deficiency: J.F. Cara, et al.; Pediatr. Clin. North Am., December, 1990, issue 37(6), pp. 1229–1254.

HASHIMOTO SYNDROME

Description Hashimoto syndrome is a major cause of hypothyroidism. In its progression it can totally destroy the thyroid gland.

Synonyms
> Hashimoto Disease
> Hashimoto Thyroiditis
> Lymphadenoid Goiter
> Struma Lymphomatosa

Signs and Symptoms The main characteristic is a painless goiter, which on palpation feels firm and either smooth or nodular. Thyroid function studies initially are normal if the disease process has not yet affected the secretion of thyroid hormone.

Etiology The cause is unknown. An autoimmune association seems certain, and there may be a familial predisposition to the disorder, but the precise factors determining the development of the disorder in certain individuals are not understood.

Epidemiology Men and women of any age can develop the syndrome, but it occurs most often in women between the ages of 30 and 50.

Related Disorders See *Graves Disease.*

Subacute thyroiditis, a fairly common inflammation of the thyroid, usually manifests about 2 weeks after a respiratory viral infection. Considerable pain and tenderness in the thyroid area accompany difficulty in swallowing. The radioiodine uptake is low, and the erythrocyte sedimentation rate is elevated. Most patients obtain relief from an analgesic or an antiinflammatory drug, and in time the thyroid levels become normal.

Riedel thyroiditis, the result of fibrous tissue formation in the thyroidal area, is very rare. The thyroid is enlarged, hard, and fixed, but nontender. Hypothyroidism results from progressive destruction of the gland.

Treatment—Standard Upon replacement of thyroid hormone, the goiter will shrink significantly, usually within 2 to 4 weeks. Lifetime replacement therapy is necessary.

Treatment—Investigational Please contact the agencies listed under Resources,

below, for the most current information.

Resources
For more information on Hashimoto syndrome: National Organization for Rare Disorders (NORD); The Thyroid Foundation of America; The Thyroid Foundation of Canada; NIH/National Institute of Diabetes, Digestive & Kidney Diseases Information Clearinghouse.

For genetic information and genetic counseling referrals: March of Dimes Birth Defects Foundation; NIH/National Center for Education in Maternal and Child Health (NCEMCH).

References
Harrison's Principles of Internal Medicine, 12th ed.: J.D. Wilson, et al.; McGraw-Hill, 1991, pp. 1711–1712.

Internal Medicine, 3rd ed.: J.H. Stein, ed.-in-chief; Little, Brown and Company, 1990, pp. 2179–2180.

HYPOPHOSPHATASIA

Description A genetic metabolic bone disorder, hypophosphatasia is a manifestation of bony demineralization and lack of calcium deposit in the osteoid and in the cartilage of the long bones in early years. The disorder causes rachitic changes. There are 4 subdivisions: infantile (neonatal); childhood; adult; and pseudohypophosphatasia.

Synonyms
Hypercalciuric Rickets
Hypophosphatemic Rickets with Hypercalciuria, Hereditary

Signs and Symptoms In hypophosphatasia a low serum alkaline phosphatase coupled with urinary excretion of phosphoethanolamine is diagnostic.

Infantile hypophosphatasia is the most frequently encountered form of the abnormality. As a rule, onset is before age 6 months, but diagnosis prenatally is possible. Demineralization is often accompanied by increased intracranial pressure, which may cause exophthalmos. Hypercalcemia and hypercalciuria may be present; calcium in the renal tubules may cause renal failure. Weakening and bending of the bones is usual, giving a picture of rickets. Significant bone abnormalities may develop.

Onset of **childhood hypophosphatasia** is generally after age 6 months and consists of loss of newly erupted teeth, increased proneness to infection, and retarded growth. X-rays may reveal abnormalities in the epiphyses and the shafts of the long bones.

Adult hypophosphatasia is rare. The patient has a history of early loss of baby teeth and rachitic symptoms as a child. Early in adulthood, the patient's permanent teeth often loosen and fall out or require extraction. The bones are less dense than they should be, and the patient is apt to be fracture-prone.

In **pseudohypophosphatasia,** the serum alkaline phosphatase is normal. Otherwise, all or many of the other findings in hypophosphatasia are present. Patients with pseudohypophosphatasia have all or many of the manifestations of hypophosphatasia. However, blood concentrations of the enzyme alkaline phosphatase are normal.

Etiology With the exception of pseudohypophosphatase, a lack of alkaline phosphatase is responsible for the signs and symptoms of hypophosphatase. The infantile, childhood, and adult forms are hereditary; the infantile and childhood types are autosomal recessive, and the adult form is autosomal dominant.

Epidemiology All forms of hypophosphatasia affect males and females in equal numbers.

Related Disorders The hallmark of all types of rickets, either hereditary or acquired, is weakening of the bones as a result of faulty calcium metabolism. In addition, other values may be deficient. When a dietary lack of vitamin D is responsible, a supplement is curative if given before completion of bone development.

Hypophosphatemic rickets (vitamin D-resistant rickets; X-linked hypophosphatemia) is an uncommon genetic form in which impairment of phosphate transport is coupled with faulty renal metabolism of vitamin D. In addition, intestinal malabsorption of calcium and phosphate can result in bone softening. Patients become weak and experience skeletal changes and growth retardation. The disorder is usually milder in females.

A rare acquired type of the disorder may be due to a benign tumor.

In **osteomalacia,** pain of varying severity accompanies softening and bending of the bones. The bones lack calcium either because of inadequate vitamin D or a renal disorder. Osteoamalacia is more common among women than men, and onset often coincides with pregnancy. Osteomalacia can be a separate entity, but may also occur with other disorders, as in hypophosphatemic rickets.

Pseudo–vitamin D-deficiency rickets (vitamin D-dependent rickets, type 1) usually starts in early infancy and causes significant skeletal changes (such as bending of the bones) and weakness. Episodic muscle cramping may occur, and convulsions and spinal and pelvic abnormalities may develop. Hereditary abnormal vitamin D-dependent metabolism is responsible, and the disorder is autosomal recessive. The serum calcium is very low; the serum phosphate is only slightly below normal or normal. Renal dysfunction causes excessive excretion of amino acids.

See *Rickets, Vitamin D-Deficiency; Osteogenesis Imperfecta; Paget's Disease of Bone.*

Treatment—Standard Ultrasonography combined with alkaline phosphatase assay and x-ray of the fetus can make the diagnosis of hypophosphatasia prenatally in severe cases.

Vitamin D and its metabolites should be avoided in hypophosphatasia. A longterm course of oral phosphate supplements may be effective in some patients. Other treatment is symptomatic and supportive. Genetic counseling is indicated for patients' families.

Treatment—Investigational A few patients with severe cases of infantile hypophosphatasia have received transfusions of alkaline phosphatase-rich plasma to supplement the lack of alkaline phosphatase.

Please contact the agencies listed under Resources, below, for the most current information.

Resources

For more information on hypophosphatasia: National Organization for Rare Disorders (NORD); The National Arthritis and Musculoskeletal and Skin Diseases Information Clearinghouse; Research Trust for Metabolic Diseases in Children.

For genetic information and genetic counseling referrals: March of Dimes Birth Defects Foundation; National Center for Education in Maternal and Child Health (NCEMCH).

References

The Metabolic Basis of Inherited Disease, 6th ed.: C.R. Scriver, et al., eds.; McGraw-Hill, 1989, pp. 2845–2856.

Enzyme Replacement Therapy for Infantile Hypophosphatasia Attempted by Intravenous Infusions of Alkaline Phosphatase-Rich Paget Plasma: Results in Three Additional Patients: M.P. Whyte, et al.; J. Pediatr., December 1984, issue 105(6), pp. 926–933.

Infantile Hypophosphatasia: Enzyme Replacement Therapy by Intravenous Infusion of Alkaline Phosphatase-rich Plasma from Patients with Paget Bone Disease: M.P. Whyte, et al.; J. Pediatr., September 1982, issue 101(3), pp. 379–386.

Infantile Hypophosphatasia Diagnosed at 4 Months and Surviving at 2 Years: A. Albeggiani, et al.; Helv. Paediatr. Acta, 1982, issue 37(1), pp. 49–58.

LIPODYSTROPHY

Description The lipodystrophies, a cluster of rare inherited or acquired metabolic disorders, are associated with defects in adipose tissue that cause total or partial loss of body fat, irregularities of carbohydrate and lipid metabolism, marked endogenous and synthetic insulin resistance, and a malfunctioning immune system. Systemic involvement occurs in varying degrees.

The disorders are categorized into 3 forms: **total lipodystrophy** (congenital and acquired forms); **partial lipodystrophy** (acquired and familial forms, and lipoatrophic diabetes mellitus); and **localized lipodystrophy** (including mesenteric, membranous, and centrifugal forms). Categorization is made on the basis of anatomic distribution of the lipodystrophy.

Synonyms

Acquired Lipodystrophy

Acquired Partial Lipodystrophy (Cephalothoracic Lipodystrophy)

Barraquer-Simons Disease

Centrifugal Lipodystrophy

Familial Lipodystrophy of Limbs and Lower Trunk (Reverse Partial Lipodystrophy; Kobberling-Dunnigan Syndrome; Lipoatrophic Diabetes

Mellitus)
Hollaender-Simons Disease
Insulin Lipodystrophy
Leprechaunism
Membranous Lipodystrophy
Mesenteric Lipodystrophy
Nasu Lipodystrophy
Partial Lipodystrophy
Progressive Lipodystrophy
Seip Syndrome (Berardinelli Syndrome; Congenital Lipoatrophic Diabetes)
Simons Syndrome
Unilateral Partial Lipodystrophy
Whipple Disease

Signs and Symptoms Total lipodystrophy, major body-wide loss of adipose tissue, is associated with abnormal carbohydrate and lipid metabolism.

Congenital total lipodystrophy is characterized by a severe loss of subcutaneous fat in the face, trunk, and limbs. The muscles and bones stand out because of the lack of subcutaneous fat. Acanthosis nigricans may appear in the skin folds, particularly in the axillae, usually at onset of puberty. Hirsutism and skin thickening may occur. Hepatomegaly, mild-to-moderate hypertension, renal disease, and genital hypertrophy are often seen. Mental retardation may occur. Symptoms may be delayed until diabetes mellitus manifests, usually at puberty. Insulin resistance, hyperglycemia, and hypertriglyceridemia are characteristic.

When acquired, total lipodystrophy usually has its onset during childhood or adulthood with loss of adipose tissue in the same pattern as that of the inherited form. Associated abnormalities are also similar, except that liver involvement may be more severe in acquired total lipodystrophy.

Partial lipodystrophy may also be hereditary or acquired. In the inherited form the trunk and limbs are most often the sites of lipoatrophy. The muscle prominence, renal disease, and hepatomegaly of total lipodystrophy are not present. Genital enlargement and a mild acanthosis nigricans may occur. Insulin resistance, hyperglycemia, and hypertriglyceridemia are characteristic. Onset is most often at puberty but may occur in middle age.

The acquired form (cephalothoracic progressive lipodystrophy) is the most frequently encountered type of lipodystrophy. It may often occur after another illness. The face, upper trunk, and upper limbs are affected. Renal disease is moderately severe, and insulin resistance, hyperglycemia, and hypertriglyceridemia are characteristic. Muscle prominence and hypertension are not present. Hepatomegaly, genital hypertrophy, and acanthosis nigricans are rare. Associated abnormalities include central nervous system dysfunction, menstrual disorders, ovarian abnormalities, and hypogonadism. Symptoms include coldness of affected sites, abdominal discomfort, diarrhea, headaches, nervousness, and fatigue.

Lipoatrophic diabetes mellitus, which is linked to partial lipodystrophy, may accompany either the inherited or the acquired form. The familial form is characterized by lipoatrophy of the trunk and limbs, sparing the face and neck. Acanthosis nigricans and genital hypertrophy are commonly present, but hepatic and renal involvement are not. Onset usually is at puberty but may occur in middle age.

The acquired form of lipoatrophic diabetes mellitus may be generalized as well as partial. Acanthosis nigricans, hyperlipidemia, and hepatosplenomegaly are present. Consequently, lipoatrophic diabetes mellitus may be mistaken for total lipodystrophy if the pattern of lost fat tissue is generalized. Onset of acquired lipoatrophic diabetes mellitus may be in childhood or early adulthood; as a rule, it begins during adolescence or in the early adult years.

Partial lipodystrophy associated with developmental abnormalities is hereditary. The areas involved are the face and buttocks. A nonprogressive disease with onset during infancy or early childhood, its characteristics are visual problems (Rieger's anomaly), short stature, underdevelopment of the midface, hypotrichosis, and insulin-dependent diabetes. Dental malformations are also present.

Localized lipodystrophies have readily identifiable hallmarks: multiple lesions that are small, well-defined atrophic areas. A frequent association is lymphocytic panniculitis. The disorder may occur in various forms, including mesenteric **(Whipple disease)**, membranous, and centrifugal lipodystrophy.

Mesenteric lipodystrophy is characterized by small intestinal adipose tissue.

Membranous lipodystrophy is characterized by bilateral multiple cystic bone lesions that precede neuropsychiatric symptoms including dementia, seizures, and ataxia. Additionally, the ocular lens may be affected.

Centrifugal lipodystrophy is a rare localized disorder identified by a small indentation in the skin that enlarges to become a circle. Severe atrophied subcutaneous adipose tissue causes the depression in the skin.

Etiology Congenital total lipodystrophy is inherited as an autosomal recessive trait; the acquired form is sporadic.

Acquired partial lipodystrophy is usually sporadic. The inherited form is autosomal dominant, although X-linked dominant inheritance has been reported.

Localized lipodystrophy may or may not be associated with an inflammatory mechanism. Forms may also occur secondary to such events as insulin injection and diphtheria/pertussis/tetanus vaccine.

Epidemiology Males and females are equally affected in congenital total lipodystrophy; in the other forms, females are affected more often than males.

Treatment—Standard No drugs are specific for the lipodystrophies. Extended courses of pimozide, a dopamine receptor-blocking drug, have been ineffective. Diet has some benefit in metabolic disorders; small frequent feedings and partial substitution of medium-chain triglycerides for polyunsaturated fats appear practical. Implants of monolithic silicon rubber as replacement of lost soft facial tissue have been successful. Dentures may be cosmetically beneficial for some patients. Longterm treatment is usually confined to associated systemic disorders, such as renal or endocrine dysfunction.

For the patient with a genetic form of lipodystrophy, genetic counseling is recommended. Other treatment is symptomatic and supportive.

Treatment—Investigational Late stages of some cases of lipodystrophy with severe renal disease may necessitate a transplant. This experimental procedure is recommended only in patients who are refractory to more conventional treatment.

Please contact the agencies listed under Resources, below, for the most current information.

Resources

For more information on lipodystrophy: National Organization for Rare Disorders (NORD); National Lipid Diseases Foundation; Endocrine Society; National Institute of Diabetes, Digestive & Kidney Diseases Information Clearinghouse; American Diabetes Association; Research Trust for Metabolic Diseases in Children.

For genetic information and genetic counseling referrals: March of Dimes Birth Defects Foundation; National Center for Education in Maternal and Child Health (NCEMCH).

References

Mendelian Inheritance in Man, 9th ed.: V.A. McKusick; The Johns Hopkins University Press, 1990, pp. 574–575, 1475, 1662.

Familial Partial Lipodystrophy: Two Types of an X-Linked Dominant Syndrome, Lethal in the Hemizygous State: J. Kobberling, et al.; J. Med. Genet., issue 23(2), pp. 120–127.

Lipolysis. Pitfalls and Problems in a Series of 1,246 Procedures: S. Cohen; Aesthetic Plast. Surg., issue 9(3), pp. 209–214.

Membranous Lipodystrophy (Nasu Disease). Clinical and Neuropathological Study of a Case: M. Minagawa, et al.; Clin. Neuropathol., issue 4(1), pp. 38–45.

Ultrastructural Abnormalities of the Liver in Total Lipodystrophy: A. Klar, et al.; Arch. Pathol. Lab. Med., issue 111(2), pp. 197–199.

McCune-Albright Syndrome

Description McCune-Albright syndrome is a multisystem disorder in which there is polyostotic fibrous dysplasia.

Synonyms

Albright Syndrome
Fibrous Dysplasia, Monostotic
Fibrous Dysplasia, Polyostotic
Osteitis Fibrosa Disseminata

Signs and Symptoms Abnormal growth of fibrous bone tissue may be increasingly painful and crippling. Any bone may be invaded, but the lesions most often occur in the extremities, pelvis, ribs, and the base of the skull. The patient is fracture-prone. Shortening of the limbs and other osseous deformities may develop. Patchy pigmentation with large, irregular café-au-lait spots may appear. Premature puberty may manifest as early as age 3 months and is more common in females than males. While menses occur early, it may be years before the breasts develop and axillary hair appears. Fertility in young patients is very rare, but in adults with McCune-Albright syndrome it is normal. Acromegaly or gigantism may result from pituitary hypersecretion of growth hormone **(GH)**.

Etiology McCune-Albright syndrome is idiopathic; a genetic inheritance has been suggested. Accelerated ovarian function due to hyperthyroidism or premature activation of the hypothalamic-pituitary-ovarian axis may explain the early puberty in females with the syndrome.

Epidemiology McCune-Albright syndrome can occur in either sex. Approximately 30 percent of patients, usually females, experience early puberty. Hundreds of cases of McCune-Albright syndrome have been described in the medical literature in the United States since Albright first recognized the disorder in 1937.

Related Disorders See *Acromegaly; Neurofibromatosis.*

Treatment—Standard Treatment is symptomatic and supportive. In some severe cases, thyroidectomy may be indicated to control persistent hyperthyroidism.

Treatment—Investigational Trials of the aromatase inhibitor testolactone, which blocks the synthesis of estrogens, are ongoing in the treatment of premature puberty in females with McCune-Albright syndrome. Cortical bone grafting has been investigated for treating fibrous dysplasia.

Please contact the agencies listed under Resources, below, for the most current information.

Resources

For more information on McCune-Albright syndrome: National Organization for Rare Disorders (NORD); The National Arthritis and Musculoskeletal and Skin Diseases Information Clearinghouse; International Center for Skeletal Dysplasia.

For genetic information and genetic counseling referrals: March of Dimes Birth Defects Foundation; National Center for Education in Maternal and Child Health (NCEMCH).

References

Fibrous Dysplasia of the Femoral Neck. Treatment by Cortical Bone Grafting: W.F. Enneking, et al.; J. Bone Joint Surg. [AM], December 1986, issue 68(9), pp. 1415–1422.

Neurofibromatosis and Albright's Sundrome: V.M. Ricciardi; Dermatol. Clin., January 1987, issue 5(1), pp. 193–203.

Treatment of Precocious Puberty in the McCune-Albright Syndrome with the Aromatase Inhibitor Testolactone: J.D. Malley, et al.; N. Engl. J. Med., October 1986, issue 315(18), pp. 1115–1119.

NELSON SYNDROME

Description Nelson syndrome is marked by abnormal hormone secretion and an enlarged pituitary gland.

Synonyms

Pituitary Tumor after Adrenalectomy

Signs and Symptoms Symptoms are hyperpigmentation, headaches, visual field disturbances, and, in females, amenorrhea. The pituitary gland is enlarged, leading to the headaches and causing visceral symptoms. Laboratory tests reveal elevated levels of ACTH and beta-melanocyte–stimulating hormone (**beta-MSH**).

Etiology Nelson syndrome can develop following bilateral adrenalectomy as treatment for Cushing syndrome. Growth of a preexisting or an occult pituitary may also be responsible.

Epidemiology Nelson syndrome occurs in approximately 5 to 10 percent of patients following bilateral adrenalectomy. In contrast, tumor-induced Nelson syndrome is rare. Males and females are affected in equal numbers.

Treatment—Standard Irradiation is used to halt abnormal pituitary growth. If the gland presses on an area of brain structure, surgical removal is indicated.

Treatment—Investigational Microsurgical removal of ACTH adenomas, using the transphenoidal approach, is an experimental treatment for Nelson syndrome.

One study found that bromocriptine (a dopamine agonist) and cyproheptadine (a serotonin antagonist) caused a significant drop in plasma ACTH levels stimulated by corticotropin-releasing factor (**CRF**). After a longer course of cyproheptadine, however, plasma ACTH levels were again elevated. Consequently, the usefulness of the drug appears limited.

Please contact the agencies listed under Resources, below, for the most current information.

Resources

For more information on Nelson syndrome: National Organization for Rare Disorders (NORD); NIH/National Institute of Neurological Disorders & Stroke (NINDS).

References
Effects of Bromocriptine and Cyproheptadine on Basal and Corticotropin-Releasing Factor (CRF)-Induced ACTH Release in a Patient with Nelson's Syndrome: Y. Hirata, et al.; Endocrinol. Jpn., October 1984, issue 31(5), pp. 619–626.

Trans-Sphenoidal Microsurgical Treatment of Nelson's Syndrome: T. Fukushima; Neurosurg. Rev., 1985, issue 8(3-4), pp. 185–194.

PRECOCIOUS PUBERTY

Description True precocious puberty is the result of premature initiation of the function of the hypothalamic-pituitary axis. Premature release of the luteinizing hormone releasing hormone (**LHRH**) by the hypothalamus triggers secretion of the pituitary gonadatropin hormones. As a consequence, the gonads function at an inappropriately early age. Precocious puberty per se has many subdivisions: isosexual, heterosexual, gonadotropin-dependent (true precocious puberty), gonadotropin-independent, male-limited (familial testotoxicosis), cerebral, central, and idiopathic precocious puberty.

Synonyms

Familial Testotoxicosis
Gonadotropin-Independent Familial Sexual Precocity
Pubertas Praecox

Signs and Symptoms In females the breasts start to develop before age 8, or menarche occurs before age 10, and growth is rapid. In males, onset is before age 10; boys grow facial, axillary, and pubic hair; growth, including that of the penis, accelerates; the voice deepens; and behavior becomes aggressive. Puberty may take place before age 3 in some children.

Children with precocious puberty are taller than their peers. Since osseous maturity is usually hastened in precocious puberty, closure of the epiphyses occurs prematurely and patients are short in stature in adulthood.

In **isosexual precocious puberty**, feminizing signs appear in girls, masculinization in boys.

Heterosexual precocious puberty causes signs of virilization in girls and feminization in boys.

Cerebral precocious puberty differs in cause but mimics true precocious puberty.

Central precocious puberty is attended by changes that concern the central nervous system.

Gonadotropin-dependent precocious puberty is marked by high gonadotropin levels in girls. Girls with McCune-Albright syndrome may have this type of precocious puberty.

Gonadotropin-independent precocious puberty usually affects boys, who have low levels of gonadotropin. Girls with McCune-Albright syndrome may have this form of precocious puberty.

Idiopathic precocious puberty is associated with EEG irregularities in girls. The cause of the unusual brain waves is unclear.

Etiology Usually precocious puberty is idiopathic. In some instances, it is due to an endocrine disorder. **Cerebral precocious puberty** is associated with a brain abnormality. **Male-limited precocious puberty (familial testotoxicosis)** is considered hereditary, either X-linked autosomal dominant or X-linked recessive.

Among the uncommon underlying disorders in girls are hypothalamic neoplasm, neurofibromatosis, congenital brain lesions, postinfectious encephalitis, hydrocephalus, and craniopharyngiomas. Very rare causes are oral contraceptives, other estrogen-containing drugs, or meat with a high estrogen content. Primary hypothyroidism and McCune-Albright syndrome often accompany precocious puberty.

Other considerations are hormone-secreting ovarian or adrenal neoplasms. Possibly the most frequently seen sex steroid-secreting tumors among girls with precocious puberty are estrogen-secreting ovarian granulosa-thecal cell tumors. Some girls may have benign ovarian cysts.

Epidemiology The incidence of precocious puberty in girls is approximately twice that in boys. Approximately 80 percent of the cases in girls are idiopathic, but disease underlies 60 percent of the cases in boys.

Related Disorders See *McCune-Albright Syndrome; Adrenal Hyperplasia, Congenital; Neurofibromatosis.*

Pseudo-precocious puberty is associated with high steroid concentrations. Such levels are present because of cortocosteroid therapy, hormone-producing tumors (usually ovarian or testicular), or adrenal disorders that cause hormonal hypersecretion. Sexual development and maturity may appear normal, but ovulation or spermatogenesis may not occur because of gonadal immaturity.

Adrenogenital syndrome comprises a group of conditions due to adrenocortical hyperplasia or glandular malignancy. Virilization of women or precocious puberty in boys are hallmarks. Hypersecretions or abnormal secretions of adrenocortical steroids are present.

Treatment—Standard Therapy depends upon the cause of precocious puberty. Glucocorticoid suppression of ACTH is indicated for girls with **heterosexual precocious puberty** due to congenital adrenal hyperplasia. Girls with **precocious puberty** and **McCune-Albright syndrome** respond to the aromatase-inhibitor testolactone, a blocker of estrogen synthesis. Some hypothalamic lesions and ovarian tumors or cysts can be excised. Once identified, exogenous hormones can be eliminated. Replacement therapy with levothyroxine is indicated for girls with **precocious puberty caused by primary hypothyroidism,** in whom closure of the epiphyses is late.

Genetic counseling is recommended for families of patients with **male-limited precocious puberty** and other hereditary types of this disorder.

Treatment—Investigational A course of at least 6 months of a combination of spironolactone and testolactone has been used experimentally in males with **isosexual precocious puberty.** These patients have abnormally rapid growth, and the goal of drug therapy is to restore the rates of growth and maturation to normal prepubertal levels.

For girls with **gonadotropin-dependent precocious puberty,** intranasal administration of the hormone-suppressing drug nafarelin acetate may be useful but is not yet approved.

For children with **central precocious puberty** an orphan drug, deslorelin (Somagard), manufactured by Roberts Laboratories, Inc., is available.

Please contact the agencies listed under Resources, below, for the most current information.

Resources

For more information on precocious puberty: National Organization for Rare Disorders (NORD); NIH/National Institute of Child Health & Human Development (NICHHD); Brain and Pituitary Foundation of America.

For genetic information and genetic counseling referrals: March of Dimes Birth Defects Foundation; National Center for Education in Maternal and Child Health (NCEMCH).

900 | ENDOCRINE DISORDERS

References

CT of Cerebral Abnormalities in Precocious Puberty: K.G. Rieth, et al.; AJR, June 1987, issue 148(6), pp. 1231–1238.

Intranasal Nafarelin: An LH-RH Analogue Treatment of Gonadotropin-Precocious Puberty: T.H. Lin, et al.; J. Pediatr., December 1986, issue 109(6), pp. 954–958.

Treatment of Precocious Puberty in the McCune-Albright Syndrome with the Aromatase Inhibitor Testolactone: P.P. Feuillan, et al.; N. Engl. J. Med., October 30, 1986, issue 315(18), pp. 1115–1119.

The Treatment of Familial Male Precocious Puberty with Spironolactone and Testolactone: L. Laue, et al.; N. Engl. J. Med., February 23, 1989, issue 320(8), pp. 496–502.

RICKETS, VITAMIN D-DEFICIENCY

Description Vitamin D-deficiency rickets, which appears during infancy and childhood, is characterized primarily by bone disease, restlessness, and retarded growth. Vitamin D is needed for the metabolism of calcium and phosphorus, which in turn affects deposition of calcium in the bones.

Synonyms
Nutritional Rickets
Rickets

Signs and Symptoms Symptoms include restlessness and lack of sleep. Growth is slowed, and there is a delay in crawling, sitting, or walking. The skull is thin at the top and back (craniotabes), there is bossing, and fontanelle closure is delayed. Beading occurs where the ribs and their cartilages join (rachitic rosary).

If the disorder is not treated, the ends of the long bones may become enlarged, the legs may become bowed, and knock-knees may result. Muscles can become weak and the chest may become deformed due to the pull of the diaphragm on the ribs weakened by rickets (Harrison's groove). Abnormal development and decay of teeth may also occur.

In more severe, untreated cases of this disorder the bones may become fragile, and fractures easily occur. Convulsions, muscle twitching, and tetany spasms of the wrist and ankle joints may also be present. Occasionally, when hypocalcemia is present because of the lack of vitamin D, mental retardation may develop.

Etiology The vitamin deficiency can be caused by poor nutrition, a lack of exposure to the sun, or intestinal malabsorption syndromes.

Epidemiology Males and females are affected in equal numbers. Babies of nursing mothers themselves deficient in vitamin D can be affected.

The disorder is rare in the United States but not uncommon in certain areas of the world. However, in the United States, children who are dark-skinned and living in cloudy northern cities, as well as children on restricted diets due to cultural or religious beliefs, are more likely to develop vitamin D-deficiency rickets.

In areas of the world where cultural habits curtail exposure to sun, or the amount of sun in a day or season is otherwise limited, the disorder tends to be more prevalent. Northern Yemen and Kuwait are areas of prevalence. Rickets is also more common in regions of Asia where there is not only limited exposure to the sun, but also low intake of meat due to a vegetarian diet.

Related Disorders See *Lowe Syndrome.*

Fanconi syndrome is a rare disorder characterized by kidney dysfunction and bone abnormalities similar to those of vitamin D-deficiency rickets. Excess amounts of phosphate, amino acids (usually bicarbonate), glucose, and uric acid are eliminated in the urine. Bone symptoms include rickets in children and osteomalacia in adults. Fanconi syndrome is thought to be inherited through recessive genes. The syndrome may be associated with a variety of inherited metabolic disorders (see *Cystinosis; Tyrosinemia I; Fructose Intolerance, Hereditary; Wilson Disease; Galactosemia).* Glycogen storage disorders are also associated.

Infantile scurvy is caused by a lack of vitamin C in the diet. Symptoms include anemia, irritability, anorexia, weakness, failure to gain weight, oral lesions, loosening of the teeth, and bleeding under the tissue layer covering the bones. Scurvy is treated with large amounts of vitamin C.

Osteomalacia is characterized by a gradual softening and bending of the bones. Pain may be present in varying degrees of severity. Softening occurs because solid bones have failed to calcify as a result of a kidney dysfunction or the lack of vitamin D. The disorder is more common in females than males, and often begins during pregnancy. It can exist alone or in association with other disorders.

Hypophosphatemic rickets, a rare genetic form of rickets, is characterized by impaired transport of phosphate and diminished vitamin D metabolism in the kidneys. Calcium and phosphate are not absorbed properly in the intestines, which can lead to softening of bones. Major symptoms of this disorder include skeletal changes, weakness, and slow growth. Cases affecting females are usually less severe than those affecting males. One rare acquired form of this disorder may be associated with a benign tumor.

Pseudo–vitamin D-deficiency rickets (vitamin D-dependent rickets, Type I) is characterized by more severe skeletal changes and weakness than those of hypophosphatemic rickets. The disorder is inherited as an autosomal recessive trait, and is caused by abnormal vitamin D metabolism. This type of rickets often begins earlier than hypophosphatemic rickets. Hypocalcemia is severe, and there is aminoaciduria. Intermittent muscle cramps and convulsions may occur. Abnormalities of the spine and pelvis may also develop.

Treatment—Standard The disorder can be prevented by providing a normal balanced diet to infants and children, assuming that they are exposed to adequate amounts of sun.

Treatment is accomplished with doses of vitamin D given daily until the bone disease is cured. The dose can then be reduced to the daily recommended requirement.

In more severe cases when cramps, convulsions, muscle twitching, and tetany of the ankle and wrist joints are present, the treatment with vitamin D is supplemented with intravenous calcium salts.

Treatment—Investigational Please contact the agencies listed under Resources,

below, for the most current information.

Resources

For more information on vitamin D-deficiency rickets: National Organization for Rare Disorders (NORD); NIH/National Institute of Diabetes, Digestive and Kidney Diseases Information Clearinghouse; NIH/National Center for Education in Maternal and Child Health (NCEMCH).

References
Internal Medicine, 2nd ed.: J.H. Stein, ed.-in-chief; Little, Brown and Company, 1987, pp. 2106–2112.

The Merck Manual, 15th ed.: R. Berkow, ed.-in-chief; Merck Sharp & Dohme Research Laboratories, 1987, pp. 924–927.

Nutritional Rickets: K.W. Feldman, et al.; Am. Fam. Physicians, November 1990, issue 42(5), pp. 1311–1318.

High Prevalence of Rickets in Infants on Macrobiotic Diets: P.C. Dagnelie, et al.; Am. J. Clin. Nutr., February 1990, issue 51(2), pp. 202–208.

Nutritional Rickets in San Diego: I. Hayward, et al.; Am. J. Dis. Child, October 1987, issue 141(10), pp. 1060–1062.

Vitamin D Deficiency Rickets: D.M. Kruger, et al.; Clin. Orthop., November 1987, issue 224, pp. 277–283.

Photosynthesis of Vitamin D in the Skin: Effect of Environmental and Lifestyle Variables: M.F. Holick; Fed. Proc., April 1987, issue 46(5), pp. 1876–1882.

The Importance of Limited Exposure to Ultraviolet Radiation and Dietary Factors in the Etiology of Asian Rickets: A Risk-Factor Model: J.B. Henderson, et al.; Q. J. Med., May 1987, issue 63(241), pp. 413–425.

High Levels of Childhood Rickets in Rural North Yemen: P. Underwood, et al.; Soc. Sci. Med., 1987, issue 24(1), pp. 37–41.

Vitamin D-Deficiency Rickets in Kuwait: The Prevalence of a Preventable Disease: M.M. Lubani, et al.; Ann. Trop. Paediatr., September 1989, issue 9(3), pp. 134–139.

Osteomalacia of the Mother–Rickets of the Newborn: W. Park, et al.; Eur. J. Pediatr., May 1987, issue 146(3), pp. 292–293.

SHEEHAN SYNDROME

Description Sheehan syndrome is characterized by hypopituitarism associated with profound blood loss during and after childbirth, and consequent postpartum collapse.

Synonyms
Postpartum Hypopituitarism
Postpartum Panhypopituitarism
Postpartum Pituitary Necrosis
Simmond Disease

Signs and Symptoms The varying manifestations of Sheehan syndrome depend on the degree of hypopituitarism. The signs and symptoms correlate with the extent of the deficiency of prolactin, gonadotropins, thyroid-stimulating hormone (**TSH**), adrenocorticotropin (**ACTH**), and growth hormone (**GH**).

The fullblown condition is associated with evidence of deficient gonadotropins:

postpartum failure of lactation, amenorrhea, absence of regrowth of pubic hair, and slowly vanishing axillary hair. Breasts and genitalia atrophy.

The hallmarks of hypothyroidism, triggered by deficient TSH, usually appear gradually; myxedema, for example, may not become apparent for years or decades.

Hypoglycemia may develop in association with GH deficiency, perhaps aided by a lack of cortisol; GH deficiency is associated with increased insulin-sensitivity, some loss of muscle strength, and mild anemia.

ACTH deficiency's manifestations are chronic hypotension with fainting and proneness to infection, even from cuts and abrasions. These features usually become apparent weeks or months postpartum.

Etiology Severe arteriolar spasm in the vessels supplying the hypothalamus, occurring in shock, is considered to be the cause of Sheehan syndrome. Spasm leads to anterior pituitary ischemia. The amount of cellular damage correlates with the severity and duration of arteriolar spasm.

Epidemiology Sheehan syndrome affects women with postpartum hemorrhage and circulatory collapse.

Treatment—Standard Hormonal replacement therapy (i.e., ovarian, thyroid, and adrenocortical hormones) is indicated. The usual partial ACTH deficiency may not require continuing cortisol replacement therapy except during times of stress.

Treatment—Investigational Please contact the agencies listed under Resources, below, for the most current information.

Resources

For more information on Sheehan syndrome: National Organization for Rare Disorders (NORD); National Institute of Diabetes, Digestive and Kidney Diseases Information Clearinghouse.

STEIN-LEVENTHAL SYNDROME

Description Stein-Leventhal syndrome is characterized by amenorrhea or abnormal menses, hirsutism, obesity, and infertility.

Synonyms
> Bilateral Polycystic Ovarian Syndrome
> Ovarian Hyperthecosis
> Polycystic Bilateral Ovarian Syndrome
> Sclerocystic Ovarian Disease

Signs and Symptoms Initial symptoms usually occur soon after puberty and before age 20. If the menses have been normal, they become irregular and gradually lessen over several months until they stop. Sometimes heavy flow intervenes during stretches of amenorrhea.

Infertility or the growth of facial hair often brings the patient to the physician's office. Signs of virilization include voice changes and male-pattern hirsutism. Obesity is often present. The ovaries become polycystic and may increase in size. Frequently the uterus is undersized. The patient is anovulatory.

Etiology The cause of Stein-Leventhal syndrome is unclear. Generally, the irregularities are attributed to the hypothalamic-pituitary-ovarian axis. Occasionally, an androgen-producing ovarian tumor is responsible.

Epidemiology Stein-Leventhal syndrome occurs in young women.

Treatment—Standard For the woman who desires pregnancy, clomiphene will often produce ovulation and normal menstruation. Pregnancy occurs in about 50 percent of treated patients. If clomiphene does not produce the desired effects, gonadotropins are a 2nd choice. If neither treatment is effective, ovarian wedge resection, or removal of the cystic portions of the ovaries, can be performed. Recurrence is common, however.

Treatment with low-dosage oral contraceptives or long-acting progestins, such as medroxyprogesterone, is indicated even when pregnancy is not a goal; it is important to suppress ovarian hormone production. Otherwise irregular bleeding may be distressing. Furthermore, endometrial changes can trigger the development of premalignant or malignant disorders. Ovarian hormone production can be fully suppressed with low-dosage oral contraceptives or long-acting progestins, such as medroxyprogesterone.

Treatment—Investigational Please contact the agencies listed under Resources, below, for the most current information.

Resources
    For more information on Stein-Leventhal syndrome: National Organization for Rare Disorders (NORD); NIH/National Institute of Child Health and Human Development (NICHHD).

References
    Cecil Textbook of Medicine, 18th ed.: J.B. Wyngaarden and L.H. Smith, Jr., eds.; W.B. Saunders Company, 1988, p. 1287.

ZOLLINGER-ELLISON SYNDROME

Description Zollinger-Ellison syndrome is associated with refractory peptic ulcers, marked gastric hyperacidity, and, usually, small gastrin-secreting tumors (gastrinomas). Benign or malignant tumors develop most often in the pancreas but are also found in the stomach, duodenum, mesentery, or spleen, or the abdominal lymph nodes.

Synonyms
    Gastrinoma
    Multiple Endocrine Neoplasia, Type I
    Pancreatic Ulcerogenic Tumor Syndrome
    Partial Multiple Endocrine Adenomatosis

Signs and Symptoms Exquisite pain from ulcers in the stomach, duodenum, jejunum, and/or esophagus is likely, and diarrhea and steatorrhea are often present. The ulcers may be refractory to any type of treatment for years, during which time the serum potassium remains low. Life-threatening complications, such as obstruction, perforations, and bleeding may occur. About 40 percent of patients have tumors, and approximately 50 percent of these are malignant.

Etiology Since 1982, 2 forms of Zollinger-Ellison syndrome have been recognized: sporadic and autosomal dominant; there may be other as yet unidentified forms. Onset of the sporadic type is usually in the mature years. The autosomal dominant type is a symptom of **multiple endocrine adenomatosis.** The cause of the tumors associated with Zollinger-Ellison syndrome is unknown.

Epidemiology Onset of Zollinger-Ellison syndrome may be during the childhood years, but the time of diagnosis is most often between ages 20 to 70. Males and females are affected in equal numbers.

Related Disorders Endocrinopathy, such as **hyperparathyroidism** and **adrenal** or **pituitary adenomas** may be associated with the syndrome.

Duodenal ulcers have a high incidence. Their development may stem from a familial proneness, or a course of corticosteroids may be the trigger. Other potential factors are cirrhosis of the liver, chronic pancreatitis, cystic fibrosis, or pulmonary emphysema.

See *Cushing Syndrome.*

Treatment—Standard Control of gastric acid secretion with antacids and drugs such as cimetidine and ranitidine, with or without anticholinergic agents, has replaced gastrectomy as treatment for most patients. Higher-than-routine doses are often required. In 1989, omeprazole was approved for the treatment of Zollinger-Ellison syndrome and other severe gastric conditions. The rate of efficacy is rising, an effect of the success of imaging procedures that pinpoint the tumor site. Surgical removal in conjunction with chemotherapy may be beneficial for some patients. Genetic counseling may be helpful.

Treatment—Investigational New diagnostic tests are being developed, such as transhepatic pancreatic vein catheterization supplemented by the determination of local hormone gradients. This may permit preoperative location of even the smallest tumors; the current success rate for tumor surgery is 20 percent. Severing the vagus nerve is under investigation to interrupt the stimulation of acid-secreting tissue. Patients who require very high doses of standard drugs may be candidates for this surgery.

Please contact the agencies listed under Resources, below, for the most current information.

Resources

For more information on **Zollinger-Ellison syndrome:** National Organization for Rare Disorders (NORD); National Digestive Diseases Information Clearinghouse.

For **genetic information and genetic counseling referrals:** March of

Dimes Birth Defects Foundation; National Center for Education in Maternal and Child Health (NCEMCH).

References

Current Management of Zollinger-Ellison Syndrome: R.T. Jensen, et. al.; Drugs, August 1986, issue 32(2), pp. 188–196.
Diagnosis and Curative Therapy in Zollinger-Ellison Syndrome: W.H. Hacki; Schweiz. Med. Wochenschr., April 1985, issue 115(17), pp. 575–581.
Zollinger-Ellison Syndrome: H.D. Becker; Wien. Klin. Wochenschr., February 1984, issue 96(4), pp. 138–144.

11 | ARTHRITIS AND CONNECTIVE TISSUE DISEASES
Marc C. Hochberg, M.D., M.P.H.

Arthritis and other diseases of the musculoskeletal system, including the diffuse connective tissue diseases, comprise the most common cause of disability in the adult civilian population of the United States. They are the leading cause of mobility limitation and the second-leading cause of activity limitation among adults ages 18 and above. It is recognized that over 100 diseases can cause arthritis. An overview of the classification of the rheumatic diseases, as suggested by the Arthritis Foundation, is listed in Table 11.1.

Table 11.1. Classification of the rheumatic diseases

   I. Osteoarthritis

  II. Diffuse connective tissue diseases

 III. Seronegative spondyloarthropathies

 IV. Infectious arthritis

  V. Arthritis associated with metabolic and/or endocrine disorders

 VI. Primary bone and cartilage disorders

VII. Arthritis associated with neuropathic disorders

VIII. Neoplasms of bones and joints

 IX. Nonarticular rheumatism

  X. Miscellaneous conditions

Modified from Primer on the Rheumatic Diseases, 9th ed.: H.R. Schumacher, Jr., J.H. Klippel, and D.R. Robinson, eds.; Arthritis Foundation, 1988. Used with permission.

Diseases associated with arthritis generally present in one of three major fashions: 1) arthritis alone; 2) arthritis as the dominant clinical finding but with extraarticular lesions; or 3) arthritis as one part of a diffuse multisystem disease. The individual conditions covered in this chapter were selected as representing four major groups of "less common" arthritis and musculoskeletal diseases: the seronegative spondyloarthropathies, to be distinguished from rheumatoid arthritis (Table 11.2); the diffuse connective tissue diseases (Table 11.3); the vasculitides and related syndromes (Table 11.4); and miscellaneous orthopedic conditions producing localized musculoskeletal pain and dysfunction.

Table 11.2.
Classification of seronegative spondyloarthropathies

Ankylosing spondylitis

Reiter's syndrome

Psoriatic arthritis

Arthritis associated with inflammatory bowel disease

The first step in evaluating the patient who presents with a musculoskeletal or rheumatic complaint is the thorough history and physical examination. Most of the rheumatic diseases are more common in females than males, except for ankylosing spondylitis, Reiter's syndrome, gout, and polyarteritis nodosa. The age of the patient is also helpful. Occurrence of the rheumatic diseases can largely be subdivided into those which affect young patients (up to age 40 years), such as ankylosing spondylitis, Reiter's syndrome, gonococcal arthritis, and systemic lupus erythematosus; those which affect middle-aged patients (between 40 and 65 years), such as gout, rheumatoid arthritis, and the diffuse connective tissue diseases; and those affecting elderly patients (65 years and older), such as polymyalgia rheumatica, giant-cell arteritis, osteoarthritis, and pseudogout (calcium pyrophospate dihydrate crystal deposition disease).

It is important to identify the type and pattern of joint involvement: whether 1) the arthritis is inflammatory (accompanied by warmth, erythema, and soft tissue swelling) or noninflammatory; 2) the course has been episodic or persistent; 3) the number of joints involved is oligoarticular (fewer than five joints) or polyarticular (five or more joints); 4)

Table 11.3. Classification of diffuse connective tissue diseases

Systemic lupus erythematosus

Scleroderma (systemic sclerosis)

Polymyositis/dermatomyositis

Sjögren's syndrome

Mixed connective tissue disease

Systemic necrotizing vasculitis

the pattern of involvement has been migratory or additive; 5) the distribution of involvement is bilateral and symmetric or asymmetric; and 6) the axial skeleton, including the sacroiliac joints, is involved or uninvolved.

After a detailed review of the musculoskeletal symptoms and signs, the presence of extraarticular features and systemic manifestations must be determined. A thorough examination of the skin, eyes, blood vessels, and cardiopulmonary systems, in particular, should be performed to evaluate for evidence of multisystem involvement. The absence of such manifestations would suggest that the patient has a primarily arthritic disease; in contrast, the dominance of such manifestations would suggest the presence of a multisystem disease, particularly a diffuse connective tissue disease or systemic vasculitis.

Laboratory testing usually serves to confirm the clinical diagnosis arrived at by the above process. In patients with arthritis, sampling of synovial fluid may be diagnostic in the presence of infection or microcrystalline disease (either gout or pseudogout), and helpful in distin-

Table 11.4. Classification of systemic vasculitides

Polyarteritis nodosa

Wegener granulomatosis

Giant-cell arteritis

Takayasu's arteritis

Kawasaki syndrome

Behçet's syndrome

Beurger's disease

Relapsing polychondritis

guishing inflammatory from noninflammatory causes of arthritis. Routine hematologic tests are usually nonspecific; however, elevation of the erythrocyte sedimentation rate (ESR) indicates the presence of a systemic inflammatory process. In patients with an ESR above 100 mm/hr, the physician should consider the diagnoses of polymyalgia rheumatica and/or giant-cell arteritis, when appropriate, or conduct a further evaluation for abnormal serum proteins (multiple myeloma, macroglobulinemia), occult infection, and occult malignancy.

Serologic testing is often performed in patients with arthritis and musculoskeletal diseases. Positive tests for rheumatoid factor and antinuclear antibodies are highly sensitive for the diagnosis of rheumatoid arthritis and the presence of a diffuse connective tissue disease, respectively. However, it must be noted that both rheumatoid factor and antinuclear antibodies are present in up to 5 percent of normals, and up to 15 percent of elderly patients aged 65 and above. Therefore, the presence of these autoantibodies alone does not make a diagnosis; the diagnosis rests on the clinical presentation, which is confirmed by results of serologic testing.

In patients suspected of having a diffuse connective tissue disease, it is appropriate to characterize the positive test for antinuclear antibodies by obtaining tests for antibodies to double-stranded deoxyribonucleic acid (DNA), and extractable nuclear antigens, including nuclear ribonucleoprotein (nRNP), Sm, Ro, La, and in individuals suspected of having scleroderma, Scl-70. The presence of antibodies to double-stranded DNA and/or Sm is highly specific for a diagnosis of systemic lupus erythematosus. The presence of antibodies to nRNP is seen in patients with several connective tissue diseases, including systemic lupus erythematosus, scleroderma, and the overlap syndrome, mixed connective tissue disease. The presence of antibodies to Ro and La is seen in patients with systemic lupus erythematosus and Sjögren's syndrome. It is important that these tests be performed in reliable clinical laboratories; "false positive" tests can result in incorrect diagnostic labeling and inappropriate therapies.

Finally, because the diseases discussed in this chapter are rare, it is entirely appropriate for the primary care physician to seek consultation with a specialist, usually a rheumatologist, for a diagnostic evaluation including recommendations for medical management. Listings of rheumatologists by geographic area are available through the local chapters of the Arthritis Foundation and the American College of Rheumatology. In instances of rare orthopedic conditions producing localized musculoskeletal pain and dysfunction, consultation with an orthopedic surgeon is appropriate. It is hoped that increased awareness of the rare musculoskeletal and connective tissue diseases by the primary care physician, coupled with timely referral for subspecialty consultation, will lead to improved diagnosis, management, and outcomes for patients with these conditions.

In addition to using this resource, readers are encouraged to obtain their individual copies of the *Primer on the Rheumatic Diseases* through their local chapters of the Arthritis Foundation; this soft-cover volume provides a concise yet thorough description of the rheumatic diseases, focusing on clinical presentation, diagnosis, and management. Additional patient education materials are also readily available through local chapters of the Arthritis Foundation.

ARTHRITIS AND CONNECTIVE TISSUE DISEASES
Listings in This Section

AMYLOIDOSIS

Description Amyloidosis is the term applied to a group of metabolic disorders in which the fibrillar protein amyloid accumulates in tissue, to the extent that the function of affected organs is impaired. The accumulation may be localized, general, or systemic. Various imperfect systems are used for classifying amyloidosis. The most widely used is based on the chemistry of the fibrils.

The most common form of amyloidosis is **AL** or light-chain-related **(primary** amyloidosis). This form of the disease may occur independently of other disease, or in the presence of multiple myeloma. The tongue, thyroid gland, intestinal tract, liver, and spleen are typically affected. Cardiac involvement may result in congestive heart failure.

AA amyloidosis **(secondary** amyloidosis) is most often discovered during the course of chronic inflammatory disease, such as rheumatoid arthritis, chronic infections, and familial Mediterranean fever. Kidneys, liver, and spleen are commonly impaired by AA amyloidosis, but the adrenal glands, lymph nodes, and vascular system may be affected as well. In addition, the skin inflammation that occurs with recurrent injections seems to induce AA amyloidosis. Nephrotic syndrome and renal failure cause the most fatalities in this category. AA amyloidosis is reported in approximately one percent of cases of chronic inflammatory disease in the United States.

The amyloidosis of **aging** is observed in the heart, and, sometimes, the pancreas and brain.

Hemodialysis-associated amyloidosis is seen in patients who have experienced longterm hemodialysis.

Familial amyloidosis is found in a series of genetically transmitted diseases that typically affect the kidney, heart, skin, and other areas of the body.

Signs and Symptoms Manifestations are nonspecific. Generally, involved organs become rubbery and firm, with waxy appearance. Often they are enlarged. Biopsy is necessary for diagnosis.

Kidneys: The nephrotic syndrome is usually accompanied by proteinuria, which worsens as the disease progresses and may finally result in renal failure. The kidney becomes small, pale, and hard. Renal tubular defects, renal vein thrombosis, and hypertension may also be noted. Amyloid may accumulate in other parts of the urogenital system, such as the bladder or ureter.

Liver and spleen: Hepato- and splenomegaly are the most notable signs. The function of the liver is significantly affected only late in the course of the disease, although elevated alkaline phosphatase and other liver function abnormalities may be detected earlier. Occurrence in the spleen increases the risk of traumatic rupture.

Heart: Cardiac involvement occurs frequently and is reflected in cardiomegaly, arrhythmias, murmurs, electrocardiogram abnormalities, and, particularly, congestive failure. Nodular deposits of amyloid may be present on pericardial and endocardial surfaces, and valvular lesions may be noted.

Gastrointestinal system: Symptoms may be similar to those of gastric carcinoma and frequently develop in association with chronic diseases, including tuberculosis and granulomatous ileitis. Amyloid accumulation in the GI tract may cause motility abnormalities in the esophagus and small and large intestines. Malabsorption, ulceration, bleeding, gastric atony, pseudo-obstruction, protein loss, and diarrhea may also be noted. Infiltration of the tongue may cause macroglossia.

Skin: Microscopic or macroscopic dermal involvement occurs in at least half of primary and secondary amyloidosis cases, and in all cases of amyloid neuropathy. Waxy-looking papules appear on the face and neck; in axillary, anal, and inguinal regions; and in mucosal areas such as the ear canal or tongue. Areas of swelling, purpura, alopecia, glossitis, and xerostomia are also found.

Nervous system: Neurologic manifestations often appear in hereditary amyloidoses, and those associated with multiple myeloma. Peripheral neuropathy may be present, as well as hypohidrosis, postural hypotension, Adie's syndrome (tonic pupil), hoarseness, sphincter dysfunction, and an increase in the concentration of cerebrospinal fluid protein.

Respiratory system: Pulmonary symptoms often parallel cardiac symptoms. Air passages and ducts may be obstructed by accumulations of amyloid in the nasal sinuses, larynx, and trachea.

Other: Amyloid arthropathy, which occurs in 6 to 15 percent of multiple myeloma cases, may involve articular cartilage or the synovial membrane and fluid. Symptoms are similar to those of rheumatoid arthritis. Amyloid deposits in muscle tissue may cause pseudomyopathy. Results of hematologic involvement may include fibrinogenopenia, increased fibrinolysis, and deficiency of certain clotting factors.

Etiology Little is known about the etiology, although it appears that the various forms of amyloidosis result from different causes. Secondary amyloidosis apparently results from excessive antigenic stimuli that accompany chronic inflammatory or infectious disease. Hereditary amyloidosis is thought to be autosomal dominant, except when associated with familial Mediterranean fever, which seems to be autosomal recessive.

Treatment—Standard No uniformly effective treatment has been found to cure the disease or reverse amyloid deposition. In secondary amyloidosis, treatment of the underlying disease may control the disease adequately, if begun in time. In addition, chronic colchicine therapy appears to improve survival. Patients with AL amyloidosis, whether they have myeloma or not, may benefit from myeloma-like protocols.

Patients with cardiac involvement may experience increased sensitivity to digitalis drugs, which should therefore be used only with extreme caution.

In cases with severe renal involvement, dialysis or kidney transplantation may be necessary. Transplantation has been successful for several patients. It is thought, however, that amyloidosis will eventually recur in the transplanted kidney.

Localized amyloid tumors may be surgically removed, generally without further complications or recurrence.

The most successful treatment has been the preventive use of colchicine in patients with familial Mediterranean fever.

Treatment—Investigational Alpha-interferon is being evaluated as a treatment and trials are being conducted using colchicine in patients with AL and AA amyloidosis.

Please contact the agencies listed under Resources, below, for the most current information.

Resources

For more information on amyloidosis: National Organization for Rare Disorders (NORD); National Institute of Diabetes, Digestive & Kidney Diseases Information Clearinghouse.

For genetic information and genetic counseling referrals: March of Dimes Birth Defects Foundation; National Center for Education in Maternal and Child Health (NCEMCH).

References

Arthritis and Allied Conditions, 11th ed.: D.J. McCarty; Lea & Febiger, 1989, pp. 1273–1293.
Cecil Textbook of Medicine, 18th ed.: J.B. Wyngaarden and L.H. Smith, Jr., eds.; W.B. Saunders Company, 1988, pp. 359–360, 1198–1203.

ANKYLOSING SPONDYLITIS

Description Ankylosing spondylitis is an inflammatory arthritis affecting the sacroiliac joints, spine, and paraspinal structures.

Synonyms

Bekhterev-Strümpell Syndrome
Marie-Strümpell Disease
Spondyloarthritis

Signs and Symptoms Back pain and postures assumed in response to the arthritic vertebrae are frequent features. The pain often is worst after periods of rest and in the night, is associated with morning stiffness and gel phenomenon, and improves with exercise and use of heat.

Muscle spasm early in the course of the disease and ankylosis as the disease progresses may prevent normal flexion of the spine during bending. The advanced disease may cause immobility of the entire spine, resulting in a straight "poker spine." X-rays show sacroiliitis and may also show spinal involvement with syndesmophyte formation and fusion of apophyseal joints.

Symptoms involving peripheral joints, including hips and shoulders, are the first to appear in 20 percent of cases. Neck movement may become limited.

About one-third of patients develop iritis. Respiratory capacity may be decreased as a result of the fixed position of the chest cage due to costovertebral joint involvement. Neurologic complications include incontinence and absence of ankle jerks due to compression of the cauda equina. In fewer than 10 percent of cases, the heart is involved, causing heartblock, arrhythmias, and/or aortic insufficiency after longstanding disease.

Etiology Though the cause of ankylosing spondylitis is unknown, familial clustering and the association with HLA-B27 strongly indicate a genetic basis. Evidence suggests that the disease occurs when a genetically predisposed person is affected by a bacterium, virus, or other environmental factor, not yet identified.

Epidemiology Ankylosing spondylitis usually begins between the ages of 20 and 40. The disorder occurs more often among whites than blacks and is at least 3 times more common in men than in women, who usually experience milder symptoms.

Related Disorders See *Psoriatic Arthritis; Reiter's Syndrome.*

Treatment—Standard Most patients respond well to medications given to reduce pain and inflammation, combined with exercises to improve posture and strengthen muscle groups to counteract potential deformity. This is particularly true for patients who contract ankylosing spondylitis early in life and for whom treatment begins early in the course of the disease.

Nonsteroidal antiinflammatory drugs are effective in treating patients; the most effective appear to be indomethacin and related compounds. Other nonsteroidal antiinflammatory drugs may also be helpful. Narcotics and systemic corticosteroid are to be avoided.

Exercises should emphasize back movements, especially extension, straightening of the thoracic vertebrae, and deep breathing. The patient should get ample rest, sleeping on his or her back on a firm mattress with a flat pillow or none at all. Some persons benefit from back braces. Swimming is an excellent exercise.

Therapeutic measures usually eliminate the need for surgery to straighten the spine.

Treatment—Investigational Please contact the agencies listed under Resources, below, for the most current information.

Resources

For more information on ankylosing spondylitis: National Organization for Rare Disorders (NORD); Ankylosing Spondylitis Association; Arthritis Foundation; The National Arthritis and Musculoskeletal and Skin Diseases Information Clearinghouse.

References
Arthritis and Allied Conditions, 11th ed.: D.J. McCarty; Lea & Febiger, 1989, pp. 934–943.
Cecil Textbook of Medicine, 18th ed.: J.B. Wyngaarden and L.H. Smith, Jr., eds.; W.B. Saunders Company, 1988, pp. 1968, 2006–2007.

ARTERITIS, GIANT-CELL

Description Giant-cell arteritis is part of a generalized vascular disorder displaying granulomatous inflammation. The chronic inflammation is so frequently confined to the aortic arch branches, principally the temporal arteries, that it is designated as a distinct entity. The disorder is a panarteritis; the greatest changes show focal necrosis and granulomatous inflammation with giant cells. Any of the large arteries are susceptible. Venous involvement is extremely rare.

Synonyms
Cranial Arteritis
Granulomatous Arteritis
Temporal Arteritis

Signs and Symptoms Onset may either be acute or gradual, with flu-like symptoms such as low-grade fever and severe stiffness. A few patients experience respiratory tract symptoms including cough, sore throat, and hoarseness. Such manifestations may direct attention away from the underlying arteritis.

Headache is a common and early symptom. Severe throbbing and boring or stabbing temporal pain is often accompanied by redness, swelling, tenderness, pulsations, and knotting of the temporal artery. The scalp may be tender.

Frequent involvement of the temporal arteries results in ophthalmic and retinal vessel disease. Half the patients have visual symptoms, but only 10 percent experience visual loss. Early diagnosis and treatment are important in preventing permanent visual loss. The process may involve other vessels such as the coronary, carotid, subclavian, pulmonary, renal, and mesenteric arteries. The disorder has serious complications including a potential for cerebral vascular accident, coronary artery occlusion, and arterial insufficiency of the extremities, as well as blindness. Angiograms show smooth, tapered arterial occlusions or stenosis.

Polymyalgia rheumatica involving the trunk, neck, shoulders, and hips accompanied by synovitis, especially of the knees, is common.

Etiology The cause is unknown. A genetic predisposition has been suggested. The immune system has been implicated in recent data, but a causal relationship has not been established.

Epidemiology Incidence is approximately 24:100,000 persons aged 50 and above. The disease develops from age 50 to age 90 years, with average onset at about 70 years. Women are affected twice as often as men. Whites are affected more often than blacks or other ethnic/racial groups.

Related Disorders See *Polymyalgia Rheumatica.*

Treatment—Standard As soon as diagnosis is suspected, treatment should begin in order to avoid serious complications such as coronary occlusion and blindness. High doses of corticosteroids (60 to 80 mg/day) control initial local and systemic symptoms. Prednisone may be given in large doses until symptoms cease and laboratory findings (elevated erythrocyte sedimentation rate) return to normal. This process usually lasts for 2 to 4 weeks. Initial therapy is followed by giving a gradually reduced dosage (about 10 percent per month) for 2 years or longer to prevent recurrence. The disease is monitored by checking the sedimentation rate. A rise in the rate along with temporal or polymyalgia symptoms heralds a return of the illness.

Treatment—Investigational Please contact the agencies listed under Resources, below, for the most current information.

Resources
   For more information on giant-cell arteritis: National Organization for Rare Disorders (NORD); NIH/National Heart, Lung and Blood Institute.

References
   Textbook of Rheumatology, 3rd ed.: W.N. Kelley, et al.; W.B. Saunders Company, 1989, pp. 1200–1208.

ARTERITIS, TAKAYASU'S

Description Takayasu's arteritis is an inflammation of the large elastic arteries and the aorta. The disorder is a progressive polyarteritis resulting in the reduction of blood flow to the head and arms, and loss of the major pulses. Irregular segmental stenosis of the large arteries and aortic regurgitation are also likely to be part of the clinical picture.

Synonyms
   Aortic Arch Syndrome
   Pulseless Disease

Signs and Symptoms Prodromes mimic acute febrile illness with systemic manifestations of fever, anorexia, malaise, myalgias, and arthralgias. Progressive obstructive arterial disease and arterial stenosis follow the acute period of the disease. When the aorta and carotid arteries are involved, the patient experiences lightheadedness, dizziness, and syncope, which is probably the result of cerebral ischemia. Carotid and superficial temporal pulses may be lost. Most patients develop cardiac and cerebral insufficiencies. There may be a ruptured aneurysm, aphasia, and episodes of blindness, dim vision, and photophobia. Brachial involvement symptoms include extremity weakness and claudication, cool skin, and the absence of radial pulses. Blood pressure may be imperceptible. Raynaud's phenomenon is regularly observed. Additional symptoms include systolic murmurs, erythema nodosum, fever, atrophy of facial muscles and soft tissues, and premature cataracts. Prognosis is more favorable when the disease progresses more slowly and the patient has the opportunity to develop adequate collateral or secondary circulation.

Etiology The cause is unclear. Certain evidence (e.g., elevated globulins levels, the presence in serum of antiaorta antibodies) suggests an immunologic process and possibly an autoimmune association, not contradicted by the familial and racial incidence associations as discussed below. Studies have shown increased frequency in Asians of HLA-Bw52; and increased frequency in North Americans of HLA-DR4. An infectious etiology has not been proved.

Epidemiology The disease is common in Japan, and occurs throughout the Orient. It has been seen in India and is reported to occur frequently in South America.

Females are primarily affected (80 to 90 percent of cases), generally between 10 and 30 years of age.

Related Disorders See *Arteritis, Giant-Cell; Polymyalgia Rheumatica.*

Treatment—Standard As soon as diagnosis is suspected, treatment should begin in order to avoid serious complications such as arterial occlusion and blindness. High doses of corticosteroids control initial local and systemic symptoms. Prednisone may be given in large doses until symptoms cease and laboratory findings return to normal. This process usually lasts 2 to 4 weeks. Initial therapy is followed by giving a gradually reduced dosage (about 10 percent/month) for 2 years or longer to prevent recurrence. The disease is monitored by checking the sedimentation rate. A rise in the rate along with recurrence of symptoms heralds a return of the illness.

Reconstructive vascular surgery may be helpful in selected patients with inactive disease.

Treatment—Investigational Please contact the agencies listed under Resources, below, for the most current information.

Resources

For more information on Takayasu's arteritis: National Organization for Rare Disorders (NORD); NIH/National Heart, Lung and Blood Institute.

References

Mendelian Inheritance in Man, 9th ed.: V.A. McKusick; The Johns Hopkins University Press, 1990, p. 1037.

Textbook of Rheumatology, 3rd ed.: W.N. Kelley, et al.; W.B. Saunders Company, 1989, pp. 1190–1192.

BEHÇET'S SYNDROME

Description Behçet's syndrome is a chronic relapsing inflammatory disorder marked by eye inflammation, oral and genital ulcers, and certain other skin lesions, as well as varying multisystem involvement including the joints, blood vessels, central nervous system, and gastrointestinal tract.

Signs and Symptoms The most frequent initial sign is aphthous stomatitis, the lesions healing in a few days to a month, but recurring. Similar genital lesions recur less frequently.

Ocular symptoms include posterior uveitis, iridocyclitis, a transient hypopyon iritis, and chorioretinitis. Although the ocular lesions may resolve, chronic recurrence of the inflammation may result in partial loss of vision or complete blindness after 4 to 8 years.

Cutaneous hypersensitivity is seen in most Behçet patients, with a pustule and erythema developing within 24 hours at the site of a pinprick into sterile skin. The skin lesions typically resemble erythema nodosum, most commonly over the lower legs.

At least 50 percent of patients develop arthralgia or a polyarthritis before, during, or after the onset of Behçet's syndrome. The arthritis usually affects large joints, ranges from mild to severe in nature, and occasionally becomes chronic. Joint damage is rarely permanent.

Vascular involvement includes thrombophlebitis of the large veins and arterial occlusion and aneurysm. Rarely, pulmonary embolism occurs.

The lesions of aphthous stomatitis may be found elsewhere in the gastrointestinal tract. Symptoms vary from mild abdominal discomfort to ulcerative colitis or regional enteritis and malabsorption problems.

The central nervous system becomes involved in about 10 percent of patients. Symptoms are first seen on the average of 16 months after initial Behçet symptoms onset. Recurrent attacks of meningoencephalitis or meningitis result in neurologic damage with such manifestations as ocular and pseudobulbar palsies and cerebellar ataxia.

Etiology The cause of Behçet's syndrome is unclear. Genetic predisposition, autoimmune mechanisms, and viral infection are under consideration.

Epidemiology Seen most frequently in the Middle East and Asia, especially Japan, the syndrome occurs twice as often in men between 20 and 30 years old than in women, and is a leading cause of blindness. However, in the United States and Australia it is more prevalent in women than in men and less severe. In the United States about 15,000 persons may be affected.

Related Disorders See *Reiter's Syndrome; Stevens-Johnson Syndrome.*

Treatment—Standard Attacks often remit spontaneously. Topical corticosteroids may relieve the pain of oral lesions, and lidocaine mouthwash also will alleviate pain. Chronic therapy with colchicine is effective in preventing recurrent attacks of oral and genital ulcers. Joint, skin, and mucosal inflammation may be reduced with high-dose oral glucocorticoids, but there is some question as to their use in posterior uveitis. Chlorambucil has been successful in treating uveitis and meningoencephalitis, but the possible toxic effects of this drug must be considered in its use.

Treatment—Investigational A study of 96 Japanese patients reported in The Lancet, May 20, 1989, indicates that cyclosporine treatment for oral ulcers, skin lesions, and optic inflammation may be beneficial. Additional studies in the United States, Israel, and Japan also suggest that the use of cyclosporine may lessen or prevent the occurrence of uveitis. Toxic effects of cyclosporine include nephrotoxicity, and it also has been reported that disease activity resumes quickly when the drug is stopped.

Azathioprine as well as chlorambucil (mentioned above) has been used to control the symptoms of eye disease in persons with Behçet's syndrome. Further research is needed.

Thalidomide, an orphan drug, is being tested for its effectiveness in treatment; this drug, however, should not be used in pregnant women because of its known ability to cause severe birth defects. Physicians wishing to inquire about testing thalidomide should contact Pediatric Pharmaceutical, 379 Thornall Street, Edison,

New Jersey, 08837.
Please contact the agencies listed under Resources, below, for the most current information.

Resources
For more information on Behçet's syndrome: National Organization for Rare Disorders (NORD); American Behçet's Association; Arthritis Foundation; J.D. Duffy, M.D., Mayo Clinic Behçet's Clinic.

References
Textbook of Rheumatology, 3rd ed.: W.N. Kelley, et al.; W.B. Saunders Company, 1989, pp. 1209–1214.
Cecil Textbook of Medicine, 18th ed.: J.B. Wyngaarden and L.H. Smith, Jr., eds.; W.B. Saunders Company, 1988, pp. 2048–2049, 1609, 2026.
Cyclosporine in Behçet's Disease Resistant to Conventional Therapy: Laura E. Caspers-Velu, et al.; Ann. of Ophthalmology, 1989.

BUERGER'S DISEASE

Description Buerger's disease is an occlusive and inflammatory disorder affecting the peripheral blood vessels. The clinical and pathologic manifestations are severe pain, Raynaud's phenomenon, venous thrombosis, and ulcerations.

Synonyms
Thromboangiitis Obliterans
Occlusive Peripheral Vascular Disease

Signs and Symptoms Intermediate and small-sized arteries and veins are affected, with chronic inflammation and thrombosis. Major vessels are only occasionally involved.

Coldness in the extremities is usually the first complaint, and pain in the affected areas is nearly intolerable. Digital ulcers may be present, as may hyperhidrosis. Red and tender raised areas abruptly appear in the skin near the valves of superficial veins, resolve gradually over several weeks, and reappear. Remissions and exacerbations up to a month long are typical, with occluded areas eventually outstripping collateral circulation, and resulting in ischemia.

In advanced Buerger's disease there may be gangrene, and intermittent claudications that mimic arteriosclerosis obliterans.

Etiology The cause is unknown; however, cigarette smoke seems to be primarily associated. Repeated blunt injury to the hand or fingers may contribute to the development of the disease.

Epidemiology Males are affected more often than females in a ratio of 75:1. The greatest incidence is between 20 and 45 years of age, and in men who smoke and are of Jewish or Oriental heritage.

Related Disorders See *Polyarteritis Nodosa; Arteritis, Takayasu; Vasculitis.*

Treatment—Standard Discontinuing the use of nicotine relieves vasoconstriction and improves circulation. Skin ulcerations should be treated immediately. Calcium channel blockers, pentoxifylline, thromboxane inhibitors, and epoprostenol may relieve symptoms. Surgery has been used to treat the pain but does not change the course.

Treatment—Investigational Preganglionic sympathectomy is recommended by some when vasospasm is excessive in advancing thromboangiitis obliterans, but not in mild cases or when gangrene is widespread. The surgical intervention is still under debate.

Revascularization combined with pharmacologic therapy using heparin, urokinase, and PGE1, is being investigated as a means to enhance circulation.

Please contact the agencies listed under Resources, below, for the most current information.

Resources

For more information on Buerger's disease: National Organization for Rare Disorders (NORD); NIH/National Heart, Lung and Blood Institute (NHLBI).

References
Buerger's Disease (Thromboangiitis Obliterans): J.W. Joyce; Rheum. Dis. Clin. North Am., 1990, vol. 16, pp. 463–470.
Fate of the Ischemic Limb in Buerger's Disease: T. Ohta, et al.; Br. J. Surg., March 1988, issue 75(3), pp. 259–262.
Thromboangiitis Obliterans (Buerger's Disease) of the Temporal Arteries: J.T. Lie, et al.; Hum. Path., May 1988, issue 19(5), pp. 598–602.
Thromboangiitis Obliterans (Buerger's Disease) in a Saphenous Vein Arterial Graft: J.T. Lie; Hum. Path., April 1987, issue 18(4), pp. 402–404.

EHLERS-DANLOS SYNDROMES (EDS)

Description EDS comprise a diverse group of inherited systemic connective tissue disorders whose major features relate to the joints and the skin. The various forms are labeled I through X to XI, depending on the categorization.

Synonyms
Arthrochalasia Multiplex Congenita
Cutis Hyperelastica
India Rubber Skin
Meekeren-Ehlers-Danlos Syndrome
Van Meekeren I Syndrome

Signs and Symptoms The clinical picture varies considerably. Characteristics in general include hyperelastic, fragile skin, hyperextensibility of joints with frequent luxations, a tendency toward bleeding and bruising, soft pseudotumors, calcified cysts and atrophic scars, and visceral anomalies. Intelligence is usually normal. Facial characteristics may be normal in appearance or may include widely spaced eyes with epicanthal folds, a broad nasal bridge, and "lop" ears.

Most striking is the soft, velvety skin that can be pulled away from underlying structures and will then return to its original position. Although hyperelastic, the skin is abnormally fragile, which is reflected in easily formed hematomas and soft pseudotumors. Minor trauma may cause gaping wounds and be difficult to suture, and surgical complications may also arise because of the deep tissue frailty. The elbows, knees, shins, and other bony prominences may have paper-thin, red-brown shiny scars. Legs and forearms may have subcutaneous nodules that move and often calcify. "India rubber men" or "human pretzels" display the abnormal positioning of the joint hyperextensibility.

Ocular symptoms include strabismus, which occurs frequently, a blue membrane around the sclera, perforation of the globe, diminished cornea, and myopia with associated glaucoma.

Other characteristics include gastrointestinal hernias and diverticula and synovial effusion. Premature birth can occur as a result of maternal tissue extensibility and fetal membrane fragility. Congenital hip dislocations and clubfeet are due to the loose-jointedness.

Diagnosis usually can be confirmed by 2 or more of the following cardinal features being present: cutaneous hyperelasticity, joint hyperextensibility, easy bruising, atrophic scars and pseudotumors, and calcified subcutaneous cysts.

Etiology Ehlers-Danlos syndromes are inherited as autosomal dominant, autosomal recessive, or X-linked recessive traits.

Epidemiology The syndromes are most prevalent among white persons of European ancestry, but may occur in dark-skinned individuals. Men and women are equally affected. Joint and skin symptoms most often are seen at an early age, but in some cases are not evident until adulthood.

Treatment—Standard Treatment is essentially supportive. Care should be taken to avoid lacerations and trauma to the joints. Homeostasis must be maintained during surgical procedures, and any time suturing is required, tissue tension should be minimized. Careful obstetric supervision must be observed during pregnancy and delivery to prevent premature birth and hemorrhaging.

Treatment—Investigational Please contact the agencies listed under Resources, below, for the most current information.

Resources
For more information on Ehlers-Danlos syndrome: National Organization for Rare Disorders (NORD); Ehlers-Danlos National Foundation; The National Arthritis and Musculoskeletal and Skin Diseases Information Clearinghouse.

References
Arthritis and Allied Conditions, 11th ed.: D.J. McCarty; Lea & Febiger, 1989, pp. 1337–1340.

Textbook of Rheumatology, 3rd ed.: W.N. Kelley, et al.; W.B. Saunders Company, 1989, pp. 1698–1703.

Mendelian Inheritance in Man, 9th ed.: V.A. McKusik; Johns Hopkins University Press, 1990, pp. 283–287, 1158–1161, 1589.

FAMILIAL MEDITERRANEAN FEVER (FMF)

Description The salient features of FMF are recurrent attacks of fever accompanied by self-limiting peritonitis, pleuritis, and, sometimes, arthritis.

Synonyms
Recurrent Polyserositis

Signs and Symptoms Symptoms of recurrent FMF attacks typically include fever, and polyserositis causing severe abdominal and pleuritic pain; the abdominal pain may mimic appendicitis. The abdominal attacks generally last up to 24 hours but may continue for 4 days. Almost three-quarters of patients have attacks of arthritis that are exquisitely painful and accompanied by some swelling and by limitation of motion. They usually end within 7 days, with joint function restored, but can continue for several weeks or months. There may be painful, erythematous, and swollen skin lesions on the lower legs.

Amyloidosis occurs in almost half of those patients who are Sephardic Jews, but less often in those of other cultures. Amyloid nephropathy may be fatal. Intestinal obstruction and meningitis may be complications.

Etiology The disease is inherited as an autosomal recessive trait.

Epidemiology The disease generally begins in childhood or the teen years and continues intermittently throughout life. Males are affected more often than females, and the majority of those affected have their origins in the Mediterranean Sea region, and include Sephardic and Iraqi Jews, Turks, Levantine Arabs, and Armenians.

Treatment—Standard Although the reason is not understood, colchicine seems to prevent attacks of FMF as well as amyloidosis. If an attack is ongoing, large doses of colchicine will halt the symptoms. Corticosteroids have not proved effective. Narcotics should be used judiciously because the intense pain requires large doses.

If the kidneys are involved by amyloidosis, renal dialysis or transplantation may be necessary.

Treatment—Investigational Please contact the agencies listed under Resources, below, for the most current information.

Resources
For more information on familial Mediterranean fever: National Organization for Rare Disorders (NORD); National Institute of Diabetes, Digestive & Kidney Diseases Information Clearinghouse; March of Dimes Birth Defects Foundation; National Center for Education in Maternal and Child Health (NCEMCH).

References
Arthritis and Allied Conditions, 11th ed.: D.J. McCarty; Lea & Febiger, 1989, pp. 995–998.
Cecil Textbook of Medicine, 18th ed.: J.B. Wyngaarden and L.H. Smith, Jr., eds.; W.B. Saunders Company, 1988, pp. 147, 795, 1196–1199.

FELTY'S SYNDROME

Description Felty's syndrome is an unusual complication of rheumatoid arthritis (**RA**) in which patients have splenomegaly and granulocytopenia. The syndrome occurs in approximately one percent of patients with RA.

Synonyms
> Splenomegaly with Rheumatoid Arthritis

Signs and Symptoms Characteristics include leukopenia associated with recurrent infections; thrombocytopenia; splenomegaly; and a yellowish-brown skin discoloration over the lower extremities. Leg ulcers, stomatitis, anemia, vasculitis, swelling of lymph nodes, and fever also may occur.

Etiology The cause of the granulocytopenia in patients with Felty's syndrome is not clear at this time. It is believed to be multifactorial, involving antigranulocyte antibodies and/or other unknown immunologic disturbance. The granulocytopenia is associated with frequent infections, most commonly involving the skin and respiratory tract.

Epidemiology The syndrome seems to occur mostly in middle-aged and elderly women, although it has been reported in men as well.

Related Disorders Rheumatoid arthritis usually occurs in middle-aged and older persons, mostly women, but can also affect children. It is characterized by pain, stiffness, swelling, and joint deformities. The hands, wrists, knees, feet, ankles, and shoulders are most commonly affected. Felty's syndrome occurs in about one percent of patients with RA.

Treatment—Standard Splenectomy for serious or recurrent infections arising from Felty's syndrome, is successful in about half of the patients. Other therapies are those used for RA, such as antiinflammatory drugs including gold, penicillamine, or methotrexate. Anemia associated with Felty's syndrome can be treated with blood transfusions or erythropoietin. The prognosis is generally uncertain and depends on several variables, including the general health of the patient and the combination of symptoms occurring in a patient.

Treatment—Investigational Lithium has been used experimentally to treat Felty's syndrome. Preliminary studies appear positive.

Please contact the agencies listed under Resources, below, for the most current information.

Resources

For more information on Felty's syndrome: National Organization for Rare Disorders (NORD); Arthritis Foundation; The National Arthritis and Musculoskeletal and Skin Diseases Information Clearinghouse.

References
Felty's Syndrome: An Analytical Review: J.L. Spivak; Johns Hopkins Med. J., 1977, vol. 141, pp. 156–162.

Lithium Carbonate Therapy in Severe Felty's Syndrome: M.J. Mant, et al.; Arch. Intern. Med., 1986, vol. 146, pp. 277–280.

Felty's Syndrome in a Child: A.M. Rosenberg, et al.; J. Rheumatol., December 1984, issue 11(6), pp. 835–837.

KAWASAKI SYNDROME

Description Kawasaki syndrome is a childhood illness characterized by fever, lymphadenopathy, rash, polyarteritis, and vasculitis.

Synonyms
Mucocutaneous Lymph Node Syndrome

Signs and Symptoms The fever typically begins abruptly and lasts for about 2 weeks but may be sustained over a month. Other symptoms occurring in the first 5 days of Kawasaki disease include bilateral conjunctivitis, stomatitis, cervical adenopathy, and rash. The palms of the hands and soles of the feet become erythematous, and in about 7 days after onset the hands and feet are edematous; in a few more days the ends of the fingers and toes are desquamative. A painful arthritis may occur at this time, usually symmetric and involving large and small joints. Thrombocytosis may develop about 10 days after onset of fever, and not disappear for a few weeks.

Cardiac complications occur in about one-third to one-half of cases, and include aneurysms, myocarditis, coronary vasculitis, pericardial effusions, arrhythmias, and, rarely, congestive heart failure and valvular disease.

Other complications include diarrhea, vomiting, hepatitis, gallbladder disease; cough; and depression and seizures.

Etiology Recent research suggests that the syndrome may be caused by a retrovirus. The virus has not yet been identified, but antibodies to retroviruses have been found in the white blood cells of Kawasaki patients.

Epidemiology The disease is seen predominantly in children under the age of 5. Extremely rare occurrences have been reported in the 20s. There is a slight prevalence of males over females, with serious complications found more often in males. Kawasaki syndrome has been reported throughout the world.

Treatment—Standard Early high-dose intravenous gamma globulin along with low-dose aspirin may reduce the development of coronary artery complications, and will reduce fever and inflammation of the respiratory tract mucous membranes, central nervous system, joints, and skin. Treatment with corticosteroids is not recommended.

The duration of aspirin therapy for prevention of coronary aneurysm is relative to the disease course, and regularly lasts over a period of several months. With the onset of an aneurysm, the aspirin therapy is continued as an anticoagulant, and bypass surgery may be indicated.

Close longterm follow-up is essential. Frequent electrocardiogram evaluation is recommended. Two-dimensional echocardiography with appropriate coronary angiography is suggested if coronary aneurysm is suspected.

Treatment—Investigational Please contact the agencies listed under Resources, below, for the most current information.

Resources
   For more information on Kawasaki syndrome: National Organization for Rare Disorders (NORD); NIH/National Institute of Allergy and Infectious Diseases (NIAID); Centers for Disease Control (CDC).

References
   Kawasaki Syndrome: D.W. Wortmann and A.M. Nelson; Rheum. Dis. Clin. North Am., 1990, vol. 16, pp. 363–375.
   Cecil Textbook of Medicine, 18th ed.: J.B. Wyngaarden and L.H. Smith, Jr., eds.; W.B. Saunders Company, 1988, pp. 1523, 2323–2324.

KIENBOECK DISEASE

Description In Kienboeck disease, derangements of the lunate bone, acquired during inflammation or injury, occur that may limit the extent of motion in the wrist.

Synonyms
   Lunatomalacia

Signs and Symptoms Degenerative changes in the lunate result in softening, deterioration, fragmentation, or compression of the affected bone. Symptoms are recurrent tenderness and pain, and thickening, swelling, and stiffness of the soft tissues overlying the lunate. Range of motion in the wrist usually is compromised. Formation of new bone will resolve the disorder.
   Diagnostic procedures include arthroscopy, CT scan, and radiography.

Etiology Kienboeck disease is caused by inflammation or injury to the wrist.

Epidemiology Onset is usually in childhood, and females are affected more often than males.

Related Disorders See *Carpal Tunnel Syndrome.*
   Juvenile osteoporosis is a porous or atrophic condition of the bony tissue that may cause fractures or pain in various bones, including the wrist. Onset is before or during puberty, with spontaneous remission occurring within several years. The cause is unknown.
   Sudeck atrophy, or posttraumatic osteoporosis, is acute atrophy of bone tissue following a seemingly minor injury, such as a sprain. Bones in the wrists and ankles are the most frequently affected.

Treatment—Standard Surgical intervention for Kienboeck disease may be necessary. Inflammation may require the use of drugs. Other treatment is symptomatic and supportive.

Treatment—Investigational Please contact the agencies listed under Resources, below, for the most current information.

Resources
  For more information on Kienboeck disease: National Organization for Rare Disorders (NORD); NIH/National Institute of Arthritis, Musculoskeletal and Skin Diseases (NIAMS) Clearinghouse.

References
  Excision of the Lunate in Kienboeck's Disease. Results After Long-Term Follow-Up: H. Kawai, et al.; J. Bone Joint Surg. (Br.), March 1988, issue 70(2), pp. 287–292.
  Ulna-Minus Variance and Kienboeck's Disease: P.A. Nathan, et al.; J. Hand Surg., September 1987, issue 12(5), pp. 777–778.

KÖHLER'S DISEASE

Description Köhler's disease is a rare foot disorder in which progressive degeneration of the navicular bone causes pain and swelling of the foot.

Synonyms
  Navicular Osteochondrosis

Signs and Symptoms The affected foot is swollen and particularly tender along the length of the arch. Walking and other weight-bearing cause further discomfort and a limp. The bone eventually regenerates and heals itself.

Etiology The cause is unknown. The disease is apparently not hereditary or caused by injury.

Epidemiology Males are affected more often than females. The disease usually occurs in children between the ages of 3 and 5.

Related Disorders See *Tarsal Tunnel Syndrome; Erythromelalgia.*
  Burning feet syndrome (Gopalan syndrome) is marked by burning, aching pain and cramps in the soles of the feet and sometimes palms of the hands. A deficiency of a B vitamin is suspected.
  Freiberg's disease (see also *Osteonecrosis),* characterized by foot pain that is exacerbated by weight-bearing or walking, is caused by progressive osteonecrosis of the head of the 2nd metatarsal. Treatment may require surgery.

Treatment—Standard Recovery is aided by avoiding weight-bearing on the affected foot, or supporting the weight-bearing with short-leg plaster casts or specially designed shoes. Recovery usually occurs in less than a year, rarely taking more than 2 years. Patients permanently regain full function of the foot.

Treatment—Investigational Please contact the agencies listed under Resources, below, for the most current information.

Resources
   For more information on Köhler's disease: National Organization for Rare Disorders (NORD); The National Arthritis and Musculoskeletal and Skin Diseases Information Clearinghouse.

References
Dorsiflexion Osteotomy in Freiberg's Disease: P. Kinnard and R. Lirette; Foot, Ankle, April 1989, issue 9(5), pp. 226–231.
Freiberg's Infraction of the Second Metatarsal Head with Formation of Multiple Loose Bodies: G. Scartozzi, et al.; J. Foot Surg., May–June 1989, issue 28(3), pp. 195–199.
Köhler's Disease of the Tarsal Navicular: G.A. Williams and H.R. Cowell; Clin. Orth., July–August 1981, issue 158, pp. 53–58.
Köhler's Disease of the Tarsal Navicular. Long-Term Follow-Up of Twelve Cases: E. Ippolito, et al.; J. Ped. Orth., August 1984, issue 4(4), pp. 416–417.
Köhler's Osteochondrosis of the Tarsal Navicular. Case Report with Twenty-Eight Year Follow-Up: K.M. Devine and R.E. Van Demark, Sr.; S.D.J. Med., September 1989, issue 42(9), pp. 5–6.

LEGG-CALVÉ-PERTHES SYNDROME

Description Legg-Calvé-Perthes syndrome affects the hip joint, with abnormalities in bone growth during the early years that may result in permanent deformity of the hip joint in young adulthood.

Synonyms
   Coxa Plana
   Slipped Capital Femoral Epiphysis

Signs and Symptoms Without warning, mild aching in the hip may occur, followed by inability to move the affected leg normally. Hip pain may increase in intensity and muscle spasms develop. The bone may shorten enough to cause an obvious limp. Osteonecrosis of the femoral head may be seen in persons with Legg-Calvé-Perthes syndrome.

Etiology The syndrome is thought to be inherited as an autosomal dominant trait. Damage to the early developing hip joint bone is caused by reduced vascular supply to the femur.

Epidemiology Onset of the disorder is between 6 and 12 years of age. Males are affected more often than females.

Related Disorders Juvenile (rheumatoid) arthritis may have symptoms similar to Legg-Calvé-Perthes syndrome.

Treatment—Standard Antiinflammatory medication and analgesics are the primary choices for patient management. Non–weight-bearing with crutch walking may be necessary for several months. Additional treatment is symptomatic and supportive.

Treatment—Investigational Please contact the agencies listed under Resources,

below, for the most current information.

Resources

For more information about Legg-Calvé-Perthes syndrome: National Organization for Rare Disorders (NORD); Arthritis Foundation; NIH/National Arthritis, Musculoskeletal and Skin (NIAMS) Information Clearinghouse; March of Dimes Birth Defects Foundation; NIH/National Center for Education in Maternal and Child Health (NCEMCH).

References

Mendelian Inheritance in Man, 9th ed.: V.A. McKusick; The Johns Hopkins University Press, 1990, pp. 563–564.

Long-Term Follow-Up of Legg-Calvé-Perthes Disease: M.P. McAndrew, et al.; J. Bone Joint Surg. (AM), July 1984, issue 66(6), pp. 860–869.

Legg-Calvé-Perthes Disease in a Family: Genetic or Environmental: M. O'Sullivan, et al.; Clin. Orth., October 1985, issue 199, pp. 179–181.

Lesions of the Femoral Neck in Legg-Perthes Disease: F.N. Silverman, AJR, June 1985, issue 144(6), pp. 1249–1254.

MISCELLANEOUS ORTHOPEDIC DISEASES

DUPUYTREN'S CONTRACTURE

Description Dupuytren's contracture commonly involves an abnormal fibrotic process of the palmar fascia that results in flexor contracture of the fingers, pain, and loss of function. Rarely, the feet are affected.

Signs and Symptoms Abnormal contractile connective tissues consisting of nodules and bands form in the palmar fascia. Initially, nodular thickening and dimpling of the skin are seen. Further growth of nodules and thickening of fascial cords develop, resulting in contracture. The disorder is usually bilateral, affecting the ring finger most often. Pain may be felt in the fingers and palm. Eventually the contractures may become disabling.

Etiology An autosomal dominant inheritance with variable penetrance has been suggested. Dupuytren's contracture seems to be associated with several diseases, including Peyronie's disease, diabetes mellitus, epilepsy, alcoholism, and rheumatoid arthritis. Injury to the hand has been reported to be a precipitating factor.

Epidemiology Caucasians are primarily affected, especially Northern Europeans. The disorder is rarely seen in children and does not occur in persons of pure African and Asian heritage. Men afflicted with Peyronie disease may also have Dupuytren's contracture.

Related Disorders Interphalangeal nodules of new growth of fibrous tissue may occur. They are most likely genetic in origin.

Treatment—Standard Pain is treated with analgesics, local heat, and corticosteroid injections into the lesion. Physical therapy is useful for preventing atrophy of the unused hand and forearm muscles. Surgical intervention has been recommended, even early intervention to prevent deformity, but procedures are complicated by such factors as neurovascular involvement with the fibrotic mass, and recurrence of contractures due to remaining abnormal connective tissue bands.

Genetic counseling may be beneficial to some patients and their families.

Treatment—Investigational Please contact the agencies listed under Resources, below, for the most current information.

Resources

For more information on Dupuytren's contracture: National Organization for Rare Disorders (NORD); National Arthritis and Musculoskeletal and Skin Diseases Information Clearinghouse.

For genetic information and genetic counseling referrals: March of Dimes Birth Defects Foundation; NIH/National Center for Education in Maternal and Child Health (NCEMCH).

References
Mendelian Inheritance in Man, 9th ed.: V.A. McKusick; The Johns Hopkins University Press, 1990, pp. 272, 273.

Arthritis and Allied Conditions, 11th ed.: D.J. McCarty; Lea & Febiger, 1989, pp. 1475–1477.

Cytogenetic Studies in Dupuytren's Contracture: D.H. Wurster-Hill, et al.; Am. J. Hum. Genet., September 1988, issue 43(3), pp. 285–292.

Dupuytren's Contracture, Alcohol Consumption, and Chronic Liver Disease: P. Attali, et al.; Arch. Int. Med., June 1987, issue 146(6), pp. 1065–1067.

Salvage of Severe Recurrent Dupuytren's Contracture on the Ring and Small Fingers: H.K. Watson, et al.; J. Hand Surg., March 1987, issue 12(2), pp. 287–289.

Dupuytren's Disease in Blacks: M.V. Makhlouf, et al.; Ann. Plast. Surg., October 1987, issue 19(4), pp. 334–336.

MIXED CONNECTIVE TISSUE DISEASE (MCTD)

Description The syndrome of MCTD encompasses an overlap of the symptoms and signs of systemic lupus erythematosus **(SLE),** scleroderma, and polymyositis. Salient features of the syndrome are sequential manifestations of symptoms and high titers of antibodies to a ribonuclease-sensitive extractable nuclear antigen (anti-RNP antibodies).

Signs and Symptoms Early symptoms and signs include fever of unknown origin, Raynaud's phenomenon, edematous hands, fatigue, and nondeforming arthritis.

The overlapping features develop sequentially over several years. Arthritis occurs in almost every case of MCTD, but rarely results in deformities similar to those seen in rheumatoid arthritis. Muscle pains occur commonly, and an inflammatory myopathy may be present that is indistinguishable clinically and histologically from polymyositis. Skin changes also are universal, and include those of SLE, including malar rash and discoid plaques, as well as those of scleroderma. In addition, mucosal ulcerations in the mouth and sicca symptoms may be present.

Pulmonary and cardiac involvement includes pulmonary hypertension and an associated pericarditis, both of which can be asymptomatic for years. Involvement of the gastrointestinal tract includes esophageal and bowel dysmotility. Renal involvement in patients with MCTD is rare; its occurrence indicates the presence of another primary connective tissue disease, especially SLE. Hematologic disorders, including anemia and leukopenia, may develop. Neurologic complications, only seen in about 10 percent of patients, include trigeminal neuropathy.

Etiology The cause is not known; however, an immunologic association is well documented. All patients have high titers of antibodies to nuclear RNP, resulting in a positive test for antinuclear antibodies in a speckled pattern. Patients lack antibodies to double-stranded DNA and the Sm antigen.

Epidemiology Onset is known to be from 4 to 80 years, with the most predominant group being in the late 30s. Nearly all of the patients are women. The disease is not associated with any specific geographic area.

Related Disorders The clinical syndrome of mixed connective tissue disease overlaps a multitude of other illnesses. See *Raynaud's Disease and Phenomenon; Systemic Lupus Erythematosus; Scleroderma; Polymyositis/Dermatomyositis.*

Treatment—Standard Many symptoms of MCTD respond in some degree to corticosteroids. Mild forms may be helped by nonsteroidal antiinflammatory drugs, antimalarials, or low doses of corticosteroids.

Treatment—Investigational Please contact the agencies listed under Resources, below, for the most current information.

Resources
For more information on MCTD: National Organization for Rare Disorders (NORD); Arthritis Foundation; Scleroderma Society; United Scleroderma Foundation; Scleroderma Information Exchange; Scleroderma Research Foundation; Sjögren's Foundation; National Lupus Foundation; Lupus Foundation of America Inc.; Systemic Lupus Erythematosus Foundation; The National Arthritis and Musculoskeletal and Skin Diseases Information Clearinghouse.

References
Textbook of Rheumatology, 3rd ed.: W.N. Kelley, et al.; W.B. Saunders Company, 1989, pp. 1148–1165.

OLLIER DISEASE

Description Ollier disease is a skeletal dysplasia usually of childhood onset, affecting the long bones and cartilage in joints of the arms and legs.

Synonyms
Multiple Cartilaginous Enchondroses

Signs and Symptoms Onset during childhood is gradual. Involvement may be either uni- or bilateral.

The head and upper body are normal. If just one leg is affected, the patient may limp; if the disease is bilateral, short stature may result. Deformities may develop in the wrists and ankles. Dislocation of the elbows or other joints with resulting fractures may occur.

The abnormal growth of bone and cartilage eventually stops. Rare associations with chondrosarcoma and ovarian juvenile granulosa cell tumor have been reported.

Etiology The cause is unknown. Overgrowth of cartilaginous cells in some skeletal and joint areas may result in cortex thinning and distortion of growth in the metaphyses.

Epidemiology Males and females are equally affected.

Related Disorders See *Maffucci Syndrome,* an autosomal dominant congenital disorder in which hemangiomas as well as enchondromas are present.

Exostosis, an epiphyseal growth abnormality inherited as a dominant trait, is an extremely rare condition, occurring chiefly among natives of Micronesia. Although usually symptom-free, the patient may experience pain because of pressure from benign exostoses. The disorder is most frequent and severe in males.

Treatment—Standard Surgical extension of the affected limb has been helpful, as has prosthetic joint replacement when appropriate. Fractures routinely heal without unusual complications.

Treatment—Investigational Please contact the agencies listed under Resources, below, for the most current information.

Resources

For more information on Ollier disease: National Organization for Rare Disorders (NORD); National Institute of Diabetes, Digestive and Kidney Diseases Information Clearinghouse.

References

Treatment of Multiple Enchrondromatosis (Ollier's Disease) of the Hand: J.F. Fatti, et al.; Orthopedics, April 1986, issue 9(4), pp. 512–518.

Ollier's Disease. An Assessment of Angular Deformity, Shortening, and Pathological Fracture in Twenty-One Patients: F. Shapiro; J. Bone Surg. (Am.), January 1982, issue 64-A(1), pp. 95–103.

Multiple Chondrosarcomas in Dyschondroplasia (Ollier's Disease): S.R. Cannon, et al.; Cancer, February 15, 1985, issue 55(4), pp. 836–840.

OSGOOD-SCHLATTER DISEASE

Description Osgood-Schlatter disease is a nonprogressive, self-limited, inflammatory condition associated with abnormal bone and cartilage formation in the tibia.

Synonyms
　　Osteochondrosis, Tibial Tubercle

Signs and Symptoms The typical symptoms, swelling accompanied by tenderness and pain, worsen with increased exercise or stretching. The disease is bilateral in about half of patients. Osgood-Schlatter disease runs a limited course (weeks to months), and the affected area will usually regenerate. Longterm effects are uncommon, although tibial fractures and joint pain have been documented years after the initial diagnosis of the disease.

Etiology The cause is unknown. Precipitating factors may include traumatic injury, chronic irritation, and misuse of immature bone or of the quadriceps.

Epidemiology Adolescent males who are athletically active are the most frequently affected.

Treatment—Standard Treatment consists initially of immobilization of the affected leg with a cast. If this is not adequate, complete bed rest is necessary. Surgery for grafting or removal of debris has been required in some cases. Any other treatment is supportive and symptomatic.

Treatment—Investigational Please contact the agencies listed under Resources, below, for the most current information.

Resources
　　For more information on Osgood-Schlatter disease: National Organization for Rare Disorders (NORD); The National Arthritis and Musculoskeletal and Skin Diseases Information Clearinghouse; Arthritis Foundation.

References
Avulsion Fracture of the Tibial Tuberosity in Late Adolescence: P. Nimityongskul, et al.; J. Trauma, April 1988, issue 28(4), pp. 505–509.

Management of Sports Injuries in Children and Adolescents: C. Stanitski; Orth. Clin. N. Amer., October 1988, issue 19(4), pp. 689–698.

Tibial Sequestrectomy in the Management of Osgood-Schlatter Disease: I. Trail; J. Ped. Orth., September–October 1988, issue 8(5), pp. 554–557.

The Sequelae of Osgood-Schlatter's Disease in Adults: J. Hogh, et al.; Int. Orth., 1988, issue 12(3), pp. 213–215.

OSTEONECROSIS

Description Osteonecrosis, a slowly progressive disorder of bone destruction, is most often due to inadequate blood supply to a bone. Most commonly affected are the ends of long bones such as the femoral heads and condyles and humeral heads. This produces pain in the hips, knees, and shoulders, respectively.

Synonyms
　　Avascular Necrosis of Bone
　　Ischemic Necrosis of Bone

Signs and Symptoms Pain usually occurs when standing, walking, or lifting, becoming more intense when pressure is exerted on the bones or joints. The pain may progress, eventually occurring while at rest or even disturbing sleep. Other symptoms include muscle spasms, joint stiffness, and limitation of range of motion.

Etiology Conditions that affect the vascular supply to bone can cause osteonecrosis. Trauma that results in dislocation or fracture of the neck of the femur is a common cause. Certain drugs (e.g., glucocorticoids), radiation, and chemotherapy can also adversely affect the blood supply to bone, as can kidney transplantation, sickle cell disease, and alcoholism, all of which can be associated with osteonecrosis.

Epidemiology Osteonecrosis can occur at any age, but is most prevalent in persons between 30 and 60 years. Males are affected more by osteonecrosis of the hip; females, of the knee. The disease is also more common in persons with rheumatic diseases, especially those treated with glucocorticoids (e.g., rheumatoid arthritis, systemic lupus erythematosus); other patients treated with steroids (e.g., asthmatics); alcoholics; diabetics; and skin divers who have experienced the bends.

Related Disorders Osteonecrosis may be produced by a wide variety of diseases, disorders, and traumatic situations. See *Vasculitis; Sickle Cell Disease; Legg-Calvé-Perthes Syndrome; Gaucher Disease; Polycythemia Vera.*

Caisson disease (decompression sickness; the bends), caused by the formation of nitrogen bubbles in the tissues and blood, occurs from a very rapid reduction of air pressure after rising quickly from deep water with high atmospheric pressure, to normal air pressure. Caisson disease is characterized by painful joints, osteonecrosis, chest tightness, giddiness, abdominal pain, vomiting, and visual difficulties. Convulsions and paralysis may also occur.

The **osteopetroses** are a group of rare inherited disorders marked by increased bone density, brittleness of bone, and in some cases skeletal abnormalities.

Treatment—Standard Diagnosis of the underlying cause is the primary basis for establishing treatment. X-rays are useful in diagnosing osteonecrosis and determining the extent of bone damage. However, when x-rays are normal, bone scans and magnetic resonance imaging may reveal the diagnosis.

Limiting weight-bearing activities, standing, and walking, and avoiding alcohol may help the recovery process. Pain is relieved with aspirin or other nonsteroidal antiinflammatory medications. Core decompression may help relieve pain in early osteonecrosis. Joint replacement surgery may be necessary when there is a fracture, or when the bone has collapsed.

Bones damaged by osteonecrosis will usually undergo progressive remodeling with the development of secondary osteoarthritis of the contiguous joint. Surgical management, either core decompression or joint arthroplasty, is often required.

Treatment—Investigational Please contact the agencies listed under Resources, below, for the most current information.

Resources

For more information on osteonecrosis: National Organization for Rare Disorders (NORD); Arthritis Foundation; NIH/National Arthritis, Musculoskeletal and Skin Diseases Information Clearinghouse.

References

Ischemic Necrosis of Bone: T.M. Zizic and D. Hungerford; *in* Harris, et al.: Textbook of Rheumatology, 3rd ed., W.B. Saunders Company, 1990.

Cecil Textbook of Medicine, 18th ed.: J.B. Wyngaarden and L.H. Smith, Jr., eds.; W. B. Saunders Company, 1988. p. 1517.

Osteonecrosis of the Hip in the Sickle Cell Diseases. Treatment and Complications: G. Hanker, et al.; J. Bone Surg. (AM), April 1988, issue 70(4), pp. 499–506.

Influence of Alcohol Intake, Cigarette Smoking, and Occupational Status on Idiopathic Osteonecrosis of the Femoral Head: K. Matsuo, et al.; Clin. Orth., September 1988, issue 234, pp. 115–123.

Osteonecrosis of the Femoral Head. Pathogenesis and Long-Term Results of Treatment: M. Meyers; Clin. Orth., June 1988, issue 231, pp. 51–61.

PAGET'S DISEASE OF BONE

Description Paget's disease of bone is a chronic, slowly progressive skeletal condition of abnormally rapid bone destruction and reformation in which the new bone is structurally abnormal, and dense and fragile. The areas most frequently affected are the spine, skull, pelvis, thighs, and lower legs.

Synonyms

Hyperostosis Corticalis Deformans

Osteitis Deformans

Signs and Symptoms Early symptoms include bone pain, joint pain (especially back, hips, and knees), and headache. Physical signs include enlargement and bowing of the thighs (femurs) and lower legs (tibias), and frontal bossing with enlargement of the skull.

As the disease progresses, other signs and symptoms may appear: further bowing of the affected limb; a waddling gait; muscle and sensory disturbances; and hearing loss. High-output congestive heart failure may occur. Osteogenic sarcoma is a rare complication.

Most cases are asymptomatic and mild and identified on pelvic x-rays. When symptoms occur, they are often vague and hard to distinguish from those of many other diseases, including lumbar spine disease and osteoarthritis.

Differential diagnosis includes normal serum calcium and phosphorous and elevated serum alkaline phosphatase as compared with other osteitis conditions that usually do not have the elevated serum alkaline phosphatase, and the characteristic lesions of the occiput and femur on x-ray.

Etiology The disease may be hereditary, but the actual cause has not been confirmed. Recent research implicates a slow virus. Pain is caused by direct bone involvement, osteoarthritis due to abnormal joint restructuring, and nerve root impingement.

Epidemiology Persons between 50 and 70 years of age are most frequently affected, although young adults have been diagnosed with the disease. Males are affected more often than females. Because so many cases are mild and go undiagnosed and untreated, the estimate of three million cases in the United States is considered below the actual incidence. Paget's disease of bone is more prevalent in those with Western European heritage.

Treatment—Standard Treatment is symptomatic and focuses on relieving pain and preventing deformity, fractures, and loss of mobility.

Diphosphonates are effective and are given intermittently for periods not exceeding 6 months, with observation of the alkaline phosphatase level. In patients who do not respond to diphosphonates, calcitonin is often used (see below, under Treatment—Investigational).

Treatment—Investigational There is ongoing research in the areas of bone tissue; the effect of Paget's disease on collagen synthesis; the action of calcitonin, parathyroid, and other hormone secretions; and the assessment of bone regeneration.

For research on using calcitonin in patients who have side effects or are resistant to diphosphonates, please contact Roy D. Altman, M.D., University of Miami School of Medicine, Division of Arthritis, (VA111) P.O. Box 016960, Miami, Florida 33101, (305) 547-5735.

For research studying etiology of the disease, and clinical studies on possible viral causes, please contact Robert Canfield, M.D., Ethel Siris, M.D., Thomas Jacobs, M.D., Columbia Presbyterian Hospital Department of Medicine, 630 W. 168th Street, New York, NY, (212) 694-3526 or 5731.

Please contact the agencies listed under Resources, below, for the most current information.

Resources

For more information on Paget's disease of bone: National Organization for Rare Disorders (NORD); The Paget's Disease Foundation, Inc.; The National Arthritis and Musculoskeletal and Skin Diseases Information Clearinghouse.

References

Mendelian Inheritance in Man, 9th ed.: V.A. McKusick; The Johns Hopkins University Press, 1990, p. 703.

Textbook of Rheumatology, 3rd ed.: W.N. Kelley, et al.; W.B. Saunders Company, 1989, pp. 1742–1743.

POLYARTERITIS NODOSA (PAN)

Description PAN is an inflammatory necrotizing systemic vascular disease having nodules along the length of small and medium-sized arteries. In varying degrees, the lesions involve most of the arteries throughout the body, and are segmental. The clinical picture is polymorphic, with many manifestations seemingly unrelated.

Synonyms
>Necrotizing Angiitis
>Periarteritis
>Periarteritis Nodosa
>Polyarteritis

Signs and Symptoms Initial symptoms and signs include fever, chills, fatigue, and weight loss. Systemic manifestations include abdominal pain, combined motor and sensory peripheral neuropathy, skin lesions, arthritis, muscle pain, and testicular pain. Gastrointestinal bleeding may occur.

The inflammatory vascular process causes arterial constriction resulting in tissue ischemia, thrombosis, occasional aneurysms, and an increased potential for arterial rupture. The kidneys are most often involved, and hypertension is common. Disease severity ranges from mild to rapidly fatal. The course is usually acute; most deaths due to vasculitis occur within a year of onset.

Diagnosis is confirmed by either biopsy or visceral angiography demonstrating aneurysms.

Etiology There is no one apparent cause, and the majority of patients have no predisposing event or circumstance. The disorder has been observed in drug abusers, particularly those using amphetamines, and in hepatitis-B patients. Research suggests that polyarteritis nodosa is an autoimmune disease possibly initially triggered by a viral infection.

Epidemiology Most often polyarteritis nodosa affects men between 40 and 60 years of age, but it has been seen in every age group. Approximately 1:100,000 persons is affected, with males having the disease 2 to 3 times more frequently than females.

Related Disorders The clinical symptoms of polyarteritis may be produced by a wide variety of related disorders, requiring a comprehensive process of differential diagnosis. See *Churg-Strauss Syndrome; Arteritis, Giant-Cell; Arteritis, Takayasu's; Wegener Granulomatosis.*

Treatment—Standard Primary treatment consists of high-dose corticosteroids (60 to 80 mg/day) such as prednisone for the relief of inflammation and immunosuppression. Cyclophosphamide in doses of 1 to 2 mg/kg/day has also been found to be effective. If indicated, aggressive treatment for hypertension should be part of the management program. Surgery is required where gastrointestinal problems such as perforation and bleeding indicate such intervention. Additional treatment is supportive and symptomatic.

Treatment—Investigational Please contact the agencies listed under Resources, below, for the most current information.

Resources
For more information on polyarteritis nodosa: National Organization for Rare Disorders (NORD); NIH/National Institute for Allergy and Infectious Dis-

eases (NIAID).

References

Textbook of Rheumatology, 3rd ed.: W.N. Kelley, et al.; W.B. Saunders Company, 1989, pp. 1172–1179.

Pulmonary Diseases and Disorders, 2nd ed.: A.P. Fishman; McGraw-Hill, 1988, pp. 1127–1128.

Clinical Findings and Prognosis of Polyarteritis Nodosa and Churg-Strauss Angiitis. A Study in 165 Patients: L. Guillevin, et al.; British J. of Rheum., August 1988, issue 27(4), pp. 258–264.

Immunosuppressive and Corticosteroid Therapy of Polyarteritis Nodosa: E.S. Leib, et al.; JAMA, December 1979, issue 67(6), pp. 941–947.

POLYMYALGIA RHEUMATICA

Description Polymyalgia rheumatica is marked by muscular pain and stiffness and generalized symptoms that include fatigue and fever. The disorder is comparatively benign and exquisitely responsive to treatment, and rarely results in permanent muscle weakness or atrophy.

Synonyms

> Anarthritic Syndrome
> Anarthritic Rheumatoid Disease

Signs and Symptoms Onset is typically abrupt, with pain and stiffness in the neck, shoulders, upper arms, low back, hips, and thighs. Distal extremities usually are not affected. The stiffness and pain are bilateral, and are most severe in the morning and after long periods of rest and inactivity. Muscle tenderness and weakness may occur, but examination of the muscles usually does not reveal any abnormality. Low-grade fever, anorexia, weight loss, fatigue, malaise, and depression may be among the initial symptoms. A peripheral rheumatoid-like arthritis occurs in about one-third of patients.

The sedimentation rate is markedly elevated, often above 100 mm/hr. Also increased are serum albumin, globulins, and fibrinogen. A nonhemolytic anemia may be present. The disease has remissions and exacerbations; however, permanent disability, even after months or years of disease, is unusual.

Etiology The cause is not known. An immunologic association and genetic predisposition have been suggested.

Epidemiology Prevalence is about 50:100,000 persons aged 50 or older.

Related Disorders Polymyalgia rheumatica and giant-cell arteritis occur in the same patient population, and often both are present in the same individual. See *Arteritis, Giant-Cell; Polymyositis/Dermatomyositis.*

Treatment—Standard Nonsteroidal antiinflammatory drugs may be used for patients without vascular symptoms or signs. If those are not effective, low-to-moderate doses of prednisone up to 20 mg/day are used. In patients with cranial symptoms suggestive of giant-cell arteritis, high-dose corticosteroids, particularly prednisone, are given. Rapid improvement in symptoms of polymyalgia rheumatica usually results within a few days after beginning prednisone. After symptoms resolve, the gradual reduction in dosage for maintenance at a rate of 10 percent per month over months is begun. Occasionally, patients require treatment for several years. Side effects of prednisone must be carefully monitored, with further reduction in dosage or even discontinuation if side effects persist.

Treatment—Investigational Please contact the agencies listed under Resources, below, for the most current information.

Resources
For more information on polymyalgia rheumatica: National Organization for Rare Disorders (NORD); Arthritis Foundation; The National Arthritis and Musculoskeletal and Skin Diseases Information Clearinghouse.

References
Textbook of Rheumatology, 3rd ed.: W.N. Kelley, et al.; W.B. Saunders Company, 1989, pp. 1200–1208.

POLYMYOSITIS/DERMATOMYOSITIS

Description Polymyositis is marked by inflammatory and degenerative changes in the muscle fibers and the supporting collagen connective tissue, resulting in muscle weakness.

Dermatomyositis is identical to polymyositis, but with the addition of a characteristic rash.

In childhood, dermatomyositis is more common than polymyositis alone.

Signs and Symptoms Typically, muscle weakness has an insidious onset, occurring primarily in the neck, trunk, and proximal extremities. The hands, feet, and facial muscles usually escape involvement. Eventually, it becomes difficult for the patient to rise from a sitting position, climb stairs, lift objects, or reach overhead. Late in the chronic stage, muscle atrophy and contractures of the extremities may develop. Occasionally, joint pain and tenderness are present. In about one-third of patients, the polyarthralgia may be accompanied by swelling and other signs of nondeforming arthritis.

Interstitial pneumonitis, manifested by dyspnea and coughing, may be an early symptom. Raynaud's phenomenon is usually limited to the fingers, and does not always occur. Numb and shiny red areas around and under the nailbeds may also appear.

Gastrointestinal involvement is essentially confined to the upper esophagus; the pharynx is involved as well. Dysphagia is a common symptom and may result in aspiration pneumonia. Abdominal symptoms, most often seen in children with juvenile dermatomyositis, include melena and hematemesis arising from gastrointestinal ulcerations.

Cardiac irregularities evident on electrocardiogram have been reported, as has acute renal failure due to excess muscle protein (myoglobin) in the urine during rhabdomyolysis. Associated malignancy, usually carcinoma, occurs in about 15 percent of patients aged 45 and over with new-onset polymyositis.

In **dermatomyositis,** cutaneous lesions may appear before muscle involvement. There may be periorbital edema, a patchy facial erythema, and erythematous dermatitis over the extensor surfaces of the joints, particularly the hands. The lesions usually fade completely, leaving a brownish pigmentation, atrophy, or vitiligo. In some patients, cutaneous changes are similar to scleroderma, especially the distribution of subcutaneous calcification seen in children. Particularly in untreated patients, the calcinosis universalis tends to be more comprehensive than in scleroderma.

Etiology The cause is not known. Immunologic mechanisms and a genetic influence have been suggested. Viral infections and toxoplasmosis have also been implicated.

Epidemiology Polymyositis and dermatomyositis may appear at any age, although 60 percent of cases occur between the ages of 30 and 60. Females are affected twice as often as males.

Childhood dermatomyositis occurs most often between 5 and 15 years of age. Dermatomyositis in adults aged 45 and above is more commonly associated with malignancy than is polymyositis.

Treatment—Standard Initial treatment is with high-dose corticosteroids such as prednisone. Muscle enzyme activity (i.e., creatine phosphokinase levels) is measured to gauge treatment effectiveness. Generally, the enzymes return to normal ranges within 6 to 12 weeks, followed by increased muscular strength. At that time, corticosteroid dosage can be gradually reduced. However, in some cases of adult polymyositis, there is either a poor response to prednisone or a need for indefinitely prolonged treatment with prednisone. In such instances, the immunosuppressive drugs methotrexate and azathioprine have been beneficial for those failing to respond to corticosteroids.

Surgical intervention is required if gastrointestinal perforation occurs.

In patients with dermatomyositis, antimalarials (e.g., hydroxychloroquine) may be helpful for control of skin rash.

Treatment—Investigational At the NIH, cyclophosphamide in combination with mesna is being tested in severely afflicted patients who are unresponsive to steroid therapy. Other investigational protocols involve the use of cyclosporine. Efficacy has not yet been determined for either of these approaches.

Please contact the agencies listed under Resources, below, for the most current information.

Resources

For more information on polymyositis and dermatomyositis: National Organization for Rare Disorders (NORD); The National Arthritis and Musculoskeletal and Skin Diseases Information Clearinghouse; Arthritis Foundation; The National Support Group for Dermatomyositis.

References
Arthritis and Allied Conditions, 11th ed.: D.J. McCarty; Lea & Febiger, 1989, pp. 1092–1117.
Textbook of Rheumatology, 3rd ed.: W.N. Kelley, et al.; W.B. Saunders Company, 1989, pp. 1265–1273, 1274–1275.

PSORIATIC ARTHRITIS

Description Psoriatic arthritis is an arthritic condition that is associated with psoriasis of the skin and/or nails and a negative test for rheumatoid factor (RF).

Synonyms
> Arthropathic Psoriasis
> Psoriatic Spondyloarthritis

Signs and Symptoms The characteristic symptoms are inflammation of the joints and surrounding tissues accompanied by psoriasis of the nails and psoriatic plaques on the scalp, elbows, knees, and lower spine. The psoriasis usually precedes joint involvement (80 percent of cases); in 20 percent of cases the joint involvement appears first.

The psoriasis is seen as erythematous, silvery-gray, sharply demarcated spots or plaques that usually appear on the scalp, behind the ears, on the elbows and knees, and on the skin over the sacrum.

The joints most commonly affected are the distal interphalangeal **(DIP)** joints of the hands and feet, as well as the wrists, knees, and ankles. Rheumatoid nodules are not present. Exacerbations and remissions tend to occur, as in patients with rheumatoid arthritis **(RA);** however, progression to chronic arthritis and severe deformities is less common than in patients with RA.

There are 5 clinical subtypes of psoriatic arthritis: 1) "classical," with involvement limited to the DIP joints of the hands and feet; 2) an asymmetric oligoarthritis usually involving knees, ankles, wrists, and feet; 3) a symmetric polyarthritis resembling RA; 4) an axial arthritis (ankylosing spondylitis) usually involving sacroiliac joints and lumbar and cervical spine; and 5) arthritis mutilans.

X-rays show DIP joint involvement. Destruction of large and small joints may occur with joint fusion. Laboratory findings reveal the presence of HLA-B27 antigen in the blood of most patients with psoriatic arthritis with axial involvement.

Patients with inflammatory polyarthritis testing negative for rheumatoid factor should be examined for undetected or minimal psoriasis.

Etiology The cause is unknown.

Epidemiology Between 5 to 30 percent of patients with psoriasis have psoriatic arthritis. The disorder is more common in women and usually first appears between the ages of 20 and 30 years. However, onset can occur at any age.

Related Disorders The clinical symptoms of psoriatic arthritis are similar to a variety of diseases and syndromes. See *Reiter's Syndrome.* **Rheumatoid arthritis (RA)** is characterized by symmetric joint inflammation. The skin is not involved. **Acute gouty arthritis** attacks are accompanied by great pain; the big toe is a frequent site. The disorder usually is self-limiting and lasts, untreated, about 1 to 2 weeks.

Treatment—Standard Treatment is similar to that of RA (including rest, joint protection, appropriate exercises), but with some significant differences. All patients should be treated with nonsteroidal antiinflammatory drugs (NSAIDs). The most effective NSAIDs for patients with psoriatic arthritis include diclofenac, sulindac, tolmetin, and indomethacin.

The cutaneous lesions of psoriatic arthritis are treated as for psoriasis.

Use of antimalarial medications is generally discouraged.

For severely affected patients, folic acid antagonists and immunosuppressive drugs, particularly methotrexate, have been effective in relieving psoriatic lesions and joint inflammation in patients; *meticulous care should be exercised in the use of methotrexate because of its potential toxicity.* Physical and occupational therapy, tailored for the individual patient, should be encouraged. Patients who fail to respond to NSAIDs alone should be referred to a rheumatologist for further treatment.

Treatment—Investigational Please contact the agencies listed under Resources, below, for the most current information.

Resources

For more information on psoriatic arthritis: National Organization for Rare Disorders (NORD); National Psoriasis Foundation; Psoriasis Research Association; Arthritis Foundation; The National Arthritis and Musculoskeletal and Skin Diseases Information Clearinghouse.

References
Arthritis and Allied Conditions, 11th ed.: D.J. McCarty; Lea & Febiger, 1989, pp. 954–971.
Cecil Textbook of Medicine, 18th ed.: J.B. Wyngaarden and L.H. Smith, Jr., eds.; W.B. Saunders Company, 1988, p. 2327.

RAYNAUD'S DISEASE AND PHENOMENON

Description Raynaud's disease, characterized by episodes of vasospasm in the fingers and skin, is considered to be the benign primary form of **Raynaud's phenomenon,** which occurs in association with systemic disorders.

Synonyms
Raynaud's Syndrome

Signs and Symptoms Usually sequential phases of pallor, cyanosis, and rubor are seen, but a dramatic stark white pallor of the affected fingers and toes may be the only element of the triad to occur. The initial pallor may be the result of vasospasm of the digital arteries or arterioles; cyanosis is probably due to stasis in affected venules and capillaries; and after a time, ranging from minutes to hours, hyperemia causes a striking rubor.

Initially, only 1 or 2 fingertips may be involved. As the disorder progresses, all the fingers in their entirety, except the thumbs, may be affected. Symptoms vary and may include feelings of numbness or cold, severe aching or pain, tingling or throbbing, a sensation of tightness, pins and needles, and severe paresthesias. Over an extended period of time, trophic changes may occur, and severe cases may develop fingertip ulcerations or gangrene. Sometimes progression is more rapid.

The possibility of associated disease should be explored, e.g., systemic lupus erythematosus, systemic sclerosis, and other connective tissue diseases. Differential diagnosis should rule out other causes of digital ischemia such as frostbite, vibration-induced trauma, atherosclerotic or Buerger's disease, and cervical rib syndrome. Unilateral symptoms are likely to be a different entity. If patients present with single limb involvement, structural arterial disease of that limb should be investigated.

Etiology The cause is uncertain. There is discussion as to whether sympathetic nervous system hyperactivity or local arterial abnormalities are the explanation for the clinical findings. Genetic inheritance has not been ruled out. Precipitating factors include stress and exposure to cold.

Epidemiology Women, especially those 30 years and older, are the largest segment of affected population. Recent studies suggest that up to 5 percent of women may have Raynaud's disease.

Related Disorders Raynaud's phenomenon may be an early presenting symptom of several diseases and disorders. See *Scleroderma; Systemic Lupus Erythematosus; Mixed Connective Tissue Disease; Polymyositis/Dermatomyositis.* Digital pain is also seen in Fabry disease and carpal tunnel syndrome (see *Fabry Disease; Carpal Tunnel Syndrome).* Other associated conditions include some manifestations of vasculitis, neurogenic lesions, drug intoxications with ergot and methysergide, dysproteinemias, myxedema, and primary pulmonary hypertension.

Treatment—Standard Basic management includes avoidance of exposure to cold and of other vasoconstrictive factors such as smoking and certain drugs. An alpha-adrenoceptor blocker (e.g., prazosin) or a calcium blocker (e.g., nifedipine) may be beneficial. Biofeedback has been useful in some instances.

Any underlying disorder of Raynaud's phenomenon must be diagnosed and treated. Sympathectomy is generally more effective for patients with Raynaud's disease who do not respond to other therapies, than for those with Raynaud's phenomenon.

Treatment—Investigational Ketanserin, a serotonin antagonist manufactured by Janssen Pharmaceutica Inc., is being investigated for digital vascular symptoms of Raynaud's disease.

An orphan drug, iloprose, manufactured by Berlex Laboratories, Inc., is being studied for the treatment of Raynaud's phenomenon with digital ulcers when it occurs with scleroderma.

Captopril (Bristol-Myers Squibb) and thymoxamine (Parke-Davis) are being tested for treating Raynaud's disease.

Please contact the agencies listed under Resources, below, for the most current information.

Resources

For more information on Raynaud's disease and phenomenon: National Organization for Rare Disorders (NORD); NIH/National Heart, Lung, and Blood Institute; The Raynaud's Association Trust; Scleroderma Society; American Heart Association.

References

Mendelian Inheritance in Man, 9th ed.: V.A. McKusick; The Johns Hopkins University Press, 1990, p. 825.

Internal Medicine, 3rd ed.: J.H. Stein, ed.-in-chief; Little, Brown and Company, 1990, p. 223.

Cecil Textbook of Medicine, 18th ed.: J.B. Wyngaarden and L.H. Smith, Jr., eds.; W.B. Saunders Company, 1988, pp. 369, 375–377.

REITER'S SYNDROME

Description Reiter's syndrome (one form of **reactive arthritis**) is characterized by a triad of arthritis, nongonococcal urethritis, and conjunctivitis, and by lesions of the skin and mucosal surfaces. An enteric initiating component has been recognized in some patients. Symptoms may not appear simultaneously; they may alternate, and there may be spontaneous remissions and recurrences.

Synonyms

Feissinger-Leroy-Reiter's Syndrome

Signs and Symptoms Although the initial symptoms are urethritis or enteritis, with arthritis and other symptoms appearing 4 days to 4 weeks later, the patient may not request help from the physician until the arthritis appears. The initial symptoms may be revealed only after some questioning, either because the patient did not make the connection or was embarrassed.

The initial urethritis may be painful, and a purulent discharge and hematuria may be present. Cultures of the genitourinary discharge do not reveal *Neisseria gonorrhoeae* but may demonstrate *Chlamydia* organisms. The enteric organisms involved are discussed below.

Arthritis usually begins abruptly, affects more than one joint, and is asymmetric. Joints of the legs and feet are involved most often; small joints of the hands are almost never affected. Joints are warm, red, swollen, and painful. Although episodes of arthritis usually last at least 2 to 4 months, symptoms may begin to subside within 2 to 6 weeks. Remission in the setting of treatment often occurs within the first year, but some attacks last several years. In such cases, the involved joints may be permanently damaged.

Extraarticular musculoskeletal findings include tendinitis (often involving the Achilles tendon), plantar fasciitis resulting in pain at the bottom of the heel, dactylitis (sausage toes), and a diffuse enthesitis involving insertions of tendons to bone. Ankylosing spondylitis develops in 10 to 20 percent of patients with sacroiliac and lumbar spine involvement.

Conjunctivitis is most often mild and bilateral, lasting a few days; however, it often recurs. Occasionally, the uvea also becomes inflamed (uveitis or iritis), with symptoms of increased sensitivity to light (photophobia); glaucoma, cataracts, and blindness may rarely develop in severe cases (approximately 5 percent).

Mucocutaneous vesicular lesions develop on the glans penis, palmar surfaces, and soles of the feet, and in the mouth, urethra, and bladder. They become eroded and erythematous but cause little pain and resolve quickly. The lesions of **keratoderma blennorrhagica,** found on the hands, arms, and trunk, are scaly and crusty and resemble pustular psoriasis, eventually peeling off. The fingernails also become brittle, thick, and opaque.

Rarely, patients develop cardiac abnormalities, including an incompetent aortic valve and cardiac conduction defects.

Laboratory findings include anemia, elevated levels of white blood cells in the blood and synovial fluids, and an elevated erythrocyte sedimentation rate. Tests for rheumatoid factor are negative. HLA-B27 is found in two-thirds to three-quarters of patients.

Etiology The precipitating event for sexually acquired Reiter's syndrome is urethritis from *Chlamydia trachomatis* or *Ureaplasma urealyticum.* Infectious agents causing enteric reactive arthritis include *Shigella flexneri,* salmonella, yersinia, and campylobacter. The HLA-B27 antigen is a predisposing factor. Recently, Reiter's syndrome has been recognized to occur in men with symptomatic HIV infection and AIDS, probably because of their increased risk of exposure to the above organisms.

Epidemiology Sexually acquired Reiter's syndrome is seen almost exclusively in males between 20 to 40 years of age. Enteric reactive arthritis is seen equally in males and females, and occasionally in children.

Related Disorders Reiter's syndrome may be mimicked by arthritis with coexistent gonorrheal urethritis. Behçet syndrome has symptoms of oral and genital lesions, uveitis, and arthritis, but they are distinctly different from those of Reiter's syndrome.

Treatment—Standard Treatment is symptomatic. Nonsteroidal antiinflammatory drugs (NSAIDs) such as indomethacin, diclofenac, tolmetin, sulindac, or phenylbutazone usually relieve the arthritis. In severe cases, folic acid antagonists such as methotrexate may relieve joint inflammation. *Methotrexate must be used with caution because of its potential toxicity.* Physical therapy may be useful during recovery from arthritis.

Urethritis should be treated with tetracycline. An appropriate antibiotic can be used to treat the enteric pathogens.

Treatment—Investigational Please contact the agencies listed under Resources, below, for the most current information.

Resources

For more information on Reiter's syndrome: National Organization for

Rare Disorders (NORD); The Arthritis Foundation; The National Arthritis and Musculoskeletal and Skin Diseases Information Clearinghouse.

References
Arthritis and Allied Conditions, 11th ed.: D.J. McCarty; Lea & Febiger, 1989, pp. 944–953.

RELAPSING POLYCHRONDRITIS

Description Relapsing polychondritis is a clinical syndrome characterized by inflammation and degeneration of the body's cartilaginous framework. Included are the nose, ears, joints, and the laryngotracheobronchial tree. Occasionally, the aortic valve is affected.

Signs and Symptoms The course is marked by exacerbations and remissions. Fever and leukocytosis may be present. Episcleritis is a common symptom.

In one or both ears, pain, tenderness, and swelling of the cartilage may occur suddenly and then spread to the fleshy portion of the outer ear. Cartilaginous destruction may follow recurrences, leaving the ears with a drooping appearance. Middle ear inflammation is likely to lead to eustachian tube obstruction, and recurrent attacks may cause hearing loss. Attacks vary in severity and in duration, lasting from days to weeks.

Joint involvement may range from mild arthralgia to severe synovitis.

Two-thirds of patients develop nasal chondritis. Again, recurrent episodes may lead to cartilage destruction and collapse of the nasal bridge, resulting in nasal congestion and a saddlenose deformity.

Collapse of the tracheal or bronchial wall may lead to speech difficulties, respiratory complications, and even death. In rare instances, heart valve abnormalities and kidney inflammation and dysfunction develop.

Etiology The cause is unknown; an immunologic mechanism is suspected.

Epidemiology The illness occurs equally in both sexes, usually from 40 to 60 years of age. All races are affected, but the syndrome predominantly affects whites.

Treatment—Standard Treatment usually is with nonsteroidal antiinflammatory drugs (NSAIDs) and corticosteroids. In severe cases, azathioprine, cyclophosphamide, and 6-mercaptopurine have been found to be useful immunosuppressants. The most severe cases may require heart valve replacement or a tracheostomy.

Treatment—Investigational Some cases may remit after use of the immunosuppressant, cyclosporine-A. Continued research is necessary to fully evaluate the safety and effectiveness of this treatment.

Please contact the agencies listed under Resources, below, for the most current information.

Resources
    For more information on relapsing polychrondritis: National Organization

for Rare Disorders (NORD); Arthritis Foundation; NIH/National Institute of Arthritis, Musculoskeletal and Skin (NIAMS) Information Clearinghouse; Polychrondritis and Rheumatoid Arthritis Clinic, Beth Israel Hospital.

References

Textbook of Rheumatology, 3rd ed.: W.N. Kelley, et al.; W.B. Saunders Company, 1989, pp. 1513–1521.

Cardiac Involvement in Relapsing Polychondritis: A. Balsa-Criado, et al.; J. Int. Cardiol., March 1987, issue 14(3), pp. 381–383.

Relapsing Polychondritis. Survival and Predictive Role of Early Disease Manifestations: C.J. Michet, et al.; Ann. Int. Med., January 1986, issue 104(1), pp. 74–78.

Pulmonary Function in Relapsing Polychondritis: W.S. Krell, et al.; Am. Rev. Respir. Dis., June 1986, issue 133(6), pp. 1120–1123.

SCLERODERMA

Description Scleroderma is a connective tissue disorder characterized by skin thickening, Raynaud's phenomenon, and a spectrum of systemic disorders.

Synonyms
> CREST Syndrome
> Dermatosclerosis
> Systemic Sclerosis

Signs and Symptoms Clinical manifestations in early stages vary considerably, and the classical cutaneous lesions may appear later. Arthralgia, morning stiffness, fatigue, and weight loss are common features. Raynaud's phenomenon is an early and frequent complaint (see *CREST syndrome,* below).

Leathery indurations of the skin are widespread and symmetrical, succeeded by atrophy and pigmentation. **Morphea,** seen usually between ages 20 to 50 years, begins with an inflammatory stage. Firm, hard, oval-shaped plaques with ivory centers and encircled by a violet ring on the trunk, face, and extremities follow the first stage. Many patients improve spontaneously. Generalized morphea is more rare and serious, and involves the dermis but not the internal organs. **Linear scleroderma** appears as a band-like thickening of skin on the arm or leg. It is most likely to be unilateral but may be bilateral. Generally surfacing in young children, the first sign is failure of one limb to grow as rapidly as its counterpart. The band may extend from the hip to heel or shoulder to hand, and have a loss of deep tissue.

Systemic manifestations of scleroderma encompass a wide range of disturbances, including inflammatory myopathy (see *Polymyositis/Dermatomyositis);* edema of the fingers and hands; and microvascular, pulmonary (progressive interstitial fibrotic lung disease), renal (rapidly progressive renal failure), cardiovascular (myocardial accelerated hypertension), gastrointestinal (esophageal and colonic dysmotility), and immunologic abnormalities.

CREST syndrome is an acronym for **c**alcinosis, **R**aynaud's phenomenon, **e**sophageal dysfunction, **s**clerodactyly and **t**elangiectasia. Calcium salts accumulate subcutaneously and in many organs. Raynaud's phenomenon affects symmetrical digits, and may lead to digital ulcers and autoamputation. Dysfunction of the lower esophagus results in acid reflux and esophageal scarring; strictures may occur. Loss of peristalsis in the small intestine causes malabsorption and increased bacterial growth. Sclerodactyly results in decreased function of the fingers and toes. Telangiectasia, while not debilitating, are unsightly. Patients with the CREST syndrome are at increased risk of developing pulmonary hypertension.

Etiology The cause is unknown. The immune and vascular systems and connective tissue metabolism are known to play some part in the disease process.

Epidemiology It is estimated that between 50,000 and 100,000 persons are presently affected with scleroderma in the United States. The disease is 3 to 4 times more common in women than men. All ages are susceptible, but onset is highest in midlife.

Related Disorders See *Mixed Connective Tissue Disease; Systemic Lupus Erythematosus; Polymyositis/Dermatomyositis.*

Treatment—Standard Treatment is supportive and symptomatic. Fibrosis of the skin and internal organs is treated with D-penicillamine. Other skin care includes lubricating creams and antibiotic ointments for ulcerations. If Raynaud's phenomenon is present, nifedipine, diltiazem, verapamil, and/or prazosin may be useful. Rarely, calcinosis requires surgical intervention. For arthralgia or arthritis, nonsteroidal antiinflammatory agents are generally given, although some patients may require low-dose corticosteroids.

Symptomatic management of pulmonary hypertension involves supplemental oxygen. The treatment of choice for renal involvement and hypertension is captopril and enalapril. Nifedipine and dipyridamole may be tried when myocardial perfusion abnormalities are present. Nonsteroidal antiinflammatory drugs and corticosteroids are used to treat the symptoms of pericarditis.

When the esophagus and gastrointestinal tract are inflamed or ulcerated, treatment of choice is H_2 blockers such as cimetidine or ranitidine; omeprazole may also be used. Metoclopramide has been found to be beneficial for dysmotility. Acid reflux can be partially controlled by dietary measures. Several small and frequent meals per day lighten the work of the gastrointestinal system. Sitting upright for at least 2 hours after eating aids digestion.

Treatment—Investigational Several experimental treatments are currently being evaluated. Early steps in the cellular synthesis of excess collagen have been blocked by retinoids for some types of scleroderma. Recombinant gamma-interferon has been shown to inhibit oversynthesis of collagen. Ketanserin, a serotonin antagonist, may be successful for treating Raynaud's phenomenon. Cyclosporine has potential in the treatment of dermatologic disorders, including those seen in collagen vascular diseases. Chlorambucil and photophoresis are also being evaluated for effectiveness.

Please contact the agencies listed under Resources, below, for the most current information.

Resources
   For more information on scleroderma: National Organization for Rare Disorders (NORD); United Scleroderma Foundation, Inc.; Scleroderma Society; Scleroderma Research Foundation; Scleroderma Information Exchange, Inc.; The National Arthritis and Musculoskeletal and Skin Diseases Information Clearinghouse.

References
   Textbook of Rheumatology, 3rd ed.: W.N. Kelley, et al.; W.B. Saunders Company, 1989, pp. 1215–1244.
   Arthritis and Allied Conditions, 11th ed.: D.J. McCarty; Lea & Febiger, 1989, pp. 460–461, 1142–1144.

SJÖGREN'S SYNDROME (SjS)

Description Sjögren's syndrome, an autoimmune disorder characterized by degeneration of the mucous-secreting glands, particularly the lacrimal and salivary glands, is also associated with rheumatic disorders such as rheumatoid arthritis.

Synonyms
   Keratoconjunctivitis Sicca
   Sicca Syndrome

Signs and Symptoms Primary SjS is characterized solely by keratoconjunctivitis sicca and xerostemia. In **secondary SjS,** keratoconjunctivitis sicca and/or xerostomia occur in the setting of a connective tissue disease, most often rheumatoid arthritis **(RA).**

   Most patients with Sjögren's syndrome have primary SjS. Symptoms onset is insidious. Decreased production of saliva and consequent dry mouth make chewing and swallowing food difficult. The lack of saliva causes particles of food to stick to the cheeks, gums, and throat. Teeth decay easily, leading to dental caries, gingivitis, and pyorrhea.

   As the lacrimal glands atrophy, tears decrease, causing keratoconjunctivitis sicca and leaving the patient with a feeling of grittiness and burning in the eyes. The eyelids may stick together.

   Dryness may extend to the skin and to the mucous membranes of the nose, throat, and vagina.

   In secondary SjS, patients may experience arthritis, rash (palpable purpura on the lower extremities, photosensitive dermatitis on the face, arms, and other sun-exposed areas), fever, and neurologic involvement. The latter may involve seizures, psychosis, dementia, and stroke-like syndromes. Patients with systemic disease usually have positive blood tests for antinuclear antibodies and antibodies to Ro and La antigens.

   A number of tests are available for the diagnosis of SjS: 1) Eye examination, including Schirmer's test (measurement of tear production) and rose bengal staining (looking for keratitis); 2) Measurement of saliva production after stimulation with lemon juice; 3) Examination of cells from the lip (minor salivary gland biopsy) to determine whether lymphocytes are present in the salivary glands; and 4) Blood tests, including ANA (anti-nuclear antibody) and anti-Ro and anti-La antibodies.

All patients suspected of having SjS should be examined by an ophthalmologist. Patients with SjS who have positive blood tests for anti-Ro antibodies should be evaluated by a rheumatologist for evidence of extraglandular involvement.

Etiology The cause is unknown. Sjögren's syndrome is an autoimmune disorder that is known to have a genetic predisposition (HLA-DR3) and often occurs in patients with rheumatoid arthritis, systemic lupus erythematosus, and other connective tissue diseases.

Epidemiology The syndrome affects 9 females to every male. Ninety percent of persons with the disorder are postmenopausal women, although symptoms may be apparent at an earlier age. Recent data suggest that men with symptomatic HIV infection may develop a syndrome similar to Sjögren's.

Related Disorders See *Systemic Lupus Erythematosus.*

Rheumatoid arthritis (RA), an inflammatory autoimmune disorder of unknown etiology, is characterized by morning stiffness and polyarthritis (chiefly the hands, wrists, knees, feet, shoulders, and hips). Once affected, a joint may remain painful and swollen for weeks, months, and even years. About 25 percent of RA patients also have SjS.

Treatment—Standard Treatment depends on symptoms. No specific therapy, however, presently restores glandular secretion.

Ocular symptoms may be relieved by the use of artificial tears and lubricating creams at bedtime.

For oral symptoms, artificial saliva can be used to wet the mouth. Patients may benefit from chewing sugarless gum or using sugarless hard candies.

Systemic medication such as corticosteroids and hydroxychloroquine and other immunosuppressive agents are occasionally needed for certain complications (the extraglandular features described above).

All patients should be routinely checked by ophthalmologists and dentists. Patients with extraglandular features should be under the care of rheumatologists.

Treatment—Investigational The National Institute of Dental Research (NIDR) is conducting studies on several drugs for treatment of SjS. For more information, please contact Alice Macynski, R.N., NIDR, 9000 Rockville Pike, Building 10, Room 1B-21, Bethesda, Maryland 20892, (301) 496-4371.

Bromhexine is an orphan drug being tested as a treatment for mild-to-moderate keratoconjunctivitis sicca. It is manufactured by Boehringer Ingelheim Pharmaceuticals, Inc.

Please contact the agencies listed under Resources, below, for the most current information.

Resources

For more information on Sjögren's syndrome: National Organization for

Rare Disorders (NORD); Sjögren's Syndrome Foundation; National Sjögren's Syndrome Association; The Arthritis Foundation; NIH/National Institute of Dental Research (NIDR); NIH/National Arthritis and Musculoskeletal and Skin Diseases Information Clearinghouse.

References
Cecil Textbook of Medicine, 18th ed.: J.B. Wyngaarden and L.H. Smith, Jr., eds.: W.B. Saunders Company, 1988, pp. 2024–2025.

SYSTEMIC LUPUS ERYTHEMATOSUS (SLE)

Description Systemic lupus erythematosus is a multisystem inflammatory disease of connective tissue involving immunologically mediated tissue injury. Many abnormalities are associated.

Synonyms
Disseminated Lupus Erythematosus

Signs and Symptoms Fatigue is an early and frequent feature. Other constitutional symptoms include fever, swollen glands, anorexia, weight loss, headaches, alopecia, and edema.

Arthritis, arthralgia, and myalgia occur in over 90 percent of patients, in some cases preceding the onset of systemic disease by months or years. The arthritis is often migratory, is symmetric, and occurs most often in the knees and finger and wrist joints. Joint involvement is usually nonerosive.

Dermatologic manifestations occur in over 80 percent of patients. Photosensitive lesions include both annular, discoid lesions and bullae. The classic erythematous butterfly rash across the bridge of the nose and cheeks appears in about 50 percent of patients, often lasting hours or days. Lesions of the mucous membranes occur in about 35 percent of patients.

Vascular involvement includes telangiectasia, Raynaud's phenomenon, and vasculitis. Pulmonary involvement includes pleurisy, cough, and pneumonitis. Cardiovascular abnormalities include pericarditis, myocarditis, and coronary artery disease. Hematologic abnormalities include anemia, leukopenia, lymphocytopenia, and thrombocytopenia in addition to the lymphadenopathy often seen early in the disease.

Renal abnormalities associated with SLE include proteinuria, interstitial nephritis, and diffuse proliferative and membranous glomerulonephritis. Neuropsychiatric symptoms include depression, anxiety, psychosis, seizures, stroke, neuropathy, and meningitis.

Tentative diagnosis can be made if 4 of the following criteria are present (using the ARA Revised Criteria for the Classification of SLE): arthritis involving 2 or more joints; malar rash; discoid rash; oral or nasal ulcers; photosensitivity; pleuritis or pericarditis; positive LE cell test, presence of anti-DNA or anti-Sm, or a chronic false-positive serologic test for syphilis; proteinuria over 0.5 g/day, cellular casts in the urine; seizures or psychosis; hemolytic anemia, leukopenia, lymphopenia, or thrombocytopenia; and an abnormal antinuclear antibody titer.

The SLE patient may experience 1 or 2 exacerbations (flares) of symptoms a year, which can be triggered by such factors as stress, infections, and exposure to sunlight.

Etiology The cause is still unknown. Immunologic, genetic, environmental, hormonal, and infectious factors have all been implicated.

SLE-like symptoms have also been induced by some drugs, including hydralazine, procainamide, isoniazid, methyldopa, and chlorpromazine.

Epidemiology Ninety percent of SLE cases occur in women, at any age, although the peak incidence is between 15 and 55 years. Black women are affected 3 times as often as white women, and the disorder also is commonly seen in Chinese women. Estimates of the prevalence in the United States vary considerably; however, most reliable estimates are about 50:100,000.

Related Disorders See *Scleroderma; Polymyositis/Dermatomyositis; Polyarteritis Nodosa; Hashimoto Syndrome; Sjögren Syndrome; Raynaud's Disease and Phenomenon; Purpura, Thrombotic Thrombocytopenic.*

Treatment—Standard Symptoms such as joint pain and fever commonly respond to aspirin or other nonsteroidal antiinflammatory agents. Anti-malarial drugs (hydroxychloroquine and chloroquine) treat skin lesions effectively, although side effects such as visual disturbances and nausea may occur during prolonged treatment. Standard treatment for more severe manifestations of SLE is corticosteroid therapy; in particular, high dosages of prednisone or its equivalent. Initial treatment and maintenance dosages vary according to organ system involvement, response, side effects, and duration of use. Corticosteroid creams and lotions effectively control rashes and skin irritation, but should be used with caution on the face and in the presence of skin infection. Since infections are a leading cause of death in SLE patients, their management should be aggressive.

Treatment—Investigational Although immunosuppressive treatment has been in use for several years, it is still considered experimental. It is thought that suppression of the immune system will also suppress the formation of harmful immune complexes appearing to cause widespread organ and tissue destruction. Unfortunately, such therapy increases the risk of infections. Drugs used with the corticosteroids are cyclophosphamide or azathioprine.

Other investigational management includes the use of corticosteroids via intravenous bolus ("pulse steroids"), and attempts to physically remove the immune complexes from the circulation by plasmapheresis or lymphoplasmapheresis.

Researchers studying cyclophosphamide, also used in the therapy of some malignancies, are treating patients with lupus nephritis as well as some severe cases of CNS lupus that do not respond to steroids, with intravenous boluses of cyclophosphamide given at 4-week intervals. Side effects and longterm efficacy are still under investigation.

Please contact the agencies listed under Resources, below, for the most current information.

Resources
For more information on SLE: National Organization for Rare Disorders, Inc. (NORD); Lupus Foundation of America, Inc.; Systemic Lupus Erythematosus Foundation, Inc.; National Lupus Foundation; The National Arthritis and Musculoskeletal and Skin Diseases Information Clearinghouse.

References
Textbook of Rheumatology, 3rd ed.: W.N. Kelley, et al.; W.B. Saunders Company, 1989, pp. 1101–1146.
Arthritis and Allied Conditions, 11th ed.: D.J. McCarty; Lea & Febiger, 1989, pp. 1022–1079.

TIETZE'S SYNDROME

Description Tietze's syndrome affects the upper costal cartilages, usually the 2nd, with tenderness, pain, and swelling.

Synonyms
Costochondritis

Signs and Symptoms Pain, tenderness, and fusiform or spindle-shaped swelling occur in one or more of the 4 upper ribs. The tenderness and swelling are localized. The pain may have a sudden or gradual onset, and may be mild or severe, dull or sharp, gripping, or neuralgic in nature. Sudden coughing or deep breathing accentuates the pain, and often precedes the swelling. The pain typically diminishes after a few weeks or months, but the swelling may persist.

Etiology The cause is unknown.

Epidemiology The syndrome usually affects older children and young adults. Males and females are affected in equal numbers.

Related Disorders Benign and malignant tumors and **angina pectoris** may mimic this syndrome.

Spinal root lesions or compression may cause chest pain similar to that seen in Tietze's syndrome. The pain develops after sudden movement of the body such as straining, coughing, sneezing, or laughing.

Chest wall pain is a broad term given to several conditions characterized by noncardiac anterior chest wall pain. A dull, aching pain results after straining, poor posture, or inflammation or infiltration of the chest muscles, ligaments, or cartilage. Chest wall pain may also arise from irritation of a nerve root in the upper spine or neck, or a fractured rib. Tietze's syndrome is included in this group of ailments.

Costal chondritis (costochondritis), inflammation of rib cartilage, is characterized by pain, sometimes radiating, of the chest wall that may be similar to that of Tietze's syndrome. However, the swelling seen in Tietze's is absent.

Treatment—Standard Treatment consists of local heat and antiinflammatory or analgesic medication. Usually the pain subsides after a few weeks or months.

Swelling may remain for a longer period of time.

Treatment—Investigational Please contact the agencies listed under Resources, below, for the most current information.

Resources

For more information about Tietze's syndrome: National Organization for Rare Disorders (NORD); National Arthritis, Musculoskeletal and Skin (NIAMS) Information Clearinghouse.

References

Musculoskeletal Chest Wall Pain: A.G. Fam, et al.; J. Can. Med. Assn., September 1, 1985, issue 133(5), pp. 379–389.

Internal Medicine, 2nd ed.: J.H. Stein, ed.-in-chief; Little, Brown and Company, 1987, p. 610.

VASCULITIS

Description Vasculitis, a vascular inflammatory disorder, may occur alone or in conjunction with allergic and rheumatic diseases.

Synonyms

Angiitis

Signs and Symptoms Inflammation of the vascular walls constricts the blood vessels and may cause ischemia, necrosis, thrombosis, and, rarely, an aneurysm. Any size vessel and any part of the vascular system may be affected, with symptoms being localized or striking larger areas of the body. Vasculitis may be the primary disorder, or secondary to other disease processes.

Because of the varied situations in which vasculitis can arise, symptoms and signs are relative to the system involved. Nonspecific symptoms may include fever, headache, weight loss, anorexia, lethargy, and weakness. Abdominal pain and diarrhea, hypertension, renal failure, and joint and muscle pain may be present. Osteonecrosis can occur when blood flow has been obstructed to the bone.

Respiratory symptoms include sinusitis, rhinorrhea, asthma, hemoptysis, dyspnea, epistaxis, and pleuritis. Rarely, inflammation of the eye, blurred vision, and, in severe cases, blindness, can be present with ocular vasculitis. Dermal vasculitis may involve nodules, macules, or purpura on any area of the body, but typically on the back, hands, buttocks, the inner aspects of the forearms, and the lower extremities. The lesions may occur just once, or recur at regular intervals. They remain for several weeks, and leave darkened spots or scarring when the inflammation subsides. In some cases urticaria, vesicles, bullae, or frank ulcerations are present.

Specific diagnosis requires an extensive and specific history and physical examination, and usually an angiogram and/or a biopsy of the affected organ or tissue.

Etiology The diverse forms that vasculitis takes have many causes, some of which are autoimmune reactions, or allergic response or hypersensitivity to medications, toxins, or environmental irritants. Other types of vasculitis are the result of fungal, viral, or parasitic infections. In some cases, the etiology cannot be determined.

Epidemiology Men and women are affected equally, with the senior years being the predominant age group.

Related Disorders Vasculitis may be either a primary disorder (see *Polyarteritis Nodosa; Wegener Granulomatosis; Lymphomatoid Granulomatosis; Arteritis, Giant-Cell; Arteritis, Takayasu's; Goodpasture Syndrome; Kawasaki Syndrome; Schoenlein-Henoch Purpura; Buerger's Disease [Thromboangiitis Obliterans]; Churg-Strauss Syndrome)* or occur in association with another disease (see *Behçet's Syndrome; Systemic Lupus Erythematosus)*. **Rheumatoid arthritis** is also an example of a condition in which vasculitis is associated with an underlying disease.

Cutaneous (dermal) necrotizing vasculitis, a vascular inflammatory disease that also affects the skin, may occur alone or in conjunction with infectious, allergic, or rheumatic illnesses. Males and females are affected equally. Inflamed vessel walls and skin lesions appear primarily on the back, buttocks, interior forearms, hands, and lower extremities. The lesions may be nodular, macular, or purpural, and may persist for several weeks and leave darkened spots and scarring. Some lesions are annular. Ulcers, vesicles, or bullae are signs of greater severity. Malaise, fever, and muscle and joint pain may be present.

Disorders with similarities to cutaneous necrotizing vasculitis include cutaneous polyarteritis, hypersensitivity vasculitis, Schoenlein-Henoch purpura, Kawasaki syndrome, and lupus erythematosus.

The cause of cutaneous necrotizing vasculitis is uncertain. Allergic reaction or hypersensitivity to medications such as sulfa and penicillins, toxins, and inhaled environmental irritants may be involved. The disorder may be associated with fungal, parasitic, or viral infections. Some cases may involve autoimmune reactions to invasive organisms. Treatment must first identify and remove any possibly precipitating factors.

Treatment—Standards Medical management is directly related to the etiology and symptoms of the underlying disease. Prednisone is effective for autoimmune forms of cutaneous vasculitis. Corticosteroids should not be used in treating Kawasaki syndrome. Immunosuppressive medications should not be used in cutaneous vasculitis alone. Other treatment is supportive and symptomatic. (See chapters on specific types of vasculitis for treatment recommendations.)

Treatment—Investigational High-dose intravenous gamma-globulin is under study for some forms of vasculitis. Other research involves the use of cytotoxic agents and steroids. Plasmapheresis may be of some benefit. To date, none of these studies is conclusive.

Please contact the agencies listed under Resources, below, for the most current information.

Resources

For more information on vasculitis: National Organization for Rare Disorders (NORD); NIH/National Heart, Lung and Blood Institute.

References

Internal Medicine, 3rd ed.: J.H. Stein, ed.-in-chief; Little, Brown and Company, 1990, pp. 1746–1756.

Arthritis and Allied Conditions, 11th ed.: D.J. McCarty; Lea & Febiger, 1989, 1166–1188.

Diagnostic Studies for Systemic Necrotizing Vasculitis. Sensitivity, Specificity, and Predictive Value in Patients With Multisystem Disease: P.J. Dahlberg, et al.; Arch. of Int. Med., January 1989, issue 149(1), pp. 161–165.

Severe Leukocytoclastic Vasculitis of the Skin in a Patient With Essential Mixed Cryoglobulinemia Treated With High-Dose Gamma-Globulin Intravenously: B.W. Boom, et al.; Arch. Dermatol., October 1988, issue 124(10), p. 1550.

Vasculitis in Older Patients: Presentations and Significance: A. Montonaro; Geriatrics, March 1988, issue 43(3), pp. 75–76, 79–83, 86.

Urticarial Vasculitis Progressing to Systemic Lupus Erythematosus: E. Bisaccia, et al.; Arch. of Dermatol., July 1988, issue 124(7), pp. 1088–1090.

12 OPHTHALMOLOGIC DISORDERS
By Richard Alan Lewis, M.D., M.S.

The evaluation of a child with a visual disability or a developmental abnormality of the visual system must depend heavily on the diligence, the prudence, and the accuracy of the complete ophthalmologic evaluation. Unfortunately, some ophthalmologists focus intently on the eyes and ocular adnexa and disregard other obvious facial and cranial defects and other systemic dysmorphic features. Nonetheless, the ophthalmologist provides key information to the thorough evaluation of a dysmorphic individual, including a unique knowledge and analysis of visual embryology, of ocular and systemic pathology, of the natural history and prognosis of visual disorders, and of the burden of ocular diseases.

Primary physicians who must evaluate, diagnose, and manage children with craniofacial defects involving the visual system should befriend an ophthalmologist, perhaps a pediatric ophthalmologist, who has demonstrated devotion to thoroughness and accuracy and who is willing to explore the patient's immediate and extended family members for variable signs of hereditary disorders. Since many heritable diseases occur with predictable mendelian patterns of inheritance, the ophthalmologist must also acknowledge that his responsibility often extends beyond the individual patient and that he is obligated to search for other affected family members and to educate individuals at risk for the disorder or for bearing affected offspring.

As in all other realms of human genetics, the primary obligation of the ophthalmologist and primary physician is to establish a diagnosis. That diagnosis must be specific rather than symptomatic. A clinical diagnosis of "nystagmus" is not acceptable, since numerous defects in the development and organization of the central nervous system, the optic nerve, or the retina, let alone defects in the anterior segment of the globe, can result in nystagmus. Nystagmus is a sign, not a unique diagnosis. The primary physician should advise the ophthalmologist about other dysmorphic features with which visual handicaps appear to be associated.

As in other genetic disease, the evaluation of the proband may involve recovery of previous written records of the patient's evaluation, copies of personal or family photographs or paintings, prior neuro-imaging studies, fundus photographs and fluorescein angiograms, and the records of electrodiagnosis. Usually, the recovery of reports is *not* adequate, since, for example, neuroradiologists may attend cranial defects or anomalies of brain structure and ignore aberrations in the anterior visual pathways, orbit, or globes. The verbal report of a previously "normal computerized tomography **(CT)** scan" may change dramatically when one finds that the actual films demonstrate only normal intracranial contents and that no views record the anterior visual pathways and orbits. Additional studies, reconstructions, or, preferably, magnetic resonance imaging **(MRI)** scans, may be necessary to complete the diagnostic assessment.

The ascertainment and personal examination of at-risk relatives may also prove extremely important. Those examinations may include siblings (for recessive disorders) or both parents (for dominant or X-linked ones) for discovery of minor manifestations. Physicians may recover photographs to look for variable facial features, previous CT or MRI scans, pathology slides, and other biochemical or chromosomal studies. For example, the evaluation of children with congenital cataracts mandates the thorough examination of both parents for minor manifestations of autosomal dominant cataracts with variable expressivity. To counsel an adult in the reproductive age group about a childhood disorder, it may be necessary to recover documents to establish an historical diagnosis that the parents retain by memory. For example, I recently counseled a 21-year-old young woman who was a survivor of unilateral retinoblastoma. Recovery and review of the original histopathology slides established a diagnosis of persistent hyperplastic primary vitreous **(PHPV),** and showed no evidence of intraocular tumor. Nonetheless, the parents had believed firmly for 20 years that the enucleated eye had contained a malignant embryonal tumor. The recurrence risk for PHPV is extremely low, whereas the recurrence risk for retinoblastoma depends substantially on other clinical and genetic parameters!

The investigation of the family history must be meticulous. That family history should ascertain the parentage and may investigate consanguinity, incest, and non-paternity. Even in the absence of known consanguinity by descent, the geographic origin of the parents, particularly if not born in the United States, or the geographic proximity of their places of birth may imply consanguinity by geography even if language differences, lack of records, and verbal history fail to establish it.

The absence of a family history of a specific disorder does not exclude the possibility of affected individuals. In the presence of a disease that can be transmitted as an autosomal dominant trait, recall and examination of both parents is mandatory, to exclude minimal manifestations. A child with profound colobomatous microphthalmia and no "family history" may have a minimally affected parent with anterior stromal hypoplasia in the characteristic inferior nasal meridian of one iris or a minor choroidal coloboma at the equator of one ocular fundus which is detectable only by biomicroscopy or indirect ophthalmoscopy by a careful and comprehensive ophthalmologist.

Ancillary diagnostic studies may include chromosome analysis, biochemical tests, molecular studies, audiometry, ultrasound of the orbit or globe, and neuro-imaging. High resolution chromosome analysis may be appropriate in any high-risk multisystem disorder. For ophthalmologists, the two key indications are unexplained mental retardation with ocular findings that are not necessarily associated, and any multisystem anomalies where the eye and the central nervous system are involved simultaneously. Of course, chromosome analysis is mandatory in known embryonal malignancies, such as retinoblastoma or aniridia–Wilms tumor.

The primary physician should engage the ophthalmologist in the contemplation of contiguous gene syndromes, when one disease of a known single gene inheritance is associated with other unexplained features or diseases. The recent association of choroideremia with microcephaly, severe neurosensory hearing impairment, short stature, obesity, and developmental delay may lead to discovery of a visible or molecular deletion on chromosome Xq21. Chromosome analysis may also be important when individuals with a female appearance present with X-linked traits, such as color blindness, which classically afflict "only" males. Examples of Turner syndrome with color vision deficiency or testicular feminization with color vision deficiency have been recorded.

Still, one may need to explain the isolated case, the infant, child, or even adolescent who is the only individual in the family afflicted with an apparent genetic disorder. The primary physician and the ophthalmologist should consider the possibility that this individual represents the new mutation, the first individual in the family to have the disease. For example, nearly one-half of individuals with classical neurofibromatosis, NF 1, are the first individuals afflicted with the disorder in their families. Once the mutation has occurred, however, the recurrence risk for offspring and subsequent generations of this individual follows a classical autosomal dominant pattern. If a new mutation for an autosomal dominant is considered, the physicians should inquire about the paternal age at the time the child was born. There is an increasing risk of new mutation, single gene, autosomal dominant disorders in the offspring of older-age-group fathers. The possibility that a person is the only affected individual in the family with a disorder would raise the prospect that the disorder is recessive and thus determined by the coincident inheritance of a recessive gene from each (normal-appearing) carrier parent. Thus, a search for parental consanguinity, the classic features of a common geographic, religious, or family background, would be appropriate.

Sometimes the isolated case does not represent a genetic or inherited disorder, but rather a somatic mutation. There is reasonable evidence that segmental neurofibromatosis (and perhaps even unilateral retinoblastoma) is not strictly speaking a germinal mutation, but rather a post-zygotic somatic event. Are the physicians certain that the parents are accurately identified? Rarely, parents will adopt a child and never admit in the child's presence that he or she has been adopted, until well after the recognition of a heritable disorder later. Non-penetrance or minimal expressivity of either a dominant or an X-linked trait can be resolved by diligent investigation of parents and other relatives or of an obligate carrier mother. Lastly, a child may be an isolated case of an apparently genetic disorder because the diagnosis is not correct. Drugs, prenatal infections, and other environmental insults can create dysmorphisms which distantly resemble genetic disease. For example, congenitally deaf, nonverbal children with pigmentary retinopathy may have Usher syndrome type I, or might have congenital rubella syndrome.

The ophthalmologist must be sensitive to these vagaries and must be willing to extend his search beyond the affected patient to the immediate family, including siblings and both parents. Information which the ophthalmologist can provide in these situations will amplify tremendously the abilities of the primary physicians to sort a clinical problem and to establish a firm diagnosis, as the basis for counseling the individual and the family about recurrence risks, natural history and outcomes, and reproductive choices.

OPHTHALMOLOGIC DISORDERS
Listings in This Section

ANIRIDIA (AN)

Description Aniridia, a genetic disorder of vision and ocular structure, is characterized by partial or nearly complete agenesis of the iris in one or both eyes. Four forms (**AN-I, AN-II, AN-III, AN-IV**) have been characterized and their signs distinguished. Type IV, the **WAGR syndrome,** consists of Wilms tumor, aniridia, gonadoblastoma, and mental retardation.

Synonyms
Irideremia

Signs and Symptoms Vision is preserved in some mild cases. **AN-I** is marked by variable expression of the disorder. Hypoplasia of the iris is rarely unilateral. In **AN-II,** abnormalities of the iris may occur alone or in combination with other disorders such as cataracts, glaucoma, nystagmus, corneal pannus, and underdevelopment of the fovea.

A 3rd type of aniridia, **AN-III,** is associated with mental retardation. The 4th type, **AN-IV (WAGR syndrome),** occurs with Wilms tumor and genitourinary abnormalities. In most cases there is also delayed mental development. The ocular abnormalities may include congenital cataracts, nystagmus, and ptosis. Other abnormalities such as micrognathia, growth deficiency, and microcephaly may be present.

Etiology AN-I has been assigned to chromosome 2 and is transmitted as am autosomal dominant trait. AN-II is thought to result from defects on the short arm of chromosome 11. It is inherited as an autosomal dominant trait, although some cases appear to be genetic mutations. An autosomal recessive inheritance is suspected in AN-III. WAGR syndrome always results from deletion at 11p13.

Epidemiology All types of aniridia affect males and females in equal numbers. The incidence is approximately 1:100,000 to 1:200,000 live births in the United States.

Related Disorders In **iridogoniodysgenesis,** a genetic eye structure disorder in newborns, the defect is underdevelopment of the stroma of the iris.

Rieger syndrome (iridogoniodysgenesis with umbilicus cutis and anomalies of the teeth, jaw, and extremities) consists of defective embryonic development of the middle layers of the iris and abnormalities in the pupil. The edges of the cornea may be clouded at birth; glaucoma also occurs.

Hereditary juvenile glaucoma, which must be distinguished from autosomal recessive congenital glaucoma, may be present at birth, but onset of symptoms may be delayed until childhood or adolescence. Other cases may represent an early onset of some other forms of glaucoma.

Treatment—Standard Treatment is usually directed toward improvement of useful vision. If there is a refractive error, a patient may benefit from corrective lenses. Drugs may be helpful in control of glaucoma. Surgery may be necessary for cataracts. Genetic counseling is recommended for all patients, regardless of the type of aniridia. Patients with AN-IV should be evaluated with karyotype for a developing Wilms tumor, either by abdominal sonogram, CT scan, or laparotomy with renal biopsy. Other treatment is symptomatic and supportive.

Treatment—Investigational Please contact the agencies listed under Resources, below, for the most current information.

Resources

For more information on aniridia: National Organization for Rare Disorders (NORD); Vision Foundation, Inc; National Association for Parents of the Visually Impaired, Inc.; National Association for the Visually Handicapped.

For genetic information and genetic counseling referrals: March of Dimes Birth Defects Foundation; National Center for Education in Maternal and Child Health (NCEMCH).

References

Mendelian Inheritance in Man, 9th ed.: V.A. McKusick; The Johns Hopkins University Press, 1990, pp. 69–71.

11p13 Deletion, Wilms' Tumour, and Aniridia: Unusual Genetic, Non-Ocular and Ocular Features of Three Cases: V. Jotterand, et al.; Br. J. Ophthalmol., 1990, vol. 74, pp. 568–570.

Familial Isolated Aniridia Associated with a Translocation Involving Chromosomes 11 and 22 [t (11;22) (p13;q12.2)]: J.W. Moore, et al.; Hum. Genet., April 1986, vol. 72(4), pp. 297–302.

Family with Aniridia, Microcornea, and Spontaneously Reabsorbed Cataract: Y. Yamamoto; Arch. Ophthalmol., April 1988, vol. 106, pp. 502–504.

Long Range Physical Map of the Wilms' Tumor-Aniridia Region on Human Chromosome 11: D.A. Compton, et al.; Cell, December 2, 1988, vol. 55, pp. 827–836.

Two Anonymous DNA Segments Distinguish the Wilms' Tumor and Aniridia Loci: L.M. Davis, et al.; Science, August 1988, vol. 241, pp. 840-842.

Wilms' Tumor Detection in Patients with Sporadic Aniridia. Successful Use of Ultrasound: A.L. Friedman; Am. J. Dis. Child, February 1986, vol. 140(2), pp. 173–174.

Wilms' Tumor with Aniridia/Iris Dysplasia and Apparently Normal Chromosomes: V.M. Riccardi, et al.; J. Pediatr., April 1982, vol. 100(4), pp. 574–577.

BROWN SYNDROME

Description This congenital or acquired disorder is due to an abnormality of the tendon sheath of the superior oblique muscle that mechanically limits eye elevation.

Synonyms

Superior Oblique Tendon Sheath Syndrome
Tendon Sheath Adherence

Signs and Symptoms Signs include squinting, ptosis, and backward head tilt. No imbalance in the lower field or overaction of the ipsilateral superior oblique muscle occurs. Fusion and stereopsis are good at near. Corrected visual acuity is also good. Hypotropia is present in the affected eye in the primary position and elevation in the nasal field is absent or severely limited. Limitation of elevation decreases as the involved eye is abducted with full elevation occurring upon completed abduction. Upon adduction of the affected eye, "downshoot" of depression of that eye occurs and the palpebral fissure widens. Temporal excursions of the involved eye are normal.

Etiology The disorder is due to a shortened tendon sheath of the superior oblique muscle, a thickening of the sheath that restricts its passage through the trochlea, or an abnormal insertion of the tendon. The condition may be congenital or may result from trochlear inflammation or from surgical or nonsurgical trauma.

Epidemiology The disorder occurs equally in both males and females.

Treatment—Standard Usually nothing is done. However, the most common surgical revision is tenectomy of the superior oblique muscle.

Treatment—Investigational Please contact the agencies listed under Resources, below, for the most current information.

Resources
    For more information on Brown syndrome: National Organization for Rare Disorders (NORD).

CHOROIDEREMIA

Description Choroideremia is an X-linked disorder of vision characterized by a typical ophthalmoscopic appearance of extensive peripheral atrophy of the retinal pigment epithelium and choriocapillaris.

Synonyms
    Choroidal Sclerosis
    Progressive Choroidal Atrophy
    Progressive Tapetochoroidal Dystrophy

Signs and Symptoms Night blindness, usually occurring in childhood, is often the first noticeable symptom. Degeneration of the vessels of the choroid and functional damage to the retina occur later in life and usually lead to progressive peripheral vision field loss and eventual blindness.

Etiology The X-linked trait has been mapped to Xq21.

Epidemiology Usually males are affected; females are carriers. Occasionally, however, older females may present severe manifestations of the carrier state and be symptomatic.

Related Disorders See *Retinitis Pigmentosa.*
    Gyrate atrophy of the choroid and retina is an autosomal recessive disorder characterized by a peripheral circular-patterned degeneration of the choroid and retina, and by hyperornithinemia caused by defects in ornithine aminotransferase.

Treatment—Standard Treatment is supportive. Organizations providing services to sight-impaired individuals may be helpful. Genetic counseling is recommended.

Treatment—Investigational Please contact the agencies listed under Resources, below, for the most current information.

Resources

For more information on choroideremia: National Organization for Rare Disorders (NORD); National Retinitis Pigmentosa Foundation Fighting Blindness; National Federation of the Blind; American Council of the Blind; American Foundation for the Blind; Vision Foundation, Inc.; American Council of the Blind Parents; National Association for Parents of the Visually Impaired, Inc. (NAPVI); National Association for the Visually Handicapped (NAVH); National Library Service for the Blind and Physically Handicapped.

For genetic information and genetic counseling referrals: March of Dimes Birth Defects Foundation; National Center for Education in Maternal and Child Health (NCEMCH).

References

Choroideremia and Deafness with Stapes Fixation: A Contiguous Gene Deletion Syndrome in Xq21: D.E. Merry, et al.; Am. J. Hum. Genet., vol. 45, 1989, pp 530–540.

Choroideremia: Further Evidence for Assignment of the locus to Xq13-Xq21: M. Schwartz, et al.; Hum. Genet., 1986, vol. 74, pp. 449–452..

Choroideremia-Locus Maps Between DXS3 and DXS11 on Xq: A. Gal, et al.; Hum. Genet., June 1986, vol. 73(2), pp. 123–126.

Histopathologic Observations in Choroideremia with Emphasis on Vascular Changes of the Uveal Tract: J.D. Cameron, et al.; Ophthalmology, February 1987, vol. 94(2), pp. 187–196.

Mendelian Inheritance in Man, 9th ed.: V.A. McKusick; Johns Hopkins University Press, 1990, pp. 1573–1575.

Multipoint Linkage Analysis of Loci in the Proximal Long Arm of the Human X Chromosome: Application of Mapping the Choroideremia Locus: J.G. Lesko, et al.; Am. J. Hum. Genet., April 1987, vol. 40(4), pp. 303–311.

DUANE SYNDROME

Description Duane syndrome is an inherited congenital ocular disorder characterized by limited horizontal motility.

Synonyms

Eye Retraction Syndrome

Retraction Syndrome

Stilling-Turk-Duane Syndrome

Signs and Symptoms The syndrome is generally unilateral. On attempted adduction, the affected eye displays retraction of the globe with narrowing of the palpebral fissure, and minimal restriction on versions and forced duction. On attempted abduction, the fissure is widened but abduction does not occur or is limited to a few degrees past midline. There is minimal to substantial face turn to the side of the affected eye. Fusion is good. Visual acuity is normal, and the involved globe is otherwise healthy. The disorder is not progressive.

Etiology The syndrome may be supranuclear in origin or may occur when horizontal rotators (one or both) are replaced with inelastic bands of fibrous tissue. Extremely rare examples of purported dominant families have been reported. Electromyography suggests some cases are caused by co-contraction of both lateral and medial rectus muscles alone or in combination with abnormality of extraocular muscle.

Epidemiology Males are affected more frequently than females.

Treatment—Standard Surgery may be performed if the patient has a cosmetic face turn, or for maximal recession of the medial rectus in the involved eye.

Treatment—Investigational Please contact the agencies listed under Resources, below, for the most current information.

Resources
   For more information on Duane syndrome: National Organization for Rare Disorders (NORD).
   For genetic information and genetic counseling referrals: March of Dimes Birth Defects Foundation; National Center for Education in Maternal and Child Health (NCEMCH).

References
   Mendelian Inheritance in Man, 9th ed.: V.A. McKusick; The Johns Hopkins University Press, 1990, pp. 271–272.

EPITHELIOPATHY, ACUTE POSTERIOR MULTIFOCAL PLACOID PIGMENT

Description Acute posterior multifocal placoid pigment epitheliopathy, a rare, acquired ocular disorder, is characterized by sudden onset of vision and inflammation of the outer retina and retinal pigment epithelium.

Signs and Symptoms A rapid but temporary loss of vision that often subsides without treatment is characteristic. Multiple yellow-white placoid lesions appear in the posterior pole of the retina in each eye. After resolution of the plaques, pigment alterations are usually permanent. The vision loss may be permanent if the plaques occur subfoveally, but more than 90 percent of patients recover 20/30 or better visual acuity within a few months of onset.

Etiology A viral etiology is suspected, but none has been isolated.

Epidemiology Males and females are affected in equal numbers. The disorder is rare in children under 10 years of age.

Related Disorders **Multifocal evanescent white dot syndrome (MEWDS)** and **acute retinal pigment epitheliitis** may be confused. These and other disorders share the common denominators of abnormal choroidal perfusion and focal retinal pigment epithelial infarction.

Treatment—Standard Treatment is minimal, symptomatic, and supportive. Rarely, anterior uveitis may require temporary suppression with topical corticosteroids and mydriatics.

Treatment—Investigational Please contact the agencies listed under Resources, below, for the most current information.

Resources

For more information on acute posterior multifocal placoid pigment epitheliopathy: National Organization for Rare Disorders (NORD); Vision Foundation, Inc.

References

Long-term Visual Function in Acute Posterior Multifocal Placoid Pigment Epitheliopathy: M.D. Wolf, et al.; Arch. Ophthalmol., 1991, vol. 109, pp. 800–803.

Long-term Follow-up of Acute Multifocal Posterior Placoid Pigment Epitheliopathy: D.F. Williams and W.F. Mieler; Br. J. Ophthalmol., December 1989, vol. 73(12), pp. 985–990.

Acute Posterior Multifocal Placoid Pigment Epitheliopathy and Cerebral Vasculitis: C.A. Wilson, et al.; Arch. Ophthalmol., June 1988, vol. 106, pp. 796–800.

Acute Posterior Multifocal Placoid Pigment Epitheliopathy Associated with Diffuse Retinal Vasculitis and Late Haemorrhagic Macular Detachment: M. Isashiki, et al.; Br. J. Ophthalmol., April 1986, vol. 70(4), pp. 255–259.

Acute Posterior Multifocal Placoid Pigment Epitheliopathy: T. Autzen, et al.; Acta Ophthalmol., June 1986, vol. 64(3), pp. 267–270.

KERATOCONUS

Description Keratoconus is a change (steepening) in the curved transparent outer layer of collagenous tissue constituting the cornea. The resulting cone-shaped cornea causes substantial problems with refraction of light. The disorder progresses slowly and occurs in 3 forms: keratoconus posticus circumscriptus; autosomal dominant keratoconus; autosomal recessive keratoconus.

Synonyms

Conical Cornea

Congenital Keratoconus

Signs and Symptoms Inherited forms of this abnormality usually begin after puberty. Symptoms may be unilateral initially and may later become bilateral. Patients frequently need a change in prescription for eye glasses; astigmatism is common, probably caused by the ectasia of the cornea. In keratoconus posticus circumscriptus, mental and physical retardation can occur.

Etiology The causes are unknown. Both autosomal dominant and recessive inheritances have been suggested.

Epidemiology Keratoconus occurs in females slightly more often than males. Onset is more frequent in adolescence than adulthood. One longterm study in the United States indicated a prevalence of 54.5 diagnosed cases of keratoconus per

100,000 population and unilateral involvement in 41 percent and bilateral disease in 59 percent at diagnosis.

Related Disorders Keratoconus may occur alone or in conjunction with other disorders, including Noonan syndrome, Down syndrome, Ehlers-Danlos syndrome, and Leber's congenital amaurosis.

Treatment—Standard Treatment of the visual defect may involve the use of hard contact lenses as a temporary measure. The only "cure" is corneal transplant (penetrating keratoplasty or epikeratoplasty). In some cases, progression may slow enough to obviate treatment. Genetic counseling may be of benefit for patients with an inherited form of keratoconus.

Treatment—Investigational Please contact the agencies listed under Resources, below, for the most current information.

Resources

For more information on keratoconus: National Organization for Rare Disorders (NORD); NIH/National Eye Institute; Eye Bank Association of America; Vision Foundation, Inc.; National Association for the Visually Handicapped (NAVH).

For genetic information and genetic counseling referrals: March of Dimes Birth Defects Foundation; NIH/National Center for Education in Maternal and Child Health (NCEMCH).

References

A 48-Year Clinical and Epidemiologic Study of Keratoconus: R.H. Kennedy, et al.; Am. J. Ophthalmol., March 15, 1986, vol. 101(3), pp. 267–273.

Contact Lens Fitting Relation and Visual Acuity in Keratoconus: K. Zadnik, et al.; Am. J. Optom. Physiol. Opt., September 1987, vol. 64(9), pp. 698–702.

Corneal Regrafts: F. Bigar, et al.; Dev. Ophthalmol., 1987, vol. 14, pp. 117–120.

Electrosurgical Keratoplasty. Clinicopathologic Correlation: P.J. McDonnell, et al.; Arch. Ophthalmol., February 1988, vol. 106(2), pp. 235–238

Long-term Comparison of Epikeratoplasty and Penetrating Keratoplasty for Keratoconus: R.F. Steinert, et al.; Arch. Ophthalmol., April 1988, vol. 106(4), pp. 493–496.

Mendelian Inheritance in Man, 9th ed.: V.A. McKusick; The Johns Hopkins University Press, 1990, p. 1286.

KERATOCONJUNCTIVITIS, VERNAL

Description A noncontagious manifestation of a seasonal allergy, vernal conjunctivitis usually affects susceptible individuals in the spring or during warm weather.

Synonyms

Seasonal Conjunctivitis

Spring Ophthalmia

Signs and Symptoms Symptoms include conjunctival inflammation, causing redness and perhaps blurred vision; cobblestone-like changes appear in the upper palpebral conjunctiva. The eyes become sensitive to light, and itching is intense. Usually the irritation is bilateral. A gelatinous nodule may develop in the limbus.

Etiology Vernal keratoconjunctivitis is thought to be an ocular hypersensitivity or allergic reaction to airborne allergens.

Epidemiology Males and females are affected equally.

Related Disorders Conjunctivitis (pink eye) is a highly contagious bacterial or viral infection of the outer lining of the eye and eyelids. The eyes become red, irritated, and burning; a scratchiness, as if caused by sand, is experienced. A cold or sore throat may precede the infection, which is most common in children. Sticky mucus is visible in the eye and can cause the eyelids to stick together.

Treatment—Standard Treatment is symptomatic and supportive. It is essential to treat any causative allergy.

Treatment—Investigational The use of cromolyn sodium in the treatment of ocular allergies such as vernal keratoconjunctivitis is being studied. The orphan drug levocabastine (Iolab Pharmaceuticals, 500 Iolab Drive, Claremont, California 91711) is being used experimentally in the treatment of vernal keratoconjunctivitis.

Please contact the agencies listed under Resources, below, for the most current information.

Resources
    For more information on vernal keratoconjunctivitis: National Organization for Rare Disorders (NORD); NIH/National Eye Institute; National Institute of Allergy & Infectious Diseases (NIAID).

References
    Ocular Allergy and Mast Cell Stabilizers: M.R. Allansmith, et al.; Surv. Ophthalmol., January–February, 1986, vol. 30(4), pp. 229–244.
    Vernal Keratoconjunctivitis: New Corneal Findings in Fraternal Twins: W.N. Rosenthal, et al.; Cornea, 1984–1985, vol. 3(4), pp. 288–290.

MACULAR DEGENERATION

Description Macular degeneration is the descriptive term for many forms of deterioration of the central area of vision (macula) from a previous state of normality. Subtypes of the disorder include Stargardt's disease and fundus flavimaculatus (occurring in juveniles); and disciform macular degeneration (termed senile macular degeneration, and, previously, Kuhnt-Junius disease).

Synonyms
    Age-Related Macular Degeneration

Signs and Symptoms Central vision is impaired or absent; peripheral vision is normal. Metamorphopsia and central scotoma are associated with the disorder. The condition may progress to a central or scarred stage and then become static.

Etiology There are genetic, environmental (including toxic), and age-related causes. Age-related macular degeneration has no clearly detectable genetic pattern. Juvenile forms are usually autosomal recessive.

Epidemiology Onset of juvenile macular dystrophy (Stargardt's disease; fundus flavimaculatus) is between ages 6 and 15. Age-related macular degeneration occurs in and after the 6th decade.

Treatment—Standard Monitoring of the status of the disorder is indicated. Genetic counseling may be helpful for those with clearly defined variants (e.g., Stargardt's disease); examination of siblings is essential.

Treatment—Investigational Laser treatment may be useful in early stages of age-related disciform disease.

Inherited retinal diseases are being studied at the Cullen Eye Institute of the Baylor College of Medicine in Houston, Texas. Families with at least 2 affected members and both parents living are needed to participate in this program.

Please contact the agencies listed under Resources, below, for the most current information.

Resources
For more information on macular degeneration: National Organization for Rare Disorders (NORD); American Foundation for the Blind; Association for Macular Diseases, Inc.; Schepens Eye Research Institute of Retina Foundation, Macular Disease Research Center; NIH/National Eye Institute; National Association for the Visually Handicapped; Vision Foundation, Inc.

References
Aging Macular Degeneration: J.C. Folk; Ophthalmology, vol. 92, May 1985, pp. 594–602.

Risk Factors in Age-Related Maculopathy Complicated by Choroidal Neovascularization: M.S. Blumenkranz, et al.; Ophthal., vol. 93, May 1986, pp. 552–558.

The Second Eye of Patients with Senile Macular Degeneration: E.R. Strahlman, et al.; Arch. Ophthalmol., vol. 101, August 1983, pp. 1191 ff.

Argon Laser Photocoagulation for Neovascular Maculopathy: Mac. Photocoag. Study Group., Arch. Ophthalmol., vol. 104, May 1986, pp. 694–701.

Recurrent Choroidal Neovascularization After Argon Laser Photocoagulation for Neovascular Maculopathy: Mac. Photocoag. Study Group., Arch. Ophthalmol., vol. 104, April 1986, pp. 503–512.

Krypton Laser Photocoagulation for Idiopathic Neovascular Lesions: Mac. Photocoag. Study Group., Arch. Ophthalmol., vol. 108, June 1990, pp. 832–837.

NORRIE DISEASE

Description Norrie disease is an X-linked hereditary disorder characterized by bilateral blindness at birth.

Synonyms
> Anderson-Warburg Syndrome
> Atrophia Bulborum Hereditaria
> Fetal Iritis Syndrome
> Oligophrenia-Microphthalmos
> Whitnall-Norman Syndrome

Signs and Symptoms Lens opacities and atrophy of the iris may be found in early infancy. Cataracts develop followed by phthisis bulbi, which is usually apparent by age 1 year. Typical findings are a small anterior chamber and a pupil without light reflex; the iris tends to adhere abnormally to the crystalline lens. A gray membrane or gray-yellow opaque mass with blood vessels is evident behind the lens, and elongated cilia are often visible on the opposite side of the pupil. Retinal folds and detached retinas may develop. By age 5 years, the lens is usually cataractous.

Mental deficiency occurs in about 50 percent of affected patients. The deficiency becomes apparent in the first 2 years of life. A progressive hearing loss may not be evident until about age 20 years. Diabetes has occurred in some patients. Nonocular symptoms and signs range from the milder (normal intelligence, normal growth, mild hearing loss) to profound mental retardation, short stature, and deafness.

Etiology The disease is inherited as an X-linked trait, mapped to Xp11.3-21.1.

Epidemiology The disease affects only males. Carrier females have no phenotypic features.

Related Disorders See *Trisomy 13 (Patau Syndrome); Usher Syndrome; Retinitis Pigmentosa.*

Retinal dysplasia is a hereditary disorder in which an elevated retinal fold arises from the optic disc, covering the macular area and widening toward the temporal fundus. This encroachment may cause blindness.

Other related disorders include **familial exudative vitreoretinopathy** and **retinopathy of prematurity.**

Treatment—Standard Surgical reattachment of the retina has been attempted but is never successful. Agencies that provide services for vision- and hearing-impaired individuals may be of benefit, as may genetic counseling.

Treatment—Investigational Please contact the agencies listed under Resources, below, for the most current information.

Resources
For more information on **Norrie disease:** National Organization for Rare Disorders (NORD); Eye Research Institute of Retina Foundation; American Council of the Blind; American Foundation for the Blind; Vision Foundation, Inc.; National Association for Parents of the Visually Impaired, Inc. (NAPVI); National Federation of the Blind.

For **braille or recorded publications:** National Library Service for the Blind and Physically Handicapped; Retinitis Pigmentosa Foundation Fighting Blindness; National Association for the Visually Handicapped (NAVH).

For genetic information and genetic counseling referrals: March of Dimes Birth Defects Foundation; NIH/National Center for Education in Maternal and Child Health (NCEMCH).

References
Mendelian Inheritance in Man, 9th ed.: V.A. McKusick; The Johns Hopkins University Press, 1990, pp. 1693–1695.

Norrie Disease Gene Is Distinct from the Monoamine Oxidase Genes: K.B. Sims, et al.; Am. J. Hum. Genet., 1989, vol. 45, pp. 424–424.

Recombinational Event Between Norrie Disease and DXS7 Loci: J.T. Ngo, et al.; Clin. Gen., 1988, vol. 34, pp. 43–47.

Norrie Disease Caused by a Gene Deletion Allowing Carrier Detection and Prenatal Diagnosis: A. de la Chapelle, et al.; Clin. Genet., October 1985, vol. 28(4), pp. 317–320.

PAPILLITIS

Description Papillitis, a progressive inflammation of all or part of the optic nerve, can cause loss of vision. The disorder is usually unilateral but may be bilateral, depending on the etiology.

Synonyms
Optic Neuritis

Signs and Symptoms The primary symptom is a rapid loss of vision, which can occur within 1 to 2 days of onset and last for months. Movement of the eyes increases pain, which is routinely present. Recovery may be spontaneous, but permanent loss of vision is possible if the underlying causes remain undiagnosed and consequently untreated.

An elderly patient with giant-cell arteritis may have headaches and fatigue as well as unilateral loss of vision. In some cases, the other eye may become involved, leading to bilateral blindness.

Etiology There are many causes. A viral illness or other inflammatory disease may precede development of papillitis. It may be part of a demyelinating process occurring after or accompanying multiple sclerosis or be due to an occlusive disease affecting the ciliary vessels, such as giant-cell arteritis. Toxins or chemicals, such as lead or ethanol, or even a bee sting may be responsible. Papillitis may occur during meningitis or after syphilis. Metastasis of a tumor to the optic nerve head may be the underlying disorder. In some cases, there may be no apparent cause.

Epidemiology The disease is equally likely to occur in males and females and at any age.

Related Disorders See *Arteritis, Giant-Cell; Multiple Sclerosis.*

Retrobulbar neuritis, an inflammation of the portion of the optic nerve that lies behind the eyeball, is usually unilateral and is characterized by pain on movement of the eye, headache, and a rapid and progressive loss of vision. Retrobulbar neuritis can be associated with multiple sclerosis or viral or infectious diseases; in most cases there is no apparent cause.

Treatment—Standard If spontaneous remission does not occur, the disease is usually treated with prednisone or methylprednisolone. A major national collaborative trial (the Optic Neuritis Treatment Trial—ONTT) began in 1988 a 3-year recruitment of subjects to determine what, if any, role corticosteroids should play. For further information, please contact Roy W. Beck, M.D., University of South Florida, Department of Ophthalmology, 12901 N. Bruce B. Downs Boulevard, Tampa, Florida 33612; (813) 974-4810.

Treatment—Investigational Please contact the agencies listed under Resources, below, for the most current information.

Resources
   For more information on papillitis: National Organization for Rare Disorders (NORD); NIH/National Eye Institute; Vision Foundation, Inc.

References
   Causes and Workup of Optic Neuropathy: J.A. McCrary III *in* Walsh & Hoyt's Clinical Neuro-Ophthalmology, vol. 1, 4th ed.: N.R. Miller, ed.; Williams and Wilkins, pp. 213–328.
   Internal Medicine, 2nd ed.: J.H. Stein, ed.-in-chief; Little, Brown and Company, 1987, p. 2171.
   Optic Neuritis in Children and its Relationship to Multiple Sclerosis: A Clinical Study in 21 Children: R. Riikonen, et al.; Dev. Med. Child Neurol., June 1988, vol. 30(3), pp. 349–359.
   Optic Neuritis in the Elderly. Prognosis for Visual Recovery and Long-Term Follow-Up: D. Jacobsen, et al.; Neurology, December 1988, vol. 38(12), pp. 1834–1837.
   Recovery After Optic Neuritis in Childhood: A. Kriss, et al.; J. Neurosurg. Psychiatry, October 1988, vol. 51(10), pp. 1253–1258.
   The Optic Neuritis Treatment Trial: R.W. Beck (Editorial); Arch. Ophthalmol., August 1988, vol. 106, pp. 1051–1053.
   Transverse Myelitis and Optic Neuritis in Systemic Lupus Erythematosus. A Case Report with Resonance Imaging Findings: J. Kenik, et al.; Arthritis Rheum., August 1987, vol. 30(8), pp. 947–950.
   Treatment of Optic Neuritis with Intravenous Megadose Corticosteroids. A Consecutive Series: T. Spoor, et al.; Ophthalmology, January 1988, vol. 95(1), pp. 131–134.

PERIPHERAL UVEITIS (PARS PLANITIS)

Description Peripheral uveitis is a vision disorder characterized by inflammation of the peripheral retina and pars plana due to infiltration by cells that produce a snowbank of debris in the vitreous humor and peripheral retina. Disorder severity is greater when symptoms begin in the first decade of life, and less when onset is in the 2nd to 4th decades.

Synonyms
   Pars Planitis
   Peripheral Retinal Inflammation

Signs and Symptoms Typical of the condition is unilateral or bilateral blurred or poor night vision. Intraocular edema, particularly on the peripheral retina or macula, can occur. Glaucoma, phthisis, or other eye complications may develop. With bilateral peripheral uveitis, the involvement of each eye may differ in severity.

Etiology The cause is unknown; autoimmune and genetic mechanisms have been suggested. Symptoms and signs are the result of inflammation of the peripheral retina and/or pars plana.

Epidemiology The more severe early-onset form of the disorder occurs in about 10 percent of cases. Males and females are affected in equal numbers.

Related Disorders **Cystoid macular edema** may be a complication of peripheral uveitis. It is characterized by edema of the central retina as a result of abnormal leakage of fluid from capillaries.

Ocular hypotension refers to hypotension in the veins or capillaries in intraocular tissue, which may cause visual disturbances similar to those of peripheral uveitis.

Treatment—Standard The usual therapy is a course of corticosteroids to reduce inflammation. Surgery may be recommended in refractory cases. Diathermy or cryotherapy may be used to seal blood vessels and stop leakage.

Treatment—Investigational Please contact the agencies listed under Resources, below, for the most current information.

Resources

For more information on peripheral uveitis (pars planitis): National Organization for Rare Disorders (NORD); Association for Macular Diseases; NIH/National Eye Institute.

References

The Enigma of Pars Planitis (Editorial): T.M. Aaberg; Am. J. Ophthalmol., June 1987, pp. 828–829.

The Significance of the Pars Plana Exudate in Pars Planitis: D.E. Henderly, et al.; Am. J. Ophthalmol., May 1987, vol. 103(5), pp. 669–671.

Pars Planitis and Autoimmune Endotheliopathy: A.A. Khodadoust, et al.; Am. J. Ophthalmol., November 1986, vol. 102(5), pp. 633–639.

RETINITIS PIGMENTOSA (RP)

Description Retinitis pigmentosa can be associated with deafness and other malfunctions, central nervous system and metabolic disorders, and chromosomal abnormalities.

Synonyms

Graefe-Sjoegren Syndrome

Signs and Symptoms Night blindness is an early symptom with onset between ages 10 and 40, slowly followed by tunnel vision. The rate and extent of progression are widely variable. When other members of a family are affected, the rates of progression are usually similar within that family.

Some individuals with RP are also born deaf (Usher syndrome Type I), or hearing-impaired (Usher syndrome Type II). (See *Usher Syndrome*).

Etiology Most cases are isolated, but RP may be recessive, autosomal dominant, or X-linked. At least 32 systemic disorders show some type of retinal involvement similar to RP.

In 1989, mutations of the rhodopsin locus were shown to be associated with 20 percent of families of autosomal dominant RP. The gene responsible for early-onset autosomal dominant RP is different from the gene that causes late-onset RP. Scientists have also found recessive genes that cause disorders similar to RP in mice, and it is hoped that this knowledge will lead to benefits for patients with rapidly progressive recessive RP.

Epidemiology The prevalence of RP is between 1:3000 and 1:5000.

Treatment—Standard Affected relatives should be examined to determine the pattern of inheritance, the basis for diagnosis, prognosis, and genetic counseling.

No cure for RP is available. When cataracts significantly interfere with vision, surgical removal may be advisable. Whether surgery improves vision often depends on the extent of retinal change.

Optical, nonoptical, and electronic vision aids allow individuals to make the maximum use of their remaining vision.

Treatment—Investigational Please contact the agencies listed under Resources, below, for the most current information.

Resources
For more information on retinitis pigmentosa: National Organization for Rare Disorders (NORD); Retinitis Pigmentation Foundation Fighting Blindness; NIH/National Eye Institute.

For genetic information and genetic counseling referrals: National Center for Education in Maternal and Child Health (NCEMCH); March of Dimes Birth Defects Foundation.

For service organizations for the blind: American Council of the Blind, Inc. (ACB); American Foundation for the Blind (AFB); American Printing House for the Blind; National Association for Parents of the Visually Impaired (NAPVI); National Association for the Visually Handicapped (NAVH); National Federation of the Blind (NFB); National Library Service for the Blind and Physically Handicapped; Recording for the Blind, Inc. (RFB).

References
Linkage to D3S47 (C17) in One Large Autosomal Dominant Retinitis Pigmentosa Family and Exclusion in Another: Confirmation of Genetic Heterogeneity: D.H. Lester, et al.; Am. J. Hum. Genet., 1990, vol. 47, pp. 536–541.
Prevalence of Retinitis Pigmentosa In Maine: C.H. Bunker, et al.; Am. J. Ophthalmol., 1984, vol. 97, pp. 357–365.
Retinitis Pigmentosa: R.A. Pagon; Survey of Ophthalmology, November–December 1988, vol. 33(3), pp. 137–177.

RETINOBLASTOMA

Description Retinoblastoma is a congenital malignant tumor, often bilateral, that develops in the ocular nerve cell layers (retina) and seems to originate from primitive photoreceptors.

Signs and Symptoms Unilateral retinoblastoma is usually diagnosed by 2 years of age; bilateral involvement, by about 8 months. A cat's eye reflex in the pupil is often the first sign. Strabismus related to loss of vision, glaucoma, and ocular inflammation also are indicative. The tumor on examination is white and varies in size. Calcifications are seen in three-quarters of cases in the globe.

Other malformations have been reported in patients with a chromosomal deletion of 13q, including cleft palate, broad nasal bridge, bulbous nose, and prominent earlobes.

Etiology Most retinoblastomas appear as isolated defects, but about 30 to 40 percent behave as autosomal dominant traits with variable expressivity. If a child inherits 2 copies of a predisposing gene, development of the disorder depends on a precipitating event, the nature of which is unknown. The retinoblastoma gene, located on chromosome 13, has been identified and cloned, and procedures developed that in some cases can predict the risk of hereditary retinoblastoma.

Epidemiology The incidence of retinoblastoma is 1:15,000 to 1:30,000 live births. It is the most common form of ocular malignancy in children. Surviving children with retinoblastoma appear to be prone to osteosarcoma, because the same gene is involved in both disorders.

Treatment—Standard Unilateral retinoblastoma is usually managed by enucleation of the eye. In instances of extremely small tumors, radiation may be tried. With bilateral retinoblastoma, the more involved eye often is enucleated and the other eye treated by photocoagulation, cryotherapy, radiation, and possibly chemotherapy. Often a combination of these treatments is used. Reexamination is usually required at 2-month intervals. Radiologic surveys for bony metastases and studies of spinal fluid and bone marrow for malignant cells may be done until all viable tumor is destroyed. Examination of siblings and other family members is indicated. Between 15 and 50 percent of retinoblastoma survivors are at lifelong risk of 2nd embryonal malignancies.

Treatment—Investigational Please contact the agencies listed under Resources, below, for the most current information.

Resources

For more information on retinoblastoma: National Organization for Rare Disorders (NORD); NIH/National Eye Institute; New England Retinoblastoma Support Group; American Cancer Society; NIH/National Cancer Institute Physician Data Query (PDQ) phoneline.

For genetic information and genetic counseling referrals: March of Dimes Birth Defects Foundation; National Center for Education in Maternal and

Child Health (NCEMCH).

References
Altered Expression of the Retinoblastoma Gene Product in Human Sarcomas: W.G. Cance, et al.; N. Engl. J. Med., 1990, vol. 323, pp. 1457–1462.
Parental Origin of Mutations of the Retinoblastoma Gene: T.P. Dryja, et al.; Nature, June 15, 1989, vol. 339, pp. 556–558.
The Incidence of Retinoblastoma in the United States: 1974 Through 1985: A. Tamboli, et al.; Arch. Ophthalmol., January 1990, vol. 108, pp. 128–132.
Oncogenic Point Mutations in the Human Retinoblastoma Gene; Their Application to Genetic Counseling: D.W. Yandell, et al.; N. Engl. J. Med., 1989, vol. 321, pp. 1689–1695.
Recent Studies of the Retinoblastoma Gene (Editorial): Arch. Ophthalmol., February 1988, vol. 106, pp. 181–182.
Prediction of the Risk of Hereditary Retinoblastoma, Using DNA Polymorphisms Within the Retinoblastoma Gene: J. Wiggs, et al.; N. Engl. J. Med., 1988, vol. 318, pp. 151–157.
Predicting the Risk of Hereditary Retinoblastoma: J.L. Wiggs and T.P. Dryja; Am. J. of Ophthalmol., 1988, vol. 106, pp. 346–351.
Incidence of Second Neoplasms in Patients with Bilateral Retinoblastoma, J.D. Roarty, et al.; Ophthalmology, November 1988, vol. 95, pp. 1583–1587.

RETINOSCHISIS

Description Retinoschisis, the splitting of the retina into 2 layers, in its various forms (typical, juvenile, senile) can be inherited or acquired. The disorder is characterized by a slow progressive loss of parts of the field of vision corresponding to the areas of the retina which have become split. Often, the condition is associated with the development of retinal cysts.

Synonyms
> Congenital Retinal Cyst
> Congenital Vascular Veils in the Retina
> Giant Cyst of the Retina
> Vitreoretinal Dystrophy

Signs and Symptoms In typical retinoschisis (Blessig cysts, Iwanoff cysts, peripheral cystoid degeneration of the retina), splitting of the retina frequently occurs bilaterally and symmetrically. Splitting may begin in the lower or upper quarter of the retina toward the temples. Vision is impaired correspondingly. The lesion is a thin, transparent, veil-like membrane, which contains the retinal blood vessels and often opacities; dome-like, it extends into the vitreous. Hemeralopia may occur. The progression of splitting and loss of vision often ceases for many years; in some cases, however, progression may be more rapid.

Senile retinoschisis is similar to typical retinoschisis but usually occurs in older patients, often without symptoms. It is bilateral in 90 percent of cases. Coalescence of peripheral sacs (Blessig cysts, Iwanoff cysts) may produce symptoms. In the early stage, the cystic space is spanned by thin gray fibers which gradually break, allowing the inner and outer leaves of the retina to separate and form an elevated cyst. In the senile form, the split may extend around the retinal perimeter; it does not usually progress to the back of the retina, and it may remain unchanged for many years.

Juvenile X-linked retinoschisis (congenital retinoschisis) is the most severe form. It is slowly progressive, and the split often extends back over the macula and may affect the fovea. In the early stages, the retinal areas that are splitting often exhibit large holes in the inner layer between blood vessels. If breaks develop in both the front and the back layers of the schisis cavity, a true retinal detachment may occur causing loss of parts of the field of vision. A scotoma with a sharp edge in the area of the schisis appears in the patient's visual field. An electroretinogram shows B-waves which are significantly lower than normal but not obliterated. Cystic macular degeneration, which causes additional loss of vision, always accompanies juvenile retinoschisis.

Diagnosis can be made through various tests, including electroretinography and fundus photography, and by examination of less severely afflicted family members.

Etiology Retinoschisis is usually hereditary. Typical retinoschisis is most often an autosomal dominant disorder; senile retinoschisis is most commonly autosomal recessive, and juvenile retinoschisis is X-linked. A similar, milder, autosomal recessive form exists (familial foveal retinoschisis). Acquired cases of retinoschisis occur with aging for unknown reasons.

Epidemiology Typical retinoschisis usually occurs in hyperopic young males. Senile retinoschisis usually affects persons in the 5th, 6th, or 7th decades. It affects males and females in equal numbers. Juvenile retinoschisis affects only boys, with one exception: it has occurred in a female whose mother is a carrier and whose father is affected.

Related Disorders See *Macular Degeneration.*

Treatment—Standard Typical and senile retinoschisis usually do not require medical treatment. In juvenile retinoschisis in which there is intraocular bleeding, vitrectomy and retinal detachment repair may be necessary. Later, photocoagulation or cryotherapy can close off the damaged area of the retina. Genetic counseling is recommended.

Treatment—Investigational Please contact the agencies listed under Resources, below, for the most current information.

Resources

For more information on retinoschisis: National Organization for Rare Disorders (NORD); The Association for Macular Diseases; NIH/National Eye Institute; National Association for the Parents of the Visually Impaired, Inc. (NAPVI); National Association for the Visually Handicapped (NAVH); Eye Research Institute of Retina Foundation; Retinitis Pigmentosa Foundation Fighting Blindness; Vision Foundation, Inc.; American Foundation for the Blind.

For genetic information and genetic counseling referrals: March of Dimes Birth Defects Foundation; National Center for Education in Maternal and Child Health (NCEMCH).

References

Linkage Relationship of X-Linked Juvenile Retinoschisis with Xp22.1-p22.3 Probes: P.A. Sieving, et al.; Am. J. Hum. Genet., 1990, vol. 47, pp. 616–621.

Linkage Relationships and Gene Order around the Locus for X-Linked Retinoschisis: T. Alitalo, et al.; Am. J. Hum. Genet., 1988, vol. 43, pp. 476–483.

Vascularized Vitreous Membranes in Congenital Retinoschisis: D.F. Arkfeld, et al.; Retina, Spring 1987, issue 7(1), pp. 20–23.

X-Linked Retinoschisis is Closely Linked to DXS41 and DXS16 but not DXS85: T. Alitalo, et al.; Clin. Genet., September 1987, issue 32(3), pp. 192–195.

Long-Term Natural History Study of Senile Retinoschisis with Implications for Management: N.E. Byer; Ophthalmology, September 1986, vol. 93, pp. 1127–1137.

Degenerative Retinoschisis with Giant Outer Layer Breaks and Retinal Detachment: J.M. Sulonen, et al.; Am. J. Ophthalmol., February 1985, vol. 99(2), pp. 114–121.

Indications for Vitrectomy in Congenital Retinoschisis: J. Schulman, et al.; Br. J. Ophthalmol., July 1985, vol. 69(7), pp. 482–486.

Typical and Reticular Degenerative Retinoschisis: B.R. Straatsma and R.Y. Foos; Am. J. Ophthalmol., 1973, vol. 75, pp. 551–575.

TOLOSA-HUNT SYNDROME

Description The syndrome is characterized by severe, usually unilateral, headaches which often precede ophthalmoplegia.

Synonyms

Ophthalmoplegia, Painful
Ophthalmoplegia Syndrome

Signs and Symptoms Chronic headaches, mild fever, and impairment of vision followed by ophthalmoplegia are the major symptoms. Edema, exophthalmos, ptosis, diminished vision, and abnormal skin sensations around the eye may be associated with the paralysis. Usually symptoms are unilateral. In addition, migraine-associated symptoms (double vision, fever, malaise, nausea, and vomiting) may develop. Even after treatment, symptoms may recur spontaneously several times.

Etiology The syndrome is thought to be due to an abnormal autoimmune response coupled with an inflammation in the cavernous sinus and superior orbital fissure. Generalized inflammation and constricted or inflamed cranial blood vessels are other potential causes.

Epidemiology The syndrome occurs in males and females in equal numbers. The average age of onset is 41, although the disorder may occur at any age.

Related Disorders In **orbital cellulitis** there is inflammation of the tissues surrounding the orb. Symptoms include extreme pain, impaired eye movement, edema, fever, and malaise. Possible complications include impaired vision, venous abnormalities, and inflammation of the entire ocular area, brain, or the meninges.

Cavernous sinus thrombosis is usually caused by infection and clotting in the veins behind the eyeballs. It can be a complication of orbital cellulitis or an infection of facial skin. Signs and symptoms include edema, exophthalmos, fever, headache, and possibly convulsions. Prompt treatment with antibiotics, intravenous fluids, and bed rest is recommended.

Migraine headaches are usually unilateral. Patients may have a genetic predisposition (dominant). Often associated with these painful attacks are irritability, nausea, vomiting, constipation or diarrhea, and photosensitivity. Constriction of the cranial arteries may precede migraine headaches in some patients. Fever and ophthalmoplegia are not part of the symptom complex of migraine and may indicate Tolosa-Hunt syndrome.

Treatment—Standard A short course of corticosteroids often relieves the pain associated with Tolosa-Hunt syndrome. Pain usually subsides in untreated cases within 15 to 20 days. With drug treatment, pain may abate within 24 to 72 hours, although attacks may recur at any time.

Treatment—Investigational Please contact the agencies listed under Resources, below, for the most current information.

Resources

For more information on Tolosa-Hunt syndrome: National Organization for Rare Disorders (NORD); NIH/National Institute of Neurological Disorders & Stroke (NINDS); National Migraine Foundation.

References

A New Etiology for Visual Impairment and Chronic Headache. The Tolosa-Hunt Syndrome May be Only One Manifestation of Venous Vasculitis: J. Hannerz, et al., Cephalalgia, March 1986, vol. 6(1), pp. 59–63.

Steroid Responsive Ophthalmoplegia in a Child. Diagnostic Considerations: R.S. Kandt, et al., Arch. Neurol., June 1985, vol. 42(6), pp. 589–591.

Transient Unilateral Oculomotor Paralysis: E. Kattner, et al., Monatsschr. Kinderheilkd., March 1985, vol. 133(3), pp. 175–177.

A New Etiology for Visual Impairment and Chronic Headache. The Tolosa-Hunt Syndrome May be Only One Manifestation of Venous Vasculitis: J. Hannerz, et al., Cephalalgia, March 1986, vol. 6(1), pp. 59–63.

USHER SYNDROME

Description Usher syndrome encompasses a group of inherited disorders characterized by night blindness and vision loss similar to that seen in retinitis pigmentosa, in association with congenital hearing impairment. The syndrome is considered to be separate from other forms of retinitis pigmentosa. It occurs in 2 forms, types I and II, distinguished by age at onset and severity of the symptoms.

Synonyms

> Hereditary Deafness-Retinitis Pigmentosa
> Retinitis Pigmentosa and Congenital Deafness

Signs and Symptoms **Type I** Usher syndrome (**USH1**) has its onset in the first decade of life, some symptoms and signs first appearing in the teens. Syndrome features are profound congenital neurosensory deafness; unintelligible speech;

night blindness (nyctalopia) in the 2nd half of the 1st decade; pigmentary retinopathy; severe, progressive visual field loss; nonrecordable electroretinogram; and nonresponsive or hyporesponsive vestibular reflexes. Central visual acuity is variable (20/20 to about 20/200); blindness may occur from age 20 to 35.

Type II Usher syndrome **(USH2)** has its retinal onset in late adolescence or early adulthood. It is characterized by moderate-to-profound neurosensory hearing loss early in life; intelligible but abnormal speech; night blindness beginning in the early teens to early 20s; pigmentary retinopathy; mild-to-moderate visual field loss; a subnormal to nonrecordable electroretinogram; and usually normal vestibular responses. Central visual acuity has the same variability as in USH1, but onset of central loss is not until the mid 20s to mid 40s.

Etiology The inheritance for both USH1 and USH2 is autosomal recessive. An X-linked form has been reported but poorly substantiated. In general, severity of symptoms is symmetrical in affected individuals within a family. The disease gene for USH2 has been mapped to chromosome 1q. These same markers do not show linkage for USH1.

Epidemiology The prevalence of Usher syndrome is approximately 4:100,000. The prevalence for USH1 has been found to be higher in persons with Acadian ancestry in Louisiana and east Texas.

Related Disorders See *Retinitis Pigmentosa.*

Hallgren syndrome (Graefe-Sjögren syndrome) is characterized by deafness at birth accompanied by progressive visual impairment, including nystagmus and cataracts. Other symptoms include psychomotor retardation, vestibulocerebellar ataxia, mental deficiency, and psychosis.

Alstrom syndrome, an inherited disorder characterized by retinal degeneration with nystagmus and loss of central vision, is associated with childhood obesity. Sensorineural hearing loss and diabetes mellitus are likely to develop after age 10.

Treatment—Standard Treatment of Usher syndrome is symptomatic and supportive. Counseling services to individuals with hearing and vision loss can be helpful; genetic counseling is recommended for patients and families. Surgery to remove cataracts in conjunction with intraocular lens implantation may improve vision in proper candidates.

Early identification of Usher syndrome in a deaf child is essential. If visual loss occurs later in life, childhood acquisition of sign language may have little communicative value in adulthood. Consequently, methods of education and options should be explored carefully during school years.

Treatment—Investigational The ongoing investigation of chromosome markers is expected to result in improved gene carrier detection and the ability to provide prenatal testing.

Please contact the agencies listed under Resources, below, for the most current information.

Resources

For more information on Usher syndrome: National Organization for Rare

Disorders (NORD); National Federation of the Blind; American Council of the Blind; American Foundation for the Blind; Retinitis Pigmentosa Foundation Fighting Blindness; NIH/National Eye Institute; Alexander Graham Bell Association for the Deaf; American Humane Association (for trained hearing dogs); Deafness Research Foundation; National Information Center on Deafness; American Society for Deaf Children; NIH/National Institute of Deafness & Other Communication Disorders (NIDCD).

For genetic information and genetic counseling referrals: March of Dimes Birth Defects Foundation; National Center for Education in Maternal and Child Health (NCEMCH).

References

Mapping Recessive Ophthalmic Diseases: Linkage of the Locus for Usher Syndrome Type II to a DNA Marker on Chromosome 1q: R.A. Lewis, et al.; Genomics, 1990, vol. 7, pp. 250–256.

Mendelian Inheritance in Man, 9th ed.: V.A. McKusick; The Johns Hopkins University Press, 1990, pp. 1522–1524, 1714.

Cataract Extraction and Intraocular Lens Implantation in Patients with Retinitis Pigmentosa or Usher's Syndrome: D.A. Newsome, et al.; Arch. Ophthalmol., June 1986, vol. 104(6), pp. 852–854.

Radiation Sensitivity of Fibroblast Strains from Patients with Usher's Syndrome, Duchenne Muscular Dystrophy, and Huntington's Disease: J. Nove, et al.; Mutat. Res., July 1987, vol. 184(1), pp. 29–38.

Usher's Syndrome, Ophthalmic and Neuro-Otologic Findings Suggesting Genetic Heterogenicity: G.A. Fishman, et al.; Arch. Ophthalmol., September 1983, vol. 101(9), pp. 1367–74.

13 | ENVIRONMENTAL/TOXIC DISORDERS
By Robert H. Gray, Ph.D.

Perhaps it takes an illness, such as the rare thyroid condition, Graves disease, diagnosed in President and Mrs. George Bush, to emphasize the importance of environmental and occupational medicine. The diagnosis of this rare disease has prompted officials to analyze the water supply in the White House and other presidential residences. Graves disease has been reported to be associated with water containing lithium and/or iodine. The chances of two non-blood-related individuals having the same thyroid disease are said to be one in three million. The incident has highlighted the need for a greater awareness of environmental factors in rare diseases. The Institute of Medicine report of 1989 points out that the current shortage of environmental and occupational physicians is between 1,600 and 3,500. These shortages should stimulate all physicians to increase their awareness of rare diseases of environmental and occupational origin.

Rare toxic disorders in humans can occur following exposures to a large spectrum of occupational or environmental toxic agents. The origin of toxic agents may be chemical, physical, or biological. Symptoms produced by such exposures are not always easily traced to the source of the problem. Exposure to some occupational agents is characterized by a latent interval between exposure and onset of the clinical symptoms. Latent periods are highly variable, but can be up to 20 years or longer. In addition, the combination of exposures to multiple toxic compounds may mask or alter the expected symptoms once the suspected agent is identified. Enumeration of a comprehensive list of toxic agents or conditions that produce toxic responses in humans is beyond the scope of this section. Here, the focus is on selected rare disorders resulting from occupational and environmental exposures.

In this section, selected rare toxic/environmental disorders of chemical, physical, or biological origin are described. Exposures of occupational origin include poisoning by selected heavy metals, including beryllium, aluminum, antimony, arsenic, cadmium, chromium, cobalt, copper, gold, lead, lithium, manganese, mercury, molybdenum, silver, vanadium, and zinc. Formaldehyde exposure is included as a different type of a toxic chemical. Radiation exposure is discussed as an example of a toxic physical agent. Two environmental disorders, acute mountain sickness (altitude sickness) and an unusual toxin of biological (fish) origin, ciguatera, are described.

Care should be exercised while investigating and diagnosing symptoms associated with rare toxic/environmental disorders. The investigation and diagnosis of such disorders requires that the physician exhibit extensive "peripheral vision" regarding the characterization of the symptoms being investigated. An acute awareness of the environment in which the patient has been living requires thorough scrutiny. A profile of the patient's workplace, home living conditions, associations with friends and co-workers, leisure time activities and social habits, and the general health of the individual can be helpful in narrowing the range of suspected problems. The patient's occupational health history should be carefully examined and documented to identify suspected toxic agent exposures and the lengths of such exposures. If occupational exposures are suspected, attempts should be made to document the route (oral, dermal, inhalation, etc.) of exposure, the estimated concentration of the toxin, and the duration of the exposure.

The following patient information may be useful in making a clinical diagnosis.

Comprehensive occupational history including jobs held and their durations.

Is the patient aware of exposure to suspected toxic agents (solvents, dust, etc.)? If so, what agents, when did the exposure take place, and what was its duration?

How long have the current symptoms been evident? Have the symptoms appeared and then disappeared?

Was protective equipment recommended in the patient's job? If so, was the equipment used?

Have the patient's co-workers experienced similar symptoms? If so, how many and how long?

Are there known sources of pollution (air or water) with potential harmful health effects near the patient's residence?

Have other members of the patient's family or those living near the patient exhibited similar symptoms? If so, when were the symptoms first observed and how long did they last?

Have there been any new construction or renovation projects initiated, or any new or seasonal maintenance procedures performed in the workplace or at home involving new materials such as plywood, carpets, or solvents, or recent applications of pesticides or herbicides? In the past, have solvents, pesticides, or herbicides been stored for extended periods near current living areas or working areas? Have there been any recent ventilation or air conditioning system modifications?

What is the smoking history of the patient? If the patient has been a smoker, how many years? Packs per day? If the patient has quit smoking, how long ago?

Has the patient's diet changed within the last week?

Answers to these questions and to others, as more is known about a suspected toxic agent exposure, should aid in eliminating some types of agents and bring one closer to identifying the causal toxic agent. Attempts have been made during the preparation of this chapter to incorporate recent findings from medical literature on the toxic agents covered. New information is, however, continually becoming available. For example, data on radiation sickness is appearing slowly from the aftermath of the Chernobyl accident in 1986. International agencies, such as the World Health Organization, are now initiating studies on the longterm health effects of radiation from the accident. The latter will provide new data in the future on short- and longterm effects of radiation exposure. Additional information on other rare forms of toxic/environmental disorders can be obtained from local poison control centers, the National Institute for Environmental Health Science (NIEHS), or the Food and Drug Administration (FDA).

ENVIRONMENTAL/TOXIC DISORDERS
Listings in This Section

ACUTE MOUNTAIN SICKNESS

Description Acute mountain sickness is a syndrome that may occur in some unacclimated persons who ascend rapidly to altitudes higher than 7000 to 9000 feet (2200 to 2743 meters).

Synonyms
> High-Altitude Illness
> Mareo
> Mountain Sickness
> Puna
> Soroche

Signs and Symptoms The syndrome may occur during the first 8 to 24 hours after a person reaches a high altitude. Severity and duration of the symptoms vary with the rate of climbing and the ascent height, as well as with the individual's susceptibility. Headache, fatigue, difficulty sleeping, anorexia, nausea, and vomiting may occur, as well as rales, retinal bleeding, and peripheral edema. Oliguria, ataxia, tachycardia, and impaired thinking may also result.

Etiology Symptoms occur because of the decrease in available oxygen to the tissues at high altitudes. Decompression-inducible platelet aggregation (DIPA) leading to vascular occlusion has been suggested as an etiologic factor in acute mountain sickness.

Epidemiology Acute mountain sickness affects males and females in equal numbers. Susceptible persons include those who require more than the normal amount of oxygen, or those who are particularly intolerant of decreased oxygen levels. Individuals who urinate infrequently appear to be particularly susceptible.

Related Disorders Subacute infantile mountain sickness is a severe disorder of infants that may occur when they are born at low altitudes and then taken to higher elevations. Thickening of the pulmonary arteries and enlargement of the cavities of the heart have been seen with this disorder.

High-altitude pulmonary edema is a severe complication of acute mountain sickness caused by the development of hypoxia at altitudes greater than 9000 feet. Findings include headaches, vomiting, dyspnea, coughing, rales, tachycardia, and cyanosis. Retinal bleeding, papilledema, problems of memory and orientation, and loss of consciousness may also occur.

High-altitude cerebral edema, also a severe consequence of acute mountain sickness, is characterized by headaches, diplopia, visual and auditory hallucinations, loss of consciousness, and ataxia.

Treatment—Standard Prompt descent is the most successful treatment for acute mountain sickness. For mild cases, rest coupled with light activity, frequent small meals, no alcohol, and acetaminophen for headache may be all the supportive care that will be needed. For more severe cases, dexamethasone can be used for its antiinflammatory properties, and acetazolamide for edema, although care should be taken to replace fluids in the sometimes already dehydrated patients.

To prevent acute mountain sickness, a slow staged ascent, remaining 2 to 5 days at a middle altitude, or prophylactic use of dexamethasone or acetazolamide may be recommended.

Treatment—Investigational Researchers are further investigating oxygen therapy and the combination of dexamethasone and acetazolamide for the treatment of acute mountain sickness.

Please contact the agencies listed under Resources, below, for the most current information.

Resources

For more information on acute mountain sickness: National Organization for Rare Disorders (NORD); NIH/National Institute of Environmental Health Sciences (NIEHS).

References

Acute Mountain Sickness, a Vascular Occlusive Disease: M. Murayama; Medical Hypotheses, March 1990, vol. 31(3), pp. 189–195.

Current Concepts: Acute Mountain Sickness: T.S. Johnson, et al.; N. Engl. J. Med., September 29, 1988, vol. 319(13), pp. 841–845.

High Altitude Cerebral Oedema: C. Clarke; Int. J. Sports Med., April 1988, vol. 9(2), pp. 170–174.

Clinical Features of Patients with High-Altitude Pulmonary Edema in Japan: T. Kobayashi et al.; Chest, November 1987, vol. 92(5), pp. 814–821.

BERYLLIOSIS

Description Berylliosis, the result of inhalation of beryllium dust or fumes, may affect the lungs, skin, eyes, or blood. It can occur acutely or after longterm exposure. Some cases may be delayed as long as 20 years after exposure.

Beryllium is used in the refining of precious metals, in structural materials in the spacecraft industry, in supersonic jets, and in certain components of the space shuttle. Reclaiming beryllium from discarded electronic components and other materials is a separate industry. Beryllium smelter workers may be exposed to high levels of the metal as it is crushed, milled, screened, and melted. Even though the workers are required to wear respirators, contamination may occur, and if dust on their clothes is brought home, other members of their families may develop the condition.

Synonyms

Beryllium Granulomatosis
Beryllium Pneumonosis
Beryllium Poisoning

Signs and Symptoms Acute berylliosis primarily affects the respiratory system. Chronic exposure is characterized by the formation of pulmonary granulomas, nodular accumulations, or inflammatory cells. Coughing, which is dry at first, later becomes violent and exhausting. Dyspnea and hemoptysis, weight loss, chest pain, and fatigue may develop.

An allergic reaction to beryllium can be manifested as an erythematous, vesicular rash on the face, neck, arms, or hands. Lymphadenopathy may be noted near the affected skin areas.

With prolonged exposure, berylliosis may become chronic. Cyanosis, accompanied by fever and weight loss, may develop, as well as orthopnea. Fingernails may become clubbed, and corneal lesions may be found. It is difficult to distinguish chronic beryllium disease from miliary tuberculosis and sarcoidosis, although central nervous system or salivary gland involvement is more typical of sarcoidosis.

Research indicates that the peripheral blood lymphocyte transformation test may be used to identify berylliosis in its early stages.

Etiology Researchers believe that the symptoms of berylliosis are caused by the processes of cell-mediated immunity, including the release of lymphocytes and lymphokines. Beryllium-specific T cells are thought to be involved.

Epidemiology Persons at risk for developing berylliosis include those employed in the aerospace, aviation, or nuclear weapons and power industries; those involved in beryllium mining and processing; and those exposed to fluorescent lamp manufacture between 1943 and 1955. In some cases, the families of these employees also may have been exposed, particularly anyone who launders the worker's clothes. Persons living in the vicinity of beryllium refineries have also been affected.

Related Disorders See *Alveolitis, Extrinsic Allergic.*

Treatment—Standard Exposure to beryllium fumes or dust should be removed. In single-exposure acute cases, treatment is symptomatic since the effects are short-term and usually reversible. In chronic cases, corticosteroid therapy may be helpful if begun early in the course of the disease. Bronchoalveolar lavage may be useful in chronic cases, both to confirm the diagnosis and to help remove inorganic particles from the lungs.

Treatment—Investigational Longterm intermittent chelation with EDTA is being evaluated.

Please contact the agencies listed under Resources, below, for the most current information.

Resources

For more information on berylliosis: National Organization for Rare Disorders (NORD); American Lung Association; NIH/National Institute of Allergy and Infectious Diseases (NIAID); Centers for Disease Control (CDC); NIH/National Institute of Environmental Health Sciences (NIEHS).

References

Internal Medicine, 3rd ed.: J.H. Stein, ed.-in-chief; Little, Brown and Company, 1990, p. 706.

Mitogenic Effect of Beryllium Sulfate on Mouse B Lymphocytes but not T Lymphocytes in Vitro: L.S. Newmann and P.A. Campbell; Int. Arch. Allergy Appl. Immunol., 1987, vol. 84(3), pp. 223–227.

Screening Blood Test Identifies Subclinical Beryllium Disease: K. Kreiss, et al.; J. Occup. Med., July 1989, vol. 31(7), pp. 603–608.

Chronic Beryllium Disease: Diagnosis, Radiographic Findings, and Correlation with Pulmonary Function Tests: J.M. Aronchick, et al.; Radiology, June 1987, vol. 163(3), pp. 677–682.

Transmission of Occupational Disease to Family Contacts: B. Knishkowy, et al.; Am. J. Ind. Med., 1986, vol. 9(6), pp. 543–550.

Chronic Beryllium Disease in a Precious Metal Refinery. Clinical Epidemiologic and Immunologic Evidence for Continuing Risk from Exposure to Low Level Beryllium Fumes: M.R. Cullen, et al.; Am. Rev. Respir. Dis., January 1987, vol. 135(1), pp. 201–208.

CIGUATERA FISH POISONING

Description Gastrointestinal, neurologic, and muscular symptoms occur after ingestion of certain tropical and subtropical fish contaminated with ciguatoxins. More than 400 species of fish have been implicated, including many that are otherwise considered edible, such as snapper, sea bass, and perch. The disease has been occurring more frequently in the United States during the past few years.

Synonyms
Fish Poisoning
Ichthyosarcotoxism

Signs and Symptoms Symptoms of acute ciguatera poisoning may begin as soon as 30 minutes after exposure. Typical initial findings include itching, tingling, and numbness of the lips, tongue, hands, and feet. Other symptoms that also may occur during the first 6 to 17 hours are abdominal cramps, nausea, vomiting, diarrhea, and pruritus. Chills, weakness, restlessness, dizziness, wheezing, myalgias, and arthralgias may develop. Acute symptoms generally resolve within a few days, but disabling neurologic symptoms may continue for several months. In severe cases, there may be rapid progression to dyspnea and muscular paralysis. Death may occur within 24 hours, from respiratory arrest or convulsions.

Etiology Ciguatera fish poisoning is caused by toxins contained in tropical fish at certain times of the year. There is no test for the detection of the toxin, and no known method of cooking the fish can eradicate the toxin.

Epidemiology Incidence of ciguatera fish poisoning is highest in tropical countries, particularly those in the Pacific.

The presence of ciguatoxin has been reported in both semen (producing symptoms in females after sexual intercourse) and breast milk.

Related Disorders **Tetraodon poisoning** results from eating puffer fish that contain the tetraodon toxin. Symptoms are similar to those of ciguatera poisoning, but mortality may be as high as 50 percent. **Scombroid poisoning** is caused by a toxin formed during bacterial decay of fish, and is usually associated with inadequate refrigeration. Symptoms generally begin soon after ingestion and resemble those of a histamine reaction, with flushing, dizziness, urticaria, nausea, and vomiting.

Treatment—Standard Gastric lavage should be instituted as soon as possible, and the effects of persistent nausea and vomiting must be treated. Appropriate measures for shock, convulsions, or respiratory failure should begin promptly if these developments occur.

Treatment—Investigational Successful treatment of acute ciguatera poisoning with an intravenous infusion of mannitol has recently been reported.

Please contact the agencies listed under Resources, below, for the most current investigation.

Resources

For more information on ciguatera fish poisoning: National Organization for Rare Disorders (NORD); Centers for Disease Control (CDC).

For immediate help: Contact the local poison control center listed in the telephone directory.

References

Cecil Textbook of Medicine, 18th ed.: J.B. Wyngaarden and L.H. Smith, Jr., eds.; W.B. Saunders Company, 1988, p. 786.

Ciguatera and Mannitol: Experience with a New Treatment Regimen: J.H. Pearn, et al.; Med. J. Australia, July 17, 1989, vol. 151(2), pp. 77–80.

Successful Treatment of Ciguatera Fish Poisoning with Intravenous Mannitol: N.A. Palafox, et al.; JAMA, May 13, 1988, vol. 259(18), pp. 2740–2742.

Can Ciguatera Be a Sexually Transmitted Disease?: W.R. Lange, et al.; J. Toxicol. Clin. Toxicol., 1989, vol. 27(3), pp. 193–197.

Mother's Milk Turns Toxic Following Fish Feast (letter): D.G. Blythe and D.P. de Sylva; JAMA, October 24–31, 1990, vol. 264(16), p. 2074.

FORMALDEHYDE POISONING

Description Formaldehyde poisoning, which results from breathing the fumes of formaldehyde, can occur while a person is working directly with the chemical, using equipment cleaned with it, or handling materials made from it.

Synonyms

Formaldehyde Exposure
Formaldehyde Toxicity
Formalin Intoxication
Formalin Toxicity

Signs and Symptoms Findings are varied. Eye, nose, and throat irritation, headaches, and dermal injury may occur. If formaldehyde is swallowed, it will burn the esophagus and stomach. Acute hemolysis has occurred when patients undergo dialysis on machines cleaned with formaldehyde. In extreme cases, formaldehyde poisoning may result in hypotension, arrhythmias, irregular breathing, restlessness, unconsciousness, and coma.

Formaldehyde exposure in mainstream tobacco smoke is suspected of increasing the risk of cancer in smokers. Other recent studies have implicated formaldehyde as a possible human carcinogen; the results do not appear definitive as yet.

Etiology Causes are varied and include the handling of products made with formaldehyde, such as chip board and foam insulation; accidental ingestion of formaldehyde; or breathing the vapors given off by the chemical itself. Poisoning may also occur when the chemical is being administered as formalin-soaked packs for cysts, or when formalin is used as a cleaning agent for hospital equipment and is not completely removed.

Epidemiology Males and females are affected in equal numbers, and in many industrial settings. In occupational settings, poisoning has occurred even with appropriate air filtering equipment. Formaldehyde is also a component of mainstream cigarette smoke, and it may contribute to carcinogenesis among smokers.

Related Disorders See *Heavy Metal Poisoning; Berylliosis.*

Treatment—Standard Treatment primarily consists of identification of the source and removal of the chemical from the occupational, domestic, or general environment. Other treatment is symptomatic and supportive.

Treatment—Investigational Please contact the agencies listed under Resources, below, for the most current information.

Resources

For more information on formaldehyde poisoning: National Organization for Rare Disorders (NORD); American Academy of Environmental Medicine; NIH/National Institute of Environmental Health Sciences (NIEHS).

References
Mortality From Lung Cancer Among Workers Employed in Formaldehyde Industries: A. Blair, et al.; Am. J. Ind. Med., 1990, vol. 17(6), pp. 683–699.

Quantitative Cancer Risk Estimation for Formaldehyde: T.B. Starr; Risk Analysis, March 1990, vol. 10(1), pp. 85–91.

Formaldehyde Exposures From Tobacco Smoke: A Review: T. Godish; Am. J. Public Health, August 1989, vol. 79(8), pp. 1044–1045.

Formaldehyde: AMA Council on Scientific Affairs; Conn. Med., April 1989, vol. 53(4), pp. 229–235.

Formaldehyde: Council on Scientific Affairs; JAMA, February 24, 1989, vol. 261(8), pp. 1183–1187.

Cancer Risks due to Occupational Exposure to Formaldehyde: Results of a Multi-Site Case-Control Study in Montreal: M. Gerin, et al.; Int. J. Cancer, July 15, 1989, vol. 44(1), pp. 53–58.

Formaldehyde-Related Health Complaints of Residents Living in Mobile and Conventional Homes: I.M. Ritchie, et al.; Am. J. Public Health, March 1987, vol. 77(3), pp. 323–328.

Formaldehyde-Induced Corrosive Gastric Cicatrization: Case Report: R. Kochhar, et al.; Hum. Toxicol., December 1986, vol. 5(6), pp. 381–382.

Acute Intravascular Hemolysis Due to Accidental Formalin Intoxication During Hemodialysis: K.K. Pun, et al.; Clin. Nephrol., March 1984, vol. 21(3), pp. 188–190.

Formalin Toxicity in Hydatid Liver Disease: A.R. Aggarwal, et al.; Anaesthesia, July 1983, vol. 38(7), pp. 662–665.

HEAVY METAL POISONING

Description Heavy metal poisoning today is generally caused by industrial exposure, although environmental exposure to toxins (e.g., aluminum, arsenic, cadmium, lead, mercury) still occurs. Depending on the type and duration of exposure, the injury may be pulmonary, neurologic, cutaneous, or gastrointestinal.

One particular syndrome, **metal fume fever,** results when a volatilized heavy metal is inhaled. This is an acute, flulike illness characterized by abrupt onset of fever, shaking chills, headache, and cough. Treatment is supportive; the illness is usually brief and self-limited. Occasionally there may be sequelae, however, such as pulmonary edema.

Signs, Symptoms, and Treatment Signs and symptoms of heavy metal poisoning vary according to the type of metal overexposure involved.

Aluminum containers used in the manufacture and processing of some foods, cosmetics, and medicines, and also aluminum used for water purification, can cause poisoning. Aluminum phosphide, used as a grain preservative, has been associated with serious cardiac disturbances. Workers exposed to aluminum ore suffer inhalation injury that may lead to pulmonary changes including emphysema. Aluminum poisoning also occurs among patients with chronic renal failure undergoing dialysis, leading to encephalopathy and osteomalacia. Deferoxamine mesylate has been used as a chelating agent, with improved symptoms and bone histology; ocular, auditory, and infectious adverse effects have been reported.

Antimony, used for hardening lead and in the manufacture of batteries and cables, may cause pulmonary injury and skin cancer, especially in individuals who smoke. Cardiac arrhythmias have also been seen following antimony exposure. Chelation therapy with dimercaprol is recommended.

Arsenic is used in the manufacture of pesticides and in other industrial settings, and also may be found in common substances such as insecticides, and, rarely, in environmental situations such as private wells. Overexposure may cause gastrointestinal disturbances, headache, drowsiness, confusion, delirium, seizures, and death. In cases of chronic poisoning, hyperkeratosis of the palms of the hands, weakness, muscle aches, chills, fever, and anemia may develop, as well as cognitive impairment and apparent psychological disturbances. Exposure to arsenic also is associated with an increased risk of cutaneous, tracheal, and bronchogenic carcinoma, and hepatic hemangiosarcoma. Chelation therapy with dimercaprol or D-penicillamine is recommended. Arsenical neuropathy does not respond well to chelation.

Beryllium (see *Berylliosis.*)

Cadmium is used for many items, including electroplating, storage batteries, vapor lamps, and in some solders. Cadmium is also present in fertilizers and sewage sludge. Overexposure may cause emphysema, fatigue, headache, vomiting, anemia, anosmia, renal dysfunction, and osteopenia. There also appears to be an association with prostatic cancer and neuropsychological impairment among cadmium workers. Dimercaprol is contraindicated for chelation therapy. Recent studies on new compounds, such as dithiocarbamate derivatives, give promise of development of useful and safe therapeutic chelating agents.

Chromium is used in the manufacture of cars, glass, pottery, and linoleum. Acute exposure is associated with gastroenteritis, shock, and toxic nephritis. Chronic exposure can cause perforation of the nasal septum. Overexposure to chromium also is associated with an incidence of respiratory tract cancer 15 to 20 times that found in the general population. Chelation therapy with calcium disodium edetate or dimercaprol is recommended.

Cobalt, used in making jet engines, and in other occupations such as diamond polishing, may be associated with gastrointestinal disturbances, tinnitus, neuropathy, respiratory diseases and bronchial hyperreactivity, thyroid dysfunction, cardiomyopathy, and nephrotoxicity. Chelation therapy with dimercaprol is recommended.

Copper, used in the manufacture of electrical wires, may cause metal fume disease, gastrointestinal disturbances, hepatic and renal failure, emphysema, and, it is suggested, hypertension in blacks. Chelation with dimercaprol and possibly D-penicillamine is recommended.

Gold is widely used in treatment of rheumatoid arthritis, Sjögren's syndrome, and nondisseminated lupus erythematosus. Overexposure to gold may cause dermatitis, headache, vomiting, bone marrow depression, the nephrotic syndrome, jaundice, cholestasis, pneumonitis, gastrointestinal bleeding, and ocular chrysiasis. Gold therapy is usually discontinued when such symptoms occur. Chelation therapy with dimercaprol is recommended.

Lead production workers, battery plant workers, welders, and solderers may be overexposed to lead if proper precautions are not taken. Environmental exposure, such as from paint and leaded gasoline, and leaching from certain imported dishware, is becoming less common but still exists. Lead poisoning may cause miscarriage, birth defects, hearing and eye-hand coordination defects, anemia, abdominal pain ("lead colic"), decreased male fertility, decreased muscular strength and endurance, nephrotoxicity, peripheral neuropathy with wrist drop, hostility, depression, and anxiety. There also may be cognitive and behavioral changes. Chelation therapy with dimercaprol and calcium disodium edetate is recommended.

Lithium is widely used in therapeutic management of psychiatric disorders, but also is found in some industrial applications. Overexposure generally occurs during therapeutic usage, when blood levels of the drug increase.

Central nervous system effects include hand tremor, parkinsonism, and memory impairment. Severe gastroenteritis may occur, and arrhythmias, hypotension, the nephrotic syndrome, and renal failure may develop. Nystagmus, carpal tunnel syndrome, a Creutzfeldt-Jakob–like syndrome, and fetal polyhydramnios have been reported.

Manganese is used as a purifying agent in the production of several metals. Acute exposure can cause metal fume fever. Chronic exposure among miners has been described as causing psychiatric disturbances that resemble schizophrenia and neurologic disturbances that resemble parkinsonism. An association between prostatic cancer and manganese exposure has been suggested.

Mercury exposure occurs most commonly among dental and chemical workers.

Exposure to this metal also may occur from its presence in dental filling amalgam and in some latex paints, and from the ingestion of seafood with high mercury levels. Pulmonary effects may include dyspnea, coughing, and chest pain. In severe cases, interstitial pneumonitis and pulmonary edema may develop. Mercury poisoning also may lead to behavioral and neurologic changes, gastrointestinal disturbances, nephrotoxicity, dehydration, and shock. Mercury pigmentation and possible neuropsychiatric symptoms were reported in an Australian case in which an over-the-counter mercury-containing cosmetic cream was used. Chelation therapy with dimercaprol or D-penicillamine is recommended.

Molybdenum is used in the hardening of steel. Overexposure may cause copper depletion, liver and kidney damage, weight loss, and central nervous system changes.

Silver exposure may be dental-related or may include working in the manufacture of precious metal powders or chemicals such as silver nitrate. Overexposure may cause fume fever, gastroenteritis, and argyria. Chelation is ineffective.

Vanadium exposure in the workplace includes the manufacture of vanadium pentoxide from magnetite ore. Overexposure may result in metal fume fever, anorexia, throat pain, nasal irritation, and acute bronchitis. Psychiatric disturbances and renal dysfunction have also been noted. A further characteristic finding is a greenish-black discoloration of the tongue. Chelation therapy with calcium disodium edetate is recommended.

Zinc is found in paints, enamels, wood preservatives, and rodenticides. Cutaneous reactions have been reported. Inhalation overexposure may lead to metal fume fever, gastrointestinal disturbances, and liver dysfunction. Chelation therapy with edetic acid or dimercaprol is recommended.

Etiology Heavy metal poisoning is a result of overexposure from industrial sites, polluted air or water, or contaminated food or cookware.

Epidemiology Industrial workers, members of their families, and others living near industrial sites are most commonly exposed to heavy metals.

Related Disorders See *Anemia, Fanconi; Wilson Disease.*

Treatment—Standard Occupational exposure to heavy metals requires careful prevention through the use of masks and protective clothing.

Treatment consists of various chelating agents as noted above. Gastric lavage is used to remove ingested materials. In the case of inhalation injury, the patient should be removed from the contaminated environment and respiration supported. Bronchodilators may be needed. In case of cerebral edema, treatment with mannitol and corticosteroid drugs, along with intracranial monitoring, is required. If kidney failure develops, hemodialysis may be needed. Treatment is otherwise symptomatic and supportive.

Treatment—Investigational Newer chelating agents are being investigated, such as dimercaptosuccinic acid for arsenic exposure, and dithiocarbamate derivatives for cadmium toxicity.

Please contact the agencies listed under Resources, below, for the most current

information.

Resources

For more information on heavy metal poisoning: National Organization for Rare Disorders (NORD); NIH/National Institute of Environmental Health Sciences (NIEHS); Food and Drug Administration (FDA).

References

The Metal in Our Mettle: R.W. Miller, FDA Consumer; December 1988–January 1989, pp. 24–27.

Aluminum:

Aspects of Aluminum Toxicity: C.D. Hewitt, et al.; Clin. Lab. Med., June 1990, vol. 10(2), pp. 403–422.

Aluminum Toxicity and Alzheimer's Disease. Is There a Connection?: R.C. Handy; Postgrad. Med., October 1990, vol. 88(5), pp. 239–240.

Aluminum Toxicity in Mammals: A Minireview: J.B. Cannata and J.L. Domingo; Vet. Hum. Toxicol., December 1989, vol. 31(6), pp. 577–583.

Cardiovascular Complications of Aluminum Phosphide Poisoning: S.N. Khosla, et al.; Angiology, April 1988, vol. 39(4), pp. 355–359.

Deferoxamine for Aluminum Toxicity in Dialysis Patients: P. Hernandez and C.A. Johnson; ANNA J., June 1990, vol. 17(3), pp. 224–228.

Complexation of Labile Metal Ions and Effect on Toxicity: A.E. Martell; Biol. Trace Elem. Res., July–September 1989, vol. 21, pp. 295–303.

Aluminum and Chronic Renal Failure: Sources, Absorption, Transport, and Toxicity: M.R. Wills and J. Savory; Crit. Rev. Clin. Lab. Sci., 1989, vol. 27(1), pp. 59–107.

Antimony:

Oral Antimony Intoxications in Man: L.F. Lauwers, et al.; Crit. Care Med., March 1990, vol. 18(3), pp. 324–326.

Arsenic:

Hematologic Effects of Heavy Metal Poisoning: Q.S. Ringenberg, et al.; South. Med. J., September 1988, vol. 81(9), pp. 1132–1139.

Acute Arsenic Intoxication: J.P. Campbell and J.A. Alvarez; Am. Fam. Physician, December 1989, vol. 40(6), pp. 93–97.

Encephalopathy: An Uncommon Manifestation of Workplace Arsenic Poisoning?: W.E. Morton and G.A. Caron; Am. J. Ind. Med., 1989, vol. 15(1), pp. 1–5.

Acute Arsenic Intoxication from Environmental Arsenic Exposure: A. Franzblau and R. Lilis; Arch. Environ. Health, November–December 1989, vol. 44(6), pp. 385–390.

Acute Lead Arsenate Poisoning: G.A. Tallis; Austral. New Z. J. Med., December 1989, vol. 19(6), pp. 730–732.

Acute Arsenic Toxicity—An Opaque Poison: J.R. Gray, et al.; Can. Assoc. Radiol. J., August 1989, vol. 40(4), pp. 226–227.

Arsenic-Induced Skin Toxicity: R.L. Shannon and D.S. Strayer; Hum. Toxicol., March 1989, vol. 8(2), pp. 99–104.

Cadmium:

The Search for Chelate Antagonists for Chronic Cadmium Intoxication: M.M. Jones and M.G. Cherian; Toxicology, May 14, 1990, vol. 62(1), pp. 1–25.

A Quantitative Study of Iliac Bone Histopathology on 62 Cases with Itai-Itai Disease: M. Noda and M. Kitagawa; Calcif. Tissue Int., August 1990, vol. 47(2), pp. 66–74.

Neuropsychological Effects of Occupational Exposure to Cadmium: R.P. Hart, et al.; J. Clin. Exp. Neuropsychol., December 1989, vol. 11(6), pp. 933–943.

Progress of Renal Dysfunction in Inhabitants Environmentally Exposed to Cadmium: T. Kido, et al.; Arch. Environ. Health, May–June 1988, vol. 43(3), pp. 213–217.

Chromium:

Environmentally Related Diseases of the Urinary Tract: R.A. Goyer; Med. Clin. N. Am., March 1990, vol. 74(2), pp. 377–389.

Review of Occupational Epidemiology of Chromium Chemicals and Respiratory Cancer: R.B. Hayes; Sci. Total Environ., June 1, 1988, vol. 71(3), pp. 331–339.

CT Findings of the Nose and Paranasal Sinuses in Chromium Intoxication: M.J. Kim, et al.; Yonsei Med. J., September 1989, vol. 30(3), pp. 305–309.

Cobalt:

Rapidly Fatal Progression of Cobalt Lung in a Diamond Polisher: B. Nemery, et al.; Am. Rev. Respir. Dis., May 1990, vol. 141(5 Pt. 1), pp. 1373–1378.

The Respiratory Effects of Cobalt: D.W. Cugell, et al.; Arch. Intern. Med., January 1990, vol. 150(1), pp. 177–183.

Evaluation of Right and Left Ventricular Function in Hard Metal Workers: S.F. Horowitz, et al.; Br. J. Ind. Med., November 1988, vol. 45(11), pp. 742–746.

Hard Metal Asthma: Cross Immunological and Respiratory Reactivity Between Cobalt and Nickel?: T. Shirakawa, et al.; Thorax, April 1990, vol. 45(4), pp. 267–271.

Copper:

Cadmium Fume Inhalation and Emphysema [in copper-cadmium alloy manufacturing]: A.G. Davison, et al.; Lancet, March 26, 1988, vol. 1(8587), pp. 663–667.

Hypertension: Heavy Metals, Useful Cations and Melanin as a Possible Repository: C.C. Pfeiffer and R.J. Mailloux; Med. Hypotheses, June 1988, vol. 26(2), pp. 125–130.

Gold:

Leucopenia in Rheumatoid Arthritis: Relationship to Gold or Sulphasalazine Therapy: R.S. Amos and D. E. Bax; Br. J. Rheumatol., December 1988, vol. 27(6), pp. 465–468.

Cholestasis and Pneumonitis Induced by Gold Therapy: J.M. Farre, et al.; Clin. Rheumatol., December 1989, vol. 8(4), pp. 538–540.

Ocular Chrysiasis: D.W. Tierney; J. Am. Optom. Assoc., December 1988, vol. 59(12), pp. 960–962.

Cutaneous Reactions to Drugs Used for Rheumatologic Disorders: D.E. Roth, et al.; Med. Clin. N. Am., September 1989, vol. 73(5), pp. 1275–1298.

Lead:

Lead-Induced Anemia: Dose-Response Relationships and Evidence for a Threshold: J. Schwartz, et al.; Am. J. Pub. Health, February 1990, vol. 80(2), pp. 165–168.

Neurobehavioral Estimation of Children with Life-Long Increased Lead Exposure: A. Benetou-Marantidou, et al.; Arch. Environ. Health, November–December 1988, vol. 43(6), pp. 392–395.

The Persistent Threat of Lead: Medical and Sociological Issues: H.L. Needleman; Curr. Probl. Pediatr., December 1988, vol. 18(12), pp. 697–744.

Lead Toxicity: From Overt to Subclinical to Subtle Health Effects: R.A. Goyer; Environ. Health Perspect., June 1990, vol. 86, pp. 177–181.

Occupational Lead Exposure and Pituitary Function: A. Gustafson, et al.; Int. Arch. Occup. Environ. Health, 1989, vol. 61(4), pp. 277–281.

Thyroid Function as Assessed by Routine Laboratory Tests of Workers with Long-Term Lead Exposure: M. Tuppurainen, et al.; Scand. J. Work Environ. Health, June 1988, vol. 14(3), pp. 175–180.

Lithium:

The Use of Lithium in the Medically Ill: K. DasGupta and J.W. Jefferson; Gen. Hosp. Psychiatry, March 1990, vol. 12(2), pp. 83–97.

Focal Segmental Glomerulosclerosis in Patients Receiving Lithium Carbonate: R.N. Santella, et al.; Am. J. Med., May 1988, vol. 84(5), pp. 951–954.

Lithium-Induced Nephrotic Syndrome: I.K. Wood, et al.; Am. J. Psychiatry, January 1989, vol. 146(1), pp. 84–87.

Lithium-Induced Downbeat Nystagmus: D.P. Williams, et al.; Arch. Neurol., September 1988, vol. 45(9), pp. 1022–1023.
Lithium-Induced Carpal Tunnel Syndrome: M.P. Deahl; Br. J. Psychiatry, August 1988, vol. 153, pp. 250–251.
A Creutzfeldt-Jakob–Like Syndrome due to Lithium Toxicity: S.J. Smith and R.S. Kocen; J. Neurol. Neurosurg. Psychiatry, January 1988, vol. 51(1), pp. 120–123.
Maternal Lithium Therapy and Polyhydramnios: M.S. Ang, et al.; Obstet. Gynecol., September 1990, vol. 76(3 Pt. 2), pp. 517–519.

Manganese:
Epidemiological Survey Among Workers Exposed to Manganese: Effects on Lung, Central Nervous System, and some Biological Indices [published erratum appears in Am. J. Med., 1987, vol. 12(1), pp. 119–120]: H. Roels, et al.; Am. J. Med., 1987, vol. 11(3), pp. 307–327.
Manganese-Induced Parkinsonism: An Outbreak due to an Unrepaired Ventilation Control System in a Ferromanganese Smelter: J.D. Wang, et al.; Br. J. Ind. Med., December 1989, vol. 46(12), pp. 856–859.
The Health Implications of Increased Manganese in the Environment Resulting from the Combustion of Fuel Additives: A Review of the Literature: W.C. Cooper; J. Toxicol. Environ. Health, 1984, vol 14(1), pp. 23–46.
A Clustering of Prostatic Cancer in an Area with Many Manganese Mines: H. Watanabe, et al.; Tohoku J. Exp. Med., December 1981, vol. 135(4), pp. 441–442.

Mercury:
Were the Hatters of New Jersey "Mad"?: R.P. Wedeen; Am. J. Ind. Med., 1989, vol. 16(2), pp. 225–233.
The Relationship Between Mercury from Dental Amalgam and Mental Health: R.L. Siblerud; Am. J. Psychother., October 1989, vol. 43(4), pp. 575–587.
Cutaneous Manifestations of Acrodynia (Pink Disease): S.M. Dinehart, et al.; Arch. Dermatol., January 1988, vol. 124(1), pp. 107–109.
Mercury Excretion and Occupational Exposure of Dental Personnel: A. Jokstad; Community Dent. Oral Epidemiol., June 1990, vol. 18(3), pp. 143–148.
Mercury Pigmentation and High Mercury Levels from the Use of a Cosmetic Cream: D.J. Dyall-Smith and J.P. Scurry; Med. J. Australia, October 1, 1990, vol. 153(7), pp. 409–410, 414–415.
Possible Foetotoxic Effects of Mercury Vapour: A Case Report: S. Gelbier and J. Ingram; Public Health, January 1989, vol. 103(1), pp. 35–40.

Molybdenum:
Trace Elements and Public Health: E.J. Calabrese, et al.; Annu. Rev. Public Health, 1985, vol. 6, pp. 131–146.

Silver:
Connective Tissue Responses to Some Heavy Metals. III. Silver and Dietary Supplements of Ascorbic Acid. Histology and Ultrastructure: G. Ellender and K.N. Ham; Br. J. Experim. Pathol., February 1989, vol. 70(1), pp. 21–39.
Potential Nephrotoxic Effects of Exposure to Silver: K.D. Rosenman, et al.; Br. J. Ind. Med., April 1987, vol. 44(4), pp. 267–272.

Vanadium:
Urinary Vanadium as a Biological Indicator of Exposure to Vanadium: T. Kawai, et al.; Int. Arch. Occup. Environ. Health, 1989, vol. 61(4), pp. 283–287.
Vanadium-Induced Impairment of Haem Synthesis: C. Missenard, et al.; Br. J. Ind. Med., October 1989, vol. 46(10), pp. 744–747.
Vanadium and Manic-Depressive Psychosis: G.J. Naylor; Nutr. Health, 1984, vol. 3(1–2), pp. 79–85.

Zinc:
Acute Lung Reaction due to Zinc Inhalation: J.L. Malo, et al.; Eur. Respir. J., January 1990, vol. 3(1), pp. 111–114.

Cutaneous Reaction to Zinc—A Rare Complication of Insulin Treatment. A Case Report: M. Sandler and H.F. Jordaan; S. Afr. Med. J., April 1, 1989, vol. 75(7), pp. 342–343.
Zinc-Induced Copper Deficiency: H.N. Hoffman, 2d, et al.; Gastroenterology, February 1988, vol. 94(2), pp. 508–512.

RADIATION SYNDROMES

Description The radiation syndromes encompass the various types of tissue injury that result from exposure to ionizing radiation. In general, the potentially harmful effects relate to the total dose and dose rate of radiation received, as well as the specific tissues involved.

Synonyms
>Radiation Disease
>Radiation Effects
>Radiation Illness
>Radiation Injuries
>Radiation Reaction
>Radiation Sickness

Signs and Symptoms The effects of radiation may be acute, delayed, or chronic, and certain tissues are more sensitive to these effects. In general, tissues with rapid cell turnover, such as lymphoid cells, gonad cells, bone marrow, and enteric mucosa are the most susceptible to radiation injury. Nerve, bone, muscle, and connective tissues are less radiosensitive.

The overall amount of tissue exposed and the rate of exposure are other important factors in determining the severity of injury. A whole-body dose of 200 **rads** (radiation absorbed dose) is not likely to be fatal, while a whole-body dose of 600 rads may be fatal if the total dose is received over a short period of time. In contrast, a far higher total dose of radiation may be tolerated (as in cancer therapy) if only a small area of tissue is irradiated, and if the dose is given over an extended period of time.

Whole-body acute irradiation, such as might occur following an accident at a nuclear power reactor, is associated with 3 distinct syndromes. The **hematopoietic syndrome** may arise following exposure of 200 to 1000 rads. Symptoms of nausea, vomiting, anorexia, and apathy peak 6 to 12 hours after exposure, and then subside. At 24 to 36 hours postexposure, the victim appears to improve, but atrophy of the lymph nodes, spleen, and bone marrow has begun, with direct cytotoxic effects as well as inhibition of cell regeneration. Pancytopenia follows, with immediate lymphopenia, later neutropenia, and at 3 to 4 weeks postexposure, thrombocytopenia. Death usually occurs within 4 weeks, from superinfection or hemorrhage.

The gastrointestinal syndrome typically develops following exposure of 400 rads or more, and results from atrophy of the gastrointestinal mucosa. This syndrome is characterized by nausea, vomiting, and diarrhea, followed by dehydration, diminished plasma volume, and vascular collapse. Death generally occurs within 3 to 10 days.

The cerebral syndrome results from very high levels of exposure (3,000 rads or more). Early symptoms include nausea and vomiting, with rapid progression to listlessness, drowsiness, and prostration. Within a few hours, tremors, convulsions, and death ensue.

A further acute syndrome is sometimes seen following therapeutic irradiation for cancer. **Acute radiation sickness** occurs most commonly after abdominal irradiation. Symptoms include nausea, vomiting, headache, malaise, and tachycardia. The etiology is unknown, but the condition is self-limiting within hours or days.

Exposure to **low-level radiation** is associated with delayed effects including amenorrhea, decreased fertility, cataracts, and hematologic abnormalities. Longterm findings include the development of various types of malignancies, as well as a nonspecific shortening of life.

Local radiation injury also may lead to various clinical abnormalities. If the bone marrow is exposed to radiation, red and white cell counts may be depressed, and prolonged aplasia may occur. Abdominal radiation may cause diarrhea, ascites, edema, proteinuria, hypertension, and renal failure. Cutaneous radiation injury may result in erythema, telangiectasia, desquamation, and chronic ulceration. Symptoms of thoracic radiation injury include dyspnea and cyanosis; radiation pneumonitis, pericarditis, and myocarditis may also develop. Exposure of the gonads may lead to aspermia or amenorrhea. Ingestion of radium salts has led to the development of osteosarcomas.

The maximum permitted occupational exposure in the United States is currently 5 **rems** (roentgen-equivalent–man) per year. Workers at several nuclear-weapons manufacturing plants, including the Oak Ridge National Laboratory in Tennessee, have been found to have higher-than-normal rates of certain types of cancer, such as leukemia and multiple myeloma. Further investigations are being undertaken to ascertain whether the 5-rem limit should be lowered. Information on maximum permissible dose levels and other important data are available in *Basic Radiation Criteria,* NCRP Report No. 39, published by the National Council on Radiation Protection and Measurements, P.O. Box 30175, Washington, DC 20014.

Diagnosis of chronic or low-level exposure may be difficult, and if suspected, serial hematologic and bone marrow studies and cataract examinations are recommended.

Etiology Cellular exposure to radiation causes DNA breakage that may be cytotoxic, mutagenic, or carcinogenic.

Exposure may derive from background ultraviolet radiation; medical use of x-rays and radiotherapy; industrial settings such as the Three Mile Island and Chernobyl nuclear power plants; and military situations such as the explosions over Japan in 1945 and fallout from the Nevada testing site between 1951 and 1958.

There is also current concern about the effects of electromagnetic radiation from household appliances and wiring, and power transmission lines. Conflicting evidence has been seen in epidemiologic studies, and the public health implications are as yet unclear.

Treatment—Standard Initial general measures to be taken following acute radiation exposure include removal of all radioactivity through wound irrigation with water and chelating solutions; induction of emesis if radioactive material was ingested; and possible blockage of thyroid uptake with Lugol's solution or saturated solution of potassium iodide. Monitoring includes urine and breath analysis.

Management of the hematopoietic syndrome involves strict isolation and aseptic techniques because of the likelihood of infection and other complications. Treatment measures include platelet transfusions and the administration of antibiotics and fresh blood. Bone-marrow–suppressing agents are usually avoided.

Management of the gastrointestinal syndrome involves replacement of fluid, electrolytes, and plasma as determined by the severity of physical findings. Antiemetics and sedatives are administered as required.

Because the cerebral syndrome is rapidly fatal, treatment is palliative. Routine measures are taken for pain, anxiety, shock, anoxia, and convulsions.

Treatment of the delayed and late effects of chronic low-level radiation exposure requires various approaches, including surgery, whole-blood transfusions, and platelet transfusions.

Treatment—Investigational Bone-marrow transplantation has been used as treatment for high-dose whole-body irradiation. This procedure was performed on 13 of the approximately 200 individuals who were exposed to radiation following the accident at the Chernobyl nuclear power station in the Soviet Union. Two patients remained alive 3 years later. Some patients apparently succumbed to graft-versus-host disease, but others died of burns and other direct radiation effects.

Transplantation of fetal hepatocytes into the bone marrow is being investigated as an alternative for bone marrow transplantation, especially in young children whose immune systems have totally failed. Following transplantation, the hepatocytes begin to function like bone marrow cells. There is less likelihood of graft-versus-host disease with this procedure than with bone marrow transplantation, but more research is needed before this approach can be considered safe and effective.

Investigations are also under way to determine the potential hematopoietic benefits of the use of cloned hematopoietic growth factors such as granulocyte or granulocyte-macrophage colony-stimulating factors. Of 8 Brazilian patients with radiation sickness treated with this approach, 4 showed significant improvement. Further research is needed to evaluate safety and effectiveness.

Please contact the agencies listed under Resources, below, for the most current information.

Resources

For more information on radiation syndromes: National Organization for Rare Disorders (NORD); National Association of Radiation Survivors (NARS); National Council on Radiation Protection and Measurements; American Cancer Society; Leukemia Society of America; NIH/National Cancer Institute Physician Data Query (PDQ) phoneline.

References

Basic Radiation Protection Criteria; Recommendations of the National Council on Radiation Protection and Measurements, National Council on Radiation Protection and Measurements, 1984.

Bone Marrow Transplantation After the Chernobyl Accident: Alexander Baranov, et al.; N. Engl. J. Med., July 27, 1989, issue 321(4), pp. 205–212.

Leukemia in Utah and Radioactive Fallout from the Nevada Test Site: A Case-Control Study: W. Stevens, et al.; JAMA, August 1, 1990, vol. 264(5), pp. 585–591.

Cancer Risk Among Atomic Bomb Survivors: The RERF Life Span Study: Y. Shimizu, et al.; JAMA, August 1, 1990, vol. 264(5), pp. 601–604.

Use of Recombinant Granulocyte-Macrophage Colony Stimulating Factor in the Brazil Radiation Accident: A. Butturini, et al.; Lancet 1988, vol. 2, pp. 471–475.

Comparison of Isoeffect Relationships in Radiotherapy: E.O. Voit and P.N. Yi; Bull. Math. Biol., 1990, vol. 52(5), pp. 657–675.

Microelectronics, Radiation, and Superconductivity: M. Gochfeld; Environ. Health Perspect., June 1990, vol. 86, pp. 285–289.

Health Effects of Nonionizing Radiation: G.M. Wilkening and C.H. Sutton; Med. Clin. North Am., March 1990, vol. 74(2), pp. 489–507.

Health Effects of Ionizing Radiation: R.J. Fry and S.A. Fry; Med. Clin. North Am., March 1990, vol. 74(2), pp. 475–488.

Evolving Perspectives on the Concept of Dose in Radiobiology and Radiation Protection: A.C. Upton; Health Physics, October 1988, vol. 55(4), pp. 605–614.

14 | MASTER RESOURCES LIST

In the preceding chapters, each listing for a specific disorder contains resources that physicians or patients may wish to consult for further information or support. The resources range from individual experts to volunteer organizations to research centers. All are listed with addresses and telephone numbers in the following master resources list.

About Face
99 Crowns Lane
Toronto, Ontario M6R 3P4
Canada
(416) 944-3223

Acne Research Institute
1236 Somerset Lane
Newport Beach, CA 92260
(914) 722-1805

Acoustic Neuroma Association
P.O. Box 12402
Atlanta, GA 30355
(404) 237-8023

Addison's Disease
see: National Addison's Disease
Foundation

**Adrenal Hyperplasia (Congenital)
Support Group**
see: Congenital Adrenal Hyperplasia
Support Group

Adrenoleukodystrophy (ALD) Project
Hugo W. Moser, M.D.
John F. Kennedy Institute
707 North Broadway
Baltimore, MD 21205
(410) 550-9000

Aicardi Syndrome Newsletter, Inc.
5115 Troy Urbana Road
Casstown, OH 45312-9711
(513) 339-6033

AIDS Information Clearinghouse
(An electronic information service available
through AT&T's ACCUNET packet or AT&T
Mail)

**AIDS information on privately funded
clinical trials, including Spanish-
speaking information specialists:**
(800) TRIALS-A
(800) 243-7012 (for the hearing-impaired)

**AIDSLINE (National Library
of Medicine)**
(800) 638-8480

AIDS
see also:
American Foundation for AIDS Research
Centers for Disease Control
National Institute of Allergy and Infectious
Diseases
National Sexually Transmitted Diseases
Hotline

Albinism
see: National Organization for Albinism and
Hypopigmentation

Alcohol Abuse
see: Fetal Alcohol Education Program
National Clearinghouse for Alcohol & Drug
Information
National Institute on Alcohol Abuse and
Alcoholism
Check also with local Alcoholics
Anonymous groups

ALD Project
see: Adrenoleukodystrophy (ALD) Project

**Alexander Graham Bell Association
for the Deaf**
3417 Volta Place NW
Washington, DC 20007
(202) 337-5220

Richard Allen, M.D.
Pediatric Neurology Service, 0800/C7123
Outpatient Building
University Hospitals
Ann Arbor, MI 48109-0800
(313) 763-4697
(For information on Aicardi Syndrome)

**Allergy and Asthma Foundation
of America**
see: Asthma and Allergy Foundation
of America

Allergy Testing
118-21 Queens Boulevard
Forest Hills, NY 11375
(718) 261-3663

**Allergy/Asthma Association
Information**
65 Tromley Drive, Suite 10
Etobicoke, Ontario, M9B SY7
Canada
(416) 244-9312/8585

**Alopecia Areata International
Research, Inc. (AARF)**
P.O. Box 1875
Thousand Oaks, CA 91358
(805) 494-4903
see: National Alopecia Areata Foundation

**Alpha-1-Antitrypsin National
Association**
1829 Portland Avenue
Minneapolis, MN 55404
(612) 871-7332

Alpha-1-Antitrypsin Deficiency Registry
The Cleveland Clinic Foundation
David P. Meeker, M.D.
Department of Pulmonary Diseases
9500 Euclid Avenue
Cleveland, OH 44195
(216) 444-6505

Alpha-1 News
c/o Peter Smith
819 Bayview Road
Neenah, WI 54956
(414) 727-4576

Alport Syndrome Study
c/o C.L. Atkin, M.D. and
    M.C. Gregory, M.D.
Department of Internal Medicine
University of Utah
Salt Lake City, UT 84132
(801) 581-6709

Alzheimer Disease and Related Disorders Association, Inc.
National Headquarters
919 North Michigan Avenue, Suite 1000
Chicago, IL 60611
(312) 335-8700

American Academy of Environmental Medicine
P.O. Box 16106
Denver, CO 80216
(303) 622-9755

American Anorexia/Bulimia Association
418 E. 76th Street
New York, NY 10021
(212) 734-1114

American Association of Kidney Patients
111 S. Parker Street, Suite 405
Tampa, FL 33606
(813) 251-0725
(800) 749-2257

American Behçet's Association
P.O. Box 54063
Minneapolis, MN 55454-0063
(507) 281-3059
(800)-7-BEHCETS (723-4238)

American Brain Tumor Association
3725 N. Talman Avenue
Chicago, IL 60618
(312) 286-5571

American Cancer Society
1599 Clifton Road NE
Atlanta, GA 30329
(404) 320-3333
(800) 227-2345

American Carpal Tunnel Syndrome Association
P.O. Box 6730
Saginaw, MI 48608
(517) 792-1337

American Celiac Society
see: Celiac Sprue Association/USA
Gluten Intolerance Group

American Chronic Pain Association, Inc.
P.O. Box 850
Rocklin, CA 95677
(916) 632-0922

American Cleft Palate Cranial Facial Association
1218 Granview Avenue
Pittsburgh, PA 15211
(412) 481-1376
For information for parents on local support
    and information groups:
(800) 24-CLEFT (242-5338)

American Council of the Blind, Inc.
1155 15th Street, N.W., Suite 720
Washington, DC 20005
(202) 467-5081
(800) 424-8666

American Council of Blind Parents
see: Council of Families with Visual
    Impairment

American Diabetes Association
National Service Center
1660 Duke Street
Alexandria, VA 22314
(703) 549-1500
(800) 232-3472

American Encephalomyelitis Society
see: Myalgic Encephalomyelitis Association

American Foundation for the Blind
15 West 16th Street
New York, NY 10011
(212) 620-2000
Regional offices:
Atlanta, GA (404) 525-2303
Chicago, IL (312) 269-0095
Dallas, TX (214) 352-7222
San Francisco, CA (415) 392-4845

American Foundation for AIDS Research
733 Third Avenue, 12th Floor
New York, NY 10017
(212) 682-7440

American Heart Association
7320 Greenville Avenue
Dallas, TX 75231
(214) 748-7212

American Hirschsprung Disease Association
22½ Spruce Street
Brattleboro, VT 05301
(802) 257-0603

American Kidney Fund
6110 Executive Boulevard, Suite 1010
Rockville, MD 20852
(301) 881-3052
(800) 638-8299
(800) 492-8361 (In Maryland)

American Liver Foundation
1425 Pompton Avenue
Cedar Grove, NJ 07009
(201) 857-2626
(800) 223-0179

American Lupus Society
3914 Del Amo Blvd., Suite 922
Torrance, CA 90503
(213) 933-4667
(800) 331-1802
    see also: Systemic Lupus Erythematosus
    Foundation, Inc.

American Lung Association
1740 Broadway
New York, NY 10019
(212) 315-8700

American Narcolepsy Association, Inc.
425 California Street, Suite 201
San Francisco, CA 94104
    or
P.O. Box 26230
San Francisco, CA 94126
(415) 788-4793

American Paraplegia Society
75-20 Astoria Blvd.
Jackson Heights, NY 11370-1177
(718) 803-3782

American Porphyria Foundation
P.O. Box 1075
Santa Rosa Beach, FL 32459
(904) 654-4754

American Printing House for the Blind
P.O. Box 6085
Louisville, KY 40206-0085
(502) 895-2405

American Reye Syndrome Association:
    see: National Reye Syndrome Foundation

American Society for Deaf Children
814 Thayer Avenue
Silver Spring, MD 20910
(301) 585-5400
(800) 942-ASDC

American Society of Hypertension
515 Madison Avenue, 21st Floor
New York, NY 10022
(212) 644-0650

American Society of Parenteral & Enteral Nutrition (ASPEN)
8630 Fenton Street, #412
Silver Springs, MD 20910
(301) 587-6315

American Speech-Language-Hearing Association
10801 Rockville Pike
Rockville, MD 20852
(301) 897-5700

American Spinal Injury Association
250 East Superior Street, Room 619
Chicago, IL 60611
(312) 908-3425

American Syringomyelia Alliance Project, Inc.
P.O. Box 1586
Longview, TX 75606
(903) 236-7079

American Tinnitus Association
P.O. Box 5
Portland, OR 97207
(503) 248-9985
    see also: E.A.R. Foundation
    Vestibular Disorders Association

The Amyotrophic Lateral Sclerosis Association
21021 Ventura Boulevard, Suite 321
Woodland Hills, CA 91364
(818) 340-7500

Anemia
see: Aplastic Anemia Foundation of America
Cooley's Anemia Foundation, Inc.
Fanconi Anemia Research Fund, Inc.
Fanconi Anemia Support Group
International Fanconi Registry
National Association for Sickle Cell Disease, Inc.
National Heart, Lung and Blood Institute
Sickle Cell Association of Ontario

Anencephaly
see: Fighters for Encephaly Support

Angelman Syndrome Foundation, Inc.
Department of Pediatrics/Genetics
P.O. Box 100296 - UFHSC
Gainesville, FL 32610-0296
(904) 392-4104

Angelman Syndrome Support Group
c/o Mrs. Sheila Woolven
15 Place Crescent
Waterlooville, Hampshire PO7 5UR
England
Tel: 0705-264-224

Ankylosing Spondylitis Association
511 North La Cienega, Suite 216
Los Angeles, CA 90048
(213) 652-0609
(800) 777-8189

Anorexia and Bulimia Treatment and Education Center (ABTEC)
621 S. Newballas, Suite 7019B
St. Louis, MO 63141
(314) 569-6898

Anorexia Nervosa and Associated Disorders, Inc.
P.O. Box Seven
Highland Park, IL 60035
(708) 831-3438

Anorexia Nervosa and Related Eating Disorders, Inc.
P.O. Box 5102
Eugene, OR 97405
(503) 344-1144
see also: American Anorexia/Bulimia Association
National Anorexic Aid Society, Inc.

Anxiety Disorders Association of America
6000 Executive Boulevard, Suite 513
Rockville, MD 20852
(301) 231-9350

Aplastic Anemia Foundation of America
P.O. Box 22689
Baltimore, MD 21203
(800) 747-2820

The Arc
(formerly, Association for Retarded Citizens)
500 East Border Street
Suite 300
Arlington, TX 76010
(817) 261-6003

Arnold-Chiari Family Network
67 Spring Street
Weymouth, MA 02188
(617) 337-2368

Arthritis Foundation
1314 Spring Street N.W.
Atlanta, GA 30309
(404) 872-7100
see also: National Arthritis, Musculoskeletal and Skin Disorders Information Clearinghouse

Arthrogryposis
see: Support Group for Arthrogryposis Multiplex Congenita
AVENUES, a National Support Group for Arthrogryposis

Association for Brain Tumor Research
see: American Brain Tumor Association

Association for Children and Adults with Learning Disabilities
see: Learning Disabilities Association of America (LDA)

Association for Children with Down Syndrome
2616 Martin Avenue
Bellmore, NY 11710
(516) 221-4700

Association of Children's Prosthetic and Orthotic Clinics
222 South Prospect Avenue
Park Ridge, IL 60068
(708) 698-1632

Association for Children with Russell-Silver Syndrome
22 Hoyt Street
Madison, NJ 07940
(201) 377-4531

Association for Glycogen Storage Diseases
Box 896
Durant, IA 52747
(319) 785-6038

Association for Macular Diseases, Inc.
210 East 64th Street
New York, NY 10021
(212) 605-3719

Association for Neurometabolic Disorders
5223 Brookfield Lane
Sylvania, OH 43506-1809
(419) 885-1497

Association for Retarded Citizens
see: The Arc

Asthma and Allergy Foundation of America
1125 15th Street N.W., Suite 502
Washington, DC 20005
(202) 466-7643
see also: Allergy/Asthma Association Information

Ataxia
see: National Ataxia Foundation

Ataxia Telangiectasia Research Foundation
344 Copa de Oro Road
Los Angeles, CA 90077
(213) 476-1218

Attention Deficit Disorders
see: CH.A.D.D., Children with Attention Deficit Disorders

Autism Society of America
National Chapter
8601 Georgia Avenue, Suite 503
Silver Springs, MD 20910
(301) 565-0433

AVENUES, a National Support Group for Arthrogryposis
P.O. Box 5192
Sonora, CA 95370-5192
(209) 928-3688

William Balistreri, M.D.
Director, Division of Pediatric Gastroenterology and Nutrition
Children's Hospital Medical Center
Elland and Bethesda Avenues
Cincinnati, OH 45229
(513) 559-4200

Batten Disease Support and Research Association
National Batten Disease Registry
13378 Palmer Road S.W.
Reynoldsburg, OH 43068
(800) 448-4570

Eugene Bauer, M.D.
Stanford University Medical Center
Department of Dermatology
Edwards Bldg., Room 144
Stanford, CA 94305
(415) 723-2300
(For information on epidermolysis bullosa)

Beckwith-Wiedemann Support Group
3206 Braeburn Circle
Ann Arbor, MI 48108
(313) 973-0263
see also: Barbara Biesecker

Behçet's Association
see: American Behçet's Association
J. Desmond O'Duffy, M.D., Mayo Clinic

Benign Essential Blepharospasm Research Foundation, Inc.
P.O. Box 12468
Beaumont, TX 77726-2468
(409) 832-0788

Barbara Biesecker
Molecular Medicine and Genetics
2570 MSRB II, Box 0674
University of Michigan Medical Center
Ann Arbor, MI 48109
(313) 764-8064
(For information on Beckwith-Wiedmann Syndrome)

Edward D. Bird, M.D., Director
Brain Tissue Resource Center
Mailman Research Center
McLean Hospital
115 Mill Street
Belmont, MA 02178
(617) 855-2400

Blindness
see: Eye Disorders

Bloom Syndrome Registry
Laboratory of Human Genetics
The New York Blood Center
310 E. 67th Street
New York, NY 10021
(212) 570-3075

**Brain and Pituitary Foundation
of America**
281 East Moody Avenue
Fresno, CA 93720-1524
(209) 434-0610

British Organic Acidemia Association
see: Organic Acidemia Association

British Polio Fellowship
Bell Close West End Road
Ruislip, Middlesex
England HA4 6LP
Telephone: 0895-675-515

Saul Brusilow, M.D.
301 Children's Medical and Surgical Center
Johns Hopkins Hospital
600 North Wolfe Street
Baltimore, MD 21205
(301) 955-5000

Canadian Hemophilia Society
1450 City Councillors Street, Suite 840
Montreal, Quebec H3A 2E6
Canada
(514) 848-0503

The Canadian Sickle Cell Society
see: Sickle Cell Association of Ontario

Cancer Information Service
Physician Data Query
National Cancer Institute
9000 Rockville Pike, Building 31, Room 1A2A
Bethesda, MD 20892
(800) 4-CANCER
In Washington, DC, and suburbs in MD
and VA: 806-5700
In Alaska: (800) 638-6070
In Oahu, HI: (800) 524-1234
(Neighbor islands, call collect)

Cancer
see: American Cancer Society
American Brain Tumor Association
Hairy Cell Leukemia Foundation
Leukemia Society of America
National Cancer Institute
The Skin Cancer Foundation

C.A.N.D.L.E.
(Childhood Aphasia, Neurological Disorders,
Landau-Kleffner Syndrome, and Epilepsy)
4414 McCampbell Drive
Montgomery, AL 36106
(205) 271-3947

Cardiac Disorders
see: Heart Disorders

Carpal Tunnel Syndrome
see: American Carpal Tunnel Syndrome
Association

Ben Carson, M.D.
Chief of Pediatric Neurosurgery
Children's Center
Johns Hopkins Hospital
Baltimore, MD 21205
(410) 955-7888
(For information on Rasmussen encephalitis)
see also: Theodore Rasmussen, M.D.

Cataplexy
see: Narcolepsy and Cataplexy Foundation
of America

**CCHS (Congenital Central
Hypoventilation Syndrome)
Parent Network**
see: Congenital Central Hypoventilation
Syndrome Parent Network

Stephen Cederbaum, M.D.
Professor of Psychiatry & Pediatrics
UCLA Medical School
Los Angeles, CA 90024
(310) 825-0402

Cerebral Palsy
see: United Cerebral Palsy Associations,
Inc.

Celiac Sprue Association/USA
P.O. Box 31700
Omaha, NE 68131-0700
(402) 558-0600
see also: Gluten Intolerance Group

Centers for Disease Control (CDC)
1600 Clifton Road, NE
Atlanta, GA 30333
(404) 639-3534

CH.A.D.D.
Children with Attention Deficit Disorders
499 N.W. 70th Avenue, Suite 308
Plantation, FL 33317
(305) 587-3700

Charcot-Marie-Tooth Association
Crozer Mills Enterprise Center
600 Upland Avenue
Upland, PA 19015
(215) 499-7486

Charcot-Marie-Tooth International
One Spring Bank Drive
St. Catherine's, Ontario
Canada L2S 2K1
(416) 687-3630

**Chemosensory Clinical Research
Center of Connecticut**
Department of BioStructure
University of Connecticut Health Center
Farmington, CT 06032
(203) 679-2459

**Children's Association for Research
on Mucolipidosis IV**
see: The Mucolipidosis IV Foundation

**Children's Brain Diseases Foundation
for Research**
350 Parnassus, Suite 900
San Francisco, CA 94117
(415) 566-5402; 565-6259; 566-4402

**Children's Craniofacial Association
(CCA)**
10210 North Central Expressway LB37
Dallas, TX 75231
(800) 535-3643

Children's Liver Foundation
14245 Ventura Boulevard
Sherman Oaks, CA 91423
(818) 906-3021

Children's PKU Network
10525 Vista Sorrento Pkwy, Suite 204
San Diego, CA 92121
(619) 587-9421

**The Chromosome 18 Registry and
Research Society**
6302 Fox Head
San Antonio, TX 78247
(512) 657-4968

**Chronic Fatigue & Immune
Dysfunction Syndrome Society
(CFIDS)**
P.O. Box 230108
Portland, OR 97223
(800) 442-3437
see also: National Chronic Fatigue
Syndrome Association, Inc.

Cleft Palate Foundation
(Teaching arm of American Cleft Palate
Craniofacial Association, with the same
address)

**Clinical Smell and Taste Research
Center**
see: Smell and Taste Research Center

Closer Look Information Center
see: National Information Center for
Children and Youth with Disabilities

Colitis and Ileitis
see: Crohn's and Colitis Foundation of
America, Inc.

**Congenital Adrenal Hyperplasia
Support Group**
10 County Highway, #4
Wrenshall, MN 55797
(218) 384-3863

**Congenital Central Hypoventilation
Syndrome Parent Network**
71 Maple Street
Oneonta, NY 13820

**Connecticut Chemosensory Clinical
Research Center**
see: Chemosensory Clinical Research
Center of Connecticut

Cooley's Anemia Foundation, Inc.
105 East 22nd Street
New York, NY 10010
(212) 598-0911
(800) 522-7222 (New York State)
(800) 221-3571

**Cornelia de Lange Syndrome
Foundation**
International Headquarters
60 Dyer Avenue
Collinsville, CT 06022
(203) 693-0159

Corporation for Menkes Disease
5720 Buckfield Court
Fort Wayne, IN 46804
(219) 436-0137

**Council of Families with Visual
Impairment**
(formerly, American Council of Blind Parents)
6212 W. Franklin Street
Richmond, VA 23226
(804) 288-0395

Council of Guilds for Infant Survival
PO Box 3586
Davenport, IA 52808
(319) 322-4870

Craniofacial Centre Children's Hospital
300 Longwood Avenue
Boston, MA 02115
(617) 735-6309

Craniofacial Disorders
see also: About Face
American Cleft Palate Cranial Facial
   Association
Children's Craniofacial Association (CCA)
Craniofacial Centre Children's Hospital
Craniofacial Family Association
FACES—National Association for the
   Craniofacially Handicapped
Forward Face
Hemifacial Microsomia Family Support
   Network
Hemifacial Microsomia/Goldenhar
   Syndrome Family Support Network
Institute of Reconstructive Plastic Surgery
National Foundation for Facial
   Reconstruction
National Institute of Dental Research
Orofacial Guild of Orange County

Cri-du-Chat Society
Department of Human Genetics
Medical College of Virginia
Box 33, MCV Station
Richmond, VA 23298
(804) 786-9632

Crohn's and Colitis Foundation of America, Inc.
444 Park Avenue South
New York, NY 10016
(212) 685-3440

Cystic Fibrosis Foundation
6931 Arlington Road
Bethesda, MD 20814
(800) FIGHT CF

Cystinosis Foundation, Inc.
17 Lake Avenue
Piedmont, CA 94611
(510) 601-6940

Deafness
see: Hearing Impairment

Deafness Research Foundation
9 East 38th Street
New York, NY 10016
(212) 684-6556

DEBRA (England)
see: Dystrophic Epidermolysis Bullosa
   Research Association (DEBRA)

DEBRA (United States)
see: Dystrophic Epidermolysis Bullosa
   Research Association of America, Inc.

Dental Disorders
see: National Foundation of Dentistry for
   the Handicapped
National Institute of Dental Research

Dermatomyositis Support Group
see: The National Support Group for
   Dermatomyositis

Diabetes
see: American Diabetes Association
National Institute of Diabetes, Digestive and
   Kidney Diseases Information
   Clearinghouse

Diamond-Blackfan Anemia Registry
Dr. Adrianna Vlachos
Mount Sinai Medical Center
One Gustave Levy Place
Box 1208
New York, NY 10029-6574
(212) 241-6031

Diamond-Blackfan Anemia Support Group
Dr. Ted Gordon-Smith
11 Hollyfield Avenue
London N11 3BY
Telephone: 81-784-2645
FAX: 81-672-4864

Angelo M. DiGeorge, M.D.
Professor of Pediatrics
Temple University School of Medicine
Section of Endocrinology and Metabolism
St. Christopher's Hospital for Children
Erie Avenue at Front Street
Philadelphia, Pennsylvania 19134
(215) 427-5173

DiGeorge Syndrome
see: Angelo M. DiGeorge, M.D.
Frank Greenberg, M.D.
Craig B. Langman, M.D., and Samuel S.
   Gidding, M.D.

Dissatisfied Parents Together
128 Branch Road
Vienna, VA 22180
(703) 938-3783
FAX: (703) 594-3847
(A group of parents whose children have had
severe adverse reactions to childhood
vaccines)

**Dizziness and Balance Disorder
Association**
see: Vestibular Disorders Association

Down Syndrome Association
155 Mitcham Road
Tooting
London SW17 9PG
England
Telephone: 081 682-4001
see also: Association for Children with
Down Syndrome
National Down Syndrome Congress
National Down Syndrome Society
also Mental Retardation

J. Desmond Duffy, M.D.
specialist in Behçet's syndrome
Mayo Clinic
Division of Rheumatology
200 First Street S.W.
Rochester, MN 55905
(507) 284-2964

Dysautonomia Foundation, Inc.
20 East 46th Street, Room 302
New York, NY 10017
(212) 949-6644

**Dystonia Medical Research
Foundation**
8383 Wilshire Boulevard, Suite 800
Beverly Hills, CA 90211
(213) 852-1630

**Dystrophic Epidermolysis Bullosa
Research Association (DEBRA)**
One Kings Road
Crowthorne
Berkshire RG11 7BG
England
Telephone: 0344 771961

**Dystrophic Epidermolysis Bullosa
Research Association of America,
Inc. (DEBRA)**
141 Fifth Avenue, Suite 7-South
New York, NY 10010
(212) 995-2220

E.A.R. Foundation
Attention: Meniere Network
2000 Church Street
Nashville, TN 37236
(615) 329-7808 (Voice and TDD)

Easter Seal Society
see: The National Easter Seal Society, Inc.

**Eczema Association for Science and
Education**
1221 South West Yamhill, Suite 303
Portland, OR 97205
(503) 228-4430

Ehlers-Danlos National Foundation
P.O. Box 1212
Southgate, MI 48195
(313) 282-0180

Encephalomyelitis
see: Myalgic Encephalomyelitis Association

The Endocrine Society
9650 Rockville Pike
Bethesda, MD 20814
(301) 571-1802

Epidermolysis bullosa
see: Dystrophic Epidermolysis Bullosa
Research Association of America, Inc.
(DEBRA)
Eugene Bauer, M.D.

Environmental Disorders
see: American Academy of Environmental
Medicine
National Association of Radiation Survivors
National Council on Radiation Units and
Measurements, Inc.
National Institute of Environmental Health
Sciences

Epilepsy Foundation of America
4351 Garden City Drive
Landover, MD 20785
(301) 459-3700
(800) 332-1000

**Erythromelalgia and Related
Disorders Association of America,
Inc.**
c/o Delia Steelman
P.O. Box 4046
Portland, OR 97208

Eye Disorders
see: American Council of the Blind, Inc.
American Council of Blind Parents
American Foundation for the Blind
American Printing House for the Blind
Association for Macular Diseases, Inc.
National Association for Parents of the
  Visually Impaired, Inc.
National Association for the Visually
  Handicapped
National Eye Institute
National Library Service for the Blind and
  Physically Handicapped
National Federation of the Blind
National Retinitis Pigmentosa Foundation
  Fighting Blindness
National Society to Prevent Blindness
Vision Foundation, Inc.

Eye Research Institute of Retina Foundation
see: Schepens Eye Research Institute of
  Retina Foundation

FACES—National Association for the Craniofacially Handicapped
P.O. Box 11082
Chattanooga, TN 37401
(615) 266-1632

Fahr Disease Registry
Parkinson's Disease and Movement Disorders
  Clinic
Bala V. Manyam, M.D.
Southern Illinois University School of
  Medicine
P.O. Box 19230
Springfield, IL 62794-9230
(217) 785-8684

Familial Polyposis Registry
Department of Colorectal Surgery
Cleveland Clinic Foundation
9500 Euclid Avenue
Cleveland, OH 44195-5001
(216) 444-6470

Families with Maple Syrup Urine Disease
Route 2, Box 24-A
Flemingsburg, KY 41041
(606) 849-4679

Families of Spinal Muscular Atrophy
P.O. Box 1465
Highland Park, IL 60035
(708) 432-5551

Fanconi Anemia Research Fund Inc.
Fanconi Anemia Support Group
66 Club Road, Suite 390
Eugene, OR 97401
(503) 687-4658

Fetal Alcohol Education Program
Boston University School of Medicine
Seven Kent Street
Brookline, MA 02146
(617) 232-7557; 739-1424

Fighters for Encephaly Support
3032 Brereton Street
Pittsburgh, PA 15219
(412) 687-6437

David B. Flannery, M.D., Director
Division of Medical Genetics
Department of Pediatrics BG-121
Medical College of Georgia
Augusta, GA 30912
(404) 721-2809
(For information on Joubert syndrome)

5p- Society
11609 Oakmont
Overland Park, KS 66210
(913) 469-8900

Food and Drug Administration (FDA)
Office of the Commissioner
Office of Orphan Products
5600 Fishers Lane (HF-35; Room 8-73)
Rockville, MD 20857
(301) 443-4903

Forward Face
317 East 34th Street, Suite 901
New York, NY 10016
(212) 263-5205
(800) 422-FACE

Foundation for Ichthyosis and Related Skin Types (F.I.R.S.T.)
P.O. Box 20921
Raleigh, NC 27619-0921
(919) 782-5728
(800) 545-3286

Fragile X Association of Michigan
1786 Edinborough Drive
Rochester Hills, MI 48306
(313) 373-3043

Fragile X Foundation
see: Institute for Basic Research in
  Developmental Disabilities

Fragile X Support Group
c/o Jackie Franklin
1380 Huntington Drive
Mundelein, IL 60060
(708) 680-3317

Freeman-Sheldon Parent Support Group
1459 East Maple Hills Drive
Bountiful, UT 84010
(801) 298-3149

Frontier's International Vitiligo Foundation
see: National Vitiligo Foundation

Galactomsemia
see: Parents of Galactosemic Children, Inc.

Gaucher Disease
see: National Gaucher Foundation

Gluten Intolerance Group of North America
P.O. Box 23053
Seattle, WA 98102-0353
(206) 325-6980
see also: Celiac Sprue Association/USA

Glycogen Storage Disease
see: Association for Glycogen Storage Disease

Frank Greenberg, M.D.
Baylor College of Medicine
Molecular Genetics
Texas Children's Hospital, Room 0154
6621 Fannin Road
Houston, TX 77030
(713) 798-4951

Guillain-Barré Syndrome
Support Group International
P.O. Box 262
Wynnewood, PA 19096
(215) 667-0131

The Haemophilia Society
P.O. Box 9
16 Trinity Street
London SE1 1DE
England
Telephone: 71-407-1010

Hairy Cell Leukemia Foundation
P.O. Box 72
Newtonville, MA 02160
(617) 244-8478

Hallermann-Streiff Parent Association
1367 Beulah Park
Lexington, KY 40597
(606) 273-6928

Mark Hallet, M.D.
National Institute of Neurological Disorders and Stroke
9000 Rockville Pike
Bldg. 31, Room 8A06
Bethesda, MD 20892
(301) 496-5751
(For information on stiff man syndrome)

Frances Harley, M.D.
Department of Pediatrics, 2C359 WMC
8440 112 Street
University of Alberta
Edmonton, Alberta T6G 2R7
Canada
(403) 492-6631
(For information on intestinal pseudoobstruction)

Hearing Impairment
see: Alexander Graham Bell Association for the Deaf
American Humane Association (For trained hearing dogs)
American Society for Deaf Children
American Speech-Language-Hearing Association
American Tinnitus Association
Deafness Research Foundation
National Association of the Deaf
National Information Center on Deafness
Self-Help for Hard-of-Hearing People, Inc.

Heart Disorders
see: American Heart Association
National Heart, Lung and Blood Institute

HEATH Resource Center (Higher Education and the Handicapped)
One Dupont Circle NW
Washington, DC 20036
(800) 544-3284

Help Alopecia International Research, Inc. (HAIR)
(Alopecia Areata International Research, Inc.)
P.O. Box 1875
Thousand Oaks, CA 91358
(805) 494-4903

Help for Incontinent People (HIP)
P.O. Box 544
Union, SC 29379
(803) 579-7900

The Hemifacial Microsomia Family Support Network
Six Country Lane Way
Philadelphia, PA 19115
(215) 677-4787

The Hemifacial Microsomia/ Goldenhar Syndrome Family Support Network
c/o Cynthia Fishman, R.N.
6 Country Lane Way
Philadelphia, PA 19115
(215) 677-4787

Hemochromatosis Research Foundation
P.O. Box 8569
Albany, NY 12208
(518) 489-0972
   see also: Iron Overload Diseases
      Association
   National Institute of Diabetes, Digestive &
      Kidney Diseases

Hemophilia
   see: The Haemophilia Society
   Canadian Hemophilia Society
   National Heart, Lung and Blood Institute
   National Hemophilia Foundation
   World Federation of Hemophilia

Hepatic Disorders
   see: Liver Disorders

The Hereditary Disease Foundation
1427 Seventh Street, Suite 2
Santa Monica, CA 90401
(213) 458-4183

Hereditary Hemorrhagic Telangiectasis Registry
(Osler-Weber-Rendu Syndrome Registry)
c/o Robert I. White, Jr., M.D.
Yale School of Medicine
Department of Diagnostic Radiology
333 Cedar Street
P.O. Box 3333
New Haven, CT 06510
(203) 785-6938

Herpes Support Group at Help South Bay
(408) 296-1444

M. Hershfield, M.D.
Duke University Medical Center
Box 3049
Room 418, Sands Building
Durham, NC 27710
(919) 684-4184
FAX: (919) 684-4168
(For information on severe combined
immunodeficiency)

Hirschsprung Disease Association
   see: American Hirschsprung Disease
      Association

Histiocytosis-X Association
609 New York Road
Glassboro, NJ 08028
(609) 881-4911
   see also: Diane Komp, M.D.

Human Growth Foundation
7777 Leesburg Pike
P.O. Box 3090
Falls Church, VA 22043
(703) 883-1773
(800) 451-6434

Huntington's Disease Society of America
140 W. 22nd Street, 6th Floor
New York, NY 10011
(212) 242-1968

Huntington Society of Canada
13 Water Street North, No. 3
PO Box 333
Cambridge, Ontario NIR 5TB
Canada
(519) 622-1002

Hydrocephalus Association
2040 Polk Street, Box 342
San Francisco, CA 94109
(415) 776-4713
   see also: National Hydrocephalus
      Foundation

Hypercalcemia
   see: Infantile Hypercalcaemia Foundation
      Ltd.

Ichthyosis
   see: Foundation for Ichthyosis and Related
      Skin Types (F.I.R.S.T.)

Immune Deficiency Foundation
PO Box 586
Columbia, MD 21045
(301) 461-3127

Infantile Hypercalcaemia Foundation Ltd.
37 Mulberry Green
Old Harlow, Essex
England CM17 OEY
Telephone: 279-272-14

Info-Line
(800) 222-LUNG

Institute for Basic Research in Developmental Disabilities
1050 Forest Hill Road
Staten Island, NY 10314
(718) 494-0600

Institute of Reconstructive Plastic Surgery
NYU Medical Center
550 First Avenue
New York, NY 10016
(212) 263-6656

International Association of Parents of the Deaf
see: American Society for Deaf Children

International Bundle Branch Block Association
6631 West 83rd Street
Los Angeles, CA 90045-2899
(213) 670-9132

International Center for Skeletal Dysplasia
St. Joseph Hospital
7620 York Road
Towson, MD 21204
(301) 337-1250

International Fanconi Registry
The Rockefeller University
c/o Arleen Auerbach, Ph.D.
1230 York Avenue
New York, NY 10021
(212) 570-7533

International FOP (Fibrodysplasia Ossificans Progressiva) Organization
910 North Jericho
Casselberry, FL 32707
(407) 365-4194

International Joseph Diseases Foundation, Inc.
P.O. Box 2550
Livermore, CA 94551-2550
see also Roger N. Rosenberg, M.D.

International Rett Syndrome Association
8511 Rose Marie Drive
Fort Washington, MD 20744
(301) 248-7031

International Tremor Foundation
360 West Superior Street
Chicago, IL 60610
(312) 664-2344

Iron Overload Diseases Association
433 Westwind Drive
West Palm Beach, FL 33408
(407) 840-8512
see also: Hereditary Hemochromatosis Research Foundation
National Institute of Diabetes, Digestive & Kidney Diseases

Jewish National Foundation for Genetic Diseases
see: National Foundation for Jewish Genetic Diseases

Joseph Disease
see: International Joseph Disease Foundation, Inc.
Roger N. Rosenberg, M.D.

Kidney Disorders
see: American Kidney Foundation
Hereditary Nephritis Foundation
National Association of Patients on Hemodialysis and Transplantation
National Institute of Diabetes, Digestive and Kidney Diseases
National Kidney Foundation
National Kidney and Urologic Diseases Information Clearinghouse
Polycystic Kidney Disease Research Foundation

Klinefelter Syndrome & Associates
P.O. Box 119
Roseville, CA 95661-0119

Klippel-Trenaunay Syndrome Support Group
4610 Wooddale Avenue
Minneapolis, MN 55424
(612) 925-2596

Diane Komp, M.D.
Yale University School of Medicine
Department of Pediatrics
P.O. Box 333
New Haven, CT 06510
(203) 785-4640
(For information on histiocytosis-X)

Lactic Acidosis Support Group
1620 Marle Avenue
Denver, CO 80229
(303) 837-2117; or 287-4953

Bert N. La Du, M.D.
Department of Pharmacology
6322 Medical Sciences, Bldg. 1
University of Michigan School of Medicine
Ann Arbor, MI 48109-0626
(313) 763-6429
(Specialist in alcaptonuria and a rare drug
reaction to succinylcholine)

**Craig B. Langman, M.D. and
Samuel S. Gidding, M.D.**
Children's Memorial Hospital
Pediatrics/Nephrology, Mail #37
2300 Children's Plaza
Chicago, IL 60614
(312) 880-4000

**Learning Disabilities Association
of America (LDA)**
4156 Library Road
Pittsburgh, PA 15234
(412) 341-1515
(412) 341-8077
    see: National Network of Learning-Disabled
    Adults, Inc.
Orton Dyslexia Society

Mark Lebwohl, M.D.
PXE Research Project, Department of
    Dermatology
Mount Sinai School of Medicine
Fifth Avenue & 100th Street
New York, NY 10029
(212) 876-7199

Leprosy
    see: National Hansen Disease Center

Leukemia Society of America
733 Third Avenue
New York, NY 10017
(212) 573-8484

Leukodystrophy
    see: United Leukodystrophy Foundation

Richard A. Lewis, M.D.
Professor
Depts. of Ophthalmology, Medicine,
    Pediatrics, and the Institute for Molecular
    Genetics
Baylor College of Medicine
6501 Fanin, NC 206
Houston, TX 77030
(713) 798-3030

Lissencephaly
    see: Support Network for Lissencephaly

Little People of America, Inc.
c/o Jean Elmendorf
P.O. Box 9897
Washington, DC 20016
(301) 589-0730

Liver Disorders
    see: American Liver Foundation
    Children's Liver Foundation
    United Liver Foundation

Lowe Syndrome Association
222 Lincoln Street
West Lafayette, IN 47906
(317) 743-3634

Lung Disorders
    see: American Lung Association
    National Heart, Lung and Blood Institute

Lupus Foundation of America, Inc.
National Headquarters
4 Research Place, Suite 180
Rockville, MD 20850-3226
(301) 670-9292
(800) 558-0121

Lupus Foundation of America, Inc.
(Chapters in most states)
    see also: American Lupus Society
    Systemic Lupus Erythematosus
    Foundation, Inc.

William L. Nyhan, M.D.
Professor of Pediatrics
U.C. School of Medicine, San Diego
La Jolla, CA 92093-0609
(619) 534-4150

Lyme Borreliosis Foundation, Inc.
P.O. Box 462
Tolland, CT 06084
(203) 871-2900

Lyme Disease Clinic
Dana Medical Center, 3rd Floor
789 Howard Avenue
New Haven, CT 06504
(203) 785-7032

Lyme Disease Clinic
Marshfield Clinic
1000 North Oak Avenue
Marshfield, WI 54449
(715) 387-5511

Lymph Disorders
see: National Heart, Lung and Blood
    Institute
National Lymphatic & Venous Diseases
    Foundation, Inc.
National Lymphedema Network

Malignant Hyperthermia Association of the United States
P.O. Box 191
Westport, CT 06881-0191
(203) 655-3007
see also: Malignant Hyperthermia Clinics
Malignant Hyperthermia Emergencies
The North American Malignant
    Hyperthermia Registry

Malignant Hyperthermia Emergencies:
Medic Alert Foundation International
(209) 634-4917
Ask for INDEX ZERO, Malignant
    Hyperthermia Consultant List

Malignant Hyperthermia Clinics:
Rochester:
Mayo Clinic
Department of Anesthesiology
200 First Street SW
Rochester, MN 55905
(507) 285-5601
Houston:
Thomas E. Nelson, M.D.
University of Texas Health Center
Medical School, Dept. of Anesthesiology
6431 Fannin Street, MSB-5020
Houston, TX 77030
(713) 792-5566
Philadelphia:
Hahnemann University Medical School
Department of Anesthesiology, Mail Stop 310
Broad and Vine Streets
Philadelphia, PA 19102
(215) 448-7960
Boston:
Massachusetts General
Department of Anesthesiology
John Ryan, M.D. (for information only)
Room ACC3
Fruit Street
Boston, MA 02114
(617) 726-8800

Maple Syrup Urine Disease
see: Families with Maple Syrup Urine
    Disease

March of Dimes Birth Defects Foundation
1275 Mamaroneck Avenue
White Plains, NY 10605
(914) 428-7100

Marfan Syndrome
see: National Marfan Foundation

Medic Alert Foundation International
see: Malignant Hyperthermia Emergencies

Meniere Disease
see: E.A.R. Foundation

Mental Health
see: National Institute of Mental Health
National Mental Health Association

Mental Retardation
see: The Arc
National Institute of Mental Retardation
    (Canada)

Migraine
see: National Headache Foundation

Hugo W. Moser, M.D.
Adrenoleukodystrophy (ALD) Project
John F. Kennedy Institute
707 North Broadway
Baltimore, MD 21205
(410) 550-9000

The Mucolipidosis IV Foundation
6 Concord Drive
Monsey, NY 10952
(914) 425-0639

Mucopolysaccharidosis (MPS)
see: Mucopolysaccharidoses (MPS)
    Research Funding Center, Inc.
National MPS Society
Society of MPS Diseases
Society of MPS Diseases, Inc.
Society of Mucopolysaccharide Disease,
    Inc.

Mucopolysaccharidoses (MPS) Research Funding Center, Inc.
3260 Old Farm Lane
Wall Lake, MI 48390
(313) 363-4412

Joseph Muenzer, M.D.
University of Michigan Medical Center
Ann Arbor, MI 48109
(For information on Hunter syndrome)

Multiple Sclerosis Society
see: National Multiple Sclerosis Society

Muscular Atrophy
see: Families of Spinal Muscular Atrophy

Muscular Dystrophy Association
3561 E. Sunrise Drive
Tuscon, AZ 85718
(602) 529-2000
see also: Society for Muscular Dystrophy
International

**Muscular Dystrophy Group of Great
Britain and Northern Ireland**
Nattrass House
35 Macaulay Road
London, England SW4 OQP
Telephone: 071-720-8055

Musculoskeletal Disorders
see: Association of Children's Prosthetic
and Orthotic Clinics
National Arthritis, Musculoskeletal and Skin
Disorders Information Clearinghouse

**Myalgic Encephalomyelitis
Association**
Stanhope House
High Street
Essex SS17 OHA
England
Telephone: 37-564-2466

Myasthenia Gravis Foundation, Inc.
53 West Jackson Boulevard, Suite 660
Chicago, IL 60604
(312) 427-6252
(800) 541-5454

**Myeloproliferative Disease
Foundation**
2220 Tiemann Avenue
Baychester, NY 10469
(212) 697-5252

Myoclonus
see: National Myoclonus Foundation

Narcolepsy
see: American Narcolepsy Association, Inc.
Narcolepsy and Cataplexy Foundation of
America
Narcolepsy Network

**Narcolepsy and Cataplexy
Foundation of America**
445 East 68th Street, #12L
New York, NY 10021
(212) 628-6315

Narcolepsy Institute
Montefiore Medical Center
111 East 210th Street
Bronx, NY 10467
(212) 920-6799

Narcolepsy Network
Box 1365, FDR Station
New York, NY 10150
(415) 591-7884
(914) 834-2855

**National Addison's Disease
Foundation**
505 Northern Boulevard, Suite 200
Great Neck, NY 11021
(516) 487-4992

National Alopecia Areata Foundation
710 C Street, Suite 11
San Rafael, CA 94901
(415) 456-4644

National Anorexic Aid Society, Inc.
1925 East Dublin Granville Road
Columbus, OH 43229
(614) 436-1112

**National Arthritis, Musculoskeletal
and Skin Diseases Information
Clearinghouse**
Box AMS
9000 Rockville Pike
Bethesda, MD 20892
(301) 496-8188

**National Association for the
Craniofacially Handicapped—
FACES**
P.O. Box 11082
Chattanooga, TN 37401
(615) 266-1632

National Association of the Deaf
814 Thayer Avenue
Silver Spring, MD 20910
(301) 587-1788

**National Association for Parents of
the Visually Impaired, Inc.**
2180 Linway Drive
Beloit, WI 53511
(608) 362-4945
(800) 562-6265

**National Association of Patients on
Hemodialysis and Transplantation**
see: American Association of Kidney
Patients

National Association for Pseudoxanthoma Elasticum
c/o Diane Clancy
82-B Phillips Street
Albany, NY 12202
(518) 426-0451

National Association of Radiation Survivors
P.O. Box 20749
Oakland, CA 94620
(510) 655-4886

National Association for Retarded Citizens
see: The Arc

National Association for Sickle Cell Disease, Inc.
3345 Wilshire Blvd., Suite 1106
Los Angeles, CA 90010
(213) 736-5455
(800) 421-8453

National Association for the Visually Handicapped
22 West 21st Street, 6th Floor
New York, NY 10010
(212) 889-3141
and
3201 Balboa Street
San Francisco, CA 94121
(415) 221-8753

National Ataxia Foundation
600 Twelve Oaks Center
15500 Wayzata Boulevard
Wayzata, MN 55391
(612) 473-7666

National Cancer Institute
Physician Data Query
Cancer Information Service
9000 Rockville Pike, Building 31, Room 1A2A
Bethesda, MD 20892
(800) 4-CANCER
In Washington, DC, and suburbs in MD and
  VA: 806-5700
In Alaska: (800) 638-6070
In Oahu, HI: (800) 524-1234 (Neighbor
  islands, call collect)

National Center for Down Syndrome
see: Down Syndrome Association

National Center for Education in Maternal and Child Health
38th and R Streets, NW
Washington, DC 20057
(202) 625-8400

National Chronic Fatigue Syndrome Association
3521 Broadway, Suite 222
Kansas City, MO 64111
(816) 931-4777
  see also Chronic Fatigue Syndrome Society

National Chronic Pain Outreach Association
7979 Old Georgetown Road, Suite 100
Bethesda, MD 20814
(301) 652-4948

National Clearinghouse for Alcohol & Drug Information
P.O. Box 2345
Rockville, MD 20847
(301) 468-2600

National Cleft Palate Association
see: About Face
American Cleft Palate Association

National Congenital Port Wine Stain Foundation
125 East 63rd Street
New York, NY 10021
(212) 755-3820
HOTLINE (516) 623-4962

National Council on Radiation Units and Measurements, Inc.
7910 Woodmont Avenue, Suite 800
Bethesda, MD 20814
(301) 657-2652

National Craniofacial Foundation
see: Children's Craniofacial Association
  (CCA)

National Cushing Syndrome Association
4645 Van Nuys Blvd., Suite 104
Sherman Oaks, CA 91403
(818) 788-9239

National Diabetes Information Clearinghouse
9000 Rockville Pike
Box NDIC
Bethesda, MD 20892
(301) 468-2162

National Digestive Diseases Information Clearinghouse
9000 Rockville Pike
Box NDDIC
Bethesda, MD 20892
(301) 468-6344

National Down Syndrome Congress
1800 Dempster
Park Ridge, IL 60068
(800) 232-NDSC

National Down Syndrome Society
666 Broadway, Suite 810
New York, NY 10012
(212) 460-9330
(800) 221-4602

National Easter Seal Society, Inc.
70 East Lake Street
Chicago, IL 60601
(312) 726-6200 (voice)
(312) 726-4258 (TDD)

National Eye Institute
9000 Rockville Pike
Bethesda, MD 20892
(301) 496-5248

National Federation of the Blind
1800 Johnson Street
Baltimore, MD 21230
(301) 659-9314
(800) 638-7518

**National Foundation of Dentistry
for the Handicapped**
1600 Stout Street, Suite 1420
Denver, CO 80202
(303) 573-0264

**National Foundation for Ectodermal
Dysplasias**
219 E. Main Street
Mascoutah, IL 62258
(618) 566-2020

**National Foundation for Facial
Reconstruction**
317 East 34th Street, Room 901
New York, NY 11016
(212) 263-6656

**National Foundation for Ileitis and
Colitis, Inc.**
see: Crohn's and Colitis Foundation of
America, Inc.

**National Foundation for Jewish
Genetic Diseases**
250 Park Avenue, Suite 1000
New York, NY 10177
(212) 371-1030

**National Foundation for Vitiligo
and Pigment Disorders**
c/o Sandy Werner
9032 South Normandy Lane
Centerville, OH 45459
(513) 885-5739

National Gaucher Foundation
19241 Montgomery Village Avenue, Suite E21
Gaithersburg, MD 20879
(301) 990-3800

National Gay & Lesbian Task Force
1734 14th Street N.W.
Washington, DC 20009
(202) 332-6483

National Gay Task Force Crisis Line
(Provides information for both medical
   professionals and nonmedical persons,
   including patients, their families, etc.)
Monday through Friday, 3 PM to 9 PM,
   Eastern time
(800) 221-7044

National Graves Disease Foundation
c/o Nancy H. Patterson, President
320 Arlington Road
Jacksonville, FL 32211
(904) 724-6744

National Hansen Disease Center
United States Public Health Service Hospital
5445 Point Claire Road
Carville, LA 70721-9607
(504) 642-4740
(800) 642-2477

National Headache Foundation
5252 North Western Avenue
Chicago, IL 60625
(800) 843-2256

**National Heart, Lung and Blood
Institute**
P.O. Box 30105
Bethesda, MD 20824-0105
(301) 496-4236

National Hemophilia Foundation
The Soho Building
110 Greene Street, Suite 303
New York, NY 10012
(212) 219-8180

National Hospice Organization
1901 Fort Myer Drive, Suite 902
Arlington, VA 22209
(703) 243-5900

National Hydrocephalus Foundation
400 North Michigan Avenue, Suite 1102
Chicago, IL 60611-4012
(815) 467-6548

National Ichthyosis Foundation
see: Foundation for Ichthyosis and Related
    Skin Types

**National Information Center on
    Deafness**
Gallaudet University
800 Florida Avenue N.E.
Washington, DC 20002
(202) 651-5051 (Voice and TDD)

**National Information Center for
    Children & Youth With Disabilities
    (NICHCY)**
PO Box 1492
Washington, DC 20013
(703) 893-6061
(800) 999-5599
(703) 893-8614 (TDD)

National Institute on Aging
9000 Rockville Pike
Bldg. 31, Rm. 5-C27
Bethesda, MD 20892
(301) 496-1752

**National Institute on Alcohol Abuse
    and Alcoholism**
5600 Fishers Lane
Rockville, MD 20857
(301) 443-3885

**National Institute of Allergy and
    Infectious Diseases (NIAID)**
9000 Rockville Pike
Bethesda, MD 20892
(301) 396-5717

**National Institute of Child Health and
    Human Development**
9000 Rockville Pike, Building 31, Room 2A-32
Bethesda, MD 20892
(301) 496-5133

**National Institute of Deafness &
    Other Communication Disorders**
see: National Institute of Neurological
    Disorders & Stroke

National Institute of Dental Research
9000 Rockville Pike
Bldg. 31, Rm. 2C33, NIH/HIDR
Bethesda, MD 20892
(301) 496-4261

**National Institute of Diabetes,
    Digestive and Kidney Diseases**
Box NDIC
9000 Rockville Pike
Bethesda, MD 20892
(301) 496-3583

**National Institute of Environmental
    Health Sciences**
Public Affairs Office
P.O. Box 12233
Research Triangle Park, NC 27709
(919) 541-3345

National Institute of Mental Health
5600 Fishers Lane, Room 15C-05
Rockville, MD 20857
(301) 443-4513

**National Institute of Mental
    Retardation
    (Canadian Association for the
    Mentally Retarded)**
York University
Kinsmen NIMR Building
4700 Keele Street, North York
Toronto, Ontario M3J 1P3
Canada
(416) 661-9611

**National Institute of Neurological,
    Disorders & Stroke**
9000 Rockville Pike, Bldg. 31, Rm 8A-16
Bethesda, MD 20892
(301) 496-5751

National Kidney Foundation
30 East 33rd Street, 11th Floor
New York, NY 10016
(212) 889-2210

**National Kidney and Urologic
    Diseases Information
    Clearinghouse**
Box NKUDIC
Bethesda, MD 20892
(301) 468-6345

**National Leigh Disease Foundation,
    Inc.**
601 Taylor Street
Corinth, MS 38834
(601) 287-8069

**National Library Service for the Blind
    and Physically Handicapped**
Library of Congress
1291 Taylor Street NW
Washington, DC 20542
(202) 707-5100

1034 | MASTER RESOURCES LIST

National Lipid Diseases Foundation
1201 Corbin Street
Elizabeth, NJ 07201
(908) 527-8000

National Lupus Foundation
see: American Lupus Society

National Lymphatic & Venous Diseases Foundation, Inc.
Attention of Mary Bellini
218 Monsignor O'Brien Highway
Cambridge, MA 02141
(800) 225-2292

National Lymphedema Network
2211 Post Street, Suite 404
San Francisco, CA 94115
(800) 541-3259

National Marfan Foundation
382 Main Street
Port Washington, New York 11050
(516) 883-8712

National Mental Health Association
1021 Prince Street
Alexandria, VA 22314
(703) 684-7722

National Migraine Foundation
see: National Headache Foundation

National Mucopolysaccharidosis (MPS) Society
17 Kramer Street
Hicksville, NY 11801
(516) 931-6338

National Multiple Sclerosis Society
National Headquarters
733 Third Avenue, 6th Floor
New York, NY 10017
(212) 986-3240
(800) 624-8236 (TDD)
(800) 227-3166 (Voice)

National Myoclonus Foundation
845 Third Avenue
New York, NY 10022
(212) 758-5656

National Network of Learning-Disabled Adults, Inc.
c/o Bill Butler
P.O. Box 32611
Phoenix, AZ 85064-2611
(602) 941-5112

National Neurofibromatosis Foundation, Inc.
141 Fifth Avenue
New York, NY 10010
(212) 460-8980

National Organization for Albinism and Hypopigmentation
1500 Locust Street
Philadelphia, PA 19107
(215) 545-2322

National Organization for Rare Disorders (NORD)
P.O. Box 8923
New Fairfield, CT 06812
(203) 746-6518

National Phenylketonuria (PKU) Foundation
6301 Tejas Drive
Pasadena, TX 77503
(713) 487-4802

National PKU News
c/o Virginia Schuett
7760 Ridge Drive, N.E.
Seattle, WA 98115

National Psoriasis Foundation
6443 SW Beaverton Highway
Suite 210
Portland, OR 97221
(503) 297-1545

National Retinitis Pigmentosa Foundation Fighting Blindness
P.O. Box 17279
1401 Mt. Royal Avenue, 4th Floor
Baltimore, MD 21217-4245
(410) 225-9400
(800) 683-5555
(410) 225-9409 (TDD)

National Reye Syndrome Foundation
P.O. Box 829
Bryan, Ohio 43506
(419) 636-2679

National Scoliosis Foundation, Inc.
72 Mount Auburn Street
Watertown, MA 02172
(617) 926-0397

National Sexually Transmitted Diseases Hotline
(800) 227-8922

National Sjögren Syndrome Association
3201 West Evans Drive
Phoenix, AZ 85023
(602) 993-7227

National Society for Children and Adults with Autism
see: Autism Society of America

National Society to Prevent Blindness
500 East Remington Road
Schaumburg, IL 60173
(708) 843-2020
(800) 221-3004 (National Center for Sight)

National Spasmodic Torticollis Association, Inc.
P.O. Box 476
Elm Grove, WI 53122
(800) HURTFUL

National Spinal Cord Injury Association
149 California Street
Newton, MA 02158

National Subacute Sclerosing Panencephalitis Registry
University of South Alabama School of
  Medicine
c/o Paul Dyken, M.D.
Department of Neurology
2451 Fillingim Street
Mobile, AL 36617
(205) 471-7834

National Sudden Infant Death Syndrome (SIDS) Resource Center
8201 Greenboro Drive, Suite 600
McLean, VA 22102
(703) 821-8955

National Sudden Infant Death Syndrome Foundation
see: SIDS Alliance

The National Support Group for Dermatomyositis
1119 Spring Garden Street
Bethlehem, PA 18017
(215) 974-9832

National Support Group for Exstrophy of the Bladder
Group for Exstrophy of the Bladder
5075 Medhurst Street
Solon, OH 44139
(216) 248-6851

National Tay-Sachs & Allied Diseases Association
2001 Beacon Street, Suite 304
Brookline, MA 02146
(617) 277-4463

National Tuberous Sclerosis Association, Inc.
8000 Corporate Drive, Suite 120
Landover, MD 20785
(301) 459-9888
(800) 225-NTSA

National Urea Cycle Disorders Foundation
1306 45½ Avenue North East
Minneapolis, MN 55421

National Vitiligo Foundation
P.O. Box 6337
Tyler, TX 75711
(903) 534-2925
  see also: National Foundation for Vitiligo
  and Pigment Disorders

National Women's Health Network
1325 G Street NW, Lower Level B
Washington, DC 20005
(202) 347-1140

Kenneth H. Nelder, M.D.
PXE Research Program
Department of Dermatology
Health Sciences Center
Texas Tech University
Lubbock, TX 79430
(806) 743-2456

Neurofibromatosis, Inc.
3401 Woodridge Court
Mitchellville, MD 20721-2817
(301) 577-8984
(410) 461-5213 (TDD)
(800) 942-6825
  see also The National Neurofibromatosis
  Foundation, Inc.

Neurofibromatosis Clinical Facilities: Boston:
Massachusetts General Hospital
Neurofibromatosis Clinic
Department of Neurosurgery
15 Parkman Street, Room 312
Boston, MA 02114
(617) 726-3776
Attention of Robert Marthuza, M.D.
(cont.)

Neurofibromatosis Clinical Facilities:
(cont.)
Washington:
Children's Hospital
Neurofibromatosis Clinic, Genetics
    Department
111 Michigan Avenue NW
Washington, D.C. 20010
(202) 745-2187
Attention of Kenneth Rosenbaum, M.D.
Philadelphia:
Children's Hospital
Neurofibromatosis Clinic
34th Street and Civic Center Boulevard,
    Room 9028
Philadelphia, PA 19104
(215) 596-9645
Attention of Anna Meadows, M.D.
New York:
Mount Sinai School of Medicine
Neurofibromatosis Clinic
100th Street and Madison Avenue
New York, NY 10029
(212) 650-6500
Attention of Alan Rubinstein, M.D.

Neurological Research Bank
    see: Wallace W. Tourtelotte, M.D.

**New York State Institute for Basic
    Research in Development
    Disabilities**
    see: Institute for Basic Research in
    Development Disabilities

Noonan Syndrome Support Group
1278 Pine Avenue
San Jose, CA 95125
(408) 723-5188

**North American Malignant
    Hyperthermia Registry**
Department of Anesthesia
Penn State College of Medicine
P.O. Box 850
Hershey, PA 17033
(717) 531-8521

**North American Pediatric
    Pseudoobstruction Society**
P.O. Box 772
Medford, MA 02155
(617) 395-4255

**Obsessive-Compulsive Foundation,
    Inc.**
P.O. Box 9573
New Haven, CT 06535
(203) 772-0565

J.M. Opitz, M.D.
Shodar Children's Hospital
P.O. Box 5539
Helena, MT 59604
(For information on Smith-Lemli-Opitz
    syndrome)

Organic Acidemia Association, Inc.
c/o Elizabeth Webb Beyer
522 Lander Street
Reno, NV 89509
(702) 322-5542

Orofacial Guild of Orange County
c/o Jane Schrenzel or Valerie Young
22832 Larkin Street
Lakeforest, CA 92630
(714) 558-1739
(714) 597-1475

Orton Dyslexia Society
Chester Bldg., Suite 382
8600 LaSalle Road
Baltimore, MD 21204-6020
(301 296-0232

**Osler-Weber-Rendu Syndrome
    Registry**
    see: Hereditary Hemorrhagic Telangiectasis
    Registry

Osteogenesis Imperfecta Foundation
5005 West Laurel Street, Suite 210
Tampa, FL 33607-3836
(813) 282-1161
    see also: Michael P. White, M.D., Shriners'
    Hospital

Ostomy Association
    see: Support Group for Parents of Ostomy
    Children
    United Ostomy Association

**The Oxalosis and Hyperoxaluria
    Foundation**
P.O. Box 1632
Kent, WA 98035
(206) 631-0386

Pachygyria
    see: Support Network for Lissencephaly

The Paget's Disease Foundation, Inc.
165 Cadman Plaza East, Room 202
Brooklyn, NY 11201
(718) 596-1043

Pain
see: American Chronic Pain Association, Inc.
National Chronic Pain Outreach Association

Charles Y.C. Pak, M.D.
U. of Texas South Western Medical Center
5323 Harry Hines Boulevard
Dallas, TX 75235
(214) 688-3111

Paraplegia
see: American Paraplegia Society

Parenteral & Enteral Nutrition
see: American Society of Parenteral &
Enteral Nutrition (ASPEN)

Parents of Galactosemic Children, Inc.
c/o Linda Manis
209-81 Solano Way
Boca Raton, FL 33433
(407) 852-0266

Parkinson Disease Foundation
William Black Medical Research Building
640 West 168th Street
New York, NY 10032
(212) 923-4700
see also: United Parkinson Foundation

Parkinson Disease and Movement Disorders Clinic
Bala V. Manyam, M.D.
Southern Illinois University School of
Medicine
P.O. Box 19230
Springfield, IL 62794-9230
(217) 782-3318

Phenylketonuria (PKU) Parents
8 Myrtle Lane
San Anselmo, CA 94960
(415) 457-4632

Phenylketonuria (PKU) Collaborative Study
Children's Hospital of Los Angeles
P.O. Box 54700
Los Angeles, CA 90054
(213) 669-2152
see also: Children's PKU Network
National PKU News

Physician Data Query
Cancer Information Service
National Cancer Institute
9000 Rockville Pike, Building 31, Room 1A2A
Bethesda, MD 20892
(800) 4-CANCER
In Washington, DC, and suburbs in MD and
VA: (301) 496-4000
In Alaska: (800) 638-6070
In Oahu, HI: (808) 524-1234 (Neighbor
islands, call collect)

Polio Information Center
510 Main Street, Suite A446
Roosevelt Island, NY 10044
(212) 223-0353
see also: British Polio Fellowship
Post-Polio National, Inc.

Polychondritis & Rheumatoid Arthritis Clinic
David Trentham, M.D., Chief, Division of
Rheumatology
Beth Israel Hospital
330 Brookline Avenue
Boston, MA 02215
(617) 735-2560

Polycystic Kidney Research Foundation
922 Walnut, Suite 411
Kansas City, MO 64106
(816) 421-1869

Porphyria
see: American Porphyria Foundation

Port Wine Stain Foundation
see: The National Congenital Port Wine
Stain Foundation

Post-Polio National, Inc.
(Post-Polio League for Information and
Outreach, Polio Society)
4200 Wisconsin Avenue N.W., Suite 106273
Washington, DC 20016
(301) 897-8180

Prader-Willi Syndrome Association
6490 Excelsior Boulevard, E-102
St. Louis Park, MN 55426
(612) 926-1947

Primary Biliary Cirrhosis Patient Support Network
Box 177
Tamworth, Ontario KOK 3GO
Canada
(613) 379-2534

The Progeria Foundation
see: Institute for Basic Research in
Developmental Disabilities
Sunshine Foundation (for children with
progeria)

The Progeria International Registry
New York State Institute for Basic Research in
Developmental Disabilities
W. Ted Brown, M.D., Ph.D.
1050 Forest Hill Road
Staten Island, NY 10314
(718) 494-5363

**Progressive Supranuclear Palsy
Research Fund**
Department of Neurology, Room 408
UMDNJ-Robert Wood Johnson Medical
School
CN19
New Brunswick, NJ 08903
(908) 937-7728
see also: Society for Progressive
Supranuclear Palsy

Pseudoobstruction Society
see: North American Pediatric
Pseudoobstruction Society

Pseudoxanthoma Elasticum (PXE)
see: Mark Lebwohl, M.D. (PXE Research
Project, New York)
National Association for Pseudoxanthoma
Elasticum
Kenneth H. Nelder, M.D. (PXE Research
Program, Texas)

Psoriasis Research Association
107 Vista del Grande
San Carlos, CA 94070
(415) 593-1394
see also: National Psoriasis Foundation

Pull-Through Network
1126 Grant Street
Wheaton, IL 60187
(708) 665-1268

Pulmonary Disorders
see: Lung Disorders

Pulmonary Hypertension
see: American Society of Hypertension

Radiation Disease
see: Environmental Disorders

Theodore Rasmussen, M.D.
Montreal Neurological Hospital
3801 University Street
Montreal H3A 2B4
Canada
(514) 398-6644
(For information on Rasmussen encephalitis)
see also: Ben Carson, M.D.

Raynaud's Scleroderma Association
112 Crewe Road
Alsager, Cheshire ST7 2JA
England
Telephone: 027-087-2776

**Reflex Sympathetic Dystrophy
Syndrome Association**
P.O. Box 821
Haddonfield, NJ 08033
(609) 858-6553

Renal Disorders
see: Kidney Disorders

**Research Trust for Metabolic
Diseases in Children**
Golden Gate Lodge
Weston Road
Crewe, Cheshire CW1 1XN
England
Telephone: 2027-025-0221

**Retinitis Pigmentosa Foundation
Fighting Blindness**
see: National Retinitis Pigmentosa
Foundation Fighting Blindness

Rett Syndrome
see: International Rett Syndrome
Association

Reye Syndrome
see: National Reye Syndrome Foundation

David Robertson, M.D.
Director of Clinical Research Center
Vanderbilt University
Nashville, TN 37232-2195
(615) 343-6499
(For information on orthostatic hypotension)

Roger N. Rosenberg, M.D.
Abe (Bunky) Morris & William Zale Chairman
in Neurology
Professor of Neurology and Physiology
University of Texas Southwestern Medical
School
5323 Harry Hines Boulevard
Dallas, TX 75235-9036
(214) 688-4800
(For information on Joseph disease)

Rubinstein-Taybi Case Documentation:
Jack H. Rubinstein, Director
Cincinnati Center for Developmental
Disorders, Pavilon Bldg.
Ell and Bethesda Avenues
Cincinnati, OH 45229-2899
(513) 559-4688

Rubinstein-Taybi Parent Support Group
414 E. Kansas
Smith Center, KS 66967
(913) 282-6237

Rubinstein-Taybi Support Group
Barbara Baron
46 Windsor Road
Great Harwood
Blackburn, Lancashire BB6 7RR
England
0254-889-122

Russell-Silver Syndrome
see: Association for Children with
Russell-Silver Syndrome

Schepens Eye Research Institute of Retina Foundation
Macular Disease Research Center
20 Staniford Street
Boston, MA 02114
(617) 742-3140

Scleroderma Federation
1182 Teaneck Road
Teaneck, NJ 07666
(201) 837-9826
see also: United Scleroderma Foundation

Scleroderma Information Exchange, Inc.
150 Hines Farm Road
Cranston, RI 02921
(401) 943-3909

Scleroderma Research Foundation
Pueblo Medical Commons
2320 Bath Street, Suite 307
Santa Barbara, CA 93105
(805) 563-9133

Scoliosis
see: National Scoliosis Foundation, Inc.

Self-Help for Hard-of-Hearing People, Inc.
7800 Wisconsin Avenue
Bethesda, MD 20814
(301) 657-2248

Short Stature Foundation
17200 Jamboree Blvd., Suite J
Irvine, CA 92714
(714) 474-4554
(800) 24-DWARF
see also: Little People of America

Shy-Drager Syndrome Support Group
1607 Silver Avenue S.E.
Albuquerque, NM 87106
(505) 243-5118

Sickle Cell Association of Ontario
55 Gateway Blvd.
Don Mills, Ontario M3C 1B4
Canada
(416) 674-6916

Sight Impairment
see: Eye Disorders

Simon Foundation
P.O. Box 815
Wilmette, IL 60091
(708) 864-3913

Sjögren Syndrome Foundation
382 Main Street
Port Washington, NY 11050
(516) 767-2866
see also: National Sjögren Syndrome
Association

Skin Cancer Foundation
245 Fifth Avenue, Suite 2402
New York, NY 10016
(212) 725-5176

James Skare, M.D.
Boston University School of Medicine
Center for Human Genetics
Boston, MA 02118
(617) 638-7086
(For information on participation in genetic
studies concerning X-linked
lymphoproliferative syndrome)

Gary R. Skuse, Ph.D.
University of Rochester Medical Center
Division of Genetics
601 Elmwood Avenue, Box 641
Rochester, NY 14642
(716) 275-3463

Sleep Disorders
see: American Narcolepsy Association, Inc.
Narcolepsy

Alfred Slonim, M.D.
Department of Pediatric Endocrinology
300 Community Drive
North Shore University Hospital
Manhasset, NY 11030
(516) 562-4635

Smell and Taste Research Center
University of Pennsylvania Hospital
3400 Spruce Street, G1
Philadelphia, PA 19104
(215) 662-2653
    see: Clinical Smell and Taste Research
    Center

Smith-Lemli-Opitz Syndrome:
Contact Dr. Opitz at
Shodar Children's Hospital
P.O. Box 5539
Helena, MT 59604
(406) 444-7500

Society of MPS Diseases
7 Chessfield Park
Buckinghamshire HP6-6RU
England

**Society of Mucopolysaccharide
Diseases, Inc.**
c/o Sheila Lee/President
204-4912 Ross Street
Red Deer, Alberta
Canada T4N 1X7

**Society for Muscular Dystrophy
International**
P.O. Box 479
Bridgewater, Nova Scotia
Canada B4V 2X6
(902) 429-6322

**Society for Progressive Supranuclear
Palsy**
2904-B Marnat Road
Baltimore, MD 21209
(301) 484-8771

**Society for the Rehabilitation of the
Facially Disfigured, Inc.**
    see: National Foundation for Facial
    Reconstruction

Sotos Syndrome:
Juan Sotos, M.D.
Children's Hospital, C-404
700 Children's Drive
Columbus, OH 43205
(614) 461-2000

**Sotos Syndrome Support Group of
Great Britain**
c/o Child Growth Foundation
4 Mayfield Avenue
London W4 1PW
England
Telephone: 081-995-0257

Sotos Syndrome USA Support Group
2333 West El Moro
Mesa, AZ 85202
(602) 890-1722

**Spasmodic Torticollis Association,
Inc.**
    see: National Spasmodic Torticollis
    Association, Inc.

**Spastic Dysphonia Support Group/Our
Voice**
156 Fifth Avenue, Suite 1033
New York, NY 10010-7002
(212) 929-4299

Spina Bifida Association of America
1700 Rockville Pike, Suite 250
Rockville, MD 20852
(301) 770-SBAA
(800) 621-3141

Spina Bifida Association of Canada
220 388 Donald Street
Winnipeg, Manitoba
Canada R3B 2J4
(204) 957-1784

Spinal Cord Injury Hotline
American Paralysis Association
2201 Argonne Drive
Baltimore, MD 21218
(800) 526-3456
    see also: American Paraplegia Society
    American Spinal Injury Association
    National Spinal Cord Injury Association
    Spinal Cord Injury (24-hour hotline)
    Spial Cord Society

Spinal Cord Injury
2201 Argonne Drive
Baltimore, MD 21218
(800) 638-1733 (In Maryland)
24-hour hotline: (800) 526-3456

Spinal Cord Society
Wendell Road
Fergus Falls, MN 56537
(218) 739-5252
    see also: American Paraplegia Society
    American Spinal Injury Association

Stiff Man Syndrome
see: Mark Hallet, M.D.

Sturge-Weber Foundation
P.O. Box 460931
Aurora, CO 80046
(303) 360-7290
(800) 627-5482

Subacute Sclerosing Panencephalitis
see: National SSPE Registry

Sudden Infant Death Syndrome (SIDS) Alliance
10500 Little Patuxent Parkway, Suite 420
Columbia, MD 21044
(800) 221-SIDS
see also: National SIDS Resource Center

Sunshine Foundation
4010 Levick Street
Philadelphia, PA 19135
(215) 335-2622
(Funds are raised to bring all children with progeria together each year so that their progress can be studied while the children socialize in a vacation atmosphere.)

Support Group for Parents of Ostomy Children
Division of United Ostomy Association
11385 Cedarbrook Road
Roscoe, IL 61073
(815) 623-8034

Support Organization for Trisomy 18/13 (S.O.F.T.) and Other Related Disorders
c/o Barbara Van Herreweghe
2982 S. Union Street
Rochester, NY 14624
(716) 594-4621

Support Group for Arthrogryposis Multiplex Congenita (AVENUES)
P.O. Box 5192
Sonora, CA 95370
(209) 928-3688

Support Network for Lissencephaly
c/o Dianna Fitzgerald
7121 Bear Road
Fort Wayne, IN 46809
(219) 747-1075

Syringomyelia
see: American Syringomyelia Alliance Project, Inc.

Systemic Lupus Erythematosus Foundation, Inc.
149 Madison Avenue, Suite 608
New York, NY 10016
(212) 685-4118
see also: Lupus Foundation of America
National Lupus Foundation

Tardive Dyskinesia/Tardive Dystonia National Association
4244 University Way N.E.
P.O. Box 45732
Seattle, WA 98145-0732
(206) 522-3166

Taste and Smell Research Center
see: Clinical Smell and Taste Research Center

Tay-Sachs Disease
see: National Foundation for Jewish Genetic Diseases
National Tay-Sachs/Allied Diseases Association

Jess Thoene, M.D.
Department of Pediatrics
University of Michigan Medical School
2612 SPH I
109 Observatory
Ann Arbor, Michigan 48109-2029
(313) 763-3427

Thrombocytopenia-Absent Radius Syndrome Association (TARSA)
212 Sherwood Drive
R.D. 1
Linwood, NJ 08221-9745
(609) 927-0418
(This organization will answer question on TAR syndrome only; it does not provide information on other forms of thrombocytopenia.)

The Thyroid Foundation of America, Inc.
Massachusetts General Hospital
Ruth Sleeper Hall, Room 350
Boston, MA 02114
(617) 726-8500

The Thyroid Foundation of Canada
CD/Box 1597
Kingston, Ontario
Canada K7L 5C8
(613) 542-8330

Tinnitus
see: American Tinnitus Association
E.A.R. Foundation
Vestibular Disorders Association

Tourette Syndrome Association
42-40 Bell Boulevard
Bayside, NY 11361
(718) 224-2999
(800) 237-0717

Wallace W. Tourtelotte, M.D.
Director, National Neurological Research
Bank
Neurology Research (W127A)
Veterans Administration
Wadsworth Medical Center
Los Angeles, CA 90073
(213) 824-4307

Toxic Epidermal Necrolysis Clinical Facilities:
St. Louis:
Washington University School of Medicine
Department of Dermatology
St. Louis, MO 63110
(314) 362-5000
New York:
Rockefeller University Hospital
Department of Investigative Dermatology
1230 York Avenue
New York, NY 10021
(212) 570-8000
Philadelphia:
Children's Hospital
Department of Pediatric Dermatology
Dermatology Clinic
34th and Civic Center Boulevard
Philadelphia, PA 19104
or
University of Pennsylvania (diagnosis only)
Dermatology Clinic
34th and Spruce Streets
Philadelphia, PA 19104
(215) 662-6535

Treacher Collins Foundation
c/o Hope Charkins-Drazin
P.O. Box 683
Norwich, VT 05055
(802) 649-3020

Tremor
see: International Tremor Foundation

Trigeminal Neuralgia Association
National Headquarters
P.O. Box 785
Barnegat Light, NJ 08006
(609) 361-1014

Trisomies and Related Disorders
see: Support Group for Trisomy 18/13 and
Other Related Disorders

Tuberous Sclerosis
see: National Tuberous Sclerosis
Association, Inc.

Turner Syndrome Society of Canada
7777 Keel Street, Floor 2
Concord, Ontario
Canada L4K 1Y7
(416) 660-7766

Turner Syndrome Society of the United States
Suite 768-214
12 Oaks Center
15500 Wayzata Blvd.
Wayzata, MN 55391
(612) 475-9944

Turner Syndrome Support Group of New England
170 Maple Street
Malden, MA 02148
(617) 322-4892

United Cerebral Palsy Associations, Inc. (main office)
1522 K Street N.W., Suite 1112
Washington, DC 20005
(202) 842-1266
(800) USA-1UCP

United Leukodystrophy Foundation
2304 Highland Drive
Sycamore, IL 60178
(815) 895-3211

United Liver Foundation
11646 West Pico Boulevard
Los Angeles, CA 90064
(213) 445-4204; 445-4200

United Ostomy Association
36 Executive Park, Suite 120
Irvine, CA 92714
(714) 660-8624

United Parkinson Foundation
360 West Superior Street
Chicago, IL 60610
(312) 664-2344

United Scleroderma Foundation, Inc.
P.O. Box 399
Watsonville, CA 94077-0350
(408) 728-2202
(800) 722-HOPE (outside CA)

United SIDS Awareness, Inc.
see: Sudden Infant Death Alliance

Urea Cycle Disorders
see: National Urea Cycle Disorders
Foundation
Organic Acidemia Association, Inc.

**U.S. Department of Health
and Human Services**
Public Health Service
Alcohol, Drug Abuse, and Mental Health
Administration
National Institute on Alcohol Abuse and
Alcoholism
5600 Fishers Lane
Rockville, MD 20857
(301) 443-3783
(800) 729-6686

Vaccines
see: Dissatisfied Parents Together
(re adverse reactions)

Vestibular Disorders Association
1015 N.W. 22nd Avenue, D-230
Portland, OR 97210-3079
(503) 229-7705
see also: American Tinnitus Association;
E.A.R. Foundation

Visual Impairment
see: Eye Disorders

Vision Foundation, Inc.
818 Mt. Auburn Street
Watertown, MA 02172
(617) 926-4232
(800) 852-3029 (within MA)

Vitiligo
see: National Foundation for Vitiligo
and Pigment Disorders

**VOCAL (Voluntary Organization for
Communication and Language)**
336 Brixton Road
London SW9
England
Telephone: 071-274-4029

Wegeners Foundation, Inc.
c/o Judith Williams
9000 Rockville Pike
Building 31A, Room B1W30
Bethesda, MD 20892
(301) 496-8331

**Wegeners Granulomatosis
Support Group**
National Chapter
P.O. Box 1518
Platte City, MO 64079
(816) 431-2096; 431-5469

Michael P. White, M.D.
Medical Director
Metabolic Research Unit
Shriners' Hospital for Crippled Children
2001 S. Lindbergh Boulevard
St. Louis, MO 63131
(314) 432-3600

Williams Syndrome Association
P.O. Box 178373
San Diego, CA 92177-8373
(314) 227-4411

Wilson's Disease Association
P.O. Box 75324
Washington, D.C. 20013
(202) 208-0934

World Federation of Hemophilia
4616 St. Catherine's Street West
Montreal, Quebec H3Z 1S3
Canada
(514) 933-7944

World Health Organization
525 23rd Street NW
Washington, DC 20037
(202) 861-3200
(202) 861-3305 (Library)

Xeroderma Pigmentosum Registry
c/o Department of Pathology
Room 520, Medical Science Building
UMDNJ—New Jersey Medical School
185 South Orange Avenue
Newark, NJ 07103
(201) 456-6255

X-Linked Lymphoproliferative Syndrome

For information on participation in genetic studies:

James Skare, M.D.
Boston University School of Medicine
Center for Human Genetics
80 East Concord Street
Boston, MA 02118
(617) 638-8000

15 | DIRECTORY OF ORPHAN DRUGS APPROVED AND IN DEVELOPMENT

This directory of orphan drugs has been compiled from data supplied by the researchers and manufacturers as of January 1992. Because the Food and Drug Administration makes every effort to expedite approval of orphan drugs, the status may have changed when you consult the listings. For complete information, call the Contact listed in the far right column.

Condition/Use	Drug Name	Status/Phase	Sponsor/Contact Person
Acne rosacea	metronidazole [topical] gel (Metrogel)	Approved for marketing	Curatek Pharmaceuticals, Inc. 1965 Pratt Blvd., Ste. 101 Elk Grove Village, IL 60007 John Presutti (800) 332-7680
Adenocarcinoma (See also Cancer, Carcinoma) Colorectal metastatic	fluorouracil (Adrucil) For use in combination with leucovorin	NDA supplement submitted	Lederle Laboratories Pearl River, NY 10965 G.W. McCarl, MD (201) 831-4617
	anti-tap-72 immunotoxin (Xomazyme-791)	Investigational	Xoma Corporation 2910 7th Street Berkeley, CA 94710 Carol DeGuzman (510) 644-1178
Ovarian advanced	altretamine (Hexalen)	Approved for marketing	U.S. Bioscience, Inc. 100 Front Street West Conshohocken, PA 19428 William McCulloch, M.R.C.P. (215) 832-4506
Adrenal cortical imaging	iodine-131-68-iodomethyl 19-norcholesterol [NP-59]	Phase III	University of Michigan 1500 E. Medical Center Dr. Ann Arbor, MI 48109-0028 David E. Kuhl, M.D. (313) 936-5388
AIDS	azido 2',3' dideoxyuridine	Phase II	Berlex Laboratories 1401 Harbor Bay Parkway Alameda, CA 94501 Lewis P. Chapman (510) 769-5200
	zidovudine (Retrovir)	Approved for marketing Exclusive approval	Burroughs Wellcome 3030 Cornwallis Rd. Research Triangle Park, NC 27709 Drug Information Serv. (800) 722-9292
	human immunodeficiency virus immune globulin	Investigational Studies in progress Phase I	Abbott Laboratories Diagnostics Division Abbott Park, IL 60064 David Nevalainen, Ph.D. (708) 937-7495

Condition/Use	Drug Name	Status/Phase	Sponsor/Contact Person
AIDS, *cont.*	Poly I: poly C_{12U} (Ampligen)	Phase II/III	HEM Pharmaceuticals Corp. 1617 JFK Boulevard Philadelphia, PA 19103 John R. Rapoza (215) 988-0080
Treatment of patients with CMV retinitis being treated with ganciclovir	filgrastim (Neupogen)	Phase II	Amgen, Inc. Amgen Center Thousand Oaks CA 91320-1789 Mark Brand (805) 499-5725
AIDS & AIDS-related complex (ARC)	dideoxycytidine, ddC	Phase III Clinical trials NDA submitted	Hoffmann-LaRoche 340 Kingsland St. Nutley, NJ 07110-1199 Darien E. Wilson (201) 235-4381
ARC	zidovudine (Retrovir)	Approved for marketing Exclusive approval	Burroughs Wellcome 3030 Cornwallis Rd. Research Triangle Park, NC 27709 Drug Information Serv. (800) 722-9292
Alpha-fetoprotein-producing germ cell tumors Detection	alpha-fetoprotein radio-immunodetection with Tc-99m (ImmuRAID-AFP-Tc-99m)	IND filed	Immunomedics, Inc. 150 Mt. Bethel Rd. Warren, NJ 07060 Kenneth Chang, Ph.D. (908) 647-5400
	iodine 1 123 murinemonoclonal antibody to alpha-fetoprotein	Inactive	Immunomedics, Inc. 150 Mt. Bethel Rd. Warren, NJ 07060 Kenneth Chang, Ph.D. (908) 647-5400
Alpha-1-Proteinase inhibitor Replacement therapy in congenital deficiency state (ATT deficiency related emphysema)	alpha-1-proteinase inhibitor [human] (Prolastin)	FDA approval (Orphan drug status)	Cutter Biological/Miles 400 Morgan Lane West Haven, CT 06516 Rene McRogers (203) 498-6444
Alternating hemiplegia	flunarizine (Sibelium)	Phase III Available on compassionate basis	Janssen Research Fdtn. 40 Kingsbridge Rd. Piscataway, NJ 08855-3998 Richard C. Meibach, Ph.D. (908) 524-9245

Condition/Use	Drug Name	Status/Phase	Sponsor/Contact Person
Amenorrhea Primary hypothalmic	luteinizing hormone-releasing hormone, GnRh (Lutrepulse)	Approved	Ortho Biotech Route 202, P.O. Box 300 Raritan, NJ 08869-0602 Dr. Robert Murphy (908) 218-6892
Amytrophic lateral sclerosis (ALS)	l-threonine (Threostat)	Approved for marketing	Tyson and Associates 12832 Chadron Avenue Hawthorne, CA 90250 Donald R. Tyson, Chairman (213) 675-1080
	myotrophin	IND to be submitted	Cephalon, Inc. 145 Brandywine Pkwy. West Chester, PA 19380 Nicole Vitullo (215) 344-0200
Anemia Associated with CRF	epoetin alfa (Epogen)	Approved for marketing Exclusive approval	Amgen, Inc. Amgen Center Thousand Oaks,CA 91320-1789 Mark Brand (805) 499-5725
Associated with HIV, ESRD, prematurity	erythropoietin [recombinant human] (Procrit)	Varies by indication Contact company	Ortho Biotech Route 202,P.O. Box 300 Raritan, NJ 08869-0602 Dr. Linda Dujack (908) 704-5057
Anorexia Associated with positive lab findings for HIV or a confirmed diagnosis of AIDS	megestrol acetate (Megace)	Clinical studies complete; analyzing study data	Bristol-Myers Squibb 2400 W. Lloyd Expressway Evansville, IN 47721-0001 Department of Medical Serv. (812) 429-5000
Antipyrine test As an index of hepatic drug-metabolizing capacity	antipyrine	Investigational	Upsher-Smith 14905–23rd Ave., N. Minneapolis, MN 55447 Lee Mork (800) 328-3344
Antithrombin III deficiency Prevention and treatment in	antithrombin III, human (ATnativ)	Approved for marketing	Baxter Healthcare Corp. 550 N. Brand Blvd Glendale, CA 91203 Michael Herrera (818) 507-5451

Condition/Use	Drug Name	Status/Phase	Sponsor/Contact Person
Asthma Severe steroid-requiring	troleandomycin	Phase II	Stanley J. Szefler, M.D. 1400 Jackson St. Denver, CO 80206 (303) 398-1379
Blepharospasm	botulinum toxin- type A (Oculinum)	FDA approved	Allergan Pharmaceuticals 2525 Dupont Drive Irvine, CA 92715 Steven Carlson (800) 347-4500
Bone marrow transplant With or without reconstruction of marrow PBSC	filgrastim (Neupogen)	Phase II	Amgen, Inc. Amgen Center Thousand Oaks CA 91320-1789 Mark Brand (805) 499-5725
For ex vivo treatment to eliminate mature T-cells from potential bone marrow grafts and in bone marrow recipients to prevent graft rejection and graft-vs.-host disease (GVHD)	CD5-T lymphocyte immunotoxin (Xomazyme-H65)	Investigational	Xoma Corporation 2910 7th Street Berkeley, CA 94710 Carol DeGuzman (510) 644-1178
Oral complications of chemotherapy in transplant patients	sucralfate suspension	Phase II	Naska Pharmacal Riverview Rd. P.O. Box 898 Lincolnton, NC 28093 Arthur H. Goldberg, Ph.D. (516) 536-3636
Stimulates white blood cell growth in bone marrow transplant patients	sargramostim GMCSF (Prokine)	Approved for marketing	Hoechst-Roussel Route 202-206 No. Somerville, NJ 08876 Susan Sutch (800) 445-4774
Brain malignancies To selectively increase blood flow and delivery of chemotherapy to brain tumor tissue	adenosine, MEDR-340	IND approved, Phase II Trials initiated	Medco Research, Inc. 8544 Beverly Blvd, Suite 308 Los Angeles, CA 90048 Roger D. Blevins, Pharm.D. (213) 966-4148

Condition/Use	Drug Name	Status/Phase	Sponsor/Contact Person
Burns Severe, in-hospital, for enhancement of nitrogen retention	somatropin (Saizen)	Preclinical	Serono Laboratories, Inc. 100 Longwater Circle Norwell, MA 02061 Gina Cella (617) 723-1300
Severe, requiring hospitalization	poloxamer 188 (Rheothrx Copolymer)	Phase I	Burroughs Wellcome 3030 Cornwallis Rd. Research Triangle Pk. NC 27709 Drug Information Serv. (800) 722-9292
Cachexia Associated with positive laboratory findings for HIV or confirmed diagnosis of AIDS	megestrol acetate (Megace)	Clinical studies complete analyzing study data	Bristol-Myers Squibb 2400 West Lloyd Expressway Evansville, IN 47721-0001 Department of Medical Serv. (812) 429-5000
Calculi, renal and bladder of the apatite or struvite variety	citric acid, glucono-delta-lactone and mag carbonate (Renacidin Irrigation)	Approved for marketing Exclusive approval	United Guardian, Inc P. O. Box 2500 Smithtown, NY 11787 Robert Rubinger (516) 273-0900
Cancer (See also Adenocarcinoma, Carcinoma) Bladder, superficial	porfimer sodium (Photofrin)	Investigational Phase III	Lederle Laboratories QLT Pearl River, NY 10965 G.W. McCarl, MD (201) 831-4617
Colorectal, carcinoembryonic antigen (CEA) producing Detection of recurrence or metastasis	(ImmuRAID-CEA-Tc-99m)	Orphan status pending PLA filed April 1991	Immunomedics, Inc. 150 Mt. Bethel Rd. Warren, NJ 07060 Kenneth Chang, Ph.D. (908) 647-5400
Colorectal, metastatic	1-leucovorin for use in combination with 5-fluorouracil	Phase III	Lederle Laboratories Pearl River, NY 10965 G.W. McCarl, MD (201) 831-4617

Condition/Use	Drug Name	Status/Phase	Sponsor/Contact Person
Esophogeal, obstructing	porfimer sodium (Photofrin)	Investigational Phase III	Lederle Laboratories QLT Pearl River, NY 10965 G.W. McCarl, MD (201) 831-4617
Lung, nonsmall cell Detection and staging, by imaging	technetium Tc 99M anti-nonsmall cell lung cancer murine monoclonal antibody (OncoTrac Nonsmall Cell Lung Cancer Imaging Kit)	Orphan status pending Phase III	NeoRx Corporation 410 W. Harrison Seattle, WA 98119 Dr. Darrell Salk (206) 281-7001
Lung, small cell	N901-blocked ricin	Phase I/II	ImmunoGen, Inc. 148 Sydney St. Cambridge, MA 02139 Carol Epstein, MD (617) 661-9312
Lung, small cell Detection and staging, by imaging	technetium Tc 99M anti-small cell lung cancer murine monoclonal antibody (OncoTrac Small Cell Lung Cancer Imaging Kit)	Orphan status pending PLA pending (Phase: FDA)	NeoRx Corporation 410 W. Harrison Seattle, WA 98119 Dr. Darrell Salk (206) 281-7001
Pain in patients tolerant to, or unresponsive to intraspinal opiates	clonidine hydrochloride	In development	Fujisawa Pharm. & Co. 3 Parkway Center. N. Deerfield, IL 60015 D.S. Ebersman (708) 317-8647
Carcinoma (See also Cancer, Adenocarcinoma) Colorectal Advanced	anti-TAP-72 immunotoxin (Xomazyme-791)	Investigational	Xoma Corporation 2910 7th Street Berkeley, CA 94710 Carol DeGuzman (510) 644-1178
	5-fluorouracil [5-Fu] use in combination with alpha-2-A, recombinant (Roferon-A)	Phase III Clinical trials	Hoffmann-LaRoche 340 Kingsland St. Nutley, NJ 07110-1199 Darien E. Wilson (201) 235-4381

Condition/Use	Drug Name	Status/Phase	Sponsor/Contact Person
Colorectal, *cont.*	leucovorin leucovorin calcium For use in combination with 5-fluorouracil	NDA supplement submitted	Lederle Laboratories Pearl River, NY 10965 G. W. McCarl, MD (201) 831-4617
Detection of suspected and previously unidentified tumor foci of recurrent colorectal cancer	111-indium murine anti-CEA monoclonal antibody	In research	Hybritech, Incorporated P.O. Box 269006 San Diego, CA 92196-9006 (619) 455-6700
Esophageal	fluorouracil [5-Fu] In combination with interferon alpha-2A, recombinant (Roferon-A)	Phase II Clinical trials	Hoffmann-LaRoche 340 Kingsland St. Nutley, NJ 07110-1199 Darien E. Wilson (201) 235-4381
Hepatocellular and hepatoblastoma detection	iodine I 123 murine monoclonal antibody to alpha-fetoprotein	Inactive	Immunomedics, Inc. 150 Mt. Bethel Rd. Warren, NJ 07060 Kenneth Chang, Ph.D. (908) 647-5400
	alpha-fetoprotein radio-immunodetection with Tc-99m (ImmuRAID-AFP-Tc-99m)	Phase I/II	Immunomedics, Inc. 150 Mt. Bethel Rd. Warren, NJ 07060 Kenneth Chang, Ph.D. (908) 647-5400
Ovarian As chemoprotective agent for cyclophosphamide	amifostine (Ethyol)	NDA submitted	U.S. Bioscience, Inc. 100 Front Street West Conshohocken, PA 19428 William McCulloch, M.R.C.P. (215) 832-4506
As chemoprotective agent for cisplatin	amifostine (Ethyol)	NDA submitted	U.S. Bioscience, Inc. 100 Front Street West Conshohocken PA 19428 William McCulloch, M.R.C.P. (215) 832-4506
Detection	indium IN 111 murine non- clonal antibody B72.3 (OncoScint OV103)	Application submitted	Cytogen Corporation 600 College Rd., East Princeton, NJ 08540 Cheryl Shipley Coyle Marketing Director (609) 987-8221

Condition/Use	Drug Name	Status/Phase	Sponsor/Contact Person
Ovarian, *cont.* Treatment	yttrium-labeled MAb (OncoRad OV103)	Phase II	Cytogen Corporation 600 College Rd., East Princeton, NJ 08540 Cheryl Shipley Coyle Marketing Director (609) 987-8221
Renal Cell	poly I: poly C12U	Phase II	HEM Pharmaceuticals Corp 1617 JFK Boulevard, Inc. Philadelphia, PA 19103 John R. Rapoza (215) 988-0080
Metastatic	interleukin-2	Phase II Clinical trials	Hoffmann-LaRoche 340 Kingsland St. Nutley, NJ 07110-1199 Darien E. Wilson (201) 235-4381
	interferon alfa-2-A (Roferon-A) concomitant administration with Interleukin-2	Phase II Clinical trials	Hoffmann-LaRoche 340 Kingsland St. Nutley, NJ 07110-1199 Darien E. Wilson (201) 235-4381
Testicular (refractory)	ifosfamide (Ifex)	Approved for marketing	Bristol-Myers Squibb 2400 West Lloyd Expressway Evansville, IN 47721-0001 Department of Medical Serv. (812) 429-5000
Cardioverter defibrillation therapy To lower defibrillation energy requirement sufficiently to allow automatic implantable therapy in patients who could not otherwise use the device	N-acetyl- procainamide (Napa)	IND approved Clinical trials not initiated	Medco Research, Inc. 8544 Beverly Blvd, Suite 308 Los Angeles, CA 90048 Roger Blevins, Pharm.D. (213) 966-4148
Carnitine deficiency	l-carnitine (Vita Carn)	Oral approved for marketing	McGaw, Inc. 2525 McGaw Ave. Irvine, CA 92714 Order Services (800) 624-2963
Primary, systemic	l-carnitine (Carnitor)	Approved for marketing Exclusive approval	Sigma Tau Pharmaceuticals 200 Orchard Ridge Drive Gaithersburg, MD 20878 Edward Helton, Director Research & Regulatory Aff. (301) 948-1041

Condition/Use	Drug Name	Status/Phase	Sponsor/Contact Person
Secondary	l-carnitine (Carnitor)	Application submitted	Sigma Tau Pharmaceuticals 200 Orchard Ridge Drive Gaithersburg, MD 20878 Edward Helton, Director Research & Regulatory Aff. (301) 948-1041
Treatment in patients with endstage renal disease who require dialysis	l-carnitine (Carnitor)	IND Phase III	Sigma Tau Pharmaceuticals 200 Orchard Ridge Drive Gaithersburg, MD 20878 Edward Helton, Director Research & Regulatory Aff. (301) 948-1041
Central precocious puberty	histrelin	Under review	Ortho Pharmaceutical Corp. Route 202,P.O. Box 300 Raritan, NJ 08869-0602 Dr. Robert Murphy (908) 218-6892
Cerebral palsy	botulinum toxin-type A (Oculinum)	Studies in progress	Allergan Pharmaceuticals 2525 Dupont Drive Irvine, CA 92715 Steven Carlson (800) 347-4500
Cervical dystonia	botulinum toxin-type A (Oculinum)	Approval pending	Allergan Pharmaceuticals 2525 Dupont Drive Irvine, CA 92715 Steven Carlson (800) 347-4500
Congenital coagulopathies Indicated in patients with hemophilia for short-term use (2-8 days) to reduce or prevent hemorrhage and reduce need for replacement therapy during and following tooth extraction	tranexamic acid (Cyklokapron)	Approved for marketing	Kabi Pharmacia 800 Centennial Ave. Piscataway, NJ 08855 (800) 526-3610
Congenital factor XIII deficiency	factor XIII [placenta-derived] (Fibrogammin)	IND to private physician	Hoechst-Roussel Route 202-206 No. Somerville, NJ 08876 Susan Sutch (800) 445-4774

Condition/Use	Drug Name	Status/Phase	Sponsor/Contact Person
Corneal erosion Recurrent	dehydrex (DEHYDREX)	IND II & III	Holles Labs 30 Forest Notch Cohasset, MA 02025 Peter Lelecas (617) 383-0741
Corneal transplant Acceleration of corneal epithelial regeneration and healing of stromal incisions	epidermal growth factor [human]	Phase II	Chiron Ophthalmics 9342 Jeronimo Irvine, CA 92718 Judy Gordon (714) 768-4690
High risk procedure	cyclosporine ophthalmic	Phase II	Sandoz Pharmaceuticals Route 10 Hanover, NJ 07936 Ronald VanValen, MRA (201) 503-7646
Corneal ulcers Treatment of nonhealing ulcers or epithelial defects which have been unresponsive to conventional therapy and the underlying cause has been eliminated	fibronectin [human plasma]	Phase III	New York Blood Center 310 E. 67th Street New York, NY 10021 Dr. Marilyn Horowitz (212) 570-3418
Cushing syndrome For use in differentiating pituitary and ectopic production of ACTH in patients with ACTH- dependent Cushing syndrome	ovine corticotropin- releasing hormone (Acthrel)	FDA approval	Ferring Labs, Inc. 400 Rella Blvd. Suffern, NY 10901 Daniel M. Linkie, Ph.D. (800) 445-3690
Cutaneous fistulas Adjunct to non-operative management in the stomach, duodeneum, small intestine (jejunum and ileum) or pancreas	somatostatin (Zecnil)	Phase III	Ferring Labs, Inc. 400 Rella Blvd. Suffern, NY 10901 Daniel M. Linkie, Ph.D. (800) 445-3690
Cystic fibrosis (CF)	amiloride *aerosolized	Phase III clinical trials	Glaxo, Inc. 5 Moore Drive Triangle Park, NC 27709 Drug Infoline (800) 334-0089

Condition/Use	Drug Name	Status/Phase	Sponsor/Contact Person
Cystic fibrosis (CF) *cont.* Reduce viscosity and enable clearance of airway secretions in patients with CF	rDNase	Phase III	Genentech, Inc. 460 Point San Bruno So. San Francisco, CA 94080 Public Relations Dept. (415) 266-2222
Treatment and prevention pulmonary infections due to Pseudomonas aeruginosa in patients with CF	mucoid exopolysac- charide pseudomonas hyperimmune globulin	Phase I	Univax Corporation 12280 Wilkins Avenue Rockville, MD 20852 Scott Harkonen, MD (301) 770-3099
Cystine nephrolithiasis Prevention of cystine kidney stone formation in patients with homozygous cystinuria who are prone to stone development	dimercapto- succinic acid (Chemet)	Approved for marketing	McNeil Consumer Products Camp Hill Road Fort Washington, PA 19034
Prevention in patients with homozygous cystinuria	tiopronin (Thiola)	Exclusive approval	Mission Pharmacal Company 2391 N.E. Loop 410 Suite 109 San Antonio, TX 78217 Urological Products Div. (800) 531-3333 (800) 292-7364 (In Texas)
Cystinosis	phospho- cysteamine	Phase III Clinical trials	Medea Research Laboratories 200 Wilson Street Pt. Jefferson Sta., NY 11776 Olga Lockhart (516) 331-0563
Nephropathic	cysteamine [2-amino- ethanethiol]	IND Phase II	Jess G. Thoene, M.D. University of Michigan 2612 SPH I 109 Observatory Ann Arbor, MI 48109-2029 (313) 763-3427
Cystitis Hemorrhagic Ifosfamide-induced For use as a prophy- lactic agent in treatment	mesna (Mesnex)	Approved for marketing	Bristol-Myers Squibb 2400 West Lloyd Expressway Evansville, IN 47721-0001 Department of Medical Serv. (812) 429-5000

Condition/Use	Drug Name	Status/Phase	Sponsor/Contact Person
Cystitis, *cont.* Interstitial	sodium pentosan polysulphate (Elmiron)	Phase III-Clinical trials complete NDA submitted	Baker-Norton Pharmaceuticals 8800 N.W. 36th Street Miami, FL 33078 Fred Sherman, M.D. (800) 347-4774
Cytomegalovirus (CMV) retinitis In immunocompromised individuals, including patients with AIDS	ganciclovir sodium (Cytovene)	Approved for marketing	Syntex (USA) , Inc. 3401 Hillview Ave. Palo Alto, CA 94304 Linda Thomas (415) 852-1321
Digitalis intoxication Potentially life-threatening in patients who are refractory to management by conventional therapy	digoxin immune fab [ovine] (Digibind)	Approved for marketing Exclusive approval	Burroughs-Wellcome 3030 Cornwallis Rd. Research Triangle Park, NC 27709 Drug Information Serv. (800) 722-9292
Donor organ tissue protection From damage or injury mediated by oxygen-derived free radicals generated during necessary periods of ischemia (hypoxia, anoxia) , and especially reperfusion, associated with the surgery	superoxide dismutase [human]	On hold	Pharmacia-Chiron 4560 Horton Street Emeryville, CA 94608 Alan Russell (510) 655-8730
Duchenne muscular dystrophy (DMD)	mazindol (Sanorex)	Investigational	Platon J. Collipp, M.D. 176 Memorial Drive Jesup, GA 31545 (912) 427-9378
Eaton-Lambert myasthenic syndrome	dynamine	Phase II	Mayo Medical Ventures 200 S. W. 1st Ave. Rochester, MN 55905 Scott Kaese (507) 284-9390
Epikeratophakia Acceleration of corneal epithelial healing	epidermal growth factor [human]	Phase I	Chiron Ophthalmics 9342 Jeronimo Irvine, CA 92718 Judy Gordon (714) 768-4690

Condition/Use	Drug Name	Status/Phase	Sponsor/Contact Person
Epilepsy Drug-resistant generalized tonic-clonic (GTC) in adults	antiepilepsirine	Pending approval	Children's Hospital 700 Children's Drive Columbus, OH 43205 Philip Walson (614) 461-2256
Esophageal varices	terlipressin (Glypressin)	Phase III	Ferring AB Soldattorspvagen 5, Box 30651 200 62 Malmo, Sweden
Bleeding	ethanolamine oleate (Ethamolin)	Approved for marketing	Reed & Carnrick Pharmaceuticals Division of Block Drug Co. 257 Cornelison Ave. Jersey City, NJ 07302 Richard J. Brown, MD (201) 434-3000
Falciparummalaria Chloroquine-resistant	mefloquine HCL (Mephaquin)	Clinical studies on hold (May be discontinued)	Martec Pharmaceutical 1800 N. Topping Kansas City, Mo 64120 Paul Sudhakar (816) 241-4144
Farbry disease	ceramide trihexosidase/ alpha- galactosidase A	Preclinical	Genzyme One Kendall Square Cambridge, MA 02139 Dr. Scott Furbish (617) 252-7614
Gallbladder disease Dissolution of cholesterol gallstones retained in the common bile duct	monoctanoin (Moctanin)	Approved for marketing Exclusive approval	Ethitek 7855 Gross Pt. Rd., Unit L Skokie, IL 60077 Irving Udell (708) 675-6616
Patients with radiolucent stones in well opacifying gall bladders in whom elective surgery would be undertaken except for presence of increased surgical risk due to systemic disease or age	chenodiol (Chenix)	Approved for marketing Exclusive approval	Solvay Pharmaceuticals 901 Sawyer Road Marietta, GA 30062 Laurie Downey, M.D. (404) 578-9000

Condition/Use	Drug Name	Status/Phase	Sponsor/Contact Person
Gaucher disease	l-cycloserine (Levcycloserine)	Investigational	City Univ., NY Medical School Convent Ave. at 138 St. New York, NY 10031 Dr. Meir Lev (212) 650-7788
Replacement therapy-Type 1	glucocerebrosidase-beta glucosidase [placenta derived] (Ceredase) alglucenase inject.	Approved for marketing	Genzyme One Kendall Square Cambridge, MA 02139 Dr. Scott Furbish (617) 252-7614
Glioma Recurrent malignant For localized placement in the brain	biodegradable polymer implant containing carmustine (Gliadel)	Investigational Phase III	Nova Pharmaceutical Corp. 6200 Freeport Centre Baltimore, MD 21224-6522 Ms. Maria Berkheimer (410) 558-7000
Graft-vs.-host disease (GVHD) Prevention of acute, in allogenic bone marrow transplantation	ST1-RTA immunotoxin [SR-44163]	Phase IIb/III Clinical trials conducted in U.S. U.K. and France	Sanofi Pharmaceuticals 40 E. 52nd St., 13th Fl. New York, NY 10022 Dr. Thomas C. Wicks (212) 754-4700
Prevention and treatment of GVHD in patients receiving bone marrow transplantation (BMT)	CD5-T lymphocyte immunotoxin (Xomazyme-H65)	Investigational PLA filed December 1988	Xoma Corporation 2910 7th Street Berkeley, CA 94710 Carol DeGuzman (510) 644-1178
Prevention and treatment of GVHD in patients receiving bone marrow transplantation	thalidomide	Phase III IND	Andrulis Research Corp 4600 East-West Hgwy. S-900 Bethesda, MD 20814 Nala Fernando (301) 953-1003
Granulomatous disease Chronic (CGD)	interferon gamma 1-B (Actimmuse)	Approved for marketing	Genentech, Inc. 460 Point San Bruno So. San Francisco, CA 94080 Public Relations Dept. (415) 266-2222

Condition/Use	Drug Name	Status/Phase	Sponsor/Contact Person
Growth and puberty Constitutional delay	sublingual testosterone (Androtest-SL)	Phase II	Gynex Pharmaceuticals 1175 Corporate Woods Pkwy Vernon Hills, IL 60061 Robert E. Dudley, Ph.D. (708) 913-1144
	oxandrolone (Oxandrin)	Phase III (Placebo-controlled and treatment IND)	Gynex Pharmaceuticals 1175 Corporate Woods Pkwy Vernon Hills, IL 60061 Robert E. Dudley, Ph.D. (708) 913-1144
Growth failure Idiopathic or organic growth hormone deficiency (GHD) in children with growth failure	sermorelin acetate (Geref)	Phase III	Serono Laboratories, Inc. 100 Longwater Circle Norwell, MA 02061 Gina Cella (617) 723-1300
	somatropin (Saizen)	NDA submitted	Serono Laboratories, Inc. 100 Longwater Circle Norwell, MA 02061 Gina Cella (617) 723-1300
Long-term treatment in children due to a lack of adequate endogenous growth hormone secretion	somatropin (Humatrope)	Approved for marketing Exclusive approval	Eli Lilly & Company Lilly Corporate Center Indianapolis, IN 46285 Medical Dept. (317) 276-3714
	somatropin (Norditropin)	NDA submitted	Novo Nordisk Princeton, NJ 08540-7810 Nathan H. Block (609) 987-5822
	somatrem human growth hormone recombinant (Protropin)	Approved for marketing	Genentech, Inc. 460 Point San Bruno So. San Francisco, CA 94080 Public Relations Dept. (415) 266-2222
	SK&F 110679	Phase II trials	SmithKline Beecham P.O. Box 7929 Philadelphia, PA 19101 Anthony Murabito, RPHMS (800) 366-8900, Ext 5231

Condition/Use	Drug Name	Status/Phase	Sponsor/Contact Person
Growth retardation Associated with chronic renal failure	human growth hormone, recombinant	Phase III	Genentech, Inc. 460 Point San Bruno So. San Francisco, CA 94080 Public Relations Dept. (415) 266-2222
HCG-producing tumors Detection of, i.e., germ cell and trophoblastic cell tumors	HCG radioimmunodetction with Tc-99m (ImmuRAID-HCG-Tc-99m)	IND 1992	Immunomedics, Inc. 150 Mt. Bethel Rd. Warren, NJ 07060 Kenneth Chang, Ph.D. (908) 647-5400
Treatment of HCG-producing tumors, i.e., germ cell and trophoblastic cell	iodine 1 131 murine monoclonal antibody to HCG	IND 1992	Immunomedics, Inc. 150 Mt. Bethel Rd. Warren, NJ 07060 Kenneth Chang, Ph.D. (908) 647-5400
Hemodialysis Replacement of heparin in patients who are at increased risk of hemorrhage	epoprostenol, prostacyclin (Flolan)	NDA submitted	Burroughs Wellcome 3030 Cornwallis Rd. Research Triangle Park, NC 27709 Drug Information Serv. (800) 722-9292
Hemophilia Hemophilia A Mild von Willebrand disease	d-8 arginine vasopressin [desmopressin] high concentration (DDAVP HC)	In clinical development	Armour Pharmaceutical Co. 920A Harvest Drive Suite 200 Blue Bell PA 19422 Garrett E. Bergman, MD (215) 540-8122
Prophylaxis and treatment of bleeding episodes/surgery	recombinate antihemophilic factor VIII (Kogenate)	Pending FDA release (Orphan Drug status)	Cutter Biological/Miles 400 Morgan Lane West Haven, CT 06516 Rene McRogers (203) 498-6444
Hemophilia B Factor IX (human replacement factor)	Factor IX (human) Monoclonal antibody purified (Mononine)	Pending FDA approval	Armour Pharmaceutical Co. 928A Harvest Drive Suite 200 Blue Bell, PA 19422 Garrett E. Bergman, MD (215) 540-8122

Condition/Use	Drug Name	Status/Phase	Sponsor/Contact Person
Hepatic metastases In patients with colorectal adenocarcinoma	disaccharide tripeptide (ImmTher)	Phase II/III	ImmunoTherapeutics, Inc. 3505 Riverview Circle Moorhead, MN 56560 Gerald Vosika (701) 232-9575
Hereditary angioneurotic edema	tranexamic acid (Cyklokapron)	Not approved On hold	Kabi Pharmacia 800 Centennial Ave. Piscataway, NJ 08855 (800) 526-3610
Herpes simplex encephalitis In individuals afflicted with AIDS	PR-225 (redox-acyclovir)	Preclinical	Pharmatec, Inc. P.O. Box 730 Alachua, FL 32615 K.S. Estes, Ph.D. (904) 462-1210
HIV wasting syndrome	oxandrolone (Oxandrin)	Phase II	Gynex Pharmaceuticals 1175 Corporate Woods Pkwy Vernon Hills, IL 60061 Robert E. Dudley, Ph.D. (708) 913-1144
Hyaline membrane disease (HMD) (Also known as Infant respiratory distress syndrome [IRDS])	surfactant [human] [amniotic fluid derived] (Human Surf)	Phase III	University of California Davis Medical Center 2615 Stockton Blvd. Sacramento, CA 95817 Allen T. Merritt, MD (916) 734-2011
Prevention of HMD, in infants born at 32 weeks gestation or less	synthetic pulmonary surfactant (Exosurf)	Approved for marketing	Burroughs Wellcome 3030 Cornwallis Rd. Research Triangle Park, NC 27709 Drug Information Serv. (800) 722-9292
Prevention and treatment in premature newborns	berectant intratracheal suspension [modified bovine lung surfactant extract] (Survanta)	Approved Currently marketed	Ross Laboratories 625 Cleveland Ave. Columbus, OH 43216 J. Harry Gunkel, MD (614) 227-3333

Condition/Use	Drug Name	Status/Phase	Sponsor/Contact Person
Hyaline membrane disease (HMD), *cont.*			
Treatment in premature newborns	human lung surfactant	Preclinical	Genentech, Inc. 460 Point San Bruno So. San Francisco, CA 94080 Public Relations Dept. (415) 266-2222
Treatment of established HMD at all gestational ages	synthetic pulmonary surfactant (Exosurf)	Approved	Burroughs Wellcome 3030 Cornwallis Rd. Research Triangle Park, NC 27709 Drug Information Serv. (800) 722-9292
Hyperammonemia Urea cycle enzymopathies	10% sodium benzoate and 10% sodium phenylacetate (Ucephan)	Oral form approved for marketing	McGaw, Inc. 2525 McGaw Ave. Irvine, CA 92714 Order Services (800) 624-2963
Hyperbilirubimenia In newborn infants unresponsive to phototherapy	flumecinol (Zixoryn)	Phase II	Farmacon 90 Grove Street, Suite 109 Ridgefield, CT 06877 (203) 438-7331
Hypercalcemia Of malignancy	gallium nitrate (Ganite)	Approved for marketing	Fujisawa Pharm. & Co. 3 Parkway Center. N. Deerfield, IL 60015 D.S. Ebersman (708) 317-8647
Hypercalciuria, absorptive Control and prevention of type I with calcium nephrolithiasis	cellulose sodium phosphate (Calcibind)	Approved for marketing Exclusive approval	Mission Pharmacal Company 2391 N.E. Loop 410 Suite 109 San Antonio, TX 78217 Urological Products Div. (800) 531-3333 (800) 292-7364 (In Texas)
Hyperphosphatemia In endstage renal disease (ESRD)	calcium acetate (PhosLo)	Approved for marketing	Braintree Laboratories 60 Columbian St., PO Box 361 Braintree, MA 02184 Peter Kenney (617) 843-2202

Condition/Use	Drug Name	Status/Phase	Sponsor/Contact Person
Hyperphosphatemia, *cont.*	calcium acetate	On hold	Pharmedic Company 417 Harvester Ct. Wheeling, IL 60090 Ragab El Rashiky, Ph.D. (708) 215-6603
Hypocalcemia Diagnostic agent for use in patients with clinical and laboratory evidence of hypocalcemia due to hypoparathyroidism or pseudohypoparathyroidism	teriparatide (Parathar)	Approved for marketing Exclusive approval	Armour Pharmaceutical Co. 920A Harvest Drive Suite 200 Blue Bell, PA 19422 Garrett E. Bergman, MD (215) 540-8122
Hypocitraturia Prevention and control of calcium renal stones	potassium citrate (Urocit-K)	Approved for marketing Exclusive approval	Mission Pharmacal Company 2391 N.E. Loop 410 Suite 109 San Antonio, TX 78217 Urological Products Div. (800) 531-3333 (800) 292-7364 (In Texas)
Hypotension Idiopathic orthostatic	midodrine HCL (Amatine)	NDA filed April 1988 Under review	Roberts Pharmaceuticals Meridian Center III 6-G Industrial Way, W. Eatontown, NJ 07724 Drew Karlan (908) 389-1182
Infertility Adjunct to gonadotropin therapy in induction of ovulation in women with anovulatory or oligoovulatory infertility who fail to ovulate in response to adequate treatment with clomiphene citrate alone and gonadotropin therapy alone	semorelin acetate (Geref)	Phase II/III	Serono Laboratories, Inc. 100 Longwater Circle Norwell, MA 02061 Gina Cella (617) 723-1300
Kaposi's sarcoma AIDS-related	interferon alfa-2-A [recombinant] (Roferon-A)	Approved for marketing	Hoffmann-LaRoche 340 Kingsland St. Nutley, NJ 07110-1199 Darien E. Wilson (201) 235-4381

Condition/Use	Drug Name	Status/Phase	Sponsor/Contact Person
Keratoconjunctivitis Vernal (VRC)	cromolyn sodium 4% ophthalmic solution (Opticrom 4% Ophthalmic Sol.)	Approved for marketing *Currently unavailable	Fisons Corporation P.O. Box 1766 Rochester, NY 14603 Elizabeth Dauley-Likly (716) 274-5955
	levocabastine ophthalmic suspension 0.05%	Phase III Application submitted	Iolab Pharmaceuticals 500 Iolab Drive Claremont, CA 91711 Mirta Negroni (800) 468-2002
Keratoconjunctivitis sicca Severe associated with Sjögren's syndrome	cyclosporine ophthalmic	Phase II	Sandoz Pharmaceuticals Route 10 Hanover, NJ 07936 Ronald G. Van Valen, MRA (201) 503-7646
Kidney stones Control and prevention of infection	acetohydroximic acid (Lithostat)	Approved for marketing Exclusive approval	Mission Pharmacal Company 2391 N.E. Loop 410 Suite 109 San Antonio, TX 78217 Urological Products Div. (800) 531-3333 (800) 292-7364 (In Texas)
Laryngeal (respiratory) papillomatosis	interferon alfa-NL (Wellferon)	PLA submitted	Burroughs Wellcome 3030 Cornwallis Rd. Research Triangle Park, NC 27709 Drug Information Serv. (800) 722-9292
Lead poisoning— children	dimercapto- succinic acid	NDA approved	McNeil Consumer Products Camp Hill Road Fort Washington, PA 19034 Medical Department (215) 233-7000
Leukemia	mitoxantrone HCL (Novantrone)	Approved for marketing Exclusive approval	Lederle Laboratories Pearl River, NY 10965 G.W. McCarl, MD (201) 831-4617
Acute	doxycytidine	IND filed Protocol amended 1991	Pharmachemie, USA, Inc. P.O. Box 145 Oradell, NJ 07649 J. David Hayden, Pres. (201) 265-1942

Condition/Use	Drug Name	Status/Phase	Sponsor/Contact Person
Leukemia, *cont.*			
Acute lymphocytic (ALL)	pegaspargase (PEG-I-asparaginase)	PLA filed Jan. 91	Enzon, Inc. 40 Cragwood Rd. S. Plainfield, NJ 07080 Zelda Wildman (908) 668-1800
I.V. therapy of B-cell ALL and non-Hodgkins lymphoma (NHL)	anti-B-4-blocked racin (Oncolysin B)	Phase II	ImmunoGen, Inc. 148 Sidney St. Cambridge, MA 02139 Carol Epstein, MD (617) 661-9312
Non-T-cell (ALL) Ex vivo purging of leukemic cells from bone marrow	anti-B-4-blocked ricin (Oncolysin B)	Phase I/II	ImmunoGen, Inc. 148 Sydney St. Cambridge, MA 02139 Carol Epstein, MD (617) 661-9312
Pediatric (ALL)	idarubicin	Investigational	Adria Laboratories P.O. Box 16529 Columbus, OH 43216-6529 Mirjam C. Gerber (614) 764-8155
Refractory childhood	teniposide	NDA submitted currently under review	Bristol-Myers Squibb 2400 West Lloyd Expressway Evansville, IN 47721-0001 Department of Medical Serv. (812) 429-5000
Acute myeloid (AML) also called acute nonlymphocytic (ANLL) In adults	idarubicin (Idamycin)	Approved	Adria Laboratories P.O. Box 16529 Columbus, OH 43216-6529 Robert P. Fudge (614) 764-8384
In ex vivo treatment of autologous bone marrow and subsequent reinfusion, in patients with AML/ANLL	4-hydroperoxy-clophosphamide 4-HC perfosfamide (Pergamid)	Investigational*/III *A treatment IND approved for AML patients in second or subsequent remission	Nova Pharmaceutical Corp. 6200 Freeport Centre Baltimore, MD 21224-6522 Jan Peterson (410) 558-7000
Acute myelocytic Ex vivo purging of leukemic cells from the bone marrow of acute patients	anti-MY9-blocked ricin	Phase I/II	ImmunoGen, Inc. 148 Sydney St. Cambridge, MA 02139 Carol Epstein, MD (617) 661-9312

Condition/Use	Drug Name	Status/Phase	Sponsor/Contact Person
Leukemia, *cont.*			
Acute myelogenous, undergoing bone marrow transplant	monoclonal antibodies PM-81 and AML 2-23	Phase I/II	Medarex, Inc. 12 Commerce Ave. West Lebanon, NH 03784 Marcia Young (603) 298-8456
Acute promyelocytic	all-trans retinoic acid	Phase II Clinical trials	Hoffmann-LaRoche 340 Kingsland St. Nutley, NJ 07110-1199 Darien E. Wilson (201) 235-4381
Chronic lymphocytic	2-chlorodeoxy-adenosine	Ongoing research	Ortho Biotech Route 202 Raritan, NJ 08869-0602 Dr. Linda Dujack (908) 704-5057
	fludarabine monophosphate	Phase III/IV	Berlex Laboratories 1401 Harbor Bay Parkway Alameda, CA 94501 Lewis P. Chapman (510) 769-5200
Hairy cell	pentostatin		Warner-Lambert 2800 Plymouth Rd. Ann Arbor, MI 48105 Mark Meyer, Pharm.D, M.S. (800) 521-8999
Lymphocytic, B-cell Detection	(ImmuRAID-LL-2-Tc-99m)	Orphan designation pending	Immunomedics, Inc. 150 Mt. Bethel Rd. Warren, NJ 07060 Kenneth Chang, Ph.D. (908) 647-5400
Myelocytic, acute & chronic I.V. therapy to treat AML patients and CML patients in blast crisis	anti-MY9-blocked ricin	Phase I/II	ImmunoGen, Inc. 148 Sydney St. Cambridge, MA 02139 Carol Epstein, MD (617) 661-9312
Lymphoma B-Cell	monoclonal antibodies [mu-rine or human] B-cell lymphoma (Specifid)	Phase II/III	IDEC Pharmaceuticals Corp 291 N. Bernardo Ave. Mountain View, CA 94043 Bridget Binko (415) 940-1200

Condition/Use	Drug Name	Status/Phase	Sponsor/Contact Person
Lymphoma, *cont.*			
Detection	(ImmuRAID-LL-2-Tc-99m)	Orphan designation pending Phase I/II	Immunomedics, Inc. 150 Mt. Bethel Rd. Warren, NJ 07060 Kenneth Chang, Ph.D. (908) 647-5400
Radioimmunotherapy (also leukemias)	iodine 131 murine monoclonal antibody IGG2A to B cell (ImmuRAIT-LL-2-1-131)	Phase I/II	Immunomedics, Inc. 150 Mt. Bethel Rd. Warren, NJ 07060 Kenneth Chang, Ph.D. (908) 647-5400
B-cell I.V. therapy of non-Hodgkins lymphoma (NHL)	anti-B-4-blocked ricin (Oncolysin B)	Phase II	ImmunoGen, Inc. 148 Sidney St. Cambridge, MA 02139 Carol Epstein, MD (617) 661-9312
Non-Hodgkins	fludarabine monophosphate	Phase II	Berlex Laboratories 1401 Harbor Bay Parkway Alameda, CA 94501 Lewis P. Chapman (510) 769-5200
	prednimustine (Sterecyt)	Compassionate IND	Kabi Pharmacia 800 Centennial Ave. Piscataway, NJ 08855 Gary Britton, Ph.D. (908) 457-8265
Malaria Prevention of chloroquine-resistant falciparum malaria	mefloquine HCL (Mephaquin)	Clinical studies On hold (May be discontinued)	Martec Pharmaceutical 1800 N. Topping Kansas City, Mo 64120 Paul Sudhakar (816) 241-4144
Treatment and prophylaxis and plasmodium	mefloquine HCL (Larium)	Approved for marketing	Hoffmann-LaRoche 340 Kingsland St. Nutley, NJ 07110-1199 Darien E. Wilson (201) 235-4381
Malignancies Treatment of patients treated with chemotherapy or chemoradiotherapy	filgrastim (Neupogen)	Phase II	Amgen, Inc. Amgen Center Thousand Oaks CA 91320-1789 Mark Brand (805) 499-5725

Condition/Use	Drug Name	Status/Phase	Sponsor/Contact Person
Mastocytosis	cromolyn sodium (Gastrocrom)	Approved for marketing	Fisons Corporation P.O. Box 1766 Rochester, NY 14603 James McGuire (716) 274-5976
Melanoma Metastatic As chemoprotective agent for cisplatin	amifostine (Ethyol)	NDA submitted	U.S. Bioscience, Inc. 100 Front Street West Conshohocken PA 19428 William McCulloch, M.R.C.P. (215) 832-4506
Detecting, by imaging	technetium Tc 99M anti-melanoma murine monoclonal antibody (OncoTrac Melanoma Imaging Kit)	PLA pending (Phase: FDA) Orphan status granted	NeoRx Corporation 410 W. Harrison Seattle, WA 98119 Dr. Darrell Salk (206) 281-7001
Metastatic, malignant	recombinant human inter-leukin-2 In combination with Roferon-A	Phase II Clinical trials	Hoffmann-LaRoche 340 Kingsland St. Nutley, NJ 07110-1199 Darien E. Wilson (201) 235-4381
	interleukin-2	Phase II Clinical trials	Hoffmann-LaRoche 340 Kingsland St. Nutley, NJ 07110-1199 Darien E. Wilson (201) 235-4381
Nodal, diagnostic use in imaging systemic and nodal metastasis	indium IN 111 antimelanoma antibody XMME-0001-DTPA (Indium IN 111 Antimelanoma Antibody XMME-0001-DTPA)	Investigational	Xoma Corporation 2910 7th Street Berkeley, CA 94710 Carol DeGuzman (510) 644-1178
Stage III not amenable to surgical resection	antimelanoma immunotoxin XMMME-Investigational 001-RTA (Xomozyme-Mel)	Investigational	Xoma Corporation 2910 7th Street Berkeley, CA 94710 Carol DeGuzman (510) 644-1178

Condition/Use	Drug Name	Status/Phase	Sponsor/Contact Person
Melanoma, *cont.*			
Stage III-IV	melanoma theraccine [therapeutic vaccine] (Melacine)	Phase III Multi-center controlled, randomized human clinical study	Ribi ImmunoChem Research P.O. Box 1409 Hamilton, MT 59840 Jon A. Rudbach, Ph.D. (406) 363-6214
Multiple sclerosis	interferon beta, recombinant human (Betaseron)	Phase III	Berlex Laboratories 1401 Harbor Bay Parkway Alameda, CA 94501 Lewis P. Chapman (510) 769-5200
	copolymer 1 [cop 1]	Phase III	Tag Pharmaceuticals c/o Lemmon Company Sellersville, PA 18960 Dr. Stanley Scheindlin (800) 523-6542
Relief of symptoms	4-aminopyridine	Phase II active	Rush-Presby-St. Luke's 1753 West Congress Pkwy Chicago, IL 60612 Multiple Sclerosis Center D. Stefoski, MD (312) 942-8011
Mycobacterium avium (MAC) complex Prevention of MAC in patients with AIDS and with CD4 counts less than 200/MM3	rifabutin	Investigational	Adria Laboratories P.O. Box 16529 Columbus, OH 43216-6529 Dr. Beverley Wynne (614) 764-8159
Treatment of MAC in patients with AIDS	rifabutin	Investigational	Adria Laboratories P.O. Box 16529 Columbus, OH 43216-6529 Dr. Beverley Wynne (614) 764-8159
Myelodyplastic syndrome Treatment	filgrastim (Neupogen)	Phase III	Amgen, Inc. Amgen Center Thousand Oaks, CA 91320-1789 Mark Brand (805) 499-5725

Condition/Use	Drug Name	Status/Phase	Sponsor/Contact Person
Myoclonus, postanoxic intention	l-5 hydroxytrypto-phan [l-5HTP]	Phase II	Bolar Pharmaceutical Co., Inc 33 Ralph Avenue Copiague, NY 11726 Joyce Del Gaudio (516) 841-8383
Myxedema coma	Cytomell/IV	Phase III trials (late)	SmithKline Beecham P. O. Box 7929 Philadelphia, PA 19101 Anthony Murabito, RPHMS (800) 366-8900, Ext 5231
Narcolepsy And auxiliary symptoms of cataplexy, sleep paralysis, hypnagogic hallucinations, and automatic behavior	sodium oxybate (gammahydroxy-butyrate)	Phase II Clinical trials	Biocraft Laboratories 18-01 River Road Fairlawn, NJ 07410 Debi Parker (201) 703-0400
Nephrotoxicity Cyclosporine-induced, in organ transplant	ketoconazole (Nizoral)	On hold	Pharmedic Company 417 Harvester Ct. Wheeling, IL 60090 Ragab El Rashiky, Ph.D. (708) 215-6603
Neurosyphilis AIDS-associated	PR-239 (redox penicillin)	Preclinical	Pharmatec, Inc. P.O. Box 730 Alachua, FL 32615 K.S. Estes, Ph.D. (904) 462-1210
Neutropenia Treatment of severe chronic	filgrastim (Neupogen)	Phase III	Amgen, Inc. Amgen Center Thousand Oaks CA 91320-1789 Mark Brand (805) 499-5725
Panencephalitis (SSPE) Subacute sclerosing	inosine pranobex inosine dimepranol acedoben (Isoprinosine)	Orphan drug designation	SysteMed, Inc. 140 Columbia Laguna Hills, CA 92656-1469 Jean Dreyer (714) 362-1330

Condition/Use	Drug Name	Status/Phase	Sponsor/Contact Person
Parkinson disease Adjuvant to levodopa and carbidopa treatment of idiopathic Parkinson disease (paralysis agitans), postencephalitic parkinsonism, and symptomatic parkinsonism	selegiline HCL (Eldepryl)	Approved for marketing	Somerset Pharmaceuticals 777 South Harbour Island Blvd., Suite 880 Tampa, FL 33602 Dana Barnett (813) 223-7677
Penicillin hypersensitivity Assessing risk of administering when it is the preferred drug of choice in adults who have a history of clinical hypersensitivity	benzylpenicillin, benzyl-penicilloic, benzylpenilloic acid (MDM)	Phase III	Schwarz Pharma P.O. Box 2038 Milwaukee, WI 53201 Carole DeRoche (414) 354-4300
Pheochromocytoma/ neuroblastoma diagnostic adjunct	iodine-131 metaiodobenzyl guanidine [m1BG]	Orphan Drug NDA filed	CIS-US, Inc. 10 DeAngelo Drive Bedford, MA 01730 David B. Reader, Exec. VP (800) 221-7554
Pituitary gland Diagnostic measure of capacity of pituitary gland to release growth hormone	NG-29 (Somatrel)	Phase III	Ferring Labs, Inc. 400 Rella Blvd. Suffern, NY 10901 Daniel M. Linkie, Ph.D. (800) 445-3690
Pneumocystis carinii pneumonia (PCP)	566C80	Treatment IND	Burroughs Wellcome 3030 Cornwallis Rd. Research Triangle Park, NC 27709 Drug Information Serv. (800) 722-9292
	pentamidine isethionate (Pentam 300)	Approved for marketing	Fujisawa Pharm. & Co. 3 Parkway Center. N. Deerfield, IL 60015 D.S. Ebersman (708) 317-8647

Condition/Use	Drug Name	Status/Phase	Sponsor/Contact Person
Pneumocystis carinii pneumonia (PCP), *cont.*			
Prevention, in patients at high risk	pentamidine isethionate [inhalation] (Pneumopent)	Pending approval NDA	Fisons Corporation P.O. Box 1766 Rochester, NY 14603 John McGinnis (716) 274-5958
Prevention, in patients at high risk of developing PCP	pentamidine isethionate (Nebupent)	Approved for marketing	Fujisawa Pharm. & Co. 3 Parkway Center, N. Deerfield, IL 60015 D.S. Ebersman (708) 317-8647
Treatment and prevention in AIDS patients	clindamycin (Cleocin)	Early development	The Upjohn Company 700 Portage Road Kalamazoo, MI 49001 James Van Sweden (800) 253-8600
Poisoning Methanol or ethylene glycol 2-butoxy ethanol 2-methoxy ethanol	4-methylpyrazole	Phase I/Phase II	LSU Medical Center Dept. of Pharmacology 151 King's Highway Shreveport, LA 71130-3932 Dr. Kenneth McMartin (318) 674-7850
Polycystic ovarian disease Induction of ovulation in patients who have an elevated LM/FSH ratio and have failed to respond to adequate clomiphene citrate therapy	urofollitropin (Metrodin)	Approved for marketing	Serono Laboratories, Inc. 100 Longwater Circle Norwell, MA 02061 Gina Cella (617) 723-1300
Polycythemia vera	anagrelide	Phase III	Roberts Pharmaceuticals Meridian Center III 6-G Industrial Way, W Eatontown, NJ 07724 Drew Karlan (908) 389-1182

Condition/Use	Drug Name	Status/Phase	Sponsor/Contact Person
Porphyria Acute, intermittent (AIP) Amelioration of recurrent attacks temporarily related to the menstrual cycle in susceptible women and similar symptoms which occur in other patients with AIP, porphyria variegata, and hereditary coproporphyria	hemin (Panhematin)	Approved for marketing Exclusive approval	Abbott Laboratories Pharmaceutical Products Div. North Chicago,IL 60064 Roland Catherall (708) 937-7495
Precocious puberty	leuprolide acetate (Lupron Depot)	Phase III Clinical trials	Tap Pharmaceuticals, Inc. 2355 Waukegan Road Deerfield, IL 60015 Medical Services (800) 622-2011
	nafarelin acetate (Synarel)	NDA Pending	Syntex (USA) , Inc. 3401 Hillview Ave. Palo Alto, CA 94304 Linda Thomas (415) 852-1321
Central precocious puberty	deslorelin (Somagard)	Phase III clinical studies Approved by FDA for sale on cost recovery basis in open Phase III protocol for CPP	Roberts Pharmaceuticals Meridian Center III 6-G Industrial Way, W Eatontown, NJ 07724 Drew Karlan (908) 389-1182
Primary pulmonary hypertension (PPH)	epoprostenol (Flolan)	Phase III	Burroughs Wellcome 3030 Cornwallis Rd. Research Triangle Park, NC 27709 Drug Information Serv. (800) 722-9292
Prostate Treatment of patients undergoing prostatectomy where hemorrhage or risk of hemmorhage as result of increased fibrinolysis or fibrinogenolysis exists	tranexamic acid (Lyklokapron)	Not approved On hold	Kabi Pharmacia 800 Centennial Ave. Piscataway, NJ 08855 (800) 526-3610

Condition/Use	Drug Name	Status/Phase	Sponsor/Contact Person
Pseudomembranous enterocolitis Caused by toxins A and B elaborated by clostridium difficile	bacitracin (Altracin)	In clinical trials	A. L. Laboratories, Inc. 1 Executive Drive P. O. Box 1299 Fort Lee, NJ 07024 Dr. Bernard Brown (201) 947-7774
Respiratory failure Treatment and prevention, due to pulmonary surfactant deficiency	surface active extract of saline lavage of bovine lungs (Infasurf)	IND	Ony, Inc. 1576 Sweet Home Rd. Amherst, NY 14228 Edmund Egan, MD (716) 636-9096
Retinitis pigmentosa	gangliosides as sodium salts (Cronassial)	Phase II	Fidia Pharmaceutical Corp. 1775 K Street, N.W. Washington, DC 20006 Jeanne Wadsworth-Hla (202) 466-7066
	(VisionAid)	Investigational Orphan drug and IND submitted	Platon J. Collipp, M.D. 176 Memorial Drive Jesup, GA 31545 (912) 427-9378
Sarcoma Bone	ifosfamide (Ifex)	Clinical studies ongoing No NDA submitted at this time	Bristol-Myers Squibb 2400 West Lloyd Expressway Evansville, IN 47721-0001 Department of Medical Serv. (812) 429-5000
Osteogenic	methotrexate sodium (Methotrexate)	Approved for marketing Exclusive approval	Lederle Laboratories Pearl River, NY 10965 G.W. McCarl, MD (201) 831-4617
	leucovorin calcium For use in combination with methotrexate	Approved for marketing Exclusive approval	Lederle Laboratories Pearl River, NY 10965 G.W. McCarl, MD (201) 831-4617
	1-leucovorin for use in combination with methotrexate	NDA submitted	Lederle Laboratories Pearl River, NY 10965 G.W. McCarl, MD (201) 831-4617

Condition/Use	Drug Name	Status/Phase	Sponsor/Contact Person
Sarcoma, *cont.*			
Soft tissue	ifosfamide (Ifex)	Clinical studies ongoing No NDA submitted at this time	Bristol-Myers Squibb 2400 West Lloyd Expressway Evansville, IN 47721-0001 Department of Medical Serv. (812) 429-5000
Severe combined immunodeficiency disease (SCID) ADA-deficiency related	pegademase bogine (Adagen Injection)	Approved March 1990	Enzon, Inc. 40 Cragwood Rd. S. Plainfield, NJ 07080 Zelda Wildman (908) 668-1800
Sickle cell disease	BW 12C	Phase II	Burroughs Wellcome 3030 Cornwallis Road Research Triangle Park, NC 27709 Drug Information Serv. (800) 722-9292
Crisis	poloxamer 188 (Rheothrx Copolymer)	Phase I	Burroughs Wellcome Co. 3030 Cornwallis Rd. Research Triangle Pk. NC 27709 Drug Information Serv. (800) 722-9292
	cetiedil citrate	Phase III Clinical trials in process	Baker-Norton Pharmaceuticals 8800 N.W. 36th Street Miami, FL 33078 Fred Sherman, M.D. (800) 347-4774
Spasticity Severe, chronic of spinal cord origin	baclofen [intrathecal] (Lioresal) (Lioresal Injection)	Treatment IND	Medtronic Neurological Div. 800 53rd Ave., N.E. Minneapolis, MN 55421 Rita Hirsch (800) 328-0810
Status epilepticus Grand mal type, emergency rescue treatment	PR-122 (redox-phenytoin)	Preclinical	Pharmatec, Inc. P.O. Box 730 Alachua, FL 32615 K.S. Estes, Ph.D. (904) 462-1210

Condition/Use	Drug Name	Status/Phase	Sponsor/Contact Person
Status epilepticus, *cont.*	PR-320 (Molecusol carbamazepine)	Preclinical	Pharmatec, Inc. P.O. Box 730 Alachua, FL 32615 K.S. Estes, Ph.D. (904) 462-1210
Streptococcal infection Treatment in neonates with disseminated Group B infection	group B streptococcus immune globulin	Phase I	Univax Biologics, Inc. 12280 Wilkins Avenue Rockville, MD 20852 Scott Harkonen, MD (301) 770-3099
Toxoplasmosis In pregnancy	spiramycin (Rovamycin)	Compassionate use study	Rhone-Poulenc Rorer, Inc. 500 Arcola Road Collegeville, PA 19426 Elizabeth Sanguinetti (215) 454-5214
Thrombocythemia Essential	anagrelide	Phase III	Roberts Pharmaceuticals Meridian Center III 6-G Industrial Way, W Eatontown, NJ 07724 Drew Karlan (908) 389-1182
Thrombocytosis In chronic myelogenous leukemia	anagrelide	Phase III	Roberts Pharmaceuticals Meridian Center III 6-G Industrial Way, W Eatontown, NJ 07724 Drew Karlan (908) 389-1182
Thrombosis Prevention and treatment in patients with hereditary AT-III deficiency In connection with surgical or obstetrical procedures or thromboembolus	Antithrombin III human (ATnativ)	Approved for marketing Exclusive approval	Baxter Healthcare Corp. 550 N. Brand Blvd Glendale, CA 91203 Michael Herrera (818) 328-5451
In thrombosis and pulmonary emboli	antithrombin III (Thrombate III)	Pending FDA release	Cutter Biological/Miles 400 Morgan Lane West Haven, CT 06516 Rene McRogers (203) 498-6444

Condition/Use	Drug Name	Status/Phase	Sponsor/Contact Person
Toxoplasmosis	566C80	Phase III	Burroughs Wellcome Co. 3030 Cornwallis Rd. Research Triangle Pk. NC 27709 Drug Information Serv. (800) 722-9292
Trypanosoma brucei Gambiense sleeping sickness	eflornithine HCL [DFMO] (Ornidyl)	Approved for marketing	Marion Merrell Dow Research P.O. Box 6300 Cincinnati, OH 45215 James Elberfeld (513) 948-6040
Tuberculosis Short course	rifampin, isoniazid pyrazinamide (Rifader V)	On hold	Marion Merrell Dow Pharm. 10123 Alliance Rd. Cincinnati, OH 45242 Dr. Robert Robinson (513) 948-7751
When use of oral form of drug is not feasible	rifampin (Rifadin I.V.)	Approved for marketing	Marion Merrell Dow Pharm. 10123 Alliance Rd. Cincinnati, OH 45242 Dr. Robert Robinson (513) 948-7751
Treatment and prophylaxis	aconiazide	Approved IND Human trials in progress	Lincoln Diagnostics P. O. Box 1139 Decatur, IL 62525 Gary L. Hein, President (217) 877-2531
Turner syndrome	ethinyl estradiol, USP (Estrafem)	Phase III	Gynex Pharmaceuticals 1175 Corporate Woods Pkwy Vernon Hills, IL 60061 Robert E. Dudley, Ph.D. (708) 913-1144
	oxandrolone (Oxandrin)	Phase III (Placebo-controlled and open-labeled)	Gynex Pharmaceuticals 1175 Corporate Woods Pkwy Vernon Hills, IL 60061 Robert E. Dudley, Ph.D. (708) 913-1144
Treatment of short stature associated	somatropin (Humatrope)	In clinical trials	Eli Lilly and Company Lilly Corporate Center Indianapolis, IN 46285 Medical Dept. (317) 276-3714

Condition/Use	Drug Name	Status/Phase	Sponsor/Contact Person
Treatment of short stature associated, *cont.*	human growth hormone recombinant	Phase III	Genentech, Inc. 460 Point San Bruno So. San Francisco, CA 94080 Public Relations Dept. (415) 266-2222
Ulcerative colitis Treatment of active phase, with involvement restricted to left side of colon	short chain fatty acid solution	Investigational	Richard Breuer, M.D. 2500 Ridge Avenue Evanston, IL 60201 (708) 869-5636
Mild to moderate, in patients intolerant to sulfasalazine	4-aminosalicylic acid	Undergoing evaluation	Warren L. Beeken, MD University of Vermont College of Medicine Given Building C-317 Burlington, VT 05405 (802) 656-2554
Uremic osteodystrophy	dihydroxycholecal ciferol	Phase III	Tag Pharmaceuticals c/o Lemmon Company Sellersville, PA 18960 Dr. Stanley Scheindlin (800) 523-6542
Uric acid Dissolution and control of uric acid and cystine calculi in the urinary tract	potassium citrate and citric acid (Polycitra-K)	Approved for marketing	Willen Drug Company 18 North High St. Baltimore, MD 21202 Joseph Weiner (410) 752-1865
Uric acid nephrolithiasis Prevention and control	potassium citrate (Urocit-K)	Approved for marketing Exclusive approval	Mission Pharmacal Company 391 N.E. Loop 410 Suite 109 San Antonio, TX 78217 Urological Products Div. (800) 531-3333 (800) 292-7364 (In Texas)
Urolithiasis Avoidance of complication of calcium stone formation	potassium citrate (Urocit-K)	Approved for marketing	Mission Pharmacal Company 2391 N.E. Loop 410 Suite 109 San Antonio, TX 78217 Urological Products Div. (800) 531-3333 (800) 292-7364 (In Texas)

Condition/Use	Drug Name	Status/Phase	Sponsor/Contact Person
Ventricular fibrillation Treatment and prevention of recurrence of primary	bethanidine sulfate	IND approved Clinical trials not initiated	Medco Research 8544 Beverly Blvd, Suite 308 Los Angeles, CA 90048 Roger Blevins, Pharm.D. (213) 966-4148
von Willebrand disease Mild	D-8 arginine vasopressin [desmopressin] high concentration (DDAVP HC)	In clinical development	Armour Pharmaceutical Co. 920A Harvest Drive Suite 200 Blue Bell, PA 19422 Garrett E. Bergman, MD (215) 540-8122
Wilson disease	zinc acetate	Phase III NDA in preparation	Lemmon Company Sellersville, PA 18960 Dr. Stanley Scheindlin (800) 523-6542
In patients intolerant of, or inadequately responsive to penicillamine	trientine HCL (Syprine)	Approved for marketing Exclusive Approval	Merck Sharp and Dohme West Point, PA 19486 Pat Graham Research Laboratories (215) 661-7300
Xeroderma pigmentosum Prevention of cutaneous neoplasms and other skin abnormalities	endonuclease V, liposome encapsulated [T4N5]	Pre-IND	Applied Genetics, Inc. 205 Buffalo Ave. Freeport, NY 11520 Dr. Daniel Yarosh (516) 868-9026

INDEX OF SYMPTOMS AND KEY WORDS

Neurofibromatosis (NF)
Bilateral acoustic neuroma. *See* Acoustic
neuroma
Bilateral polycystic ovarian syndrome. *See* Stein-
Leventhal syndrome
Bilateral renal agenesis. *See* Amniotic bands
Bilateral rightsidedness sequence. *See* Ivemark
syndrome
Bile ducts of liver, abnormalities of, Meckel
syndrome and, 94
Biliary atresia, 803, 804, **809-10**
See also Hepatitis, neonatal
Bilirubin encephalopathy. *See* Kernicterus
Billowing posterior mitral leaflet syndrome. *See*
Mitral valve prolapse syndrome (MVPS)
Binge eating
anorexia nervosa and, 296
bulimia and, 326
Binswanger disease, **324-25**
Binswanger encephalopathy. *See* Binswanger
disease
Biodegradable polymer implant containing
carmustine (Gliadel), 1060
Biotinidase deficiency. *See* Multiple carboxylase
deficiency
Birth defects, lead poisoning and, 1004
Birth weight
large, Sotos syndrome and, 126
low
bilateral renal agenesis and, 852
congenital rubella and, 695
Cornelia de Lange syndrome and, 44
cri du chat syndrome and, 46
Dubowitz syndrome and, 57
fetal alcohol syndrome and, 61
Freeman-Sheldon syndrome and, 65
Prader-Willi syndrome and, 113
Roberts syndrome and, 116
Smith-Lemli-Opitz syndrome and, 125
Tay syndrome and, 795
Williams syndrome and, 152
Wolf-Hirschhorn syndrome and, 154
Bis(monoacylglycero)-phosphate, increased
amounts in large thoracic and abdominal
organs, Niemann-Pick disease and, 237
Biventricular fibrosis, 479
B-K mole syndrome. *See* Dysplastic nevus
syndrome
Black fever. *See* Rocky Mountain spotted fever
(RMSF)
Black hairy tongue. *See* Hairy tongue
Black measles. *See* Rocky Mountain spotted fever
(RMSF)
Blackouts, sleep apnea and, 299
Bladder
enlarged (in female), Beckwith-Wiedemann
syndrome and, 30
impaired control of
cerebral palsy and, 330
Devic disease and, 344
spina bifida occulta and, 438
missing, sirenomelia sequence and, 124
paralysis of, syringomyelia and, 444
Bladder and bowel dysfunction
multiple sclerosis (MS) and, 386
Shy-Drager syndrome and, 435
Bladder cancer, orphan drugs for, 1051
Blastomycosis, **637-38**
Bleeding
into epidermis and mucous membranes,
aplastic anemia and, 523
essential thrombocythemia and, 603

excessive
from cuts and injuries, Bernard-Soulier
syndrome and, 540
on injury, Chédiak-Higashi syndrome and,
542
from mouth during dental work, May-
Hegglin anomaly and, 579
familial polyposis and, 817
gastrointestinal
gold poisoning and, 1004
idiopathic thrombocytopenic purpura (ITP)
and, 591
polyarteritis nodosa (PAN) and, 940
von Willebrand disease and, 607
Wiskott-Aldrich syndrome and, 721
Zellweger syndrome and, 275
genitourinary, idiopathic thrombocytopenic
purpura (ITP) and, 591
internal
alpha-1-antitrypsin deficiency and, 175
slow, factor XIII deficiency and, 547
uncontrolled, without apparent cause,
hemophilia and, 560
in nose, prolonged, von Willebrand disease
and, 607
Peutz-Jeghers syndrome and, 827
rectal
familial polyposis and, 817
Gardner syndrome and, 818
subcutaneous, thrombasthenia and, 601-2
from umbilical cord, factor XIII deficiency and,
547
vaginal, idiopathic thrombocytopenic purpura
(ITP) and, 591
See also Hemorrhage
Bleeding diathesis, 512
cholestasis and, 814
TORCH syndrome and, 704
Bleeding tendency, 511-13
Ehlers-Danlos syndromes (EDS) and, 924
hereditary fructose intolerance and, 195
Schwachman syndrome and, 596
thrombasthenia and, 601-2
Blepharophimosis
cerebro-oculo-facio-skeletal (COFS) syndrome
and, 331
Dubowitz syndrome and, 57
Blepharospasm. *See* Benign essential
blepharospasm (BEB)
Blepharospasm oromandibular dystonic
syndrome. *See* Meige syndrome
Blessig cysts, 984
Blindness
Alpers disease and, 291
Behçet's syndrome and, 921
congenital toxoplasmosis and, 708
cortical
Sturge-Weber syndrome and, 132
subacute sclerosing panencephalitis (SSPE)
and, 701
infantile metachromatic leukodystrophy and,
376
Krabbe leukodystrophy and, 374
Maroteaux-Lamy syndrome and, 222
olivopontocerebellar atrophy III and, 410
papillitis and, 979
Reiter's syndrome and, 948
temporary
conversion disorder and, 338
Takayasu's arteritis and episodes of, 920
vasculitis and, 957
See also Color blindness; Night blindness

Brachydactyly
  oral-facial-digital syndrome and, 103
  Saethre-Chotzen syndrome and, 121
  with webbing, Carpenter syndrome and, 33
Bradycardia
  fever and, Dengue fever and, 651
  Guillain-Barré syndrome and, 357
  infantile apnea and, 298
Bradykinesia
  progressive supranuclear palsy (PSP) and, 427
  vitamin E deficiency and, 271
Brain
  absence of brain tissue, anencephaly and, 22
  nevi in, blue rubber bleb nevus and, 32
  uneven atrophy of, Pick's disease and, 423
Brain abscesses
  nocardiosis and, 679
  predisposition to, atrial septal defects and, 469
Brain damage
  osteopetrosis and, 106
  propionic acidemia and, 169
Brain demyelination
  Baló disease and, 318
  childhood ALD and, 171
  neonatal ALD and, 171
Brain hernia, Roberts syndrome and, 116
Brain malignancies, orphan drugs for, 1050
Brain stem, compression of, achondroplasia and, 15
Brain tumor. See Astrocytoma, benign
Branched chain ketonuria. See Maple syrup urine disease
Brancher deficiency. See Andersen disease
Branchio-oto-renal syndrome, 853
Brandt syndrome. See Acrodermatitis enteropathica (AE)
Brandywine type dentinogenesis imperfecta. See Dentinogenesis imperfecta, type III
Brazilian trypansomiasis. See Chagas disease
Breakbone fever. See Dengue fever
Breast(s)
  absent or abnormally developed
    with normal nipple development in women, Tay syndrome and, 795
    Poland syndrome and, 112
  atrophy, Sheehan syndrome and, 903
  development before age 8, precocious puberty and, 898
  enlarged, in men, and secreting milk, Forbes-Albright syndrome and, 881
  late development of, McCune-Albright syndrome and, 895
Breastbone, depression of, 18p- syndrome and, 12
Breath
  shortness of
    alpha-1-antitrypsin deficiency and, 174
    eosinophilic gastroenteritis (EG) and, 820
    lymphangiomyomatosis and, 572-73
    thrombotic thrombocytopenic purpura (TTP) and, 594
  urine-like odor, Alport syndrome and, 839
Breathing
  difficulties
    during activity or feeding, ventricular septal defects and, 499-501
    exertion-produced, warm-antibody hemolytic anemia and, 531
    Farber disease and, 192
    Guillain-Barré syndrome and, 357
    histiocytosis X and, 564
    megaloblastic anemia and, 532

  sideroblastic anemia and, 534
  due to spasms of tongue, throat, and respiratory tract, Meige syndrome and, 381
  inability, except when sitting upright, mitral valve prolapse syndrome (MVPS) and, 485
  irregular, formaldehyde poisoning and, 1001
  labored, hemolytic-uremic syndrome (HUS) and, 843
  noisy
    Hurler syndrome and, 209
    Maroteaux-Lamy syndrome and, 222
  periods of deep, abnormal (in infants), Joubert syndrome and, 364
  rapid
    pheochromocytoma and, 588
    and shallow, ventricular septal defects and, 499
    and shallow, with moderate exercise, fibrosing alveolitis and, 466
  temporary cessation of
    grand mal seizures and, 348
    infantile apnea and, 298
Breda's disease. See Yaws
Breech birth
  bilateral renal agenesis and, 852
  Smith-Lemli-Opitz syndrome and, 125
Brissaud II. See Tourette syndrome
Brittle bone disease. See Osteogenesis imperfecta (OI)
Broad beta disease, **471-72**
Broad thumb-hallux syndrome. See Rubinstein-Taybi syndrome
Brocq-Duhring disease. See Dermatitis herpetiformis (DH)
Bronchial hyperreactivity, cobalt poisoning and, 1004
Bronchiectasis, 79-80
  central, allergic bronchopulmonary aspergillosis and, 631
  Kartagener syndrome and, 79
  paroxysmal coughing and, pertussis and, 682
Bronchiolar constriction, anaphylaxis and, 630
Bronchitis
  frequent, precipitating heart failure
    atrioventricular septal defect and, 470-71
    cor triatriatum and, 474
  vanadium poisoning and, 1005
  See also Alpha-1-antitrypsin (AAT) deficiency; Pertussis
Bronchopleural fistula, pulmonary mycetoma and, 631
Bronchopneumonia, Moebius syndrome and, 97
Bronchopulmonary dysplasia, 494
Bronze diabetes. See Hemochromatosis, hereditary
Brown enamel, hereditary. See Amelogenesis imperfecta
Brown-Séquard syndrome, 397
Brown syndrome, **970-71**
Brown teeth, hereditary. See Dentinogenesis imperfecta, type I
Brucellosis, **640-42**
  See also Typhoid
Bruegel syndrome. See Meige syndrome
Bruising, bruisability
  alpha-1-antitrypsin deficiency and, 175
  easy
    with bruises lingering, Bernard-Soulier syndrome and, 540
    Chédiak-Higashi syndrome and, 542
    Ehlers-Danlos syndromes (EDS) and, 924

Chest cage, large, spondyloepiphyseal dysplasia tarda and, 130
Chest cavity, bell-shaped, asphyxiating thoracic dystrophy and, 28
Chest muscles and cartilage, absent or abnormally developed, Poland syndrome and, 112
Chest pain
    acanthocheilonemiasis and, 619
    achalasia and, 807
    atypical, mitral valve prolapse syndrome (MVPS) and, 485
    berylliosis and, 999
    Chagas disease and, 643
    eosinophilic gastroenteritis (EG) and, 820
    fibrosing alveolitis and, 466
    leptospirosis and, 675
    lymphomatoid granulomatosis and, 484
    mercury poisoning and, 1005
    nocardiosis and, 679
    panic-anxiety syndrome and, 414
    pulmonary paracoccidioidomycosis and, 681
    resembling angina, exertion-caused, sideroblastic anemia and, 534
    vague, fibrosing alveolitis and, 466
    ventricular septal defects and, 499-500
Chest retractions, infant respiratory distress syndrome (IRDS) and, 494
Chest wall
    cystic hygroma originating at, 48
    limited motion of, eosinophilic gastroenteritis (EG) and, 820
Chest wall pain, 956
Chest x-ray
    patchy infiltrates on, Stevens-Johnson syndrome and, 700
    presence of cavity on, tuberculosis (TB) and, 710
Chewing
    fatigue in muscles employed in, myasthenia gravis (MG) and, 395
    slowness in, Thomsen disease and, 447
Chiari-Frommel syndrome, 870, **875**
    See also Forbes-Albright syndrome
Chiari I syndrome. *See* Chiari-Frommel syndrome
Chickenpox, 665-66
Chikungunya, **644**
Chilblains. *See* Perniosis
Childhood ALD, 170-71
Childhood hypophosphatasia, 890
Childhood muscular dystrophy. *See* Muscular dystrophy, Duchenne (DMD)
Childhood tuberculosis (primary TB), 711
Childish behavior, Binswanger disease and, 325
Chills
    acquired agranulocytosis and, 520
    angioimmunoblastic with dysproteinemia lymphadenopathy (AILD) and, 570
    arsenic poisoning and, 1003
    blastomycosis and, 637-38
    ciguatera fish poisoning and, 1000
    extrinsic allergic alveolitis and, 465
    glucose-6-phosphate dehydrogenase (G6PD) deficiency and, 552
    leptospirosis and, 675
    polyarteritis nodosa (PAN) and, 940
    Q fever and, 685
    shaking, metal fume fever and, 1003
    Weber-Christian disease and, 800
Chin
    H-shaped dimple on, Freeman-Sheldon

syndrome and, 65
    pointed, leprechaunism and, 87
    prominent, Coffin-Lowry syndrome and, 41
    receding
        bilateral renal agenesis and, 853
        11q- syndrome and, 9
        Hutchinson-Gilford syndrome and, 74
        Tay syndrome and, 795
        Treacher Collins syndrome and, 136
        small, cri du chat syndrome and, 46
Chloracne, 732, 733
2–Chlorodeoxyadenosine, 1067
Choanal atresia
    Antley-Bixler syndrome and, 25
    CHARGE association and, 35
Choking
    ataxia telangiectasia and, 312
    Friedreich ataxia and, 309
    Marie ataxia and, 311
    Rubinstein-Taybi syndrome and, 118
Cholelithiasis
    hereditary spherocytic hemolytic anemia and, 529
    thalassemia major and, 600
Cholera, **645-46**
Cholestasis, 803, **813-15**
    gold poisoning and, 1004
    neonatal hepatitis and, 670
    See also Vitamin E deficiency
Cholestasis-lymphedema syndrome, 808
Cholestasis with peripheral pulmonary stenosis. *See* Alagille syndrome
Cholesterol
    elevated level of, broad beta disease and, 471-72
    increased amounts in large thoracic and abdominal organs, Niemann-Pick disease and, 237
    low plasma
        acanthocytosis and, 517
        Tangier disease and, 265
Chondrodysplasia, Murk-Jansen type. *See* Metaphyseal chondrodysplasia, Jansen type
Chondrodysplasia punctata. *See* Conradi-Hünermann syndrome
Chondrodysplasia (rhizomelic type), 43
Chondrodystrophia calcificans congenita. *See* Conradi-Hünermann syndrome
Chondrodystrophic myotonia. *See* Schwartz-Jampel syndrome
Chondrodystrophy
    with clubfeet. *See* Diastrophic dysplasia
    epiphyseal. *See* Dysplasia epiphysealis hemimelica
    hypochondroplasia, 75
    See also Achondroplasia
Chondroectodermal dysplasia, 28
Chondrosarcoma, 545
    Maffucci syndrome and, 89
    Ollier disease and, 935
Chorea
    Kufs disease and, 369
    olivopontocerebellar atrophy I and, 410
    rheumatic fever and, 688
    tardive dyskinesia and, 445
    See also Myoclonus
Chorea minor. *See* Sydenham chorea
Choreic movements, chronic, glutaricaciduria I and, 199
Choreiform movements, Huntington disease and, 359

13q- syndrome and, 10
Clitoris, small, Robinow syndrome and, 117
Clitoromegaly
    Beckwith-Wiedemann syndrome and, 30
    3–Beta-HSD deficiency and, 867
    Fraser syndrome and, 64
    21–hydroxylase deficiency and, 868
    leprechaunism and, 87
Clonidine hydrochloride, 1052
Clotting, blood. See Blood clotting mechanisms,
    disruptions of
Clubbing
    of fingernails, berylliosis and, 999
    of fingers
        Graves disease and, 883
        hereditary hemorrhagic telangiectasia and,
            562
        ventricular septal defects and, 500
    of fingertips
        atrial septal defects and, 469
        tetralogy of Fallot and, 497
    of toes, Graves disease and, 883
Clubfoot, 38-39
    acanthocytosis and, 517
    amniotic bands and, 20
    cri du chat syndrome and, 46
    diastrophic dysplasia and, 53
    Ehlers-Danlos syndromes (EDS) and, 925
    Freeman-Sheldon syndrome and, 65
    Gordon syndrome and, 68
    Larsen syndrome and, 84
    Moebius syndrome and, 97
    trisomy 18 syndrome and, 144
    See also Amniotic bands
Clumsiness, Sydenham chorea and, 442
Cluster headache, 337-38
Clutaricaciduria II. See Medium-chain acyl-CoA
    dehydrogenase (MCAD) deficiency
Cluttering, fragile X syndrome and, 62
Coagulation factor in blood, reduced levels of,
    acanthocytosis and, 517
Coagulation system, disorders of, 510-11
Cobalt poisoning, 1004
Coccygeal region, cystic hygroma originating at,
    48
Coccyx, malformed, diastrophic dysplasia and, 53
Cockayne syndrome, 39-40
Coffin-Lowry syndrome, 40-41
Coffin-Siris syndrome, 42
Coffin syndrome. See Coffin-Lowry syndrome
Cold, increased sensitivity to, hereditary
    hemochromatosis and, 556
Cold agglutinin disease. See Anemia, hemolytic,
    cold-antibody
Cold-antibody disease. See Anemia, hemolytic,
    cold-antibody
Cold-induced vascular disease. See Perniosis
Cold intolerance
    Addison disease and, 866
    congenital adrenal hyperplasia (CAH) and, 867
    empty sella syndrome and, 346
Coldness
    in extremities, Buerger's disease and, 923-24
    in fingers, Raynaud's disease and phenomenon
        and, 946
    lipodystrophy and, 893
Colic, polycystic kidney diseases (PKD) and, 851
Collagen diseases, 461
Collodion baby. See Ichthyosis congenita
Coloboma
    Aicardi syndrome and, 288
    CHARGE association and, 35

of choroid and optic nerve, nevoid basal cell
    carcinoma syndrome and, 585
13q- syndrome and, 10
trisomy 13 syndrome and, 143
Wolf-Hirschhorn syndrome and, 154
Coloboma of iris-anal atresia syndrome, 64, 141,
    853
Colon, palpable, Hirschsprung disease and, 822
Colon cancer, Gardner syndrome and, 818
Colonic adenomas, multiple, Gardner syndrome
    and, 818-19
Color blindness
    testicular feminization with, 964
    Turner syndrome with, 964
Colorectal adenocarcinoma, orphan drugs for,
    1062
Colorectal cancer, orphan drugs for, 1051
Colorectal carcinoma, orphan drugs for, 1052-53
Colorectal metastatic adenocarcinoma, orphan
    drugs for, 1047
Coma
    argininosuccinic aciduria and, 179
    carbamyl phosphate synthetase deficiency and,
        182
    citrullinemia and, 186
    formaldehyde poisoning and, 1001
    hereditary carnitine deficiency syndromes and,
        184
    hereditary fructose intolerance and, 195
    herpetic encephalitis and, 655
    isovaleric acidemia and, 166
    maple syrup urine disease and, 221
    medium-chain acyl-CoA dehydrogenase
        (MCAD) deficiency and, 225
    methylmalonic acidemia and, 167
    ornithine transcarbamylase (OTC) deficiency
        and, 240
    propionic acidemia and, 169
    Reye syndrome and, 686
    Rocky Mountain spotted fever (RMSF) and,
        691
    simian B virus infection and, 699
    thrombotic thrombocytopenic purpura (TTP)
        and, 594
Common purpura, 593
Common ventricle (cor triloculare biatriatum).
    See Ventricular septal defects
Communicating hydrocephalus, 362
Complement-mediated urticaria angioedema. See
    Angioedema, hereditary
Complete anodontia. See Anodontia
Complete heart block, congenital, 460
Complex carbohydrate intolerance. See Glucose-
    galactose malabsorption
Compulsive behaviors, obsessive-compulsive
    disorder and, 409
Computerized tomography (CT), 278
Concentrating, difficulty in
    in adolescence, familial dysautonomia and, 353
    Alzheimer disease and, 291
    celiac sprue and, 813
    Creutzfeldt-Jakob disease and, 339
    18p- syndrome and, 12
    myalgic encephalomyelitis and, 659
    polycythemia vera and, 589
Concentric sclerosis. See Baló disease
Confusion
    acute intermittent porphyria and, 248
    Addison disease and, 866
    Alzheimer disease and, 292
    arsenic poisoning and, 1003
    benign astrocytoma and, 305

Roberts syndrome and, 116
Robinow syndrome and, 117
Rubinstein-Taybi syndrome and, 118
Russell-Silver syndrome and, 120
Seckel syndrome and, 122
Smith-Lemli-Opitz syndrome and, 125
Tay syndrome and, 795
13q- syndrome and, 10
trisomy 13 syndrome and, 143
trisomy 18 syndrome and, 144
Wolf-Hirschhorn syndrome and, 154
X-linked ichthyosis and, 773
Cubitum valgum, Noonan syndrome and, 102
Cupulolithiasis. *See* Benign paroxysmal positional
  vertigo (BPPV)
Curly hair osteosclerosis. *See* Trichodentoosseous
  syndrome (TDOS)
Curschmann-Batten-Steinert syndrome. *See*
  Myotonic dystrophy
Cushing syndrome, **877-78**
  orphan drugs for, 1056
  See also Amenorrhea, primary; Zollinger-
    Ellison syndrome
Cutaneous (dermal) necrotizing vasculitis, 958
Cutaneous fistulas, orphan drugs for, 1056
Cutaneous inflammatory bowel disease (Crohn's
  disease). *See* Hidradenitis suppurativa
Cutaneous mastocytosis. *See* Mastocytosis
Cutaneous TB, 711
Cutis hyperelastica. *See* Ehlers-Danlos
  syndromes (EDS)
Cutis laxa, **742-43**
Cyanosis, 460
  atrial septal defects and, 469
  berylliosis and, 999
  during exertion, Eisenmenger syndrome and,
    476
  extrinsic allergic alveolitis and, 465
  hereditary hemorrhagic telangiectasia and, 562
  infantile apnea and, 298
  infant respiratory distress syndrome (IRDS)
    and, 494
  Ivemark syndrome and, 77
  lissencephaly and, 377
  mild, atrioventricular septal defect and, 470-71
  Pierre Robin syndrome and, 111
  primary pulmonary hypertension (PPH) and,
    490
  Raynaud's disease and phenomenon and, 945
  at rest or with crying, tetralogy of Fallot and,
    497
  thoracic radiation injury and, 1010
  ventricular septal defects and, 499
Cyclic edema. *See* Idiopathic edema
Cyclic hematopoiesis. *See* Cyclic neutropenia
Cyclic neutropenia, 507-8, **543-44**
  See also Sutton disease II
Cyclosporine ophthalmic, 1056, 1065
Cyklokapron, 1055, 1062
Cyprus fever. *See* Brucellosis
Cystathionine beta-synthase deficiency. *See*
  Homocystinuria
Cystathioninuria, 207
Cysteamine (2-amino-ethanethiol), 1057
Cysticercosis, **649-50**
Cystic fibrosis (CF), 887
  orphan drugs for, 1056-57
  See also Schwachman syndrome
Cystic hygroma, **48-49**

Cystic lymphangioma. *See* Cystic hygroma
Cystic macular degeneration, juvenile
  retinoschisis and, 985
Cystine nephrolithiasis, orphan drugs for, 1057
Cystine storage disease. *See* Cystinosis
Cystinosis, **187-89**, 836
  orphan drugs for, 1057
  See also Fanconi syndrome; Lowe syndrome;
    Renal glycosuria
Cystinuria, **189-91**, 836
  See also Lowe syndrome
Cystitis, orphan drugs for, 1057-58
Cystoid macular edema, 981
Cysts
  calcified, Ehlers-Danlos syndromes (EDS)
    and, 924
  extradural, hereditary lymphedema and, 574
  multiple, on head and face, nevoid basal cell
    carcinoma syndrome and, 585
  retinal, retinoschisis and, 984
Cytogenic anemia. *See* Anemia, pernicious
Cytomegalovirus (CMV) retinitis
  orphan drugs for, 1058
  for patients being treated with ganciclovir,
    1048
Cytomegalovirus infection
  acquired immune deficiency syndrome (AIDS)
    and, 621
  Nezelof syndrome and, 586
  TORCH syndrome and, 703-5
Cytomell/IV, 1071
Cytovene, 1058

D-8 arginine vasopressin [desmopressin] high
  concentration (DDAVP HC), 1080
Dactylitis (sausage toes)
  Reiter's syndrome and, 947
  sickle cell disease and, 597
Danbolt-Closs syndrome. *See* Acrodermatitis
  enteropathica (AE)
Dandy fever. *See* Dengue fever
Dandy-Walker cysts. *See* Dandy-Walker
  syndrome
Dandy-Walker deformity. *See* Dandy-Walker
  syndrome
Dandy-Walker syndrome, **341**, 362
  See also Coffin-Siris syndrome; Joubert
    syndrome
Darier disease, **743-45**
  See also Epidermolytic hyperkeratosis;
    Erythrokeratodermia symmetrica
    progressiva; Erythrokeratodermia
    variabilis; Erythrokeratolysis hiemalis;
    Ichthyosis; Ichthyosis, X-linked;
    Pemphigus; Sjögren-Larsson syndrome
Davidenkov's syndrome (Kaeser syndrome
  neurogenic scapuloperoneal amyotrophy),
  433
Davies disease. *See* Endomyocardial fibrosis
  (EMF)
Daydreaming, petit mal seizures misdiagnosed as,
  349
DDAVP HC, 1080
Deafness
  acoustic nerve or cochlear, Alport syndrome
    and, 839
  Arnold-Chiari syndrome and, 303
  conductive
    Klippel-Feil syndrome and, 81

Saint Louis, 656
  severe, simian B virus infection and, 699
  toxoplasmosis in immunosuppressed patient
    and, 708
  West Nile, 656
Encephalitis periaxialis concentrica. *See* Baló
    disease
Encephalitis periaxialis diffusa. *See*
    Adrenoleukodystrophy (ALD)
Encephalocele, posterior, Meckel syndrome and,
    93
Encephalofacial angiomatosis. *See* Sturge-Weber
    syndrome
Encephalomyelitis, acute disseminated, 344
Encephalomyelitis, myalgic (ME), **658-60**
Encephalomyelopathy. *See* Leigh disease
Encephalopathy among dialysis patients,
    aluminum poisoning and, 1003
Encephalotrigeminal angiomatosis. *See* Sturge-
    Weber syndrome
Enchondromatosis, Maffucci syndrome and, 89
Enchondromatosis with multiple cavernous
    hemangiomas. *See* Maffucci syndrome
Endemic syphilis. *See* Bejel
Endocardial dysplasia. *See* Endocardial
    fibroelastosis (EFE)
Endocardial fibroelastosis (EFE), **477-79**
Endocardial sclerosis. *See* Endocardial
    fibroelastosis (EFE)
Endocarditis
  brucellosis and, 641
  localized listeria infection and, 677
  Q fever and, 685
  rheumatic fever and, 688
Endocardium, milky-white thickening of,
    endocardial fibroelastosis (EFE) and, 478
Endochondral bone formation, achondroplasia
    and impairment of, 15
Endocrine tumors. *See* Carcinoid syndrome
Endolymphatic hydrops. *See* Meniere disease
Endomyocardial fibrosis (EMF), **479-80**
Endonuclease V, liposome encapsulated [T4N5],
    1080
Endothelioma, diffuse, of bones. *See* Ewing
    sarcoma
End-stage renal failure, polycystic kidney diseases
    (PKD) and, 851
Engelmann disease, **58-59**
Enlarged tongue. *See* Macroglossia
Enteric fever. *See* Typhoid
Enteritis
  CMV, acquired immune deficiency syndrome
    (AIDS) and, 621
  regional, Behçet's syndrome and, 922
  Reiter's syndrome and, 947
Enterocolitis, acute. *See* Typhoid
Enterovirus infection, primary
    agammaglobulinemias and, 519
Enthesitis, Reiter's syndrome and, 947
Environment, extreme reaction to rearrangement
    of objects in, autism and, 316
Eosinophilia
  allergic bronchopulmonary aspergillosis and,
    631
  asymptomatic, in tourist returning from trip,
    acanthocheilonemiasis and, 619
  thrombocytopenia-absent radius syndrome
    and, 134
  toxocariasis and, 706
Eosinophilic gastroenteritis. *See* Gastroenteritis,
    eosinophilic (EG)
Eosinophilic granuloma. *See* Histiocytosis X

Eosinophilic pneumonia. *See* Aspergillosis
Eosinophils, lung tissue infiltrations by, Churg-
    Strauss syndrome and, 472
Epibulbar dermoid, Goldenhar syndrome and, 67
Epicanthal folds
  broad or beaked, Wolf-Hirschhorn syndrome
    and, 154
  cri du chat syndrome and, 46
  Down syndrome and, 55
  Ehlers-Danlos syndromes (EDS) and, 925
  18p- syndrome and, 11
  18q- syndrome and, 11
  Lowe syndrome and, 219
  Moebius syndrome and, 97
  Noonan syndrome and, 102
  oral-facial-digital syndrome and, 103
  prominent, bilateral renal agenesis and, 853
  Smith-Lemli-Opitz syndrome and, 125
  trisomy 18 syndrome and, 144
  Zellweger syndrome and, 275
Epidemic cholera. *See* Cholera
Epidemic myalgic encephalomyelitis. *See*
    Encephalomyelitis, myalgic (ME)
Epidemic neuromyasthenia. *See*
    Encephalomyelitis, myalgic (ME)
Epidermal growth factor, 1056, 1058
Epidermal scaly patch, Bowen disease and, 739-
    40
Epidermis
  bleeding into, aplastic anemia and, 523
  brown or black precancerous spot, irregular in
    shape resembling freckle, malignant
    melanoma and, 576
  hemorrhagic purplish patches in, chronic
    myelogenous leukemia and, 568
  thickened and papillomatous, acanthosis
    nigricans and, 731
  See also Skin
Epidermolysis bullosa acquisita, 783, 786
Epidermolysis bullosa (EB), **750-52**
  See also Pemphigus; Toxic epidermal necrolysis
    (TEN)
Epidermolytic hyperkeratosis, **752-53**
  See also Erythrokeratodermia symmetrica
    progressiva; Erythrokeratodermia
    variabilis; Erythrokeratolysis hiemalis;
    Ichthyosis; Ichthyosis, harlequin type;
    Ichthyosis, lamellar recessive; Ichthyosis,
    X-linked; Ichthyosis congenita; Ichthyosis
    hystrix, Curth-Macklin type; Ichthyosis
    vulgaris; Pemphigus; Sjögren-Larsson
    syndrome
Epididymal disease, blastomycosis and, 637
Epididymitis, filariasis and, 661
Epiduritis, 302, 428
Epigastric cramping, giardiasis and, 663
Epigastric pain, fascioliasis and, 660
Epikeratophasia, orphan drugs for, 1058
Epilepsy, **347-50**
  Aicardi syndrome and, 288
  Angelman syndrome and, 23
  contralateral, Parry-Romberg syndrome and,
    109
  focal, vascular malformations of the brain and,
    456
  grand mal or Jacksonian seizures, agenesis of
    the corpus callosum (ACC) and, 287
  Landau-Kleffner syndrome and, 372
  orphan drugs for, 1059
  progressive myoclonic, 399
  startle, 366
  See also Alpers disease; Autism;

Hyperchylomicronemia
Fats, inability to metabolize well, acanthocytosis and, 517
Fatty liver with encephalopathy. *See* Reye syndrome
Fatty tissue
  excess, Lowe syndrome and, 219
  painful, irregularly shaped, soft deposits, Dercum disease and, 878
  See also Subcutaneous fat
Favism, 552-53
Fear of impending doom, unreasonable, panic-anxiety syndrome and, 414
Febrile mucocutaneous syndrome. *See* Stevens-Johnson syndrome
Febrile neutrophilic dermatosis, acute. *See* Sweet syndrome
Febris melitensis. *See* Brucellosis
Febris sudoralis. *See* Brucellosis
Febris undulans. *See* Brucellosis
Feeding
  difficulties with
    atrioventricular septal defect and, 470-71
    CHARGE association and, 35
    Coffin-Lowry syndrome and, 41
    due to fatigue, ventricular septal defects and, 499-501
    harlequin type ichthyosis and, 769
    of infant with nipple, cerebro-costo-mandibular syndrome and, 34
    lissencephaly and, 377
    Menkes disease and, 226
    Tay-Sachs disease and, 266
    Zellweger syndrome and, 275
  poor, in full-term infants, kernicterus and, 368
Feeding problems
  alpha-1-antitrypsin deficiency and, 174
  Coffin-Siris syndrome and, 42
  Cornelia de Lange syndrome and, 44
  macroglossia and, 88
  maple syrup urine disease and, 221
  nonketotic hyperglycinemia and, 239
  phenylketonuria and, 242
  Rubinstein-Taybi syndrome and, 118
  Sandhoff disease and, **259-60**
Feet, foot
  burning feet syndrome, 447, 930
  burning pain and redness of, worsening during hot weather, erythromelalgia and, 758
  burning tingling or numbness in, tarsal tunnel syndrome and, 446
  clubfoot, 38-39
  cold, von Hippel-Lindau syndrome and, 148
  deformities of
    bilateral renal agenesis and, 853
    fiber type disproportion, congenital (CFTD) and, 354
    leprosy and, 673
  dragging of
    primary lateral sclerosis and, 426
    torsion dystonia and, 449, 450
  edema on backs of, hereditary angioedema and, 536
  enlargement of, gradual, acromegaly and, 863
  flat
    Aarskog syndrome and, 13
    cri du chat syndrome and, 46
    Marfan syndrome and, 92
    phenylketonuria and, 242
  high-arched, with hyperextension of big toe, Friedreich ataxia and, 309
  large

with cold and bluish color, Cockayne syndrome and, 40
Klippel-Trenaunay syndrome and, 83
leprechaunism and, 87
Sotos syndrome and, 126
more bluish than hands, Eisenmenger syndrome and, 476
paralytic episodes involving, moyamoya disease and, 385
rocker-bottom, cerebro-oculo-facio-skeletal (COFS) syndrome and, 331
short, broad and flat, Aarskog syndrome and, 13
short and stubby, with broad, short nails, acrodysostosis and, 16
small
  Cornelia de Lange syndrome and, 44
  disproportionately, hypochondroplasia and, 75
18p- syndrome and, 12
swollen
  cholinergic urticaria and, 715
  and tender along length of arch, Köhler's disease and, 930-31
  vesicular lesions on, hand-foot-mouth syndrome and, 665
  See also Soles of feet
Feissinger-Leroy-Reiter's syndrome. *See* Reiter's syndrome
Felty's syndrome, **927-28**
  See also Banti syndrome
Femoral head
  aseptic necrosis of, sickle cell disease and, 597
  malformed, diastrophic dysplasia and, 53
  osteonecrosis of, Legg-Calvé-Perthes syndrome and, 931
Femur
  bowing and fractures of, Antley-Bixler syndrome and, 25
  changed shape and density, Fairbank disease and, 60
  painful tumor in, Ewing sarcoma and, 544
  pain in, Engelmann disease and, 59
Fertility, decreased
  lead poisoning and, 1004
  low-level radiation exposure and, 1010
Fetal activity or movement
  decreased, Prader-Willi syndrome and, 113
  weak, trisomy 18 syndrome and, 144
Fetal alcohol syndrome (FAS), **61-62**
Fetal cystic hygroma. *See* Cystic hygroma
Fetal endomyocardial fibrosis. *See* Endocardial fibroelastosis (EFE)
Fetal face syndrome. *See* Robinow syndrome
Fetal iritis syndrome. *See* Norrie disease
Fetal polyhydramnios, lithium poisoning and, 1004
Fetal toxoplasmosis, 708
Fetal warfarin syndrome, 43
Fetus, amniotic bands constraining, 20-21
Fever
  accompanied by headache, sore throat, and conjunctivitis, 33toxic shock syndrome (TSS) and, 705
  acquired agranulocytosis and, 520
  acquired immune deficiency syndrome (AIDS) and, 620
  acute, angioimmunoblastic with dysproteinemia lymphadenopathy (AILD) and, 570
  Addison disease and, 866
  arsenic poisoning and, 1003

oval or round hairless areas on, alopecia areata
    and, 737
round and smaller than normal, Fahr disease
    and, 351
small
    lissencephaly and, 377-78
    Williams syndrome and, 152
    tendency to rotate to one side, spasmodic
        torticollis and, 436
Headache
    acute mountain sickness and, 997
    Arnold-Chiari syndrome and, 303
    arsenic poisoning and, 1003
    botulism and, 638
    brain abscesses and, nocardiosis and, 679
    brucellosis and, 641
    cadmium poisoning and, 1003
    cerebral cysticercosis and, 649
    Chiari-Frommel syndrome and, 875
    chikungunya and, 644
    chronic, Tolosa-Hunt syndrome and, 986
    cluster, **337-38**
    cold-antibody hemolytic anemia and, 527
    cranial AVM and, 468
    cryptococcosis and, 648
    cystinosis and, 188
    empty sella syndrome and, 346
    epilepsy and, 348
    essential thrombocythemia and, 603
    after exposure to cold
        paroxysmal cold hemoglobinuria (PCH) and,
            558
        and pruritis or angioedema, cold urticaria
            and, 716
    following exertion, aplastic anemia and, 523
    formaldehyde poisoning and, 1001-2
    Frölich syndrome and, 882
    generalized, worse in the morning, and
        accompanied by vomiting, malignant
        astrocytoma and, 307
    giant-cell arteritis and, 917
    gold poisoning and, 1004
    hereditary spherocytic hemolytic anemia and,
        529
    herpetic encephalitis and, 654
    at high altitude, acute mountain sickness and,
        997
    hydrocephalus and, 362
        Dandy-Walker syndrome and, 341
    idiopathic edema and, 567
    lipodystrophy and, 893
    malignant astrocytoma and, 307
    malignant hyperthermia and, 90
    May-Hegglin anomaly and, 579
    metal fume fever and, 1003
    migraine, 337, 987
    mild and resistant to analgesics, pseudotumor
        cerebri and, 428
    morning, sleep apnea and, 299
    moyamoya disease and, 385-86
    myalgic encephalomyelitis and, 659
    myelitis and, 397
    myelofibrosis-osteosclerosis (MOS) and, 583-
        85
    Nelson syndrome and, 897
    Oroya fever, 635
    Paget's disease of bone and, 938
    painful in morning, accompanied by vomiting
        but rarely nausea, glioblastoma
        multiforme and, 550
    pheochromocytoma and, 588
    polycythemia vera and, 589

rash on hands, feet, and in mouth, hand-foot-
    mouth syndrome and, 665
recurrent, benign astrocytoma and, 305
severe
    arachnoiditis and, 302
    Dengue fever and, 651
    leptospirosis and, 675-76
    loss of vision in one eye and, Wyburn-Mason
        syndrome and, 155
    to point of immobilization, chikungunya and,
        644
    Rocky Mountain spotted fever (RMSF) and,
        690
    simian B virus infection and, 699
    sudden
        Japanese encephalitis and, 656
        Q fever and, 685
    systemic lupus erythematosus (SLE) and, 954
    thrombotic thrombocytopenic purpura (TTP)
        and, 594
    typhoid and, 713
    vasculitis and, 957
    venous malformations of the brain and, 456
    von Hippel-Lindau syndrome and, 148
    Waldenstrom macroglobulinemia and, 718
Hearing, highly sensitive, Williams syndrome
    and, 152
Hearing defects, lead poisoning and, 1004
Hearing loss
    acoustic neuroma and, 285
    cerebro-costo-mandibular syndrome and, 34
    childhood ALD and, 171
    conductive, Crouzon disease and, 47
    Cornelia de Lange syndrome and, 44
    hereditary lymphedema and, 574
    high-tone, Alport syndrome and, 839
    Hunter syndrome and, 208
    intermittent, Meniere disease and, 383
    Kartagener syndrome and, 79
    mannosidosis and, 220
    Morquio disease and, 228
    Norrie disease and, 978
    osteogenesis imperfecta and, 104, 105
    Paget's disease of bone and, 938
    relapsing polychrondritis and, 949
    sensorineural
        kernicterus and, 368
        Klippel-Feil syndrome and, 81
    tinnitus and, 449
    Waldenstrom macroglobulinemia and, 718
    See also Deafness
Heart
    enlarged
        endocardial fibroelastosis (EFE) and, 478
        and inflamed cardiac wall, Kearns-Sayre
            syndrome and, 367
        persistent truncus arteriosus and, 498
    nodular growth around valves, Farber disease
        and, 192
    right-sided positioning of, dextrocardia with
        situs inversus and, 474-75
    sounds emanating more clearly from right
        chest, dextrocardia with situs inversus and,
        474
Heart beat
    irregular
        gallop rhythm, endocardial fibroelastosis
            (EFE) and, 478
        Kugelberg-Welander syndrome and, 371
        mastocytosis and, 578
        thrombotic thrombocytopenic purpura
            (TTP) and, 594

Tay syndrome and, 794-95
X-linked, **773-74**
 See also Ichthyosis congenita; Keratosis
  follicularis spinulosa decalvans; Sjögren-
  Larsson syndrome
 See also Erythrokeratodermia symmetrica
  progressiva; Erythrokeratodermia
  variabilis; Erythrokeratolysis hiemalis
Ichthyosis congenita, **767-68**
 See also Epidermolytic hyperkeratosis;
  Erythrokeratodermia symmetrica
  progressiva; Erythrokeratodermia
  variabilis; Erythrokeratolysis hiemalis;
  Ichthyosis, harlequin type; Ichthyosis,
  lamellar recessive; Ichthyosis, X-linked;
  Ichthyosis hystrix, Curth-Macklin type;
  Ichthyosis vulgaris; Keratosis follicularis
  spinulosa decalvans; Netherton syndrome;
  Sjögren-Larsson syndrome; Tay syndrome
Ichthyosis congenita, harlequin fetus type. *See*
 Ichthyosis, harlequin type
Ichthyosis hystrix, Curth-Macklin type, **769-71**
 See also Epidermolytic hyperkeratosis;
  Erythrokeratodermia variabilis;
  Erythrokeratodermia symmetrica
  progressiva; Erythrokeratolysis hiemalis;
  Ichthyosis, harlequin type; Ichthyosis,
  lamellar recessive; Ichthyosis, X-linked;
  Ichthyosis vulgaris; Sjögren-Larsson
  syndrome
Ichthyosis linearis circumflexa, Netherton
 syndrome and, 781
Ichthyosis simplex. *See* Ichthyosis vulgaris
Ichthyosis vulgaris, **772-73**
 Kufs disease and, 369
 See also Erythrokeratodermia variabilis;
  Ichthyosis congenita; Ichthyosis hystrix,
  Curth-Macklin type
Icterohemorrhagic leptospirosis. *See* Weil
 syndrome
I-cycloserine (Levcycloserine), 1060
Idarubicin (Idamycin), 1066
Idiopathic brachial plexus neuropathy. *See*
 Parsonnage-Turner syndrome
Idiopathic cardiomyopathy, 478
Idiopathic edema, **566-67**
Idiopathic growth delay. *See* Growth delay,
 constitutional
Idiopathic hemochromatosis, 535
Idiopathic infantile hypercalcemia, 153
Idiopathic neonatal hepatitis. *See* Hepatitis,
 neonatal
Idiopathic orthostatic hypotension, 487
Idiopathic precocious puberty, 898
Idiopathic pulmonary hemosiderosis, 481
Idiopathic refractory sideroblastic anemia. *See*
 Anemia, sideroblastic
Idiopathic renal hematuria. *See* IgA nephropathy
Idiopathic short stature. *See* Growth delay,
 constitutional
Idiopathic thrombocythemia. *See*
 Thrombocythemia, essential
Idiosyncratic porphyria. *See* Porphyria cutanea
 tarda (PCT)
Ifosfamide (Ifex), 1054, 1075, 1076
IgA, markedly reduced serum, Waldmann disease
 and, 831
IgA deficiency, 519
IgA nephropathy, **848-49**
 See also Hematuria, benign familial
IgE, elevated serum, allergic bronchopulmonary
 aspergillosis and, 631

IgG
 around keratinocytes in skin in areas of blisters,
  pemphigus and, 785
 markedly reduced serum, Waldmann disease
  and, 831
IgG subclass deficiencies, 519
IgM, elevated monoclonal (over 3 gm/dl),
 Waldenstrom macroglobulinemia and, 718
IgM deficiency, 519
Ileum, lesions in, Maffucci syndrome and, 89
Ileus, botulism and, 638
Iliac spurs, nail-patella syndrome and, 98
Iliopsoas, nocardiosis and, 679
Ilium, flared, Melnick-Needles syndrome and, 95
Imaging, 3
Imitation of another person's movements,
 uncontrollable, Tourette syndrome and,
 452
Immotile cilia syndrome. *See* Kartagener
 syndrome; Polynesian bronchiectasis
ImmTher, 1062
Immune system impairment, multiple
 carboxylase deficiency and, 234
Immunization, antibodies not formed after,
 severe combined immunodeficiency
 (SCID) and, 697
Immunoblastic lymphadenopathy. *See*
 Lymphadenopathy, angioimmunoblastic
 with dysproteinemia (AILD)
Immunodeficiency with ataxia telangiectasia. *See*
 Ataxia telangiectasia
Immunodeficiency with thrombocytopenia and
 eczema. *See* Wiskott-Aldrich syndrome
Immunoglobulin deficiency. *See*
 Agammaglobulinemias, primary
ImmuRAID-AFP-Tc-99m, 1048, 1053
ImmuRAID-CEA-Tc-99m, 1051
ImmuRAID-LL-2-Tc-99m, 1067, 1068
ImmuRAIT-LL-2-1-131, 1068
Imperforate anus, **76-77**
 partial trisomy 22 and, 141
 sirenomelia sequence and, 124
 VACTERL association and, 146
Impulsiveness, attention deficit hyperactivity
 disorder (ADHD) and, 314
Inattention, attention deficit hyperactivity
 disorder (ADHD) and, 314
Inborn errors of urea synthesis. *See* Arginase
 deficiency; Argininosuccinic aciduria;
 Carbamyl phosphate synthetase (CPS)
 deficiency; Citrullinemia; N-acetyl
 glutamate synthetase (NAGS) deficiency;
 Ornithine transcarbamylase (OTC)
 deficiency
Inclusion-body encephalitis, 702
Inclusion body myositis. *See* Myositis inclusion
 body (IBM)
Inclusion cell disease. *See* Mucolipidosis II (ML
 II)
Incontinence
 acute intermittent porphyria and, 247
 ankylosing spondylitis and, 917
 benign astrocytoma and, 305
 Binswanger disease and, 325
 exstrophy of the bladder and, 841
 fecal, myelitis and, 397
 frontal lobe tumors and, 384
 urinary, spinal stenosis and, 439
Incontinentia pigmenti, **775-76**
Incontinentia pigmenti achromians, 775
Incoordination. *See* Coordination, difficulty with
Indian childhood cirrhosis, 226

Leg ulcers
  Felty's syndrome and, 927
  hereditary spherocytic hemolytic anemia and, 529
  pyoderma gangrenosum and, 790
  pyruvate kinase deficiency and, 257
  sickle cell disease and, 597
  thalassemia major and, 600
Leigh disease, **216-17**
  See also Alpers disease; Pyruvate dehydrogenase (PDH) deficiency
Leigh necrotizing encephalopathy. *See* Leigh disease
Leiner disease, **777-79**
  See also Sweet syndrome
Leiner-Moussous desquamative erythroderma. *See* Leiner disease
Le jeune syndrome. *See* Cri du chat syndrome
Lens
  gray membrane or gray-yellow opaque mass with blood vessels behind, Norrie disease and, 978
  opacification or displacement in early infancy, Norrie disease and, 978
  Sturge-Weber syndrome and, 132
Lenticonus, Alport syndrome and, 839
Lenticular degeneration, progressive. *See* Wilson disease
Lentigines, LEOPARD syndrome and, 779
LEOPARD syndrome, **779-80**
Lepoutre's syndrome. *See* Hyperoxaluria, primary (PH)
Lepra. *See* Leprosy
Leprechaunism, **87-88**
  See also Lipodystrophy
Lepromatous disease, 673
Leprosy, **672-75**
  See also Lymphocytic infiltrate of Jessner; Mycosis fungoides
Leptomeningeal angiomas, Sturge-Weber syndrome and, 132
Leptomeningioma. *See* Meningioma
Leptomeningitis, 302
Leptospiral jaundice. *See* Weil syndrome
Leptospirosis, **675-76**
  Weil syndrome and, 719-21
Lermoyez syndrome. *See* Meniere disease
Leroy disease. *See* Mucolipidosis II (ML II)
Lesch-Nyhan syndrome, 158, **217-18**
Lesion(s)
  bluish or red-brown ulcerated, measuring 1 to 15 cm in diameter, mycosis fungoides and, 582
  eruptive xanthomas, hyperchylomicronemia and, 211
  gray, pink, or yellow, cavernous lymphangioma and, 571
  multiple, on face, neck, chest, and back, nevoid basal cell carcinoma syndrome and, 584
  raised red or purplish, vascular malformations of the brain and, 456
  smooth, pink or red, sometimes clear in center, lymphocytic infiltrate of Jessner and, 575
  on tongue, bleeds easily, fails to heal, tongue carcinoma and, 606
  See also Skin lesion(s)
Lethal midline granuloma. *See* Wegener granulomatosis
Lethargy
  aplastic anemia and, 523
  argininosuccinic aciduria and, 179
  benign astrocytoma and, 305

carbamyl phosphate synthetase deficiency and, 182
Castleman disease and, 541
  in full-term infants, kernicterus and, 368
  hereditary spherocytic hemolytic anemia and, 529
  21–hydroxylase deficiency and, 868
  isovaleric acidemia and, 166
  listeria meningoencephalitis and, 677
  maple syrup urine disease and, 221
  medulloblastoma and, 380
  methylmalonic acidemia and, 167
  phenylketonuria and, 242
  propionic acidemia and, 168, 169
  pure red cell aplasia and, 590
  Sandhoff disease and, 259
  vasculitis and, 957
  Wilms tumor and, 610
Letterer-Siwe disease. *See* Histiocytosis X
Leucine, high blood levels of, maple syrup urine disease and, 221
Leucovorin calcium for use in combination with 5-fluorouracil, 1053
Leucovorin calcium for use in combination with methotrexate, 1075
1–Leucovorin for use in combination with 5-Fluorouracil, 1051
1–Leucovorin for use in combination with methotrexate, 1075
Leukemia, 513
  acute, 506
    sideroblastic anemia and, 535
  Bloom syndrome and, 31
  chronic lymphatic, 531
  chronic lymphocytic, 582
    vaccinia necrosum and, 647
    See also Waldenstrom macroglobulinemia
  chronic myelogenous, **567-69**
    thrombocytosis in, orphan drugs for, 1077
  Down syndrome and, 56
  Fanconi anemia and, 525
  hairy cell, **569-70**
    orphan drugs for, 1067
  orphan drugs for, 1065-67
  plasma cell, 581
  Wiskott-Aldrich syndrome and, 721
  See also Polycythemia vera
Leukemic reticuloendotheliosis. *See* Leukemia, hairy cell
Leukocytes
  cystine crystals in, cystinosis and, 188
  reduced number of, Chédiak-Higashi syndrome and, 542
Leukocytic anomaly albinism. *See* Chédiak-Higashi syndrome
Leukocytic inclusions with platelet abnormality. *See* May-Hegglin anomaly
Leukocytopenia, Aase-Smith syndrome and, 14
Leukocytosis
  chronic granulomatous disease and, 554
  cold urticaria and, 716
  relapsing polychondritis and, 949
Leukodystrophy, Canavan, **373-74**
  See also Adrenoleukodystrophy (ALD); Alexander disease; Leukodystrophy, Krabbe; Leukodystrophy, metachromatic (MLD); Pelizaeus-Merzbacher brain sclerosis
Leukodystrophy, globoid cell. *See* Leukodystrophy, Krabbe
Leukodystrophy, Krabbe, **374-75**
  See also Alexander disease; Leukodystrophy,

metachromatic (MLD); Pelizaeus-
Merzbacher brain sclerosis
Leukodystrophy, metachromatic (MLD), **375-77**
progressive multifocal leukoencephalopathy,
702
Waldenstrom macroglobulinemia and, 718
See also Adrenoleukodystrophy (ALD);
Alexander disease; Multiple sulfatase
deficiency; Pelizaeus-Merzbacher brain
sclerosis; Seitelberger disease
Leukodystrophy with rosenthal fibers. *See*
Alexander disease
Leukoencephalitis periaxialis concentrica. *See*
Baló disease
Leukoencephalopathy. *See* Leukodystrophy,
metachromatic (MLD)
Leukopenia
babesiosis and, 633
Felty's syndrome and, 927
mixed connective tissue disease (MCTD) and,
934
severe combined immunodeficiency (SCID)
with, 697
systemic lupus erythematosus (SLE) and, 954
Leukoplakia, keratosis on precancerous,
cutaneous squamous cell carcinoma and,
598
Leuprolide acetate (Lupron Depot), 1074
Levcycloserine, 1060
Levocabastine ophthalmic suspension 0.05%,
1065
Levulosuria. *See* Fructosuria
Leyden-Moebius muscular dystrophy, 355, 390
Libido, decreased
empty sella syndrome and, 346
Forbes-Albright syndrome and, 881
hereditary hemochromatosis and, 556
sleep apnea and, 299
Lichen sclerosus et atrophicus (LSA), **780-81**
Lifting, weakness in, myotonic dystrophy and,
404
Lightheadedness
congenital heart block and, 482
after sudden standing, orthostatic hypotension
and, 486
Takayasu's arteritis and, 920
Lignac-Fanconi syndrome. *See* Cystinosis
Limb-girdle muscular dystrophy. *See* Leyden-
Moebius muscular dystrophy
Limbs
abnormal movements of, Gaucher disease and,
198
long, Marfan syndrome and, 92
reduction in size of, amniotic bands and, 20
short
achondroplasia and, 15
McCune-Albright syndrome and, 895
See also Arm(s); Extremities; Leg(s)
Limbus, gelatinous nodule in, vernal
keratoconjunctivitis and, 975, 976
Limit dextrinosis. *See* Forbes disease
Limp
intermittent, spinal stenosis and, 439
Köhler's disease and, 930-31
Legg-Calvé-Perthes syndrome and, 931
Ollier disease and, 935
Linear scleroderma, 950
Lingua nigra. *See* Hairy tongue
Lingua plicata, Melkersson-Rosenthal syndrome
and, 382
Lioresal Injection, 1076
Lipidemia, von Gierke disease and, 272

Lipid histiocytosis. *See* Niemann-Pick disease
Lipid storage, prenatal, Niemann-Pick disease
and, 237
Lipid storage diseases, 506
Gaucher disease, 197-99
Lipodystrophy, **892-95**
Lipofuscin accumulation in brain, Kufs disease
and, 369
Lipofuscinosis, generalized. *See* Kufs disease
Lipoid hyperplasia, congenital, 867
Lipomas, Proteus syndrome and, 115
Lips
biting of, Lesch-Nyhan syndrome and, 218
brown-to-black macules around, Peutz-Jeghers
syndrome and, 827
cleft, 36-38
ectropion of, lamellar recessive ichthyosis and,
771
edema in
hereditary angioedema and, 536
Melkersson-Rosenthal syndrome and, 382
full
Waardenburg syndrome and, 149
Williams syndrome and, 152
patulous, acquired immunodeficiency
dysmorphic syndrome and, 628
prominent upper, Blackfan-Diamond anemia
and, 524
retracted upper, fetal alcohol syndrome and, 61
short philtrum, Wolf-Hirschhorn syndrome
and, 154
smacking of, epilepsy and, 348
sucking and smacking of, tardive dyskinesia
and, 445
swollen, cholinergic urticaria and, 715
thick
Coffin-Lowry syndrome and, 41
Coffin-Siris syndrome and, 42
mannosidosis and, 220
thin, downturned, Cornelia de Lange
syndrome and, 44
thin upper, and long philtrum,
trichorhinophalangeal syndrome and, 138
triangular groove in upper, acquired
immunodeficiency dysmorphic syndrome
and, 628
Lip span, wide, flat, Miller-Dieker syndrome and,
377
Lisch nodules, 2
in iris, neurofibromatosis and, 100
Lissencephaly, **377-78**
Listeria meningoencephalitis, 677
Listeria sepsis, 677
Listeriosis, **676-78**
Listlessness
citrullinemia and, 186
classic galactosemia and, 196
frontal tumors and, 384
isovaleric acidemia and, 166
nonketotic hyperglycinemia and, 239
radiation exposure and, cerebral radiation
syndrome and, 1010
Reye syndrome and, 686
Lithium poisoning, 1004
Lithostat, 1065
Little's disease. *See* Cerebral palsy
Liver
angiomatous tumors in, von Hippel-Lindau
syndrome and, 148
deeply pigmented, Dubin-Johnson syndrome
and, 816-17
enlarged

individuals and, 708
Waldenstrom macroglobulinemia and, 718
X-linked lymphoproliferative (XLP) syndrome and, 612
Lymphadenopathy, angioimmunoblastic with dysproteinemia (AILD), **570-71**
Lymphangiectatic protein-losing enteropathy. *See* Waldmann disease
Lymphangioleiomatosis. *See* Lymphangiomyomatosis
Lymphangioma
cavernous, **571-72**
Proteus syndrome and, 115
Lymphangiomyomatosis, **572-73**
Lymphangiosarcomas, Maffucci syndrome and, 89
Lymphangitis, filariasis and, 661
Lymphedema, hereditary, **573-74**
See also Lymphangioma, cavernous
Lymphedema tarda, 574
Lymph glands, shrunken, Nezelof syndrome and, 586
Lymph nodes
abnormal development or nondevelopment of peripheral, ataxia telangiectasia and, 313
atrophy of, hematopoietic syndrome and, 1009
enlarged or swollen
angioimmunoblastic with dysproteinemia lymphadenopathy (AILD) and, 570
Chédiak-Higashi syndrome and, 542
Felty's syndrome and, 927
Gianotti-Crosti syndrome and, 760
Hodgkin disease and, 565
mastocytosis and, 578
tongue carcinoma and, 606
Weber-Christian disease and, 800
lacking in lymphocytes, severe combined immunodeficiency (SCID) and, 697
nodules in, Farber disease and, 192
Lymphocytes, reduced or absent T and B, severe combined immunodeficiency (SCID) and, 697
Lymphocytic infiltrate of Jessner, **575-76**
See also Mycosis fungoides
Lymphocytic panniculitis, lipodystrophy and, 894
Lymphocytoma cutis, 575
Lymphocytopenia, systemic lupus erythematosus (SLE) and, 954
Lymphocytosis, pertussis and, 682
Lymphoma
B-cell, orphan drugs for, 1067, 1068
higher-than-normal incidence of, ataxia telangiectasia and, 313
orphan drugs for, 1067-68
Wiskott-Aldrich syndrome and, 721
X-linked lymphoproliferative (XLP) syndrome and, 612
Lymphomatoid granulomatosis, **484-85**
See also Vasculitis
Lymphopenia
hematopoietic syndrome and, 1009
Nezelof syndrome and, 586
Waldmann disease and, 831
Lymph varices, filariasis and, 662
Lysinuria, 189, 190
Lysosomal alpha-D-mannosidase deficiency. *See* Mannosidosis
Lysosomal alpha-glucosidase deficiency. *See* Pompe disease
Lysosomal inclusions, abnormal, mucolipidosis IV and, 231

McArdle disease, **223-24**
See also Glycogen storage disease VII (GSD VII); Pompe disease
McCune-Albright syndrome, **895-96**
Gonadotropin-dependent precocious puberty and, 898
See also Acromegaly
Machado disease, 363-64
Macrocephaly
Greig cephalopolysyndactyly syndrome and, 70
Maroteaux-Lamy syndrome and, 222
Morquio disease and, 227
osteopetrosis and, 106
Proteus syndrome and, 115
Robinow syndrome and, 117
Macroglobulinemia. *See* Waldenstrom macroglobulinemia
Macroglossia, **88-89**
amyloidosis and, 916
Beckwith-Wiedemann syndrome and, 29
Hurler syndrome and, 209
Pompe disease and, 245
Macrostomia, Goldenhar syndrome and, 66
Macular degeneration, **976-77**
See also Retinoschisis
Macules
bright red spots in, Niemann-Pick disease and, 238
brown-to-black, Peutz-Jeghers syndrome and, 827
intraocular edema on peripheral, peripheral uveitis and, 981
leprosy and, 673
pruritic, erythematous, 2 to 5 cm in diameter, cholinergic urticaria and, 715
reddish-brown, pruritic, urticaria pigmentosa and, 798
vasculitis and, 957
Maffucci syndrome, **89-90**
See also Blue rubber bleb nevus; Ollier disease; Proteus syndrome
Magersucht. *See* Anorexia nervosa
Magnetic resonance imaging (MRI), 278-79
Malabsorption
acanthocytosis and, 517
amyloidosis and, 916
Behçet's syndrome and, 922
celiac sprue and, 812
congenital sucrose-isomaltase, 830-31
Cronkhite-Canada disease and, 815
giardiasis and, 663
glucose-galactose, 821-22
megaloblastic anemia and, 532
mild-to-moderate, eosinophilic gastroenteritis (EG) and, 820
retractile mesenteritis and, 678
scleroderma and, 950-51
Maladie de tics. *See* Tourette syndrome
Malaise
babesiosis and, 633
Chagas disease and, 642
Churg-Strauss syndrome and, 472
erythema multiforme and, 753
after exposure to cold, paroxysmal cold hemoglobinuria (PCH) and, 558
hairy cell leukemia and, 569
herpetic encephalitis and, 654
lymphomatoid granulomatosis and, 484
myalgic encephalomyelitis and, 659
myelitis and, 397
pertussis and, 682
polycythemia vera and, 589

polymyalgia rheumatica and, 941
and rash on hands, feet, and in mouth, hand-
    foot-mouth syndrome and, 665
retractile mesenteritis and, 678
simian B virus infection and, 699
sweet syndrome and, 793
Takayasu's arteritis and, 920
thalassemia major and, 600
Tolosa-Hunt syndrome and, 986
toxoplasma infections in immunocompetent
    individuals and, 708
typhoid and, 713
Weber-Christian disease and, 800
Wegener granulomatosis and, 609
Malar hypoplasia
Goldenhar syndrome and, 66
Treacher Collins syndrome and, 136
Malaria, orphan drugs for, 1068
    See also Babesiosis; Typhoid
Mal del pinto. See Pinta
Male-limited precocious puberty (familial
    testotoxicosis), 898
Malignancies, orphan drugs for, 1068
    See also Blastomycosis
Malignant anemia. See Anemia, pernicious
Malignant carcinoid syndrome. See Carcinoid
    syndrome
Malignant fever. See Malignant hyperthermia
Malignant hyperphenylalaninemia. See
    Tetrahydrobiopterin deficiencies
Malignant hyperpyrexia. See Malignant
    hyperthermia
Malignant hyperthermia, **90-92**
central core disease and, 329
    See also Noonan syndrome
Malignant lymphangiitis and granulomatosis. See
    Lymphomatoid granulomatosis
Malignant lymphoma, 484, 541, 612
acquired immune deficiency syndrome (AIDS)
    and, 621
of the bone, 545
Malignant melanoma, **576-77**
    See also Bowen disease; Nevoid basal cell
        carcinoma syndrome; Squamous cell
        carcinoma, cutaneous; Xeroderma
        pigmentosum
Malignant neutropenia. See Agranulocytosis,
    acquired
Mallory-Weiss syndrome, **825-26**
Maltese fever. See Brucellosis
Mandible
hyperostosis of bones of, craniometaphyseal
    dysplasia and, 45
hypoplasia
    Carpenter syndrome and, 33
    Goldenhar syndrome and, 66
    Treacher Collins syndrome and, 136
prominent, Pfeiffer syndrome and, 110
protruding, Angelman syndrome and, 23
small
    Smith-Lemli-Opitz syndrome and, 125
    Turner syndrome and, 145
Mandibular incisors, lack of, tooth and nail
    syndrome and, 135
Mandibular malocclusion, craniometaphyseal
    dysplasia and, 45
Mandibular nerve, brief but intense bursts of
    pain along, 453
Mandibular prognathism, Crouzon disease and,
    47
Mandibulofacial dysostosis. See Nager acrofacial
    dysostosis; Treacher Collins syndrome

Mandibulofacial dysostosis with epibulbar
    dermoids. See Goldenhar syndrome
Mandibulo-oculo-facial dyscephaly. See
    Hallermann-Streiff syndrome
Manganese poisoning, 1004
Mannosidosis, **220-21**
Maple syrup urine disease, **221-22**, 280
    See also Acidemia, isovaleric (IVA); Nonketotic
        hyperglycinemia
Marble bones. See Osteopetrosis
Marchiafava-Micheli syndrome. See
    Hemoglobinuria, paroxysmal nocturnal
    (PNH)
Mareo. See Acute mountain sickness
Marfan syndrome, 2, **92-93**, 461
    See also Dilatation of the pulmonary artery,
        idiopathic (IDPA); Homocystinuria;
        Mitral valve prolapse syndrome (MVPS)
Marie disease. See Acromegaly
Marie-Strümpell disease. See Ankylosing
    spondylitis
Marker X syndrome. See Fragile X syndrome
Maroteaux-Lamy syndrome, **222-23**
    See also Mucolipidosis III;
        Mucopolysaccharidosis (MPS); Multiple
        sulfatase deficiency
Marrow. See Bone marrow
Martin-Bell syndrome. See Fragile X syndrome
Mass lesions, toxoplasmosis in
    immunosuppressed patient and, 708
Mast cell leukemia, 578
Mastocytosis, **577-78**
orphan drugs for, 1069
urticaria pigmentosa and, 798
Mathematical ability
autism and, 316
poor, fragile X syndrome and, 62
Maxilla
prominent
    phenylketonuria and, 242
    13q- syndrome and, 10
underdeveloped
    acrodysostosis and, 16
    Pfeiffer syndrome and, 110
Maxillary hypoplasia
Crouzon disease and, 47
Goldenhar syndrome and, 66
Treacher Collins syndrome and, 136
Maxillary nerve, brief but intense bursts of pain
    along, 453-54
May-Hegglin anomaly, **579-80**
    See also Bernard-Soulier syndrome; Chédiak-
        Higashi syndrome; Thrombasthenia;
        Thrombocytopenia, essential
Mazindol (Sanorex), 1058
Measles antibody, high serum levels of, subacute
    sclerosing panencephalitis (SSPE) and,
    701
Measles (rubeola), 691, 694
    See also Rocky Mountain spotted fever
        (RMSF); Roseola infantum; Rubella
Meckel-Gruber syndrome. See Meckel syndrome
Meckel syndrome, **93-94**
Medial canthi, lateral displacement of,
    Waardenburg syndrome and, 149
Median neuritis. See Carpal tunnel syndrome
    (CTS)
Median neuropathy. See Carpal tunnel syndrome
    (CTS)
Mediterranean anemia. See Thalassemia major
Mediterranean fever. See Brucellosis
Medium-chain acyl-CoA dehydrogenase

Nevus cavernosus. *See* Cavernous hemangioma
Nevus flammeus
  congenital, Klippel-Trenaunay syndrome and,
    82
  on forehead, thrombocytopenia-absent radius
    syndrome and, 134
  unilateral, along site of trigeminal nerve,
    Sturge-Weber syndrome and, 132
Nevus sebaceus of Jadassohn, 115
Nezelof syndrome, **586-87**
  See also Agammaglobulinemias, primary;
    DiGeorge syndrome
NG-29 (Somatrel), 1072
Nicotine, heightened reaction to, hyperhidrosis
  and, 765
Niemann-Pick disease, **237-39**
  See also Kufs disease; Sandhoff disease
Night blindness (nyctalopia)
  choroideremia and, 971
  retinitis pigmentosa (RP) and, 981
  sialidosis and, 263
  Usher syndrome and, 988
Nightsweats
  brucellosis and, 641
  chronic myelogenous leukemia and, 568
  Hodgkin disease and, 565
  tuberculosis (TB) and, 710
Night vision, poor, peripheral uveitis (pars
  planitis) and, 981
Nikolsky sign, pemphigus vulgaris, 785
Nipples
  enlarged, in girls, leprechaunism and, 87
  persistent discharge from, after childbirth,
    Chiari-Frommel syndrome and, 875
  wide apart
    Fraser syndrome and, 64
    Smith-Lemli-Opitz syndrome and, 125
Njovera. *See* Bejel
Nocardiosis, **679-80**
  See also Tuberculosis (TB)
Nocturnal myoclonus, 399
Nodular mesenteritis. *See* Mesenteritis, retractile
Nodular nonsuppurative panniculitis. *See* Weber-
  Christian disease
Nodules
  nonsuppurating subcutaneous fat, Weber-
    Christian disease and, 800
  skin, leprosy and, 673
  subcutaneous, on bony prominences,
    rheumatic fever and, 688
  subcutaneous inflamed, resembling boils,
    hidradenitis suppurativa and, 763
  vasculitis and, 957
Nonarteriosclerotic cerebral calcification. *See*
  Fahr disease
Nonclassical adrenal hyperplasia (NAH), 868
Noncommunicating hydrocephalus. *See* Dandy-
  Walker syndrome
Non-Hodgkin lymphomas, 565-66
  orphan drugs for, 1066, 1068
Nonketotic carnitine deficiency. *See* Medium-
  chain acyl-CoA dehydrogenase (MCAD)
  deficiency
Nonketotic glycinemia. *See* Nonketotic
  hyperglycinemia
Nonketotic hyperglycinemia, **239-40**
  See also Acidemia, isovaleric (IVA)
Nonne syndrome. *See* Ataxia, Marie
Nonprogressive congenital myopathy. *See* Central
  core disease
Nonpuerperal amenorrhea-galactorrhea. *See*
  Forbes-Albright syndrome

Nonpuerperal galactorrhea. *See* Forbes-Albright
  syndrome
Nonpuerperal galactorrhea-amenorrhea. *See*
  Ahumada-del Castillo syndrome
Nonsecretory myeloma, 581
Nonspecific sclerosing mesenteritis. *See*
  Mesenteritis, retractile
Nonthrombocytopenic idiopathic purpura. *See*
  Purpura, Schoenlein-Henoch
Nontropical sprue. *See* Celiac sprue
Nonvenereal syphilis. *See* Bejel
Noonan syndrome, **102-3**, 460
  See also Keratoconus; Malignant hyperthermia;
    Turner syndrome; Williams syndrome
Normal-pressure hydrocephalus, 362
Norman-Roberts syndrome, 377
Norrie disease, **977-79**
North American blastomycosis. *See* Blastomycosis
Nose
  beaked
    diastrophic dysplasia and, 53
    Rubinstein-Taybi syndrome and, 118
    Seckel syndrome and, 122
    Tay syndrome and, 795
    and thin, Werner syndrome and, 151
    Treacher Collins syndrome and, 136
  broad
    broad-based, oral-facial-digital syndrome
      and, 103
    Coffin-Siris syndrome and, 42
    and flat, Conradi-Hünermann syndrome
      and, 43
    with flattened bridge, Fraser syndrome and,
      64
    Greig cephalopolysyndactyly syndrome and,
      70
    with thick alar cartilage, Coffin-Lowry
      syndrome and, 41
    Wolf-Hirschhorn syndrome and, 154
  broad nasal tip with anteverted nostrils, Smith-
    Lemli-Opitz syndrome and, 125
  bulbous, retinoblastoma and, 983
  bulbous tip of
    Alagille syndrome and, 808
    trichorhinophalangeal syndrome and, 138
  destruction of, Gangosa and, 723
  discoloration of, alcaptonuria and, 173
  flat
    amniotic bands and, 20
    Carpenter syndrome and, 33
    cleft lip and cleft palate and, 36
    leprechaunism and, 87
    mannosidosis and, 220
    large rounded, trisomy 9p and, 141
  narrow and beaked, Hallermann-Streiff
    syndrome and, 71
  "parrot beak"
    bilateral renal agenesis and, 853
    Crouzon disease and, 47
    prominent, cri du chat syndrome and, 46
  saddlenose deformity
    relapsing polychondritis and, 949
    Wegener granulomatosis and, 609
  sharp, beaklike, Hutchinson-Gilford syndrome
    and, 74
  short
    acquired immunodeficiency dysmorphic
      syndrome and, 628
    and broad, Aarskog syndrome and, 13
    and flattened, acrodysostosis and, 16
  short upturned tip of, 11q- syndrome and, 9
  small

retroorbital, Dengue fever and, 651
in shoulder, severe, sharp, lancinating,
    Parsonnage-Turner syndrome and, 419
spinal, osteopetrosis and, 106
temporal, throbbing and boring or stabbing,
    giant-cell arteritis and, 917
testicular, polyarteritis nodosa (PAN) and, 940
tibial, Osgood-Schlatter disease and, 936
of tumor, Ewing sarcoma and, 544-45
ulcer-like, following eating, giant hypertrophic
    gastritis and, 819
unilateral and in one site, spasmodic torticollis
    and, 436
upon muscular contraction, myositis ossificans
    and, 402
in upper 4 ribs, Tietze's syndrome and, 956
when standing, walking, or lifting,
    osteonecrosis and, 937
wrist
    carpal tunnel syndrome (CTS) and, 327
    Kienboeck disease and, 929-30
See also Abdominal pain; Arthralgia; Back pain;
    Burning pain or sensations; Chest pain;
    Myalgia
Painful bruising syndrome. See Gardener-
    Diamond syndrome
Palatal myoclonus, 399
Palate
abnormalities of, cerebro-costo-mandibular
    syndrome and, 34
broad lateral ridges in, Smith-Lemli-Opitz
    syndrome and, 125
cleft, 36-38
hard, destruction of, Gangosa and, 723
high and narrow, Rubinstein-Taybi syndrome
    and, 118
high arched
    congenital fiber type disproportion and, 354
    fragile X syndrome and, 62
    Marfan syndrome and, 92
    nemaline myopathy and, 408
    Pfeiffer syndrome and, 110
high-pointed, Apert syndrome and, 26
narrow, arched, Turner syndrome and, 145
Paleness. See Pallor
Palilalia, Tourette syndrome and, 452
Pallidopyramidal syndrome. See Parkinson
    disease
Pallister-Killian syndrome, **107-8**
Pallister mosaic aneuploidy. See Pallister-Killian
    syndrome
Pallister mosaic syndrome. See Pallister-Killian
    syndrome
Pallor
Aase-Smith syndrome and, 14
atrial flutter and, 501
bone pain and, multiple myeloma and, 580
dramatic stark white, of fingers and toes,
    Raynaud's disease and phenomenon and,
    945
endocardial fibroelastosis (EFE) and, 478
Goodpasture syndrome and, 480
megaloblastic anemia and, 532
myelofibrosis-osteosclerosis (MOS) and, 583-
    85
paroxysmal nocturnal hemoglobinuria (PNH)
    and, 559
pheochromocytoma and, 588
pure red cell aplasia and, 590
thalassemia minor and, 601
thrombotic thrombocytopenic purpura (TTP)
    and, 594

of tongue and lips, sickle cell disease and, 597
urine-like breath odor in association with,
    Alport syndrome and, 839
warm-antibody hemolytic anemia and, 531
Wilms tumor and, 610-11
See also Anemia
Palmar fascia
nodules and bands in
    Dupuytren's contracture and, 932
Palms of hands
abnormally flat thenar eminence on, Holt-
    Oram syndrome and, 72
deep creases in, trisomy 8 and, 141
erythematous, Kawasaki syndrome and, 928
hyperkeratosis of, arsenic poisoning and, 1003
keratoderma on, lamellar recessive ichthyosis
    and, 771
pronounced markings, ichthyosis vulgaris and,
    772
scaling on, pityriasis rubra pilaris (PRP) and,
    788
simian creases on, 18q- syndrome and, 11
symmetrical red scaling, peeling plaques on,
    erythrokeratolysis hiemalis and, 757
thick and hard skin on, ichthyosis hystrix,
    Curth-Macklin type and, 770
xanthomas on, broad beta disease and, 471
Palpebral (eyelid) slant, antimongoloid, Noonan
    syndrome and, 102
Palpebral fissure
almond-shaped, Prader-Willi syndrome and,
    113
downslanting, Coffin-Lowry syndrome and, 41
enlarged, remaining open even during sleep,
    Bell's palsy and, 320
short, fetal alcohol syndrome and, 61
slanted, trisomy 13 syndrome and, 143
Palpitations
epilepsy and, 348
megaloblastic anemia and, 532
mitral valve prolapse syndrome (MVPS) and,
    485
panic-anxiety syndrome and, 414
pheochromocytoma and, 588
thalassemia major and, 600
warm-antibody hemolytic anemia and, 531
Palsy. See Cerebral palsy
Pancreatic adenocarcinomas, Maffucci syndrome
    and, 89
Pancreatic cholera, 645, 874
Pancreatic cysts, asphyxiating thoracic dystrophy
    and, 28
Pancreatic ulcerogenic tumor syndrome. See
    Zollinger-Ellison syndrome
Pancreatitis
hyperchylomicronemia and, 211
See also Alpha-1-antitrypsin (AAT) deficiency
Pancytopenia
hematopoietic syndrome and, 1009
osteopetrosis and, 106
Panhematin, 1074
Panic, sleep paralysis and, 405
Panic-anxiety syndrome, **413-15**
See also Depersonalization disorder
Panic disorder. See Panic-anxiety syndrome
Panmyelopathy. See Anemia, aplastic
Panmyelophthisis. See Anemia, aplastic
Papilledema
cryptococcosis and, 648
Dandy-Walker syndrome and, 341
moyamoya disease and, 385
with progressive visual loss, pseudotumor

positional vertigo (BPPV)
Posture
 contorted, autism and, 316
 slumped-forward, Kugelberg-Welander
  syndrome and, 371
 squatting, tetralogy of Fallot and, 497
 stooped, Parkinson disease and, 417
 subtle change in, metachromatic
  leukodystrophy and, 376
Posturing, abnormal, vitamin E deficiency and,
 271
Potassium, lowered blood levels of, Romano-
 Ward syndrome and, 495, 496
Potassium citrate and citric acid (Polycitra-K),
 1079
Potassium citrate (Urocit-K), 1064, 1079
Potter facies, bilateral renal agenesis and, 853
Potter syndrome, 21, 94, 853
Pott's disease, 711
PR-122 (redox-phenytoin), 1076
PR-225 (redox-acyclovir), 1062
PR-239 (redox penicillin), 1071
PR-320 (Molecusol carbamazepine), 1077
Prader-Willi syndrome, 2, 4, **113-14**
 See also Frölich syndrome; Laurence-Moon-
  Biedl syndrome (LMBS)
Precocious puberty, 120, **897-900**
 11-Beta-hydroxylase deficiency and, 868
 orphan drugs for, 1074
Prednimustine (Sterecyt), 1068
Preexcitation syndrome. *See* Wolff-Parkinson-
 White (WPW) syndrome
Pregnancy
 in bicornuate uterus, amniotic bands and, 20-
  21
 listeriosis of, 676-77
 muscle weakness and, myasthenia gravis (MG)
  and, 396
Premature aging
 ataxia telangiectasia and, 313
 Cockayne syndrome and, 39
 Werner syndrome and, 151
Premature senility syndrome. *See* Hutchinson-
 Gilford syndrome
Prematurity, trisomy 18 syndrome and, 144
Prenatal skeletal growth, lack of, triploid
 syndrome and, 140
Presenile dementia. *See* Alzheimer disease
Presenile tremor syndrome. *See* Benign essential
 tremor syndrome
Pricking sensations, panic-anxiety syndrome and,
 414
Primary adrenal insufficiency. *See* Addison
 disease
Primary anemia. *See* Anemia, pernicious
Primary B cell lymphoma of the brain, acquired
 immune deficiency syndrome (AIDS) and,
 621
Primary biliary cirrhosis, **828-30**
 See also Banti syndrome; Dubin-Johnson
  syndrome
Primary central hypoventilation syndrome. *See*
 Ondine's curse
Primary ciliary dyskinesia. *See* Kartagener
 syndrome
Primary granulocytopenia. *See* Agranulocytosis,
 acquired
Primary hemochromatosis. *See*
 Hemochromatosis, hereditary
Primary lateral sclerosis, **426-27**
 See also Amyotrophic lateral sclerosis (ALS)
Primary obliterative pulmonary vascular disease.

See Pulmonary hypertension, primary
 (PPH)
Primary optic atrophy, 434
Primary pulmonary hypertension (PPH), 459
 orphan drugs for, 1074
Primary reading disability. *See* Dyslexia
Primary thrombocythemia. *See*
 Thrombocythemia, essential
Procrit, 1049
Profound colobomatous microphthalmia, 962
Progeria, Gottron syndrome as mild form of, 69
Progeria (childhood). *See* Hutchinson-Gilford
 syndrome
Progeria of adulthood. *See* Werner syndrome
Progeroid appearance, Hallermann-Streiff
 syndrome and, 71
Progeroid nanism. *See* Cockayne syndrome
Prognathism
 acrodysostosis and, 16
 Cockayne syndrome and, 40
Progressive autonomic failure. *See* Shy-Drager
 syndrome
Progressive bulbar palsy, 294
Progressive bulbar paralysis. *See* Amyotrophic
 lateral sclerosis (ALS)
Progressive choroidal atrophy. *See* Choroideremia
Progressive diaphyseal dysplasia. *See* Engelmann
 disease
Progressive familial intrahepatic cholestasis, 808
Progressive hemifacial atrophy. *See* Parry-
 Romberg syndrome
Progressive hypoerythemia. *See* Anemia, aplastic
Progressive multifocal leukoencephalopathy, 702
Progressive muscular atrophy. *See* Amyotrophic
 lateral sclerosis (ALS)
Progressive myoclonic epilepsy, 399
Progressive pallid degeneration syndrome. *See*
 Hallervorden-Spatz disease
Progressive panacinar emphysema, alpha-1-
 antitrypsin deficiency and, 174
Progressive poliodystrophy. *See* Alpers disease
Progressive supranuclear palsy (PSP), **427-28**
Progressive tapetochoroidal dystrophy. *See*
 Choroideremia
Progressive tardive muscular dystrophy. *See*
 Muscular dystrophy, Becker (BMD)
Prokine, 1050
Prolactin, high levels of, Forbes-Albright
 syndrome and, 881
Prolastin, 1048
Proline oxidase deficiency. *See* Hyperprolinemia
 type I
Pronator quadratus syndrome, 327
Propionate, massive amount in blood, propionic
 acidemia and, 169
Propionyl-CoA carboxylase (PCC) deficiency. *See*
 Acidemia, propionic
Proprioception, loss of, malignant astrocytoma
 and, 307
Proptosis
 Antley-Bixler syndrome and, 25
 craniometaphyseal dysplasia and, 45
Prostatectomy, orphan drugs for, 1074
Prostate disease, blastomycosis and, 637-38
Prostatic cancer
 cadmium poisoning and, 1003
 manganese poisoning and, 1004
Prostration
 Dengue fever and, 651
 radiation exposure and, cerebral radiation
  syndrome and, 1010
Protein intolerance, propionic acidemia and, 168

Systemic vasculitides, classification of, 909
Systemic venous hypertension, right ventricular
    fibrosis and, 479
System vasculitis with asthma and eosinophilia.
    See Churg-Strauss syndrome

Tachycardia
    aplastic anemia and, 523
    atrial flutter and, 501
    atrioventricular septal defect and, 470-71
    cor triatriatum and, 473, 474
    Graves disease and, 883
    malignant hyperthermia and, 90
    panic-anxiety syndrome and, 414
    peripheral, at high altitudes, acute mountain
        sickness and, 997
    pernicious anemia and, 533
    stiff-man syndrome and, 441
Tachypnea
    atrioventricular septal defect and, 470-71
    cor triatriatum and, 473
    secondary pulmonary hypertension (SPH) and,
        491
Talipes calcaneus, talipes equinovarus, talipes
    equinus, talipes valgus, talipes varus. *See*
    Clubfoot
Talking, slowness in, Thomsen disease and, 447
Tall stature
    homocystinuria and, 207
    Marfan syndrome and, 92
Tandem spinal stenosis. *See* Spinal stenosis
Tangier disease, **265-66**
    See also Acanthocytosis
Tantrums, autism and, 316
Tapanui flu. *See* Encephalomyelitis, myalgic
    (ME)
Tardive dyskinesia, **445-46**
    See also Benign essential blepharospasm
    (BEB); Torsion dystonia
Tardive muscular dystrophy. *See* Muscular
    dystrophy, Émery-Dreifuss
Tardy ulnar palsy, 327
Target cell anemia. *See* Thalassemia major
Tarsal tunnel syndrome, **446-47**
    See also Köhler's disease
Tarsoepiphyseal aclasis. *See* Dysplasia
    epiphysealis hemimelica
Tarsomegaly. *See* Dysplasia epiphysealis
    hemimelica
Tarui disease. *See* Glycogen storage disease VII
    (GSD VII)
Taste, absence of sense of
    Bell's palsy and, 320
    familial dysautonomia and, 353
Taurodontia, trichodentoosseous syndrome and,
    137
Taurodontism, 19
Tay-Sachs disease, **266-67**
    See also Alpers disease; Kufs disease; Leigh
    disease; Sandhoff disease
Tay syndrome, **794-96**
    See also Ichthyosis; Netherton syndrome
T cell counts, low, Nezelof syndrome and, 586
Tear duct dysfunction
    blocked or missing, Rubinstein-Taybi
        syndrome and, 118
    Parry-Romberg syndrome and, 108
Tears
    decreased, Sjögren's syndrome (SjS) and, 952
    lack of, familial dysautonomia and, 353
Technetium Tc 99M antimelamona murine
    monoclonal antibody (Onco Trac

Melanoma Imaging Kit), 1069
Technetium Tc 99M anti-nonsmall cell lung
    cancer murine monoclonal antibody
    (Onco Trac Nonsmall Cell Lung Cancer
    Imaging Kit), 1052
Teeth
    abnormal, Gardner syndrome and, 818
    abnormal development of
        cleft lip and cleft palate and, 36
        macroglossia and, 88
        vitamin D-deficiency rickets and, 900
    abscessed during first years of life,
        trichodentoosseous syndrome and, 137
    anodontia, 24-25
    crowded
        Hutchinson-Gilford syndrome and, 74
        Marfan syndrome and, 92
    decay or loss, incontinentia pigmenti and, 775
    delayed eruption of
        Dubowitz syndrome and, 57
        growth hormone deficiency (GHD) and, 887
        hypophosphatemic rickets and, 846
        nevoid basal cell carcinoma syndrome and,
            585
    early erosion of pulp, dentinogenesis
        imperfecta, type III and, 51-52
    enamel. *See* Tooth enamel
    extra
        oral-facial-digital syndrome and, 103
        trichorhinophalangeal syndrome and, 138
    gnashing, grand mal seizures and, 348
    grinding, autism and, 316
    half-moon-shaped or obliterated pulp
        chambers, radicular dentin dysplasia and,
        50
    lack of contact between adjacent, amelogenesis
        imperfecta and, 19
    loss of, histiocytosis X and, 564
    loss of newly erupted, hypophosphatasia and,
        890
    maleruption of, causing malocclusion, Pfeiffer
        syndrome and, 110
    malformed, epidermolysis bullosa (EB) and,
        751
    misaligned
        acrodysostosis and, 16
        Hurler syndrome and, 209
        radicular dentin dysplasia and, 50
    premature eruption, histiocytosis X and, 564
    presence at birth, Hallermann-Streiff
        syndrome and, 71
    shell, 52
    snow-capped, 10
    unerupted and partially resorbed into jaws,
        amelogenesis imperfecta and, 19
    widely spaced
        acromegaly and, 863
        Hunter syndrome and, 208
        mannosidosis and, 220
        Morquio disease and, 227
        phenylketonuria and, 242
Teeth, deciduous
    brownish-blue opalescent, coronal dentin
        dysplasia and, 49
Teeth, permanent
    absence of
        except for molars, Hallermann-Streiff
            syndrome and, 71
        tooth and nail syndrome and, 135
    flame-shaped pulp chambers, coronal dentin
        dysplasia and, 50
    loosening and falling out in early adulthood,